Brief Contents

1 Introduction to Health Care Agencies, *1*

2 The Person's Rights, *12*

3 The Nursing Assistant, *21*

4 Delegation, *31*

5 Ethics and Laws, *38*

6 Student and Work Ethics, *55*

7 Communicating With the Health Team, *67*

8 Assisting With the Nursing Process, *83*

9 Understanding the Person, *92*

10 Body Structure and Function, *108*

11 Growth and Development, *126*

12 Care of the Older Person, *140*

13 Safety, *154*

14 Fall Prevention, *186*

15 Restraint Alternatives and Safe Restraint Use, *200*

16 Preventing Infection, *217*

17 Body Mechanics, *250*

18 Safely Moving the Person, *262*

19 Safely Transferring the Person, *281*

20 The Person's Unit, *303*

21 Bedmaking, *319*

22 Personal Hygiene, *335*

23 Grooming, *366*

24 Urinary Elimination, *388*

25 Urinary Catheters, *407*

26 Bowel Elimination, *422*

27 Nutrition and Fluids, *442*

28 Nutritional Support and IV Therapy, *473*

29 Measuring Vital Signs, *486*

30 Exercise and Activity, *513*

31 Comfort, Rest, and Sleep, *531*

32 Admissions, Transfers, and Discharges, *545*

33 Assisting With the Physical Examination, *561*

34 Collecting and Testing Specimens, *567*

35 The Person Having Surgery, *588*

36 Wound Care, *604*

37 Pressure Ulcers, *621*

38 Heat and Cold Applications, *634*

39 Oxygen Needs, *642*

40 Respiratory Support and Therapies, *658*

41 Rehabilitation and Restorative Nursing Care, *666*

42 Hearing, Speech, and Vision Problems, *675*

43 Cancer, Immune System, and Skin Disorders, *693*

44 Nervous System and Musculo-Skeletal Disorders, *705*

45 Cardiovascular, Respiratory, and Lymphatic Disorders, *724*

46 Digestive and Endocrine Disorders, *739*

47 Urinary and Reproductive Disorders, *749*

48 Mental Health Disorders, *757*

49 Confusion and Dementia, *769*

50 Intellectual and Developmental Disabilities, *786*

51 Sexuality, *794*

52 Caring for Mothers and Babies, *800*

53 Assisted Living, *822*

54 Basic Emergency Care, *829*

55 End-of-Life Care, *851*

56 Getting a Job, *860*

REVIEW QUESTION ANSWERS, *870*

APPENDIX A   National Nurse Aide Assessment Program (NNAAP®) Written Examination Content Outline and Skills Evaluation, *873*

APPENDIX B   Minimum Data Set—Selected Pages, *874*

APPENDIX C   Care Area Assessment (CAA)— Sample Page, *876*

APPENDIX D   Infant and Child Safety, *877*

GLOSSARY, *883*

KEY ABBREVIATIONS, *893*

INDEX, *895*

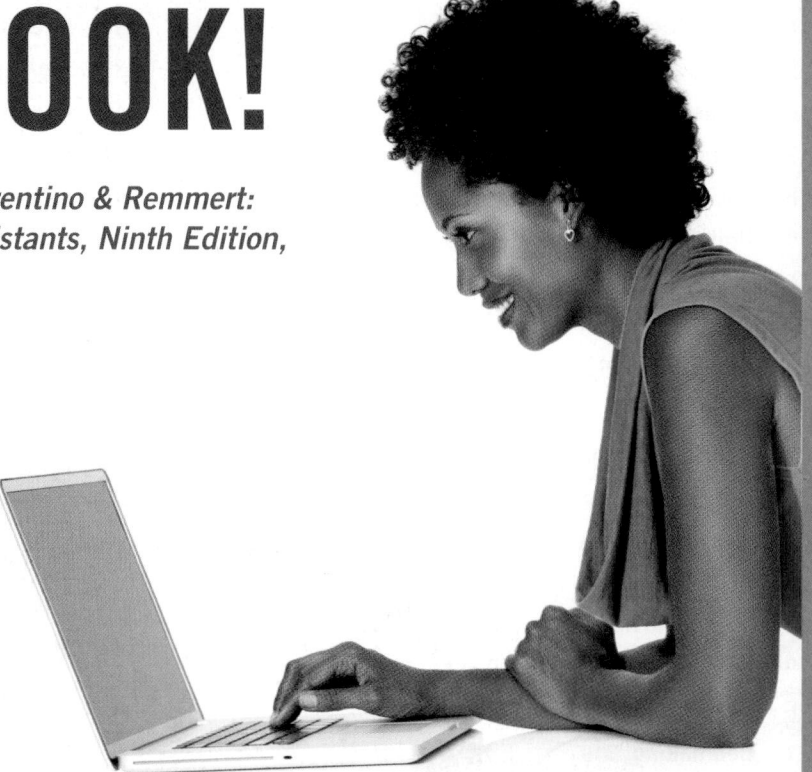

NINTH EDITION

MOSBY'S TEXTBOOK FOR

NURSING ASSISTANTS

SHEILA A. SORRENTINO, PhD, RN
Delegation Consultant
Anthem, Arizona

LEIGHANN N. REMMERT, MS, RN
Certified Nursing Assistant Instructor
Williamsville, Illinois

ELSEVIER

ELSEVIER

3251 Riverport Lane
St. Louis, Missouri 63043

MOSBY'S TEXTBOOK FOR NURSING ASSISTANTS,   ISBN: 978-0-323-31974-4 (Softcover)
NINTH EDITION   ISBN: 978-0-323-31975-1 (Hardcover)

Copyright © 2017, Elsevier Inc. All Rights Reserved.

Previous editions copyrighted 2012, 2008, 2004, 2000, 1996, 1992, 1987, and 1984.

Library of Congress Cataloging-in-Publication Data
Sorrentino, Sheila A., author.
  Mosby's textbook for nursing assistants / Sheila A. Sorrentino,
Leighann N. Remmert.—Ninth edition.
      p. ; cm.
  Textbook for nursing assistants
  Includes bibliographical references and index.
  ISBN 978-0-323-31974-4 (pbk. : alk. paper)—ISBN 978-0-323-31975-1 (hardcover : alk. paper)
  I. Remmert, Leighann N., author.   II. Title.   III. Title: Textbook for nursing assistants.
  [DNLM: 1. Nurses' Aides. 2. Nursing Care. WY 193]
  RT84
  610.7306'98—dc23
                            2015036852

Content Strategist: Nancy O'Brien
Content Development Manager: Ellen Wurm-Cutter
Senior Content Development Specialist: Maria Broeker
Publishing Services Manager: Jeff Patterson
Book Production Specialist: Bill Drone
Design Direction: Brian Salisbury

Printed in Canada

Last digit is the print number: 9 8 7 6 5 4 3 2 1

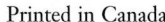

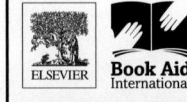

Working together to grow libraries in developing countries

www.elsevier.com • www.bookaid.org

The cycle of life, with its joys and sorrows, continues ...

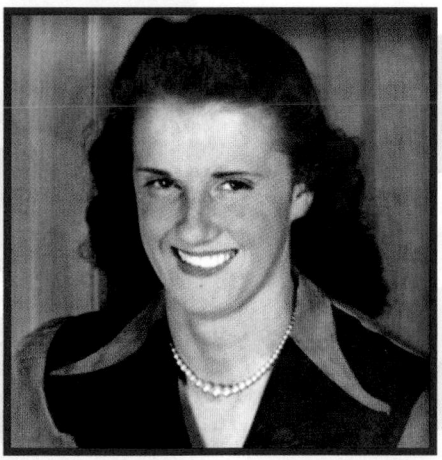

In memory of my mom
December 21, 1918—October 14, 2015
A beautiful woman with amazing inner strength
She is with my dad and their babies now
Love you, Mom
Sheila

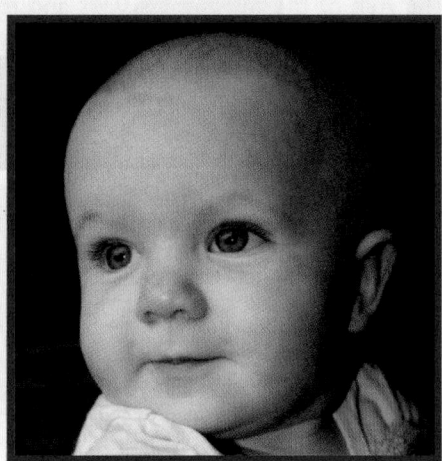

To my baby girl
Ava Leigh Remmert
Born February 18, 2015
You remind me daily how precious life is
With all my love,
Mom (Leighann)

About the Authors

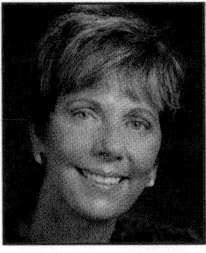

Sheila A. Sorrentino was instrumental in the development and approval of CNA-PN-ADN career-ladder programs in the Illinois community college system and has taught at various levels of nursing education—nursing assistant, practical nursing, associate degree nursing, and baccalaureate and higher degree programs. Her career includes experiences in nursing practice and higher education—nursing assistant, staff nurse, charge and head nurse, nursing faculty, program director, assistant dean, and dean.

A Mosby author and co-author of several nursing assistant titles since 1982, Dr. Sorrentino's titles include:

- *Mosby's Textbook for Nursing Assistants* (ed 1–9)
- *Mosby's Essentials for Nursing Assistants* (ed 1–5)
- *Mosby's Textbook for Long-Term Care Nursing Assistants* (ed 1–6)
- *Mosby's Textbook for Nursing Assistive Personnel* (ed 1–2)
- *Mosby's Basic Skills for Nursing Assistants*
- *Mosby's Textbook for Medication Assistants*

She was also involved in the development of an early version of *Mosby's Nursing Assistant Video Skills* and *Mosby's Nursing Video Skills*, winner of the 2003 AJN Book of the Year Award (electronic media). An earlier version of nursing assistant video skills won an International Films Award on caregiving.

Dr. Sorrentino has a Bachelor of Science degree in nursing, a Master of Arts degree in education, a Master of Science degree in nursing, and a PhD in higher education administration. She is a member of Sigma Theta Tau International, the Honor Society of Nursing. Her past community activities include the Rotary Club of Anthem (Anthem, Arizona), the Provena Senior Services Board of Directors (Mokena, Illinois), the Central Illinois Higher Education Health Care Task Force, the Iowa-Illinois Safety Council Board of Directors, and the Board of Directors of Our Lady of Victory Nursing Center (Bourbonnais, Illinois).

She received an alumni achievement award from Lewis University for outstanding leadership and dedication in nursing education. She is also a member of the Illinois State University College of Education Hall of Fame.

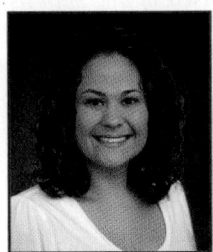

Leighann N. Remmert is a nursing assistant instructor in central Illinois. She has taught adult learners and high school nursing assistant students in the classroom and clinical settings.

Leighann has a Bachelor of Science degree in nursing from Bradley University (Peoria, Illinois) and a Master of Science degree in nursing education from Southern Illinois University Edwardsville (Edwardsville, Illinois). Leighann's clinical background includes the roles of nursing assistant/tech, nurse extern, staff nurse, charge nurse, nurse preceptor, and trauma nurse specialist. She acquired diverse clinical experience as a nursing assistant/tech and extern at St. John's Hospital (Springfield, Illinois). As an RN, Leighann concentrated in the area of emergency nursing at Memorial Medical Center (Springfield, Illinois). She is a member of Sigma Theta Tau International, the Honor Society of Nursing, and the Certified Nursing Assistant Educator's Association (Illinois, Central Region).

Leighann supervised, instructed, and evaluated student learning in various long-term care and acute care settings as a clinical nursing instructor at the Capital Area School of Practical Nursing (Springfield, Illinois). As a nursing assistant instructor, Leighann guides students in acquiring the skills and knowledge needed to succeed as nursing assistants. Through her teaching, she emphasizes the importance of professionalism and work ethics, safety, teamwork, communication, and accountability. Valuing the role of the nursing assistant and treating the person with dignity, care, and respect are integral to her instruction in the classroom and clinical settings.

Leighann is co-author of *Mosby's Textbook for Nursing Assistants* (ed 8–9), *Mosby's Essentials for Nursing Assistants* (ed 4–5), and *Mosby's Textbook for Medication Assistants*. She was a consultant on *Mosby's Textbook for Long-Term Care Nursing Assistants* (ed 6) and served as a content adviser for *Mosby's Nursing Assistant Video Skills* (version 4.0).

Leighann and her husband, Shane, have 2 daughters, Olivia and Ava. Leighann and Shane are active in various ministry areas at Elkhart Christian Church (Elkhart, Illinois). Leighann is certified as a Basic Life Support instructor and teaches CPR courses for the church and community.

Acknowledgments

Many individuals help us develop an accurate, up-to-date, and timely publication. Therefore we extend a "thank you" and appreciation to:

- Susan Morris and Katrina Walters at Heritage Health–Peru (Illinois) for reviewing selected content, answering questions, and providing clarification. Our thank you extends to Rose Mary Carrico at Illinois Valley Community Hospital (Peru, Illinois).
- Pam Randolph of the Arizona Board of Nursing for suggesting ways to strengthen content and instructor materials.
- Ray Norris (Anthem, Arizona) for clarifying aspects of military time.
- The Christian Village and Abraham Lincoln Memorial Hospital in Lincoln, Illinois, for hosting photo shoots.
- Jo Hilliard for her outstanding efforts coordinating the photo shoot at The Christian Village. Jo went above and beyond!
- Angela Stoltzenburg for coordinating the photo shoot at Abraham Lincoln Memorial Hospital. It was a pleasure to take photos at this impressive agency with such accommodating staff.
- Family, friends, and colleagues who participated in our photo shoot: Brittany Ackman, Judy Aper, Vicki Brickey, Laurie Cleary, Steven Cosby, Mary J. Dennison, Roger Dennison Sr., Charles R. Draper, Shirelle Dukes, Olivia Griesheim, Jo Hilliard, Sharon Koester, David F. Mabry, Angela Mahler, Roberta McKay, Katherine E. Parrott, Olivia Remmert, Shane C. Remmert, Jordan Rick, Debra Schmidt.

- Mike DeFilippo (St. Louis, Missouri), our favorite photographer. The things we ask Mike to do require acrobatic movements and magic!
- Anne and Jeremy Skowronski for the photo of their son, Benjamin.
- Sandy Remmert and Caitlin Remmert (parents Sean and Melissa Remmert) for allowing use of their photo.
- Gene Vogelgesang for providing the chapel photo from Illinois Valley Community Hospital (Peru, Illinois).
- The artists at Graphic World (St. Louis, Missouri) for their talented work.
- The reviewers who made comments and offered suggestions to improve our textbook. See "Reviewers" list below.
- Susan Broadhurst (New Orleans, Louisiana) for her role as copy editor. She accommodates our style well.
- Michael McConnell for his proofreading efforts. The task requires attention to detail.
- And finally the Elsevier/Mosby staff involved:
  - Nancy O'Brien, Content Strategist
  - Maria Broeker, Senior Content Development Specialist
  - Kathleen Nahm, Content Coordinator
  - Bill Drone, Book Production Specialist
  - Brian Salisbury, Designer

To all individuals who contributed to this effort in any way, we are sincerely grateful.

Sheila A. Sorrentino
Leighann N. Remmert

REVIEWERS

Sheryl L. Gray, RN, MSN, PCC
Registered Nurse
Population Care Coordinator
Ormond Beach, Florida

Brenda Hickland, BSN, RN
Virtual Learning Initiative Project Team Leader, NAA 100
Hopkinsville Community College
Hopkinsville, Kentucky

Janis Longfield McMillan, MSN, RN, CNE
Assistant Clinical Professor
School of Nursing
Northern Arizona University
Flagstaff, Arizona

**Joan K. Mooney, RN, EMT-B, BS Sec. Ed.,
MS Student Personnel and Guidance, BS Nursing**
Health Science Instructor
Texas Health Occupations Association, Board of Directors
Spring, Texas

Julie Morgan, RN, BSN, MSED
Instructor
Olean Career & Technical Center
Jamestown Community College
Olean, New York

Elizabeth Pagenkopf, RN, MSN
CNA Instructor
William Rainey Harper College
Palatine, Illinois

Jordan Rick, RN, BA
Registered Nurse, Heritage Health-Peru
Supply Sergeant, Illinois Army National Guard
Peru, Illinois

Cheryl F. Walburn, MSN, RN
Instructor, Clarkson College
Omaha, Nebraska;
Owner, Administrator, Instructor
Providence Health Career Institute
Lincoln, Nebraska

Instructor Preface

The ninth edition of *Mosby's Textbook for Nursing Assistants* serves several purposes.

- Prepares students to function as nursing assistants in nursing centers, hospitals, and home care settings.
- Assists faculty in meeting educational goals.
- Serves as a resource when preparing for the competency evaluation.
- Serves as a resource for nursing assistants wanting to review or learn new information for safe care.

The following foundational principles are presented in specific chapters while values, objectives, and organizational strategies are integrated in content and key features throughout the book. (See "Student Preface," p. xii for key features.)

- Patients and residents are *persons* with dignity having a past, a present, and a future. Such persons are physical, social, psychological, and spiritual beings with basic needs and protected rights.
- Nursing assistant roles, functions, and limitations are described in federal and state laws with dependence on effective delegation and good work ethics.
- Body structure and function, body mechanics, preventing infection, and safety and comfort measures form an essential knowledge base.
- Communication skills enhance relationships with the nursing and health teams, patients and residents, and families and visitors.
- The nursing assistant has a key role in the nursing process.

CONTENT ISSUES

Content decisions are based on changes in laws or in guidelines and standards issued by government, accrediting agencies, and national organizations. So are changes to state curricula and competency evaluations.

Student learning needs and abilities, instructor desires, work-related issues, course/program and book length, and student cost also are among the many factors considered.

New Content

Chapter 1: Introduction to Health Care Agencies
- FOCUS ON COMMUNICATION: The Health Team
- Patient Protection and Affordable Care Act of 2010
- FOCUS ON SURVEYS: Your Role

Chapter 2: The Person's Rights
- FOCUS ON SURVEYS: Resident Rights
- FOCUS ON SURVEYS: Activities

Chapter 3: The Nursing Assistant
- FOCUS ON SURVEYS: Maintaining Competence
- Nursing Assistant Job Titles

Chapter 4: Delegation *(new)*
- PROMOTING SAFETY AND COMFORT: Who Can Delegate
- Box 4-1 Examples of Tasks That Can and Cannot Be Delegated
- DELEGATION GUIDELINES: Step 2—Communication

Chapter 5: Ethics and Laws
- Wrongful Use of Electronic Communications
- Box 5-5 Electronic Communications
- FOCUS ON COMMUNICATION: Wrongful Use of Electronic Communications
- FOCUS ON SURVEYS: Reporting Abuse
- Box 5-6 Examples of Physical Abuse
- Box 5-10 Intimate Partner Violence—Risk Factors and Warning Signs
- PROMOTING SAFETY AND COMFORT: Intimate Partner Violence
- FOCUS ON CHILDREN AND OLDER PERSONS: Intimate Partner Violence

Chapter 6: Student and Work Ethics
- Burnout
- Box 6-4 Burnout—Causes, Signs, and Symptoms
- Bullying
- Unethical Student Behavior

Chapter 7: Communicating With the Health Team
- FOCUS ON MATH: Reporting and Recording Time
- FOCUS ON COMMUNICATION: Reporting and Recording Time
- Electronic Recording

Chapter 8: Assisting With the Nursing Process
- FOCUS ON SURVEYS: Planning

Chapter 9: Understanding the Person
- FOCUS ON COMMUNICATION: Communication Barriers

Chapter 11: Growth and Development
- Box 11-1 Growth and Development—Developmental Tasks
- PROMOTING SAFETY AND COMFORT: Infants (1 Month to 1 Year)
- Language Development
- Box 11-2 Language Development in Infants
- PROMOTING SAFETY AND COMFORT: Teen Dating

Chapter 12: Care of the Older Person
- Death of a Child
- Senior Citizen Housing
- Group Settings
- Adult Care Facilities

Chapter 13: Safety
- FOCUS ON SURVEYS: Safety
- FOCUS ON SURVEYS: Disasters
- Elopement

Chapter 14: Fall Prevention
- FOCUS ON SURVEYS: Fall Prevention
- FOCUS ON LONG-TERM CARE AND HOME CARE: Causes and Risk Factors for Falls
- Bed and Chair Alarms
- PRE-PROCEDURE AND POST-PROCEDURE: Using a Transfer/Gait Belt
- Moving the Person From the Floor

Chapter 15: Restraint Alternatives and Safe Restraint Use
- FOCUS ON SURVEYS: Safe Restraint Use

Chapter 16: Preventing Infection
- FOCUS ON SURVEYS: Infection
- FOCUS ON SURVEYS: Hand Hygiene
- FOCUS ON SURVEYS: Transmission-Based Precautions
- FOCUS ON SURVEYS: Laundry

Chapter 17: Body Mechanics
- FOCUS ON MATH: Fowler's Positions

Chapter 18: Safely Moving the Person (new)
- Box 18-1 Functional Status—Bed Mobility
- FOCUS ON SURVEYS: Protecting the Skin
- Box 18-2 Guidelines for Moving Persons in Bed
- FOCUS ON COMMUNICATION: Moving Persons in Bed

Chapter 19: Safely Transferring the Person (new)
- Box 19-1 Functional Status—Transfers
- FOCUS ON SURVEYS: Bed to Chair or Wheelchair Transfers
- Lateral Transfers
- TEAMWORK AND TIME MANAGEMENT: Using a Mechanical Lift
- PROCEDURE: Transferring the Person Using a Stand-Assist Mechanical Lift

Chapter 20: The Person's Unit
- FOCUS ON SURVEYS: Noise

Chapter 21: Bedmaking
- FOCUS ON SURVEYS: Linens

Chapter 22: Personal Hygiene
- PROMOTING SAFETY AND COMFORT: Personal Hygiene

Chapter 23: Grooming
- FOCUS ON SURVEYS: Grooming
- PROMOTING SAFETY AND COMFORT: Dressing and Undressing

Chapter 24: Urinary Elimination
- PROMOTING SAFETY AND COMFORT: Urinary Elimination
- Box 24-2 Incontinence—Risk Factors and Causes
- FOCUS ON SURVEYS: Managing Incontinence

Chapter 25: Urinary Catheters (new)
- FOCUS ON SURVEYS: Urinary Catheters
- PROMOTING SAFETY AND COMFORT: Urinary Catheters
- FOCUS ON MATH: Removing Indwelling Catheters

Chapter 26: Bowel Elimination
- DELEGATION GUIDELINES: Bowel Elimination
- PROMOTING SAFETY AND COMFORT: Bowel Elimination
- FOCUS ON MATH: Enemas

Chapter 27 Nutrition and Fluids
- FOCUS ON SURVEYS: Nutrition and Fluids
- Gluten-Free Diet
- Food Intake
- FOCUS ON MATH: Food Intake
- Box 27-7 I&O Converting Measures
- FOCUS ON MATH: Measuring Intake and Output
- FOCUS ON SURVEYS: Feeding the Person

Chapter 28: Nutritional Support and IV Therapy
- DELEGATION GUIDELINES: Nutritional Support and IV Therapy

Chapter 29: Measuring Vital Signs
- FOCUS ON CHILDREN AND OLDER PERSONS: Taking Temperatures
- FOCUS ON MATH: Taking Temperatures With Glass Thermometers
- FOCUS ON MATH: Taking Radial Pulses
- FOCUS ON MATH: Taking Apical and Apical-Radial Pulses
- Checking Pedal Pulses
- FOCUS ON MATH: Counting Respirations
- FOCUS ON MATH: Measuring Blood Pressure

Chapter 31: Comfort, Rest, and Sleep
- FOCUS ON SURVEYS: Pain

Chapter 32: Admissions, Transfers, and Discharges
- FOCUS ON MATH: Weight and Height

Chapter 34: Collecting and Testing Specimens
- PROMOTING SAFETY AND COMFORT: Collecting and Testing Specimens
- PROMOTING SAFETY AND COMFORT: The Midstream Specimen

Chapter 36: Wound Care
- PROMOTING SAFETY AND COMFORT: Wound Care
- Box 36-4 Diabetes Foot Care
- FOCUS ON LONG-TERM CARE AND HOME CARE: Diabetic Foot Ulcers

Chapter 37: Pressure Ulcers
- Kennedy Terminal Ulcer
- FOCUS ON SURVEYS: Prevention and Treatment

Chapter 40: Respiratory Support and Therapies
- PROMOTING SAFETY AND COMFORT: Respiratory Support and Therapies
- DELEGATION GUIDELINES: Suctioning

Chapter 42: Hearing, Speech, and Vision Problems
- Box 42-1 Hearing Loss—Signs and Symptoms

Chapter 43: Cancer, Immune System, and Skin Disorders
- Celiac Disease
- Hashimoto's Disease
- Box 43-3 AIDS—Stages and Signs and Symptoms
- PROMOTING SAFETY AND COMFORT: HIV/AIDS
- HIV Prevention

Chapter 44: Nervous System and Musculo-Skeletal Disorders
- Box 44-3 Traumatic Brain Injury—Signs and Symptoms

Chapter 45: Cardiovascular, Respiratory, and Lymphatic Disorders
- Box 45-3 Heart Failure—Signs and Symptoms
- Viral Hemorrhagic Fevers
- Ebola
- Enterovirus D68

Chapter 46: Digestive and Endocrine Disorders
- Inflammatory Bowel Disease

Chapter 47: Urinary and Reproductive Disorders
- Box 47-1 Urinary Tract Infections

Chapter 48: Mental Health Disorders
- Generalized Anxiety Disorder
- FOCUS ON CHILDREN AND OLDER PERSONS: Drug Abuse and Addiction

Chapter 49: Confusion and Dementia
- Box 49-7 Three Stages of Alzheimer's Disease
- Added to Box 49-9 Care of Persons With AD and Other Dementias:
  - Paranoia
  - Catastrophic Reactions
  - Agitation and Aggression
  - Repetitive Behaviors
  - Rummaging and Hiding Things
- FOCUS ON SURVEYS: Care of Persons With AD and Other Dementias

Chapter 50: Intellectual and Developmental Disabilities
- FOCUS ON LONG-TERM CARE AND HOME CARE: Intellectual and Developmental Disabilities
- Box 50-2 Adaptive Behaviors

Chapter 51: Sexuality
- Gender Identity

Chapter 52: Caring for Mothers and Babies
- Sudden Unexpected Infant Death
- FOCUS ON MATH: Weighing Infants

Chapter 53: Assisted Living
- FOCUS ON LONG-TERM CARE AND HOME CARE: ALR Services and Living Areas

Chapter 54: Basic Emergency Care
- FOCUS ON COMMUNICATION: Chains of Survival
- Box 54-2 Chains of Survival
- FOCUS ON CHILDREN AND OLDER PERSONS: Breathing
- FOCUS ON CHILDREN AND OLDER PERSONS: Hands-Only CPR
- FOCUS ON MATH: CPR for Children and Infants

Chapter 54: Basic Emergency Care—cont'd
- Poisoning
- Concussions
- Emergency Care for Concussions
- FOCUS ON CHILDREN AND OLDER PERSONS: Emergency Care for Concussions

Chapter 55: End-of-Life Care
- FOCUS ON SURVEYS: Advance Directives

Chapter 56: Getting a Job (new)
- Questions You Cannot Be Asked
- Box 56-4 Interview Questions Not Allowed by the EEOC
- FOCUS ON COMMUNICATION: Questions You Cannot Be Asked

New Key Terms
- Afebrile (Chapter 29)
- Antisepsis (Chapter 16)
- Arrhythmia (Chapter 45)
- Bed mobility (Chapter 18)
- Bullying (Chapter 6)
- Burnout (Chapter 6)
- Certification (Chapter 3)
- Child abuse and neglect (Chapter 5)
- Circumcised (Chapter 22)
- Code of ethics (Chapter 5)
- Competent (Chapter 4)
- Condom catheter (Chapter 25)
- Convenience (Chapter 15)
- Cross-contamination (Chapter 16)
- Discipline (Chapter 15)
- Disinfectant (Chapter 16)
- Electronic health record (Chapter 7)
- Electronic medical record (Chapter 7)
- Elopement (Chapter 13)
- Endorsement (Chapter 3)
- Entrapment (Chapter 20)
- Equivalency (Chapter 3)
- Febrile (Chapter 29)
- Functional status (Chapter 18)
- Gender identity (Chapter 51)
- Hospital bed system (Chapter 20)
- Hydration (Chapter 27)
- Infestation (Chapter 23)
- Intact skin (Chapter 37)
- Intimate partner violence (Chapter 5)
- Job application (Chapter 56)
- Job interview (Chapter 56)
- Lateral transfer (Chapter 19)
- Mole (Chapter 43)
- Opposition (Chapter 30)
- Orthotic device (Chapter 30)
- Over-active bladder (Chapter 24)
- Person's unit (Chapter 20)
- Pivot (Chapter 19)
- Pneumonia (Chapter 45)
- Prenatal care (Chapter 52)
- Pressure point (Chapter 37)

- Pulse oximetry (Chapter 39)
- Reciprocity (Chapter 3)
- Scabies (Chapter 23)
- Sexual orientation (Chapter 51)
- Skin breakdown (Chapter 37)
- Sleep deprivation (Chapter 31)
- Sleepwalking (Chapter 31)
- Surveyor (Chapter 1)
- Teen dating violence (Chapter 11)
- Uncircumcised (Chapter 22)
- Weight-bearing (Chapter 18)
- Work-related musculo-skeletal disorders (Chapter 17)

New Figures

- **Fig. 1-5** Nursing care patterns.
- **Fig. 4-1** The nurse considers the person's needs, the task, and the staff member's abilities when making delegation decisions.
- **Fig. 4-2** The delegation process has 4 steps.
- **Fig. 4-3** A nurse and nursing assistant discuss a delegated task.
- **Fig. 5-4** Some signs of elder abuse.
- **Fig. 7-1 B,** An electronic medical record.
- **Fig. 9-9** Behavior issues are a response to illness, injury, or disability. Or they are life-long.
- **Fig. 11-11** An 8-month-old uses a pincer grasp to pick up small objects.
- **Fig. 11-22** A wedding celebrates a couple's marriage.
- **Fig. 11-23** This woman enjoys time with her grandchild.
- **Fig. 13-19** Hazard Communication Standard pictograms.
- **Fig. 14-14** Moving the person from the floor using a mechanical lift.
- **Fig. 16-3** Cross-contamination. **A,** Microbes on the person's skin are transmitted to the nursing assistant's hands. **B,** Contaminated hands transmit microbes from 1 person to another.
- **Fig. 16-10** Hands are dried starting at the fingertips and working up to the forearms.
- **Fig. 16-23** Household disposable sharps container labeled with "Do Not Recycle."
- **Fig. 17-7** Measuring bed angles.
- **Fig. 19-4 A,** Moving a wheelchair up a ramp. **B,** Moving a wheelchair down a ramp.
- **Fig. 19-5 A,** Moving a wheelchair up a curb. **B,** Moving a wheelchair down a curb.
- **Fig. 19-13 A,** The wheelchair is next to the toilet.
- **Fig. 19-17 A,** Parts of a stand-assist lift.
- **Fig. 19-19** A full-sling supports the entire body.
- **Fig. 19-20** Using a stand-assist lift.
- **Fig. 21-8 A,** Cotton drawsheet. **B,** Padded waterproof drawsheet.
- **Fig. 22-30 B–C,** Cleaning the perineum. **B,** Clean the other side of the labia with a clean part of the washcloth. Use a downward stroke. **C,** Clean the vaginal area with a clean part of the washcloth. Use a downward stroke.

- **Fig. 23-23** Applying pullover garments.
- **Fig. 25-2** Parts of a Foley catheter (indwelling catheter).
- **Fig. 25-3** Parts of the urine drainage system.
- **Fig. 25-4 A,** Urine drainage bag secured to the bed frame. **B,** Urine drainage bag secured to a chair.
- **Fig. 25-5 C,** The catheter is secured to the man's thigh with a leg band.
- **Fig. 25-6** *Shading* shows the flank area.
- **Fig. 25-7** Cleaning the catheter. **A,** The catheter is cleaned with a circular motion at the meatus.
- **Fig. 25-14** A syringe is read at the top of the plunger.
- **Fig. 25-15** The balloon size marked on the catheter may not equal the amount of water in the balloon. The nurse tells you the amount.
- **Fig. 26-2** Color chart for stools.
- **Fig. 26-3** Stool shapes and consistencies.
- **Fig. 26-10** A stoma on the surface of the body.
- **Fig. 27-5** Percent of food eaten.
- **Fig. 27-6** Percents measure parts of a whole.
- **Fig. 27-9** A graduate is held at eye level to read the amount.
- **Fig. 27-10** Calculating unlabeled measurements.
- **Fig. 27-15** Water mug with straw.
- **Fig. 29-12** Values used to read thermometers.
- **Fig. 29-13** Reading thermometers.
- **Fig. 29-28** Parts of an aneroid sphygmomanometer.
- **Fig. 29-29** Reading the manometer.
- **Fig. 32-4** The names of nursing team members are posted on a marker board.
- **Fig. 34-6 A,** Stool specimen container. **B,** Stool specimen container with attached spoon.
- **Fig. 34-19** Charting sample (blood glucose).
- **Fig. 36-9** Skin protector.
- **Fig. 36-13 I,** Fungal infection of the toenail.
- **Fig. 37-3** Intact skin.
- **Fig. 37-6 A–C,** Kennedy terminal ulcer.
- **Fig. 43-4** Body parts affected by autoimmune disorders.
- **Fig. 44-5** Altered consciousness.
- **Fig. 47-3** Ileal conduit.
- **Fig. 52-7** Juvenile Products Manufacturers Association safety certification seal.

New Procedures

- PROCEDURE: Transferring the Person Using a Stand-Assist Mechanical Lift

FEATURES AND DESIGN

For features and design elements, see "Student Preface," p. xii.

May this book serve you and your students well. We aim to provide current information for teaching and learning safe and effective care during a time of dynamic change in health care.

Sheila A. Sorrentino, BSN, MA, MSN, PhD, RN
Leighann N. Remmert, BSN, MS, RN

Student Preface

This book with special features (pp. xiii-xvi) was designed to help you learn. This preface gives study guidelines to help you use the book. To study effectively, use a study system with these steps.
- Survey or preview
- Question
- Read and record
- Recite and review

SURVEY OR PREVIEW

Preview or survey the reading assignment for a few minutes. This gives an idea of what the assignment covers. It also helps you to recall what you know about the subject. Carefully look over the assignment. Preview the chapter title, objectives, key terms and abbreviations, headings, subheadings, and key ideas in italics. Also survey the boxes and chapter review questions.

QUESTION

Questioning sets a purpose for reading. Form questions to answer while reading. Questions should relate to how the information applies to care or possible test questions. Use the headings and subheadings to form questions. What, why, or how questions are helpful. Avoid questions with 1-word answers. If a question does not help you study, change the question.

READ AND RECORD

You read to:
- Gain new information.
- Connect new information to what you already know.
- Find answers to your questions.

Break the assignment into small parts. Then answer your questions as you read each part. Underline or highlight important information. This reminds you of what you need to learn. Review the marked parts later. Make notes by writing down important information in the margins or in a notebook. Use words and statements to prompt your memory about the material.

To remember what you read, organize information into a study guide. Create diagrams or charts to show relationships or steps in a process. Note taking in an outline also is very useful. For example:
1. Main heading
   A. Second level
   B. Second level
      (1) Third level
      (2) Third level

RECITE AND REVIEW

Finally, recite and review. Use your notes and study guides. Answer your questions and others from reading and answering chapter "Review Questions." Answer all questions out loud (recite).

Reviewing is more about *when* to study rather than *what* to study. You decided *what* to study during your preview, question, and reading steps. It is best to review right after the first study session, 1 week later, and before a quiz or test.

We hope you enjoy learning and your work. You and your work are important. You and the care you give make a difference in the person's life!

Sheila A. Sorrentino
Leighann N. Remmert

SPECIAL FEATURES

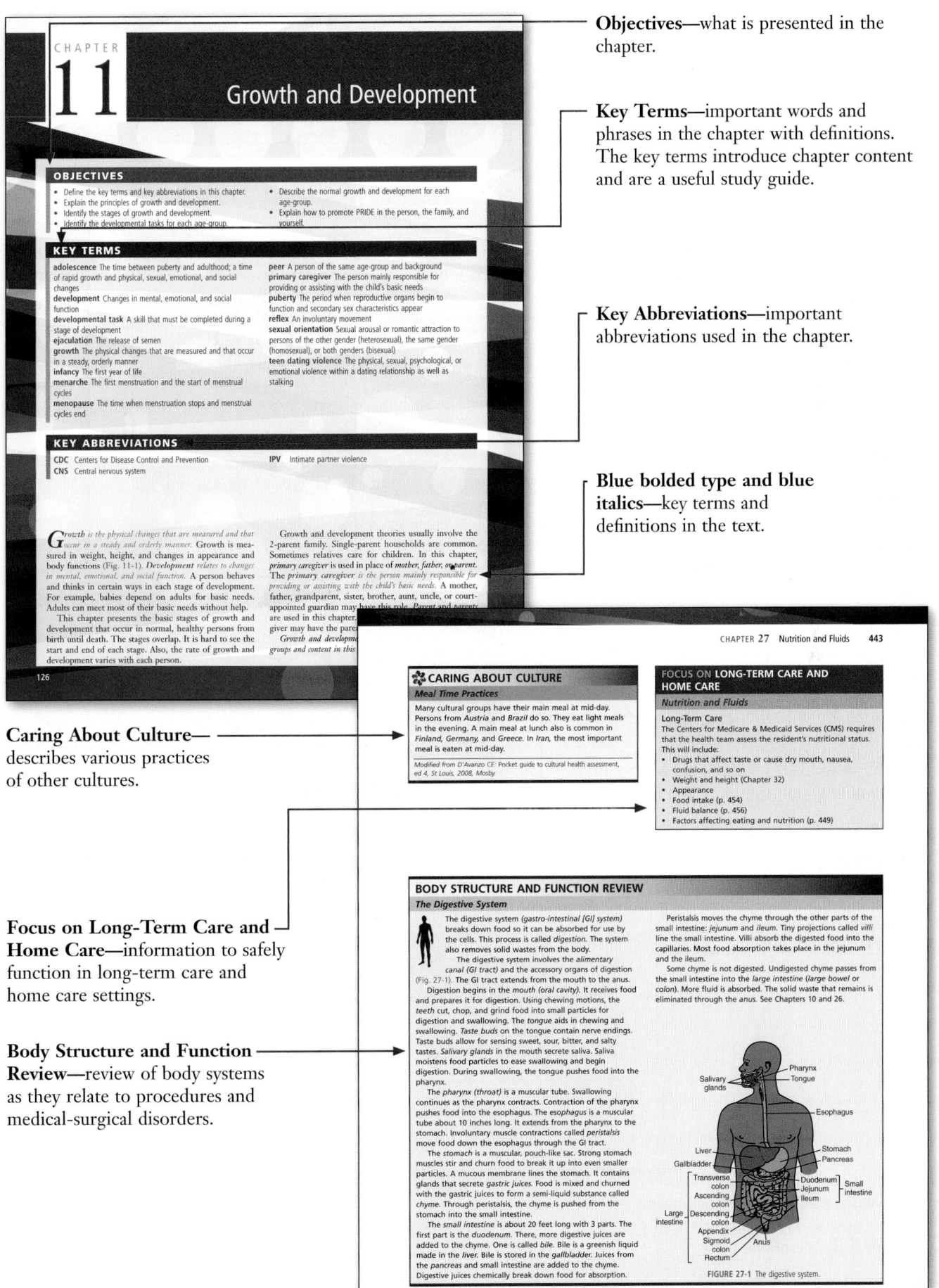

Objectives—what is presented in the chapter.

Key Terms—important words and phrases in the chapter with definitions. The key terms introduce chapter content and are a useful study guide.

Key Abbreviations—important abbreviations used in the chapter.

Blue bolded type and blue italics—key terms and definitions in the text.

Caring About Culture—describes various practices of other cultures.

Focus on Long-Term Care and Home Care—information to safely function in long-term care and home care settings.

Body Structure and Function Review—review of body systems as they relate to procedures and medical-surgical disorders.

Focus on Communication— suggest what to say and questions to ask when interacting with patients, residents, visitors, and the nursing team.

Color illustrations and photographs— visually present key ideas, concepts, and procedure steps.

Heading icons— alert to associated procedures. Procedure boxes have the same icon.

Boxes and tables— rules, principles, guidelines, signs and symptoms, nursing measures, and other information. They are useful study guides.

Focus on Math *(NEW!)*— math involved in various care measures and procedures.

Teamwork and Time Management— suggest how to work with and help nursing team members.

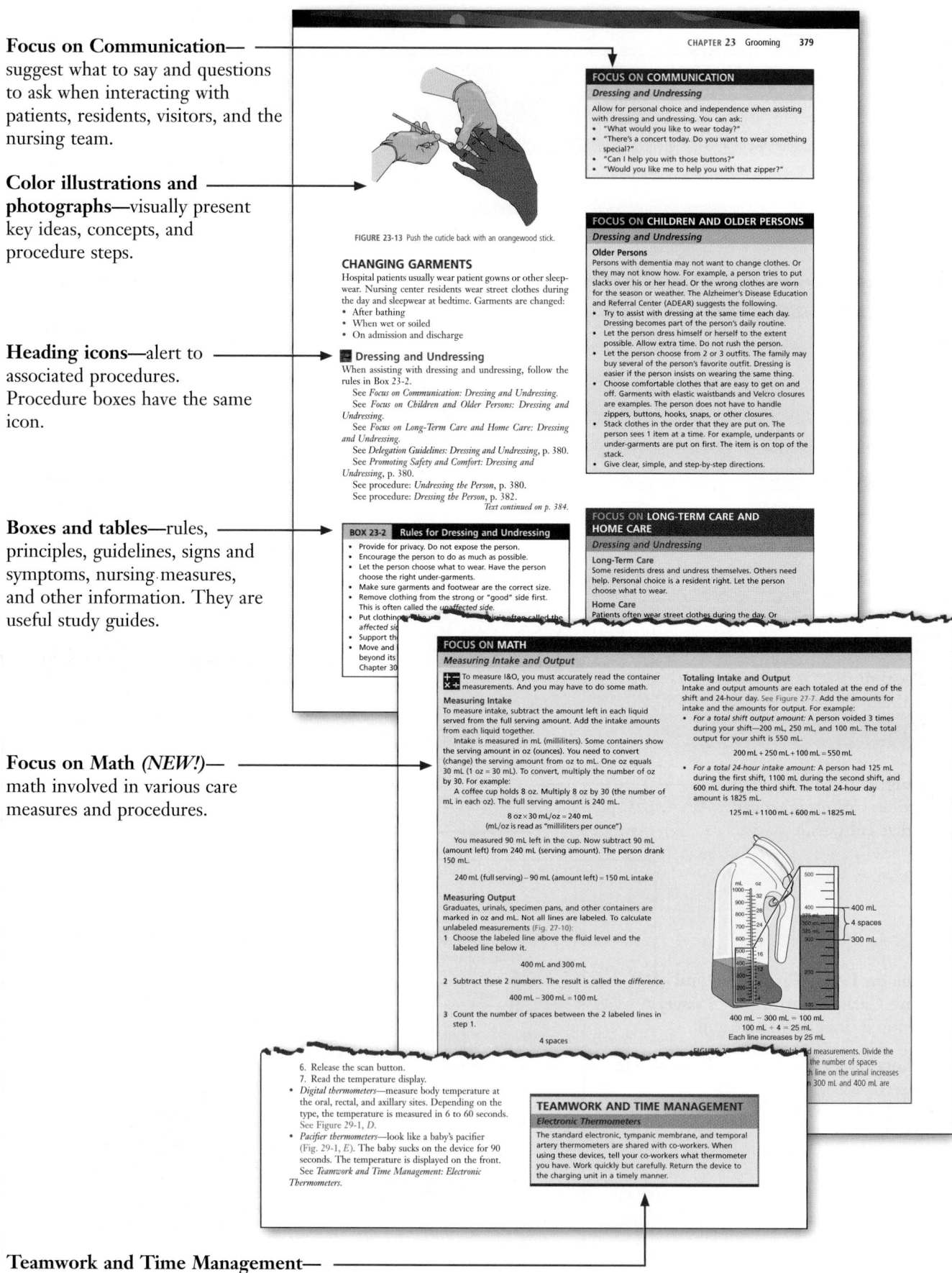

CHAPTER 23 Grooming   379

FIGURE 23-13 Push the cuticle back with an orangewood stick.

CHANGING GARMENTS
Hospital patients usually wear patient gowns or other sleepwear. Nursing center residents wear street clothes during the day and sleepwear at bedtime. Garments are changed:
- After bathing
- When wet or soiled
- On admission and discharge

Dressing and Undressing
When assisting with dressing and undressing, follow the rules in Box 23-2.

See *Focus on Communication: Dressing and Undressing.*
See *Focus on Children and Older Persons: Dressing and Undressing.*
See *Focus on Long-Term Care and Home Care: Dressing and Undressing.*
See *Delegation Guidelines: Dressing and Undressing,* p. 380.
See *Promoting Safety and Comfort: Dressing and Undressing,* p. 380.
See procedure: *Undressing the Person,* p. 380.
See procedure: *Dressing the Person,* p. 382.

Text continued on p. 384.

BOX 23-2   Rules for Dressing and Undressing
- Provide for privacy. Do not expose the person.
- Encourage the person to do as much as possible.
- Let the person choose what to wear. Have the person choose the right under-garments.
- Make sure garments and footwear are the correct size.
- Remove clothing from the strong or "good" side first. This is often called the *unaffected side.*
- Put clothing on the weak side first. This is often called the *affected side.*
- Support the ...
- Move and ... beyond its ... Chapter 30.

FOCUS ON COMMUNICATION
Dressing and Undressing

Allow for personal choice and independence when assisting with dressing and undressing. You can ask:
- "What would you like to wear today?"
- "There's a concert today. Do you want to wear something special?"
- "Can I help you with those buttons?"
- "Would you like me to help you with that zipper?"

FOCUS ON CHILDREN AND OLDER PERSONS
Dressing and Undressing

Older Persons
Persons with dementia may not want to change clothes. Or they may not know how. For example, a person tries to put slacks over his or her head. Or the wrong clothes are worn for the season or weather. The Alzheimer's Disease Education and Referral Center (ADEAR) suggests the following.
- Try to assist with dressing at the same time each day. Dressing becomes part of the person's daily routine.
- Let the person dress himself or herself to the extent possible. Allow extra time. Do not rush the person.
- Let the person choose from 2 or 3 outfits. The family may buy several of the person's favorite outfit. Dressing is easier if the person insists on wearing the same thing.
- Choose comfortable clothes that are easy to get on and off. Garments with elastic waistbands and Velcro closures are examples. The person does not have to handle zippers, buttons, hooks, snaps, or other closures.
- Stack clothes in the order that they are put on. The person sees 1 item at a time. For example, underpants or under-garments are put on first. The item is on top of the stack.
- Give clear, simple, and step-by-step directions.

FOCUS ON LONG-TERM CARE AND HOME CARE
Dressing and Undressing

Long-Term Care
Some residents dress and undress themselves. Others need help. Personal choice is a resident right. Let the person choose what to wear.

Home Care
Patients often wear street clothes during the day. Or ...

FOCUS ON MATH
Measuring Intake and Output

To measure I&O, you must accurately read the container measurements. And you may have to do some math.

Measuring Intake
To measure intake, subtract the amount left in each liquid served from the full serving amount. Add the intake amounts from each liquid together.

Intake is measured in mL (milliliters). Some containers show the serving amount in oz (ounces). You need to convert (change) the serving amount from oz to mL. One oz equals 30 mL (1 oz = 30 mL). To convert, multiply the number of oz by 30. For example:

A coffee cup holds 8 oz. Multiply 8 by 30 (the number of mL in each oz). The full serving amount is 240 mL.

8 oz × 30 mL/oz = 240 mL
(mL/oz is read as "milliliters per ounce")

You measured 90 mL left in the cup. Now subtract 90 mL (amount left) from 240 mL (serving amount). The person drank 150 mL.

240 mL (full serving) − 90 mL (amount left) = 150 mL intake

Measuring Output
Graduates, urinals, specimen pans, and other containers are marked in oz and mL. Not all lines are labeled. To calculate unlabeled measurements (Fig. 27-10):
1 Choose the labeled line above the fluid level and the labeled line below it.

400 mL and 300 mL

2 Subtract these 2 numbers. The result is called the *difference.*

400 mL − 300 mL = 100 mL

3 Count the number of spaces between the 2 labeled lines in step 1.

4 spaces

Totaling Intake and Output
Intake and output amounts are each totaled at the end of the shift and 24-hour day. See Figure 27-7. Add the amounts for intake and the amounts for output. For example:
- *For a total shift output amount:* A person voided 3 times during your shift—200 mL, 250 mL, and 100 mL. The total output for your shift was 550 mL.

200 mL + 250 mL + 100 mL = 550 mL

- *For a total 24-hour intake amount:* A person had 125 mL during the first shift, 1100 mL during the second shift, and 600 mL during the third shift. The total 24-hour day amount is 1825 mL.

125 mL + 1100 mL + 600 mL = 1825 mL

400 mL − 300 mL = 100 mL
100 mL ÷ 4 = 25 mL
Each line increases by 25 mL

FIGURE ... unlabeled measurements. Divide ... the number of spaces ... each line on the urinal increases ... 300 mL and 400 mL are ...

6. Release the scan button.
7. Read the temperature display.
- *Digital thermometers*—measure body temperature at the oral, rectal, and axillary sites. Depending on the type, the temperature is measured in 6 to 60 seconds. See Figure 29-1, *D.*
- *Pacifier thermometers*—look like a baby's pacifier (Fig. 29-1, *E*). The baby sucks on the device for 90 seconds. The temperature is displayed on the front. See *Teamwork and Time Management: Electronic Thermometers.*

TEAMWORK AND TIME MANAGEMENT
Electronic Thermometers

The standard electronic, tympanic membrane, and temporal artery thermometers are shared with co-workers. When using these devices, tell your co-workers what thermometer you have. Work quickly but carefully. Return the device to the charging unit in a timely manner.

Delegation Guidelines—information needed from the nurse and the care plan to perform a procedure. They also list the observations to report and record.

Promoting Safety and Comfort—safety and comfort measures when giving care.

Title bar icons:
- **Video clip icons**—video clips available on-line on *Evolve Student Learning Resources.*
- **Video icons**—procedures included in *Mosby's Nursing Assistant Video Skills 4.0.*
- **NATCEP icons**—skills that are part of competency evaluations.

Procedures—divided into *Quality of Life, Pre-Procedure, Procedure,* and *Post-Procedure* sections. The *Quality of Life* section lists 6 simple courtesies that show respect for the person.

Procedure icons—alert to associated content areas. Heading icons and procedure icons are the same.

Focus on Children and Older Persons—age-specific needs, considerations, and special circumstances of children and older persons, especially persons with Alzheimer's disease and other dementias.

Charting samples—recordings of care and observations.

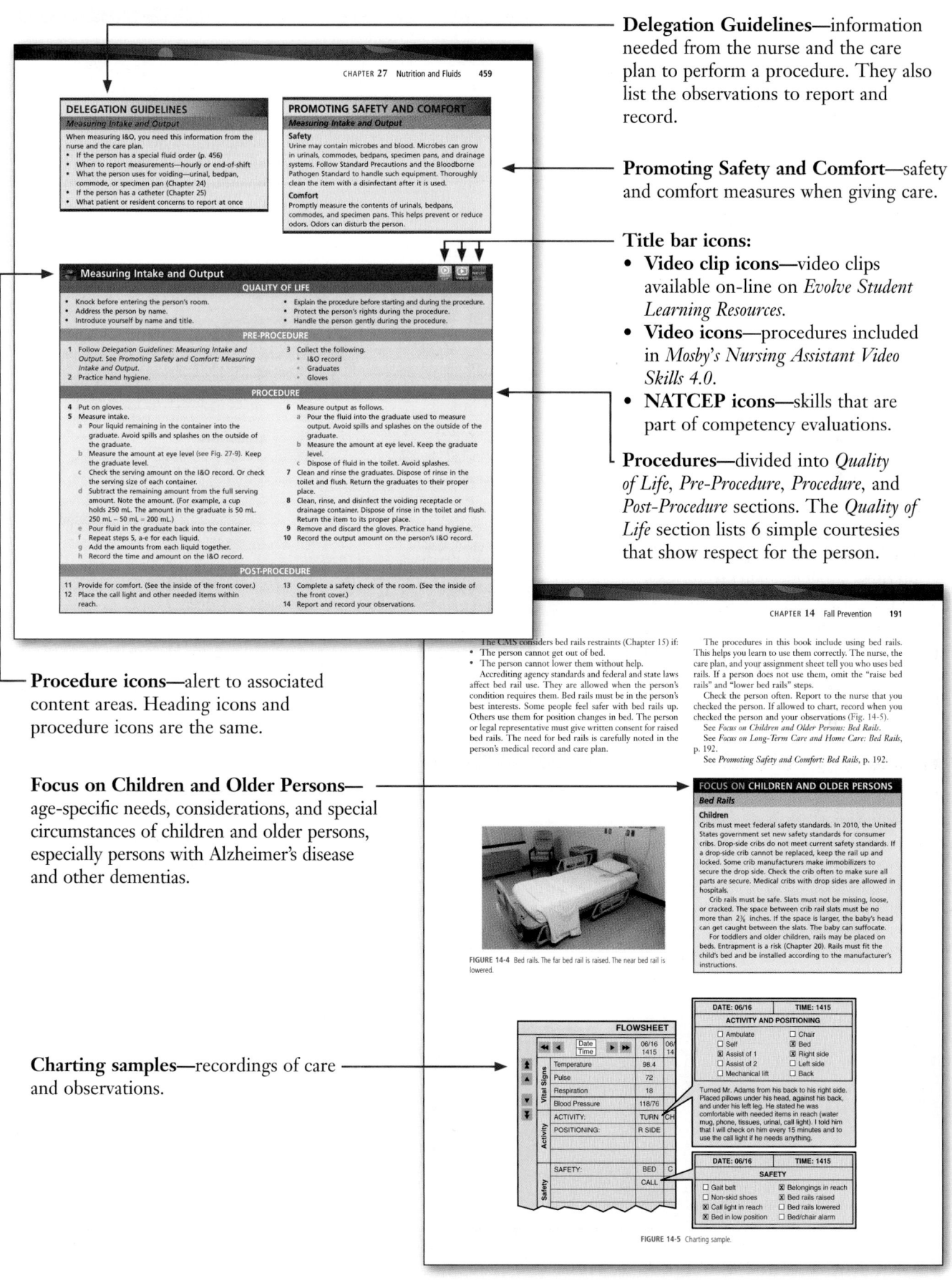

CHAPTER 27 Nutrition and Fluids   459

DELEGATION GUIDELINES
Measuring Intake and Output

When measuring I&O, you need this information from the nurse and the care plan.
- If the person has a special fluid order (p. 456)
- When to report measurements—hourly or end-of-shift
- What the person uses for voiding—urinal, bedpan, commode, or specimen pan (Chapter 24)
- If the person has a catheter (Chapter 25)
- What patient or resident concerns to report at once

PROMOTING SAFETY AND COMFORT
Measuring Intake and Output

Safety
Urine may contain microbes and blood. Microbes can grow in urinals, commodes, bedpans, specimen pans, and drainage systems. Follow Standard Precautions and the Bloodborne Pathogen Standard to handle such equipment. Thoroughly clean the item with a disinfectant after it is used.

Comfort
Promptly measure the contents of urinals, bedpans, commodes, and specimen pans. This helps prevent or reduce odors. Odors can disturb the person.

Measuring Intake and Output

QUALITY OF LIFE
- Knock before entering the person's room.
- Address the person by name.
- Introduce yourself by name and title.
- Explain the procedure before starting and during the procedure.
- Protect the person's rights during the procedure.
- Handle the person gently during the procedure.

PRE-PROCEDURE
1 Follow *Delegation Guidelines: Measuring Intake and Output.* See *Promoting Safety and Comfort: Measuring Intake and Output.*
2 Practice hand hygiene.
3 Collect the following.
   - I&O record
   - Graduates
   - Gloves

PROCEDURE
4 Put on gloves.
5 Measure intake.
   a Pour liquid remaining in the container into the graduate. Avoid spills and splashes on the outside of the graduate.
   b Measure the amount at eye level (see Fig. 27-9). Keep the graduate level.
   c Check the serving amount on the I&O record. Or check the serving size of each container.
   d Subtract the remaining amount from the full serving amount. Note the amount. (For example, a cup holds 250 mL. The amount in the graduate is 50 mL. 250 mL − 50 mL = 200 mL.)
   e Pour fluid in the graduate back into the container.
   f Repeat steps 5, a-e for each liquid.
   g Add the amounts from each liquid together.
   h Record the time and amount on the I&O record.
6 Measure output as follows.
   a Pour the fluid into the graduate used to measure output. Avoid spills and splashes on the outside of the graduate.
   b Measure the amount at eye level. Keep the graduate level.
   c Dispose of fluid in the toilet. Avoid splashes.
7 Clean and rinse the graduates. Dispose of rinse in the toilet and flush. Return the graduates to their proper place.
8 Clean, rinse, and disinfect the voiding receptacle or drainage container. Dispose of rinse in the toilet and flush. Return the item to its proper place.
9 Remove and discard the gloves. Practice hand hygiene.
10 Record the output amount on the person's I&O record.

POST-PROCEDURE
11 Provide for comfort. (See the inside of the front cover.)
12 Place the call light and other needed items within reach.
13 Complete a safety check of the room. (See the inside of the front cover.)
14 Report and record your observations.

CHAPTER 14 Fall Prevention   191

The CMS considers bed rails restraints (Chapter 15) if:
- The person cannot get out of bed.
- The person cannot lower them without help.

Accrediting agency standards and federal and state laws affect bed rail use. They are allowed when the person's condition requires them. Some people feel safer with bed rails up. Others use them for position changes in bed. The person or legal representative must give written consent for bed rails. The need for bed rails is carefully noted in the person's medical record and care plan.

The procedures in this book include using bed rails. This helps you learn to use them correctly. The nurse, the care plan, and your assignment sheet tell you who uses bed rails. If a person does not use them, omit the "raise bed rails" and "lower bed rails" steps.

Check the person often. Report to the nurse that you checked the person. If allowed to chart, record when you checked the person and your observations (Fig. 14-5).

See *Focus on Children and Older Persons: Bed Rails.*
See *Focus on Long-Term Care and Home Care: Bed Rails,* p. 192.
See *Promoting Safety and Comfort: Bed Rails,* p. 192.

FOCUS ON CHILDREN AND OLDER PERSONS
Bed Rails

Children
Cribs must meet federal safety standards. In 2010, the United States government set new safety standards for consumer cribs. Drop-side cribs do not meet current safety standards. If a drop-side crib cannot be replaced, keep the rail up and locked. Some crib manufacturers make immobilizers to secure the drop side. Check the crib often to make sure all parts are secure. Medical cribs with drop sides are allowed in hospitals.

Crib rails must be safe. Slats must not be missing, loose, or cracked. The space between crib rail slats must be no more than 2⅜ inches. If the space is larger, the baby's head can get caught between the slats. The baby can suffocate. For toddlers and older children, rails may be placed on beds. Entrapment is a risk (Chapter 20). Rails must fit the child's bed and be installed according to the manufacturer's instructions.

FIGURE 14-4 Bed rails. The far bed rail is raised. The near bed rail is lowered.

FLOWSHEET		06/16 1415	06/ 14
Date Time			
Vital Signs Temperature		98.4	
Pulse		72	
Respiration		18	
Blood Pressure		118/76	
Activity ACTIVITY:		TURN CH	
POSITIONING:		R SIDE	
Safety SAFETY:		BED C	
		CALL	

DATE: 06/16	TIME: 1415
ACTIVITY AND POSITIONING	
☐ Ambulate	☐ Chair
☐ Self	☒ Bed
☒ Assist of 1	☒ Right side
☐ Assist of 2	☐ Left side
☐ Mechanical lift	☐ Back

Turned Mr. Adams from his back to his right side. Placed pillows under his head, against his back, and under his left leg. He stated he was comfortable with needed items in reach (water mug, phone, tissues, urinal, call light). I told him that I will check on him every 15 minutes and to use the call light if he needs anything.

DATE: 06/16	TIME: 1415
SAFETY	
☐ Gait belt	☒ Belongings in reach
☐ Non-skid shoes	☒ Bed rails raised
☒ Call light in reach	☐ Bed rails lowered
☒ Bed in low position	☐ Bed/chair alarm

FIGURE 14-5 Charting sample.

Focus on Surveys *(NEW!)*—questions that surveyors may ask you or what they may observe you doing.

Focus on PRIDE: The Person, Family, and Yourself—build on chapter content to help you promote *pride* in the person, the family, and yourself. The first letter of each section spells *PRIDE*.
- *Personal and Professional Responsibility*—how to have pride in yourself through personal and professional behaviors and development.
- *Rights and Respect*—how to promote the person's rights and respect him or her as a person with dignity and value.
- *Independence and Social Interaction*—ways to help the person remain or attain independence and interact socially with others.
- *Delegation and Teamwork*—how to work efficiently with and help nursing team members.
- *Ethics and Laws*—laws affecting nursing care and doing the right thing when dealing with patients, residents, and co-workers.

Focus on PRIDE: Application *(NEW!)*—how to apply information in Focus on PRIDE. Questions are intended for personal thought or classroom discussion.

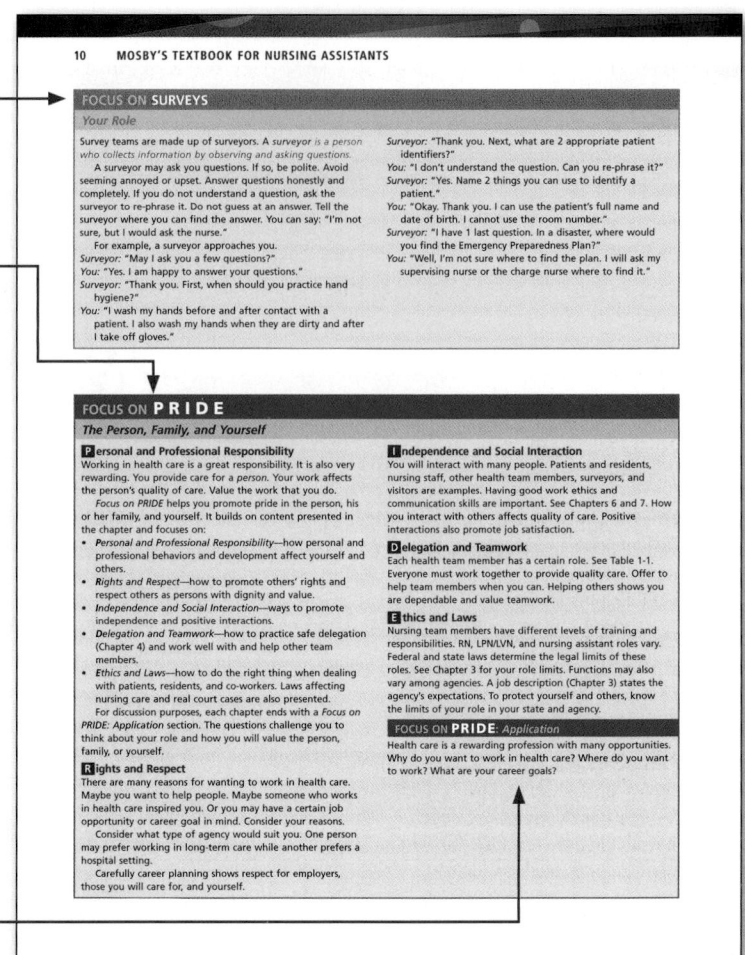

Review Questions—study guides to review what you have learned. Use them to study for a test or for the competency evaluation. Answers are at the back of the book. See p. 870.

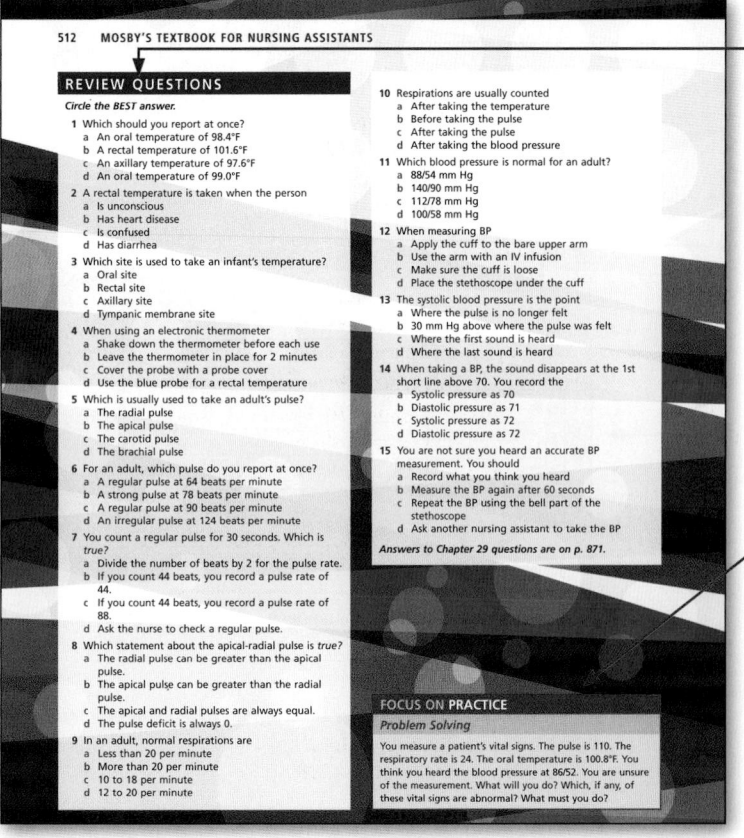

Focus on Practice: Problem Solving *(NEW!)*—follow the Review Questions. A situation is presented that you may encounter as a student or in the work setting. For classroom discussion or self-study, questions follow about what you should do, how you should act, or how you can improve the situation.

Contents

1 **Introduction to Health Care Agencies,** *1*
Agency Purposes, 1
Types of Agencies, 2
Organization, 3
The Nursing Team, 7
Nursing Care Patterns, 8
Paying for Health Care, 8
Meeting Standards, 9

2 **The Person's Rights,** *12*
Patient Rights, 12
Resident Rights, 12
Ombudsman Program, 18

3 **The Nursing Assistant,** *21*
History and Current Trends, 21
Federal and State Laws, 22
Roles and Responsibilities, 25

4 **Delegation,** *31*
Who Can Delegate, 31
Delegation Process, 32
The Five Rights of Delegation, 35
Your Role in Delegation, 35

5 **Ethics and Laws,** *38*
Ethical Aspects, 39
Legal Aspects, 40
Reporting Abuse, 44
Wills, 52

6 **Student and Work Ethics,** *55*
Health, Hygiene, and Appearance, 56
Preparing for School or Work, 57
Teamwork, 58
Managing Stress, 62
Harassment, 63
Resigning From a Job, 64
Losing a Job, 64
Drug Testing, 65
Unethical Student Behavior, 65

7 **Communicating With the Health Team,** *67*
Communication, 68
The Medical Record, 68
The Kardex or Care Summary, 72
Reporting and Recording, 72
Computers and Other Electronic Devices, 75
Phone Communications, 77
Medical Terms and Abbreviations, 77

8 **Assisting With the Nursing Process,** *83*
Assessment, 84
Nursing Diagnosis, 86
Planning, 86
Implementation, 88
Evaluation, 90
Your Role, 90

9 **Understanding the Person,** *92*
Caring for the Person, 92
Basic Needs, 93

Culture and Religion, 94
Effects of Illness and Disability, 95
Persons You Will Care For, 96
Communicating With the Person, 97
Persons With Special Needs, 103
Family and Friends, 103
Behavior Issues, 104

10 **Body Structure and Function,** *108*
Cells, Tissues, and Organs, 108
The Integumentary System, 110
The Musculo-Skeletal System, 110
The Nervous System, 113
The Circulatory System, 115
The Lymphatic System, 117
The Respiratory System, 118
The Digestive System, 119
The Urinary System, 119
The Reproductive System, 120
The Endocrine System, 122
The Immune System, 123

11 **Growth and Development,** *126*
Principles, 127
Infancy (Birth to 1 Year), 127
Toddlerhood (1 to 3 Years), 131
Preschool (3 to 6 Years), 132
School Age (6 to 9 or 10 Years), 133
Late Childhood (9 or 10 to 12 Years), 134
Adolescence (12 to 18 Years), 135
Young Adulthood (18 to 40 Years), 136
Middle Adulthood (40 to 65 Years), 137
Late Adulthood (65 Years and Older), 137

12 **Care of the Older Person,** *140*
Psychological and Social Changes, 140
Physical Changes, 142
Housing Options, 147

13 **Safety,** *154*
A Safe Setting, 155
Accident Risk Factors, 156
Identifying the Person, 156
Preventing Burns, 159
Preventing Poisoning, 159
Preventing Suffocation, 163
**Relieving Choking—Adult or Child (Over 1 Year
of Age), 166**
**Relieving Choking—In the Infant (Less Than 1 Year of
Age), 168**
Preventing Equipment Accidents, 169
Hazardous Chemicals, 171
Disasters, 173
Using a Fire Extinguisher, 176
Workplace Violence, 178
Risk Management, 181

14 **Fall Prevention,** *186*
Causes and Risk Factors for Falls, 187
Fall Prevention Programs, 188

Transfer/Gait Belts, 193
Using a Transfer/Gait Belt, 195
The Falling Person, 196
Helping the Falling Person, 197
Moving the Person From the Floor, 197

15   Restraint Alternatives and Safe Restraint Use, *200*
History of Restraint Use, 201
Restraint Alternatives, 201
Safe Restraint Use, 202
Applying Restraints, 213

16   Preventing Infection, *217*
Microorganisms, 218
Infection, 219
Medical Asepsis, 221
Hand-Washing, 225
Using an Alcohol-Based Hand Rub, 225
Isolation Precautions, 228
Donning and Removing Personal Protective Equipment, 237
Double-Bagging, 239
Bloodborne Pathogen Standard, 240
Surgical Asepsis, 244
Sterile Gloving, 246

17   Body Mechanics, *250*
Principles of Body Mechanics, 250
Work-Related Injuries, 253
Positioning the Person, 256

18   Safely Moving the Person, *262*
Preventing Work-Related Injuries, 263
Protecting the Skin, 264
Moving Persons in Bed, 265
Raising the Person's Head and Shoulders, 266
Moving the Person Up in Bed, 268
Moving the Person Up in Bed With an Assist Device, 270
Moving the Person to the Side of the Bed, 272
Turning Persons, 273
Turning and Re-Positioning the Person, 273
Logrolling the Person, 275
Sitting on the Side of the Bed (Dangling), 276
Sitting on the Side of the Bed (Dangling), 278
Re-Positioning in a Chair or Wheelchair, 279

19   Safely Transferring the Person, *281*
Wheelchair and Stretcher Safety, 283
Stand and Pivot Transfers, 286
Transferring the Person to a Chair or Wheelchair, 287
Transferring the Person From a Chair or Wheelchair to Bed, 290
Transferring the Person To and From the Toilet, 291
Lateral Transfers, 292
Moving the Person to a Stretcher, 294
Mechanical Lifts, 295
Transferring the Person Using a Stand-Assist Mechanical Lift, 297
Transferring the Person Using a Full-Sling Mechanical Lift, 299

20   The Person's Unit, *303*
Comfort, 304
Room Furniture and Equipment, 306

21   Bedmaking, *319*
Types of Beds, 319
Linens, 320
Making Beds, 322
Making a Closed Bed, 324
Making an Open Bed, 328
Making an Occupied Bed, 329
Making a Surgical Bed, 332

22   Personal Hygiene, *335*
Daily Care, 337
Oral Hygiene, 338
Assisting the Person to Brush and Floss the Teeth, 340
Brushing and Flossing the Person's Teeth, 341
Providing Mouth Care for the Unconscious Person, 343
Providing Denture Care, 345
Bathing, 346
Giving a Complete Bed Bath, 350
Assisting With the Partial Bath, 353
Assisting With a Tub Bath or Shower, 357
Perineal Care, 358
Giving Female Perineal Care, 359
Giving Male Perineal Care, 362
Reporting and Recording, 363

23   Grooming, *366*
Hair Care, 367
Brushing and Combing Hair, 370
Shampooing the Person's Hair, 373
Shaving, 374
Shaving the Person's Face With a Safety Razor, 375
Nail and Foot Care, 376
Giving Nail and Foot Care, 378
Changing Garments, 379
Undressing the Person, 380
Dressing the Person, 382
Changing a Patient Gown on a Person With an IV, 385

24   Urinary Elimination, *388*
Normal Urination, 389
Giving the Bedpan, 392
Giving the Urinal, 394
Helping the Person to the Commode, 396
Urinary Incontinence, 396
Applying Incontinence Products, 401
Bladder Training, 404

25   Urinary Catheters, *407*
Purposes and Types of Catheters, 408
Catheter Care, 408
Giving Catheter Care, 411
Urine Drainage Systems, 412
Changing a Leg Bag to a Standard Drainage Bag, 413
Emptying a Urine Drainage Bag, 415
Removing Indwelling Catheters, 416
Removing an Indwelling Catheter, 417
Applying a Condom Catheter, 419

26   Bowel Elimination, *422*
Normal Bowel Elimination, 423
Factors Affecting BMs, 425
Common Problems, 426
Checking For and Removing a Fecal Impaction, 428
Bowel Training, 430
Suppositories, 430
Enemas, 431
Giving a Cleansing Enema, 433
Giving a Small-Volume Enema, 435
Giving an Oil-Retention Enema, 436
The Person With an Ostomy, 436
Changing an Ostomy Pouch, 439

27   Nutrition and Fluids, *442*
Basic Nutrition, 444
Meeting Nutritional Needs, 448
Special Diets, 451
Food Intake, 454
Fluid Balance, 456
Measuring Intake and Output, 459
Meeting Food and Fluid Needs, 460

Preparing the Person for a Meal, 461
Serving Meal Trays, 463
Feeding the Person, 465
Providing Drinking Water, 467
Foodborne Illness, 468

28 Nutritional Support and IV Therapy, 473
Enteral Nutrition, 474
Parenteral Nutrition, 478
IV Therapy, 479

29 Measuring Vital Signs, 486
Measuring and Reporting Vital Signs, 487
Body Temperature, 488
Taking a Temperature With an Electronic
    Thermometer, 492
Taking a Temperature With a Glass Thermometer, 495
Pulse, 497
Taking a Radial Pulse, 501
Taking an Apical Pulse, 502
Taking an Apical-Radial Pulse, 503
Respirations, 504
Counting Respirations, 505
Blood Pressure, 506
Measuring Blood Pressure, 509
Pain, 511

30 Exercise and Activity, 513
Bedrest, 514
Range-of-Motion Exercises, 517
Performing Range-of-Motion Exercises, 519
Ambulation, 522
Helping the Person Walk, 524

31 Comfort, Rest, and Sleep, 531
Comfort, 532
Pain, 532
Giving a Back Massage, 537
Rest, 539
Sleep, 539

32 Admissions, Transfers, and Discharges, 545
Admissions, 546
Preparing the Room, 547
Preparing the Person's Room, 547
Admitting the Person, 550
Measuring Weight and Height, 555
Measuring Height—The Person Is in Bed, 556
Moving the Person to a New Room, 557
Moving the Person to a New Room, 557
Transfers and Discharges, 558
Transferring or Discharging the Person, 558

33 Assisting With the Physical Examination, 561
Your Role, 561
Equipment, 561
Preparing the Person, 562
Preparing the Person for an Examination, 563
Positioning and Draping, 564
Assisting With the Exam, 565

34 Collecting and Testing Specimens, 567
Urine Specimens, 568
Collecting a Random Urine Specimen, 569
Collecting a Midstream Specimen, 570
Collecting a 24-Hour Urine Specimen, 572
Collecting a Urine Specimen From an Infant or
    Child, 573
Testing Urine With Reagent Strips, 575
Straining Urine, 576
Stool Specimens, 577
Collecting and Testing a Stool Specimen, 578

Sputum Specimens, 580
Collecting a Sputum Specimen, 581
Blood Glucose Testing, 582
Measuring Blood Glucose, 584

35 The Person Having Surgery, 588
Psychological Care, 589
Pre-Operative Care, 589
The Surgical Skin Prep—Shaving the Skin, 593
Sedation and Anesthesia, 595
Post-Operative Care, 595
Applying Elastic Stockings, 599
Applying an Elastic Bandage, 600

36 Wound Care, 604
Skin Tears, 607
Circulatory Ulcers, 608
Wound Healing, 611
Dressings, 614
Applying a Dry, Non-Sterile Dressing, 617
Binders and Compression Garments, 618
Heat and Cold Applications, 619
Meeting Basic Needs, 619

37 Pressure Ulcers, 621
Pressure Ulcer Definitions, 622
Risk Factors, 623
Persons at Risk, 624
Pressure Ulcer Stages, 625
Sites, 626
Prevention and Treatment, 627
Complications, 631
Reporting and Recording, 631

38 Heat and Cold Applications, 634
Heat Applications, 635
Cold Applications, 636
Applying Heat and Cold Applications, 638
Cooling and Warming Blankets, 640

39 Oxygen Needs, 642
Factors Affecting Oxygen Needs, 643
Altered Respiratory Function, 644
Respiratory Tests, 645
Using a Pulse Oximeter, 646
Meeting Oxygen Needs, 647
Assisting With Deep-Breathing and Coughing Exercises, 649
Assisting With Oxygen Therapy, 651
Setting Up Oxygen, 655

40 Respiratory Support and Therapies, 658
Artificial Airways, 658
Suctioning, 660
Mechanical Ventilation, 662
Chest Tubes, 663

41 Rehabilitation and Restorative Nursing Care, 666
Restorative Nursing, 667
Rehabilitation and the Whole Person, 667
The Rehabilitation Team, 670
Rehabilitation Programs and Services, 671
Quality of Life, 673

42 Hearing, Speech, and Vision Problems, 675
Ear Disorders, 675
Speech Disorders, 681
Eye Disorders, 682
Caring for Eyeglasses, 689

43 Cancer, Immune System, and Skin Disorders, 693
Cancer, 693
Immune System Disorders, 699
Skin Disorders, 702

44   Nervous System and Musculo-Skeletal Disorders, *705*
Nervous System Disorders, 705
Musculo-Skeletal Disorders, 712

45   Cardiovascular, Respiratory, and Lymphatic Disorders, *724*
Cardiovascular Disorders, 725
Respiratory Disorders, 731
Lymphatic Disorders, 735

46   Digestive and Endocrine Disorders, *739*
Digestive Disorders, 739
Endocrine Disorders, 745

47   Urinary and Reproductive Disorders, *749*
Urinary System Disorders, 749
Reproductive Disorders, 754

48   Mental Health Disorders, *757*
Basic Concepts, 758
Anxiety Disorders, 758
Schizophrenia, 760
Bipolar Disorder, 761
Depression, 761
Personality Disorders, 762
Substance Abuse Disorder, 762
Eating Disorders, 764
Suicide, 765
Care and Treatment, 766

49   Confusion and Dementia, *769*
Confusion, 769
Dementia, 771
Alzheimer's Disease, 771
Care of Persons With AD and Other Dementias, 778

50   Intellectual and Developmental Disabilities, *786*
Intellectual Disabilities, 788
Down Syndrome, 788
Fragile X Syndrome, 789
Autism, 789
Cerebral Palsy, 790
Spina Bifida, 790
Hydrocephalus, 791

51   Sexuality, *794*
Sex and Sexuality, 794
Sexual Orientation, 796
Injury, Illness, and Surgery, 796
Sexuality and Older Persons, 796
Meeting Sexual Needs, 796
The Sexually Aggressive Person, 797
Sexually Transmitted Diseases, 798

52   Caring for Mothers and Babies, *800*
Safety and Security, 800
Signs and Symptoms of Illness, 804
Helping Mothers Breast-Feed, 805
Bottle-Feeding Babies, 807
Cleaning Baby Bottles, 808
Burping the Baby, 809
Diapering, 810
Diapering a Baby, 811
Umbilical Cord Care, 813
Circumcision Care, 813
Bathing an Infant, 814
Giving a Baby a Sponge Bath, 815
Giving a Baby a Tub Bath, 817

Nail Care, 817
Weighing Infants, 817
Weighing an Infant, 818
Care of the Mother, 818

53   Assisted Living, *822*
Assisted Living Residents, 823
ALR Services and Living Areas, 823
Staff Requirements, 824
Service Plans, 824
Transfer, Discharge, and Eviction, 827

54   Basic Emergency Care, *829*
Emergency Care, 829
BLS for Adults, 830
Adult CPR—1 Rescuer, 837
Adult CPR With AED—2 Rescuers, 837
BLS for Children and Infants, 838
Child CPR—1 Rescuer, 842
Child CPR With AED—2 Rescuers, 842
Infant CPR—1 Rescuer, 843
Infant CPR With AED—2 Rescuers, 843
Choking, 844
Poisoning, 844
Hemorrhage, 844
Fainting, 845
Shock, 845
Stroke, 846
Seizures, 846
Concussions, 847
Burns, 848

55   End-of-Life Care, *851*
Terminal Illness, 852
Attitudes About Death, 852
The Stages of Dying, 853
Comfort Needs, 854
The Family, 855
Legal Issues, 855
Signs of Death, 856
Care of the Body After Death, 856
Assisting With Post-Mortem Care, 857

56   Getting a Job, *860*
Sources of Jobs, 860
What Employers Look For, 860
Job Applications, 861
The Job Interview, 864
Accepting or Declining a Job Offer, 867
Drug Testing, 867

REVIEW QUESTION ANSWERS, *870*

APPENDIX A   National Nurse Aide Assessment Program (NNAAP®) Written Examination Content Outline and Skills Evaluation, *873*

APPENDIX B   Minimum Data Set—Selected Pages, *874*

APPENDIX C   Care Area Assessment (CAA)— Sample Page, *876*

APPENDIX D   Infant and Child Safety, *877*

GLOSSARY, *883*

KEY ABBREVIATIONS, *893*

INDEX, *895*

Introduction to Health Care Agencies

OBJECTIVES

- Define the key terms and key abbreviations in this chapter.
- Describe the types, purposes, and organization of health care agencies.
- Describe the members of the health team and nursing team.
- Describe the nursing service department.
- Describe 5 nursing care patterns.
- Describe the programs that pay for health care.
- Explain your role in meeting standards.
- Explain how to promote PRIDE in the person, the family, and yourself.

KEY TERMS

acute illness A sudden illness from which a person is expected to recover

assisted living residence (ALR) Provides housing, personal care, support services, health care, and social activities in a home-like setting to persons needing help with daily activities

case management A nursing case manager coordinates the care of specific groups of patients from admission through discharge and into the home or long-term care setting

chronic illness An on-going illness that is slow or gradual in onset; it has no known cure; it can be controlled and complications prevented with proper treatment

functional nursing A nursing care pattern focusing on tasks and jobs; each nursing team member has certain tasks and jobs to do

health team The many health care workers whose skills and knowledge focus on the person's total care; interdisciplinary health care team

hospice A health care agency or program for persons who are dying

licensed practical nurse (LPN) A nurse who has completed a practical nursing program and has passed a licensing test; called *licensed vocational nurse (LVN)* in California and Texas

licensed vocational nurse (LVN) See "licensed practical nurse (LPN)"

nursing assistant A person who has passed a nursing assistant training and competency evaluation program; performs delegated nursing tasks under the supervision of a licensed nurse

nursing team Those who provide nursing care—RNs, LPNs/LVNs, and nursing assistants

patient-focused care A nursing care pattern; services are moved from departments to the bedside

primary nursing A nursing care pattern; an RN is responsible for the person's total care

registered nurse (RN) A nurse who has completed a 2-, 3-, or 4-year nursing program and has passed a licensing test

surveyor A person who collects information by observing and asking questions

team nursing A nursing care pattern; a team of nursing staff is led by an RN who decides the amount and kind of care each person needs

terminal illness An illness or injury from which the person will not likely recover

KEY ABBREVIATIONS

DON	Director of nursing
LPN	Licensed practical nurse
LVN	Licensed vocational nurse

RN	Registered nurse
SNF	Skilled nursing facility

Health care agencies (Box 1-1, p. 2) vary in size, services, hours open, and staff. The *person* is always the focus of care.

Staff members have special talents, knowledge, and skills. All work to meet the person's needs.

Health care agencies must follow local, state, and federal laws and rules. This is to ensure safe care.

AGENCY PURPOSES

Services range from simple to complex. Some agencies have 1 purpose and offer 1 service. Surgery centers are an example. Surgeries and medical procedures are done in a non-hospital setting. The person returns home the same day or the next day. Other agencies have many purposes and services.

BOX 1-1	Types of Health Care Agencies

- Hospitals
- Long-term care centers (nursing homes, nursing facilities, nursing centers)
- Memory care facilities
- Home care agencies; home health care agencies
- Surgery centers
- Urgent care centers
- Adult day-care centers
- Assisted living residences
- Board and care homes
- Rehabilitation and sub-acute care facilities
- Hospices
- Doctors' offices
- Clinics
- Centers for persons with mental health disorders
- Centers for persons with intellectual and developmental disabilities
- Drug and alcohol treatment centers
- Crisis centers for rape, abuse, suicide, and other emergencies

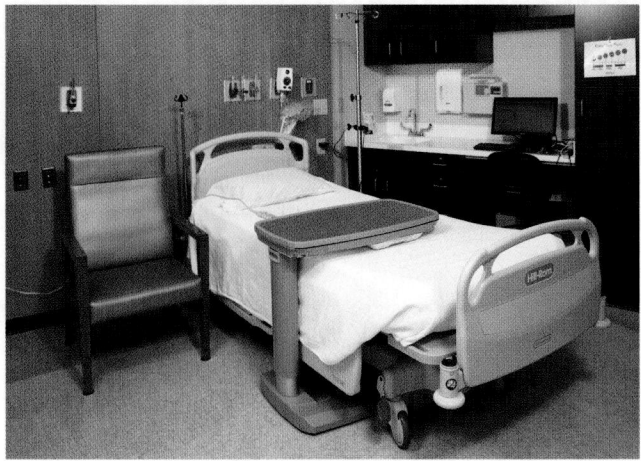

FIGURE 1-1 A hospital room.

The purposes of health care are:

- *Health promotion.* The goal is to reduce the risk of physical or mental illness. People learn about healthy living. This includes diet, exercise, and the warning signs and symptoms of illness. They learn how to manage and cope with health problems.
- *Disease prevention.* Measures are taken to reduce risk factors and prevent disease. Immunizations prevent some infectious diseases. Polio, measles, mumps, smallpox, and hepatitis B are examples. Simple life-style changes can promote health. For example, high blood pressure can cause heart attacks and strokes. Diet and exercise help to lower blood pressure.
- *Detection and treatment of disease.* This involves diagnostic tests, physical exams, surgery, emergency care, and drugs. Respiratory, physical, and occupational therapies are common. The nursing team observes signs and symptoms, gives care, and follows the doctor's orders.
- *Rehabilitation and restorative care.* This involves returning persons to their highest possible level of physical and mental functioning and to independence. *Independence* means *not relying on or needing care from others.* The process starts when the person first seeks health care. He or she learns or re-learns skills needed to live, work, and enjoy life. Maintaining function is important. Help is given to make needed changes at home.

These purposes are related. For example: having chest pain, Mr. Parker goes to a hospital emergency room. After an exam and tests, the doctor diagnoses a heart attack. Mr. Parker is admitted to the hospital for treatment. He also receives teaching and counseling about heart attack risk factors, diet, drugs, life-style, activity, and coping with fears and concerns. He begins a rehabilitation program. Activity starts slowly and may progress from walking to jogging and swimming. Successful treatment and rehabilitation promote health and may prevent another heart attack.

Student Learning

Agencies are often learning sites for students. Students assist in the purposes of health care. They are involved with and provide care.

TYPES OF AGENCIES

Nursing assistants work in many settings. Some work in doctors' offices and clinics. Most work in the following agencies.

Hospitals

Hospitals provide emergency care, surgery, nursing care, x-ray procedures and treatments, and laboratory testing. They also provide respiratory, physical, occupational, speech, and other therapies. Hospital care is either in-patient or out-patient. *In-patient care* is health care a person receives when admitted to an agency such as a hospital or skilled nursing facility. See Figure 1-1. *Out-patient (ambulatory) care* includes medical or surgical care received when a person is not admitted to an agency.

People of all ages need hospital care. They have babies, surgery, physical and mental health disorders, and broken bones. Some are dying.

Hospital patients have acute, chronic, or terminal illnesses.

- *Acute illness is a sudden illness from which the person is expected to recover.* A heart attack is an example.
- *Chronic illness is an on-going illness that is slow or gradual in onset. There is no known cure. The illness can be controlled and complications prevented with proper treatment.* Diabetes is an example.
- *Terminal illness is an illness or injury from which the person will not likely recover.* The person will die (Chapter 55). Cancers not responding to treatment are examples.

Rehabilitation and Sub-Acute Care Agencies

Hospital stays are often short. Some people do not need hospital care but are too sick or disabled to go home. Care needs fall between hospital care and long-term care. Along with rehabilitation, complex equipment and care measures are needed. See Chapter 41 for common rehabilitation programs.

Some hospitals and long-term care centers have rehabilitation and sub-acute care units. Others are separate agencies. Many persons fully recover and return home. Others need long-term care.

Long-Term Care Centers

Some persons cannot care for themselves at home but do not need hospital care. Long-term care centers are designed to meet their needs. Care needs range from simple to complex. Medical, nursing, dietary, recreation, rehabilitation, and social services are provided. So are housekeeping and laundry services.

Persons in long-term care centers are called *residents.* They are not *patients.* The center is their temporary or permanent home.

Most residents are older. Many have chronic diseases, poor nutrition, memory problems, or poor health. Not all residents are old. Some are disabled from birth defects, accidents, or disease. Hospital patients are often discharged while still recovering from illness or surgery. Some need home care. Others need long-term care until able to go home. Others need care until death.

Skilled Nursing Facilities. Skilled nursing facilities (SNFs) provide more complex care than do nursing centers. They are part of hospitals or nursing centers. SNF residents need rehabilitation or recovery time. Often they return home after a short stay. Others remain nursing center residents.

Assisted Living Residences

An *assisted living residence (ALR) provides housing, personal care, support services, health care, and social activities in a home-like setting to persons needing help with daily activities* (Chapter 53). Some ALRs are part of nursing centers or retirement communities (Chapter 12).

The person has a room or an apartment. Three meals a day and 24-hour supervision are provided. So are housekeeping, laundry, social, recreational, transportation, and some health care services. Help is given with personal care and drugs.

Mental Health Centers

Some persons have problems with life events. Others present dangers to themselves or others because of how they think and behave. Out-patient mental health care is common. Some need short-term or long-term in-patient care.

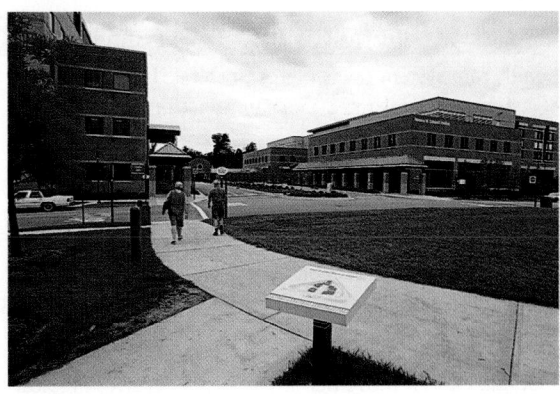

FIGURE 1-2 The hospital and doctors' offices are part of a health care system. (Courtesy Anne Arundel Health System, Inc. Annapolis, Md.)

Home Care Agencies

Health care services are provided to people where they live. Services range from health teaching and supervision to bedside nursing care. Physical therapy, rehabilitation, and food services are common. Hospitals, health care systems, public health departments, and private businesses offer home care.

People of all ages need home health care. So do some persons who are dying.

Hospices

A *hospice is a health care agency or program for persons who are dying.* Such persons no longer respond to treatments aimed at cures. Usually they have less than 6 months to live.

The physical, emotional, social, and spiritual needs of the person and family are met. The focus is on comfort, not cure. Children and pets can visit. Family and friends can assist with care.

Hospice care is provided by hospitals, nursing centers, and home care and hospice agencies.

Health Care Systems

Agencies join together as 1 provider of care. A system usually has hospitals, nursing centers, home care agencies, hospice settings, and doctors' offices (Fig. 1-2). An ambulance service and medical supply store for home care are common. The system serves a community or larger region.

The goal is to meet all health care needs. A person uses system providers as needed (Box 1-2, p. 4).

ORGANIZATION

An agency has a governing body called the *board of trustees* or *board of directors.* The board makes policies. It makes sure that safe care is given at the lowest possible cost. Local, state, and federal laws are followed.

An administrator manages the agency. He or she reports directly to the board. Directors or department heads manage certain areas (Fig. 1-3, p. 4).

See *Focus on Long-Term Care and Home Care: Organization,* p. 4.

BOX 1-2	Using a Health Care System

A health care system owns Mercy Hospital. The system also has:
- Doctors' offices
- A home care service
- An ambulance service
- A medical supply store
- A nursing center

June Adams is 78 years old. She sees Dr. Moore in his office complaining of chest pain, dizziness, and a "pounding heart." She is having a heart attack. Dr. Gills, a heart specialist, takes over her care. A few days later she has a stroke and cannot move her left side. She receives medical care. When stable, she transfers to the hospital's rehabilitation unit.

After 2 weeks on the rehabilitation unit, Mrs. Adams returns home. She needs a hospital bed, commode, bedpan, wheelchair, and other items. The family rents some items and buys others at the medical supply store.

Mrs. Adams returns home by ambulance. The system's home care agency arranges for a nursing assistant to meet daily hygiene and grooming needs. A nurse visits 3 times a week.

A month later Mrs. Adams has another stroke. She returns to the hospital by ambulance. After 8 days, she transfers again to the rehabilitation unit. The second stroke has caused more disabilities. Her doctors suggest nursing center care. Mrs. Adams and her family agree. Mrs. Adams is transferred to the nursing center by ambulance.

FOCUS ON LONG-TERM CARE AND HOME CARE

Organization

Long-Term Care

Nursing centers are usually owned by an individual or a corporation. Some are owned by county or state health departments. The U.S. Department of Veterans Affairs (Veterans Administration; VA) also has nursing centers.

Each center has an administrator. Department directors report to the administrator. Nursing centers have nursing, therapy, and food service departments. They also have housekeeping, maintenance, laundry, social service, activity, and other departments.

A human resources director handles personnel matters such as hiring staff. A finance director handles billing. A social services director meets the social needs of residents and families. An activities director plans resident activities.

By law, nursing centers must have a doctor as a medical director. This doctor consults with the staff about medical problems not handled by a resident's doctor. Guidance is given about resident care policies and programs.

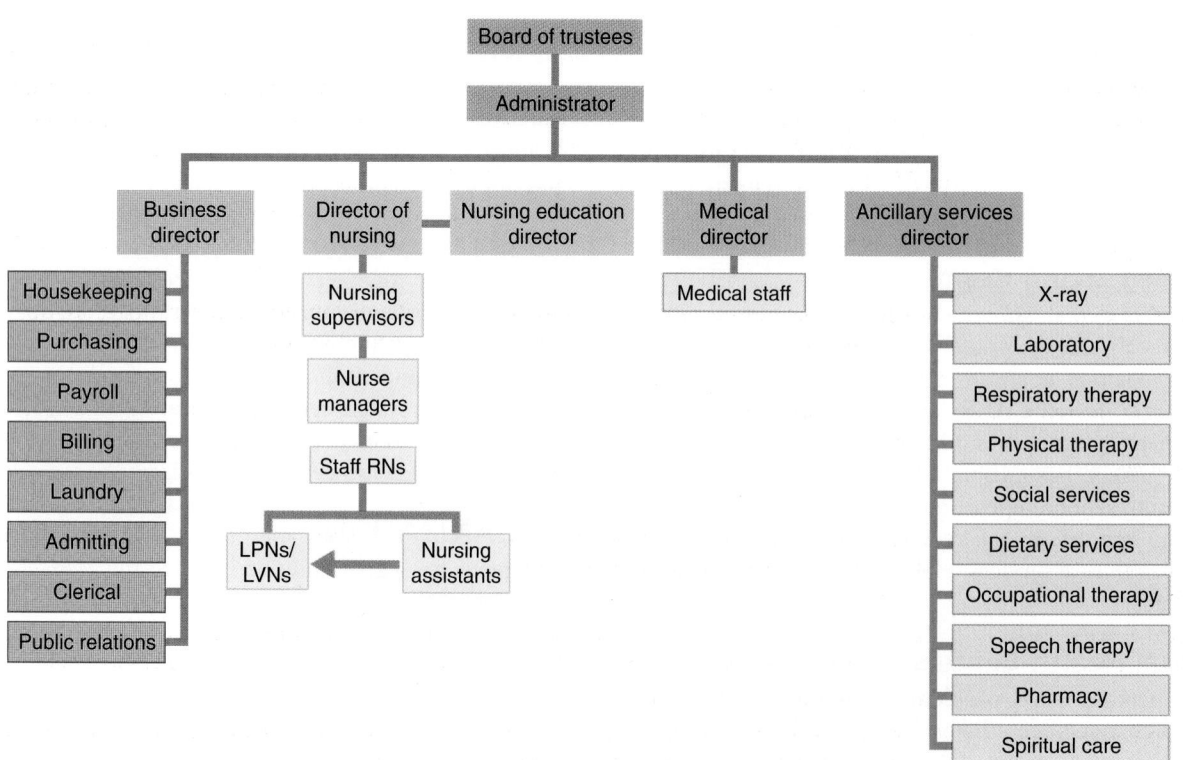

FIGURE 1-3 Sample organizational chart of a health care agency. Titles and departments may vary among states and agencies.

The Health Team

The **health team** (interdisciplinary health care team) involves the many health care workers whose skills and knowledge focus on the person's total care (Table 1-1). The goal is to provide quality care. The person is the focus of care (Fig. 1-4, p. 7).

Many team members are involved in the care of each person. Coordinated care is needed. A registered nurse (RN) leads this team.

See *Focus on Communication: The Health Team.*

TABLE 1-1	Health Team Members	
Title	**Description**	**Credentials**
Activities director/ recreational therapist	Assesses, plans, and implements recreational needs.	Bachelor's degree in most areas
Audiologist	Tests hearing; prescribes hearing aids, works with persons who are hard-of-hearing.	Doctorate in audiology; state license
Cleric (clergyman; clergywoman)	Assists with spiritual needs.	Priest, minister, rabbi, sister (nun), deacon, or other pastoral training
Clinical nurse specialist	Advanced practice RN who consults in a specialty. Geriatrics, critical care, diabetes, rehabilitation, and wound care are examples.	RN with a master's degree or doctorate in a clinical specialty
Dental hygienist	Cleans teeth and provides preventive care. Supervised by a licensed dentist.	Associate's degree in dental hygiene; state license
Dentist	Treats problems with the teeth, gums, and mouth.	Doctor of dental surgery (DDS) or doctor of dental medicine (DMD); state license
Dietitian and nutritionist	Assesses and plans for nutritional needs. Teaches about diet and healthy eating.	Bachelor's degree; registered dietitian nutritionist (RDN) credential; license, registration, or certification in most states
Homemaker/home health aide	Assists persons in home settings—laundry; bedmaking; shops for food; plans and prepares meals; assists with hygiene, dressing, and grooming.	Varies from state to state—on-the-job training or formal training (see "Nursing assistant")
Licensed practical/ vocational nurse (LPN/LVN)	Provides nursing care and gives drugs under an RN's direction.	State-approved program (usually 1 year in length); licensing exam and state license
Medical or clinical laboratory technician	Collects specimens. Performs laboratory tests on blood, urine, and other body fluids, secretions, and excretions.	Associate's degree or certificate; license/ registration in some states
Medical or clinical laboratory technologist	Performs complex laboratory tests and procedures on blood, urine, and other body fluids, secretions, and excretions; supervises medical/clinical laboratory technicians.	Bachelor's degree; license/registration in some states
Medical records and health information technician	Maintains medical records and transcribes medical reports. Codes patient information for billing purposes.	Certificate or associate's degree; certification test
Medication assistant-certified (MA-C)	Gives drugs as allowed by state law under the supervision of a licensed nurse.	Certified nursing assistant with additional education required by state law; state certification
Nurse practitioner	Advanced practice RN in a nursing specialty. Does physical exams, diagnoses common health problems, and prescribes drugs and treatments.	RN with a master's or doctorate degree in a nursing area; certification test

Modified from Bureau of Labor Statistics, U.S. Department of Labor: Occupational outlook handbook, January 8, 2014.

Continued

TABLE 1-1	Health Team Members—cont'd	
Title	**Description**	**Credentials**
Nursing assistant	Assists nurses and gives care. Supervised by a licensed nurse.	Completion of a state-approved training and competency evaluation program; state registry; state certification, license, or registration
Occupational therapist registered (OTR)	Assists persons to learn or retain skills needed for daily living.	Master's degree or doctoral degree; certification test; state license or registration
Occupational therapy assistant	Performs tasks and services supervised by an OTR.	Associate's degree; license in most states
Pharmacist	Fills drug orders written by doctors; monitors and evaluates drug interactions; consults with doctors and nurses about drug actions and interactions	Pharm.D. degree; state license
Physical therapist (PT)	Assists ill and injured persons with movement and pain management.	Doctoral degree; state license
Physical therapy assistant	Performs tasks and services supervised by a PT.	Associate's degree; license in some states
Physician (doctor)	Diagnoses and treats diseases and injuries.	Medical school graduation (MD, DO), residency, and national board certification; state license
Physician's assistant (PA)	Performs exams, diagnoses, and provides treatments under the direction of a doctor.	Master's degree; state license
Podiatrist	Prevents, diagnoses, and treats foot disorders.	Doctor of podiatric medicine (DPM); residency; state license
Radiographer/ radiologic technologist	Takes images using x-ray and other equipment.	Associate's degree; license/certification in most states
Registered nurse (RN)	Assesses, makes nursing diagnoses, plans, implements, and evaluates nursing care. Supervises LPNs/LVNs and nursing assistants.	Associate's degree, diploma, or bachelor's degree; licensing exam and state license
Respiratory therapist (RT)	Assists in treating lung and heart disorders; gives respiratory treatments and therapies.	Associate's or bachelor's degree; license in most states
Social worker	Deals with social, emotional, and environmental issues affecting illness and recovery. Coordinates community agencies to assist the person and family.	Bachelor's or master's degree; license in some states
Speech-language pathologist/speech therapist	Diagnoses and treats communication and swallowing disorders.	Master's degree; license in most states

Nursing Service

Nursing service is a large department (see Fig. 1-3). The director of nursing (DON) is an RN. (*Director of nursing services*, *chief nurse executive*, *vice president of nursing*, and *vice president of patient services* are some other titles.) Usually a bachelor's or higher degree is required. The DON is responsible for the entire nursing staff and the nursing care given.

Nursing supervisors and nurse managers (usually RNs) assist the DON. They over-see a work shift, nursing unit, or certain function. Nurse supervisors or managers are responsible for all nursing care and the actions of nursing staff in their areas.

- Shift managers coordinate nursing care for a certain shift.
- Hospital nursing areas include surgical, medical, intensive care, pediatric, and mental health units. They also include operating and recovery areas, an emergency room, and a maternity department.
- Examples of nursing functions include staff development, restorative nursing, infection control, and continuous quality care.

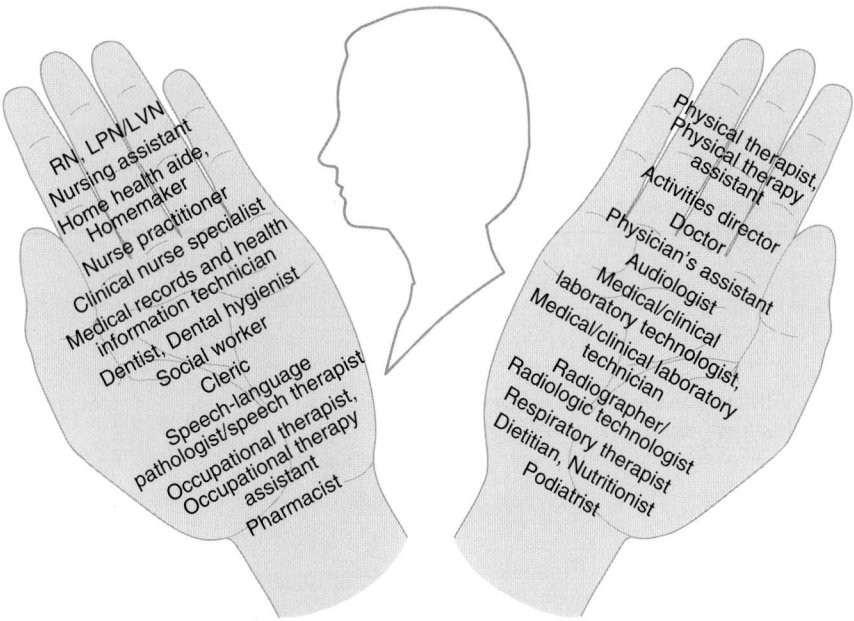

FIGURE 1-4 Members of the health team. The person is the focus of care.

Nursing units usually have charge nurses for each shift. Usually RNs, LPNs/LVNs can be charge nurses in some states. The charge nurse is responsible for all nursing care and nursing staff actions during that shift. Staff RNs report to the charge nurse. LPNs/LVNs report to staff RNs or to the charge nurse. You report to the nurse supervising your work.

Nursing education (staff development) is part of nursing service. Nursing education staff:

- Plan and present educational programs (in-service programs). This includes programs that meet federal and state educational requirements.
- Provide new and changing information.
- Show how to use new equipment and supplies.
- Review policies and procedures on a regular basis.
- Educate and train nursing assistants.
- Conduct new employee orientation programs.

THE NURSING TEAM

The *nursing team involves those who provide nursing care—RNs, LPNs/LVNs, and nursing assistants. All focus on the physical, social, emotional, and spiritual needs of the person and family.*

Registered Nurses

A *registered nurse (RN) has completed a 2-, 3-, or 4-year nursing program and has passed a licensing test.*

- Community college programs—2 years
- Hospital-based diploma programs—2 or 3 years
- College or university programs—4 years

Nursing and the social and physical sciences are studied. Graduates take a licensing test offered by their state board of nursing. They receive a license and become *registered* after passing the test. RNs must have a license recognized by the state in which they work.

RNs assess, make nursing diagnoses, plan, implement, and evaluate nursing care (Chapter 8). They provide care and delegate (Chapter 4) nursing care and tasks to the nursing team. They evaluate how nursing care affects each person. RNs teach the person and family how to improve health and independence.

RNs follow the doctor's orders. They may delegate them to other nursing team members. RNs do not prescribe treatments or drugs. However, RNs can become *clinical nurse specialists* or *nurse practitioners*. These RNs have limited diagnosing and prescribing functions.

RNs work as staff nurses, nurse supervisors or managers, DONs, agency administrators, and instructors. Other career options depend on education, abilities, and experience.

Licensed Practical Nurses and Licensed Vocational Nurses

A *licensed practical nurse (LPN) has completed a practical nursing program and has passed a licensing test.* Hospitals, community colleges, vocational schools, and technical schools offer programs. Usually 1 year in length, some programs are 10 or 18 months long. Some high schools offer 2-year programs.

Graduates take a licensing test for practical nursing. After passing the test, they have a license to practice and the title of *licensed practical nurse.* **Licensed vocational nurse (LVN)** *is used in California and Texas. LPNs/LVNs must have a license recognized by the state where they work.*

LPNs/LVNs are supervised by RNs, licensed doctors, and licensed dentists. They have fewer responsibilities and functions than RNs do. They need little supervision when the person's condition is stable and care is simple. They assist RNs with acutely ill persons and complex procedures.

Nursing Assistants

A *nursing assistant has passed a nursing assistant training and competency evaluation program (NATCEP).* Nursing assistants *perform delegated nursing tasks under the supervision of a licensed nurse.* Nursing assistants are discussed in Chapter 3.

NURSING CARE PATTERNS

The nursing care pattern used depends on how many persons need care, the staff, and the cost. See Figure 1-5.

- *Functional nursing focuses on tasks and jobs. Each nursing team member has certain tasks and jobs to do.* For example, 1 nurse gives all drugs. Another gives all treatments. Nursing assistants give baths, make beds, and serve meals.
- *Team nursing involves a team of nursing staff led by an RN.* Called the "team leader," *the RN decides the amount and kind of care each person needs.* The team leader delegates the care of certain persons to other nurses and nursing assistants. Delegation (Chapter 4) is based on the person's needs and team member abilities. Team members report observations and the care given to the team leader.
- *Primary nursing* involves total care. *The primary nurse (an RN) is responsible for the person's total care.* The nursing team assists as needed. The RN gives nursing care and makes discharge plans. If needed, home or long-term care is arranged. The RN teaches and counsels the person and family.
- *Case management. A nursing case manager coordinates the care of specific groups of patients from admission through discharge and into the home or long-term care setting.* He or she communicates with doctors and the health team. Communication also is with insurance companies and community agencies. Case managers work with certain doctors, certain age-groups, or persons with certain health problems. Heart diseases, diabetes, and cancer are examples.
- *Patient-focused care is when services are moved from departments to the bedside.* Besides nursing care, the nursing team performs basic skills usually done by other health team members. For example, an RN draws a blood sample. This reduces the number of staff involved and the care costs.

PAYING FOR HEALTH CARE

Health care is costly. Some people avoid health care because they cannot pay. Others pay doctor bills but go without food or drugs. Health insurance covers some costs. Rarely are all costs covered.

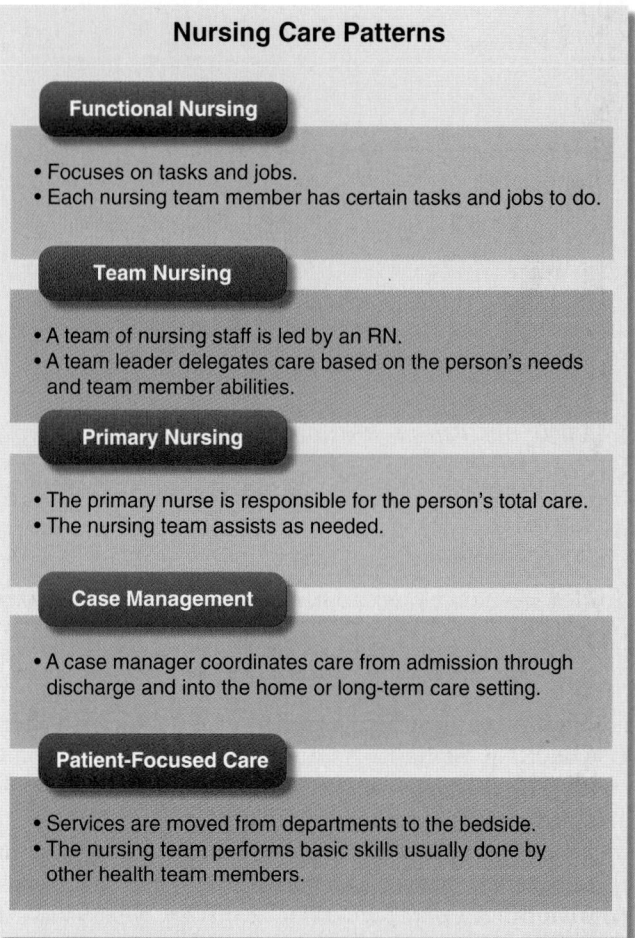

Nursing Care Patterns

Functional Nursing
- Focuses on tasks and jobs.
- Each nursing team member has certain tasks and jobs to do.

Team Nursing
- A team of nursing staff is led by an RN.
- A team leader delegates care based on the person's needs and team member abilities.

Primary Nursing
- The primary nurse is responsible for the person's total care.
- The nursing team assists as needed.

Case Management
- A case manager coordinates care from admission through discharge and into the home or long-term care setting.

Patient-Focused Care
- Services are moved from departments to the bedside.
- The nursing team performs basic skills usually done by other health team members.

FIGURE 1-5 Nursing care patterns.

These programs help pay for health care.
- *Private insurance* is bought by individuals and families.
- *Group insurance* is bought by groups or organizations for individuals. This is often an employee benefit.
- *Medicare* is a federal program for persons 65 years of age or older. Some younger people with certain disabilities qualify. Part A covers hospital, SNF, nursing home, hospice, and home care costs. Part B covers ambulance services, medical equipment, mental health, and some drugs. Part B is voluntary. The person pays a monthly premium.
- *Medicaid* is jointly funded by the federal government and the states. People and families with low incomes usually qualify. It covers children and older, blind, and disabled persons.

See *Promoting Safety and Comfort: Paying for Health Care.*

PROMOTING SAFETY AND COMFORT

Paying for Health Care

Safety

Some conditions can be prevented with proper care. Medicare pays a lower rate for such conditions if they are acquired during a hospital stay. Pressure ulcers (Chapter 37) and certain types of falls, trauma, and infections are examples. You must help prevent such conditions.

Patient Protection and Affordable Care Act of 2010

In 2010 the *Patient Protection and Affordable Care Act* (Obamacare) was signed into law. Its purpose is health insurance for all Americans. The law requires everyone to have health insurance. Persons who do not have health insurance will pay a tax.

Some people without health insurance do not qualify for Medicare or Medicaid. They can buy insurance through health insurance exchanges. These are market-places for buying health insurance. Exchanges are run by the federal government, by states, or both.

The law provides for the following.
- Up to age 26, children can be part of their parents' insurance plans.
- If a person becomes ill, the insurance company cannot limit coverage or cancel the plan.
- An insurance company cannot deny coverage for children who are chronically ill.
- Insurance companies must provide 10 essential benefits.
  - Out-patient care
  - Emergency room services
  - Hospital costs
  - Preventive and wellness care and management of chronic diseases
  - Maternity and newborn care
  - Mental health treatment including alcohol, drug, and substance abuse and addiction
  - Prescription drugs
  - Services and devices for persons with injuries, disabilities, or chronic conditions
  - Laboratory tests
  - Pediatric care

Prospective Payment Systems

Prospective payment systems (PPS) limit the amount paid by insurers, Medicare, and Medicaid. *Prospective* means *before*. The amount paid for services is determined before giving care. If costs are less than the amount paid, the agency keeps the extra money. If costs are greater, the agency takes the loss.

Different systems are used for hospitals, home health care agencies, SNFs, rehabilitation centers, and other health care agencies. Each system determines the amount paid.

MEETING STANDARDS

Health care agencies must meet standards set by federal and state governments and accrediting agencies. Standards relate to policies, procedures, and quality of care. An agency must meet standards for:
- *Licensure.* An agency must have a state license to operate and provide care.
- *Certification.* This is required to receive Medicare and Medicaid funds.
- *Accreditation.* This is voluntary. It signals quality and excellence.

The Survey Process

Surveys are done to see if standards are met. A survey team will:
- Review policies, procedures, and medical records.
- Interview staff, patients and residents, and families.
- Observe how care is given.
- Observe if dignity and privacy are promoted.
- Check for cleanliness and safety.
- Make sure staff meet state requirements. (Are doctors and nurses licensed? Are nursing assistants on the state registry?)

If standards are met, the agency receives a license, certification, or accreditation. Sometimes problems *(deficiencies)* are found. The agency usually has 60 days to correct the problem. Sometimes less time is given. The agency can be fined for uncorrected or serious deficiencies. Or it can lose its license, certification, or accreditation.

Your Role

You have an important role in meeting standards and in the survey process. You must:
- Provide quality care.
- Protect the person's rights.
- Provide for the person's and your own safety.
- Help keep the agency clean and safe.
- Act in a professional manner.
- Have good work ethics.
- Follow agency policies and procedures.
- Answer questions honestly and completely.
See *Focus on Surveys: Your Role*, p. 10.

FOCUS ON SURVEYS

Your Role

Survey teams are made up of surveyors. A *surveyor* is a person *who collects information by observing and asking questions.*

A surveyor may ask you questions. If so, be polite. Avoid seeming annoyed or upset. Answer questions honestly and completely. If you do not understand a question, ask the surveyor to re-phrase it. Do not guess at an answer. Tell the surveyor where you can find the answer. You can say: "I'm not sure, but I would ask the nurse."

For example, a surveyor approaches you.

Surveyor: "May I ask you a few questions?"
You: "Yes. I am happy to answer your questions."
Surveyor: "Thank you. First, when should you practice hand hygiene?"
You: "I wash my hands before and after contact with a patient. I also wash my hands when they are dirty and after I take off gloves."

Surveyor: "Thank you. Next, what are 2 appropriate patient identifiers?"
You: "I don't understand the question. Can you re-phrase it?"
Surveyor: "Yes. Name 2 things you can use to identify a patient."
You: "Okay. Thank you. I can use the patient's full name and date of birth. I cannot use the room number."
Surveyor: "I have 1 last question. In a disaster, where would you find the Emergency Preparedness Plan?"
You: "Well, I'm not sure where to find the plan. I will ask my supervising nurse or the charge nurse where to find it."

FOCUS ON PRIDE

The Person, Family, and Yourself

Personal and Professional Responsibility

Working in health care is a great responsibility. It is also very rewarding. You provide care for a *person.* Your work affects the person's quality of care. Value the work that you do.

Focus on PRIDE helps you promote pride in the person, his or her family, and yourself. It builds on content presented in the chapter and focuses on:

* *Personal and Professional Responsibility*—how personal and professional behaviors and development affect yourself and others.
* *Rights and Respect*—how to promote others' rights and respect others as persons with dignity and value.
* *Independence and Social Interaction*—ways to promote independence and positive interactions.
* *Delegation and Teamwork*—how to practice safe delegation (Chapter 4) and work well with and help other team members.
* *Ethics and Laws*—how to do the right thing when dealing with patients, residents, and co-workers. Laws affecting nursing care and real court cases are also presented.

For discussion purposes, each chapter ends with a *Focus on PRIDE: Application* section. The questions challenge you to think about your role and how you will value the person, family, or yourself.

Rights and Respect

There are many reasons for wanting to work in health care. Maybe you want to help people. Maybe someone who works in health care inspired you. Or you may have a certain job opportunity or career goal in mind. Consider your reasons.

Consider what type of agency would suit you. One person may prefer working in long-term care while another prefers a hospital setting.

Careful career planning shows respect for employers, those you will care for, and yourself.

Independence and Social Interaction

You will interact with many people. Patients and residents, nursing staff, other health team members, surveyors, and visitors are examples. Having good work ethics and communication skills are important. See Chapters 6 and 7. How you interact with others affects quality of care. Positive interactions also promote job satisfaction.

Delegation and Teamwork

Each health team member has a certain role. See Table 1-1. Everyone must work together to provide quality care. Offer to help team members when you can. Helping others shows you are dependable and value teamwork.

Ethics and Laws

Nursing team members have different levels of training and responsibilities. RN, LPN/LVN, and nursing assistant roles vary. Federal and state laws determine the legal limits of these roles. See Chapter 3 for your role limits. Functions may also vary among agencies. A job description (Chapter 3) states the agency's expectations. To protect yourself and others, know the limits of your role in your state and agency.

FOCUS ON PRIDE: Application

Health care is a rewarding profession with many opportunities. Why do you want to work in health care? Where do you want to work? What are your career goals?

REVIEW QUESTIONS

Circle the BEST answer.

1 Helping persons return to their highest physical and mental function is called
  a Maintaining independence
  b Promoting health
  c Preventing disease
  d Rehabilitation

2 Rehabilitation starts when the
  a Person is ready to leave the agency
  b Person first seeks health care
  c Doctor writes the order
  d Health team thinks the person is ready

3 A health care program for dying persons is a
  a Hospice
  b Home care agency
  c Skilled nursing facility
  d Hospital

4 You work in an assisted living residence. You
  a Give care in the person's home
  b Care for patients recovering from surgery
  c Help persons with their daily activities
  d Care for persons with acute illnesses

5 Who controls policy in a health care agency?
  a The survey team
  b The board of directors
  c The health team
  d Medicare and Medicaid

6 Who is responsible for the entire nursing staff and safe nursing care?
  a The case manager
  b The director of nursing
  c The charge nurse
  d The RN

7 You are a member of
  a The health team and the nursing team
  b The health team and the medical team
  c The nursing team and the medical team
  d The board of trustees

8 The nursing team includes
  a Doctors
  b Pharmacists
  c Physical and occupational therapists
  d RNs, LPNs/LVNs, and nursing assistants

9 Nursing assistants are supervised by
  a Licensed nurses
  b Other nursing assistants
  c The health team
  d The medical director

10 The nursing assistant's role is to
  a Meet Medicare and Medicaid standards
  b Perform delegated tasks
  c Follow the doctor's orders
  d Manage care

11 Nursing tasks are delegated according to a person's needs and staff member abilities. This nursing care pattern is called
  a Team nursing
  b Functional nursing
  c Case management
  d Primary nursing

12 Medicare is for persons who
  a Are 65 years of age or older
  b Need nursing center care
  c Have group insurance
  d Have low incomes

13 Which is required for an agency to operate and provide care?
  a Accreditation
  b Certification
  c A license
  d A survey

14 Which is voluntary for health care agencies?
  a Licensure
  b Certification
  c Accreditation
  d Surveys

15 Surveys are done to
  a Reduce health care costs
  b See if agencies meet set standards
  c Educate the nursing team
  d Determine the amount paid by insurers

16 A surveyor asks you some questions. You should
  a Refer all questions to the nurse
  b Answer as the DON tells you to
  c Give as little information as possible
  d Give honest and complete answers

Answers to Chapter 1 questions are on p. 870.

FOCUS ON **PRACTICE**

Problem Solving

The nurse supervising your work was supposed to return from a break 15 minutes ago. The nurse did not tell you who is supervising your work during the break. You have a question about a patient's care. What will you do? Your nursing department is organized as shown in Figure 1-3. Who should you tell about the problem?

The Person's Rights

People want to know about their health problems and treatment. They want to understand and take part in treatment decisions. As patients and residents, they have certain rights.

PATIENT RIGHTS

The Patient Care Partnership: Understanding Expectations, Rights, and Responsibilities is a document issued by the American Hospital Association. The document explains the person's rights and expectations during hospital stays. The relationship between the doctor, health team, and patient is stressed. See Box 2-1.

RESIDENT RIGHTS

The *Omnibus Budget Reconciliation Act of 1987* (OBRA) is a federal law. It applies to all 50 states. The Centers for Medicare & Medicaid Services (CMS) is responsible for enforcing OBRA.

OBRA requires that nursing centers provide care in a manner and in a setting that maintains or improves each person's quality of life, health, and safety. Nursing assistant training and competency evaluation are part of OBRA (Chapter 3). Resident rights are a major part of OBRA.

Residents have rights as United States citizens. For example, they have the right to vote. They also have rights relating to their everyday lives and care in a nursing center.

These rights are protected by federal and state laws. Nursing centers must protect and promote such rights. The center cannot interfere with a resident's rights. Some residents cannot exercise their rights. A representative (spouse, partner, adult child, court-appointed guardian) does so for them. A *representative is a person with the legal right to act on the patient's or resident's behalf when he or she cannot do so for himself or herself.*

Nursing centers must inform residents of their rights. Residents must also be informed of the rules about their conduct and responsibilities in the center. Residents are informed orally and in writing. The information is given before or during admission to the center, as needed during the person's stay, and when laws or center rules change. Resident rights and other information are given in the language the person uses and understands.

- An interpreter is used if the person speaks and understands a foreign language or communicates by sign language.
- Written translations are provided in the foreign languages common in the center's geographic area.
- Medical terms are avoided to the extent possible.
- Sign language and other communication aids are used as necessary.
- Large-print texts are available for persons with impaired vision.

BOX 2-1	The Patient Care Partnership—Understanding Expectations, Rights, and Responsibilities (A Summary)

High-Quality Care
- The hospital provides needed care with skill, compassion, and respect.
- The patient has the right to know the identities of those involved in care.
  - Doctors, nurses, and other staff
  - Students and other trainees

Clean and Safe Setting
- The hospital has policies and procedures to:
  - Avoid mistakes.
  - Prevent abuse or neglect.
- The patient is told of unexpected or significant events.
  - What happened
  - Needed changes in care

Involvement in Care
- The patient has the right to make informed decisions about treatment choices.
  - What are the benefits and risks of each treatment?
  - Is the treatment experimental or part of a research study?
  - What can be expected from treatment?
  - How might long-term effects of treatment affect quality of life?
  - What will the patient and family need to do after hospital discharge?
  - What are the costs of using uncovered services or providers?
- The patient has the right to consent to or refuse treatment. The patient is told of the effects of refusing recommended treatment.
- The patient is expected to give information about:
  - Past illnesses, surgeries, or hospital stays
  - Allergic reactions
  - Drugs or dietary supplements that are taken
  - Any health plan admission requirements
- The health team is expected to respect the patient's health care goals, values, and spiritual beliefs. The patient is responsible for sharing his or her wishes with the doctor, family, and care team.

Involvement in Care—cont'd
- The patient is expected to communicate about who makes decisions when the patient is unable.
  - The patient shares *power of attorney, living will,* or *advance directive* documents with the doctor, family, and health team (Chapter 55).
  - The hospital provides help with making difficult decisions. Counselors or chaplains are available.

Protection of Privacy
- The hospital protects the confidentiality of:
  - The patient's relationships with the doctor and health team
  - Information about the patient's health and care
- The hospital provides a "Notice of Privacy Practices" describing:
  - How patient information is used, disclosed, and protected
  - How to obtain a copy of the hospital's records about patient care

Preparing to Leave the Hospital
- The hospital helps identify sources for follow-up care. The hospital's financial interest in any referrals is disclosed.
- The hospital coordinates hospital activities with community caregivers. The hospital requests permission to share information about care.
- The hospital provides information and training about self-care in the home setting.

Help With Bills and Insurance Claims
- The hospital files insurance, Medicare, or Medicaid claims.
- Patients can contact the business office for questions about insurance coverage.
- The hospital tries to help patients find financial help or make other arrangements if the person is without health coverage. The patient provides needed information to obtain coverage or assistance.

Modified from American Hospital Association: The patient care partnership: understanding expectations, rights, and responsibilities.

Resident rights (Box 2-2, p. 14) also are posted throughout the center. Those affecting your role are described in this chapter.

See *Focus on Surveys: Resident Rights.*

FOCUS ON SURVEYS

Resident Rights

Resident rights are a major focus of surveys. Surveyors observe staff behaviors and actions. They listen to staff comments and remarks. You may not know they are doing so. What you say and do must promote the person's quality of life, health, and safety. For example, a surveyor may observe:
- How you prevent unnecessary exposure of the person's body
- How you help a person dress for the season and time of day
- How you label clothing
- If you knock on a person's door before entering the room
- If you change a person's radio or TV without permission
- If you move a person's personal items without permission
- How you address and speak to a person

You will learn how to protect the person's rights as you study this and other chapters. You must always act and speak in a professional manner.

BOX 2-2	Resident Rights

- To be treated with dignity and respect. And to receive quality care.
- To exercise his or her rights as a center resident and as a United States citizen.
- To be informed orally and in writing of his or her rights and center rules. This is done in a language the person understands.
- To access all records about himself or herself, including current clinical records.
- To obtain copies of his or her records. This is at the resident's expense.
- To refuse treatment.
- To refuse to take part in experimental research. This is the development and testing of new treatments and drugs.
- To make advance directives (Chapter 55).
- To be informed of Medicare benefits and services. This includes costs and charges covered and not covered.
- To file complaints with the appropriate state agency about abuse, neglect, and the mis-use of his or her property.
- To be informed of center services and of the charges for those services.
- To choose his or her doctor.
- To know the name, specialty, and how to contact the doctor responsible for his or her care.
- To be fully informed of his or her total health status, including his or her medical condition.
- To be informed of:
  - Any accident or injury that may need medical attention
  - A change in the person's physical, mental, or psycho-social status
  - The need to stop, change, or add a treatment
  - A decision to transfer or discharge the person
  - A change in the person's room or roommate
  - A change in the person's rights under federal or state law
- To manage his or her personal and financial affairs.
- To be fully informed in advance about his or her care and treatment. This includes changes in care and treatment.
- To privacy and confidentiality:
  - Of personal and medical records
  - Of treatment and personal care
  - Of written and phone communications
  - During visits with family and friends
  - When meeting with resident groups

- To voice grievances and have them solved promptly.
- To see the results of federal and state surveys. The person also has the right to see plans to correct problems or areas of weakness.
- To perform services for the center or to refuse to perform services.
- To send and receive mail that is not open. To buy supplies to send mail.
- To receive information from his or her doctor and community and state agencies responsible for protecting persons with intellectual and developmental disabilities and mental health disorders.
- To have and use personal items and clothing.
- To share a room with his or her spouse (husband, wife) when married residents live in the same center (Chapter 51).
- To take his or her drugs without help if able.
- To refuse to change to a different room.
- To be free from physical and chemical restraints (Chapter 15).
- To be free from abuse (verbal, sexual, physical), bodily punishment, and involuntary seclusion (Chapter 5).
- To be cared for in a manner and in a setting that maintains or enhances quality of life.
- To choose activities, schedules, and health care that meet his or her interests and needs.
- To interact with community members inside and outside the center.
- To make choices about his or her life in the center.
- To organize and take part in resident groups.
- To take part in social, religious, and community activities.
- To a setting and services that consider his or her needs and choices.
- To be informed of his or her health and medical condition in a language that he or she understands. That language is used when he or she takes part in care planning.
- To a clean, comfortable, and home-like setting. This includes temperature, lighting, and sound levels.
- To attain or maintain his or her highest level of function.
- To closet space.
- To visit with his or her spouse or partner, family, and friends at any reasonable hour.

Information

The *right to information* means access to all records about the person. They include the medical record, contracts, incident reports, and financial records. The request can be oral or written.

The person has the right to be fully informed of his or her health condition. The person must also have information about his or her doctor. This includes the doctor's name, specialty, and how to contact the doctor.

Report any request for information to the nurse. *You do not give the information described above to the person or family* (Chapter 3).

See *Focus on Communication: Information.*

FOCUS ON COMMUNICATION

Information

You may be asked about a person's care. You must not give out information. This is the nurse's responsibility. You can say: "I am sorry. I am not allowed to give information. I will report your request to the nurse." Communicate the request promptly. You can tell the person: "I told the nurse about your question. The nurse will speak with you soon."

Refusing Treatment

The person has the right to refuse treatment. *Treatment means the care provided to maintain or restore health, improve function, or relieve symptoms.* A person who does not give consent (Chapter 5) or refuses treatment cannot be treated against his or her wishes. The center must find out what the person is refusing and why. The center must:

- Find out the reason for the refusal.
- Explain the problems that can result from the refusal.
- Offer other treatment options.
- Continue to provide all other services.

Advance directives are part of the right to refuse treatment (Chapter 55). They include living wills and instructions about life support. *Advance directives* are written instructions about health care when the person is not able to make such decisions.

Report any treatment refusal to the nurse. The nurse may change the person's care plan (Chapter 8).

Privacy and Confidentiality

Residents have the *right to personal privacy*. Staff must provide care in a manner that maintains privacy of the person's body. Expose the person's body only as necessary. Only staff directly involved in care and treatment are present. Consent is needed for others to be present. For example, a student wants to observe a treatment. The person's consent is needed for the student to observe.

Privacy is maintained for all personal care measures. Bathing, dressing, and elimination are examples. Protect privacy by:

- Closing privacy curtains, doors, and window coverings.
- Removing residents from public view.
- Providing clothes or draping the person to prevent unnecessary exposure of body parts.
- Practicing the measures listed in Chapter 5. See "Invasion of Privacy" in Chapter 5.

Leaving the person without a gown, clothing, or bed covers violates the right to privacy. So does leaving the door open when the person uses the bathroom, commode, urinal, or bedpan.

Residents have the right to visit with others in private—in areas where others cannot see or hear them. If requested, the center must provide private space. Offices, chapels, dining rooms, and meeting rooms are used as needed.

Residents have the right to make phone calls in private (Fig. 2-1). The calls must not be over-heard. Therefore phones are not used in offices or at the nurses' station. Centers provide cordless phones or phone jacks in resident rooms. Phones are at the correct height for use by persons in wheelchairs. Phones for hard-of-hearing persons are also available. Some residents have their own wireless phones.

The right to privacy also involves mail. The person has the right to send and receive mail without others interfering. No one can open mail the person sends or receives without his or her consent. Un-opened mail is given to the person within 24 hours of delivery to the center. Mail the person sends is delivered to the postal service within 24 hours on days of regular delivery or pick-up services.

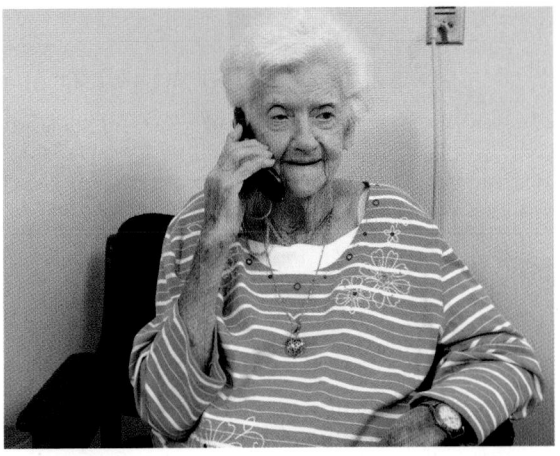

FIGURE 2-1 A resident is talking privately on her phone.

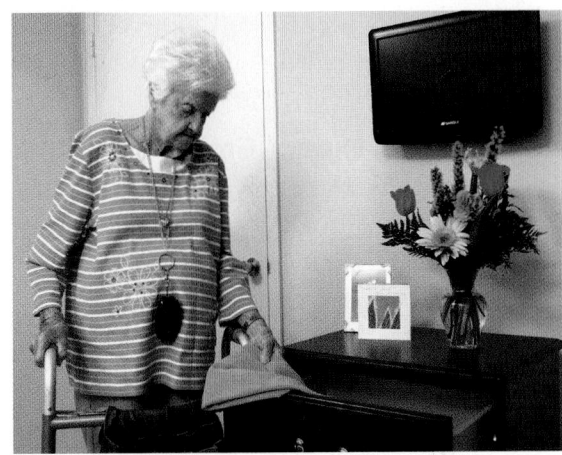

FIGURE 2-2 A resident is choosing what clothing to wear.

Information about the person's care, treatment, and condition is kept confidential. So are medical and financial records. Consent is needed to release them to other agencies or persons.

You must provide privacy and protect confidentiality. Doing so shows respect for the person. It also protects the person's dignity. Privacy and confidentiality are discussed in Chapters 5 and 6.

Personal Choice

Residents have the *right to make their own choices*. This includes:

- Choosing doctors
- Choosing friends and visitors inside and outside the center
- Helping to plan and decide about care and treatment
- Choosing activities, schedules, and care based on preferences:
  - When to go to bed and when to get up
  - What to wear (Fig. 2-2)
  - How to spend time
  - What to eat

Personal choice promotes quality of life, dignity, and self-respect. You must allow personal choice whenever safely possible.

Grievances

Residents have the *right to voice concerns, questions, and complaints about treatment and care*. The problem may involve another person. It may be about care that was given or not given. The center must promptly try to correct the matter. No one can punish the person in any way for voicing the grievance.

Work

The person does not work for care, care items or other things, or privileges. The person is not required to perform services for the center.

However, the person has the *right to work or perform services if he or she wants to do so*. Some people like to garden, repair or build things, clean, sew, mend, or cook. Other persons need work for rehabilitation or activity reasons. The desire or need for work is part of the person's care plan. Residents volunteer or are paid for their services.

Taking Part in Resident Groups

The person has the *right to form and take part in resident groups*. Families can meet with other families. These groups can plan activities, discuss concerns, and suggest center improvements. They can support and comfort group members. They can also take part in educational events.

Residents have the right to take part in social, cultural, religious, and community events. They have the right to help in getting to and from events of their choice.

Personal Items

Residents have the *right to keep and use personal items*. This includes clothing and some furnishings. The type and amount of the items allowed depend on space needs and the health and safety of others.

Treat the person's property with care and respect. The items may not have value to you but have meaning to the person. They also relate to personal choice, dignity, a home-like setting, and quality of life.

The person's property is protected. Items are labeled with the person's name. The center must investigate reports of lost, stolen, or damaged items. Sometimes the police help. The person and family are advised not to keep jewelry and costly items in the center.

Protect yourself and the center from being accused of stealing. Do not go through a person's closet, drawers, purse, or other space without the person's knowledge and consent. A nurse may ask you to inspect closets and drawers. Center policy should require that a co-worker and the person or legal representative be present. They witness your actions. Follow center policy for reporting and recording the inspection.

Freedom From Abuse, Mistreatment, and Neglect

Residents have the *right to be free from verbal, sexual, physical, and mental abuse* (Chapter 5). *Abuse* means:
- The willful infliction of injury, unreasonable confinement, intimidation (to threaten to hurt or punish), or punishment that results in physical harm, pain, or mental anguish.
- Depriving the person of the goods or services needed to attain or maintain well-being.

They also have the right to be free from *involuntary seclusion*.
- *Separating the person from others against his or her will*
- *Keeping the person to a certain area*
- *Keeping the person away from his or her room without consent*

No one can abuse, neglect, or mistreat a resident. This includes center staff, volunteers, and staff from other agencies or groups. It also includes other residents, family members, visitors, and legal representatives. Centers must investigate suspected or reported cases of abuse. They cannot employ persons who:
- Were found guilty of abusing, neglecting, or mistreating others by a court of law.
- Have a finding entered into the state's nursing assistant registry (Chapter 3) about abuse, neglect, mistreatment, or wrongful acts involving the person's money or property. A *finding* means that a state determined that the employee abused, neglected, mistreated, or wrongfully used the person's money or property.

Freedom From Restraint

Residents have the *right not to have body movements restricted*. Restraints and certain drugs can restrict body movements (Chapter 15). Some drugs are restraints because they affect mood, behavior, and mental function. Sometimes residents are restrained to protect them from harming themselves or others. A doctor's order is needed for restraint use. Restraints are not used for staff convenience or to discipline a person. They are used only if required to treat the person's medical symptoms.

Quality of Life

Residents have the *right to quality of life*. They must be cared for in a manner and in a setting that promotes dignity and respect for self. This means that staff must provide care in a manner that maintains or enhances the person's self-esteem and feelings of self-worth. Care must promote physical, mental, and social well-being. Protecting resident rights promotes quality of life. It shows respect for the person.

Speak to the person in a polite and courteous manner. Good, honest, and thoughtful care enhances the person's quality of life. Box 2-3 lists OBRA-required actions that promote dignity and privacy.

See *Focus on Communication: Quality of Life*.

BOX 2-3	OBRA-Required Actions to Promote Dignity and Privacy

Courteous and Dignified Interactions
- Use the right tone of voice.
- Use good eye contact.
- Stand or sit close enough as needed.
- Use the person's proper name and title. For example: "Mrs. Crane."
- Gain the person's attention before interacting with him or her.
- Use touch if the person approves.
- Respect the person's social status.
- Listen with interest to what the person is saying.
- Do not yell at, scold, or embarrass the person.

Privacy and Self-Determination
- Drape properly during care and procedures to avoid exposure and embarrassment.
- Drape properly in a chair.
- Use privacy curtains or screens during care and procedures.
- Close the room door during care and procedures as the person desires. Also close window coverings.
- Knock on the door before entering. Wait to be asked in.
- Close the bathroom door when the person uses the bathroom.

Personal Choice and Independence
- Person smokes in allowed areas.
- Person takes part in activities according to his or her interests.
- Person takes part in scheduling activities and care.
- Person gives input into the care plan about preferences and independence.

Personal Choice and Independence—cont'd
- Person is involved in a room or roommate change.
- The person's items are moved or inspected only with the person's consent.

Courteous and Dignified Care
- Groom hair, beards, and nails as the person wishes.
- Assist with dressing in the right clothing for time of day and personal choice.
- Promote independence and dignity in dining.
- Respect private space and property. For example, change radio or TV stations only with the person's consent.
- Assist with walking and transfers. Do not interfere with independence.
- Assist with bathing and hygiene preferences. Do not interfere with independence.
  - Appearance is neat and clean.
  - The person is clean shaven or has a groomed beard and mustache.
  - Nails are trimmed and clean.
  - Dentures, hearing aids, eyeglasses, and other devices are used correctly.
  - Clothing is clean.
  - Clothing is properly fitted and fastened.
  - Shoes, hose, and socks are properly applied and fastened.
  - Extra clothing is worn for warmth as needed. Sweaters and lap blankets are examples.

FOCUS ON COMMUNICATION

Quality of Life

Every person deserves to be addressed in a manner that conveys dignity and respect. When speaking with a patient or resident, address the person by his or her title and last name. For example: Mr. Baker, Mrs. Harty, or Dr. Collins. Do not address a person by his or her first name or another name unless the person requests it. Avoid the use of terms like *Sweetheart, Honey, Grandpa,* and *Dear.*

Activities. Residents have the *right to activities that enhance each person's physical, mental, and psycho-social well-being.* Activities promote self-esteem, pleasure, comfort, education, creativity, success, and independence. Their purpose must relate to the person's needs, interests, culture, and background. Religious services provide for spiritual health. Activities are meaningful for the person when they:
- Reflect the person's interests and life-style.
- Are enjoyed by the person.
- Help the person feel useful or produce something useful.
- Provide a sense of belonging.

Activities involve large groups (bingo) or small groups (a card game). Other activities are for 2 people. Or the person does something alone. Writing a letter and playing a computer game are examples.

You assist residents to and from activity programs. You may need to help them with activities.

See *Focus on Communication: Activities.*
See *Teamwork and Time Management: Activities*, p. 18.
See *Focus on Surveys: Activities*, p. 18.

FOCUS ON COMMUNICATION

Activities

You may need help assisting residents to and from activity programs. Politely ask a co-worker to help you. Share the following with your co-worker.
- What time you need help.
- How much of the co-worker's time you need.
- The residents you need help with.
- If the person walks or uses a wheelchair.
- What assistive devices are used. Eyeglasses, hearing aids, canes, and walkers are examples.

Always say "please" when asking for help. And thank the person for helping you. For example: "Jane, can you please help me assist 2 residents to the concert? It starts at 2:00, so I'll need your help at 1:45. Mr. Harris needs his glasses and hearing aid. He'll use a walker. Mrs. Janz uses a wheelchair. She needs her glasses and a blanket for her lap. The blanket is in her wheelchair. The concert is over at 3:00. Can you help me then, too? Thanks so much for helping me."

TEAMWORK AND TIME MANAGEMENT
Activities

Residents may need help to and from activity programs. Know when an activity begins and ends. Before assisting residents to activities:

- Assist with elimination needs and hand-washing.
- Assist with grooming measures such as brushing and combing hair. A person may want to apply perfume or make-up.
- Make sure the person wears the correct clothing and footwear for the activity.
- Provide needed assistive (adaptive) devices. Eyeglasses, hearing aids, canes, and walkers are examples.

Allow 15 to 20 minutes to assist residents to and from the activity area. Help co-workers as needed.

You may have to help residents with activities (Fig. 2-3). If not, use activity time wisely. Provide needed care and visit residents who cannot leave their rooms. You can also clean and straighten rooms, bathrooms, shower rooms, and utility rooms.

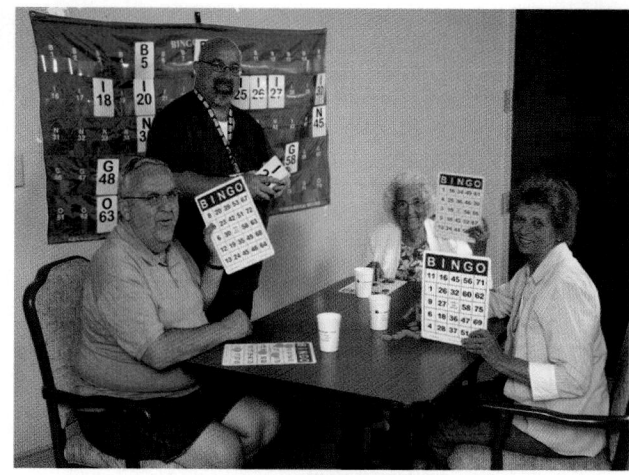

FIGURE 2-3 A nursing assistant is helping residents in an activity program.

FOCUS ON SURVEYS
Activities

Surveyors may ask you about:

- Your role in helping residents get ready for a group activity.
  - How do you make sure the person is out of bed, dressed, and ready to take part in the activity?
  - How do you provide needed transportation?
- Your role in providing help with activities of daily living during an activity. For example, does the person need to use the bathroom? Does the person need help with eating?
- Your role in helping a person with an individual activity. For example, you play cards with a person. Do you have needed supplies? Is the person properly positioned? Do you provide good lighting?
- How are activities provided when the activities staff are not available?

Environment. Residents have the *right to a safe, clean, comfortable, and home-like setting.* The person is allowed to have and use personal items to the extent possible.

The center must provide a setting and services that meet the person's needs and preferences. The setting and staff must promote the person's independence, dignity, and well-being. The center must try to change schedules, call systems, and room arrangements to meet the person's desires and needs.

For example, the center must make changes when the person:

- Refuses a bath because a shower is preferred.
- Wants a shower at a different time or day.
- Refuses a shower because of the fear of falling.
- Is uneasy about the staff giving care.
- Is worried about falling.
- Cannot reach or use the call light.
- Cannot reach personal items.
- Does not like the food served.

OMBUDSMAN PROGRAM

The Older Americans Act is a federal law. It requires a long-term care ombudsman program in every state. An *ombudsman is someone who supports or promotes the needs and interests of another person.* Long-term care ombudsmen are state employees or volunteers. They are not hospital or nursing center employees.

Ombudsmen act on behalf of persons receiving health care. They protect a person's health, safety, welfare, and rights. They:

- Investigate and resolve complaints.
- Provide services to assist the person.
- Assist with hospital access or discharge concerns.
- Provide information about long-term care services.
- Monitor nursing care and conditions.
- Provide support to resident and family groups.
- Help the person and family resolve family conflicts.
- Help the center manage difficult problems.

Residents have the right to voice grievances and disputes. They also have the right to communicate privately with anyone of their choice. They can share concerns with anyone outside the center.

Nursing centers must post the names, addresses, and phone numbers of local and state ombudsmen. The postings must be where residents can easily see them.

A resident or family may share a concern with you. Follow center policies and procedures for contacting an ombudsman. Ombudsman services are useful when:

- There is concern about a person's care or treatment.
- Someone interferes with a person's rights, health, safety, or welfare.

FOCUS ON **PRIDE**
The Person, Family, and Yourself

P ersonal and Professional Responsibility
OBRA is concerned with quality of life, health, and safety. All care must maintain or improve each person's quality of life. You are responsible for the care you give. To provide quality care:
- Protect the person's rights.
- Provide for safety (Chapter 13) and prevent falls (Chapter 14).
- Help keep the agency clean and safe.
- Act in a professional manner.
- Have good work ethics (Chapter 6).
- Follow agency policies and procedures.

Take pride in the work you do. The care you give helps improve each person's quality of life, health, and safety.

R ights and Respect
Every person has the right to refuse treatment. This does not mean that all treatment stops. The health team offers other treatment options. For example, the doctor suggests short-term placement in a nursing center. The person refuses. The family agrees to help the person at home. A social worker helps the person and family arrange for home health care and respite care. *Respite care* relieves caregivers of daily care for a short time.

When treatment is refused, the health team works with the person and family to provide care in a manner that respects the decision and promotes well-being.

I ndependence and Social Interaction
Many patients and residents feel a loss of independence and social interaction. Promote independence by having the person choose food, clothing, activities, and schedules.

Encourage social interaction by telling the person about activities and offering help to and from activities. Also respect the person's right to privacy when visiting with others and making phone calls. These actions help improve independence, self-worth, and quality of life.

D elegation and Teamwork
Health care agencies must meet the person's needs and preferences. Schedules, care assignments, and room arrangements may need to change to meet the person's needs. Flexibility, good teamwork, and communication are required to provide quality care.

For example, Mrs. Gordon needs help with bathing. She likes to bathe at night. She says bathing at night helps her rest better. However, the day shift gives baths. You share her preference with the nurse. The daytime and evening staffs work together so Mrs. Gordon can bathe when she chooses.

E thics and Laws
Every person has the right to keep his or her personal information private. This includes information about health care. The *Health Insurance Portability and Accountability Act of 1996 (HIPAA)* protects the privacy and security of a person's health information. HIPAA is discussed further in Chapter 5.

Follow agency policies and procedures for protecting health information. Only staff directly involved in the person's care can discuss the person's treatment. Direct questions to the nurse.

FOCUS ON **PRIDE**: *Application*
You have an important role in protecting the person's rights. Identify 3 ways you can promote the person's right to:
- Personal choice
- Privacy and confidentiality
- A safe, clean, and comfortable setting

REVIEW QUESTIONS
Circle T if the statement is TRUE or F if it is FALSE.

1 T F The *Patient Care Partnership: Understanding Expectations, Rights, and Responsibilities* is a federal law.

2 T F OBRA applies to all 50 states.

3 T F Nursing center residents have rights as U.S. citizens.

4 T F Residents are informed of their rights only in writing.

5 T F Residents have the right to choose their own doctors.

6 T F You should open the person's mail within 24 hours of it being delivered to the center.

7 T F A resident complains about the food. The center must try to provide desired foods.

8 T F Residents must provide some type of work for the center.

9 T F Resident groups can discuss ideas for activity programs.

10 T F An employee was found guilty of abusing a resident. The center can continue to employ the person.

11 T F You can restrain a resident to provide care.

Continued

REVIEW QUESTIONS—cont'd

Circle the BEST answer.

12 The *Patient Care Partnership: Understanding Expectations, Rights, and Responsibilities* is concerned with
   a Hospital care
   b Home care
   c Long-term care
   d All health care agencies and settings

13 These statements are about hospital care. Which is correct?
   a Patients must file their own insurance claims.
   b The health team makes care decisions when the person is unable.
   c Patients must allow students to provide care.
   d Patients have the right to make informed treatment choices.

14 A son has the legal right to act on his mother's behalf. The son is his mother's legal
   a Ombudsman
   b Representative
   c Caregiver
   d Health care provider

15 A daughter wants to read her father's medical record. What should you do?
   a Give her the medical record.
   b Ask the resident if she can read the record.
   c Tell the nurse.
   d Tell her that she cannot do so.

16 A resident refuses to have a shower. What should you do?
   a Tell her that she cannot refuse a shower.
   b Tell her daughter.
   c Comply, but tell her she must shower tomorrow.
   d Tell the nurse.

17 Which violates the person's right to privacy?
   a Closing the bathroom door when the person uses the bathroom
   b Opening window blinds when assisting with bathing
   c Covering the person for personal care
   d Asking the person's permission to observe a treatment

18 A resident has a phone and wants to make a call. What should you do?
   a Leave the room.
   b Tell the nurse.
   c Ask the person to use the phone at the nurses' station.
   d Close the privacy curtain so you can finish your tasks in the room.

19 Who decides how to style a person's hair?
   a The person
   b The nurse
   c You
   d The ombudsman

20 Residents have the right to
   a Bring weapons into the center
   b Mistreat other residents
   c Use other residents' personal items
   d Voice complaints about care

21 A resident brought furniture and other items from home. They are
   a Sent home with the family
   b Labeled with the person's name
   c Arranged as you prefer
   d Shared with the person's roommate

22 Residents have the right to be free from
   a Disease
   b Grievances
   c Involuntary seclusion
   d Rules

23 Who selects activities for a resident?
   a The nurse
   b You
   c The person's representative
   d The person

24 A nursing center must provide
   a A safe, clean, and comfortable setting
   b A private bathroom
   c A bed near a window
   d A noise-free setting

25 A long-term care ombudsman
   a Is employed by the nursing center
   b Investigates resident complaints
   c Grants a nursing center a license or certification
   d Can prevent a resident from leaving the center

26 Which action promotes dignity?
   a Restraining the person
   b Making clothing choices for the person
   c Scolding the person
   d Listening to the person

27 Which is the correct way to address a person?
   a "Hello, sweetie."
   b "Hello, Jim."
   c "Hello, Mrs. Smith."
   d "Hello, Grandpa."

28 Which promotes privacy?
   a Entering a person's room without knocking
   b Closing the privacy curtain for a procedure
   c Leaving the door open during personal care
   d Looking through the person's belongings

Answers to Chapter 2 questions are on p. 870.

FOCUS ON PRACTICE

Problem Solving

You are assisting a resident with feeding. The resident refuses to eat. What will you do? Does the resident have the right to refuse to eat? What is the nursing center's responsibility?

The Nursing Assistant

OBJECTIVES

- Define the key terms and key abbreviations in this chapter.
- Explain the history and trends affecting nursing assistants.
- Explain the laws that affect nursing assistants.
- List the reasons for denying, suspending, or revoking a nursing assistant's certification, license, or registration.
- Describe the training and competency evaluation requirements for nursing assistants.
- Identify the information in the nursing assistant registry.

- Explain how to obtain certification, a license, or registration in another state.
- Describe what nursing assistants can do and their role limits.
- Describe the standards for nursing assistants developed by the National Council of State Boards of Nursing.
- Explain why a job description is important.
- List nursing assistant job titles used in some agencies.
- Explain how to promote PRIDE in the person, the family, and yourself.

KEY TERMS

certification Official recognition by a state that standards or requirements have been met
endorsement A state recognizes the certificate, license, or registration issued by another state; reciprocity or equivalency
equivalency See "endorsement"
job description A document that describes what the agency expects you to do

nursing task Nursing care or a nursing function, procedure, activity, or work that can be delegated to nursing assistants when it does not require a nurse's professional knowledge or judgment
reciprocity See "endorsement"

KEY ABBREVIATIONS

CNA	Certified nursing assistant; certified nurse aide	**NCSBN**	National Council of State Boards of Nursing
LNA	Licensed nursing assistant	**OBRA**	Omnibus Budget Reconciliation Act of 1987
LPN	Licensed practical nurse	**RN**	Registered nurse
LVN	Licensed vocational nurse	**RNA**	Registered nurse aide
NATCEP	Nursing assistant training and competency evaluation program	**SRNA**	State registered nurse aide
		STNA	State tested nurse aide

Federal and state laws and agency policies combine to define your roles and functions. To protect patients and residents from harm, you need to know:

- What you can and cannot do
- Rules and standards of conduct affecting your work
- Your role limits

Laws, job descriptions, and the person's condition shape your work. So does the amount of supervision you need.

HISTORY AND CURRENT TRENDS

For decades, nursing assistants have helped nurses in hospitals and nursing centers with basic nursing care. Often called nurse's aides, they helped with bathing, grooming, elimination, bedmaking, and other needs. Until the 1980s, training was not required by law. Nurses gave on-the-job training. Some hospitals, nursing centers, and schools offered courses.

Before the 1980s, team nursing was common. A team leader (registered nurse; RN) assigned care to nurses and nursing assistants. Assignments depended on each person's needs and condition. It also depended on the staff member's education and experience.

Primary nursing emerged in the 1980s. RNs planned and gave care. Many hospitals hired only RNs. Meanwhile, nursing centers relied on nursing assistants for resident care.

Home care increased during the 1980s. With prospective payment systems, health care payments were limited (Chapter 1). To reduce costs, hospital stays were shorter. Discharged hospital patients often needed care at home.

Managing health care costs is a growing concern. Efforts to reduce costs include:

- *Hospital closings.* Many do not make enough money to stay open.
- *Hospital mergers.* Hospitals share resources and avoid the same costly services. For example, 1 hospital offers heart surgery. The other serves children.
- *Health care systems.* Agencies join together as 1 provider of care. See Chapter 1.
- *Managed care.* Insurers have contracts with doctors, hospitals, and health care systems for reduced rates.
- *Staffing mix.* Hospitals hire RNs, licensed practical nurses/licensed vocational nurses (LPNs/LVNs), and nursing assistants. Most hospitals require a state-approved nursing assistant training and competency evaluation for employment. More training is given for tasks not learned in the training program.
- *Patient-focused care.* Services are moved from departments to the bedside. Staff are cross-trained to perform basic skills of other health team members. For example, a blood test is ordered. The nurse tells the unit secretary, who calls the laboratory. A laboratory technician goes to the patient's room to draw the blood sample. Many people are involved. With patient-focused care, a nursing team member draws the blood. Fewer staff provide services, which lowers cost.

FEDERAL AND STATE LAWS

The U.S. Congress makes federal laws for all 50 states to follow. State legislatures make state laws. For example, the Maine legislature makes state laws for Maine. The Ohio legislature does so for Ohio. You must know the federal and state laws that affect your work. They provide direction for what you can do.

See Chapter 5 for other laws affecting your work.

Nurse Practice Acts

Each state has a nurse practice act. A nurse practice act:

- Defines RN and LPN/LVN and their scope of practice.
- Describes RN and LPN/LVN education and licensing requirements.
- Protects the public from persons practicing nursing without a license. Persons who do not meet the state's requirements cannot perform nursing functions.

The law allows for denying, revoking, or suspending a nursing license. The intent is to protect the public from unsafe nurses. Reasons include:

- Being convicted of a crime in any state
- Selling or distributing drugs
- Using a person's drugs for oneself
- Placing a person in danger from the over-use of alcohol or drugs
- Demonstrating grossly negligent nursing practice
- Being convicted of abusing or neglecting children or older persons

- Violating a nurse practice act and its rules and regulations
- Demonstrating incompetent behaviors
- Aiding or assisting another person to violate a nurse practice act and its rules and regulations
- Making medical diagnoses
- Prescribing drugs and treatments

Nursing Assistants. Nurse practice acts are used to decide what nursing assistants can do. Some also regulate nursing assistant roles, functions, education, and certification requirements. Other states have separate laws for nursing assistants.

If you do something beyond the legal limits of your role, you could be practicing nursing without a license. This means serious legal problems for you, your supervisor, and your employer.

You must be able to function with skill and safety. Like nurses, you can have your certification (license, registration) denied, revoked, or suspended. (See "Certification.")

The Omnibus Budget Reconciliation Act of 1987

The *Omnibus Budget Reconciliation Act of 1987 (OBRA)* is a federal law. It applies to all 50 states.

OBRA sets minimum requirements for nursing assistant training and evaluation. Each state must have a nursing assistant training and competency evaluation program (NATCEP). A nursing assistant must successfully complete a NATCEP to work in a nursing center, hospital long-term care unit, or home care agency receiving Medicare funds.

The Training Program. OBRA requires at least 75 hours of instruction. Some states require more hours. Classroom and at least 16 hours of supervised practical training are required (Fig. 3-1). Practical training (clinical practicum or clinical experience) occurs in a laboratory or clinical setting. Students perform nursing tasks on another person. A nurse supervises this training.

The training program includes the knowledge and skills needed to give basic nursing care. Areas of study include:

- Communication
- Infection control
- Safety and emergency procedures
- Residents' rights
- Basic nursing skills and personal care skills
- Feeding methods
- Elimination procedures
- Skin care
- Transferring, positioning, and turning methods
- Dressing
- Helping the person walk
- Range-of-motion exercises
- Signs and symptoms of common diseases
- Caring for cognitively impaired persons (those with thinking and memory problems)
  See *Focus on Communication: The Training Program.*

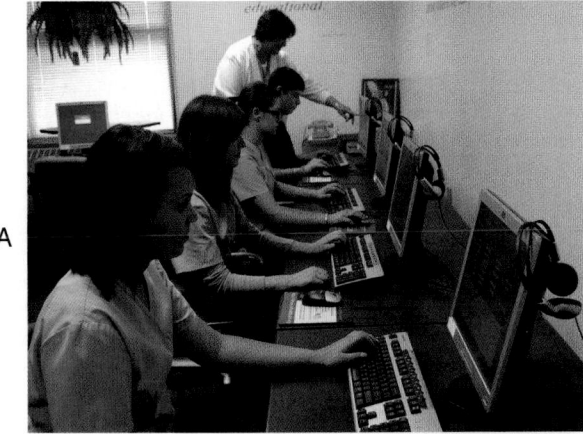

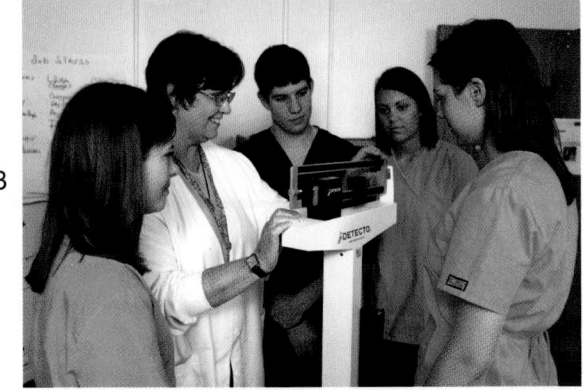

FIGURE 3-1 Nursing assistant training program. **A,** Students study in a classroom setting. **B,** An instructor demonstrates a skill in a laboratory setting.

FOCUS ON COMMUNICATION

The Training Program

Student clinical experiences commonly take place in a real clinical setting. Care is practiced on patients or residents. The patient or resident has the right to know who you are. When you meet the person, introduce yourself. Tell the person you are a student. For example: "Hello. My name is Jenna Smith. I am a nursing assistant student. I will be working with your nurse, Mr. Kline, today."

Competency Evaluation. The competency evaluation has a written test and a skills test (Appendix A, p. 873).
- The written test has multiple-choice questions. Each has 4 choices. Only 1 answer is correct. The number of questions varies from state to state.
- The skills test involves performing certain skills learned in your training program.

You take the competency evaluation after your training program. Your instructor knows the testing service used in your state and when and where the tests are given. You complete the application in writing or on-line. The evaluation has a fee. If working in a nursing center, the employer pays the fee. Otherwise you pay the fee.

You are told the place and time of the test after your application is processed. Some states give a choice of test dates and sites.

Your training prepares you for the competency evaluation. If you listen, study hard, and practice safe care, you should do well. If the first attempt was not successful, you can re-test. OBRA allows at least 3 attempts to successfully complete the evaluation.

Each testing service has a candidate handbook. Review the handbook carefully as you prepare for the competency evaluation.

Nursing Assistant Registry. OBRA requires a nursing assistant registry in each state. It is an official record or listing of persons who have successfully completed that state's approved NATCEP. The registry has information about each nursing assistant.
- Full name, including maiden name and any married names.
- Last known home address.
- Registry number and the date it expires.
- Date of birth.
- Last known employer, date hired, and date employment ended.
- Date the competency evaluation was passed.
- Information about findings of abuse, neglect, or dishonest use of property. It includes the nature of the offense and supporting evidence. If a hearing was held, the date and its outcome are included. The person has the right to include a statement disputing the finding. All information stays in the registry for at least 5 years.

Any health care agency can access registry information. You also receive a copy of your registry information. The copy is sent when the first entry is made and when information is changed or added. You can correct wrong information.

Certification. *Certification is the official recognition by a state that standards or requirements have been met.* After successfully completing your state's NATCEP, you have the title used in your state.
- Certified nursing assistant (CNA) or certified nurse aide (CNA). CNA is used in most states.
- Licensed nursing assistant (LNA). Used in Arizona, New Hampshire, and Vermont.
- Registered nurse aide (RNA). Used in West Virginia.
- State registered nurse aide (SRNA). Used in Kentucky.
- State tested nurse aide (STNA). Used in Ohio.

Nursing assistants can have their certification (licenses, registration) denied, revoked, or suspended. See Box 3-1, p. 24 for the reasons listed by the National Council of State Boards of Nursing (NCSBN).

BOX 3-1	Losing Certification, a License, or Registration

The National Council of State Boards of Nursing (NCSBN) lists these reasons for doing so.
- Substance abuse or dependency.
- Abandoning, abusing, or neglecting a person.
- Fraud or deceit. Examples are:
  - Filing false personal information
  - Providing false information when applying for initial certification, re-instatement, or renewal
- Violating professional boundaries (Chapter 5).
- Giving unsafe care.
- Performing acts beyond the nursing assistant role.
- Misappropriation (stealing, theft) or mis-using property.
- Obtaining money or property from a patient or resident. This can be done through fraud, falsely representing oneself, or by force.
- Being convicted of a crime. Examples include murder, assault, kidnapping, rape or sexual assault, robbery, sexual crimes involving children, criminal mistreatment of children or a vulnerable adult (Chapter 5), drug trafficking, embezzlement (to take a person's property for one's own use), theft, and arson (starting fires).
- Failing to conform to the standards of nursing assistants (p. 26).
- Putting patients and residents at risk for harm.
- Violating a person's privacy.
- Failing to maintain the confidentiality of patient or resident information.

Maintaining Competence. Re-training and a new competency evaluation program are required for nursing assistants who have not worked for 24 months. It does not matter how long you worked as a nursing assistant before. What matters is how long you did *not* work. States can require:
- A new competency evaluation
- Both re-training and a new competency evaluation

Agencies must provide 12 hours of educational programs to nursing assistants every year. Performance reviews also are required. That is, your work is evaluated. These requirements help ensure that you have the current knowledge and skills to give safe, effective care.

See *Teamwork and Time Management: Maintaining Competence.*

See *Focus on Surveys: Maintaining Competence.*

Working in Another State

To work in another state, you must meet that state's NATCEP requirements. First, contact the state agency responsible for NATCEPs and the nursing assistant registry. To find that agency, do 1 of the following.
- Contact your current nursing assistant registry.
- Go to the NCSBN website. Find the link to the state agency.

TEAMWORK AND TIME MANAGEMENT
Maintaining Competence

Educational programs are commonly called *in-service programs* or *in-service training*. Some are required; others are optional. Program announcements and schedules are posted on bulletin boards on nursing units, in staff locker rooms and lounges, by the time clock, and on websites. Some are included with your paycheck. Know where the agency posts in-service information. Check those areas often.

Such training is scheduled before, during, or after your shift. If before work, plan to arrive early. If after work, plan to stay late. Arrange for transportation and childcare as needed (Chapter 6).

If the program is during your shift, plan with your co-workers. Some staff stay on the unit while others attend the program. Staff on the unit tend to all patients and residents. A person may have special care while you are away. Share this information with the staff providing the care. When you return to the unit, thank your co-workers for helping you. Help your co-workers when they leave to attend in-service programs.

FOCUS ON SURVEYS
Maintaining Competence

Surveyors must make sure that nursing assistants are competent to safely care for residents. They will:
- Check if nursing assistants have completed a NATCEP.
- Ask nursing assistants:
  - Where they received their training
  - The length of their training
  - How long they have worked in the agency
- Observe if nursing assistants are able to:
  - Maintain or improve the person's independent functioning.
  - Perform range-of-motion exercises (Chapter 30).
  - Transfer the person from bed to a wheelchair (Chapter 19).
  - Observe, describe, and report the person's behavior and condition to the nurse (Chapters 7 and 8).
  - Follow instructions.
  - Practice infection control (Chapter 16) and safety measures (Chapters 13 and 14).

Then apply to the state agency for endorsement (reciprocity, equivalency) as a CNA (LNA, RNA, SRNA, STNA). *Endorsement (reciprocity, equivalency) means that a state recognizes the certificate, license, or registration issued by another state.* This mean that:
- Your application for CNA (LNA, RNA, SRNA, STNA) is reviewed to see if you meet the state's requirements.
  - Your certification (license, registration) is current and in good standing.
  - You meet that state's education, work, and legal requirements.
- Certification (a license, registration) is granted if the requirements are met.

Follow the application instructions. Expect to:
- Complete the required forms.
- Provide proof of successfully completing a NATCEP. You may need to send a copy of the certificate of course completion from your NATCEP. Do not send the original.
- Request written registry verification from the state in which you are currently certified (licensed, registered). Pay the required fee.
- Provide fingerprints.
- Pay the required application fee.

A criminal background check is done. Registry information is checked. Expect an investigation if the check shows a criminal history. Or if the registry check shows findings of abuse, neglect, dishonest use of property, or other action against you.

You must be truthful. False or misleading information may result in:
- Denial of certification (a license, registration)
- Disciplinary action
- A fine

The application review results in 1 or more of the following.
- Being granted or denied certification (a license, registration).
- Having to take a NATCEP competency test. This may be the written test, the skills test, or both.
- Having to take the entire NATCEP in that state (training program and competency test).

ROLES AND RESPONSIBILITIES

Nurse practice acts, OBRA, state laws, and legal and advisory opinions direct what you can do. To protect persons from harm, you must understand what you can do, what you cannot do, and the legal limits of your role. In some states, this is called *scope of practice*. The NCSBN calls it *range of functions*.

Licensed nurses supervise your work. You perform nursing tasks related to the person's care. A ***nursing task*** *is the nursing care or a nursing function, procedure, activity, or work that can be delegated to nursing assistants when it does not require a nurse's professional knowledge or judgment.* (See Chapter 4.) Often you function without a nurse in the room. At other times you help nurses give care. The rules in Box 3-2 will help you understand your role.

The range of functions for nursing assistants varies among states and agencies. Before you perform a nursing task make sure that:
- Your state allows nursing assistants to do so.
- It is in your job description.
- You have the necessary education and training.
- A nurse is available to answer questions and to supervise you.

BOX 3-2	Rules for Nursing Assistants

- You are an assistant to the nurse.
- A nurse assigns and supervises your work.
- You report observations about the person's physical and mental status to the nurse (Chapters 7 and 8). Report changes in the person's condition or behavior at once.
- The nurse decides what is done for a person. The nurse decides what should not be done for a person. You do not make these decisions.
- Review directions and the care plan with the nurse before going to the person.
- Perform only those nursing tasks that you are trained to do.
- Ask a nurse to supervise you if you are not comfortable performing a nursing task.
- Perform only the nursing tasks that your state and job description allow.

You perform nursing tasks to meet the person's hygiene, safety, comfort, nutrition, exercise, and elimination needs. You move and transfer persons and make observations. You measure temperatures, pulses, respirations, and blood pressures. And you help promote the person's mental comfort.

Box 3-3, p. 26 describes the limits of your role—tasks that you should never do. State laws differ. Know what you can do in the state in which you are working. For example, you move from Vermont to Texas. You must learn the laws and rules in Texas. Or you might work in 2 states. For example, you work in Illinois and Iowa. You must know the laws of both states.

State laws and rules limit nursing assistant functions. Your job description reflects those laws and rules. An agency can further limit what you can do. So can a nurse based on the person's needs. However, no agency or nurse can expand your range of functions beyond what your state's laws and rules allow.

See *Focus on Long-Term Care and Home Care: Roles and Responsibilities.*

FOCUS ON LONG-TERM CARE AND HOME CARE

Roles and Responsibilities

Home Care
You provide personal care and home services. Home services depend on the needs of the person and family. They may include:
- Laundry. You wash, iron or fold, and mend clothing and linens. This may include family laundry.
- Shopping for groceries and household items.
- Preparing and serving meals. You plan menus, follow diets, and feed the person if necessary.
- Light housekeeping. You do not do heavy housekeeping. This includes moving heavy furniture, waxing floors, shampooing carpets, washing windows, and cleaning rugs or drapes. You do not carry firewood, coal, or ash containers.

BOX 3-3	Role Limits

- **Never give drugs.** This includes drugs given:
  - Orally, rectally, vaginally, and by injection
  - By application to the skin, eyes, ears, and nose
  - Directly into the bloodstream or through an intravenous (IV) line

  Nurses give drugs. Many states allow nursing assistants to give some drugs after completing a state-approved medication assistant training program. The function must be in your job description. And you must have the necessary supervision.
- **Never insert tubes or objects into body openings. Do not remove them from the body.** You must not insert tubes into the person's bladder, esophagus, trachea, nose, ears, bloodstream, or surgically created body openings. Exceptions to this rule are the procedures you will study during your training. Giving enemas is an example. To give enemas, the task must be in your job description. And you must have the necessary supervision.
- **Never take oral or phone orders from doctors.** Politely give your name and title, and ask the doctor to wait for a nurse. Promptly find a nurse to speak with the doctor.
- **Never perform procedures that require sterile technique.** With sterile technique, all objects in contact with the person are free of microorganisms (Chapter 16). Sterile technique and procedures require skills, knowledge, and judgment beyond your training. You can assist a nurse with a sterile procedure. However, you will not perform the procedure yourself.
- **Never tell the person or family the person's diagnosis or medical or surgical treatment plans.** This is the doctor's responsibility. Nurses may clarify what the doctor has said.
- **Never diagnose or prescribe treatments or drugs for anyone.** Doctors diagnose and prescribe.
- **Never supervise others including other nursing assistants.** This is a nurse's responsibility. You will not be trained to supervise others. Supervising others can have serious legal problems.
- **Never ignore an order or request to do something.** This includes nursing tasks that you can do, those you cannot do, and those beyond your legal limits. Promptly and politely explain to the nurse why you cannot carry out the order or request. The nurse assumes you are doing what you were told to do unless you explain otherwise. You cannot neglect the person's care.

BOX 3-4	Nursing Assistant Standards

The nursing assistant:
- Performs nursing tasks within the range of functions allowed by the state's nurse practice act and its rules.
- Is honest and shows integrity in performing nursing tasks. (*Integrity* involves following a code of ethics. See Chapter 5.)
- Bases nursing tasks on his or her education and training. Also bases them on the nurse's directions.
- Is accountable for his or her behavior and actions while assisting the nurse and helping patients and residents.
- Performs delegated aspects of the person's nursing care. See Chapter 4.
- Assists the nurse in observing patients and residents. Also assists in identifying their needs.
- Communicates:
  - Progress toward completing nursing tasks
  - Problems in completing nursing tasks
  - Changes in the person's status
- Asks the nurse to clarify what is expected when unsure.
- Uses educational and training opportunities as available.
- Practices safety measures to protect the person, others, and self.
- Respects the person's rights, concerns, decisions, and dignity.
- Functions as a member of the health team. Helps implement the care plan (Chapter 8).
- Respects the person's property and the property of others.
- Protects confidential information unless required by law to share the information.

Modified from National Council of State Boards of Nursing, Inc.: Model nursing practice act and model administrative rules, Chicago, 2006, Author.

Nursing Assistant Standards

OBRA defines the basic range of functions for nursing assistants. All NATCEPs include those functions. Some states allow other functions. NATCEPs also prepare nursing assistants to meet the standards listed in Box 3-4.

Job Description

The *job description is a document that describes what the agency expects you to do* (Fig. 3-2). It also states educational requirements and your job title. (See "Nursing Assistant Job Titles," p. 29.)

Always obtain a written job description when you apply for a job. Ask questions about it during your job interview. Before accepting a job, tell the employer about:
- Functions you did not learn
- Functions you cannot do for moral or religious reasons

Clearly understand what is expected before taking a job. Do not take a job that requires you to:
- Act beyond the legal limits of your role.
- Function beyond your training limits.
- Perform acts that are against your morals or religion.

No one can force you to do something beyond the legal limits of your role. Sometimes jobs are threatened for refusing to follow a nurse's orders. Often staff obey out of fear. That is why you must understand:
- Your roles and responsibilities
- What you can safely do
- The things you should never do
- Your job description
- The ethical and legal aspects of your role

See *Focus on Communication: Job Description*, p. 29.

POSITION DESCRIPTION/PERFORMANCE EVALUATION

Job Title: LTC Certified Nursing Assistant (CNA)   Supervised by: CNA Coordinator, Charge Nurse

Prepared by: _____   Approved by: _____

Date: _____   Date: _____

Job Summary: Provides direct and indirect resident care activities under the direction of an RN or LPN/LVN. Assists residents with activities of daily living, provides for personal care and comfort, and assists in the maintenance of a safe and clean environment for an assigned group of residents.

DUTIES AND RESPONSIBILITIES:

3 = Exceeds Performance   2 = Expected Performance   1 = Needs Improvement

Demonstrates Competency in the Following Areas:

	3	2	1
Assists in the preparation for admission of residents.	3	2	1
Assists in and accompanies residents in the admission, transfer and discharge procedures.	3	2	1
Provides morning care, which may include bed bath, shower or whirlpool, oral hygiene, combing hair, back care, dressing residents, changing bed linen, cleaning overbed table and bedside stand, straightening room and other general care as necessary throughout the day.	3	2	1
Provides evening care which includes hands/face washing as needed, oral hygiene, back rubs, peri-care, freshening linen, cleaning overbed tables, straightening room and other general care as needed.	3	2	1
Notifies appropriate licensed staff when resident complains of pain.	3	2	1
Provides postmortem care and assists in transporting bodies to the morgue.	3	2	1
Assists LPN/LVN in treatment procedures.	3	2	1
Provides general nursing care such as positioning residents, lifting and turning residents, applying/utilizing special equipment, assisting in use of bedpan or commode and ambulating the residents.	3	2	1
Performs all aspects of resident care in an environment that optimizes resident safety and reduces the likelihood of medical/health care errors.	3	2	1
Supports and maintains a culture of safety and quality.	3	2	1
Takes and records temperature, pulse, respiration, weight, blood pressure and intake-output.	3	2	1
Makes rounds with outgoing shift; knows whereabouts of assigned residents.	3	2	1
Makes rounds with oncoming shift to ensure the unit is left in good condition.	3	2	1
Adheres to policies and procedures of the facility and the Nursing Department.	3	2	1
Participates in socialization activities on the unit.	3	2	1
Turns and positions residents as ordered and/or as needed, making sure no rough surfaces are in direct contact with the body. Lifts and turns with proper and safe body mechanics and with available resources.	3	2	1
Checks for reddened areas or skin breakdown and reports to RN or LPN/LVN.	3	2	1
Ensures residents are dressed properly and assists, as necessary. Ensures that used clothing is properly stored in bedside stand or on hangers in closet. Ensures that all residents are clean and dry at all times.	3	2	1
Checks unit for adequate linen. Folds neatly and arranges linen in linen closet. Cleans linen cart. Provides clean linen and clothing. Makes beds.	3	2	1
Treats residents and their families with respect and dignity.	3	2	1
Restrains residents properly, when ordered.	3	2	1
Accompanies residents to appointments, as directed.	3	2	1
Provides reality orientation in daily care.	3	2	1
Prepares residents for meals; serves and removes food trays and assists with meals or feeds residents, if necessary.	3	2	1
Distributes drinking water and other nourishments to residents.	3	2	1
Performs general care activities for residents in isolation.	3	2	1
Answers residents' call lights, anticipates residents' needs and makes rounds to assigned residents.	3	2	1
Assists residents with handling and care of clothing and other personal property (including dentures, glasses, contact lenses, hearing aids and prosthetic devices).	3	2	1
Transports residents to and from various departments, as requested.	3	2	1
Reports and, when appropriate, records any changes observed in condition or behavior of residents and unusual incidents.	3	2	1
Participates in and contributes to interdisciplinary care conferences.	3	2	1
Must be able to follow directions, both oral and written, and work cooperatively with other staff members.	3	2	1

FIGURE 3-2 A sample nursing assistant job description. Note that the job description is also a performance evaluation. (Provided by MCN Healthcare, Denver, Colo. www.MCNHealthcare.com. All rights reserved.)

Continued

POSITION DESCRIPTION/PERFORMANCE EVALUATION—cont'd

Must have the ability to acquire knowledge of and develop skills in basic nursing procedures and simple charting.	3	2	1
Establishes and maintains interpersonal relationship with residents, family members and other facility staff while assuring confidentiality of resident information.	3	2	1
Attends inservice education programs, as assigned, to learn new treatments, procedures, developmental skills, etc.	3	2	1
Practices careful, efficient and nonwasteful use of supplies and linen and follows established charge procedure for resident charge items.	3	2	1
Maintains personal health in order to prevent absence from work due to health problems.	3	2	1
Possesses a genuine interest and concern for geriatric and disabled persons.	3	2	1

Professional Requirements:

Adheres to dress code, appearance is neat and clean.	3	2	1
Completes annual education requirements.	3	2	1
Maintains regulatory requirements.	3	2	1
Maintains resident confidentiality at all times.	3	2	1
Reports to work on time and as scheduled, completes work within designated time.	3	2	1
Wears identification while on duty, uses computerized punch time system correctly.	3	2	1
Completes inservices and returns in a timely fashion.	3	2	1
Attends annual review and department inservices, as scheduled.	3	2	1
Attends at least ____ staff meetings annually, reads and returns all monthly staff meeting minutes.	3	2	1
Represents the organization in a positive and professional manner.	3	2	1
Actively participates in performance improvement and continuous quality improvement (CQI) activities.	3	2	1
Complies with all organizational policies regarding ethical business practices.	3	2	1
Communicates the mission, ethics and goals of the facility.	3	2	1

TOTAL POINTS _____ _____ _____

Regulatory Requirements:
- High School graduate or equivalent.
- Current Certified Nursing Assistant (CNA) certification in State of _____ for Long Term Care Facilities.
- Current Basic Cardiac Life Support certification within three (3) months of hire date.

Language Skills:
- Able to communicate effectively in English, both verbally and in writing.
- Additional languages preferred.

Skills:
- Basic computer knowledge.

Physical Demands:
- For physical demands of position, including vision, hearing, repetitive motion and environment, see following description.

Reasonable accommodations may be made to enable individuals with disabilities to perform the essential functions of the position without compromising patient care.

I have received, read and understand the Position Description/Performance Evaluation above.

_____   _____
Name/Signature   Date Signed

FIGURE 3-2, cont'd

FOCUS ON COMMUNICATION

Job Description

Your training prepares you to perform certain nursing tasks. The agency may not let you do everything you learned. Other agencies may want you to do things that you did not learn. Use your job description to discuss these issues with the nurse.

For example, you apply to work in a hospital. The job description includes measuring blood glucose (Chapter 34). You did not learn this skill in your training program. You can say: "I see measuring blood glucose is in the job description. I did not learn that in my training program. Will I be trained to perform this skill?"

Carefully review your job description. Know what you can and cannot do. Ask if you have questions.

Nursing Assistant Job Titles.
After successfully completing a NATCEP, you have a title used by law and the nursing assistant registry in your state (see "Certification," p. 23). For job purposes, agencies often use other titles for nursing assistants who have completed a NATCEP and are on a state registry. Your job title depends on the setting and your roles and functions in the agency. Examples are listed in Box 3-5.

BOX 3-5	Nursing Assistant Titles

State Registry Titles
- Certified nurse aide; certified nursing assistant (CNA): most states
- Licensed nursing assistant (LNA): Arizona; New Hampshire; Vermont
- Registered nurse aide (RNA): West Virginia
- State registered nurse aide (SRNA): Kentucky
- State tested nurse aide (STNA): Ohio

Agency Job Titles
- Clinical technician
- Health care assistant
- Health care technician
- Nurse technician
- Nursing care partner
- Nursing support technician
- Patient care assistant
- Patient care attendant
- Patient care monitor
- Patient care technician
- Patient care worker
- Support partner

FOCUS ON PRIDE

The Person, Family, and Yourself

Personal and Professional Responsibility
Your training program will prepare you with the knowledge and skills to be a nursing assistant. Personal and professional qualities allow you to do your job well. Examples include good communication skills, patience, compassion, and teamwork. You will learn about other qualities when you study work ethics in Chapter 6. Job descriptions often outline professional requirements. See Figure 3-2. Make an effort to develop personal and professional qualities during and after your training.

Rights and Respect
Most training programs involve practice in a real clinical setting. Sometimes a patient or resident refuses to have a student. Or the person refuses to allow a student to watch a procedure. The person's right to refuse must be respected.

If this happens to you, you may feel disappointed and rejected. Or you may feel that you did something wrong. Kindly accept the person's request. Try not to be ashamed or upset. Tell your instructor. Do not speak badly about the patient or resident. The person may have had a bad experience. This had nothing to do with you. Respect the person's right to choose who is involved in his or her care.

Independence and Social Interaction
Your training involves learning the skills needed for basic nursing care. You will practice many skills in the classroom or laboratory before going to the clinical setting. Use practice time wisely. Practice as if you were with a real patient or resident. Practice what to say and how to act. Practice the skill many times. This will better prepare you for the clinical setting. You will feel more comfortable and confident in your abilities.

Delegation and Teamwork
Delegation deals with what you are asked to do. (See Chapter 4.) To safely assist the nurse, you must know what you can and cannot do. This protects the person and you.

Do not be discouraged by what you *cannot* do. Value what you *can* do. You have a very important role. Your attitude affects the work you do. Take pride in your role.

Ethics and Laws
Some nursing assistants work in more than 1 setting. Some are also emergency medical technicians (EMTs). EMTs give emergency care outside of health care settings. State laws and rules for EMTs and nursing assistants differ. For example, you work as an EMT and a nursing assistant. Your state laws allow EMTs to start intravenous (IV) lines. Nursing assistants do not start IVs.

The ability to do something does not give the right to do so in all settings. There are legal limits to your role. Be proud of the advanced skills and training you may have. But when working as a nursing assistant, follow your state's laws and rules for nursing assistants.

FOCUS ON PRIDE: Application
Knowing what you can and cannot do prepares you to work safely. Make a list of skills you will learn in your training program. Then make a list of functions outside your role limits. Why must you work within the limits of your role?

REVIEW QUESTIONS

Circle T if the statement is TRUE or F if it is FALSE.

1 T F   OBRA requires a nursing assistant training and competency evaluation program in every state.

2 T F   You are allowed 1 attempt to pass your state's competency evaluation.

3 T F   Each state must have a nursing assistant registry.

4 T F   You have not worked for 3 years. Your certification (license, registration) is still current.

5 T F   All states have the same training and evaluation requirements.

6 T F   An agency can expand your range of functions beyond what is allowed in your state.

Circle the BEST answer.

7 Nursing practice is regulated by
   a The National Council of State Boards of Nursing
   b Nurse practice acts
   c Medicare
   d Medicaid

8 What state law affects what nursing assistants can do?
   a Standards for nursing assistants
   b Medicaid
   c OBRA
   d Nurse practice act

9 Your nursing assistant certification can be revoked for
   a Refusing a nursing task
   b Asking the nurse questions
   c Performing acts beyond your role
   d Keeping the person's information confidential

10 As a nursing assistant, you
    a Must perform all tasks as directed by the nurse
    b Make decisions about a person's care
    c Need a written job description before employment
    d Give a drug when a nurse tells you to

11 As a nursing assistant, you
    a Can take verbal or phone orders from doctors
    b Report observations to the nurse
    c Can remove tubes from the person's body
    d Can ignore a nursing task if it is not in your job description

12 Who assigns and supervises your work?
    a A nurse
    b The health team
    c Another nursing assistant
    d You

13 You are responsible for
    a Supervising other nursing assistants
    b Telling the person his or her diagnosis
    c Knowing what you can safely do
    d Deciding what treatments are needed

14 You perform a task not allowed by your state. Which is *true*?
    a If a nurse asked you to do the task, there is no legal problem.
    b You could be practicing nursing without a license.
    c You can perform the task if it is in your job description.
    d If you complete the task safely, there is no legal problem.

15 Which describes what an agency expects you to do?
    a Nurse practice act
    b Range of functions
    c Scope of practice
    d Job description

Answers to Chapter 3 questions are on p. 870.

FOCUS ON PRACTICE

Problem Solving

You are training in the clinical setting. A resident asks you to help her move from her wheelchair to bed. You have not learned how to perform transfers yet. How will you respond? What will you do? As a student, what rules must you follow to protect patients and residents?

Delegation

4

OBJECTIVES

- Define the key terms and key abbreviations in this chapter.
- Identify members of the nursing team who can delegate nursing tasks.
- Describe the 4 steps in the delegation process.
- Describe the *Five Rights of Delegation*.

- Explain your role in the delegation process.
- Describe the *Five Rights of Delegation* for nursing assistants.
- Explain how to accept or refuse a delegated task.
- Explain how to promote PRIDE in the person, the family, and yourself.

KEY TERMS

accountable Being responsible for one's actions and the actions of others who performed the delegated tasks; answering questions about and explaining one's actions and the actions of others

competent Having the necessary ability, knowledge, or skill to perform a task safely and successfully

delegate To authorize another person to perform a nursing task in a certain situation

nursing task Nursing care or a nursing function, procedure, activity, or work that can be delegated to nursing assistants when it does not require an RN's professional knowledge or judgment

responsibility The duty or obligation to perform some act or function

KEY ABBREVIATIONS

LPN	Licensed practical nurse
LVN	Licensed vocational nurse

NCSBN	National Council of State Boards of Nursing
RN	Registered nurse

Nurse practice acts give nurses certain responsibilities. They also give them the legal authority to perform nursing actions. A *responsibility is the duty or obligation to perform some act or function.* For example, RNs (registered nurses) are responsible for supervising LPNs/LVNs (licensed practical nurses/licensed vocational nurses) and nursing assistants. Only RNs can carry out this responsibility.

You perform nursing tasks. A *nursing task is the nursing care or a nursing function, procedure, activity, or work that can be delegated to nursing assistants when it does not require an RN's professional knowledge or judgment.* Nurses delegate nursing tasks. *Delegate means to authorize another person to perform a nursing task in a certain situation.* The person must be competent to perform the task in the given situation. *Competent means having the necessary ability, knowledge, or skill to perform a task safely and successfully.* For example, you know how to give a bed bath. However, Mr. Jones is a new resident. The RN wants to spend time with him and assess his nursing needs. You do not assess. Therefore the RN gives the bath.

WHO CAN DELEGATE

RNs can delegate nursing tasks to LPNs/LVNs and nursing assistants. In some states, LPNs/LVNs can delegate nursing tasks to nursing assistants. Nurses can only delegate tasks to you within your range of functions (Chapter 3). And they can only delegate tasks in your job description (Chapter 3).

A nurse's delegation decisions must protect the person's health and safety. The delegating nurse is legally accountable for the nursing tasks delegated. *Accountable means to be responsible for one's actions and the actions of others who performed the delegated tasks. It also involves answering questions about and explaining one's actions and the actions of others.*

The delegating nurse must make sure that the task was completed safely and correctly. If the RN delegates, the RN is responsible for the delegated task. If the LPN/LVN delegates, he or she is responsible for the delegated task. The RN also supervises LPNs/LVNs. Therefore the RN is legally accountable for the tasks that LPNs/LVNs delegate to nursing assistants. The RN is accountable for all nursing care.

PROMOTING SAFETY AND COMFORT
Who Can Delegate

Safety

Delegation requires a nurse's knowledge and judgment. Delegated nursing tasks must be:

- Within the nurse's scope of practice. For example, bathing is within the nurse's scope of practice. Under the right conditions, the nurse can delegate the bathing task to you. Pulling out loose teeth is not within a nurse's scope of practice. The nurse cannot tell you to pull out a person's loose tooth.
- Within the nursing assistant range of functions allowed by your state. For example, your state does not allow nursing assistants to cut toenails. The nurse cannot delegate cutting toenails to you. The nurse must know:
  - The range of functions allowed in your state
  - The content and skills learned in your nursing assistant training and competency evaluation program (NATCEP)
- Listed in your job description. For example, your state allows nursing assistants to give enemas. The task is not in your job description. The nurse cannot delegate the task to you. The nurse must know the tasks allowed by your job description.

  You must know what you can and cannot do (Box 4-1). You must refuse a task that you were not trained to do. You also must refuse a delegated task that is:

- Beyond the nurse's scope of practice
- Beyond the nursing assistant range of functions allowed by your state
- Not in your job description

  See "Refusing a Task," p. 35.

BOX 4-1   Examples of Tasks That Can and Cannot Be Delegated

Examples of Tasks That CAN Be Delegated to You:
- Measure and record temperature, pulse, respirations, and blood pressure
- Measure weight and height
- Measure intake and output
- Collect specimens
- Give bed baths, showers, or tub baths
- Give perineal care
- Provide hair care
- Provide oral hygiene
- Give a back massage
- Assist with walking
- Perform range-of-motion exercises
- Move and transfer a person
- Turn and re-position a person
- Assist with coughing and deep-breathing exercises
- Serve and remove food trays
- Answer call lights
- Clean reading glasses
- Make beds
- Straighten bed linens and the person's room
- Stock linen, supply carts, and bedside supplies
- Empty wastebaskets
- Clean over-bed tables, bedside stands, counters, and other surfaces

Examples of Tasks That CANNOT Be Delegated to You:
- Perform assessments (Chapter 8)
- Develop care plans (Chapter 8)
- Evaluate response to care (Chapter 8)
- Provide education (teaching) to the person and family
- Supervise others
- Take oral or phone orders from doctors
- Give drugs
- Perform procedures requiring sterile technique
- Insert intravenous (IV) catheters

Nursing assistants cannot delegate. You cannot delegate any task to other nursing assistants or to any other worker. You can ask someone to help you. But you cannot ask or tell someone to do your work. Also, you cannot re-delegate a task to another nursing assistant or other worker.

See *Promoting Safety and Comfort: Who Can Delegate.*

DELEGATION PROCESS

To make delegation decisions, the nurse follows a process. The person's needs, the nursing task, and the staff member doing the task must fit (Fig. 4-1). The nurse decides if the task will or will not be delegated to you. The person's needs and the task may require a nurse's knowledge, judgment, and skill. You may be asked to assist.

The nurse decides what is best for the person at the time. Do not get offended or angry if a task is not delegated to you. The nurse's decision is also best for you at the time. You must not do a task requiring a nurse's knowledge, judgment, or skill. For example, you always care for Mrs. Mills. Now she is weak and not eating well. The nurse wants to evaluate the changes in her condition. The nurse gives needed care. Mrs. Mills needs the nurse's knowledge and judgment.

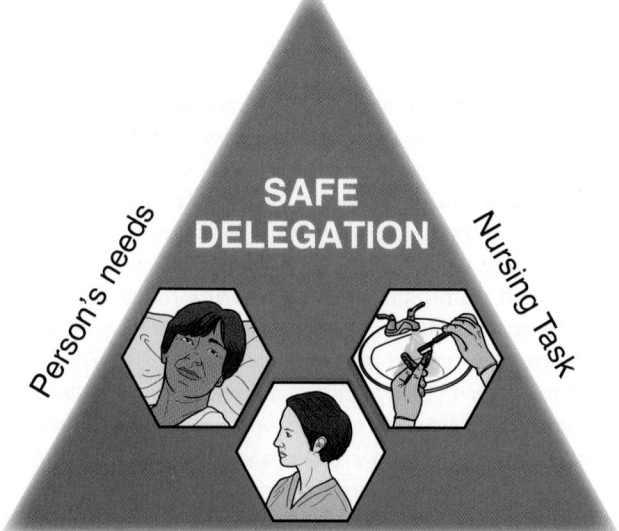

FIGURE 4-1 The nurse considers the person's needs, the task, and the staff member's abilities when making delegation decisions.

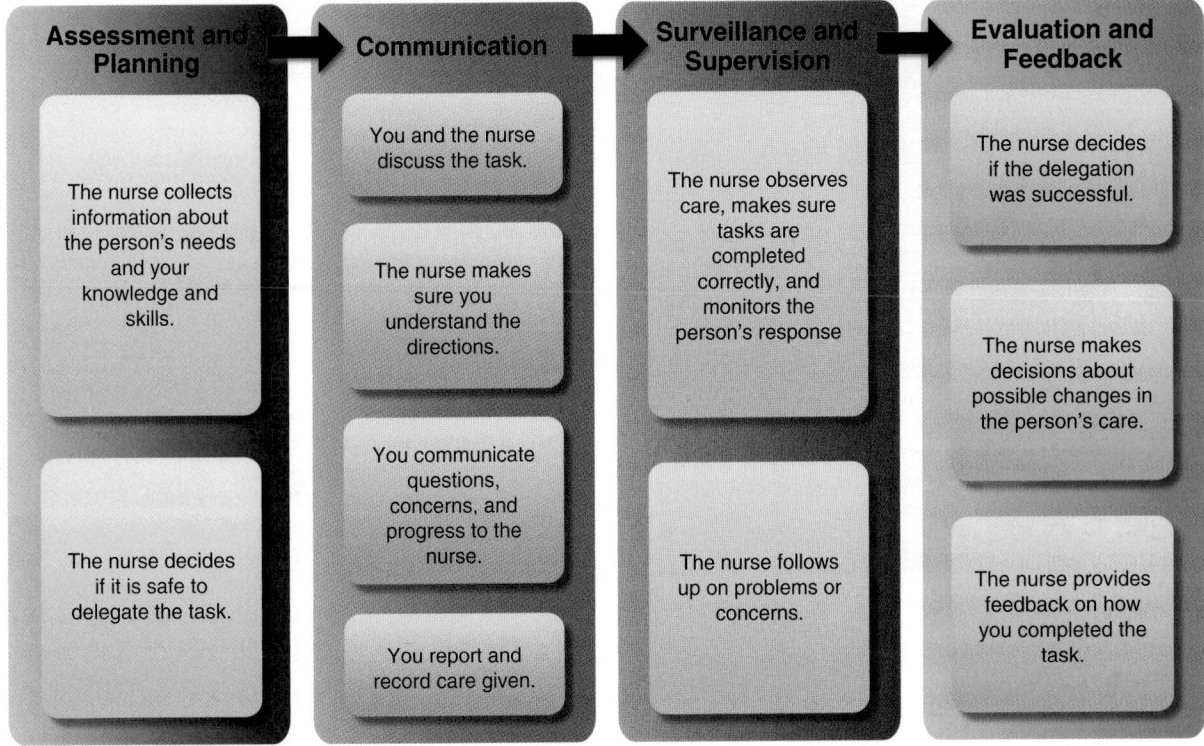

FIGURE 4-2 The delegation process has 4 steps.

The person's circumstances are central factors in delegation decisions. Delegation decisions must result in the best care for the person. Otherwise the person's health and safety are at risk. Also, the nurse may face serious legal problems. If you perform a task that places the person at risk, you may face serious legal problems.

The National Council of State Boards of Nursing (NCSBN) describes the delegation process in 4 steps (Fig. 4-2). To safely delegate nursing tasks, the nurse follows each step.

Step 1—Assessment and Planning

The nurse needs to understand the person's needs. And the nurse needs to know your knowledge, skills, and job description.

When assessing the person's needs, the nurse answers these questions.
- What are the person's needs? How complex are they? How can they vary? How urgent are the care needs?
- What are the most important long-term needs? What are the most important short-term needs?
- How much judgment is needed to meet the person's needs and give care?
- How predictable is the person's health status? How does the person respond to health care?
- What problems might arise from the task? How severe might they be?
- What actions are needed if a problem occurs? How complex are the needed actions?
- What emergencies or incidents might arise? How likely might they occur?

- How involved is the person in health care decisions? How involved is the family?
- How will delegating the task help the person? What are the risks to the person?

To assess your knowledge and skills, the nurse answers these questions.
- What knowledge and skills are needed to safely perform the task?
- What is your role in the agency? What is in your job description?
- What are the conditions under which you will perform the task?
- What is expected after completing the task?
- What problems can arise from the task? What problems might the person develop during the task?

The nurse then decides if it is safe to delegate the task. It must be safe for the person and you. If unsafe, the nurse stops the delegation process. If it is safe for the person and you, the nurse moves to step 2.

Step 2—Communication

This step involves the nurse and you. The nurse must give clear and complete directions about:
- How to perform and complete the task
- What observations to report and record
- When to report observations
- What specific patient or resident concerns to report at once
- Priorities for tasks
- What to do if the person's condition changes or needs change

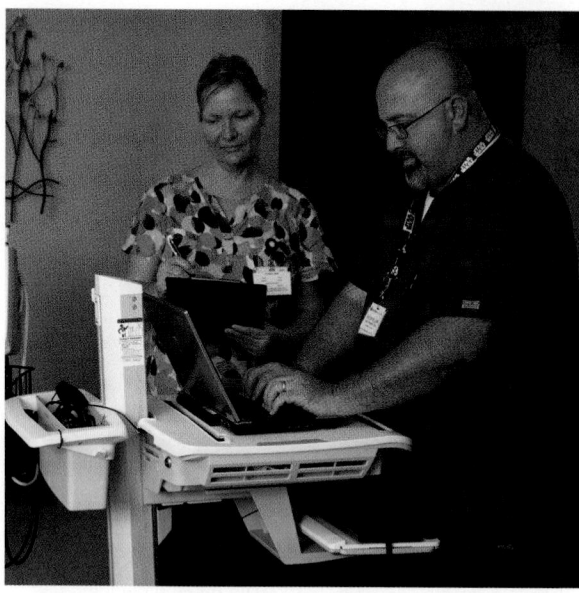

FIGURE 4-3 A nurse and nursing assistant discuss a delegated task.

The nurse must make sure that you understand the directions to give safe care. The nurse asks questions to make sure you understand. He or she may ask you to explain what you need to do. Do not be insulted by such questions. The intent is to protect the person and you.

Before performing a delegated task, it is important to discuss the task with the nurse (Fig. 4-3). Make sure that you:
- Ask questions about the task and what you are expected to do.
- Tell the nurse if you have not done the task before or not often.
- Ask for needed training or supervision.
- Re-state what is expected of you.
- Re-state what specific patient or resident concerns to report to the nurse.
- Explain how and when you will report progress in completing the task.
- Know how to contact the nurse for an emergency.
- Know what to do during an emergency.

After completing a delegated task, you report and record the care given. You also report and record your observations. See "Reporting and Recording" in Chapter 7.

See *Focus on Long-Term Care and Home Care: Step 2—Communication.*

See *Delegation Guidelines: Step 2—Communication.*

Step 3—Surveillance and Supervision

Surveillance means *to keep a close watch over someone or something. Supervise* means *to over-see, direct, or manage.* In this step, the nurse:
- Observes the care you give.
- Makes sure that you complete the task correctly.
- Observes the person's condition and response to care.

How often the nurse makes observations depends on:
- The person's health status and needs
- If the person's condition is stable or unstable
- If the nurse can predict the person's responses and risks to care
- The setting where the task occurs
- The resources and support available
- If the task is simple or complex

The nurse must follow up on problems or concerns. For example, the nurse takes action if:
- You did not complete the task in a timely manner.
- The task did not meet expectations.
- There is a change in the person's condition.

The nurse is alert for signs and symptoms that signal a possible change in the person's condition. With your help, the nurse can take action before the person's condition changes.

Sometimes problems arise during a task. By supervising you, the nurse can detect and solve problems early. This helps you complete the task safely and on time.

After you complete the task, the nurse may review and discuss what happened with you. This helps you learn. If something similar happens again, you have ideas about how to adjust.

Step 4—Evaluation and Feedback

Evaluate means *to judge*. The nurse decides if the delegation was successful. The nurse answers these questions.

- Was the task done correctly?
- Did the person respond as expected?
- Was the outcome (the result) as desired? Was the result good or bad?
- Was communication between you and the nurse timely and effective?
- What went well? What were the problems?
- Does the care plan need to change (Chapter 8)?
- Did the nurse give you the right feedback? *Feedback* means *to respond*. The nurse tells you what you did correctly and about any errors. Feedback is a way for you to learn and improve the care you give.
- Did the nurse thank you for completing the task?

THE FIVE RIGHTS OF DELEGATION

The NCSBN's *Five Rights of Delegation* is another way to view the delegation process. The nurse answers questions listed in the 4 steps described above. The *Five Rights of Delegation* are:

- *The right task.* Can the task be delegated? Is the nurse allowed to delegate the task? Is the task in your job description?
- *The right circumstances.* What are the person's physical, mental, emotional, and spiritual needs at this time?
- *The right person.* Do you have the training and experience to safely perform the task for this person?
- *The right directions and communication.* The nurse must give clear directions. The nurse tells you what to do and when to do it. The nurse tells you what observations to make and when to report back. The nurse allows questions and helps you set priorities. By setting priorities, you know what to do first, second, and so on.
- *The right supervision.* The nurse:
  - Guides, directs, and evaluates the care you give.
  - Demonstrates tasks as needed and is available for questions. The less experience you have with a task, the more supervision you need. Complex tasks require more supervision than basic tasks. Also, the person's circumstances affect how much supervision you need.
  - Assesses how the task affected the person and how well you performed the task.
  - Tells you what you did well and how to improve your work. This helps you learn and give better care.

YOUR ROLE IN DELEGATION

You perform delegated tasks for or on *a person*. You must protect the person from harm. You have 2 choices when delegated a task. You either *agree* or *refuse* to do a task. Use the *Five Rights of Delegation* in Box 4-2.

BOX 4-2	The *Five Rights of Delegation* for Nursing Assistants

The Right Task
- Does your state allow you to perform the task?
- Were you trained to do the task?
- Do you have experience performing the task?
- Is the task in your job description?

The Right Circumstances
- Do you have experience with the task given the person's condition and needs?
- Do you understand the purposes of the task for the person?
- Can you perform the task safely under the current circumstances?
- Do you have the equipment and supplies to safely complete the task?
- Do you know how to use the equipment and supplies?

The Right Person
- Are you comfortable performing the task?
- Do you have concerns about performing the task?

The Right Directions and Communication
- Did the nurse give clear directions and instructions?
- Did you review the task with the nurse?
- Do you understand what the nurse expects?

The Right Supervision
- Is a nurse available to answer questions?
- Is a nurse available if the person's condition changes or if problems occur?

Modified from National Council of State Boards of Nursing, Inc.: The five rights of delegation, Chicago, 1997, Author.

Accepting a Task

When you agree to perform a task, you are responsible for your own actions. What you do or fail to do can harm the person. *You must complete the task safely.* Ask for help if you are unsure or have questions about a task. Report to the nurse what you did and your observations.

Refusing a Task

You have the right to say "no." Sometimes refusing to follow the nurse's directions is your right and duty. You should refuse to perform a task when:

- The task is beyond the legal limits of your role. That is, the task is beyond the range of functions allowed by your state.
- The task is not in your job description.
- You were not trained to perform the task.
- The task could harm the person.
- The person's condition has changed.
- You do not know how to use the supplies or equipment.
- Directions are not ethical or legal.
- Directions are against agency policies.
- Directions are not clear or complete.
- A nurse is not available for supervision.

Use common sense. This protects you and the person. Ask yourself if what you are doing is safe for the person.

Never ignore an order or a request to do something. Tell the nurse about your concerns. For tasks within the legal limits of your role and in your job description, the nurse can help increase your comfort. The nurse can:

- Answer your questions.
- Demonstrate the task.
- Show you how to use supplies and equipment.
- Help you as needed.
- Observe you doing the task.
- Check on you often.
- Arrange for needed training.

Do not refuse a task because you do not like it or do not want to do it. You must have sound reasons. Otherwise, you place the person at risk for harm. You could lose your job.

See *Focus on Communication: Refusing a Task.*

FOCUS ON COMMUNICATION

Refusing a Task

A nurse may delegate a task that was not part of your training. The task is in your job description. You can say: "I know this task is in my job description, but I did not learn it in school. Can you show me what to do and then observe me doing it? That would really help me."

A nurse may ask you to do something that is not in your job description. With respect, you must firmly refuse the nurse's request. For example: Mr. Wey is in the bathroom when the nurse brings a drug to him. The nurse tells you to give him the drug when he comes out of the bathroom. If you give the drug, you are performing a task and responsibility outside the limits of your role. With respect, firmly refuse to follow the nurse's direction. You can say: "I'm sorry, but I cannot give Mr. Wey that drug. I was not trained to give drugs, and that task is not in my job description. I'll tell you when Mr. Wey comes out of the bathroom."

FOCUS ON PRIDE

The Person, Family, and Yourself

Personal and Professional Responsibility

You must communicate delegation concerns to the nurse. If uncertain about your ability to safely perform a delegated task, tell the nurse. Maybe you have not done the task before. Maybe the equipment is unfamiliar. Or the person's condition has changed.

Never be ashamed of refusing a task to protect the person. Take pride in protecting the person from harm.

Rights and Respect

Feedback improves delegation. Staff learn what went well and how the process can improve. Feedback should be given and received in a respectful manner. Thank the nurse for positive feedback. With corrective feedback:

- Listen carefully.
- Have good eye contact.
- Consider ways you can improve.
- Avoid arguing or being defensive.
- Thank the nurse for the feedback.

Willingly accept corrective feedback. Always strive to learn and improve.

Independence and Social Interaction

Staff relationships and interactions affect delegation outcomes. Delegation experiences are positive when staff:

- Communicate openly.
- Trust each other.
- Help and encourage each other.
- Work toward a common goal.

With positive interactions, each nursing team member is valued. And the person benefits from effective care.

The nursing team must work well together. If not, the delegation experience can be challenging and frustrating. For example, the nurse does not give clear directions or needed information about the person. You are left wondering what you need to do and when.

Delegation and Teamwork

You may be delegated several tasks at a time. This can be overwhelming. For example, you are asked to:

- Take Mr. Austin's temperature.
- Get Ms. Sams a glass of water.
- Turn and re-position Mr. Mason.
- Assist Mrs. Walters to the bathroom.

When delegated several tasks, stay calm and positive. Tell the nurse. Ask the nurse to help you set priorities. Also, good teamwork is needed. The nursing team must work together to provide care. Offer to help others. Thank others when they help you.

Ethics and Laws

Ethics involves making choices about what should and should not be done. You must choose to accept or refuse delegated tasks. For example:

- A nurse asks you to adjust Ms. Howe's oxygen flow. Your state does not allow nursing assistants to give oxygen. The nurse's directions are not legal. Refusing the task is the right thing to do.
- Mr. Flynn fell. You tell the nurse at once. The nurse says: "Take him to the dining room. I'll check him after lunch." Agency policy states that a nurse must immediately assess the resident after a fall. The nurse's directions are against agency policy. Refusing is the right thing to do.
- Your uncle is a patient on your nursing unit. He is in a coma. (He is unaware of his setting and unable to respond.) The nurse knows that your aunt wants someone else to provide personal care. The nurse says: "We are busy, so give your uncle a bed bath today. Your aunt will visit at 1:00, so be done before then." The nurse's directions are unethical. Refusing the task is the right thing to do.

Nurses are legally responsible for making safe and ethical delegation decisions. You are responsible for your decision to accept or refuse a task and how you complete the task.

FOCUS ON PRIDE: Application

What must you consider when deciding to accept or refuse a delegated task? How would you respectfully refuse? Give an example.

REVIEW QUESTIONS

Circle T if the statement is TRUE or F if it is FALSE.

1 T F   Nursing assistants can delegate.

2 T F   Nurses can delegate nursing responsibilities to you.

3 T F   A delegated task must be safe for the person.

4 T F   Delegated tasks must be in your job description.

5 T F   The nurse is responsible for delegation decisions.

6 T F   If a task is in your job description, the nurse must delegate it to you.

7 T F   You must have clear directions before performing a task.

Circle the BEST answer.

8 As a nursing assistant, you
   a Must accept all tasks delegated by the nurse
   b Make decisions about a person's care
   c Must know what tasks are in your job description
   d Give a drug when a nurse tells you to

9 You are responsible for
   a Completing delegated tasks safely
   b Assessing the person's needs
   c Supervising other nursing assistants
   d Deciding what treatments are needed

10 The communication step of the delegation process involves
   a Observing care
   b Determining who should perform a task
   c Deciding if the delegation was successful
   d Asking questions about a task

11 These statements are about surveillance and supervision. Which is correct?
   a The nurse must be with you when you provide care.
   b The nurse must make sure you complete tasks correctly.
   c Simple tasks require more supervision than complex ones.
   d Less supervision is required when the person's condition is unstable.

12 A patient begins having trouble swallowing. The nurse decides not to delegate feeding to you. Why?
   a The task is beyond the legal limits of your role.
   b You are not trained to do the task.
   c The nurse does not trust you to do the task safely.
   d The person's circumstances have changed.

13 A nurse delegates a task to you. You must
   a Complete the task
   b Delegate the task if you are busy
   c Decide to accept or refuse the task
   d Ignore the request if you do not know what to do

14 You can refuse to perform a task if
   a The task is within the legal limits of your role
   b The task is in your job description
   c You do not like the task
   d A nurse is not available to supervise you

15 You decide to refuse a task. What should you do?
   a Communicate your concerns to the nurse.
   b Delegate the task to a nursing assistant.
   c Ignore the request.
   d Talk to the director of nursing.

Answers to Chapter 4 questions are on p. 870.

FOCUS ON PRACTICE

Problem Solving

You are delegated the following tasks. Which will you accept? Which must you refuse? What will you say to the nurse when refusing a task?
- Teach a patient to use crutches.
- Collect a urine specimen.
- Measure a patient's weight.
- Insert a urinary catheter using sterile technique.
- Measure a patient's pulse and blood pressure.

Ethics and Laws

OBJECTIVES

- Define the key terms and key abbreviations in this chapter.
- Describe ethical conduct.
- Describe the rules of conduct for nursing assistants.
- Explain how to maintain professional boundaries.
- Explain how to prevent negligent acts.
- Give examples of false imprisonment, defamation, assault, battery, and fraud.

- Describe how to protect the right to privacy.
- Explain the correct use of electronic communications.
- Explain the purpose of informed consent.
- Describe elder, child, and domestic abuse.
- Explain your role in relation to wills.
- Explain how to promote PRIDE in the person, the family, and yourself.

KEY TERMS

abuse The willful infliction of injury, unreasonable confinement, intimidation, or punishment that results in physical harm, pain, or mental anguish; depriving the person (or the person's caregiver) of the goods or services needed to attain or maintain well-being

assault Intentionally attempting or threatening to touch a person's body without the person's consent

battery Touching a person's body without his or her consent

boundary crossing A brief act or behavior of being over-involved with the person; the intent of the act or behavior is to meet the person's needs

boundary sign Acts, behaviors, or thoughts that warn of a boundary crossing or boundary violation

boundary violation An act or behavior that meets your needs, not the person's

child abuse and neglect The intentional harm or mistreatment of a child under 18 years old; it involves any recent act or failure to act on the part of a parent or caregiver; it results in death, serious physical or emotional harm, sexual abuse, or exploitation; and it presents a likely or immediate risk for harm

civil law Laws concerned with relationships between people

code of ethics Rules, or standards of conduct, for group members to follow

crime An act that violates a criminal law

criminal law Laws concerned with offenses against the public and society in general

defamation Injuring a person's name and reputation by making false statements to a third person

elder abuse Any knowing, intentional, or negligent act by a caregiver or any other person to an older adult; the act causes harm or serious risk of harm

ethics Knowledge of what is right conduct and wrong conduct

false imprisonment Unlawful restraint or restriction of a person's freedom of movement

fraud Saying or doing something to trick, fool, or deceive a person

intimate partner violence (IPV) Physical, sexual, or psychological harm by a current or former partner or spouse

invasion of privacy Violating a person's right not to have his or her name, photo, or private affairs exposed or made public without giving consent

law A rule of conduct made by a government body

libel Making false statements in print, in writing (including e-mail and text messages), through pictures or drawings, through broadcast (radio, TV, or video), posted on-line on websites, or through video sites and social media sites

malpractice Negligence by a professional person

neglect The failure of responsible persons to provide food, shelter, health care, or protection for a vulnerable elder

negligence An unintentional wrong in which a person did not act in a reasonable and careful manner and a person or the person's property was harmed

professional boundary That which separates helpful behaviors from behaviors that are not helpful

professional sexual misconduct An act, behavior, or comment that is sexual in nature

protected health information Identifying information and information about the person's health care that is maintained or sent in any form (paper, electronic, oral)

self-neglect A person's behaviors and way of living that threaten his or her health, safety, and well-being

slander Making false statements through the spoken word, sounds, sign language, or gestures

standard of care The skills, care, and judgments required by a health team member under similar conditions

KEY TERMS—cont'd

tort A wrong committed against a person or the person's property

vulnerable adult A person 18 years old or older who has a disability or condition that makes him or her at risk to be wounded, attacked, or damaged

will A legal document of how a person wants property distributed after death

KEY ABBREVIATIONS

CDC Centers for Disease Control and Prevention

HIPAA Health Insurance Portability and Accountability Act of 1996

IPV Intimate partner violence

OBRA Omnibus Budget Reconciliation Act of 1987

Nurse practice acts, your training and job description, and safe delegation serve to protect patients and residents from harm (Chapters 3 and 4). Protecting them from harm also involves a complex set of rules and standards of conduct. They form the ethical and legal aspects of care.

ETHICAL ASPECTS

Ethics is knowledge of what is right conduct and wrong conduct. Morals are involved. *Morals* involve right and wrong and good and bad behavior. Ethics also deals with choices or judgments about what should or should not be done. An ethical person behaves and acts in the right way. He or she does not cause a person harm.

Ethical behavior also involves not being prejudiced or biased. To be *prejudiced* or *biased* means *making judgments and having views before knowing the facts.* Your judgments and views usually are based on your values and standards. They are based on your culture, religion, education, and experiences. The person's situation and yours may be very different. For example:

- Children think their mother needs nursing home care. In your culture, children care for older parents at home.
- A person has tattoos and body piercings. You do not like tattoos or body piercings.
- An older man does not want life-saving measures. You believe that everything must be done to save a life.

Do not judge the person by your values and standards. Do not avoid persons whose standards and values differ from your own.

Ethical problems involve making choices. What is the right thing to do? For example:

- A co-worker is in an empty room drinking from a cup. You smell alcohol on her breath. She asks you not to tell anyone.
- A resident has bruises all over her body. She told the nurse that she fell. She tells you that her son is very mean to her. She asks you not to tell the nurse.

BOX 5-1	Code of Conduct for Nursing Assistants

- Respect each person as an individual.
- Know the limits of your role and knowledge.
- Perform only those tasks within the legal limits of your role.
- Perform only those tasks that you have been trained to do.
- Perform no act that will harm the person.
- Take drugs only if prescribed and supervised by your doctor.
- Follow the directions and instructions of the nurse to your best possible ability.
- Follow agency policies and procedures.
- Complete each task safely.
- Be loyal to your employer and co-workers.
- Act as a responsible citizen at all times.
- Keep the person's information confidential.
- Protect the person's privacy.
- Protect the person's property.
- Consider the person's needs to be more important than your own.
- Report errors and incidents honestly and at once.
- Be accountable for your actions.

Codes of Ethics

Professional groups have codes of ethics. A *code of ethics has rules, or standards of conduct, for group members to follow.* The American Nurses Association (ANA) has a code of ethics for registered nurses (RNs). The National Federation of Licensed Practical Nurses has 1 for licensed practical nurses/licensed vocational nurses (LPNs/LVNs). The rules of conduct in Box 5-1 can guide your thinking and behavior. See Chapter 6 for student and work ethics.

Professional Boundaries

A *boundary* limits or separates something. For example, a fence forms a boundary. You stay inside or outside of the fenced area. As a nursing assistant, you enter into a helping relationship with patients, residents, and families. The helping relationship has professional boundaries.

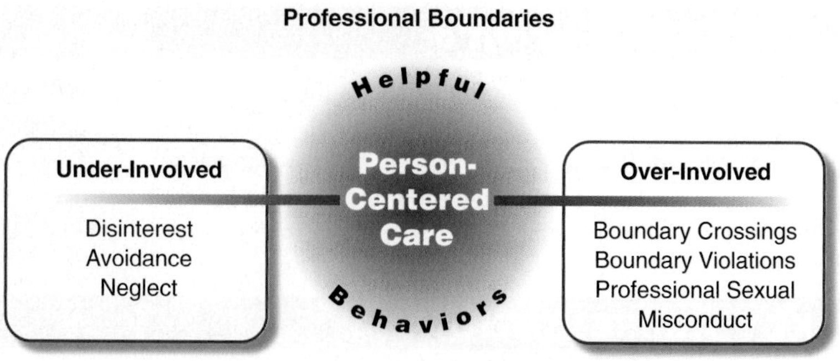

Professional Boundaries

FIGURE 5-1 Professional boundaries guide your behavior. Your focus is on helping the person. Being under-involved or over-involved is not helpful. (Modified from National Council of State Boards of Nursing, Inc.: *A nurse's guide to professional boundaries*, Chicago, 2014, Author.)

Professional boundaries separate *helpful behaviors from behaviors that are not helpful* (Fig. 5-1). The boundaries create a helpful zone. Your behavior must help the person. If you are under-involved, the following can occur.

- Disinterest—you lack interest in the person.
- Avoidance—you avoid the person.
- Neglect—you do not properly care for the person (p. 46).

If you are over-involved, the following can occur.

- *Boundary crossing is a brief act or behavior of being over-involved with the person. The intent of the act or behavior is to meet the person's needs.* The act or behavior may be thoughtless or something you did not mean to do. Or it could have purpose if it meets the person's needs. For example, you give a crying patient a hug. The hug meets the person's needs at the time. If the hug meets your needs, the act is wrong. Also, it is wrong to hug the person every time you see him or her.
- *Boundary violation is an act or behavior that meets your needs, not the person's.* The act or behavior is not ethical. It violates the code of conduct in Box 5-1. The person can be harmed. Boundary violations include:
  - Abuse (p. 44).
  - Giving a lot of information about yourself. You tell the person about your personal relationships or problems.
  - Keeping secrets with the person.
- *Professional sexual misconduct is an act, behavior, or comment that is sexual in nature.* It is sexual misconduct even if the person consents or makes the first move.

Some boundary violations and some types of professional sexual misconduct also are crimes. To maintain professional boundaries, follow the rules in Box 5-2. Be alert to boundary signs. *Boundary signs are acts, behaviors, or thoughts that warn of a boundary crossing or boundary violation* (Box 5-3).

See *Focus on Communication: Professional Boundaries.*

LEGAL ASPECTS

Ethics is about what you *should or should not do.* Laws tell you what you *can and cannot do.* A *law is a rule of conduct made by a government body.* The U.S. Congress and state legislatures make laws. Enforced by the government, laws protect the public welfare.

BOX 5-2   Maintaining Professional Boundaries

- Follow the code of conduct listed in Box 5-1.
- Talk to the nurse if you sense a boundary sign, crossing, or violation.
- Avoid caring for family, friends, and people with whom you do business. This may be hard to do in a small community. Always tell the nurse if you know the person. The nurse may change your assignment.
- Do not make sexual comments or jokes.
- Do not use offensive language.
- Use touch correctly (Chapter 9). Touch or handle sexual and genital areas only to give needed care. Such areas include the breasts, nipples, perineum, buttocks, and anus.
- Do not visit or spend extra time with a patient or resident who is not part of your assignment.
- The following apply to patients, residents, and family members.
  - Do not date, flirt with, kiss, or have a sexual relationship with them.
  - Do not discuss your sexual relationships with them.
  - Do not say or write things that could suggest a romantic or sexual relationship with them.
  - Do not accept gifts, loans, money, credit cards, or other valuables from them.
  - Do not give gifts, loans, money, credit cards, or other valuables to them.
  - Do not borrow from them. This includes money, personal items, and transportation.
  - Maintain a professional relationship at all times. Do not develop a personal relationship or friendship with them.
  - Do not share personal or financial information with them.
  - Do not help with their finances.
  - Do not take a person home with you. This includes for holidays or other events.
- Ask yourself these questions before you date or marry a person whom you cared for. Be aware of the risk for professional sexual misconduct.
  - How long ago were you involved with the person's care?
  - Was the person's care short-term or long-term?
  - What kind and how much information do you have about the person? How will that information affect your relationship with the person?
  - Will the person need more care in the future?
  - Does dating or marrying the person place the person at risk for harm?

BOX 5-3	Boundary Signs

- You think about the person when not at work.
- You organize your work and provide other care around the person's needs.
- You spend time with the person. You visit with the person during breaks, meal times, when off duty, and so on.
- You trade assignments so you provide the person's care.
- You give more care or attention to the person at the expense of others.
- You believe that you are the only person who understands the person and his or her needs.
- The person gives you gifts or money.
- You give the person gifts or money.
- You share information about yourself with the person.
- You talk about your work situation with the person.
- You flirt with the person.
- You make comments with a sexual message.
- You tell the person "off-color" jokes.
- You notice more touch between you and the person.
- You use foul, vulgar, or offensive language when talking to the person.
- You and the person have secrets.
- You choose the person's side when he or she disagrees with other staff or the family.
- You select what you report and record. You do not give complete information.
- You do not like questions about your care or your relationship with the person.
- You change how you dress or your appearance when you will work with the person.
- You receive gifts from the person after he or she leaves the agency.
- You have contact with the person after he or she leaves the agency.

FOCUS ON COMMUNICATION

Professional Boundaries

Some patients, residents, and families want to thank the staff. Some send thank-you cards and letters. Some offer gifts—candy, cookies, money, gift certificates, flowers, and so on. Accepting gifts is a boundary violation. When offered a gift, you can say:
- "Thank you so much for thinking of me. It's very kind of you. However, it is against center policy to accept gifts of any kind. I do appreciate your offer."
- "Thank you for wanting me to have the flowers from your friend. They are lovely. However, it is against hospital policy to receive gifts. Let me help you find a way to take them home."

Criminal laws *are concerned with offenses against the public and society in general. An act that violates a criminal law is called a* **crime**. A person found guilty of a crime is fined or sent to prison. Murder, robbery, stealing, rape, kidnapping, and abuse (p. 44) are crimes.

Civil laws *are concerned with relationships between people.* Examples of civil laws are those that involve contracts and nursing practice. A person found guilty of breaking a civil law usually has to pay a sum of money to the injured person.

Torts

Tort comes from the French word meaning *wrong*. Torts are part of civil law. A **tort** *is a wrong committed against a person or the person's property.* Some torts are *unintentional*. Harm was not intended. Some torts are *intentional*. The act was done on purpose and harm was intended.

Negligence and Malpractice. *Negligence is an unintentional wrong. The negligent person did not act in a reasonable and careful manner. As a result, a person or the person's property was harmed.* The person causing the harm did not intend or mean to cause harm. The person failed to do what a reasonable and careful person *would have done*. Or he or she did what a reasonable and careful person *would not have done*. The negligent person may have to pay damages (a sum of money) to the one injured.

Malpractice is negligence by a professional person. A person has professional status because of his or her education and the service provided. Nurses, doctors, dentists, and pharmacists are examples.

What you do or do not do can lead to a lawsuit if you harm a person or the property of another. **Standard of care** *refers to the skills, care, and judgments required by a health team member under similar conditions.* Standards of care come from:
- Laws, including nurse practice acts and those relating to nursing assistants.
- Textbooks.
- Agency policy books and procedure manuals (Fig. 5-2, p. 42). *Policy books* are guides for staff conduct. *Procedure manuals* explain how to perform certain procedures.
- Manufacturer's instructions for equipment and supplies.
- Job descriptions.
- Approval and accrediting agency standards.
- Standards and guidelines from government agencies.

The following actions could lead to charges of negligence.
- You fail to test the water temperature for a shower. The water is too hot. The person is burned.
- Mrs. Parks needs help to the bathroom. You do not answer her call light promptly. She gets up without help. She falls and breaks an arm.
- You do not follow the manufacturer's instructions for using a mechanical lift. Mr. Brown slips out of the lift and falls to the floor. He fractures a hip.
- Mrs. Clark complains of chest pain. You do not tell the nurse. Mrs. Clark has a heart attack and dies.
- Two residents have the same last name. You do not identify the person before a procedure. You perform the procedure on the wrong person. Both residents are harmed. One had a procedure that was not ordered. The other did not have a needed procedure.

You are legally responsible *(liable)* for your own actions. The nurse is liable as your supervisor. However, you have personal liability. Remember, sometimes refusing to follow the nurse's directions is your right and duty (Chapter 4).

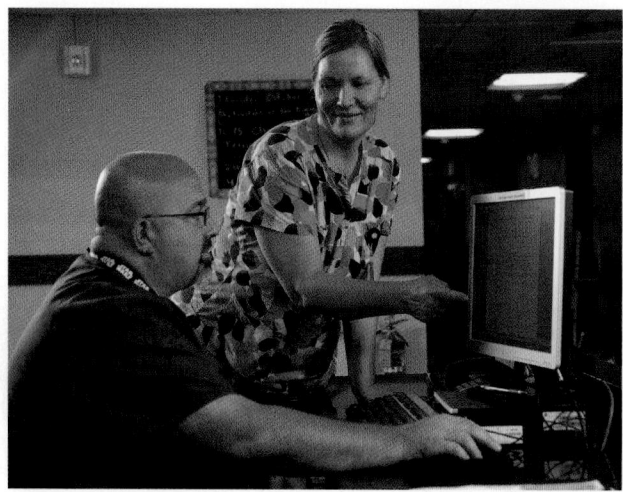

FIGURE 5-2 A nurse and a nursing assistant review an electronic policy manual.

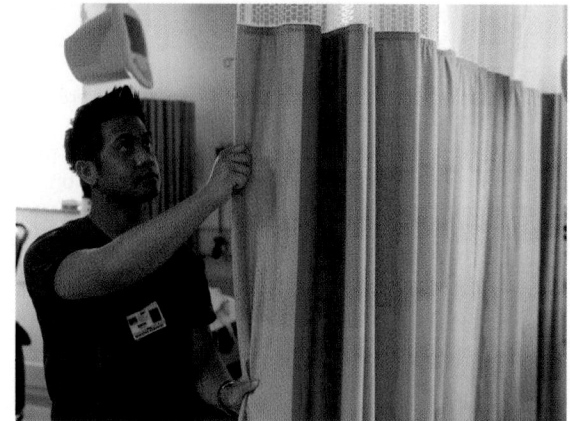

FIGURE 5-3 Pulling the privacy curtain around the bed helps protect the person's privacy.

Defamation. *Defamation is injuring a person's name and reputation by making false statements to a third person.*

- *Libel is making false statements in print, in writing (including e-mail and text messages), through pictures or drawings, through broadcast (radio, TV, or video), posted on-line on websites, or through video sites and social media sites.* See "Wrongful Use of Electronic Communications."
- *Slander is making false statements through the spoken word, sounds, sign language, or gestures.*

Examples of defamation include:
- Implying or suggesting that a person uses drugs
- Saying that a person is insane or mentally ill
- Posting on-line that a co-worker was fired for hitting a resident
- Implying or suggesting that a person steals money from the staff

To protect yourself from defamation, never make false statements about a patient, resident, family member, visitor, co-worker, or any other person. This includes:
- *Through e-mails or text messages*
- *On websites, video sites, or social media sites*
- *In newspapers, magazines, or other print sources*
- *Through broadcasts (TV, radio, or film)*
- *With words, sounds, signs, gestures, or any form of communication*

False Imprisonment. *False imprisonment is the unlawful restraint or restriction of a person's freedom of movement.* It involves:
- Threatening to restrain a person
- Restraining a person
- Preventing a person from leaving the agency

BOX 5-4	Protecting the Right to Privacy

- Keep all information about the person confidential.
- Cover the person when he or she is being moved in hallways and elevators.
- Ask visitors to leave the room when care is given.
- Screen the person. Close the privacy curtain as in Figure 5-3. Close the room door when giving care. Also close window coverings.
- Close the bathroom door when the person uses the bathroom for elimination or personal hygiene.
- Expose only the body part involved in a task.
- Do not discuss the person or the person's treatment with anyone except the nurse supervising your work. "Shop talk" is a common cause of invasion of privacy.
- Do not open the person's mail.
- Allow the person to visit with others in private.
- Allow the person to use the phone in private.
- Follow agency policies and procedures required to protect privacy.

Invasion of Privacy. *Invasion of privacy is violating a person's right not to have his or her name, photo, or private affairs exposed or made public without giving consent.* You must treat the person with respect and ensure privacy. Only staff involved in the person's care should see, handle, or examine his or her body. See Box 5-4 for measures to protect privacy.

Health Insurance Portability and Accountability Act of 1996. The *Health Insurance Portability and Accountability Act of 1996 (HIPAA)* protects the privacy and security of a person's health information. *Protected health information refers to identifying information and information about the person's health care that is maintained or sent in any form (paper, electronic, oral).* Failure to follow HIPAA rules can result in fines, penalties, and criminal actions including jail time.

To avoid HIPAA violations:

- Always follow agency policies and procedures.
- *Never take photos or videos of patients or residents or any person in the health care or home care setting.* Sharing photos or videos or posting them on video sites or social media sites is a very serious violation of HIPAA.
- *Never send an e-mail or text message or post anything on a website, video site, or social media site about a patient, resident, family member, or visitor.* Sharing information is a very serious violation of HIPAA.
- *Never write anything for a newspaper, magazine, or print source about a patient, resident, family member, or visitor.*
- *Never broadcast (through TV, radio, or video) anything about a patient, resident, family member, or visitor.*
- *Only discuss the person's health information with staff directly involved in the person's care.*
- See "Wrongful Use of Electronic Communications."

You may be asked questions about the person or the person's care. Direct any questions about the person or the person's care to the nurse. Also follow the rules for using computers and other electronic devices (Chapter 7).

Fraud. *Fraud is saying or doing something to trick, fool, or deceive a person.* The act is fraud if it does or could harm a person or the person's property. Telling a person or family that you are a nurse is fraud. So is giving wrong or incomplete information on a job application.

Assault and Battery. Assault and battery may result in both civil and criminal charges.

- *Assault is intentionally attempting or threatening to touch a person's body without the person's consent.* The person fears bodily harm. Threatening to "tie down" a person is an example of assault.
- *Battery is touching a person's body without his or her consent.* The person must consent to any procedure, treatment, or other act that involves touching the body. The person has the right to withdraw consent at any time.

Protect yourself from being accused of assault and battery. Explain to the person what you are going to do and get the person's consent. Consent may be verbal—"yes" or "okay." Or it can be a gesture—a nod, turning over for a back rub, or holding out an arm for you to take a pulse.

Wrongful Use of Electronic Communications

Electronic communications include e-mail, text messages, faxes, websites, video sites, and social media sites. Video and social media sites include Facebook, Twitter, LinkedIn, YouTube, Instagram, blogs and comments to blog postings, chat rooms, bulletin boards, and so on. Other forms of electronic communications are expected in the future.

Correct use of electronic communications is essential in your personal life and as a member of the health and

BOX 5-5	Electronic Communications

- Follow agency policies for using electronic communications.
- Remember that:
  - Anything you send or post electronically can be sent or shared with other than the intended person.
  - Deleted content can still be accessed. Electronic communications last forever. They can be retrieved for legal purposes in a court of law.
  - Private information shared with the intended person still violates the rights to privacy and confidentiality.
  - Referring to a person by nickname, room number, diagnosis, or other means but not by name is still violating the rights to privacy and confidentiality.
- Protect the person's privacy and maintain confidentiality at all times.
- Never take photos or videos of the person or any part of the person's body.
- Never transmit in any way information about the person or images (photos, videos, art) of the person.
- Never identify patients or residents by name.
- Never provide information that can lead to the person being identified.
- Maintain professional boundaries. Avoid on-line contact with patients and residents, former patients and residents, and family members.
- Do not use electronic communications to share or discuss workplace issues or co-workers.
- Tell the nurse at once if you may have violated the person's right to privacy or confidentiality. If you suspect that a co-worker has done so, also tell the nurse.
- See "Gossip" in Chapter 6.
- See "Unethical Student Behavior" in Chapter 6.
- See "Computers and Other Electronic Devices" in Chapter 7.

Modified from National Council of State Boards of Nursing: A nurse's guide to the use of social media, Chicago, 2011, Author.

nursing teams. Follow the rules in Box 5-5. Do so whether using a computer, wireless phone, camera, or other electronic device at home, at school, at work, or in any other setting. Wrongful use of electronic communications can result in job loss and loss of your certification (license, registration) for:

- Defamation
- Invasion of privacy
- HIPAA violations
- Violating the right to confidentiality (Chapter 6)
- Patient or resident abuse (p. 44)
- Unprofessional or unethical conduct

Federal laws such as HIPAA protect the person's privacy and confidentiality. So do some state laws. Wrongful use of electronic communications may be violations of federal and state laws. Besides losing your certification (license, registration), wrongful use can result in:

- Civil action resulting in a fine
- Criminal action resulting in a fine or jail time

See *Focus on Communication: Wrongful Use of Electronic Communications*, p. 44.

FOCUS ON COMMUNICATION

Wrongful Use of Electronic Communications

The following are examples of the wrongful use of electronic communications.

- Laura is a nursing assistant student. On the last day of clinical, she asks 2 residents if she can take a picture with them. Laura posts the picture on Facebook with this comment: "Done with clinical! I'll miss my residents."
- Justin works in a hospital oncology (cancer) unit. A patient, Mrs. Warner, has a blog to keep family and friends updated. Mrs. Warner posts that she had a tiring day of treatments. Justin posts: "Chemo can wear you down. Maybe the new medicine will help you rest. Hope you feel better tomorrow. See you then."
- Sara works in home care. She sends a text message to a friend that says: "I'll be done at Mr. Gentry's on Third Street at noon. Want to get lunch?"

Often wrongful use of electronic communications is not intentional. You must be very careful. Your communication must protect the person's privacy and confidentiality at all times.

FOCUS ON COMMUNICATION

Informed Consent

There are different ways to give consent.

- *Written consent.* The person signs a form agreeing to a treatment or procedure. You are not responsible for obtaining written consent.
- *Verbal consent.* The person says aloud that he or she consents. "Yes" and "okay" are examples.
- *Implied consent.* For example, you ask Mr. Jones if you can check his blood pressure. He extends his arm. His movement implies consent.

Before any procedure or task, explain the steps to the person. This is how you obtain verbal or implied consent. Also explain each step. This allows the person the chance to refuse at any time.

Informed Consent

A person has the right to decide what will be done to his or her body and who can touch his or her body. The doctor is responsible for informing the person about all aspects of treatment. Consent is informed when the person clearly understands:

- The reason for a treatment, procedure, or care measure
- What will be done
- How it will be done
- Who will do it
- The expected outcomes
- Other treatment, procedure, or care options
- The effects of not having the treatment, procedure, or care measure

Persons under legal age (usually 18 years) cannot give consent. Nor can persons who are mentally incompetent. Such persons are unconscious, sedated, or confused. Or they have certain mental health disorders. Informed consent is given by a responsible party—a wife, husband, parent, daughter, son, guardian, or legal representative.

Consent is needed when the person enters the agency. A form is signed giving general consent to treatment. Special consent forms are required before admission to a secured dementia care unit (Chapter 49). Some procedures performed by the doctor require special consents. The doctor informs the person about all aspects of the procedure. The nurse may have this responsibility.

You are never responsible for obtaining written consent. In some agencies, you can witness the signing of a consent. When a witness, you are present when the person signs the consent.

See *Focus on Communication: Informed Consent.*

REPORTING ABUSE

Some persons are mistreated or harmed on purpose. This is abuse. *Abuse is:*

- *The willful infliction of injury, unreasonable confinement, intimidation, or punishment that results in physical harm, pain, or mental anguish. Intimidation means to make afraid with threats of force or violence.*
- *Depriving the person (or the person's caregiver) of the goods or services needed to attain or maintain well-being.*

Abuse includes involuntary seclusion (Chapter 2). Abuse is a crime. It can occur at home or in a health care agency. All persons must be protected from abuse. This includes persons in a coma.

The abuser is usually a family member or caregiver—spouse, partner, adult child, and others. The abuser can be a friend, neighbor, landlord, or other person. Both men and women are abusers. Both men and women are abused.

State laws, accrediting agencies, and the *Omnibus Budget Reconciliation Act of 1987* (OBRA) do not allow agencies to employ persons who were convicted of abuse, neglect, or mistreatment. Before hiring, the agency must thoroughly check the applicant's work history. All references are checked. Efforts must be made to find out about any criminal records.

The agency also checks the nursing assistant registry for findings of abuse, neglect, or mistreatment. It also is checked for mis-using or stealing a person's property.

See *Focus on Communication: Reporting Abuse.*
See *Focus on Surveys: Reporting Abuse.*

Vulnerable Adults

Vulnerable comes from the Latin word *vulnerare*, which means *to wound*. *Vulnerable adults are persons 18 years old or older who have disabilities or conditions that make them at risk to be wounded, attacked, or damaged.* They have problems caring for or protecting themselves due to:
- A mental, emotional, physical, intellectual, or developmental disability. See Chapter 50.
- Brain damage.
- Changes from aging.

All patients and residents, regardless of age or care setting, are vulnerable. Older persons and children are at risk for abuse.

See *Focus on Long-Term Care and Home Care: Vulnerable Adults*.

Elder Abuse

An *elder* is an *older adult*. **Elder abuse** *is any knowing, intentional, or negligent act by a caregiver or any other person to an older adult. The act causes harm or serious risk of harm.* Elder abuse can take these forms. Often more than 1 form of abuse is present.

- *Physical abuse.* This involves inflicting, or threatening to inflict, physical pain or injury. See Box 5-6 for examples of physical abuse.
- *Neglect.* **Neglect** *is the failure of responsible persons to provide food, shelter, health care, or protection for a vulnerable elder.* This includes failure to provide health care or treatment, food, water, clothing, hygiene, shelter, comfort, safety, or other needs. In health care, neglect includes but is not limited to:
  - Leaving the person lying or sitting in urine or feces
  - Keeping persons alone in their rooms or other areas
  - Failing to answer call lights
- *Verbal abuse.* Verbal abuse is using oral or written words or statements that speak badly of, sneer at, criticize, or condemn the person. It includes unkind gestures, threats of harm, or saying things to frighten the person. For example, a person is told that he or she will never see family members again.
- *Involuntary seclusion.* This involves confining the person to a certain area. People have been locked in closets, basements, attics, bathrooms, and other spaces.
- *Financial exploitation or misappropriation.* To *exploit* means *to use unjustly*. *Misappropriate* means *to dishonestly, unfairly, or wrongly take for one's own use.* The older person's resources (money, property, assets) are mis-used by another person. Or the resources are used for the other person's profit or benefit. The person's money is stolen or used by another person. It is also mis-using a person's property. For example, children sell their mother's house without her consent. Other examples of exploitation or misappropriation include:
  - The person reports that someone is taking his or her money, property, or assets.
  - Withdrawing money from a bank account without permission.
  - Adding a person's name to a bank signature card without permission.
  - Using a person's credit card or debit card without permission.
  - Changing a person's will, insurance policy, or financial documents.
  - Unpaid bills.
  - Forging a person's signature on checks or other documents.

BOX 5-6	Examples of Physical Abuse
• Beating	• Hair-pulling
• Burning	• Hitting
• Corporal punishment— punishment inflicted directly on the body (beatings, lashings, whippings, and so on)	• Kicking
	• Physical or chemical restraint (Chapter 15)
	• Pinching
	• Punching
• Depriving of a basic need—food, water, shelter, and so on (Chapter 9)	• Pushing
	• Shaking
	• Shoving
	• Slapping
• Force-feeding	• Striking with or without an object
• Grabbing	

- *Emotional or mental abuse.* This involves inflicting mental pain, anguish, or distress through verbal or nonverbal acts. Humiliation, harassment, ridicule, insults, and threats of punishment are examples. It includes being deprived of needs such as food, clothing, care, a home, or a place to sleep. Treating the person like an infant or child and the "silent treatment" (not speaking to the person) are other forms of emotional or mental abuse.
- *Sexual abuse.* This is non-consensual sexual contact of any kind. *Consensual* involves *giving consent*. *Non-consensual* means *not giving consent*. Unwanted touching, forced nudity, and taking photos or videos are forms of sexual abuse. So is harassing the person about sex or attacking the person sexually. The person may be forced to perform sexual acts out of fear of punishment or physical harm.
- *Abandonment.* *Abandon* means *to leave or desert someone.* The person is deserted by someone who is supposed to provide care. Abandonment involves the following 4 points.
  - You accept an assignment to care for a person or group of persons.
  - You accept the assignment for a certain time period.
  - You remove yourself from the care setting—home, hospital, nursing center, or other agency.
  - You do not report off to a staff member who will assume responsibility for care.
    Examples of abandonment include:
  - You leave the agency before your shift ends. You did not tell the nurse that you were leaving.
  - You do not report to a home care assignment. You are the only one providing care.
  - You leave without completing a home care assignment.
  - You sleep on the job. You do not provide care.

There are many signs of elder abuse. The abused person may show only some of the signs in Box 5-7. See Fig. 5-4.

BOX 5-7	Signs of Elder Abuse

- The person reports mistreatment—abuse (physical, verbal, financial, emotional or mental, sexual), neglect, seclusion, abandonment.
- Living conditions are not safe, clean, or adequate. See *Focus on Long-Term Care and Home Care: Vulnerable Adults,* p. 45.
- Personal hygiene is lacking (Chapter 22). The person is not clean. Clothes are dirty.
- Poor oral hygiene (Chapter 22).
- Weight loss—there are signs of poor nutrition and poor fluid intake.
- Assistive (adaptive) devices are missing or broken—eyeglasses, hearing aids, dentures, cane, walker, and so on.
- Medical needs are not met.
- Frequent injuries—conditions behind the injuries are strange or seem impossible.
- Old and new injuries—bruises, pressure marks, welts, scars, fractures, punctures, and so on.
- Complaints of pain or itching in the genital or anal area.
- Bleeding and bruising around the breasts or in the genital or anal area.
- Torn, stained, or bloody undergarments.
- Burns on the feet, hands, buttocks, or other parts of the body. Cigarettes and cigars cause small circle-like burns.

- Pressure ulcers (Chapter 37) or contractures (Chapter 30).
- The person seems very quiet or withdrawn.
- Unexplained withdrawal from normal activities.
- The person seems fearful, anxious, or agitated.
- Sudden changes in alertness.
- Depression.
- Sudden changes in finances.
- The person does not want to talk or answer questions.
- The person is restrained. Or the person is locked in a certain area for long periods.
- The person cannot reach toilet facilities, food, water, and other needed items.
- Private conversations are not allowed. The caregiver is present during all conversations.
- Strained or tense relationships with a caregiver.
- Frequent arguments with a caregiver.
- The person seems anxious to please the caregiver.
- Drugs are not taken properly. Drugs are not bought. Or too much or too little of the drug is taken.
- Emergency visits may be frequent.
- The person may change doctors often. Some people do not have a doctor.

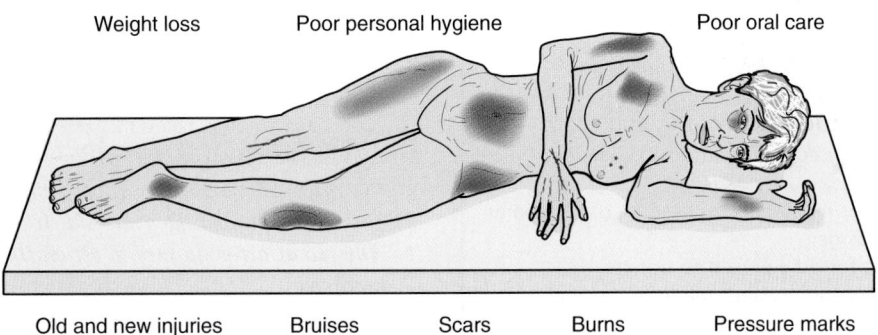

Weight loss   Poor personal hygiene   Poor oral care

Old and new injuries   Bruises   Scars   Burns   Pressure marks

FIGURE 5-4 Some signs of elder abuse.

Reporting Elder Abuse. Federal and state laws require the reporting of elder abuse. If abuse is suspected, it must be reported. Where and how to report abuse varies among states. You may suspect abuse. If so, discuss the matter and your observations with the nurse. Give as many details as possible. The nurse contacts health team members as needed.

The nurse also contacts community agencies that investigate elder abuse. They act at once if the problem is life-threatening. Sometimes the police or courts are involved.

Helping abused older persons is not always easy or possible. Some abuse is not reported or recognized. Or the investigating agency cannot gain access to the person. Sometimes older persons are abused by a spouse or adult child. A victim may want to protect the spouse or child. Some victims are embarrassed or believe abuse is deserved. A victim may fear what will happen. He or she may think

that the present situation is better than no care at all. Some people fear not being believed if they report the abuse themselves.

Examples of Elder Abuse. Box 5-8 on p. 48 lists examples of elder abuse. An investigation can lead to 1 or more of the following.

- Job loss
- Loss of certification (license, registration)
- Being convicted of a crime

See *Focus on Long-Term Care and Home Care: Examples of Elder Abuse,* p. 48.

BOX 5-8	Elder Abuse

Common Examples

- A person constantly crying out for help is taken to his room. He is left alone with the door closed.
- A person is told to be nice. Otherwise care will not be given.
- A person cannot control her bowels. She is called "dirty" and "disgusting."
- A person is turned in a rough and hurried manner.
- The nurse uses a person's phone to call a friend.
- A person lies in a wet and soiled bed all night.
- Money is taken from a person's wallet.
- A person uses the call light a lot. It is taken away from the person.
- A person's mouth is forced open. Food is forced into the person's mouth.
- A person is told that her daughter does not visit because she is so mean.

Prosecuted Cases

- A resident was complaining of pain while being cleaned. To stop him from complaining, a nursing assistant stuck a rag down his throat.
- A patient was screaming. To stop the patient from screaming, a nurse poured water down her throat.
- A nursing assistant beat and kicked a 92-year-old man who was lying on the floor.
- A nursing assistant stepped on a resident's face.
- A person was visiting his grandmother. While there, he sexually abused a patient with head injuries.
- A nursing assistant dragged a female patient in a wheelchair into a room. The nursing assistant forced the patient to have sex with him.
- A nursing assistant teased and taunted a resident with dementia.
- A health care worker repeatedly insulted an older woman because her son was gay.
- A nursing assistant forced a person to urinate in bed. Then the nursing assistant made fun of the person.
- Two older women lived in a board and care home. Both had Alzheimer's disease. They were left in a room with blood splattered on the walls. The carpet was caked with feces, vomitus, and urine. The women were partially dressed. One was tied to the bed with a sheet.
- A nursing assistant failed to feed a resident who could not feed herself. A video camera caught the nursing assistant dumping the person's food into trash cans.
- A resident could not talk. She totally depended on the staff for care. She did not have a bowel movement for 26 days. She was given a laxative every 3 days. No other treatment was given for her constipation.
- Caregivers willfully neglected to give drugs to residents.

Modified from Elder abuse and neglect: prosecution and prevention, *San Francisco, American Society on Aging.*

FOCUS ON LONG-TERM CARE AND HOME CARE

Examples of Elder Abuse

Long-Term Care

OBRA requires these actions if abuse is suspected within the center.

- The matter is reported at once to the administrator. It also is reported at once to other officials as required by federal and state laws.
- All claims of abuse are thoroughly investigated.
- The center must prevent further potential for abuse while the investigation is in progress.
- Investigation results are reported to the center administrator within 5 days of the incident. They also are reported to other officials as required by federal and state laws.
- Corrective actions are taken if the claim is found to be true.

Home Care

Abandonment is always serious. However, it is most serious in home care. Unlike hospitals and nursing centers, often you are the only caregiver in the home. If you leave before completing your assignment, there is no one else to give care. The person is left alone without needed care. Serious harm could result. You could have your certification (license, registration) revoked or suspended for abandonment in any setting.

Child Abuse and Neglect

Child abuse and neglect is the intentional harm or mistreatment of a child under 18 years old. It involves the following.

- *Any recent act or failure to act on the part of a parent or caregiver.*
- *The act or failure to act results in death, serious physical or emotional harm, sexual abuse, or exploitation.*
- *The act or failure to act presents a likely or immediate risk for harm.*

Child abuse and neglect occur at every social level. They occur in low-, middle-, and high-income families. The abuser's education level may be low or high. Often the abuser is a household member or caregiver—parent, parent's partner, brother or sister, foster parent, nanny, babysitter. Usually an abuser is someone the family knows. Risk factors for abusing children include:

- Stress
- Family crisis (divorce, unemployment, low income, moving, crowded living conditions, intimate partner violence, p. 51)
- Single-parenting
- Teenage parenting
- Several young children under 5 years of age
- Physical or mental illness, including depression
- Drug or alcohol abuse

- Abuser history of being abused or neglected as a child
- Discipline beliefs that include physical punishment
- Lack of emotional attachment to the child
- Poor parent-child relationships
- A child with birth defects, chronic illness, or a physical, intellectual, or developmental disability
- A child with a personality or behaviors that the abuser considers "different" or not acceptable
- Unrealistic expectations for the child's behavior or performance
- Lack of understanding about children's needs, child development, and parenting skills
- Families that move often and do not have family or friends nearby

Types of Child Abuse and Neglect. Child abuse and neglect have many forms. Often more than 1 type is present.

- *Physical abuse* is injuring the child on purpose. It can cause bruising, fractures, or death. Physical abuse includes striking, punching, beating, kicking, shaking, throwing, stabbing, choking, hitting, burning, or biting the child. Any action that injures the child is physical abuse.
- *Neglect* is failing to provide for a child's basic needs.
  - *Physical neglect* is failure to provide food, shelter, or supervision.
  - *Medical neglect* is failure to provide needed medical or mental health treatment. (Some religious beliefs do not allow medical care. This would not be considered medical neglect.)
  - *Educational neglect* is failure to educate a child or provide special education needs.
  - *Emotional neglect* is not meeting the child's needs for affection and attention. Letting a child use alcohol or other drugs is also emotional neglect.
- *Sexual abuse* is using, persuading, forcing, or exposing a child to engage in sexual contact, activity, or behavior. There may be oral, genital, vaginal, anal, buttock, or breast involvement.
  - *Rape or sexual assault*—forced sexual acts with a person against his or her will.
  - *Molestation*—sexual advances toward a child. It includes kissing, touching, or fondling sexual areas. The abuser may kiss, touch, or fondle the child. Or the child is forced to kiss, touch, or fondle the abuser.
  - *Incest*—sexual activity between family members. The abuser may be a parent, brother or sister, aunt or uncle, cousin, or grandparent.
  - *Child pornography*—taking photos or videos of a child involved in sexual acts or poses.
  - *Child prostitution*—forcing a child to engage in sexual acts for money. Usually the child is forced to have many sexual partners.

- *Emotional abuse* is injuring the child mentally or his or her sense of self-worth. The abuser constantly criticizes, threatens, or rejects the child. The abuser may with-hold love, support, or guidance. The child has changes in behavior, emotional responses, thinking, reasoning, learning, and so on. The child may show anxiety, depression, withdrawal, or aggressive behaviors. Emotional abuse is almost always present with other forms of abuse.
- *Substance abuse* is part of child abuse and neglect in some states. Pre-natal exposure (during pregnancy) is 1 form of substance abuse. Others involve alcohol abuse, drug abuse, and illegal drug activity. A *controlled substance* is a drug or chemical substance whose possession and use are controlled by law. Substance abuse involves:
  - Making a controlled substance in the presence of a child.
  - Making a controlled substance on the premises occupied by a child.
  - Allowing a child to be present where there are chemicals or equipment used to make or store a controlled substance.
  - Selling, distributing, or giving drugs or alcohol to a child.
  - Using a controlled substance (a caregiver) that impairs the caregiver's ability to adequately care for the child.
  - Exposing the child to equipment and supplies for using, selling, or distributing drugs.
  - Exposing the child to other drug-related activities.
- *Abandonment* is when the parent's identity or whereabouts are unknown. The child is left in circumstances where the child suffers serious harm. Or the parent fails to maintain contact with the child or provide support for the child.

Reporting Child Abuse and Neglect. Box 5-9 on p. 50 lists the signs of child abuse and neglect. Report any changes in the child's body or behavior. Child and parent behaviors may signal that something is wrong.

Child abuse is complex. Many more behaviors, signs, and symptoms are present than discussed here. You must be alert for signs and symptoms of child abuse. All states require the reporting of suspected child abuse. However, someone should not be falsely accused.

If you suspect child abuse, share your concerns with the nurse. Give as much detail as you can. The nurse contacts health team members and child protection agencies as needed.

BOX 5-9	Child Abuse and Neglect—Signs and Symptoms

General Behaviors
- **The Child**
  - Reports bad treatment or abuse by a parent or caregiver.
  - Has sudden changes in behavior.
  - Has sudden changes in school performance or grades.
  - Has learning problems or problems concentrating.
  - Has health problems that go unattended.
  - Seems watchful; seems to be waiting for something bad to happen.
  - Lacks adult supervision.
  - Is overly agreeable or obedient.
  - Is quiet, withdrawn, or uninvolved.
  - Arrives early at school or stays late.
  - Does not want to go home from school, activities, or a friend or family member's house.
  - Fears a parent or a certain person; does not want to be around a certain person.
- **The Parent**
  - Denies that the child has problems at school or home.
  - Blames the child for problems at school or home.
  - Gives different stories about what happened. Or the parent does not offer an explanation of what happened.
  - Blames injuries on play or other children.
  - Takes the child for frequent emergency room visits.
  - Uses harsh discipline. Asks the teachers or caregivers to give harsh discipline.
  - Describes the child as bad, evil, worthless, or a burden.
  - Demands physical or academic performance above what the child can achieve.
  - Shows little concern for the child.
  - Relies on the child for care, attention, or emotional satisfaction.
  - Has a history of child abuse.
  - Has a history of abusing pets or animals.
  - Abuses alcohol or drugs.
  - Has behaviors that are bizarre or not logical.
  - Limits the child's contact with other children.
  - Is secretive.
  - Is jealous or controls other family members.
- **Parent and Child**
  - Rarely touch or look at each other.
  - View their relationship as poor or bad.
  - State that they do not like each other.

Physical Abuse
- Bruises on the face (eyes, lips, mouth, cheeks), back, buttocks, abdomen, chest, or inner thighs.
- Welts on the face (lips, mouth, cheeks), back, buttocks, abdomen, chest, or inner thighs.
  - The shape of the object causing the welt may be seen. The shape may be of a belt, belt buckle, chain, clothes hanger, rope, or other object.
- Burns and scalds on the feet, hands, back, buttocks, or other body parts.
  - Intentional burns leave a pattern from the item causing the burn. Cigarettes, irons, curling irons, ropes, stove burners, and radiators are examples.
  - In scalds, the area put in hot liquid is clearly marked. For example, a scald to the hand looks like a glove. A scald to the foot looks like a sock.

Physical Abuse—cont'd
- Fractures of the nose, skull, arms, or legs.
- Bite marks.
- Abuses animals or pets.

Neglect
- Fails to gain weight.
- Shows great affection to others.
- Wants to eat large amounts of food.
- Begs or steals food or money.
- Is dirty or has a severe body odor.
- Lacks the correct clothing for the weather.
- Abuses alcohol or drugs.
- States that no one is at home to provide care.
- Is often absent from school.
- Lacks medical or dental care. Does not have needed eyeglasses.

Sexual Abuse
- Bleeding, cuts, or bruises of the genitalia, anus, breasts, or mouth.
- Trouble walking or sitting.
- Stains or blood on underclothing.
- Bedwetting.
- Sudden change in appetite.
- Painful urination.
- Signs and symptoms of urinary tract infection (Chapter 47).
- Vaginal discharge.
- Genital odor.
- Genital pain.
- Pregnancy.
- Fearful behaviors—nightmares, depression, unusual fears, attempts to run away.
- Sexual knowledge or behavior that does not fit with one's age.

Emotional Abuse
- Sudden changes in self-confidence or self-esteem.
- Headaches.
- Stomach aches.
- Abnormal fears.
- Nightmares.
- Attempts to run away.
- Extremes in behavior—overly agreeable or demanding; quiet and withdrawn or aggressive.
- Depression.
- Avoids certain situations—going to school, riding the school bus.
- Seeks affection from others.
- Has attempted suicide.
- Rocks oneself or bangs head.

Modified from Child Welfare Information Gateway: What is child abuse and neglect: recognizing the symptoms, Washington, DC, July 2013, Children's Bureau.

Intimate Partner Violence

The Centers for Disease Control and Prevention (CDC) defines *intimate partner violence (IPV)* as *physical, sexual, or psychological harm by a current or former partner or spouse.* Also called domestic abuse, domestic violence, intimate partner abuse, partner abuse, and spousal abuse—IPV occurs in relationships. IPV includes teen dating violence and dating violence. In IPV, 1 partner has power and control over the other through abuse. The abuse may range from 1 hit to chronic, severe battering. Rarely is IPV a 1-time event.

IPV causes fear and harm. Usually more than 1 type of IPV is present. The CDC describes the following.

* *Physical violence*—unwanted punching, slapping, scratching, grabbing, pushing, shoving, throwing, choking, poking, biting, shaking, pulling hair, twisting arms, or kicking. It may involve burns, weapons, or restraints. Physical injuries occur. Death is a constant threat.
* *Sexual violence*—unwanted sexual contact. The CDC describes 3 types of sexual violence.
  * Use of physical force to make a person engage in a sexual act against his or her will. The act does not have to be completed.
  * A sex act involving a person unable to understand the nature of the act, unable to decline taking part in the act, or unable to communicate that he or she is unwilling to engage in the act. The person may not be able to understand because of illness, disability, alcohol, drugs, or pressure to perform. The act does not have to be completed.
  * Abusive sexual contact.

* *Threats of physical or sexual violence*—words, gestures, or weapons are used to communicate threats of death, disability, injury, or harm.
* *Psychological and emotional violence*—acts, threats of acts, or forceful actions cause trauma to the victim. They include:
  * Humiliating the victim.
  * Controlling what the victim can and cannot do.
  * Keeping information from the victim.
  * Doing something on purpose to embarrass the victim or make him or her feel less than whole.
  * Keeping the victim away from family and friends.
  * Denying the victim money or access to other basic needs. This includes having or not having a job, paychecks, money gifts from family and friends, money for household expenses, and car use.
  * Prior physical or sexual violence. Or prior threat of physical or sexual violence.
  * Stalking—harassing or threatening behavior such as following the person, appearing at the person's home or business, phone calls, leaving messages or objects, or damaging property.

Both males and females can be victims. However, most victims are women. There is no set age, race, culture, religion, educational level, income level, or marital status for IPV. Patients and residents can suffer from IPV. For example, a husband slaps his wife during a visit. Or a wife uses her husband's money for herself rather than buying her husband's needed medicine. You, yourself, may be a victim of IPV. Box 5-10 lists the risk factors and warning signs of IPV.

BOX 5-10 Intimate Partner Violence—Risk Factors and Warning Signs

Risk Factors—The Victim or Abuser
* Low self-esteem
* Low income
* Low educational level
* Young age
* Problem behavior as a youth
* Heavy alcohol or drug use
* Depression
* Anger and hostility
* Antisocial or borderline personality traits (Chapter 48)
* History of physical abuse
* Few friends; being kept away from friends
* Unemployment
* Emotional dependence and insecurity
* Belief in strict gender roles—men are dominant and aggressive in relationships; men make family decisions; women stay at home and do not work; women are submissive (obey, follow orders) to men
* Desire for power and control in relationships

Risk Factors—The Victim or Abuser—cont'd
* Emotional aggression—unkind and hurtful remarks
* Being a victim of abuse
* Having poor parenting as a child
* Having been physically disciplined as a child
* Marital conflicts—fights, tension, other struggles
* Divorce or marital separation
* Control by 1 partner over another
* Financial stress or hardship
* Unhealthy family relationships or interactions

Warning Signs
* Unwanted physical or sexual contact
* Threats to you, your children, family members, or pets
* Threats of suicide to get you to do something
* Using or threatening to use a weapon against you
* Keeping or taking your paycheck
* Saying things to put you down or make you feel bad
* Keeping you from seeing family or friends
* Keeping you from going to work

Modified from Centers for Disease Control and Prevention: Intimate partner violence: risk and protective factors, *Atlanta, December 24, 2013, updated February 11, 2015 and* What is abuse: a warning list, *www.domestic violence.org/what-is-abuse/*

Intimate partner violence is a safety issue. Like child abuse and neglect and elder abuse, IPV is complex. The victim often hides the abuse. He or she may protect the abuser. State laws vary about reporting IPV. However, the health team has an ethical duty to give information about safety and community resources. If you suspect IPV, share your concerns with the nurse. The nurse gathers information to help the person.

See *Promoting Safety and Comfort: Intimate Partner Violence.*

See *Focus on Children and Older Persons: Intimate Partner Violence.*

See *Focus on Long-Term Care and Home Care: Intimate Partner Violence.*

WILLS

A *will is a legal document of how a person wants property distributed after death.* You can ethically and legally witness a will signing. Or you can refuse to do so without fear of a legal action.

A person may ask you to prepare a will. You must politely refuse. Explain that you do not have the legal knowledge or ability to prepare a will. Report the request to the nurse. The nurse will speak to the person or family member about contacting a lawyer.

Do not witness a will signing if you are named in the will. To do so prevents you from getting what was left to you. As a witness, be prepared to testify that:
- The person was of sound mind when the will was signed.
- The person stated that the document was his or her last will.

Many agencies do not let staff witness wills. Know your agency's policy before you agree to witness a will. If you have questions, ask the nurse. If you witness a will, tell the nurse.

PROMOTING SAFETY AND COMFORT

Intimate Partner Violence

Safety
Intimate partner violence occurs in relationships. Relationship partners may be:
- Married
- Not married but living together
- Dating
- Divorced or separated
- Female and male; male and male; female and female

If you are a victim of abuse, call 911 or the police. Tell the police everything that happened—the abuser, what happened, marks on your body, and so on. Answer their questions honestly and completely. The police can help you and your children to a safe place. They can give you information about IPV, IPV programs and shelters, and how to develop a personal safety plan.

FOCUS ON CHILDREN AND OLDER PERSONS

Intimate Partner Violence

Children
Teenagers can be victims of dating violence (Chapter 11). The CDC defines *teen dating violence as physical, sexual, or psychological or emotional violence within a dating relationship. It includes stalking.* Teen dating violence can occur:
- In person or electronically
- With a current or former dating partner

Victims of teen dating violence are at risk for poor school performance, binge drinking, suicide attempts, and fighting. They are at risk for carrying violence into future relationships.

FOCUS ON LONG-TERM CARE AND HOME CARE

Intimate Partner Violence

Long-Term Care
Under OBRA, the resident has the right to be free from abuse, mistreatment, and neglect. If a resident is abused by anyone, the abuse must be reported. This includes abuse by a partner.

FOCUS ON **PRIDE**

The Person, Family, and Yourself

Personal and Professional Responsibility
States have laws about who must report abuse and neglect. Such persons are called *mandatory reporters. Mandatory* means *required.* For example, most states require that health care providers report suspected abuse or neglect of children, vulnerable adults, and elders. Tell the nurse if you suspect abuse or neglect.

Some states require that all persons report suspected mistreatment. Other states allow voluntary reporting. You or someone you know may be in danger. Or you suspect abuse or neglect. You can use these resources for help.
- For dangerous or life-threatening situations—call 911.
- For child abuse or neglect—contact your local child protective services office or the police. Call the Childhelp National Child Abuse Hotline at 1-800-4-A-CHILD.
- For intimate partner violence—the National Domestic Violence Hotline has resources and information. You can call 1-800-799-SAFE or visit www.thehotline.org.
- For elder abuse, neglect, or exploitation—visit the National Center on Elder Abuse's website.

FOCUS ON **P R I D E—cont'd**

The Person, Family, and Yourself

R ights and Respect

Respectful treatment involves treating the person with kindness, patience, and dignity. Needed care is provided in a safe manner. Mistreatment and harm are avoided.

All persons must be protected from abuse, mistreatment, and neglect. Health care agencies have procedures for investigating suspected abuse and neglect. Be alert for signs and symptoms. If you suspect abuse or neglect, tell the nurse. Take pride in protecting persons from harm.

I ndependence and Social Interaction

You will interact closely with patients, residents, and families. You may begin to know them well. Social and professional relationships differ. To maintain professional boundaries:
- Follow the "Code of Conduct for Nursing Assistants" in Box 5-1.
- See "Maintaining Professional Boundaries" in Box 5-2.
- Monitor for "Boundary Signs." See Box 5-3.
- Ask the nurse if you have a question about an interaction.

Use good judgment when interacting with patients, residents, and families. Take pride in being professional.

D elegation and Teamwork

Working within the limits of your role protects persons from harm. You must understand your roles and responsibilities to know when a task is outside these limits. For example, the nurse asks you to obtain written consent for a procedure. You accept the task. As a result, the person is not given needed information about the procedure. The person suffers harm.

Sometimes refusing a delegated task is your right and duty. Accepting a task beyond the legal limits of your role can lead to negligence.

E thics and Laws

The following is a real account of an intentional tort committed by a nursing assistant.

A licensed nursing assistant (LNA) worked at a nursing center. Her license was suspended for using a resident's credit card. The card was used without the resident's knowledge or consent. The LNA signed the resident's name to charges totaling about $1490. The LNA also took and used a nurse's credit card. Criminal charges of false impersonation were filed against the LNA.

The LNA was charged with:
- *Failing to comply with federal or state laws and rules*
- *Abusing or neglecting a patient*
- *Misappropriating patient property (p. 46)*
- *Being unfit or incompetent to function as a nursing assistant by reason of any cause.*
- *Engaging in conduct of a character likely to deceive, defraud, or harm the public.*

The LNA's license was suspended indefinitely. This means that the LNA:
- *Had to give her license to the Board.*
- *Could ask the Board to re-instate her license, but she had to prove that:*
  - *She posed no danger to the public or the practice of nursing.*
  - *She would safely and competently perform an LNA's duties.*
  - *She meets the requirements for license renewal and re-instatement.*

(State of Vermont Board of Nursing, 2000.)

FOCUS ON **PRIDE**: *Application*

Ethics and laws deal with right and wrong conduct. A code of conduct guides your thinking and behavior. Write a personal code of conduct stating what you expect of yourself as a nursing assistant.

REVIEW QUESTIONS

Circle the BEST answer.

1 Ethics is
   a Making judgments before you have the facts
   b Knowledge of right and wrong conduct
   c A behavior that meets your needs, not the person's
   d A health team member's skill, care, and judgment

2 Which is ethical behavior?
   a Sharing information about a person with a friend
   b Accepting gifts from a resident's family
   c Reporting errors
   d Calling your family before answering a call light

3 On your days off, you call the agency to check on a patient. This is a
   a Professional boundary
   b Tort
   c Boundary violation
   d Boundary sign

4 To maintain professional boundaries, your behaviors must
   a Help the person
   b Meet your needs
   c Be biased
   d Show that you care

5 You help with a friend's hospital care. This is a
   a Professional boundary
   b Boundary crossing
   c Tort
   d Crime

6 Which is a crime?
   a Abuse
   b Slander
   c Negligence
   d Fraud

Continued

REVIEW QUESTIONS—cont'd

7 These statements are about negligence. Which is *true?*
a It is an intentional tort.
b The negligent person acted in a reasonable manner.
c The person or the person's property was harmed.
d A prison term is likely.

8 Threatening to touch the person's body without the person's consent is
a Assault
b Battery
c Defamation
d False imprisonment

9 Restraining a person's freedom of movement is
a Neglect
b Invasion of privacy
c Defamation
d False imprisonment

10 A person's photos are shown to others without consent. This is
a Battery
b Fraud
c Invasion of privacy
d Malpractice

11 Sharing a resident's photo on a social media site is
a Fraud
b Allowed with the family's consent
c A violation of HIPAA
d Allowed if you obtain informed consent

12 You tell others that you are nurse. This is
a Negligence
b Fraud
c Libel
d Slander

13 Informed consent is when the person
a Fully understands all aspects of his or her treatment
b Signs a consent form
c Is admitted to the agency
d Decides what to do with property after his or her death

14 Who is *most* at risk for being wounded, attacked, or damaged?
a A teenager
b A single mother
c A caregiver
d An older person

15 Self-neglect is when
a A caregiver harms a person
b The person's behaviors put him or her at risk for harm
c A person is deprived of food, clothing, hygiene, and shelter
d The person does not receive attention or affection

16 You scold an older person for not eating lunch. This is
a Physical abuse
b Neglect
c Battery
d Verbal abuse

17 You leave a home care patient before completing your assignment. This is abuse by
a Abandonment
b Neglect
c Involuntary seclusion
d Control

18 You fall asleep at work. This is
a Abandonment
b Neglect
c A boundary violation
d Malpractice

19 Which is a sign of elder abuse?
a Stiff joints and joint pain
b Weight gain
c Poor personal hygiene
d Forgetfulness

20 Depriving a child of food, clothing, and shelter is
a Physical abuse
b Neglect
c Abandonment
d Emotional abuse

21 An older adult has a black eye, bruises on the face, and bite marks on the arms. These are signs of
a Physical abuse
b Sexual abuse
c Neglect
d Substance abuse

22 A child is dirty and has a body odor. These are signs of
a Physical abuse
b Sexual abuse
c Neglect
d Substance abuse

23 Blood stains on a child's underpants are a sign of
a Physical abuse
b Sexual abuse
c Neglect
d Substance abuse

24 These statements are about intimate partner violence. Which is *true?*
a It always involves physical harm.
b Most victims are male.
c One partner has control over the other partner.
d Only 1 type of abuse is usually present.

25 You suspect a resident was abused. What should you do?
a Tell the nurse.
b Call the police.
c Tell the family.
d Ask the person about the abuse.

Answers to Chapter 5 questions are on p. 870.

FOCUS ON PRACTICE

Problem Solving

A resident in your nursing center asks you to visit on your day off. The resident wants you to bring your children to visit. How will you respond? How do professional boundaries protect the person? How do these actions affect professional boundaries?

Student and Work Ethics

- Define the key terms and key abbreviation in this chapter.
- Describe the qualities and traits of a successful nursing assistant.
- Describe good health and hygiene practices.
- Explain how to look professional.
- Explain how to plan for childcare and transportation.
- Describe ethical behavior on the job.
- Explain how to manage stress.

- Explain how to problem solve and deal with conflict.
- Explain the aspects of harassment.
- Explain how to resign from a job.
- Identify the common reasons for losing a job.
- Explain the reasons for drug testing.
- Describe unethical student behavior and possible consequences.
- Explain how to promote PRIDE in the person, the family, and yourself.

KEY TERMS

bullying Repeated attacks or threats of fear, distress, or harm by a bully toward a victim
burnout A job stress resulting in being physically or mentally exhausted, having doubts about your abilities, and having doubts about the value of your work
confidentiality Trusting others with personal and private information
conflict A clash between opposing interests or ideas
courtesy A polite, considerate, or helpful comment or act
gossip To spread rumors or talk about the private matters of others

harassment To trouble, torment, offend, or worry a person by one's behavior or comments
priority The most important thing at the time
professionalism Following laws, being ethical, having good work ethics, and having the skills to do your work
stress The response or change in the body caused by any emotional, physical, social, or economic factor
stressor The event or factor that causes stress
teamwork Staff members work together as a group; each person does his or her part to give safe and effective care
work ethics Behavior in the workplace

KEY ABBREVIATION

NATCEP Nursing assistant training and competency evaluation program

As a student and a nursing assistant, you must act and function in a professional manner. *Professionalism involves following laws, being ethical, having good work ethics, and having the skills to do your work.* Laws and ethics are discussed in Chapter 5. *Laws* are rules of conduct made by government bodies. *Ethics* deals with right and wrong conduct. It involves choices and judgments about what to do or what not to do. An ethical person does the right thing.

In the workplace, certain behaviors (conduct), choices, and judgments are expected. *Work ethics deals with behavior in the workplace.* Your conduct reflects your choices and judgments. Work ethics involves:
- How you look
- What you say
- How you behave
- How you treat others
- How you work with others
- The qualities and traits described in Box 6-1, p. 56 (Fig. 6-1, p. 56)

In this chapter, "work ethics" also applies to you as a student. To be a successful student, practice good work ethics in the classroom and clinical setting and in your relationships with instructors and fellow students.

BOX 6-1	Qualities and Traits for Good Work Ethics

- *Being Caring.* Have concern for the person. Help make the person's life happier, easier, or less painful.
- *Being Dependable.* Report to work on time and when scheduled. Perform delegated tasks. Keep obligations and promises.
- *Being Considerate.* Respect the person's physical and emotional feelings. Be gentle and kind toward patients, residents, families, and co-workers.
- *Being Cheerful.* Greet and talk to people in a pleasant manner. Do not be moody, bad-tempered, or unhappy while at work.
- *Having Empathy.* Empathy is seeing things from the person's point of view—putting yourself in the person's place. How would you feel if you had the person's problems?
- *Being Trustworthy.* Patients, residents, families, and staff have confidence in you. They believe you will keep information confidential. They trust you not to gossip about patients, residents, families, or the health team.
- *Being Respectful.* Patients and residents have rights, values, beliefs, and feelings. They may differ from yours. Do not judge or condemn the person. Treat the person with respect and dignity at all times. The person has the right to respectful treatment. Also show respect for the health and nursing teams.
- *Being Courteous.* Be polite and courteous to patients, residents, families, visitors, and co-workers. See p. 60 for common courtesies in the workplace.
- *Being Conscientious.* Be careful, alert, and exact in following instructions. Give thorough care. Do not lose or damage the person's property.
- *Being Honest.* Accurately report the care given, your observations, and any errors.
- *Being Cooperative.* Willingly help and work with others. Also take that "extra step" during busy and stressful times.
- *Having Enthusiasm.* Be eager, interested, and excited about your work. Your work is important.
- *Being Self-aware.* Know your feelings, strengths, and weaknesses. You need to understand yourself before you can understand patients and residents.
- *Having Patience.* Tolerate problems and delays without getting upset, annoyed, or angry. Stay calm. Do not hurry or rush the person or a co-worker.

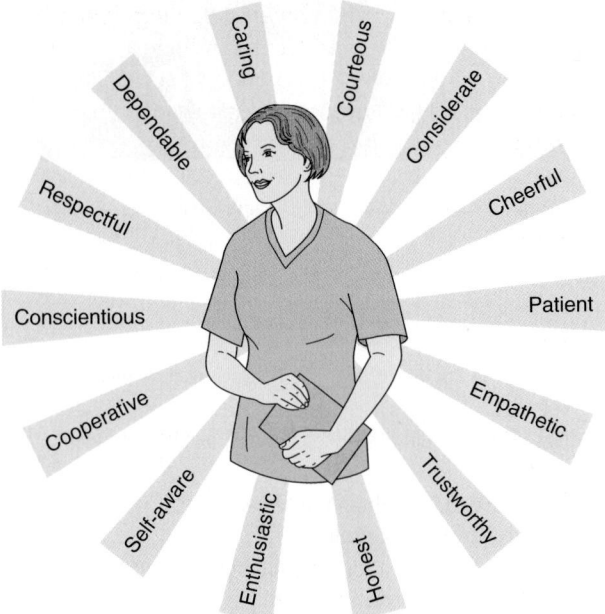

FIGURE 6-1 Good work ethics involves these qualities and traits.

Your Health

Your health is important as a student and nursing assistant. In order to learn and to give safe and effective care, you must be physically and mentally healthy. Otherwise you cannot function at your best.

- *Diet.* You need a balanced diet (Chapter 27). Eat a good breakfast. To maintain your weight, balance your calorie intake with your energy needs. To lose weight, have fewer calories than your energy needs. Avoid foods high in fat, oil, and sugar. Also avoid salty foods and "crash" diets.
- *Sleep and rest.* Most adults need 7 to 8 hours of sleep daily. Fatigue, lack of energy, and being irritable mean you need more rest and sleep.
- *Body mechanics.* You will bend, carry heavy objects, and move and turn persons. These tasks place stress and strain on your body. Use your muscles correctly (Chapter 17).
- *Exercise.* Exercise promotes muscle tone, circulation, and weight loss. Walking, running, swimming, and hiking are good forms of exercise. Regular exercise helps you feel better physically and mentally. Consult your doctor before starting a vigorous exercise program.
- *Your eyes.* You will read instructions and take measurements. Wrong readings and measurements can harm the person. Have your eyes checked. Wear needed eyeglasses or contact lenses. Have good lighting for reading and fine work.
- *Smoking.* Smoking causes lung, heart, and circulatory disorders. Smoke odors stay on your breath, hands, clothing, and hair. Hand-washing and good hygiene are needed.

HEALTH, HYGIENE, AND APPEARANCE

Patients, residents, families, and visitors expect you to look, act, and be healthy. For example, a person must stop smoking. Yet you are seen smoking. And you and your clothes smell of smoke. If you are not clean, people wonder if you give good care. Your health, hygiene, and appearance need careful attention.

- *Drugs.* Some drugs affect thinking, feeling, behavior, and function. Working under the influence of drugs affects the person's safety and yours. Take only those drugs ordered by your doctor. Take them in the prescribed way.
- *Alcohol.* Alcohol is a drug that depresses the brain. It affects thinking, balance, coordination, and alertness. Never go to work under the influence of alcohol. Do not drink alcohol while working. Like other drugs, alcohol affects the person's safety and yours.

Your Hygiene

Your hygiene needs careful attention. Bathe daily. Use a deodorant or antiperspirant to prevent body odors. Brush your teeth often—upon awakening, before meals, after meals, at bedtime. Use mouthwash to prevent breath odors. Shampoo often. Style hair in a simple, attractive way. Keep fingernails clean, short, and smoothly and neatly shaped.

Menstrual hygiene is important. Change tampons or sanitary pads often, especially for heavy flow. Wash your genital area with soap and water at least twice a day. Also practice good hand-washing.

Foot care prevents odors and infection. Wash your feet daily. Dry thoroughly between the toes. Cut toenails straight across after bathing or soaking them.

Your Appearance

How you look affects the way people think about you and the agency. When staff or students are clean and neat, people think the agency is clean and neat. They think the agency is unclean if the staff or students are messy and unkempt. People also wonder about the quality of care given.

Home and social attire is not proper at work or as a student in the clinical setting. You cannot wear jeans, halter tops, tank tops, short skirts, or low-cut tops or pants. Clothing must not be tight, revealing, or sexual. Women cannot show cleavage, the tops of breasts, or upper thighs. Men must avoid tight pants and exposing their chests. Only the top shirt button is open. Follow the practices in Box 6-2. They help you look clean, neat, and professional (Fig. 6-2, p. 58).

PREPARING FOR SCHOOL OR WORK

Being dependable is important as a student and in the workplace. As a student, you are preparing yourself for work. The classroom and clinical settings give you the chance to develop dependable behaviors. To show you are dependable:

- Be on time for class and clinical experiences. Arrive early to store your belongings, use the restroom, and gather needed items for class or clinical. Be ready when the class or clinical experience starts.
- Complete and turn in assignments on time.
- Pay attention and follow directions.
- Stay for the entire class or clinical experience.

BOX 6-2	Practices for a Professional Appearance

- Practice good hygiene.
- Follow your training program's or the agency's dress code. The dress code tells about uniform style and color, shoes, make-up, jewelry, and so on.
- Wear uniforms that fit well. They are modest in length and style. Follow the dress code.
- Keep uniforms clean, pressed, and mended. Sew on buttons. Repair zippers, tears, and hems.
- Wear a clean uniform daily.
- Wear your name badge or photo ID (identification) at all times when on duty. Make sure it can be seen. Wear it according to agency policy. It is best to wear it above your waist. Agencies may use first names only or first and last names. The agency may let you decide what to have on your name badge. For security, some staff choose the first-name-only option. As a student, your ID will include the school's name.
- Wear undergarments that are clean and fit properly. Change them daily.
- Wear undergarments in the correct color for your skin tone. Do not wear colored (red, pink, blue, and so on) ones. They can be seen through white and light-colored uniforms.
- Cover tattoos (body art). They may offend others.
- Follow the dress code for jewelry. Wedding and engagement rings may be allowed. Rings and bracelets can scratch a person. Confused or combative persons might pull on jewelry (necklaces, dangling earrings). So might young children.
- Do not wear jewelry in pierced eyebrows, nose, lips, or tongue while on duty.
- Follow the dress code for earrings. Usually small, simple earrings are allowed.
- For multiple ear piercings, usually only 1 set of earrings is allowed.
- Wear a wristwatch with a second (sweep) hand.
- Wear clean stockings and socks that fit well. Change them daily.
- Wear shoes that fit, are comfortable, give needed support, and have non-skid soles. Do not wear sandals or open-toed shoes.
- Wear clean shoes. Wash or replace shoes and laces as needed.
- Keep fingernails clean, short, and smoothly and neatly shaped. Long or jagged nails can scratch a person. Nails must be natural, not artificial.
- Do not wear nail polish. Chipped nail polish may provide a place for microbes to grow.
- Have a simple, attractive hairstyle. Hair is off your collar and away from your face. Use simple pins, combs, barrettes, and bands to keep long hair up and in place.
- Keep beards and mustaches clean and trimmed.
- Use make-up that is modest in amount and moderate in color. Avoid a painted and severe look.
- Do not wear perfume, cologne, or after-shave lotion. The scents may offend, nauseate, or cause breathing problems in patients and residents.

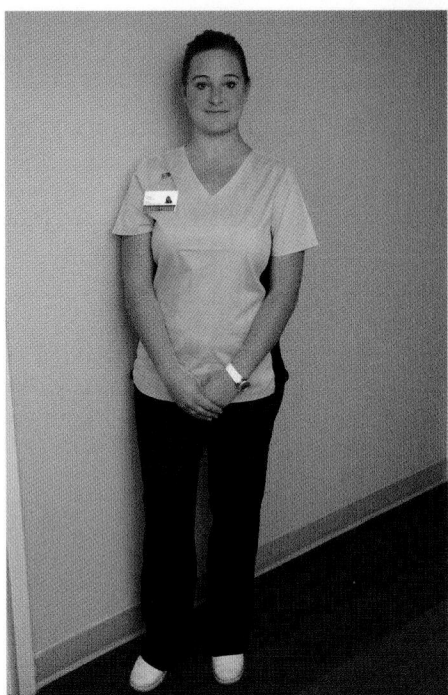

FIGURE 6-2 The nursing assistant is well groomed. Her uniform and shoes are clean. Her hair has a simple style—away from her face and off of her collar. She does not wear jewelry.

To be dependable in the work setting, you must:
* Work when scheduled.
* Get to work on time.
* Stay the entire shift.

Absences and tardiness can affect your success in school. Your state's nursing assistant training and competency evaluation program (NATCEP) requires a certain number of hours. To pass the course, you must complete the required number of hours.

Absences and tardiness are also common reasons for losing a job. Childcare and transportation issues often interfere with getting to school and work. You need to plan carefully.

Childcare

Someone needs to care for your children when you leave for school or work, while you are at school or work, and before you get home. Also plan for emergencies.
* Your childcare provider is ill or cannot care for your children that day.
* A child becomes ill or injured while you are at school or work.
* You will be late getting home from school or work.

Transportation

Plan for getting to and from school or work. If you drive, keep your car in good working order. Keep enough gas in the car. Or leave early to get gas.

Carpooling is an option. Carpoolers depend on each other. If the driver is late leaving, everyone is late for school or work. If 1 person is not ready when the driver arrives, everyone is late for school or work. Carpool with staff you trust to be ready on time. When you drive, leave and pick up others on time. As a passenger, be ready to be picked up on time. Be on time as a driver and as a passenger.

Know bus or train schedules. Know what bus or train to take if delays occur. Always carry enough money for fares to and from school or work.

Have a back-up plan for getting to school or work. Your car may not start, the carpool driver may not go to school or work, or public transportation may not run.

TEAMWORK

Teamwork means that staff members work together as a group. Each person does his or her part to give safe and effective care. Teamwork involves:
* Working when scheduled.
* Being cheerful and friendly.
* Performing delegated tasks.
* Helping others willingly.
* Being kind to others.

You are an important member of the health and nursing teams. Quality of care is affected by how you work with others and how you feel about your job. Some days it might seem that you are doing more work than others. Other days, your co-workers may feel that you are doing less than they are. Try not to compare your assignments and what you are doing to other staff. Each staff member has a role to play individually and as a team member.

Attendance

Your NATCEP or employer has an attendance policy. Be on time for class and clinical experiences.

Report to work when scheduled and on time. The entire unit is affected when just 1 person is late. Call the agency if you will be late or cannot go to work. Follow the attendance policy in your employee handbook. Poor attendance can cause you to lose your job.

Be *ready to work* when your shift starts.
* Store your belongings before your shift starts.
* Use the restroom when you arrive at the agency.
* Arrive on your nursing unit a few minutes early. This gives you time to greet others and settle yourself.

You must stay the entire shift. Prepare for childcare emergencies. Watching the clock for when your shift ends gives a bad image. You may need to work over-time. Prepare to stay longer if necessary. When it is time to leave, report off duty to the nurse.

See *Focus on Communication: Attendance.*
See *Teamwork and Time Management: Attendance.*
See *Focus on Long-Term Care and Home Care: Attendance.*

FOCUS ON COMMUNICATION
Attendance

You may have days that you cannot go to class or clinical or to work. Illness, a family death, and other emergencies are reasons. You must tell your instructor or the agency about your absence. Otherwise you could have an unexcused absence from your NATCEP. Your instructor may not allow you to make up the absence. If working, you could lose your job. To report an absence:

- *Call well before class, clinical, or your shift begins.* See the attendance policy in your student or employee handbook for when you should call. Calling at least 2 hours before the start time is common.
- *Know who to call.* As a student, call your instructor. A charge nurse, nurse manager, or supervisor often handles absences in the work setting. You may need your call transferred. For example: "Hello. This is Erin Jones. Please transfer me to the charge nurse." You must give information to the right person.
- *Give the reason for your absence.* Be honest. You can say: "I am sorry. I will be absent from work (class, clinical) today. I have a fever and a cough."
- *Tell how long you expect to be absent.* People often miss 1 or 2 days for illness or a family emergency. Longer absences or uncertain time frames require more communication.

TEAMWORK AND TIME MANAGEMENT
Attendance

Sometimes a staff member is late for work. Or someone does not show up for work. Until a replacement arrives, you and other staff have extra work. Patient and resident care cannot suffer.

To promote teamwork and manage your time:
- Ask the nurse how you can help.
- Do not complain about not having enough staff.
- Ask the nurse to list the most important tasks and care measures.

FOCUS ON LONG-TERM CARE AND HOME CARE
Attendance

Home Care
You must complete home care assignments. Never leave in the middle of an assignment. Nor should you leave before someone from the next shift arrives. Leaving before you complete an assignment is *abandonment* (Chapter 5).

Sometimes conflicts or problems occur (p. 62). Try to finish the assignment. Explain the problem to the nurse. He or she will try to make needed changes. Do not walk out on (abandon) the person. That would be unsafe for the person. Walking out (abandonment) is very unethical behavior. It also is abuse (Chapter 5).

Your Attitude

You need a good attitude (see Box 6-1). Show that you enjoy your work. Listen to others. Be willing to learn. Stay busy and use your time well.

Your work is very important. Nurses, patients, residents, and families rely on you for good care. They expect you to be pleasant and respectful. You must believe that you and your work have value.

Always think before you speak. These statements signal a bad attitude.
- "That's not my resident (patient)."
- "I can't. I'm too busy."
- "I didn't do it."
- "I don't feel like it."
- "It's not my fault."
- "Don't blame me."
- "It's not my turn. I did it yesterday."
- "Nobody told me."
- "That's not my job."
- "You didn't say that you needed it right away."
- "I did more than she (he) did."
- "I work harder than anyone else."
- "No one appreciates what I do."
- "I'm tired of this place."
- "Is it time to leave yet?"
- "Good luck. I had a horrible day."

Gossip

To *gossip means to spread rumors or talk about the private matters of others.* Gossiping is unprofessional and hurtful. To avoid being a part of gossip:
- Remove yourself from a group or setting where people are gossiping.
- Do not make or repeat any comment that can hurt a person, family member, visitor, co-worker, fellow student, instructor, or the school or agency.
- Do not make or repeat any comment that you do not know is true. Making or writing false statements about another person is defamation (Chapter 5).
- Do not talk about patients, residents, family members, visitors, co-workers, fellow students, instructors, or the school or agency at home or in social settings.
- Do not send or post hurtful, false, or private comments about others or the school or agency by e-mail, instant messaging, text messaging, video sites, or social media. See "Wrongful Use of Electronic Communications" in Chapter 5.

Confidentiality

The person's information is private and personal. *Confidentiality means trusting others with personal and private information.* The person's information is shared only among staff involved in his or her care. The person has the right to privacy and confidentiality. Agency, family, and co-worker information also is confidential. So is student information.

Share information only with the nurse or your instructor. Avoid talking about patients, residents, families, the agency, or co-workers when others are present. Do not talk about them in hallways, elevators, dining areas, or outside the agency. Others may over-hear you.

Patients, residents, and visitors are very alert to comments. They think you are talking about them or their loved ones. This leads to wrong information and wrong impressions about the person's condition. You can easily upset the person or family. Be very careful about what, how, when, and where you say things.

Do not eavesdrop. To *eavesdrop* means *to listen in or over-hear what others are saying.* It invades a person's privacy.

Many agencies have intercom systems. They allow for communication between the bedside and the nurses' station (Chapter 20). The person uses the intercom to signal for help. Someone at the nurses' station answers the intercom. The nursing team also uses the intercom to communicate with each other. Be careful what you say. The intercom is like a loud speaker. Others nearby can hear what you are saying.

See *Focus on Communication: Confidentiality.*

FOCUS ON COMMUNICATION

Confidentiality

Your family and friends may ask about patients, residents, families, or staff. For example, your mother says: "Mrs. Drew goes to our church. I heard she's in your nursing home. What's wrong with her?"

Do not share any information with your family and friends. Doing so violates the person's right to privacy and confidentiality (Chapters 2 and 5). You can say: "I'm sorry, but I can't tell you about anyone in the center. It is unprofessional and against center policies. And it violates the person's right to privacy and confidentiality. Please don't ask me about anyone in the center."

Speech and Language

Your speech and language must be professional. Words used in home and social settings may not be proper in class, the clinical setting, and at work. Words used with family and friends may offend patients, residents, families, visitors, and co-workers. Remember:

- Do not swear or use foul, vulgar, slang, or abusive language.
- Speak softly and gently. Control the volume and tone of your voice.
- Speak clearly. Hearing problems are common.
- Do not shout or yell.
- Do not fight or argue with a person, family member, visitor, co-worker, your instructor, or a fellow student.

Courtesies

A *courtesy is a polite, considerate, or helpful comment or act.* Courtesies take little time or energy. And they mean so much to people. Even the smallest kind act can brighten someone's day.

- Address others by Miss, Mrs., Ms., Mr., or Doctor. Use a first name only if the person asks you to do so. Do not call your instructor by his or her first name.
- Say "please." Begin or end each request with "please."
- Say "thank you" whenever someone does something for you or helps you.
- Apologize. Say "I'm sorry" when you make a mistake or hurt someone. Even little things—like bumping someone in the hallway—need an apology.
- Be thoughtful. Compliment others. Wish others a happy birthday, day or weekend off, or holiday.
- Wish the person and family well when they leave the agency. "Stay well" and "stay healthy" are examples.
- Hold doors open for others. If you are at the door first, open the door and let others pass through. In business, men and women hold doors open for each other.
- Hold elevator doors open for others coming down the hallway.
- Let patients, residents, families, and visitors enter elevators first.
- Stand to greet families and visitors.
- Help others willingly when asked.
- Give praise. If you see a co-worker or student do or say something that impresses you, tell that person. Also tell your co-workers or other students.
- Do not take credit for another person's deeds. Give the person credit for the action.

Personal Matters

You were hired to do a job. Personal matters cannot interfere with your job. Otherwise care is neglected. You could lose your job for tending to personal matters at work. To keep personal matters out of the workplace:

- Make phone calls during meals and breaks. Use a pay phone or your wireless phone.
- Do not let family and friends visit you on the unit. If they must see you, meet them during a meal or break.
- Make appointments (doctor, dentist, lawyer, and others) for your days off.
- Do not use agency computers, printers, fax machines, copiers, or other equipment for your personal use.
- Do not take the agency's supplies (pens, paper, and others) for your personal use.
- Do not discuss personal problems.
- Control your emotions. If you need to cry or express anger, do so in private. Get yourself together quickly and return to your work.
- Do not borrow money from or lend it to co-workers or fellow students. This includes meal money and bus or train fares. Borrowing and lending can lead to problems with co-workers and students.

- Do not sell things or engage in fund-raising. For example, do not sell your child's candy or raffle tickets to co-workers or other students.
- Turn off personal pagers and wireless phones.
- Do not send or check e-mail or text messages.

Meals and Breaks

Meal breaks are usually 30 minutes. Other breaks are usually 15 minutes. Meals and break times are scheduled so that some staff are always on the unit. Staff remaining on the unit cover for the staff on break.

Staff members depend on each other. Leave for and return from breaks on time. That way other staff can have their turn. Do not take longer than allowed. Tell the nurse when you leave and return to the unit.

Your school or agency may have break rooms for preparing and eating meals. Break rooms often have tables and chairs, a microwave, refrigerator, and sink. Some have coffee makers, cups, and utensils. Clean up after yourself before leaving the break room. Do not leave messes for other students or staff. Follow school or agency policies for keeping food and drinks in the refrigerator. Discard or take home food and food containers daily.

Job Safety

You must protect patients, residents, families, visitors, co-workers, and yourself from harm. Everyone is responsible for safety. Negligent acts affect the safety of others (Chapter 5). Safety practices are presented throughout this book. These guidelines apply to everything you do as a student and nursing assistant.

- Understand the roles, functions, and responsibilities in your job description.
- Follow agency rules, policies, and procedures in the:
  - Employee handbook
  - Policy book
  - Procedure manual
- Know what is right and wrong conduct.
- Know what you can and cannot do.
- Develop the desired qualities and traits in Box 6-1.
- Follow the nurse's directions and instructions.
- Question unclear directions and things you do not understand.
- Help others willingly when asked.
- Ask for any training you might need.
- Report accurately. This includes measurements, observations, the care given, the person's complaints, and any errors (Chapters 7 and 13).
- Accept responsibility for your actions. Admit when you are wrong or make mistakes. Do not blame others. Do not make excuses for your actions. Learn what you did wrong and why. Always try to learn from your mistakes.
- Handle the person's property carefully and prevent damage.
- Follow the safety measures in Chapter 13 and throughout this book.

Planning Your Work

You will give care and perform routine nursing unit tasks. Some tasks are done at certain times. Others are done at the end of the shift.

The nurse, the Kardex, the care plan, and your assignment sheet help you decide what to do and when (Chapters 7 and 8). This is called *priority setting*. A ***priority*** *is the most important thing at the time.* Setting priorities involves deciding:

- Which person has the greatest or most life-threatening needs.
- What task the nurse or person needs done first.
- What tasks need to be done at a certain time.
- What tasks need to be done when your shift starts.
- What tasks need to be done at the end of your shift.
- How much time it takes to complete a task.
- How much help you need to complete a task.
- Who can help you and when.

Priorities change as the person's needs change. A person's condition can improve or worsen. New patients and residents are admitted. Others are transferred to other nursing units or discharged. These and many other factors can change priorities.

Setting priorities is hard at first. It becomes easier with experience. You can ask your instructor or the nurse to help you set priorities. Plan your work to give safe, thorough care and to make good use of your time (Box 6-3).

BOX 6-3   Planning Your Work

- Discuss priorities with the nurse.
- Know the routine of your shift and nursing unit.
- Follow unit policies for shift reports.
- List tasks that are on a schedule. For example, some persons are turned or offered the bedpan every 2 hours.
- Judge how much time you need for each person and task.
- Identify tasks to do while patients and residents are eating, visiting, or involved with activities or therapies.
- Plan care around meal times, visiting hours, and therapies. Also consider recreation and social activities.
- Identify when you will need help from a co-worker. Ask a co-worker to help you.
- Give the time when you will need help and for how long.
- Schedule equipment or rooms for the person's use. The shower room is an example.
- Review delegated tasks. Gather needed supplies ahead of time.
- Do not waste time. Stay focused on your work.
- Leave a clean work area. Make sure rooms are neat and orderly. Also clean utility areas.
- Be a self-starter. Have initiative. Ask others if they need help. Follow unit routines, stock supply areas, and clean utility rooms. Stay busy.

MANAGING STRESS

Stress is the response or change in the body caused by any emotional, physical, social, or economic factor. Stress is normal. It occurs every minute of every day. It occurs in everything you do.

A *stressor is the event or factor that causes stress.* Many stressors are pleasant—watching a child play, planning a party, laughing with family and friends, enjoying a nice day. Some are not pleasant—illness, injury, family problems, death of loved ones, divorce, money concerns. Going to school and some parts of your job are stressful.

No matter the cause—pleasant or unpleasant—stress affects the whole person.

- *Physically*—sweating, increased heart rate, faster and deeper breathing, increased blood pressure, dry mouth, and so on
- *Mentally*—anxiety, fear, anger, dread, apprehension, and using defense mechanisms (Chapter 48)
- *Socially*—changes in relationships, avoiding others, needing others, blaming others, and so on
- *Spiritually*—changes in beliefs and values and strengthening or questioning one's beliefs in God or a higher power

Prolonged or frequent stress threatens physical and mental health. Some problems are minor—headaches, stomach upset, sleep problems, muscle tension, and so on. Others are life-threatening—high blood pressure, heart attack, stroke, ulcers, and so on.

Dealing with stress is important. School and job stresses affect your family and friends. Personal stress affects your studies or work. Stress affects you, the care you give, the person's quality of life, and how you relate to co-workers.

To reduce or cope with stress:

- Exercise regularly. Exercise has physical and mental benefits—cardiovascular health, weight control, tension release, emotional well-being, and relaxation.
- Get enough rest and sleep.
- Eat healthy.
- Plan personal and quiet time for you. Read, take a hot bath, go for a walk, meditate, or listen to music. Do what makes you feel good.
- Use common sense about what you can and cannot do. Do not try to do everything that family and friends ask you to do. Consider the amount of time and energy that you have.
- Do 1 thing at a time. The demands on you may seem overwhelming. List each thing that you have to do. Set priorities.
- Do not judge yourself harshly. Do not try to be perfect or expect too much from yourself.
- Give yourself praise. You do good and wonderful things every day.
- Have a sense of humor. Laugh at yourself. Laugh with others. Spend time with those who make you laugh.
- Have a social life that does not include co-workers.
- Talk to the nurse if your work or a person is causing too much stress. The nurse can help you deal with the matter.

Dealing With Conflict

People bring their values, attitudes, opinions, experiences, and expectations to school and work settings. Differences often lead to conflict. *Conflict is a clash between opposing interests or ideas.* People disagree and argue. There are misunderstandings and unrest.

Conflicts arise over issues or events. Work schedules, absences, and the amount and quality of work performed are examples. The problems must be worked out. Otherwise, unkind words or actions may occur. The learning or work setting becomes unpleasant. Care is affected.

Resolving Conflict. To resolve conflict, identify the real problem. This is part of *problem solving.* The problem solving process involves these steps.

- Step 1: Define the problem. *A nurse ignores me.*
- Step 2: Collect information about the problem. Do not include unrelated information. *The nurse does not look at me. The nurse does not talk to me. The nurse does not respond when I ask for help. The nurse does not ask me to help with tasks that require 2 people. The nurse talks to other staff members.*
- Step 3: Identify possible solutions. *Ignore the nurse. Talk to my supervisor. Talk to co-workers about the problem. Change jobs.*
- Step 4: Select the best solution. *Talk to my supervisor.*
- Step 5: Carry out the solution. *See below.*
- Step 6: Evaluate the results. *See below.*

Communication and good work ethics help prevent and resolve conflicts. Identify and solve problems before they become major issues. To deal with conflict:

- Ask your instructor or supervisor for some time to talk privately. Explain the problem. Give facts and specific examples. Ask for advice in solving the problem.
- Approach the person with whom you have the conflict. Ask to talk privately. Be polite and professional.
- Agree on a time and place to talk.
- Talk in a private setting. No one should hear you or the other person.
- Explain the problem and what is bothering you. Give facts and specific behaviors. Focus on the problem. Do not focus on the person.
- Listen to the person. Do not interrupt.
- Identify ways to solve the problem. Offer your thoughts. Ask for the other person's ideas.
- Set a date and time to review the matter.
- Thank the person for meeting with you.
- Carry out the solution.
- Review the matter as scheduled.

  See *Focus on Communication: Resolving Conflict.*

FOCUS ON COMMUNICATION

Resolving Conflict

You may find it hard to talk to someone with whom you have a conflict. This is hard for many people. However, letting the problem or issue continue only makes the matter worse. The following may help you start talking to the person.

- "You say 'no' when I ask you to help me. I help you when you ask me to. This really bothers me. Can we talk privately for a few minutes?"
- "I heard you tell John that you saw me sitting in Mrs. Gordon's room. You seemed angry when you said it. Can we talk privately? I want to explain why I was sitting and find out why that bothers you."
- "The new schedule shows me working every weekend this month. Please tell me why. The employee handbook says that we work every other weekend."
- "We were late for class 2 times this week when you drove. What can I do to help so that we are not late?"

Burnout

You must guard against burnout. *Burnout is a job stress resulting in:*
- *Being physically or mentally exhausted*
- *Having doubts about your abilities*
- *Having doubts about the value of your work*

Burnout occurs over time. Causes, signs, and symptoms are listed in Box 6-4. Burnout can lead to physical and mental health problems. They include fatigue, sleep problems, depression, anxiety, alcohol or substance abuse, heart disease, diabetes, stroke, and weight gain. Problems can develop at home and with personal relationships. To guard against burnout, see "Managing Stress."

HARASSMENT

Harassment means to trouble, torment, offend, or worry a person by one's behavior or comments. Harassment can be sexual. Or it can involve age, race, ethnic background, religion, or disability. Respect others. Do not offend others by your gestures, remarks, or use of touch. Do not offend others with jokes, photos, or other pictures (drawings, cartoons, and so on). Harassment is not legal.

You have the right not to be harassed as a student. No student, in your NATCEP or otherwise, should be allowed to harass or bully you (p. 64). The same applies to your instructor, other school instructors or staff, and staff in the clinical setting. If you believe that you are being harassed or bullied, talk to your instructor or school counselor. Follow the steps in "Resolving Conflict."

See *Focus on Communication: Harassment.*

BOX 6-4	Burnout—Causes, Signs, and Symptoms

Causes of Burnout
- Schedules, assignments, or workloads that you find difficult
- Not being comfortable with your supervisor or co-workers
- Being bullied or heavily criticized by your supervisor or a co-worker
- Conflicts with how problems and grievances are handled
- Not liking your job or the agency
- Having skills that are greater than or lesser than what the job requires
- Not having emotional support at work, at home, or socially
- Lack of balance between work and home, family, and social life

Signs and Symptoms of Burnout
- Lack of energy
- Sense of dread about going to work; not wanting to go to work
- Sleep problems
- Forgetfulness
- Problems concentrating
- Frequent illness—infection, cold, influenza
- Physical symptoms:
  - Chest pain
  - Rapid or irregular heartbeat
  - Shortness of breath
  - Gastro-intestinal pain
  - Dizziness
  - Fainting
  - Headaches
  - Loss of appetite
- Anxiety
- Anger
- Depression
- Irritability
- Wanting to be alone
- Calling in sick; going to work late

FOCUS ON COMMUNICATION

Harassment

You have the right to feel safe and not threatened. If someone's comments make you uncomfortable, you can say: "Please don't say things like that. It's unprofessional." If someone's actions make you uneasy, you can say: "Please don't do that. It's unprofessional." Leave the area. Report the person's statements or actions to the nurse.

Sexual Harassment

Sexual harassment involves unwanted sexual behaviors by another. The behavior may be a sexual advance. Or it may be a request for a sexual favor. Some remarks, comments, and touching are sexual. The behavior affects the person's work and comfort. In extreme cases, the person's job (or grade) is threatened if sexual favors are not granted.

Sexual harassment can take the form of sexting. *Sexting* combines the words *sex* and *texting*. Sexting involves creating, sending, and posting sexually aggressive text messages and photos or videos of oneself or others. Usually done using wireless phones, other electronic devices may be used.

Victims of sexual harassment may be men or women. Men harass women or men. Women harass men or women. You might feel that you are being harassed. If so, report the matter to the nurse and the human resources officer. As a student, tell your instructor and school counselor.

Be careful about what you say or do. Even innocent remarks and behaviors can be viewed as harassment. You might not be sure about your own or another person's remarks or behaviors. If so, talk to your instructor or the nurse. You cannot be too careful.

Bullying

Bullying is repeated attacks or threats of fear, distress, or harm by a bully toward a victim. Bullying can be physical (hitting, tripping), verbal (name calling, teasing), or social (rumors, leaving the person out of a group). Property damage and forcing a person to do something against his or her will are other forms of bullying.

Bullying can occur in work, classroom, clinical, or social settings. Cyber-bullying occurs through electronic means (including wireless phones)—e-mail, chat rooms, instant messaging, text messaging, videos, photos, and social media sites.

According to the Centers for Disease Control and Prevention (CDC), bullying can result in injury, emotional distress, and even death. Victims of bullying are at risk for depression, anxiety, sleep problems, and poor school or work performance. Those who bully are at risk for substance abuse, school or work problems, and violence.

Talk to your instructor or supervisor if you are being bullied. He or she will try to help you with the situation.

RESIGNING FROM A JOB

A job closer to home, better pay, or new opportunities may prompt you to leave your job. School, children, and illness are other reasons. Whatever the reason, tell your employer. Do 1 of the following.
- Give a written notice.
- Write a resignation letter.
- Complete a form in the human resources office.

BOX 6-5	Common Reasons for Losing a Job

- Poor attendance—not going to work or excessive tardiness (being late).
- Abandonment—leaving the job during your shift.
- Falsifying a record—job application or a person's record.
- Violent behavior in the workplace.
- Having weapons in the workplace—guns, knives, explosives, or other dangerous items.
- Having, using, or distributing alcohol in the work setting.
- Having, using, or distributing drugs in the work setting. This excludes having or using drugs ordered by your doctor.
- Taking a person's drugs for your own use or giving them to others.
- Harassment (p. 63).
- Using offensive speech and language.
- Stealing or destroying the agency's or a person's property.
- Showing disrespect to patients, residents, families, visitors, co-workers, or supervisors.
- Abusing or neglecting a person.
- Invading a person's privacy.
- Failing to maintain patient, resident, family, agency, or co-worker confidentiality. This includes access to computer and other electronic information.
- Wrongful use of electronic communications (Chapter 5).
- Using the agency's supplies and equipment for your own use.
- Defamation—see Chapter 5 and "Gossip" (p. 59).
- Abusing meal breaks and break time.
- Sleeping on the job.
- Violating the agency's dress code.
- Violating any agency policy or care procedure.
- Tending to personal matters while on duty.

A 2-week notice is a good practice. Do not leave a job without notice. Doing so can affect patient and resident care. Include the following in your notice.
- Reason for leaving
- The last date you will work
- Comments thanking the employer for the opportunity to work in the agency

An exit interview is common practice. You and the employer talk before you leave the agency. Or a survey may be sent to your home. The employer asks what you liked about the agency and your job. Often employees are asked how the agency can improve.

LOSING A JOB

A job is a privilege. You must perform your job well and protect patients and residents from harm. No pay raise or losing your job results from poor performance. Failing to follow agency policy is often grounds for termination. So is failure to get along with others. Box 6-5 lists the many reasons why you can lose your job. To protect your job, function at your best. Always practice good work ethics.

DRUG TESTING

Drug and alcohol use affect patient, resident, and staff safety. Quality of care suffers. Those who use drugs or alcohol are late to work or absent more often than staff who do not use such substances. Therefore drug testing policies are common. Review your agency's policy for when and how you might be tested.

UNETHICAL STUDENT BEHAVIOR

Your NATCEP and school will likely have a code of conduct. Violating the code of conduct is unethical behavior. Many of the reasons listed in Box 6-5 are violations of your school's and NATCEP's code of conduct. As a result, your school and NATCEP may take 1 or more of the following actions.

- Dismissing you from the school or NATCEP
- Issuing a failing grade
- Not recommending that you take the competency evaluation (written and skills tests)

You must act in an ethical manner at all times. Always try to do the right thing. If you do, you will be a successful nursing assistant.

FOCUS ON **PRIDE**

The Person, Family, and Yourself

Personal and Professional Responsibility

You are responsible for your behavior in the workplace. How you act makes a difference. The *Employee Handbook* of OSF Saint Francis Medical Center (Peoria, Ill.) says it well.

You are what people see when they arrive here; yours are the eyes they look into when they're frightened and lonely. Yours are the voices people hear when they ride the elevators, when they try to sleep, and when they try to forget their problems. You are what they hear on their way to appointments which could affect their destinies, and what they hear after they leave those appointments. Yours are the comments people hear when you think they can't.

Yours is the intelligence and caring that people hope they'll find here. If you're noisy, so is the medical center. If you're rude, so is the medical center. And if you're wonderful, so is the medical center.

You can help the person feel cared for, safe, and secure. By practicing good work ethics, you can make others' lives happier, easier, and less painful.

Rights and Respect

Conflict with other students and co-workers will arise. Dealing with conflict can be hard. But it must be addressed. Deal with conflict in a respectful and mature way. Do not gossip, put others down, or talk about people behind their backs. These behaviors are disrespectful and not professional.

Everyone, including you, deserves to be treated with respect. If you feel someone has wronged you, address the issue. Politely ask to talk to the person in private. Speak calmly and respectfully. Focus on the problem and the solution. Do not attack the person's character. For example, do not say: "You are so mean. I can't believe you were talking about me behind my back." Instead, you can say: "It bothers me that you didn't come to me about this. Next time could you talk to me first?" For good relationships, identify and resolve conflict in a respectful and professional manner.

Independence and Social Interaction

Social interaction is a vital part of your job. Smile and greet patients and residents by name. Politely introduce yourself. Do not appear hurried. Display a caring and friendly manner all the time. Remain calm and helpful in stressful situations. These actions promote good relationships and reflect well on you and the agency.

Delegation and Teamwork

Your work ethics affect the team. Greet co-workers pleasantly. Help others willingly. After completing tasks, ask the nurse if you can help with anything else. Be available. Stay where you can be found easily. If you will be in 1 area for a while, tell the nurse.

When you would like a break, ask the nurse. Return from breaks on time. Help others so they may take a break. Set a positive example with your behavior. Your actions help build a strong team.

Ethics and Laws

As a student and nursing assistant, you are responsible for following the ethical guidelines in this chapter. Patients, residents, families, visitors, and co-workers depend on you to give safe and effective care. You must:

- Attend clinical and work when scheduled.
- Arrive at clinical and work on time.
- Stay the entire clinical time or work shift.
- Complete your assignments.
- Work safely.
- Be pleasant and courteous.

Take pride in your work ethics. Your work affects quality of life.

FOCUS ON **PRIDE**: *Application*

Think of a person you enjoy working with. What qualities do you value in a co-worker? How will you apply these qualities in your work?

REVIEW QUESTIONS

Circle T if the statement is TRUE and F if it is FALSE.

1 T F   You wear needed eyeglasses. This helps protect the person's safety.

2 T F   Childcare requires planning before going to school.

3 T F   Being on time for work means arriving at the agency when your shift starts.

4 T F   You share confidential information with a friend. You could lose your job.

5 T F   You must be careful what you say over the intercom system.

6 T F   You do not follow the agency's dress code. You could lose your job.

7 T F   You can use the agency's computer for your homework.

8 T F   You can use your wireless phone to send text messages during clinical.

9 T F   You must know the agency's attendance policy.

10 T F   Harassment is legal in the workplace.

Circle the BEST answer.

11 Which will help you do your job well?
 a Sleeping 3 to 4 hours daily
 b Avoiding exercise
 c Using drugs and alcohol
 d Having good nutrition

12 Which is a good hygiene practice?
 a Bathing weekly
 b Wearing strongly scented perfume or cologne
 c Brushing teeth after meals
 d Having long and polished fingernails

13 You are getting ready for clinical. Which is a good practice?
 a Styling hair up and off your collar
 b Wearing jewelry
 c Wearing your name badge at waist level
 d Applying heavy make-up

14 Empathy is
 a Feeling sorry for a person
 b Seeing things from the other person's point of view
 c Being polite to others
 d Saying kind things

15 Which statement reflects a good attitude?
 a "It's not my fault."
 b "I'm sorry. I didn't know."
 c "That's not my job."
 d "I did it yesterday. It's your turn."

16 A co-worker tells you that a doctor and nurse are dating. This is
 a Gossip
 b Eavesdropping
 c Confidential information
 d Sexual harassment

17 Which is professional speech and language?
 a Using vulgar words
 b Shouting
 c Arguing
 d Speaking clearly

18 Which is a courteous act?
 a Telling a co-worker he did a good job
 b Calling a resident "Honey"
 c Taking credit for a co-worker's work
 d Closing an elevator door as a person approaches

19 You are on a meal break. Which is *true*?
 a You cannot make personal phone calls.
 b Family members cannot meet you.
 c The nurse needs to know that you are off the unit.
 d You can take a few extra minutes if needed.

20 When planning your work
 a Discuss priorities with the nurse
 b Skip the shift report to allow more time for work
 c Do not ask co-workers for help
 d Plan care so that you can watch the person's TV

21 These statements are about stress. Which is *true*?
 a Personal stress does not affect work.
 b Stress affects the whole person.
 c All stress is unpleasant.
 d Stress is abnormal.

22 Which helps to reduce stress?
 a Exercise, rest, and sleep
 b Blaming others for things you did not do
 c Putting off quiet time to get work done
 d Agreeing to do everything others ask

23 Thinking about work makes you irritable and anxious. These are
 a Normal feelings
 b Physical effects of stress
 c Healthy ways of managing stress
 d Signs of burnout

24 You have extra work because a co-worker is often late for work. To resolve the conflict
 a Explain the problem to your supervisor
 b Discuss the matter during the end-of-shift report
 c Ignore the problem
 d Complain about the person to co-workers

25 Which is *not* harassment?
 a Asking for a sexual favor
 b Joking about a person's religion
 c Using touch to comfort a person
 d Acting like a disabled person

26 Which is *not* a reason for losing your job?
 a Leaving the job during your shift
 b Using alcohol in the work setting
 c Sleeping on the job
 d Taking a meal break

Answers to Chapter 6 questions are on p. 870.

FOCUS ON **PRACTICE**

Problem Solving

A co-worker did not show up for work. You and the other staff members have extra work. How do you respond? Do you complain or keep a positive attitude? How will you plan, prioritize, and manage the extra work?

Communicating With the Health Team

OBJECTIVES

- Define the key terms and key abbreviations in this chapter.
- Explain why health team members need to communicate.
- Describe the rules for good communication.
- Explain the purpose, parts, and information found in the medical record.
- Describe the legal and ethical aspects of medical records.
- Describe the purpose of the Kardex and care summary.
- List the information you need to report to the nurse.
- List the rules for recording.

- Explain how computers and other electronic devices are used in health care.
- Explain how to protect the right to privacy when using computers and other electronic devices.
- Describe how to answer phones.
- Use the 24-hour clock, medical terminology, and medical abbreviations.
- Explain how to promote PRIDE in the person, the family, and yourself.

KEY TERMS

abbreviation A shortened form of a word or phrase

anterior At or toward the front of the body or body part; ventral

chart See "medical record"

clinical record See "medical record"

communication The exchange of information—a message sent is received and correctly interpreted by the intended person

distal The part farthest from the center or from the point of attachment

dorsal See "posterior"

electronic health record (EHR) An electronic version of a person's medical record; electronic medical record

electronic medical record (EMR) See "electronic health record"

end-of-shift report A report that the nurse gives at the end of the shift to the on-coming shift; change-of-shift report

Kardex A type of card file that summarizes information found in the medical record—drugs, treatments, diagnoses, routine care measures, equipment, and special needs

lateral Away from the mid-line; at the side of the body or body part

medial At or near the middle or mid-line of the body or body part

medical record The legal account of a person's condition and response to treatment and care; chart or clinical record

posterior At or toward the back of the body or body part; dorsal

prefix A word element placed before a root; it changes the meaning of the word

progress note Describes the care given and the person's response and progress

proximal The part nearest to the center or to the point of attachment

recording The written account of care and observations; charting, documentation

reporting The oral account of care and observations

root A word element containing the basic meaning of the word

suffix A word element placed after a root; it changes the meaning of the word

ventral See "anterior"

word element A part of a word

KEY ABBREVIATIONS

ADL	Activities of daily living		**EPHI; ePHI**	Electronic protected health information
EHR	Electronic health record		**PHI**	Protected health information
EMR	Electronic medical record			

Health team members communicate with each other to give coordinated and effective care. They share information about:

- What was done for the person
- What needs to be done for the person
- The person's response to treatment

For example, the doctor ordered a blood test for Mr. Bloom. Food and fluids affect the test results. Mr. Bloom must fast for 10 hours before the blood is drawn. A nurse tells the dietary department that Mr. Bloom will have breakfast later. She explains the breakfast delay to you and Mr. Bloom. A technician tells the nurse the blood sample was drawn. The nurse orders the meal. A dietary worker brings the tray to the nursing unit. You serve Mr. Bloom's tray. When he is done eating, you remove the tray and observe what he ate. You report your observations to the nurse. The nurse records your observations in Mr. Bloom's medical record.

Team members communicated with each other and Mr. Bloom. His care was coordinated and effective. He knew that he was not neglected or forgotten.

You need to understand the aspects and rules of communication. Then you can learn how to communicate with the nursing and health teams.

COMMUNICATION

Communication is the exchange of information—a message sent is received and correctly interpreted by the intended person. For good communication:

- Use words that mean the same thing to you and the message receiver. Avoid words with more than 1 meaning. What does "far" mean—50 feet or 100 feet?
- Use familiar words. You will learn medical terms. If someone uses a strange term, ask what it means. Or use a dictionary. You must understand the message. Otherwise communication does not occur. Also, avoid terms that the person and family do not understand.
- Be brief and concise. Do not add unrelated or unnecessary information. Stay on the subject. Do not wander in thought or get wordy.
- Give information in a logical and orderly way. Organize your thoughts. Present them step-by-step.
- Give facts and be specific. Give the receiver a clear message. You report a pulse rate of 110. It is more specific and factual than saying the "pulse is fast."

THE MEDICAL RECORD

The *medical record (chart, clinical record) is the legal account of a person's condition and response to treatment and care.* Medical records are written using paper forms or electronically through the use of computers (Fig. 7-1). An *electronic health record (EHR) or electronic medical record (EMR) is an electronic version of a person's medical record.* More and more agencies are using EHRs (EMRs). In time, all medical records will be electronic.

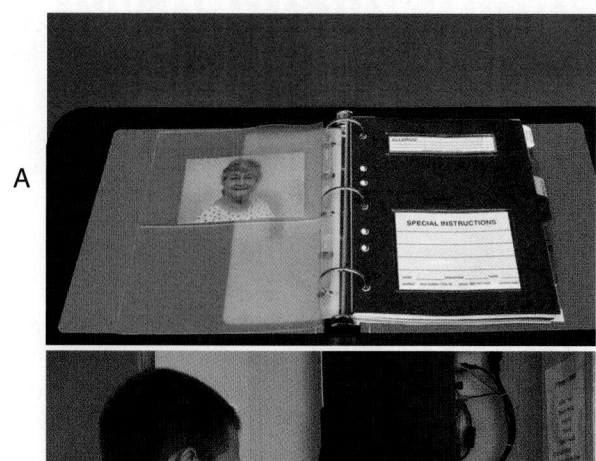
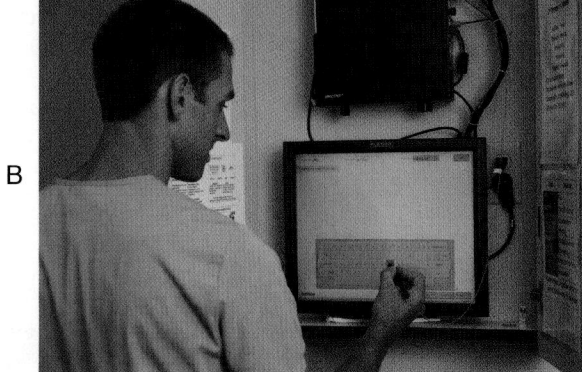

FIGURE 7-1 Medical records. A, A written medical record. **B,** An electronic medical record.

The health team uses the medical record to share information about the person. The record is a permanent legal document. Often it is used months or years later if the person's health history is needed. It can be used in court as legal evidence of the person's problems, treatment, and care.

The record is organized into sections. Each page has the person's name, room and bed number, and other identifying information. Common parts of the record include:

- Admission record
- Health history
- Physical examination results
- Doctor's orders
- Doctor's progress notes
- Progress notes (nursing team and health team)
- Graphic sheets and flow sheets
- Laboratory results
- X-ray reports
- Therapy records: intravenous (IV), respiratory, and others
- Consultation reports
- Assessments from nursing, social services, dietary services, and recreational therapy
- Special consents

The health team records on forms for their departments. Other team members read the information. It tells the care provided and the person's response.

Agencies have policies about medical records and who can see them. Policies address:
- Who records
- When to record
- Ink color to use (for paper charting)
- Abbreviations
- How to make and sign entries
- How to correct errors

Some agencies allow nursing assistants to record observations and care. Others do not. You must follow your agency's policies.

Professional staff involved in a person's care can review charts. Cooks and laundry, housekeeping, and office staff do not need to read charts. Some agencies let nursing assistants read charts. If not, the nurse shares needed information.

You have an ethical and legal duty to keep the person's information confidential. You may know someone in the agency. If not involved in the person's care, you have no right to review the person's chart. Doing so is an invasion of privacy.

Patients and residents have the right to the information in their medical records. The person or the person's legal representative may ask to see the chart. Report the request to the nurse. The nurse handles the request.

The following parts of the medical record relate to your work. They may be paper forms or electronic records.

The Admission Record

The admission record is completed when the person is admitted to the agency. It has the person's identifying information—legal name, birth date, age, gender (male or female), address, and marital status. Nearest relative and legal representative names are included. Other information includes known allergies, diagnoses, date and time of admission, and doctor's name. Religion, place of worship, and employer are often included.

Each person receives an identification (ID) number. It is on the admission record and ID bracelet (Chapter 13). So is information about advance directives. An *advance directive* is a document stating a person's wishes about end-of-life care (Chapter 55).

Use the admission record for forms needing the same information. That way the person does not have to answer the same question many times.

Health History

The health history (nursing history) is completed when the person is admitted. The nurse interviews the person. You can use the form to learn about the person's background and health history. It contains information about:
- The chief complaint—reason for seeking health care
- History of the current illness—sudden or gradual in onset, when it started, signs and symptoms, and so on
- Past health problems, surgeries, and injuries
- Childhood illnesses
- Allergies
- Current drugs
- Family health history
- Life-style—habits, diet, sleep, hobbies, and so on
- The need for dentures, eyeglasses or contact lenses, and hearing aids
- Problems with activities of daily living (ADL)
- Education and occupation

The Graphic Sheet

The graphic sheet is used to record measurements and observations made daily, every shift, or 3 to 4 times a day (Fig. 7-2, p. 70). Information includes vital signs—blood pressure, temperature, pulse, respirations. It also includes weight, intake and output (Chapter 27), bowel movements (feces), and doctor's visits.

Progress Notes

The *progress note* *describes the care given and the person's response and progress* (Fig. 7-3, p. 71). The nurse records:
- Signs and symptoms
- Information about treatments and drugs
- Information about teaching and counseling
- Procedures performed by the doctor
- Visits by other health team members
  See *Focus on Long-Term Care and Home Care: Progress Notes.*

FOCUS ON LONG-TERM CARE AND HOME CARE

Progress Notes

Long-Term Care
The nurse writes progress notes for an unusual event, a problem, or a change in the person's condition. The *Omnibus Budget Reconciliation Act of 1987 (OBRA)* requires summaries of care at least every 3 months. They reflect the person's progress toward the goals set in the care plan (Chapter 8). They also reflect the response to care. Some centers require summaries more often.

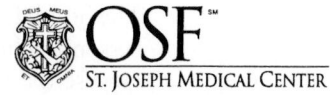

DAILY SUMMARY AND GRAPHIC

ST. JOSEPH MEDICAL CENTER
Bloomington, Illinois 61701

TEMPERATURE
Write in 105° or over

	2400	0400	0800	1200	1600	2000	2400	0400	0800	1200	1600	2000	2400	0400	0800	1200	1600	2000	2400	0400	0800	1200	1600	2000
DATE 5-7							5-8																	
HOSPITAL DAY 4							5																	
POST OP DAY																								
B/P			130/80	120/76	130/76	130/80			120/72	120/80	130/80	130/82												

TEMPERATURE

104 40
102.2 39
100.4 38
98.6 37 •
96.6 36

	2400	0400	0800	1200	1600	2000	2400	0400	0800	1200	1600	2000												
PULSE			74	80	76	74			74	74	76	72												
RESPIRATION			18	18	16	16			18	20	18	16												
WEIGHT																								
DR. VISIT	@ 0900																							

INTAKE	2300-0700	0700-1500	1500-2300	TOTAL	2300-0700	0700-1500	1500-2300	TOTAL	2300-0700	0700-1500	1500-2300	TOTAL	2300-0700	0700-1500	1500-2300	TOTAL
Oral	100	1200	800	2100	100	1050	820	1970								
IV																
Tube Feedings																
PPN/TPN/Lipids																
Blood/Blood Products																
IV Meds																
Chemotherapy																
Unreturned irr. sol.																
TOTAL INTAKE	100	1200	800	2100	100	1050	820	1970								
OUTPUT	2300-0700	0700-1500	1500-2300	TOTAL	2300-0700	0700-1500	1500-2300	TOTAL	2300-0700	0700-1500	1500-2300	TOTAL	2300-0700	0700-1500	1500-2300	TOTAL
Urine	0	1050	800	1850	200	850	750	1800								
GI																
Emesis	100			100												
Drains																
TOTAL OUTPUT	100	1050	800	1950	200	850	750	1800								
Feces		✓				✓										

FIGURE 7-2 A sample graphic sheet. (Courtesy OSF St Joseph Medical Center, Bloomington, Ill.)

Date	Time	Nursing Margin	Other Depts Margin
3-19	1700	Out with family for dinner. Jane Doe, LPN	
3-19	1930	Returned from outing accompanied by her son. States she had a pleasant time. Mary Smith, CNA	
3-20	0900	IN BED. COMPLAINS OF HEADACHE. T 98.4 ORALLY, RADIAL PULSE 72 AND REGULAR, RESPIRATIONS 18 AND UNLABORED. BP 134/84 LEFT ARM LYING DOWN. ALICE JONES, RN NOTIFIED OF RESIDENT COMPLAINT AND VITAL SIGNS. ANN ADAMS, CNA	
3-20	0910	In bed resting. States she has had a headache for about 1/2 hour. Denies nausea and dizziness. No other complaints. PRN Tylenol given. Instructed resident to use call light if headache worsens or other symptoms occur. Alice Jones, RN	
3-20	0945	Resting quietly. Denies headache at this time. T 98.4 orally, radial pulse 70 and regular, respirations 18 and unlabored. BP 132/84 left arm lying down. Alice Jones, RN	

FIGURE 7-3 Progress notes. Note that other members of the health team also can record on this form.

Flow Sheets

Flow sheets are used to record frequent measurements or observations. For example, vital signs are measured every 30 minutes. A vital signs flow sheet is used. The bedside intake and output record is another flow sheet (Chapter 27).

See *Focus on Long-Term Care and Home Care: Flow Sheets.*

FOCUS ON LONG-TERM CARE AND HOME CARE

Flow Sheets

Long-Term Care

An activities of daily living (ADL) flow sheet is used to record a person's ability to perform ADL (Fig. 7-4). This flow sheet addresses hygiene and grooming, feeding, elimination, activity and transfers, and safety.

Home Care

In home care, a weekly record has sections for each day and for care activities. There are sections for vital signs and weight, bathing, hygiene and grooming, activity, procedures, and nutrition. You record on the day care was given.

FIGURE 7-4 A sample flow sheet. This form shows some items on an activities of daily living flow sheet.

Activities of Daily Living Flow Sheet

JAN FEB (MAR) APR

ORDER/INSTRUCTION	TIME	1	2	3	4	5	6	7	8	9
Bowel Movements L = Large M = Medium S = Small IC = Incontinent	11-7	M								
	7-3			L						
	3-11									
Urinary Elimination I = Independent IC = Incontinent FC = Foley catheter	11-7	I	I	I	I					
	7-3	I	I	I	I					
	3-11	I	IC	I	I					
Weight Bearing Status TT = Toe touch AT = As tol. P = Partial F = Full NWB = No weight bearing	11-7	AT	AT	AT	AT					
	7-3	AT	AT	AT	AT					
	3-11	AT	AT	AT	AT					
Transfer Status ML = Mech lift SBA = Stand by assist; Assist of 1 or 2 (A-1, A-2)	11-7	SBA	SBA	SBA	SBA					
	7-3	SBA	SBA	SBA	SBA					
	3-11	SBA	SBA	SBA	A-1					
Activity A = Ambulate GC = Gerichair T = Turn every 2 hrs. W/C = Wheelchair	11-7	T	T	T	T					
	7-3	A	A	A	A					
	3-11	A	A	A						
Safety LT = Lap tray BR = Bed rails BA = Bed alarm SB = Seat belt	11-7									
	7-3									
	3-11									
Feeding Status I = Independent S = Set up F = Staff feed SP = Swallow precautions TL = Thickened liquids	Breakfast	S	S	S	S					
	Lunch	S	S	S	S					
	Supper	S	S	S	S					
Amount of food taken in %	Breakfast	75	100	100	75					
	Lunch	75	75	100	75					
	Supper	50	50	50	75					
Bath and Shampoo every _Monday_ & _Thursday_ on _7-3_ shift T = Tub S = Shower B = Bed bath	11-7									
	7-3	T								
	3-11									
Oral Care Own/(Dentures)/No teeth I = Independent S = Set up A = Assist	11-7	S	S	S	S					
	7-3	S	S	S	S					
	3-11	S	S	S	S					
Dressing I = Independent S = Set up A = Assist T = Total care	11-7	A	A	S	S					
	7-3									
	3-11	A	A	A	A					
Grooming: Washing Face and Hands Combing Hair I = Independent S = Set up A = Assist T = Total care	11-7	A	A	A	A					
	7-3	A	A	A	A					
	3-11	A	A	A	A					
Trim Fingernails weekly _Thursday_	11-7									
	7-3			✓						
	3-11									
Lotion Arms and Legs twice daily	11-7									
	7-3	✓	✓	✓	✓					
	3-11	✓	✓	✓	✓					
Shave Men daily	11-7									
Shave (Women) every _Monday_ & _Thursday_ on _7-3_ shift	7-3			✓						
	3-11									
Amount Between-Meal Snacks taken in %	AM	100	75	100	50					
	PM	100	100	75	75					
	HS	50	75	75	75					
Intake and Output	11-7									
	7-3									
	3-11									
Vital Signs Every _Thursday_	11-7									
	7-3			✓						
	3-11									
Weight Every _Thursday_	11-7			✓						
	7-3									
	3-11									

DIET	NOURISHMENT/SPECIAL FEEDING	INTAKE/OUTPUT
Regular	*Health shake at Bedtime*	Encourage/**Restrict** Fluids __2000__ mL/24 Hr.
Hold:		7-3 __1000__ 3-11 __800__ 11-7 __200__

FUNCTIONAL STATUS

	SELF	ASSIST	TOTAL	OTHER	SPECIFY
Feeding	☐	☒	☐	☐	
Bathing	☐	☒	☐	☐	
Toileting	☐	☒	☐	☐	
Oral Care	☐	☒	☐	☐	
Positioning	☒	☐	☐	☐	
Transferring	☒	☐	☐	☐	
Wheeling	☐	☐	☐	☐	
Walking	☒	☐	☐	☐	
	☐	☐	☐	☐	

ACTIVITIES

Bedrest & BRP _____
Bedside Commode _____
Up ad Lib __X__
Chair _____
Ambulatory __X__
Ambulate & Assist _____
Turn _____
Dangle _____
Mode of Travel _____

ELIMINATION

Urinary - Cont. (Incont.)
Catheter _____
Date Changed _____
Irrigations _____

Bowel - (Cont.) Incont.
Ostomy _____
Irrigations _____

VITALS

Temp. *daily*
Pulse *daily*
Resp. *daily*
BP *daily*
Weight *daily*
Other:
  Pulse OX
  daily

COMMUNICATION DEFICITS ☐ None

Hearing __*Hard-of-hearing*__
Vision __*Impaired*__
Speech _____
Language __*Impaired*__

PROSTHESIS ☐ None

Glasses __X__ Dentures __X__
Contacts _____ Limb _____
Hearing Aid __*L ear*__

SPECIAL CONDITIONS (Paralysis, Pressure Ulcers, Etc.)

SAFETY/SUPPORTIVE MEASURES

Bed rails: ☒ Nights Only ☐ Constant ☐ No Need
Restraints: _____
Support Devices: ☐ PRN ☐ Constant

RESPIRATORY THERAPY

Aerosol
IPPB
Ultrasonic
Rx Med _____

OXYGEN

__2__ Liter/Minute
☒ PRN ☐ Constant
___ Tent   ___ Catheter
___ Mask   __X__ Cannula

DATE	TREATMENTS

SPECIAL EQUIPMENT/PROCEDURES/ANCILLARY SERVICES/ETC.

Speech therapy 3 times/wk.

ORDERED	SCHEDULED	COMPLETED	X-RAY AND SPECIAL DIAGNOSTIC EXAMS
10-20	10-20	10-20	*Chest x-ray*

DATE	TIME	SCHEDULED MEDICATIONS	DATE	TIME	PRN MEDICATIONS
10-19		*Lasix 40 mg PO daily*			
10-19		*Lanoxin 0.25 mg PO daily*			
			MISCELLANEOUS		

ALLERGIES:	NURSING ALERTS:	EMERGENCY CONTACT:	
☒ None Known	*fall prevention*	Name: *Parker, Marie* Relationship: *Wife*	Telephone No. Home: __555-1212__ Bus: _____

ROOM	NAME	PHYSICIAN	ADMITTING DIAGNOSIS/PROBLEM	HOSP. NO.
310	*Parker, Edwin*	*Dr. S Epstein*	1. *CHF* 2. *Dementia*	*1035B*

FIGURE 7-5 A sample Kardex. (Courtesy Briggs Corporation, Des Moines, Iowa.)

THE KARDEX OR CARE SUMMARY

The **Kardex** *is a type of card file. It summarizes information in the medical record—drugs, treatments, diagnoses, routine care measures, equipment, and special needs. The Kardex is a quick, easy source of information about the person* (Fig. 7-5). *It is not part of the permanent medical record.*

With computer systems, the person's information is organized in an electronic care summary. Summaries can often be printed for reference.

REPORTING AND RECORDING

The health team communicates by reporting and recording. **Reporting** *is the oral account of care and observations.* **Recording** *(charting, documentation) is the written account of care and observations.*

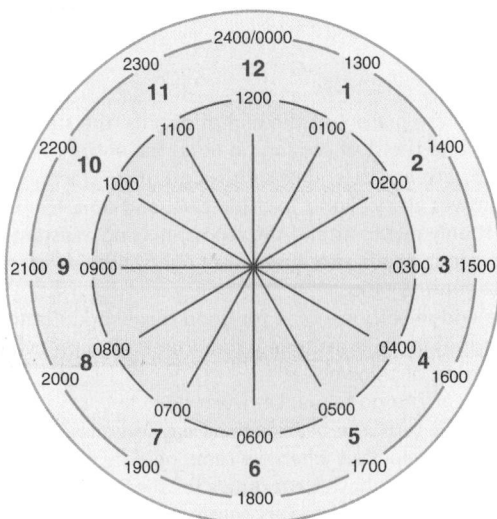

FIGURE 7-6 The 24-hour clock. The AM times are in orange. The PM times are in purple. Note: 12 noon is 1200; 12 midnight is 2400 or 0000.

BOX 7-1	24-Hour Clock		
AM		**PM**	
Conventional Time	24-Hour Time	Conventional Time	24-Hour Time
12:00 MIDNIGHT	0000 or 2400	12:00 NOON	1200
1:00 AM	0100	1:00 PM	1300
2:00 AM	0200	2:00 PM	1400
3:00 AM	0300	3:00 PM	1500
4:00 AM	0400	4:00 PM	1600
5:00 AM	0500	5:00 PM	1700
6:00 AM	0600	6:00 PM	1800
7:00 AM	0700	7:00 PM	1900
8:00 AM	0800	8:00 PM	2000
9:00 AM	0900	9:00 PM	2100
10:00 AM	1000	10:00 PM	2200
11:00 AM	1100	11:00 PM	2300

FOCUS ON MATH

Reporting and Recording Time

A *digit* is any number from 0 to 9. With conventional time, 3 or 4 digits are used. With 24-hour time, 4 digits are used. To change conventional time to 24-hour time with 4 digits, do the following.

- When an AM time has 3 digits (from 1:00 AM to 9:59 AM), remove the colon and add 0 as the first digit. For example:
  - Add 0 to 1:00 AM for 0100.
  - Add 0 to 7:30 AM for 0730.
  - Add 0 to 9:59 AM for 0959.
- When an AM or 12:00 PM time has 4 digits (10:00 AM to 12:59 PM), simply remove the colon. For example:
  - 10:00 AM becomes 1000.
  - 11:15 AM becomes 1115.
  - 12:59 PM becomes 1259.
- For PM times, remove the colon and add 1200 to the time. For example:
  - 1:00 PM becomes 1300 by adding 100 and 1200.
    (100 + 1200 = 1300)
  - 4:30 PM becomes 1630 by adding 430 and 1200.
    (430 + 1200 = 1630)
  - 10:40 PM becomes 2240 by adding 1040 and 1200.
    (1040 + 1200 = 2240)
  Some agencies use 0000 for midnight. Others use 2400.

For example:
- 12:05 AM may be written as 0005 or 2405.
- 12:58 AM may be written as 0058 or 2458.

Follow agency policy.

Reporting and Recording Time

The 24-hour clock (military time or international time) has 4 digits (Fig. 7-6). The first 2 digits are for the hours: 0100 = 1:00 AM; 1300 = 1:00 PM. The last 2 digits are for minutes: 0110 = 1:10 AM. Colons and AM and PM are not used. Box 7-1 shows how "conventional time" is written in "24-hour time."

See *Focus on Math: Reporting and Recording Time.*

See *Focus on Communication: Reporting and Recording Time.*

FOCUS ON COMMUNICATION

Reporting and Recording Time

You must use AM and PM with conventional time. Someone may forget to use AM or PM. Writing may be unclear. The correct time is not communicated. Harm to the person could result. How you read and report 24-hour time is important.
- When a 24-hour time begins with zero (0) read or say the "0" as "zero" or "oh."
- When the last 2 digits (minutes) end in "00," read or say the numbers as "hundred hours." For example:
  - 0200 is read as "zero two hundred hours" or "oh two hundred hours."
  - 1000 is read as "ten hundred hours."
- When the last 2 digits are numbers other than 2 zeros (00), read or say the first 2 numbers (hours) and the last 2 numbers (minutes). Follow the last 2 numbers with "hundred hours." For example:
  - 1215 is read as "twelve fifteen hundred hours."
  - 1620 is read as "sixteen twenty hundred hours."

Reporting

Report care and observations to the nurse:
- When there is a change from normal or a change in the person's condition. Report these changes at once.
- When the nurse asks you to do so.
- When you leave the unit for meals, breaks, or other reasons.
- Before the end-of-shift report.
  When reporting, follow the rules in Box 7-2, p. 74.
  See *Teamwork and Time Management: Reporting.*

TEAMWORK AND TIME MANAGEMENT

Reporting

The nurse needs your full attention when reporting. If distracted, you could omit or forget to report important things.

Nurses must give their full attention when receiving reports. If someone is reporting to a nurse, do not interrupt unless the matter is urgent. You must not distract the nurse.

BOX 7-2	Rules for Reporting

- Be prompt, thorough, and accurate.
- Give the person's name and room and bed number.
- Give the time your observations were made or the care was given. Use conventional time (AM or PM) or 24-hour clock time according to agency policy.
- Report only what you observed and did yourself.
- Report care measures that you expect the person to need. For example, the person may need the bedpan during your meal break.
- Report expected changes in the person's condition. For example, the person may be tired after lunch.
- Give reports as often as the person's condition requires. Or give them when the nurse asks you to.
- Report at once any changes from normal or changes in the person's condition. See Chapter 8.
- Use your written notes to give a specific, concise, and clear report (Fig. 7-7).

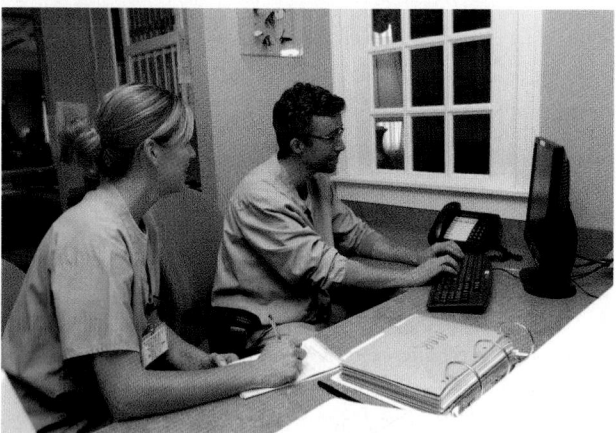

FIGURE 7-7 The nursing assistant uses notes to report to the nurse.

End-of-Shift Report. *The nurse gives a report at the end of the shift to the on-coming shift. This is called the **end-of-shift report** or change-of-shift report.* The nurse reports about:
- The care given
- The care to give during other shifts
- The person's current condition
- Likely changes in the person's condition

In some agencies, the entire nursing team hears the end-of-shift report as they come on duty. In other agencies, only nurses hear the report. After the report, information is shared with nursing assistants.

See *Teamwork and Time Management: End-of-Shift Report.*

See *Promoting Safety and Comfort: End-of-Shift Report.*

TEAMWORK AND TIME MANAGEMENT
End-of-Shift Report

Two staffs are present at the end of a shift—the staff going off duty and the staff coming on duty. The entire on-coming shift may attend the end-of-shift report. If so, staff going off duty answer all call lights, provide care, and tend to routine tasks. If only nurses attend the report, nursing assistants of the on-coming shift also answer call lights, provide care, and tend to routine tasks.

The end-of-shift is a time for good teamwork. Continue to do your job. Your attitude is important. If going off duty, avoid saying or thinking:
- "I'm ready to go home. Let them do it."
- "It's their turn. I've been here all day (evening or night)."
- "No one helped us when we came on duty."

Some agencies have clear duties for the 2 shifts. For example, those going off duty continue to answer call lights. They know about changes in the person's condition and care plan and about new orders. They also know about the care needs of new patients or residents. The on-coming shift has yet to learn this information. The on-coming shift uses this time to perform routine tasks and to collect needed supplies and equipment.

PROMOTING SAFETY AND COMFORT
End-of-Shift Report

Safety
You may not hear the end-of-shift report as you come on duty. Yet you need to answer call lights and give care before the nurse shares new information with you. To give safe care:
- Check the care plan and Kardex (care summary) before granting a request. The person's condition or care plan may have changed. There may be new doctor's orders.
- Ask a nurse about the care needs of new patients or residents. If the need is urgent, politely interrupt the end-of-shift report to ask your questions.
- Do not take directions or orders from another nursing assistant. Remember, nursing assistants cannot supervise or delegate to other nursing assistants.

Recording

When recording (documenting, charting), you must communicate clearly and thoroughly. Follow the rules in Box 7-3. The sample in Figure 7-8 shows how the rules apply for paper charting. Anyone who reads your charting should know:
- What you observed
- What you did
- The person's response

See *Focus on Communication: Recording.*

BOX 7-3 Rules for Recording

General Rules

- Follow agency policies and procedures for recording. Ask for needed training.
- Include the date and time for every recording. Use conventional time (AM or PM) or 24-hour time according to agency policy.
- Use only agency-approved abbreviations (p. 80).
- Use correct spelling, grammar, and punctuation.
- Do not use ditto marks.
- Sign or save all entries as required by agency policy.
- Check the name and identifying information on the chart. You must record on the correct chart.
- Record only what you observed and did yourself. Do not record for another person.
- Never chart a procedure, treatment, or care measure until after it is completed.
- Be accurate, concise, and factual. Do not record judgments or interpretations.
- Record in a logical manner and in sequence.
- Be descriptive. Avoid terms with more than 1 meaning.
- Use the person's exact words whenever possible. Use quotation marks ("...") to show a direct quote.
- Chart any changes from normal or changes in the person's condition. Also chart that you told the nurse (include the nurse's name), what you said, and the time you made the report.
- Do not omit information.
- Record safety measures. Examples include placing the call light within reach, assisting the person when up, or reminding a person not to get out of bed.

On Computer

- Log in using your username and password. Do not chart using another person's username.
- Check the time your entry is made. Make sure it is the right time.
- Check for accuracy. Review your entry before saving.
- Save your entries. Un-saved data will be lost.
- Follow the manufacturer's instructions for changing or un-charting a mistaken entry. Most electronic systems keep a record of an entry before a change was made. The first entry is still visible.
- Log off when done charting. This prevents others from charting under your username.
- See "Computers and Other Electronic Devices."

On Paper

- Make sure each form has the person's name and other identifying information.
- Always use ink. Use the ink color required by the agency.
- Make sure writing is readable and neat.
- Never erase or use correction fluid. Draw a line through the incorrect part. Date and initial the line. Write "mistaken entry" over it if this is agency policy. Then re-write the part. Follow agency policy for correcting errors.
- Sign your entries. Include your name and title.
- Do not skip lines. Draw a line through the blank space of a partially completed line or to the end of the page. This prevents others from recording in a space with your signature.

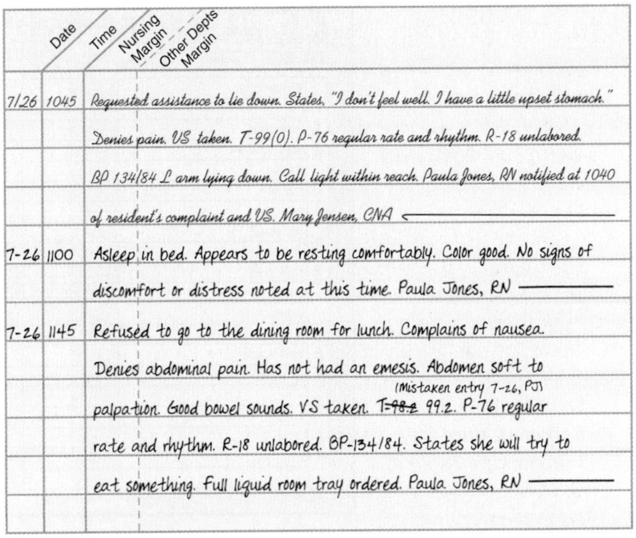

Date	Time	Nursing Margin / Other Depts Margin
7/26	1045	Requested assistance to lie down. States, "I don't feel well. I have a little upset stomach."
		Denies pain. VS taken. T-99(0). P-76 regular rate and rhythm. R-18 unlabored.
		BP 134/84 L arm lying down. Call light within reach. Paula Jones, RN notified at 1040
		of resident's complaint and VS. Mary Jensen, CNA ———
7-26	1100	Asleep in bed. Appears to be resting comfortably. Color good. No signs of
		discomfort or distress noted at this time. Paula Jones, RN ———
7-26	1145	Refused to go to the dining room for lunch. Complains of nausea.
		Denies abdominal pain. Has not had an emesis. Abdomen soft to
		palpation. Good bowel sounds. VS taken. T-~~98.2~~ (Mistaken entry 7-26, PJ) 99.2. P-76 regular
		rate and rhythm. R-18 unlabored. BP-134/84. States she will try to
		eat something. full liquid room tray ordered. Paula Jones, RN ———

FIGURE 7-8 Charting sample on paper.

FOCUS ON COMMUNICATION

Recording

"Small," "moderate," "large," "long," and "short" mean different things to different people. Is small the size of a dime? Or is it the size of a quarter? In health care, different meanings can cause serious problems. Give accurate descriptions and measurements. If you have a question, ask the nurse to look at what you are trying to describe.

Electronic Recording. Electronic health records (EHRs) and electronic medical records (EMRs) improve access to the person's medical record. In many agencies, recording is done in patients' or residents' rooms, in hallways, at the nurses' station, or on portable devices. Users log in to access the record (Fig. 7-9, p. 76). You will be trained to use your agency's system.

COMPUTERS AND OTHER ELECTRONIC DEVICES

Computer systems collect, send, record, and store information (data). Data are retrieved when needed.

Computers and faxes are used to send messages and reports to the nursing unit. This reduces clerical work and phone calls. And data are sent with greater speed and accuracy.

Each staff member using computers and other electronic devices has a username and password. They are used to access, send, receive, or store protected health information (PHI).

You must follow the agency's policies when using computers and other electronic devices. You must keep PHI and electronic protected health information (ePHI, EPHI) confidential. Follow the rules in Box 7-4 and the ethical and legal rules about privacy, confidentiality, and defamation (Chapters 5 and 6) when using computers and other electronic devices.

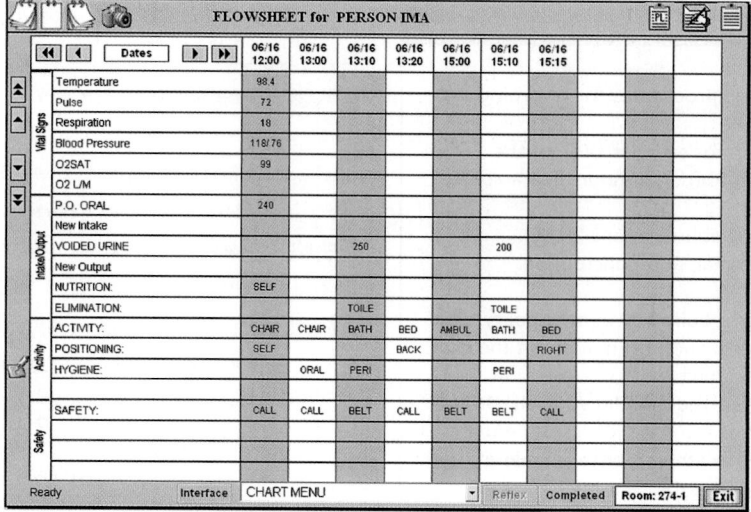

FLOWSHEET for PERSON IMA

Dates		06/16 12:00	06/16 13:00	06/16 13:10	06/16 13:20	06/16 15:00	06/16 15:10	06/16 15:15			
Vital Signs	Temperature	98.4									
	Pulse	72									
	Respiration	18									
	Blood Pressure	118/76									
	O2SAT	99									
	O2 L/M										
	P.O. ORAL	240									
Intake/Output	New Intake										
	VOIDED URINE			250			200				
	New Output										
	NUTRITION:	SELF									
	ELIMINATION:			TOILE			TOILE				
Activity	ACTIVITY:	CHAIR	CHAIR	BATH	BED	AMBUL	BATH	BED			
	POSITIONING:	SELF			BACK			RIGHT			
	HYGIENE:		ORAL	PERI			PERI				
Safety	SAFETY:	CALL	CALL	BELT	CALL	BELT	BELT	CALL			

| Ready | | Interface | CHART MENU | | Reflex | Completed | Room: 274-1 | Exit |

FIGURE 7-9 Electronic charting sample. (Courtesy Abraham Lincoln Memorial Hospital, Lincoln, Ill.)

BOX 7-4	**Computers and Other Electronic Devices**

Computers

- See "Wrongful Use of Electronic Communications" in Chapter 5.
- Do not tell anyone your username or password. If someone has your information, he or she can access, record, send, receive, or store EPHI (ePHI) under your name. It will be hard to prove that someone other than you did so.
- Do not write down, post, or expose your username or password. This is for your security. For example, do not write them on a note pad or post them at your work station.
- Change your password often. Follow agency policy.
- Do not use another person's username or password.
- Follow the rules for recording (see Box 7-3).
- Enter data carefully. Double-check your entries.
- Prevent others from seeing what is on the screen.
  - Place the monitor so the screen cannot be seen in the hallway or by others.
  - Be aware of anyone standing behind you.
  - Stand or sit with your back to the wall if using a mobile computer unit.
  - Do not leave the computer unattended.
- Log off after making an entry.
- Do not leave printouts where others can read them or pick them up.
- Shred or destroy computer-printed documents or worksheets. Follow agency policy.
- Send e-mail and messages only to those needing the information.
- Do not use e-mail for information or messages that require immediate reporting. Give the report in person. The person may not read the e-mail in a timely manner.
- Do not use e-mail or messages to report confidential information. This includes addresses, phone numbers, and Social Security numbers. The computer system may not be secure.
- Remember that any communication can be read or heard by someone other than the intended person.
- Remember that deleted communications can be retrieved by authorized staff.

Computers—cont'd

- Do not use the agency's computer for personal use. Do not:
  - Send personal e-mail messages.
  - Send or receive e-mail or messages that are offensive, not legal, or sexual.
  - Send or receive e-mail for illegal activities, jokes, politics, gambling (including football and other pools), chain letters, or other non-work activities.
  - Post information, opinions, or comments on websites or video or social media sites (Facebook, Twitter, LinkedIn, YouTube, blogs and comments to blog postings, chat rooms, bulletin boards, and so on).
  - Upload, download, or send materials containing a copyright, trademark, or patent.
- Remember that the agency has the right to monitor your use of computers or other electronic devices. This includes Internet use.
- Do not open another person's e-mail or messages.
- Follow agency policy for mis-directed e-mails.

Faxes

- See "Wrongful Use of Electronic Communications" in Chapter 5.
- Use the agency's approved "cover sheet." The sheet has instructions about:
  - The confidentiality of PHI (EPHI; ePHI)
  - The receiver's responsibilities concerning PHI (EPHI; ePHI)
  - The receiver's responsibilities if the fax is received in error (mis-directed fax)
- Complete the "cover sheet" according to agency policy. The following is common.
  - Name of the person to receive the fax
  - Receiver's fax number
  - Date
  - Number of pages being faxed
  - Department name
  - Name and phone number of the employee sending the fax
- Follow agency policy for a mis-directed fax.
- Do not leave sent or received faxes unattended in the fax machine or lying around.

Computers are used for measurements such as blood pressures, temperatures, and heart rates. The computer senses normal and abnormal measurements. When the abnormal is sensed, an alarm alerts the nursing staff. Computer monitoring is common in hospitals and in skilled nursing units.

Computers and other electronic devices save time. Quality care and safety are increased. Fewer errors are made in recording. Records are more complete. Staff are more efficient.

PHONE COMMUNICATIONS

You will answer phones at the nurses' station or in the person's room. You need good communication skills. The caller cannot see you. But you give much information by your tone of voice, how clearly you speak, and your attitude. Act as if speaking to someone face-to-face. Be professional and courteous. Also practice good work ethics. Follow the agency's policy and the guidelines in Box 7-5.

See *Focus on Long-Term Care and Home Care: Phone Communications.*

BOX 7-5 | Answering Phones

- Answer the call after the first ring if possible. Be sure to answer by the fourth ring.
- Do not answer the phone in a rushed or hasty manner.
- Give a courteous greeting. Identify the nursing unit and give your name and title. For example: "Good morning, 3 center. Mark Wills, nursing assistant."
- Write this information when taking a message.
  - The caller's name and phone number (include the area code and extension number)
  - The date and time
  - The message
- Repeat the message and phone number back to the caller.
- Ask the caller to "Please hold" if necessary. First find out who is calling and the caller's number. Then ask if the caller can hold. Do not put callers with an emergency on hold.
- Do not lay the phone down or cover the receiver with your hand when not speaking to the caller. The caller may over-hear confidential conversations.
- Return to a caller on hold within 30 seconds. Ask if the caller can wait longer or if the call can be returned.
- Do not give confidential information to any caller. Patient, resident, and employee information is confidential. Refer such calls to the nurse.
- Transfer the call if appropriate.
  - Tell the caller that you are going to transfer the call.
  - Give the name of the department or the person's name who should answer the phone if appropriate.
  - Get the caller's name and number in case the call gets disconnected.
  - Give the caller the phone number in case the call gets disconnected or the line is busy.
- End the conversation politely. Thank the person for calling and say good-bye.
- Give the message to the appropriate person.

FOCUS ON LONG-TERM CARE AND HOME CARE

Phone Communications

Home Care

When answering phones in patients' homes, simply answer with "hello." This is for everyone's safety—the person, family, and you. The caller has too much information when you give the person's name ("Price residence") or your name and title.

People call homes for many reasons. Some make sales calls or to obtain donations. Others have criminal intent. They want to know who is there. Saying that you are a home health assistant tells that an ill, older, or disabled person is in the home. It is hard for these people to protect and defend themselves. They are easy prey for criminals.

Do not give your name or the person's name until you know who is calling and why. Make sure it is someone you want to talk to—the person's family or friend, your supervisor, or a caller expected by the person.

MEDICAL TERMS AND ABBREVIATIONS

Medical terms and abbreviations are used in health care. Someone may use a word or phrase that you do not understand. If so, ask a nurse to explain its meaning. Otherwise, communication does not occur. A medical dictionary is useful to learn new words.

Like all words, medical terms are made up of *parts of words or* **word elements**—prefixes, roots, and suffixes (Box 7-6, pp. 78-79). Most are from Greek or Latin. They are combined to form medical terms. To translate a term, the word is separated into its elements.

Prefixes, Roots, and Suffixes

A **prefix** *is a word element placed before a root. It changes the meaning of the word.* The prefix *olig* (scant, small amount) is placed before the root *uria* (urine) to make *oliguria*. It means a scant amount of urine. Prefixes are used with other word elements. Prefixes are never used alone.

The **root** *is the word element that contains the basic meaning of the word.* It is combined with another root, prefixes, or suffixes. A vowel (an *o* or an *i*) is added when 2 roots are combined or when a suffix is added to a root. The vowel makes the word easier to pronounce.

A **suffix** *is a word element placed after a root. It changes the meaning of the word.* Suffixes are not used alone. When translating medical terms, begin with the suffix. For example, *nephritis* means inflammation of the kidney. It was formed by combining *nephro* (kidney) and *itis* (inflammation).

BOX 7-6	Medical Terminology		
Prefix	**Meaning**	**Root (Combining Vowel)**	**Meaning**
a-, an-	without, not, lack of	arteri (o)	artery
ab-	away from	arthr (o)	joint
ad-	to, toward, near	bronch (o)	bronchus, bronchi
ante-	before, forward, in front of	card, cardi (o)	heart
anti-	against	cephal (o)	head
auto-	self	chole, chol (o)	bile
bi-	double, two (2), twice	chondr (o)	cartilage
brady-	slow	colo	colon, large intestine
circum-	around	cost (o)	rib
contra-	against, opposite	crani (o)	skull
de-	down, from	cyan (o)	blue
dia-	across, through, apart	cyst (o)	bladder, cyst
dis-	apart, free from	cyt (o)	cell
dys-	bad, difficult, abnormal	dent (o)	tooth
ecto-	outer, outside	derma	skin
en-	in, into, within	duoden (o)	duodenum
endo-	inner, inside	encephal (o)	brain
epi-	over, on, upon	enter (o)	intestines
eryth-	red	fibr (o)	fiber, fibrous
eu-	normal, good, well, healthy	gastr (o)	stomach
ex-	out, out of, from, away from	gloss (o)	tongue
hemi-	half	gluc (o)	sweetness, glucose
hyper-	excessive, too much, high	glyc (o)	sugar
hypo-	under, decreased, less than normal	gyn, gyne, gyneco	woman
in-	in, into, within, not	hem, hema, hemo, hemat (o)	blood
inter-	between	hepat (o)	liver
intra-	within	hydr (o)	water
intro-	into, within	hyster (o)	uterus
leuk-	white	ile (o), ili (o)	ileum
macro-	large	laparo	abdomen, loin, flank
mal-	bad, illness, disease	laryng (o)	larynx
meg-	large	lith (o)	stone
micro-	small	mamm (o)	breast, mammary gland
mono-	one (1), single	mast (o)	mammary gland, breast
neo-	new	meno	menstruation
non-	not	my (o)	muscle
olig-	small, scant	myel (o)	spinal cord, bone marrow
para-	beside, beyond, after	necro	death
per-	by, through	nephr (o)	kidney
peri-	around	neur (o)	nerve
poly-	many, much	ocul (o)	eye
post-	after, behind	oophor (o)	ovary
pre-	before, in front of, prior to	ophthalm (o)	eye
pro-	before, in front of	orth (o)	straight, normal, correct
re-	again, backward	oste (o)	bone
retro-	backward, behind	ot (o)	ear
semi-	half	ped (o)	child, foot
sub-	under, beneath	pharyng (o)	pharynx
super-	above, over, excess	phleb (o)	vein
supra-	above, over	pnea	breathing, respiration
tachy-	fast, rapid	pneum (o)	lung, air, gas
trans-	across	proct (o)	rectum
uni-	one (1)	psych (o)	mind
		pulmo	lung
Root (combining vowel)	**Meaning**	py (o)	pus
abdomin (o)	abdomen	rect (o)	rectum
aden (o)	gland	rhin (o)	nose
adren (o)	adrenal gland	salping (o)	eustachian tube, fallopian tube
angi (o)	vessel	splen (o)	spleen

BOX 7-6 Medical Terminology—cont'd

Root (Combining Vowel)	Meaning
sten (o)	narrow, constriction
stern (o)	sternum
stomat (o)	mouth
therm (o)	heat
thoraco	chest
thromb (o)	clot, thrombus
thyr (o)	thyroid
toxic (o)	poison, poisonous
toxo	poison
trache (o)	trachea
urethr (o)	urethra
urin (o)	urine
uro	urine, urinary tract, urination
uter (o)	uterus
vas (o)	blood vessel, vas deferens
ven (o)	vein
vertebr (o)	spine, vertebrae

Suffix	Meaning
-algia	pain
-asis	condition, usually abnormal
-cele	hernia, herniation, pouching
-centesis	puncture and aspiration of
-cyte	cell
-ectasis	dilation, stretching
-ectomy	excision, removal of
-emia	blood condition
-genesis	development, production, creation
-genic	producing, causing
-gram	record

Suffix	Meaning
-graph	a diagram, a recording instrument
-graphy	making a recording
-iasis	condition of
-ism	a condition
-itis	inflammation
-logy	the study of
-lysis	destruction of, decomposition
-megaly	enlargement
-meter	measuring instrument
-oma	tumor
-osis	condition
-pathy	disease
-penia	lack, deficiency
-phagia	to eat or consume, swallowing
-phasia	speaking
-phobia	an exaggerated fear
-plasty	surgical repair or re-shaping
-plegia	paralysis
-ptosis	falling, sagging, dropping down
-rrhage, rrhagia	excessive flow
-rrhaphy	stitching, suturing
-rrhea	flow, discharge
-scope	examination instrument
-scopy	examination using a scope
-stasis	maintenance, maintaining a constant level
-stomy, -ostomy	creation of an opening
-tomy, -otomy	incision, cutting into
-uria	condition of the urine

Forming Medical Terms. Medical terms are formed by combining word elements. Remember, prefixes always come before roots. Suffixes always come after roots. A root can be combined with prefixes, roots, and suffixes. For example:

- The prefix *dys* (difficult) is combined with the root *pnea* (breathing). This forms *dyspnea*. It means difficulty breathing.
- The root *mast* (breast) combined with the suffix *ectomy* (excision or removal) forms *mastectomy*. It means removal of a breast.
- Endocarditis has the prefix *endo* (inner), the root *card* (heart), and the suffix *itis* (inflammation). *Endocarditis* means inflammation of the inner part of the heart.

Abdominal Regions

The abdomen is divided into regions (Fig. 7-10, p. 80). They are used to describe the location of body structures, pain, or discomfort. The regions are:

- Right upper quadrant (RUQ)
- Left upper quadrant (LUQ)
- Right lower quadrant (RLQ)
- Left lower quadrant (LLQ)

Directional Terms

Certain terms describe the position of 1 body part in relation to another. These terms give the direction of the body part when a person is standing and facing forward (Fig. 7-11, p. 80).

- *Anterior (ventral)—at or toward the front of the body or body part*
- *Posterior (dorsal)—at or toward the back of the body or body part*
- *Proximal—the part nearest to the center or to the point of attachment*
- *Distal—the part farthest from the center or from the point of attachment*
- *Lateral—away from the mid-line; at the side of the body or body part*
- *Medial—at or near the middle or mid-line of the body or body part*

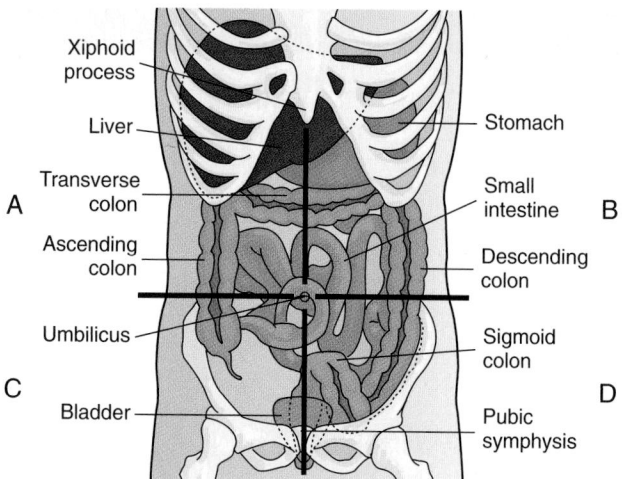

FIGURE 7-10 The 4 abdominal regions. **A,** Right upper quadrant. **B,** Left upper quadrant. **C,** Right lower quadrant. **D,** Left lower quadrant.

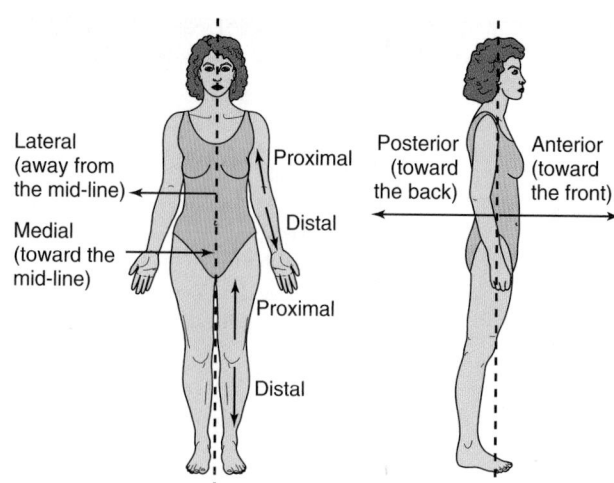

FIGURE 7-11 Directional terms describe the position of 1 body part in relation to another.

Abbreviations

Abbreviations are shortened forms of words or phrases. They save time and space when recording. Each agency has a list of accepted abbreviations. Obtain the list when you are hired. Use only those on the list. If not sure about using an abbreviation, write the term out in full. This promotes accurate communication.

Common abbreviations are on the inside of the back cover for easy use.

Common Terms and Phrases

Some terms and phrases apply to basic care and safety. Because they are used throughout this book, they are defined in Box 7-7. Some are presented as key terms in other chapters.

BOX 7-7	Common Health Care Terms and Phrases
abnormal	Different from what is normal or usual
activities of daily living (ADL)	The activities usually done during a normal day in a person's life
assistive (adaptive) device	Any item used by the person or staff to promote the person's function or safety (hand rails, grab bars, transfer lifts, canes, walkers, wheelchairs, and so on)
atrophy	The decrease in size or the wasting away of tissue
call light	Part of the call system allowing the person to signal the nurses' station for help
care plan	A written guide about the person's care
chronic	A disease or disorder lasting a long time, often for the rest of the person's life
cognitive function	Involves memory, thinking, reasoning, understanding, judgment, and behavior
contracture	The lack of joint mobility caused by abnormal shortening of a muscle
dementia	The loss of cognitive and social function caused by changes in the brain; the loss of cognitive function
drug	A substance taken by mouth, injected, or applied to treat or prevent a disease or condition; medication, medicine
dysphagia	Difficulty *(dys)* swallowing *(phagia)*
dyspnea	Difficult, labored, or painful *(dys)* breathing *(pnea)*
feces	The semi-solid mass of waste products in the colon that are expelled through the anus
fever	Elevated body temperature
Fowler's position	A semi-sitting position; the head of the bed is raised between 45 and 60 degrees
incontinence	Not being able to control urination (urinary incontinence) or bowel movements (fecal incontinence)
orientation; oriented	Awareness of one's self and others, one's location, and time; or awareness of one's surroundings
perineal	The genital and anal areas
pressure ulcer	A localized injury to the skin and/or underlying tissue usually over a bony prominence resulting from pressure or pressure in combination with shear; any lesion caused by unrelieved pressure that results in damage to underlying tissues
semi-Fowler's position	The head of the bed is raised 30 degrees; or the head of the bed is raised 30 degrees and the knee portion is raised 15 degrees
supine	The back-lying or dorsal recumbent position
vital signs	Temperature, pulse, respirations, and blood pressure (and pain in some agencies)
voiding	Emptying urine from the bladder; urinating, urination

FOCUS ON **PRIDE**

The Person, Family, and Yourself

Personal and Professional Responsibility

You are responsible for the information you report and record. It must be accurate. False or incomplete information can harm the person. If your agency allows nursing assistants to chart:

- Chart what you do. If not charted, there is no proof that you completed a task.
- Never falsify charting. Never chart that something was done when it really was not.
- Only chart after completing a task. If events change, your charting is wrong.
- Ask the nurse if you have questions about what or how to chart.

Rights and Respect

Many agencies conduct employee satisfaction surveys. The surveys allow you to share thoughts about your job with supervisors and co-workers. Surveys often ask about interactions with the health team.

You have the right to voice your true thoughts on a survey. When filling out a survey:

- Be honest. Positive and negative comments are important.
- Take the survey seriously. Do not rush. Answer the questions completely.
- Complete and return the form in a timely manner.

Surveys are 1 way agencies show respect for employees. Comments are used to make changes and improve communications with the health team. Take pride in your ideas. Your thoughts matter.

Independence and Social Interaction

Communication with the health team is not limited to reporting and recording. You interact in the nurses' station, hallways, break room, cafeteria, parking lot, and so on. Informal interactions carry over into working relationships. Treat co-workers with kindness and respect. Have a good attitude. Be someone others enjoy working with!

Delegation and Teamwork

You are responsible for your speech, actions, and charting. This is called being accountable. For example, you are delegated a task. You must complete the task and report or record its completion. If you do not complete the task, you are still held accountable. You must tell the nurse why it was not done. Or you must complete the task.

Do not be offended when asked if you completed a task or charted. This is part of accountability. The nurse must know what was done and what was not done. Show you are accountable by:

- Completing tasks in a timely manner
- Recording accurately
- Reporting when you complete a task
- Telling the nurse if a task was not done and why

Ethics and Laws

Truthful recording is taken seriously. Legal action can be taken against persons who record false information. For example:

A licensed nursing assistant (LNA) worked at a home health and hospice agency. On November 9, 2001, she recorded on a time sheet that she was in a patient's home for about 30 minutes. However, the patient was in the hospital from November 8 through November 14, 2001.

The LNA admitted to unprofessional conduct. Her conduct violated Administrative Rules of the Board of Nursing for:

- *Making inaccurate or misleading entries*
- *Failing to comply with federal or state laws or rules*
  The LNA was given a reprimand by the Board.
  (State of Vermont Board of Nursing, 2003.)

A *reprimand* means that the Board considered her conduct to be improper. However, the Board did not limit her right to work as an LNA.

You are accountable for the information you record. Take pride in honest and accurate recording.

FOCUS ON **PRIDE**: *Application*

Explain why accurate and timely reporting and recording are important. Make a list of ways to stay organized for prompt and accurate reporting and recording.

REVIEW QUESTIONS

Circle T if the statement is TRUE or F if it is FALSE.

1 T F Medical records communicate information about patients and residents.

2 T F Medical records are often electronic.

3 T F You help with Mrs. Gordon's care. Recording on her medical record violates her right to privacy.

4 T F Medical records can be used as evidence of the care given.

5 T F You can access all medical records in the agency.

6 T F When using a computer, the person's privacy must be protected.

7 T F You can give information about the person over the phone.

8 T F You should leave faxes in the fax machine for the nurse to read.

Continued

REVIEW QUESTIONS—cont'd

Circle the BEST answer.

9 To communicate well, you should
   a Use terms with many meanings
   b Give long descriptions
   c Use unfamiliar terms
   d Give facts and be specific

10 A person is discharged from the agency. His medical record is
   a Destroyed
   b Sent home with the family
   c Permanent
   d No longer private

11 You need to know if a resident uses a hearing aid. You should
   a Check the Kardex
   b Read the progress notes
   c Check the graphic sheet
   d Interrupt the end-of-shift report to ask the nurse

12 Where does the nurse describe the nursing care given?
   a Admission record
   b ADL flow sheet
   c Progress notes
   d Kardex

13 When recording,
   a Use pencil
   b Include the date and time
   c Erase errors
   d Sign entries with your first name only

14 These statements are about recording. Which is *true*?
   a Avoid using the person's exact words.
   b Record only what you did and observed.
   c Use correction fluid to cover a mistaken entry.
   d Chart a procedure before completing it.

15 In the evening, the clock shows 9:26. In 24-hour clock time this is
   a 9:26 PM
   b 1926
   c 0926
   d 2126

16 In the morning, the clock shows 7:45. In 24-hour clock time this is
   a 0745
   b 1945
   c 745
   d 7:45 AM

17 A suffix is
   a Placed at the beginning of a word
   b Placed after a root
   c A shortened form of a word or phrase
   d The main meaning of the word

18 Which word means a blood condition involving too much sugar?
   a Hepat-itis
   b Tachy-cardia
   c Hyper-glyc-emia
   d A-phasia

19 Which word means an excessive flow of blood?
   a Hemi-plegia
   b Cyan-osis
   c Laparo-scopy
   d Hemo-rrhage

20 You are asked to complete a task *stat*. "Stat" means
   a At once, immediately
   b As desired
   c Without moving the person
   d When necessary, as needed

21 Which definition below is *correct*?
   a *Contracture* is the decrease in size or wasting away of tissue.
   b *Dysphagia* is difficulty swallowing.
   c *Supine* is a sitting position with the head of the bed raised 45 degrees.
   d *Dyspnea* means elevated body temperature.

22 Which term relates to the side of the body?
   a Anterior
   b Lateral
   c Posterior
   d Proximal

23 You have access to the agency's computer. Which is *true*?
   a You should log off after making an entry.
   b E-mail is used for reports the nurse needs at once.
   c You can use another person's username if yours does not work.
   d You can use the computer for your personal needs.

24 A resident asks you to answer her phone. How should you answer?
   a "Good morning. Mrs. Park's room."
   b "Good morning. Third floor."
   c "Good morning. Tammy Brown, nursing assistant, speaking."
   d "Hello."

Answers to Chapter 7 questions are on p. 870.

FOCUS ON PRACTICE

Problem Solving

A resident tells you she has a headache. You tell the nurse. What do you record in the person's chart? What rules must you follow when reporting and recording? You made a mistake while recording. How do you correct the error?

Assisting With the Nursing Process

OBJECTIVES

- Define the key terms and key abbreviations in this chapter.
- Explain the purpose of the nursing process.
- Describe the 5 steps of the nursing process.
- Explain your role in each step of the nursing process.
- Explain the difference between objective data and subjective data.

- Identify the observations that you need to report to the nurse.
- Explain the purpose of care conferences.
- Explain how to use assignment sheets.
- Explain how to promote PRIDE in the person, the family, and yourself.

KEY TERMS

assessment Collecting information about the person; a step in the nursing process

evaluation To measure if goals in the planning step were met; a step in the nursing process

goal That which is desired for or by a person as a result of nursing care

implementation To perform or carry out nursing interventions (nursing measures or nursing actions) in the care plan; a step in the nursing process

medical diagnosis The identification of a disease or condition by a doctor

nursing care plan A written guide about the person's nursing care; care plan

nursing diagnosis Describes a health problem that can be treated by nursing measures; a step in the nursing process

nursing intervention An action or measure taken by the nursing team to help the person reach a goal; nursing action, nursing measure

nursing process The method nurses use to plan and deliver nursing care; its 5 steps are assessment, nursing diagnosis, planning, implementation, and evaluation

objective data Information that is seen, heard, felt, or smelled by an observer; signs

observation Using the senses of sight, hearing, touch, and smell to collect information

planning Setting priorities and goals; a step in the nursing process

signs See "objective data"

subjective data Things a person tells you about that you cannot observe through your senses; symptoms

symptoms See "subjective data"

KEY ABBREVIATIONS

BMs	Bowel movements	**MDS**	Minimum Data Set
CAA	Care Area Assessment	**OASIS**	Outcome and Assessment Information Set
CMS	Centers for Medicare & Medicaid Services	**RN**	Registered nurse
IDCP	Interdisciplinary care planning		

Nurses communicate with each other about the person's strengths, problems, needs, and care. This information is shared through the nursing process. The *nursing process is the method nurses use to plan and deliver nursing care. It has 5 steps.*

- *Assessment*
- *Nursing diagnosis*
- *Planning*
- *Implementation*
- *Evaluation*

The nursing process focuses on the person's nursing needs. The person and nursing team need good communication.

Each step is important. With good communication, nursing care is organized and has purpose. All nursing team members do the same things for the person. They have the same goals. The person feels safe and secure with consistent care.

The nursing process is used in all health care settings and for all age-groups. It is on-going. New information is gathered and the person's needs may change. However, the steps are the same. You will see how the nursing process is continuous as each step is explained (Fig. 8-1, p. 84).

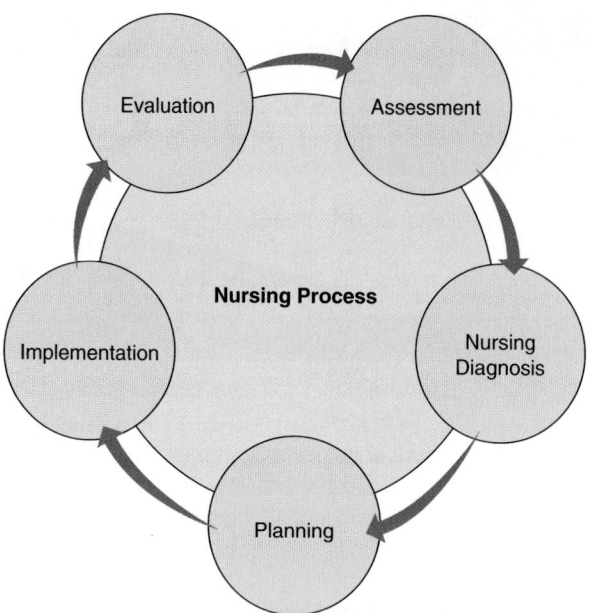

FIGURE 8-1 The nursing process is continuous.

- A change in the person's ability to respond
  - A responsive person no longer responds.
  - A non-responsive person now responds.
- A change in the person's mobility
  - The person cannot move a body part.
  - The person can now move a body part.
- Complaints of sudden, severe pain
- A sore or reddened area on the person's skin
- Complaints of a sudden change in vision
- Complaints of pain or difficulty breathing
- Abnormal respirations
- Complaints of or signs of difficulty swallowing
- Vomiting
- Bleeding
- Dizziness
- Vital signs outside their normal ranges—temperature, pulse, respirations, and blood pressure (Chapter 29)

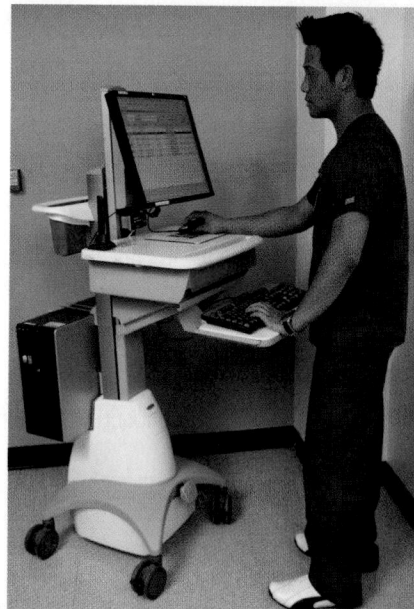

FIGURE 8-2 The nursing assistant uses an electronic device to note observations.

ASSESSMENT

Assessment involves collecting information about the person. The nurse takes a health history about current and past health problems. The family's health history is important. Many diseases are genetic. That is, the risk for certain diseases is inherited from parents. For example, a mother had breast cancer. Her daughters are at risk. The nurse reviews information from the doctor, test results, and past medical records.

An RN (registered nurse) assesses the person's body systems and mental status. You play a key role in assessment. You make many observations as you give care and talk to the person.

Observation is using the senses of sight, hearing, touch, and smell to collect information.

- You *see* how the person lies, sits, or walks. You see flushed or pale skin. You see red and swollen body areas.
- You *listen* to the person breathe, talk, and cough. You use a stethoscope to listen to the heartbeat and to measure blood pressure.
- Through *touch*, you feel if the skin is hot or cold, or moist or dry. You use touch to take the person's pulse.
- *Smell* is used to detect body, wound, and breath odors. You also smell odors from urine and bowel movements (BMs).

Objective data (signs) are seen, heard, felt, or smelled by an observer. You can feel a pulse. You can see urine color. *Subjective data (symptoms) are things a person tells you about that you cannot observe through your senses.* You cannot feel or see the person's pain, fear, or nausea.

Box 8-1 lists the observations to report at once. Box 8-2 lists the basic observations you need to make and report to the nurse. Make notes of your observations. Use them to report and record observations. Carry a note pad and pen in your pocket. Note your observations as you make them. The agency may provide electronic devices for recording (Fig. 8-2).

You do not assess. You are responsible for reporting and recording observations. The nurse assesses.

The assessment step never ends. New information is collected with every patient or resident contact. New observations are made. The person shares more information. Often the family adds more information.

See *Focus on Long-Term Care and Home Care: Assessment,* p. 86.

BOX 8-2	Basic Observations

Ability to Respond

- Is the person easy or hard to wake up?
- Can the person give his or her name, the time, and location when asked?
- Does the person identify others correctly?
- Does the person answer questions correctly?
- Does the person speak clearly?
- Are instructions followed correctly?
- Is the person calm, restless, or excited?
- Is the person conversing, quiet, or talking a lot?

Movement

- Can the person squeeze your fingers with each hand?
- Can the person move arms and legs?
- Are movements shaky or jerky?
- Does the person complain of stiff or painful joints?

Pain or Discomfort

- Where is the pain located? (Ask the person to point to the pain.)
- Does the pain go anywhere else?
- How does the person rate the severity of the pain—mild, moderate, severe?
- How does the person rate the pain on a scale of 0 to 10 (Chapter 31)?
- When did the pain begin?
- What was the person doing when the pain began?
- How long does the pain last?
- How does the person describe the pain?
  - Sharp
  - Severe
  - Knife-like
  - Dull
  - Burning
  - Aching
  - Comes and goes
  - Depends on position
- Was a pain-relief drug given?
- Did the pain-relief drug relieve pain? Is the pain still present?
- Is the person able to sleep and rest?
- What is the position of comfort?

Skin

- Is the skin pale or flushed?
- Is the skin cool, warm, or hot?
- Is the skin moist or dry?
- Does the skin appear mottled (blotchy, spotted with color)?
- What color are the lips and nail beds?
- Is the skin intact? Are there broken areas? If so, where?
- Are sores or reddened areas present? If yes, where?
- Are bruises present? Where are they located?
- Does the person complain of itching? If yes, where?

Eyes, Ears, Nose, and Mouth

- Is there drainage from the eyes? What color is the drainage?
- Are the eyelids closed? Do they stay open?
- Are the eyes reddened?
- Does the person complain of spots, flashes, or blurring?
- Is the person sensitive to bright lights?
- Is there drainage from the ears? What color is the drainage?
- Can the person hear? Is repeating necessary? Are questions answered correctly?

Eyes, Ears, Nose, and Mouth—cont'd

- Is there drainage from the nose? What color is the drainage?
- Can the person breathe through the nose?
- Is there breath odor?
- Does the person complain of a bad taste in the mouth?
- Does the person complain of painful gums or teeth?
- Do the person's gums bleed with oral hygiene (Chapter 22)?

Respirations

- Do both sides of the person's chest rise and fall with respirations?
- Is breathing noisy?
- Does the person complain of pain or difficulty breathing?
- What is the amount and color of sputum?
- What is the frequency of the person's cough? Is it dry or productive?

Bowels and Bladder

- Is the abdomen firm or soft?
- Does the person complain of gas?
- Which does the person use: toilet, commode, bedpan, or urinal?
- What are the amount, color, and consistency of bowel movements (BMs)?
- What is the frequency of BMs?
- Can the person control BMs?
- Does the person have pain or difficulty urinating?
- What is the amount of urine?
- What is the color of urine?
- Is the urine clear? Are there particles in the urine?
- Does urine have a foul smell?
- Can the person control the passage of urine?
- What is the frequency of urination?

Appetite

- Does the person like the food served?
- How much of the meal is eaten?
- What foods does the person like?
- Can the person chew food?
- What is the amount of fluid taken?
- What fluids does the person like?
- How often does the person drink fluids?
- Can the person swallow food and fluids?
- Does the person complain of nausea?
- What is the amount and color of vomitus?
- Does the person have hiccups?
- Is the person belching?
- Does the person cough when swallowing?

Activities of Daily Living

- Can the person perform personal care without help?
  - Bathing?
  - Brushing teeth?
  - Combing and brushing hair?
  - Shaving?
- Does the person feed himself or herself?
- Can the person walk?
- What amount and kind of help is needed?

Bleeding

- Is the person bleeding from any body part? If yes, where and how much?

NURSING DIAGNOSIS

The RN uses assessment information to make a nursing diagnosis. A *nursing diagnosis describes a health problem that can be treated by nursing measures.* See Box 8-3 for examples. The problem may exist or develop.

Nursing diagnoses and medical diagnoses are not the same. A *medical diagnosis is the identification of a disease or condition by a doctor.* Doctors use drugs, therapies, and surgery to cure or heal.

A person can have many nursing diagnoses. They deal with the total person—physical, emotional, social, and spiritual needs. Nursing diagnoses may change as assessment information changes. Or new ones are added. For example, "Pain: Acute" is added after surgery.

PLANNING

Planning involves setting priorities and goals. Nursing interventions (nursing measures or nursing actions) are chosen to help the person meet the goals. The person, family, and health team help the RN plan care.

Priorities relate to what is most important for the person. Maslow's theory of basic needs is useful for setting priorities (Chapter 9). The needs are arranged in order of importance. Some needs are required for life and survival (oxygen, water, and food). They must be met before all other needs. They have priority and must be done first.

Goals are then set. A *goal is that which is desired for or by a person as a result of nursing care.* Goals are aimed at the person's highest level of well-being and function—physical, emotional, social, and spiritual. Goals promote health and prevent health problems. They also promote rehabilitation.

BOX 8-3	Nursing Diagnoses Approved by the North American Nursing Diagnosis Association International (NANDA-I)

- Activity Intolerance; Activity Intolerance, Risk for
- Airway Clearance, Ineffective
- Anxiety
- Aspiration, Risk for
- Bleeding, Risk for
- Body Temperature, Risk for Imbalanced
- Breathing Pattern, Ineffective
- Comfort: Impaired, Readiness for Enhanced
- Communication: Readiness for Enhanced
- Confusion: Acute, Chronic, Risk for Acute
- Constipation; Constipation: Perceived, Risk for
- Dentition, Impaired
- Diarrhea
- Elimination: Impaired Urinary, Readiness for Enhanced Urinary
- Falls, Risk for
- Fatigue
- Fear
- Incontinence, Bowel
- Incontinence, Urinary: Functional; Overflow; Reflex; Stress; Urge; Urge, Risk for
- Infection, Risk for
- Injury, Risk for
- Insomnia

- Memory, Impaired
- Mobility: Impaired Bed, Impaired Physical, Impaired Wheelchair
- Nausea
- Nutrition, Imbalanced: Less Than Body Requirements
- Obesity
- Oral Mucous Membrane, Impaired
- Overweight; Overweight, Risk for
- Pain: Acute, Chronic
- Self-Care Deficit: Bathing, Dressing, Feeding, Toileting
- Self-Care, Readiness for Enhanced
- Skin Integrity: Impaired, Risk for Impaired
- Sleep Pattern, Disturbed
- Stress, Overload
- Suffocation, Risk for
- Suicide, Risk for
- Surgical Recovery, Delayed
- Swallowing, Impaired
- Tissue Integrity, Impaired
- Transfer Ability, Impaired
- Urinary Retention
- Walking, Impaired
- Wandering

Nursing interventions are chosen after goals are set. An *intervention* is an *action or measure*. A ***nursing intervention*** *(nursing action, nursing measure) is an action or measure taken by the nursing team to help the person reach a goal.* A nursing intervention does not need a doctor's order. However, some nursing measures come from a doctor's order. For example, a doctor orders that Mrs. Lange walk 50 yards 2 times a day. The nurse includes this order in the care plan.

The ***nursing care plan*** *(care plan) is a written guide about the person's nursing care.* It has the person's nursing diagnoses and goals. It also has the nursing measures or actions for each goal. The care plan is a communication tool.

- It communicates what care to give.
- It helps ensure that nursing team members give the same care.

Each agency has a care plan form. It is found in the medical record, on the Kardex, or on a computer (Fig. 8-3).

See *Focus on Surveys: Planning.*

FOCUS ON SURVEYS

Planning

During a survey, you may be asked about the person's care plan. Give honest and complete answers. You may be asked about:

- The person's goals
- Care measures
- How the care measures are carried out
- How you give input about the person's care needs and your observations

Nursing Diagnosis	Goal	Intervention
Constipation related to lack of privacy as evidenced by no BM for 5 days.	Patient will have regular BMs by 6/30.	Ask patient to use call light when urge to have BM is felt. Answer call light promptly. Assist patient to bathroom. Close bathroom door for privacy. Leave the room if the patient can be alone; tell the patient you are leaving and that you will return when the call light is on.
Insomnia related to noisy environment as evidenced by patient complaints of noise and lack of sleep.	Patient will report a restful sleep by 6/29.	Perform any necessary care measures before bedtime. Close the door to the patient's room. Turn off television or radio or keep volume low if patient prefers. Ask staff to avoid unnecessary talking outside the patient's room. Ask staff to speak in low voices. Turn off unneeded equipment.

FIGURE 8-3 Nursing care plan. Each nursing diagnosis has a goal. There are nursing interventions (nursing measures or nursing actions) for each goal.

Care Conferences

The RN may conduct a care conference to share information and ideas about the person's care. The purpose is to develop or revise the person's nursing care plan. Effective care is the goal. Nursing assistants usually take part in the conference.

The care plan is carried out. It may change as the person's nursing diagnoses change.

See *Focus on Communication: Care Conferences.*

See *Focus on Long-Term Care and Home Care: Care Conferences.*

IMPLEMENTATION

To *implement* means *to perform or carry out. The step of performing or carrying out nursing interventions (nursing measures or nursing actions) is called* **implementation.** Care is given.

Nursing care ranges from simple to complex. The nurse delegates tasks within your legal limits and job description. The nurse may ask you to assist with complex measures.

You report the care given to the nurse. In some agencies, you record the care given. Report and record *after* giving care, not before. Also report and record your observations. The nurse uses them for assessment. New observations may change the nursing diagnoses and the care plan. To give correct care, you must know about changes in the care plan.

FOCUS ON COMMUNICATION

Care Conferences

You see what patients and residents like and do not like. You see what they can and cannot do. Patients and residents talk to you. They tell you about their families and interests. You make observations every time you are with them. Share this information during care conferences. Also share ideas about the person's care. For example, you can say:
- "Mr. Antonio misses the fresh green beans and broccoli from his garden. Can he have those more often?"
- "Mrs. Clark can use her feet to propel her wheelchair. Why do we push her wheelchair?"
- "Miss Walsh never talks when her family visits. Yet she talks to her roommate all the time."

FOCUS ON LONG-TERM CARE AND HOME CARE

Care Conferences

Long-Term Care
The CMS requires 2 types of resident care conferences.
- *Interdisciplinary care planning (IDCP) conferences.* These are held to form care plans for new residents. They are also held regularly to review and update care plans. The RN, doctor, and other health team members attend.
- *Problem-focused conferences.* These are used when 1 problem affects a person's care. Only staff involved with the problem attend.

The person and family have the right to take part in planning conferences. The person may refuse actions suggested by the health team.

Problems identified on the MDS give *triggers* (clues) for the Care Area Assessments (CAAs) (Appendix C, p. 876).

CMS requires a *comprehensive care plan.* Like the nursing care plan, it is a written guide about the person's care. Developed by the health team, the person and family give input. The care plan has the person's problems, nursing diagnoses, and goals. It has the actions to help the person.

For example, Mr. Woo is weak from illness and no exercise. The MDS shows that he cannot do activities of daily living (ADL). This triggers the CAAs. A care plan is developed to solve the problem. The goal is for Mr. Woo to do his own ADL. Actions to help Mr. Woo reach the goal are:
- Occupational therapy to work with Mr. Woo on ADL daily
- Physical therapy to work with Mr. Woo on exercises daily
- Nursing staff to walk Mr. Woo 20 yards twice daily

The care plan also has the person's strengths. For example, Mr. Woo can feed himself. This strength increases his independence. The health team helps Mr. Woo continue to feed himself.

Assignment Sheet

Date: _9–10_
Shift: _Day_
Nursing assistant: _John Reed_
Supervisor: _Mary Adams, RN_

Breaks: _1000_   _1400_
Lunch: _1230_
Unit Tasks: _Pass drinking water at 0900_
Clean utility room at 1430

Check the care plan for other care measures and information

Room # _501A_ Name: _Mrs. Ann Lopez_ ID Number: _S1514491530_ Date of birth: _11/04/1925_ VS: _Daily at 0700_ T _____ P _____ R _____ BP _____ Wt: _Weekly (Monday at 0700)_ _____ Intake _____ Output _____ BM _____ Bath: Portable tub Shampoo Bed rails	**Functional status/other care measures and procedures** Total assist with ADL Stand-pivot transfers Uses w/c Incontinent of bowel and bladder – uses briefs Bilateral passive ROM exercises to extremities twice daily Turn and re-position q2h when in bed Wears eyeglasses and dentures Diet: High fiber (Total Assist)
Room # _510B_ Name: _Mr. Mark Lee_ ID Number: _D4468947762_ Date of birth: _12/29/1926_ VS: _2 times daily, at 0700 and 1500_ 0700: T _____ P _____ R _____ BP _____ 1500: T _____ P _____ R _____ BP _____ Wt: _Daily at 0700_ Intake _____ Output _____ BM _____ Bath: Shower	**Functional status/other care measures and procedures** Independent with ADL Independent with ambulation Attends exercise group every morning Continent of bowel and bladder – q4h bathroom schedule to maintain continence Wears eyeglasses Coughing and deep-breathing exercises q4h Diet: Sodium-controlled (Independent)

FIGURE 8-4 A sample assignment sheet. Note: This assignment sheet is a computer printout.

Assignment Sheets

The nurse communicates delegated tasks to you. An assignment sheet is used for this purpose (Fig. 8-4). The assignment sheet tells you about:

- Each person's care.
- What measures and tasks need to be done.
- Which nursing unit tasks to do. Cleaning utility rooms and stocking shower rooms are examples.

Talk to the nurse about an unclear assignment. Also check the care plan and Kardex or care summary if you need more information.

See *Focus on Communication: Assignment Sheets.*
See *Teamwork and Time Management: Assignment Sheets.*

TEAMWORK AND TIME MANAGEMENT

Assignment Sheets

Use your assignment sheet to organize your work and set priorities.

- What do you need to do first?
- What can you do while the person is having a meal?
- What can you do when the person is at an activity or a therapy (physical, occupational, and so on)?
- Do you need to reserve a room (shower room, tub room) or equipment (portable tub, shower chair)?
- What do you need help with?
- How many co-workers are needed to complete tasks such as turning and transferring a person?
- Ask a co-worker to help you. Tell what you need help with, when you need the help, and how long the task will take.
- Check off tasks as you complete them.

FOCUS ON **COMMUNICATION**

Assignment Sheets

Assignment sheets provide a summary of the information you need to care for your patients and residents. The sheets communicate information clearly and in an organized way. See Figure 8-4.

Use your assignment sheets to receive a report from the nurse. Add new information. Ask the nurse if you have questions. For example: "I have a question about Mr. Lee. My assignment sheet does not mention assistive devices. Last week physical therapy was helping him use a walker instead of his cane. Which is he using now?"

EVALUATION

Evaluate means *to measure*. The **evaluation** *step involves measuring if the goals in the planning step were met.* Progress is evaluated. Goals may be met totally, in part, or not at all. Assessment information is used for this step. Changes in nursing diagnoses, goals, and the care plan may result.

YOUR ROLE

The nursing process never ends. Nurses constantly collect information about the person. Nursing diagnoses, goals, and the care plan may change as the person's needs change.

You have a key role in the nursing process. Your observations are used for nursing diagnoses and planning. You may help develop care plans. In the implementation step, you perform tasks in the care plan. Your assignment sheet tells you what to do. Your observations are used for the evaluation step.

FOCUS ON **PRIDE**

The Person, Family, and Yourself

Personal and Professional Responsibility

In Chapter 29, you will learn how to measure vital signs—temperature, pulse, respirations, and blood pressure. Chapter 30 is about assisting with range-of-motion exercises and walking. And Chapter 34 is about collecting specimens. These are some ways that you assist with the nursing process.

How you perform these actions affects the person's care. You are responsible for doing these skills correctly. You will practice skills in your training. Practice them until you feel comfortable. Ask your instructor if you have questions about a skill. Take pride in learning to do your job well. Take your skills training seriously.

Rights and Respect

The person has the right to take part in care planning. The person also has the right to refuse actions suggested by the health team. The team works with the person to agree upon a plan of care that meets the person's needs and preferences.

For example, the health team suggests applying elastic stockings (Chapter 35) on Mr. Barton's legs to prevent blood clots. Mr. Barton says they are "too tight" and "uncomfortable." He refuses to wear them. The nurse speaks with Mr. Barton about trying a sequential compression device (Chapter 35) instead. The nurse explains that adjustable sleeves are placed on the lower legs. The sleeves attach to a pump. The pump inflates and deflates 1 sleeve at a time. Mr. Barton agrees to try the device.

Independence and Social Interaction

Patients and residents often feel a loss of independence. Being involved in care planning can help them feel in control of their care. Care planning begins when the person is admitted to the agency. The plan is focused on the person's needs. The plan is modified as needs change. It is an on-going process. The person is involved the whole time.

To help the person feel involved, you can:
- Listen to the person's needs and concerns.
- Ask about the person's preferences.
- Tell the nurse about your observations and ideas to improve care.

Delegation and Teamwork

Assignment sheets communicate the care and unit tasks delegated to you. If you have a problem with an assignment or task, politely tell the nurse. Do not complain. Give the reason. Not liking an assignment or task is not a good reason. The nurse will decide if a change is needed.

Ethics and Laws

Assignment sheets contain confidential information. Always keep your sheets with you. Do not leave them lying around for others to find. This violates the *Health Insurance Portability and Accountability Act of 1996* (Chapter 5). Before leaving work, place your assignment sheets in a wastebasket marked CONFIDENTIAL INFORMATION for shredding. Take pride in protecting the privacy and security of protected health information.

FOCUS ON **PRIDE**: *Application*

Explain the importance of your role in the nursing process. How do your observations, input, and care affect the person?

REVIEW QUESTIONS

Circle the BEST answer.

1 Which is a step in the nursing process?
   a Observation
   b Reporting
   c Evaluation
   d Assignment

2 The nursing process
   a Involves guidelines for care plans
   b Is a care conference
   c Involves an assignment sheet
   d Is the method nurses use to plan and deliver nursing care

3 What happens during assessment?
   a Goals are set.
   b Information is collected.
   c Nursing measures are carried out.
   d Progress is evaluated.

4 Which is a symptom?
   a Redness
   b Vomiting
   c Pain
   d Pulse rate of 78

5 Which is a sign?
   a Nausea
   b Headache
   c Dizziness
   d Dry skin

6 Which should you report at once?
   a The person had a bowel movement.
   b The person complains of sudden, severe pain.
   c The person does not like the food served for lunch.
   d The person complains of stiff, painful joints.

7 Which should you report at once?
   a The person can no longer move a body part.
   b The person answers questions correctly.
   c The person has a breath odor.
   d The person walked to the dining room.

8 Measures in the care plan are carried out. This is
   a A nursing diagnosis
   b Planning
   c Implementation
   d Evaluation

9 Which statement about the nursing process is *true*?
   a It is done without the person's input.
   b You are responsible for it.
   c It is used to communicate the person's care.
   d Steps can be done in any order.

10 Which statement about care conferences is *true*?
   a The person's family is not involved.
   b Any staff member can attend.
   c You do not share ideas about the person's care.
   d The person can refuse suggested actions.

11 The care plan is
   a Written by the doctor
   b The measures to help the person
   c The same for all persons
   d Also called the Kardex

12 To communicate delegated tasks to you, the nurse uses
   a The care plan
   b The Kardex
   c An assignment sheet
   d Care conferences

13 Which is a nursing diagnosis?
   a Cancer
   b Heart attack
   c Kidney failure
   d Chronic pain

14 Your role in the nursing process involves
   a Reporting observations
   b Making nursing diagnoses
   c Writing the care plan
   d Evaluating if goals are met

Answers to Chapter 8 questions are on p. 870.

FOCUS ON PRACTICE

Problem Solving

Mrs. Trent had a stroke. She cannot speak and needs help with ADL. You finish brushing her hair. Her daughter enters the room and says: "No one does Mom's hair the way she likes it." How will you respond?

Mrs. Trent's daughter often tells you about her mother's preferences. Should these comments be shared? Explain the family's role in planning care. Explain your role.

Understanding the Person

OBJECTIVES

- Define the key terms in this chapter.
- Identify the parts that make up the whole person.
- Explain how to properly address the person.
- Explain Abraham Maslow's theory of basic needs.
- Explain how culture and religion influence health and illness.
- Identify the emotional and social effects of illness.
- Describe the persons cared for in health care agencies.
- Identify the elements needed for good communication.
- Describe how to use verbal and nonverbal communication.

- Explain the methods and barriers to good communication.
- Explain how to communicate with persons who have disabilities or who are comatose.
- Explain why family and visitors are important to the person.
- Identify courtesies given to the person, family, and friends.
- Explain how to communicate with persons who have behavior problems.
- Explain how to promote PRIDE in the person, the family, and yourself.

KEY TERMS

bariatrics The field of medicine focused on the treatment and control of obesity

body language Messages sent through facial expressions, gestures, posture, hand and body movements, gait, eye contact, and appearance

comatose Being unable to respond to stimuli

culture The characteristics of a group of people—language, values, beliefs, habits, likes, dislikes, customs—passed from 1 generation to the next

disability Any lost, absent, or impaired physical or mental function

esteem The worth, value, or opinion one has of a person

geriatrics The field of medicine concerned with the problems and diseases of old age and older persons

holism A concept that considers the whole person; the whole person has physical, social, psychological, and spiritual parts that are woven together and cannot be separated

morbid obesity The person weighs 100 pounds or more over his or her normal weight

need Something necessary or desired for maintaining life and mental well-being

nonverbal communication Communication that does not use words

obesity Having an excess amount of total body fat; body weight is 20% or more above what is normal for the person's height and age

obstetrics The field of medicine concerned with the care of women during pregnancy, labor, and childbirth and for 6 to 8 weeks after birth

optimal level of function A person's highest potential for mental and physical performance

paraphrasing Re-stating the person's message in your own words

pediatrics The field of medicine concerned with the growth, development, and care of children—newborns to teenagers

psychiatry The field of medicine concerned with mental health disorders

religion Spiritual beliefs, needs, and practices

self-actualization Experiencing one's potential

self-esteem Thinking well of oneself and seeing oneself as useful and having value

verbal communication Communication that uses written or spoken words

The patient or resident is the most important person in the agency. Age, religion, and nationality make each person unique. So do culture, education, occupation, and life-style. Each person is special and has value. The person is treated with respect—as someone who thinks, acts, feels, and makes decisions.

CARING FOR THE PERSON

For effective care, you must consider the whole person. *Holism* means *whole*. *Holism is a concept that considers the whole person. The whole person has physical, social, psychological, and spiritual parts. These parts are woven together and cannot be separated* (Fig. 9-1).

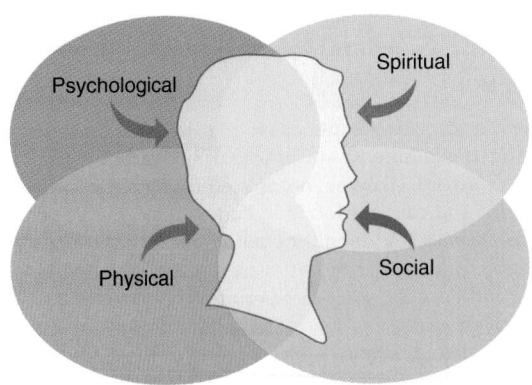

FIGURE 9-1 A person is a physical, psychological, social, and spiritual being. The parts overlap and cannot be separated.

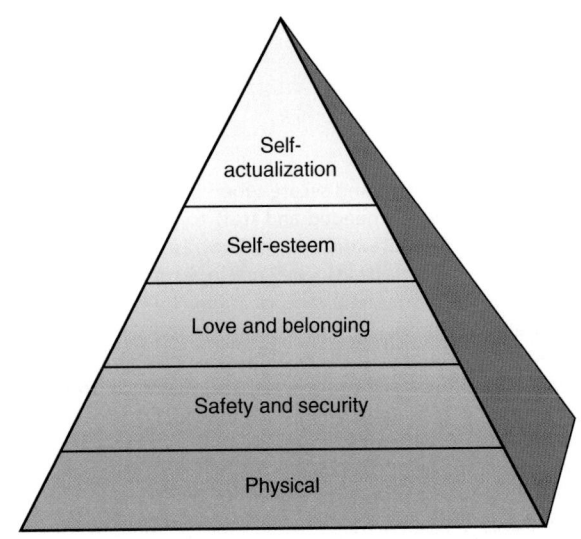

FIGURE 9-2 Basic needs for life as described by Maslow. (Redrawn from Maslow AH, Frager RD (Editor), Fadiman J (Editor): *Motivation and personality*, ed 3. © 1987. Reprinted with permission of Ann Kaplan.)

Each part relates to and depends on the others. As a social being, a person speaks and communicates with others. Physically, the brain, mouth, tongue, lips, and throat structures must function for speech. Communication is also psychological. It involves thinking and reasoning.

Holistic care involves the whole person. To consider only the physical part is to ignore the person's ability to think, make decisions, and interact with others. It also ignores the person's experiences, life-style, culture, religion, joys, sorrows, and needs.

Disability and illness affect the whole person. For example, Mrs. Beal had a stroke. She needs help with physical needs in a nursing center. She had to leave her home. Relationships with her husband and children are changed. She is angry with God for letting this happen to her. The health team plans care to help her deal with her problems.

Addressing the Person

You must know and respect the whole person for effective, quality care. Too often a person is referred to as a room number. For example: "12A needs the bedpan" rather than "Mrs. Brown in 12A needs the bedpan." This strips the person of his or her identity. It reduces the person to a "thing."

Patients and residents are not "things." They are not your family or children. They are complex human beings. To address patients and residents with dignity and respect:
- Use their titles—Mrs. Jones, Mr. Smith, Miss Turner, Ms. Norris, or Dr. Gonzalez.
- Do not call them by their first names or any other name unless they ask you to.
- Do not call them Grandma, Papa, Sweetheart, Honey, or other names.

BASIC NEEDS

A *need is something necessary or desired for maintaining life and mental well-being.* According to Abraham Maslow, a famous psychologist, basic needs must be met for a person to survive and function. In this theory, needs are arranged in order of importance (Fig. 9-2). Lower-level needs must be met before higher-level needs. Basic needs, from the lowest level to the highest level, are:
- Physical needs
- Safety and security needs
- Love and belonging needs
- Self-esteem needs
- The need for self-actualization

People normally meet their own needs. Disease, injury, or advanced age may prevent them from doing so. Ill or injured persons usually seek health care.

Physical Needs

Oxygen, food, water, elimination, rest, and shelter are needed to live and survive. A person dies within minutes without oxygen. Without food or water, weakness and illness occur within a few hours. The kidneys and intestines must function. If not, poisonous wastes build up in the blood and can cause death. Without enough rest and sleep, a person becomes very tired. Without shelter, the person is exposed to extremes of heat and cold.

Safety and Security Needs

The person needs to feel safe from harm, danger, and fear. Many people are afraid of health care agencies. Some care involves strange equipment. Some care causes pain or discomfort. People feel safe and more secure if they know what will happen. For every task, even a simple bath, the person should know:
- Why it is needed
- Who will do it
- How it will be done
- What sensations or feelings to expect

See *Focus on Long-Term Care and Home Care: Safety and Security Needs*, p. 94.

Safety and Security Needs

Long-Term Care

Some people feel safe and secure when in a nursing center. They have help when needed and staff to protect them. Others do not feel safe and secure. They are not in their usual, secure home settings. They are in a strange place with strange routines. Strangers care for them. Some become scared and confused.

Show new residents their setting. Listen to their concerns. Explain all routines and procedures. You may have to repeat information often—sometimes for many days or weeks until the person feels safe and secure. Be patient, kind, and understanding.

Love and Belonging Needs

Love and belonging needs (emotional needs) relate to love, closeness, and affection. They also involve meaningful relationships with others. Some people become weaker or die from the lack of love and belonging. This is seen in children and in older persons who have out-lived family and friends. Family, friends, and the health team can meet love and belonging needs.

Self-Esteem Needs

Esteem is the worth, value, or opinion one has of a person. *Self-esteem means to think well of oneself and to see oneself as useful and having value.* People often lack self-esteem when ill, injured, older, or disabled. For example:

- An older man built his home and worked a farm. He supported and raised a family. Now he cannot dress or feed himself.
- A woman lost her hair from cancer treatments. She does not feel attractive or whole.
- A person has a slow, crippling disease.
- A person had a leg amputated.

You must treat all persons with respect. While it takes more time, encourage them to do as much for themselves as possible. This helps increase self-esteem.

The Need for Self-Actualization

Self-actualization means experiencing one's potential. It involves learning, understanding, and creating to the limit of a person's ability. This is the highest need. Rarely, if ever, is it totally met. Most people constantly try to learn and understand more. This need can be postponed and life will continue.

CULTURE AND RELIGION

Culture is the characteristics of a group of people—language, values, beliefs, habits, likes, dislikes, and customs. They are passed from 1 generation to the next. The person's culture influences health beliefs and practices. Culture also affects thinking and behavior during illness and when in a hospital or nursing center.

✿ CARING ABOUT CULTURE

Health Care Beliefs

Some *Mexican Americans* believe that illness is caused by prolonged exposure to hot or cold. If hot causes illness, cold is used for cure. Likewise, hot is used for illnesses caused by cold. Hot and cold are found in body organs, medicines (drugs), the air, and food. Hot conditions include fever, infection, rashes, sore throat, diarrhea, and constipation. Cold conditions include cancer, joint pain, earache, and stomach cramps.

The hot-cold balance is also a belief of some *Vietnamese Americans*. Illnesses, food, drugs, and herbs are hot or cold. Hot is given to balance cold illnesses. Cold is given for hot illnesses.

Modified from Giger JN: Transcultural nursing: assessment and intervention, ed 6, St Louis, 2013, Mosby.

✿ CARING ABOUT CULTURE

Sick Care Practices

Folk practices are common among some *Vietnamese Americans*. They include *cao gio* ("rub wind")—rubbing the skin with a coin to treat the common cold. Skin pinching (*bat gio*—"catch wind") is for headaches and sore throats. Herbs, oils, and soups are used for many signs and symptoms.

Some *Russian Americans* practice folk medicine. Herbs are taken through drinks or enemas. For headaches, an ointment is placed behind the ears and temples and at the back of the neck. Treatment for back pain involves placing a dough of dark rye flour and honey on the spine.

Some *Mexican Americans* use folk healers. A *yerbero* uses herbs and spices to prevent or cure disease. A *curandero* (*curandera* if female) deals with serious physical and mental illnesses. Witches use magic. A *brujos* is a male witch. A *brujas* is a female witch.

Modified from Giger JN: Transcultural nursing: assessment and intervention, ed 6, St Louis, 2013, Mosby.

People come from many cultures, races, and nationalities. Their family practices and food choices may differ from yours. So might their hygiene habits and clothing styles. Some speak a foreign language. Some cultures have beliefs about what causes and cures illness. (See *Caring About Culture: Health Care Beliefs.*) They may perform rituals to rid the body of disease. (See *Caring About Culture: Sick Care Practices.*) Many cultures have health beliefs and rituals about dying and death (Chapter 55). Culture also is a factor in communication.

Religion relates to spiritual beliefs, needs, and practices. Religions may have beliefs about daily living, behaviors, relationships with others, diet, healing, days of worship, birth and birth control, drugs, and death.

Many people find comfort and strength from religion during illness. They may want to pray and observe religious practices. Hospitals and nursing centers offer religious services. Many have chapels or meditation areas for prayer (Fig. 9-3). Assist the person to attend services as needed. Some residents leave nursing centers to worship.

A person may want to see a cleric (Chapter 1). If so, tell the nurse. Make sure the room is neat and orderly. Have a chair ready for the cleric. Provide privacy during the visit.

The nursing process reflects the person's culture and religion. The care plan includes the person's cultural and religious practices.

You must respect the person's culture and religion. You will meet people from many cultures and religions. Learn about their beliefs and practices. This helps you understand the person and give better care.

A person may not follow all the beliefs and practices of his or her culture or religion. Some people do not practice a religion. Each person is unique. Do not judge the person by your standards. And do not force your ideas on the person.

See *Focus on Communication: Culture and Religion.*

See *Focus on Long-Term Care and Home Care: Culture and Religion.*

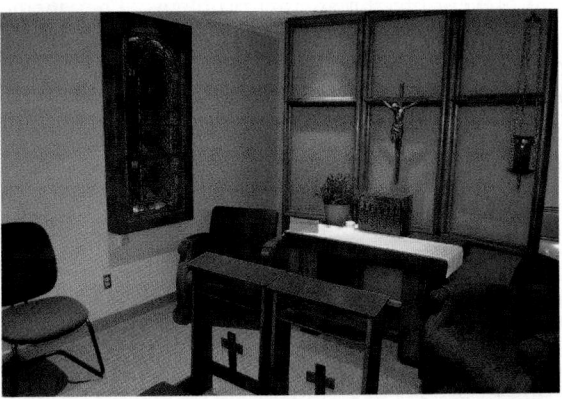

FIGURE 9-3 A hospital chapel provides a quiet area for prayer. (Courtesy Gene Vogelgesang, Illinois Valley Community Hospital, Peru, Illinois.)

EFFECTS OF ILLNESS AND DISABILITY

People do not choose illness or injury. Physical, psychological, and social effects occur. Disabilities may result. A *disability is any lost, absent, or impaired physical or mental function.* It may be temporary or permanent.

Normal activities—work, driving, fixing meals, yard work, hobbies—may be hard or impossible. Daily activities bring pleasure, worth, and contact with others. People often feel angry, upset, and useless when unable to perform them. These feelings may increase if help is needed with routine functions.

Fears of death, disability, chronic illness, and loss of function are common. Some people explain why they are afraid. Others do not share feelings. Some fear being laughed at for being afraid. A person with a broken leg may fear having a limp or not walking again. Surgery may bring fears of cancer. These feelings are normal and expected. You need to understand the effects of illness and disability. How would you feel and react if you had the person's problems?

Sometimes recovery is delayed or does not occur. Then the psychological and social effects of illness or disability become greater.

Anger is a common response to illness and disability. Persons needing nursing center care are often angry. They may direct anger at you. However, they are usually angry at the situation. You might have problems dealing with a person's anger. If so, ask the nurse for help. (See "Behavior Issues," p. 104.)

You can help the person feel safe, secure, and loved. Take an extra minute to "visit," to hold a hand, or to give a hug. (Remember to maintain professional boundaries. See Chapter 5.) Show that you are willing to help with personal needs. Respond promptly. Treat each person with respect and dignity.

See *Focus on Long-Term Care and Home Care: Effects of Illness and Disability.*

FOCUS ON **COMMUNICATION**

Culture and Religion

Hospitals and nursing centers ask about culture and religion on admission. The care plan communicates practices to include in the person's care. Check the care plan for the person's preferences. You can also ask: "Do you have any cultural or religious practices that should be part of your care?"

FOCUS ON **LONG-TERM CARE AND HOME CARE**

Culture and Religion

Home Care
Culture is reflected in the home. Homes vary in size, neatness, and furnishings. Some are expensive. Others reflect poverty. Whether rich or poor, treat each person and family with respect, kindness, and dignity. Do not judge the person's life-style, habits, religion, or culture.

FOCUS ON **LONG-TERM CARE AND HOME CARE**

Effects of Illness and Disability

Long-Term Care
Some people feel alone and isolated after out-living family and friends. Those with disabilities or chronic illnesses may have fears and concerns about nursing centers. They may feel alone and abandoned by family and friends. They may fear care from strangers. Many fear increasing loss of function. Some express their fears. Others do not or cannot.

Optimal Level of Function

Patients and residents are helped to maintain their *optimal level of function*. *This is the person's highest potential for mental and physical performance.* Encourage the person to be as independent as possible. Always focus on the person's abilities. Do not focus on disabilities.

Hospital patients are often treated as sick, dependent people. Promoting this "sick role" in a nursing center reduces quality of life. The health team focuses on improving the person's quality of life. You must help each person regain or maintain as much physical and mental function as possible.

PERSONS YOU WILL CARE FOR

People are often grouped in health care by their problems, needs, and age.

- *Mothers and newborns.* **Obstetrics** *is the field of medicine concerned with the care of women during pregnancy, labor, and childbirth and for 6 to 8 weeks after birth* (Chapter 52). They receive pre-natal (before birth) care in clinics or doctors' offices. When labor begins, mothers are admitted to hospital obstetrics (maternity) units. Pregnancy, labor, and childbirth are normal and natural events. However, problems can occur during and after pregnancy and childbirth.

- *Children.* **Pediatrics** *is the field of medicine concerned with the growth, development, and care of children—newborns to teenagers* (usually to age 16). Pediatric units are designed and equipped for the needs of children and parents. The nursing staff meets the child's physical, safety, and emotional needs (Fig. 9-4).

- *Adults with medical problems.* Medical problems are illnesses, diseases, and injuries not needing surgery. There are acute, chronic, and terminal illnesses. Examples are infections, arthritis, and high blood pressure.

- *Persons having surgery.* Care is given before and after surgery (Chapter 35). Surgeries range from simple to very complex. Appendix removal (appendectomy) is a simple surgery. Heart and brain surgeries are complex. Before surgery, the person is prepared for the surgery and for what happens after it. This includes addressing fears and concerns. Needs after surgery relate to relieving pain, preventing complications, and adjusting to body changes.

- *Persons with mental health disorders.* **Psychiatry** *is the field of medicine concerned with mental health disorders* (Chapter 48). Problems vary from mild to severe. Some persons need help coping with life stresses. Others are severely disturbed. They cannot do simple things—eat, bathe, or get dressed. Some persons present dangers to themselves or others. They need special care and treatment.

- *Persons needing bariatric care.* **Bariatrics** *is the field of medicine focused on the treatment and control of obesity.* **Obesity** *is having an excess amount of total body fat. Body weight is 20% or more above what is normal for that person's height and age.* Some people are morbidly obese. (*Morbid* means *diseased.*) **Morbid obesity** *means that the person weighs 100 pounds or more over his or her normal weight.* Persons with bariatric needs are at risk for many serious health problems. They include heart disease, high blood pressure, stroke, cancer, diabetes, skin problems, and depression. The person has many physical and emotional needs.

- *Persons in special care units.* Some people are seriously ill or injured. Special care units are designed to treat and prevent life-threatening problems. They include emergency rooms and intensive care, coronary care, burn, and kidney dialysis units (Fig. 9-5).

- *Persons needing sub-acute care or rehabilitation.* Some persons need more recovery time than hospital care allows. Others need rehabilitation (Chapter 41). They need to regain functions lost from surgery, illness, or accidents.

- *Older persons.* **Geriatrics** *is the field of medicine concerned with problems and diseases of old age and older persons.* Aging is a normal process (Chapter 12). It is not an illness or disease. Many older persons enjoy good health. Others have acute or chronic illnesses. Body changes normally occur with aging. Social and psychological changes also occur. (See *Focus on Long-Term Care and Home Care: Persons You Will Care For.*)

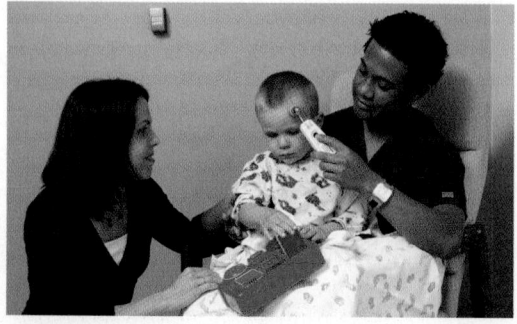

FIGURE 9-4 The nursing assistant gives care to a sick child.

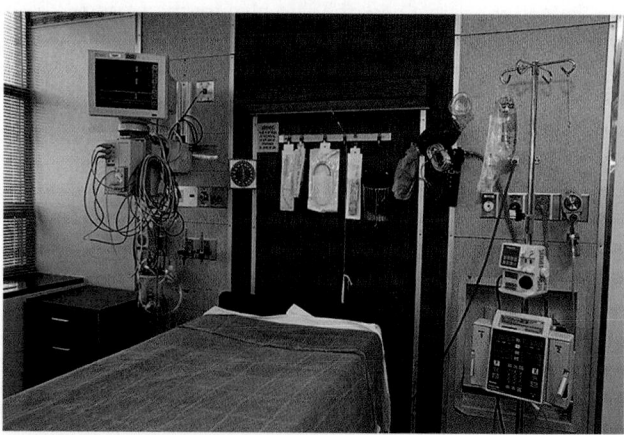

FIGURE 9-5 A room in an intensive care unit.

Persons You Will Care For

Long-Term Care

Most residents are older. Their problems and care needs vary.

- *Alert, oriented persons.* They know who they are and where they are. They have physical problems. The amount of care required depends on the degree of disability.
- *Confused and disoriented persons.* These persons are mildly to severely confused and disoriented. The problem may be temporary. For others, confusion and disorientation are permanent and become worse (Chapter 49).
- *Persons needing complete care.* They are very disabled, confused, or disoriented. They need total help with all activities of daily living (ADL). They cannot meet their own needs. Some cannot say what they need or want.
- *Short-term residents.* These people are recovering from fractures, acute illness or surgery, and other injuries. Often they are younger than most residents. Some may need tube feedings, wound care, or other treatments. Others need therapy programs—physical, occupational, speech and language, or respiratory. The goal is to regain optimal level of function to go home.

Long-Term Care—cont'd

- *Persons needing respite care.* Some people living at home go to nursing centers for short stays. This is *respite care*. *Respite* means *rest* or *relief*. The caregiver can take a vacation, tend to business, or simply rest. Respite care may be a few days to several weeks.
- *Life-long residents.* Birth defects and childhood injuries and diseases can cause disabilities. Disabilities may be physical impairments, intellectual impairments, or both. The person needs life-long assistance, support, and special devices.
- *Residents with mental health disorders.* Behavior and function are affected. In severe cases, self-care and independent living are impaired. Some persons have both physical and mental health disorders. (See Chapter 48.)
- *Terminally ill residents.* Terminally ill persons are dying. The goal is to provide quality end-of-life care (Chapter 55).

COMMUNICATING WITH THE PERSON

You communicate with the person every time you give care. You give information to the person. The person gives information to you. Your body sends messages all the time—at the bedside, in hallways, at the nurses' station, in the dining room, and elsewhere. The person and family are aware of what you say and do. Good work ethics and understanding the person are needed for good communication. What you say and what you do are also important.

Effective Communication

For effective communication between you and the person, you must:

- Follow the rules of communication (Chapter 7).
  - Use words that have the same meaning for you and the person.
  - Avoid medical terms and words not familiar to the person.
  - Communicate in a logical and orderly manner. Do not wander in thought.
  - Give facts and be specific.
  - Be brief and concise.
- Understand and respect the patient or resident as a person.
- View the person as a physical, psychological, social, and spiritual human being.
- Appreciate the person's problems and frustrations.
- Respect the person's rights, religion, and culture.
- Give the person time to understand the information that you give.

Effective Communication

Communicating with persons who have dementia is often hard. The Alzheimer's Disease Education and Referral Center (ADEAR) recommends the following. Also see Chapter 49.

- Gain the person's attention before speaking. Call the person by name. Make eye contact.
- Choose simple words and short sentences.
- Use a gentle, calm voice.
- Do not talk to the person as you would a baby.
- Do not talk about the person as if he or she is not there.
- Keep distractions and noise to a minimum.
- Help the person focus on what you are saying.
- Allow the person time to respond. Do not interrupt.
- Try to provide the word the person is struggling to find.
- State questions and instructions in a positive way.

- Repeat information as often as needed. Repeat what you said. Use the exact same words. Do not give the person a new message to process. If the person does not seem to understand after repeating, try re-phrasing the message. This is very important for persons with hearing problems.
- Ask questions to see if the person understood you.
- Be patient. People with memory problems may ask the same question many times. Do not say that you are repeating information.
- Include the person in conversations when others are present. This includes when a co-worker is assisting with care.

See *Focus on Communication: Effective Communication.*

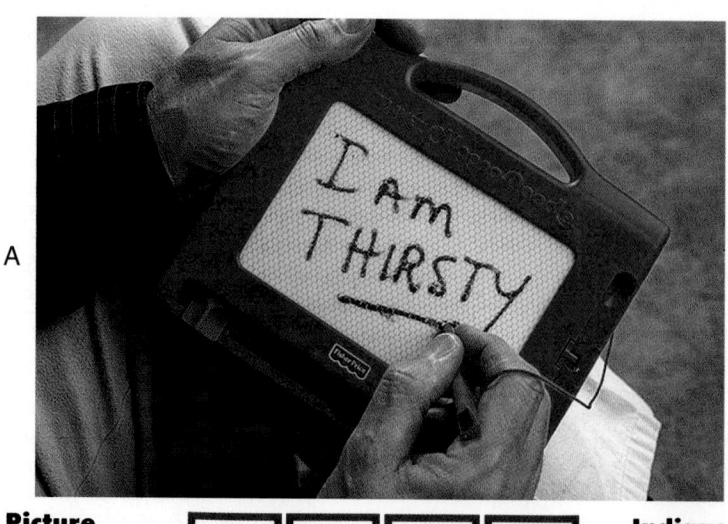

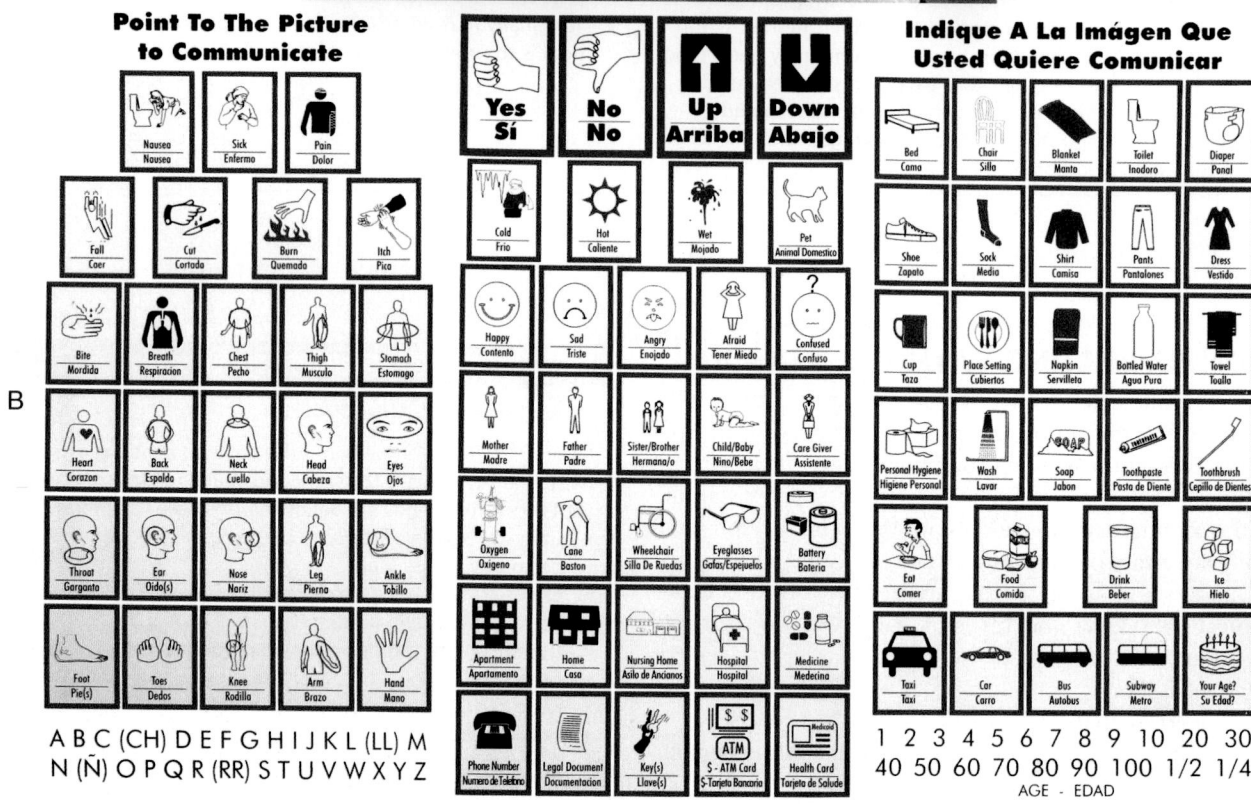

FIGURE 9-6 Communication aids. **A,** Magic Slate. **B,** Picture board in English and Spanish.

Verbal Communication

Verbal communication uses written or spoken words. You talk to the person. You share information and find out how the person feels. Most verbal communication involves the spoken word. Follow these rules.

- Face the person. Look directly at the person.
- Position yourself at the person's eye level. Sit or squat by the person as needed.
- Control the loudness and tone of your voice.
- Speak clearly, slowly, and distinctly.
- Do not use slang or vulgar words.
- Repeat information as needed.
- Ask 1 question at a time. Wait for an answer.
- Do not shout, whisper, or mumble.
- Be kind, courteous, and friendly.

You use the written word when the person cannot speak or hear but can read. The nurse and care plan tell you how to communicate with the person. The devices shown in Figure 9-6 are often used. The person may have poor vision. When writing messages:

- Keep them simple and brief.
- Use a black felt pen on white paper.
- Print in large letters.

Some persons cannot speak or read. Ask questions that have "yes" or "no" answers. The person can nod, blink, or use other gestures for "yes" and "no." Follow the care plan. A picture board may be helpful (Fig. 9-7).

Persons who are deaf may use sign language. See Chapter 42.

● ESTOY/TENGO
I AM

○ Dificultad para respirar
Short Of Breath

○ Frustrado/a
Frustrated

○ Náuseas
Nauseous

○ Ansiedad
Anxious

○ Decepcionado/a
Disappointed

○ Cansado/a
Tired

○ Somnoliento/a
Drowsy

○ Mejor
Better

○ Sed
Thirsty

○ Calor
Hot

○ Frío
Cold

○ Inseguro/a (con lo que está sucediendo)
Unsure (Of What Is Happening)

○ Arcadas
Gagging

○ Dolor
In Pain

○ Mareado/a
Light Headed

○ Miedo
Afraid

○ Solo/a
Lonely

○ Enfadado/a
Angry

○ Mojado/a
Wet

○ Peor
Worse

○ Hambre
Hungry

● QUIERO
I WANT

EZ BOARD DE VIDATAK
SISTEMA INNOVADOR DE COMUNICACIÓN PARA PACIENTES

EZ BOARD BY VIDATAK
AN INNOVATION IN PATIENT COMMUNICATION

○ Que me hagan una succión
Suctioned

○ Sentarme
To Sit Up

○ Agua
Water

○ Bañarme
Bath

○ Anteojos
Eyeglasses

○ Calcetines
Socks

○ Hacer una llamada
Make A Call

○ Darme vuelta a la derecha
To Turn Right

○ Que apaguen la luz
Lights Off

○ En silencio
It Quiet

○ Más control
More Control

○ Recostarme
To Lie Down

○ Hielo
Ice

○ Champú
Shampoo

○ Un cepillo para el pelo
Hairbrush

○ Un orinal
Urinal

○ Llamar a la enfermera, Ver TV
Call Light, TV

○ Darme vuelta a la izquierda
To Turn Left

○ Que bajen las luces
Lights Dim

○ Dormir
To Sleep

○ Sentirme reconfortado/a
To Be Comforted

○ Orar
Prayer

○ Ejercicio físico
Exercise

○ Crema para el cuerpo
Lotion

○ Masaje
Massage

○ Chata para orinar
Bedpan

○ Almohada
Pillow

○ Enciendan la luz
Lights On

○ Cobija
Blanket

○ Descansar
To Rest

● QUIERO VER A UN/A
I WANT TO SEE

○ Médico
Doctor

○ Enfermera
Nurse

○ Asistente
Assistant

○ Terapeuta respiratorio
Respiratory Therapist

○ Terapeuta físico
Physical Therapist

○ Trabajador social
Social Worker

○ Capellán
Chaplain

○ Mi familia
My Family

● QUIERO LIMPIARME
I WANT TO CLEAN

○ La boca
Mouth

○ La nariz
Nose

○ Los dientes
Teeth

○ Las manos
Hands

○ La cara
Face

○ El cabello
Hair

!	1	2	3	4	5	6	7	8	9	0	-	+	=	¡Gracias!

Q W E R T Y U I O P [ ] ¡Te quiero mucho!

A S D F G H J K L : ' I Love You

Z X C V B N M , . ?

SPACE

VIDATAK EZ BOARD

Para prevenir infecciones, se ruega no usar esta pizarra con diferentes pacientes. For infection control purposes, please do not reuse this board between patients.

FIGURE 9-6, cont'd C, Communication board in Spanish.

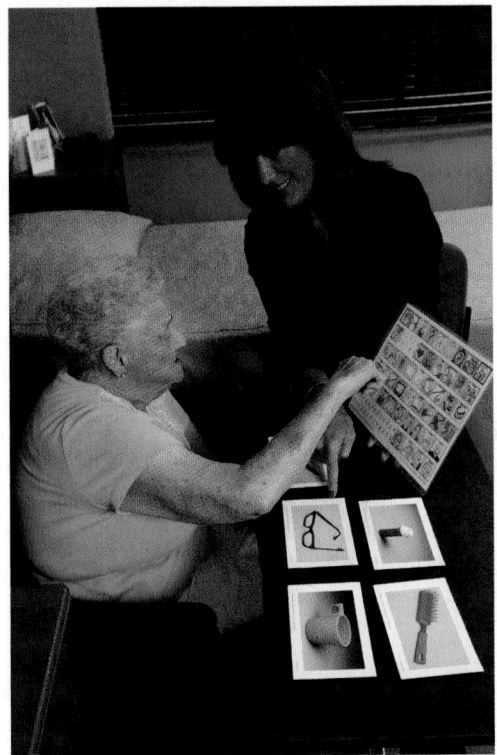

FIGURE 9-7 A therapist helps a resident use a picture board and picture cards to communicate.

Nonverbal Communication

Nonverbal communication does not use words. Messages are sent with gestures, facial expressions, posture, body movements, touch, and smell. Nonverbal messages more accurately reflect a person's feelings than words do. They are usually involuntary and hard to control. A person may say one thing but act another way. Watch the person's eyes, hand movements, gestures, posture, and other actions. They may tell you more than words.

Touch. Touch is a very important form of nonverbal communication. It conveys comfort, caring, love, affection, interest, trust, concern, and reassurance. Touch means different things to different people. The meaning depends on age, gender (male or female), experiences, and culture.

Cultural groups have rules or practices about touch. They relate to who can touch, when it can occur, and where to touch the body. (See *Caring About Culture: Touch Practices,* p. 100.)

Some people do not like being touched. However, stroking or holding a hand can comfort a person. Touch should be gentle—not hurried, rough, or sexual. To use touch, follow the person's care plan. Remember to maintain professional boundaries.

See *Focus on Children and Older Persons: Touch,* p. 100.

❊ CARING ABOUT CULTURE

Touch Practices

Touch practices vary among cultural groups. Touch is a friendly gesture in the *Philippine* culture. Touch is often used in *Mexico*. Some people believe that using touch while complimenting a person is important. It is thought to neutralize the power of the evil eye *(mal de ojo)*.

Persons from the *United Kingdom* tend to reserve touch for persons they know well. Within limits, touch is acceptable in *Poland*. Its use depends on age, gender, and relationship.

In *India,* men shake hands with other men but not with women. For women, they place their palms together and bow slightly. As a sign of respect or to seek a blessing, people touch the feet of older adults.

In *Vietnam,* a person's head is touched by others. It is considered the center of the soul. Men do not touch women they do not know. Men commonly shake hands with men.

People from *China* do not like touching by strangers. A nod or slight bow is given during introductions. Health care workers of the same gender are preferred.

In *Ireland,* a firm handshake is preferred. Only family and close friends are embraced.

Modified from D'Avanzo CE: Pocket guide to cultural health assessment, ed 4, St Louis, 2008, Mosby.

❊ CARING ABOUT CULTURE

Facial Expressions

Through facial expressions, Americans communicate:
* *Coldness*—there is a constant stare. Face muscles do not move.
* *Fear*—eyes are wide open. Eyebrows are raised. The mouth is tense with the lips drawn back.
* *Anger*—eyes are fixed in a hard stare. Upper lids are lowered. Eyebrows are drawn down. Lips are slightly compressed.
* *Tiredness*—eyes are rolled upward.
* *Disapproval*—eyes are rolled upward.
* *Disgust*—narrowed eyes. The upper lip is curled. There are nose movements.
* *Embarrassment*—eyes are turned away or down. The face is flushed. The person pretends to smile. He or she rubs the eyes, nose, or face. He or she twitches the hair, beard, or mustache.
* *Surprise*—direct gaze with raised eyebrows.

Italian, Jewish, African-American, and *Hispanic* persons smile readily. They use many facial expressions and gestures for happiness, pain, or displeasure. *Irish, English,* and *Northern European* persons tend to have less facial expression.

In some cultures, facial expressions mean the opposite of what the person feels. For example, *Asians* may conceal negative emotions with a smile.

Modified from Giger JN: Transcultural nursing: assessment and intervention, ed 6, St Louis, 2013, Mosby.

FOCUS ON CHILDREN AND OLDER PERSONS

Touch

Children

Touch soothes and comforts infants and young children. They like to be held, stroked, rocked, patted, and cuddled. Older children and teenagers like to give and receive hugs.

Contact must be professional, casual, and with consent. It must not be sexual or involve sexual areas.

Body Language. People send messages through their *body language.*
* *Facial expressions* (see *Caring About Culture: Facial Expressions*)
* *Gestures*
* *Posture*
* *Hand and body movements*
* *Gait*
* *Eye contact*
* *Appearance* (dress, hygiene, jewelry, perfume, cosmetics, body art and piercings, and so on)

Many messages are sent through body language. Slumped posture may mean the person is not happy or not feeling well. A person may deny pain. Yet he or she protects the affected body part by standing, lying, or sitting in a certain way. Your actions, movements, and facial expressions send messages. So do how you stand, sit, walk, and look at the person. Your body language should show interest, caring, respect, and enthusiasm.

Often you will need to control your body language. Control reactions to odors from body fluids, secretions, excretions, or the person's body. The person cannot control some odors. Embarrassment increases if you react to odors.

Communication Methods

Certain methods help you communicate with others. They result in better relationships. More information is gained for the nursing process.

Listening. Listening means to focus on verbal and non-verbal communication. You use sight, hearing, touch, and smell. You focus on what the person is saying. You observe nonverbal clues. They can support what the person says. Or they can show other feelings. For example, Mrs. Hayes says: "I want to stay here. That way my son won't have to care for me." You see tears and she looks away from you. Her verbal says *happy.* Her nonverbal shows *sadness.*

Listening requires that you care and have interest. Follow these guidelines.
* Face the person.
* Have good eye contact with the person. See *Caring About Culture: Eye Contact Practices.*
* Lean toward the person (Fig. 9-8). Do not sit back with your arms crossed.
* Respond to the person. Nod your head. Say: "uh huh," "mmm," and "I see." Repeat what the person says. Ask questions.
* Avoid the communication barriers (p. 102).

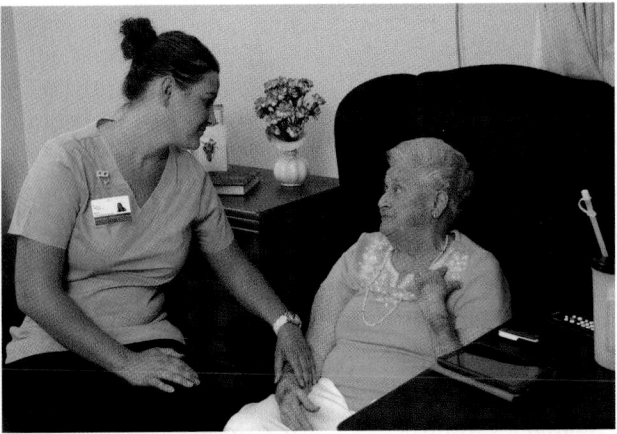

FIGURE 9-8 Listen by facing the person. Have good eye contact. Lean toward the person.

✿ CARING ABOUT CULTURE

Eye Contact Practices

In the *American* culture, eye contact signals a good self-concept. It also shows openness, interest in others, attention, honesty, and warmth. Lack of eye contact can mean:

- Shyness
- Lack of interest
- Humility
- Guilt
- Embarrassment
- Low self-esteem
- Rudeness
- Dishonesty

For some *Asian* and *American Indian* cultures, eye contact is impolite. It is an invasion of privacy. In certain *Indian* cultures, eye contact is avoided with persons of higher or lower socio-economic class. It is also given a special sexual meaning.

In *Iraq*, men and women avoid direct eye contact. Long, direct eye contact is rude in *Mexico*. In rural parts of *Vietnam*, it is not respectful to look at another person while talking. Blinking means that a message is received. In the *United Kingdom*, looking directly at a speaker means the listener is paying attention.

Modified from Giger JN: Transcultural nursing: assessment and intervention, ed 6, St Louis, 2013, Mosby. Modified from D'Avanzo CE: Pocket guide to cultural health assessment, ed 4, St Louis, 2008, Mosby.

Paraphrasing. *Paraphrasing is re-stating the person's message in your own words.* You use fewer words than the person did. Paraphrasing:

- Shows you are listening.
- Lets the person see if you understand the message.
- Promotes more communication.

The person usually responds to your statement. For example:

Mrs. Hayes: My son was crying after talking to the doctor. I don't know what they said.

You: Your son was crying?

Mrs. Hayes: The doctor must have told him about my tumor.

Direct Questions. Direct questions focus on certain information. You ask the person what you need to know. Some direct questions have "yes" or "no" answers. Others require more information. For example:

You: Mrs. Hayes, do you want to shower this morning?

Mrs. Hayes: Yes.

You: Mrs. Hayes, when would you like to do that?

Mrs. Hayes: Could we start in 15 minutes? I want to call my son first.

You: Yes, we can start in 15 minutes. Did you have a bowel movement today?

Mrs. Hayes: No.

You: You said you didn't eat well this morning. What did you eat?

Mrs. Hayes: I had toast and coffee. I didn't feel like eating this morning.

Open-Ended Questions. Open-ended questions lead or invite the person to share thoughts, feelings, or ideas. The person chooses what to talk about. He or she controls the topic and the information given. Answers require more than a "yes" or "no." For example:

- "What do you like about living with your son?"
- "What was your husband like?"
- "What do you like about being retired?"

Clarifying. Clarifying lets you make sure that you understand the message. You can ask the person to repeat the message, say you do not understand, or re-state the message. For example:

- "Could you say that again?"
- "I'm sorry, Mrs. Hayes. I don't understand what you mean."
- "Are you saying that you want to go home?"

Focusing. Focusing is dealing with a certain topic. It is useful when a person rambles or wanders in thought. For example, Mrs. Hayes talks at length about food and places to eat. You need to know why she did not eat much breakfast. To focus on breakfast you say: "Let's talk about breakfast. You said you didn't feel like eating."

Silence. Silence is a very powerful way to communicate. Sometimes you do not need to say anything. This is true during sad times. Just being there shows you care. At other times, silence gives time to think, organize thoughts, or choose words. Silence is useful when making decisions. It also helps when the person is upset and needs to gain control. Silence on your part shows caring and respect for the person's situation and feelings.

Sometimes pauses or long silences are uncomfortable. You do not need to talk when the person is silent. The person may need silence. Dealing with silence gets easier as you gain experience in your role.

See *Caring About Culture: The Meaning of Silence*, p. 102.

✿ CARING ABOUT CULTURE
The Meaning of Silence

In the *English* and *Arabic* cultures, silence is used for privacy. Among *Russian, French,* and *Spanish* cultures, silence means agreement between parties. In some *Asian* cultures, silence is a sign of respect, particularly to an older person.

Modified from Giger JN: Transcultural nursing: assessment and intervention, ed 6, St Louis, 2013, Mosby.

Communication Barriers

Communication barriers prevent the sending and receiving of messages. Communication fails. You must avoid these barriers.

- *Unfamiliar language.* You and the person must use and understand the same language. If not, messages are not accurately interpreted. See *Evolve Student Learning Resources* for useful Spanish Vocabulary and Phrases.
- *Cultural differences.* The person may attach different meanings to verbal and nonverbal communication. See *Caring About Culture: Communicating With Persons From Other Cultures.*
- *Changing the subject.* Someone changes the subject when the topic is uncomfortable. Avoid changing the subject when possible.
- *Giving your opinion.* Opinions involve judging values, behaviors, or feelings. Let others express feelings and concerns without adding your opinion. Do not make judgments or jump to conclusions.
- *Talking a lot when others are silent.* Talking too much is usually because of nervousness and discomfort with silence. Silences have meaning. They show acceptance, rejection, and fear. They also show the need for quiet and time to think.
- *Failure to listen.* Do not pretend to listen. It shows lack of interest and caring. This causes poor responses. You miss important complaints of pain, discomfort, or other symptoms that you must report to the nurse.
- *Pat answers.* "Don't worry." "Everything will be okay." "Your doctor knows best." These make the person feel that you do not care about his or her concerns, feelings, and fears.
- *Illness and disability.* Speech, hearing, vision, cognitive function, and body movements are often affected. Verbal and nonverbal communication is affected.
- *Age.* Values and communication styles vary among age-groups. See *Focus on Communication: Communication Barriers.*

✿ CARING ABOUT CULTURE
Communicating With Persons From Other Cultures

To communicate with persons from other cultures:
- Ask the nurse about the beliefs and values of the person's culture. You can also ask the person and family. Learn as much as you can about the person's culture.
- Do not judge the person by your attitudes, values, beliefs, and ideas.
- Follow the person's care plan. It includes the person's cultural beliefs and customs.
- Do the following when communicating with foreign-speaking persons.
  - Convey comfort by your tone of voice and body language.
  - Do not speak loudly or shout. It will not help the person understand English.
  - Speak slowly and distinctly.
  - Keep messages short and simple.
  - Be alert for words the person seems to understand.
  - Use gestures and pictures.
  - Repeat the message in other ways.
  - Avoid using medical terms and abbreviations.
  - Be alert for signs the person is pretending to understand. Nodding and answering "yes" to all questions are signs that the person does not understand what you are saying.

Modified from Giger JN: Transcultural nursing: assessment and intervention, ed 6, St Louis, 2013, Mosby.

FOCUS ON COMMUNICATION
Communication Barriers

Persons from different cultures may speak a language you do not understand. This is a communication barrier. Such persons may normally have family or friends translate. In the health care setting, the nurse may prefer to use a translator from the agency.

Trained translators know medical terms. Family or friends may not know a term. They may state something other than what was meant. There is a risk of giving wrong information. Also, having family or friends translate violates the right to privacy. The *Health Insurance Portability and Accountability Act of 1996* (HIPAA) protects the right to privacy and security of a person's health information (Chapter 5). Privacy is protected when using a translator from the agency.

PERSONS WITH SPECIAL NEEDS

Each person is unique. Special knowledge and skills may be required to meet the person's needs.

Persons With Disabilities

A person may acquire a disability any time from birth through old age. For example, children can develop hearing problems from ear infections. Head injuries can impair cognitive function. Spinal cord injuries can affect movements. And loud noise (music, machines) is linked to hearing loss. The cause or the age of onset does not matter. The person does not choose to have a disability. The person has to adjust. For many people, this can be long and hard (Chapter 41).

Your attitude is important for effective communication. People with disabilities have the same basic needs as you and everyone else. They feel joy, sorrow, happiness, sadness, and other emotions just like you and everyone else. They laugh, cry, have families, go to school, work, get married, and pay bills just like you and everyone else. And they have the right to dignity and respect just like you and everyone else.

To communicate with persons who have disabilities, see persons:

- Who have speech disorders—Chapter 42
- Who are hard-of-hearing—Chapter 42
- Who are blind—Chapter 42
- Who are confused—Chapter 49
- With Alzheimer's disease and other dementias—Chapter 49

Common courtesies and manners (*etiquette*) apply to any person with a disability. See Box 9-1 for disability etiquette.

The Person Who Is Comatose

Comatose means being unable to respond to stimuli. The person who is comatose is unconscious. The person cannot respond to others. Often the person can hear and can feel touch and pain. Pain may be shown by grimacing or groaning. Assume that the person hears and understands you. Use touch and give care gently. Practice these measures.

- Knock before entering the person's room.
- Tell the person your name, the time, and the place every time you enter the room.
- Give care on the same schedule every day.
- Explain what you are going to do. Explain care measures step-by-step as you do them.
- Tell the person when you are completing care.
- Use touch to communicate care, concern, and comfort.
- Tell the person what time you will be back to check on him or her.
- Tell the person when you are leaving the room.

BOX 9-1	Disability Etiquette

- Extend the same courtesies to the person as you would to anyone else.
- Provide for privacy.
- Do not hang on or lean on a person's wheelchair.
- Treat adults as adults. Use the person's first name only if he or she asks you to do so.
- Do not pat a person who is in a wheelchair on the head.
- Speak directly to the person. Do not address questions for the person to his or her companion.
- Do not be embarrassed if you use words relating to the disability. For example, you say: "Did you see that?" to a person with a vision problem.
- Sit or squat to talk to a person in a wheelchair or in a chair. This puts you and the person at eye level.
- Ask the person if help is needed before acting. If the person says "no," respect the person's wishes. If the person wants help, ask what to do and how to do it.
- Think before giving directions to a person in a wheelchair. Think about distances, weather conditions, stairs, curbs, steep hills, and other obstacles.
- Allow the person extra time to say or do things. Let the person set the pace in walking, talking, or other activities.

Modified from Easter Seals, Disability etiquette, *2015.*

FAMILY AND FRIENDS

Family and friends help meet basic needs. They offer support and comfort. They lessen loneliness. Some also help with the person's care. This helps both the person and family. The family knows the person's physical and emotional needs are met. The presence or absence of family or friends affects the person's quality of life.

The person has the right to visit with others in private and without unnecessary interruptions. You may need to give care when visitors are there. Protect the right to privacy. Do not expose the person's body in front of them. Politely ask them to leave the room. Show them where to wait. Promptly tell them when they can return. A partner or family member may want to help you. If the patient or resident consents, you can let the person stay.

Treat family and friends with courtesy and respect. They have concerns about the person's condition and care. They need support and understanding. However, do not discuss the person's condition with them. Refer their questions to the nurse.

Visiting rules depend on agency policy and the person's condition. Parents can visit with children whenever they want. Dying persons usually can have family present all the time. Know your agency's visiting policies and what is allowed for the person.

Visitors may have questions about the chapel, gift shop, lounge, dining room, or business office. Know the location, special rules, and hours of these areas.

✿ CARING ABOUT CULTURE

Family Roles in Sick Care

In *Vietnam*, family members are involved in the person's hospital care. They stay at the bedside and sleep in the person's bed or on straw mats. In *Vietnam* and *China*, family members provide food, hygiene, and comfort.

In *Pakistan*, hospitals have different sections for females and males. Adult family members of the opposite sex are not allowed to stay overnight.

Modified from D'Avanzo CE: Pocket guide to cultural health assessment, ed 4, St Louis, 2008, Mosby.

FOCUS ON CHILDREN AND OLDER PERSONS

Family and Friends

Older Persons
Sometimes older brothers, sisters, and cousins live together. They provide companionship and share living expenses. They care for each other during illness or disability.

Some older people live with their children—in the child's home or the parent's home. The older parent may be healthy, need some supervision, or be ill or disabled. Living with a child can help the older person feel safe and secure. Often the adult child gives care to the parent.

Adult children often need to work. Adult day-care centers provide meals, supervision, and supervised activities for older persons. Cards, board games, movies, crafts, dancing, walks, and lectures are common. Help is given as needed. Some provide transportation from home to the center.

See "Living With Family" in Chapter 12.

FOCUS ON LONG-TERM CARE AND HOME CARE

Family and Friends

Home Care
Family personalities and attitudes affect the mood in the home. Many families are happy and supportive. Others have poor relationships. Mental or physical illness, drug or alcohol abuse, unemployment, and delinquency may affect the family. Some families have problems coping with or accepting the person's illness or disability.

Your supervisor explains family problems to you. Do not get involved. Be professional and have empathy. Do not give advice, take sides, or make judgments about family conflicts. Maintain professional boundaries at all times.

A visitor may upset or tire a person. Report your observations to the nurse. The nurse will speak with the visitor about the person's needs.

See *Caring About Culture: Family Roles in Sick Care.*

See *Focus on Children and Older Persons: Family and Friends.*

See *Focus on Long-Term Care and Home Care: Family and Friends.*

BEHAVIOR ISSUES

Many patients, residents, and families accept illness, injury, and disability. Others do not adjust well. They have some of the following behaviors (Figure 9-9). These behaviors are new for some people. For others, they are life-long. They are part of one's personality.

- *Anger.* Anger is a common emotion. Causes include fear, pain, and dying and death. Loss of function and loss of control over health and life are causes. Anger is a symptom of some diseases that affect thinking and behavior. Some people are generally angry. Anger is communicated verbally and nonverbally. Verbal outbursts, shouting, raised voices, and rapid speech are common. Some people are silent. Others are not cooperative. They may refuse to answer questions. Nonverbal signs include rapid movements, pacing, clenched fists, and a red face. Glaring and getting close to you when speaking are other signs. Violent behaviors can occur.

- *Demanding behavior.* Nothing seems to please the person. The person is critical of others. He or she wants care given at a certain time and in a certain way. Loss of independence, loss of health, and loss of control of life are causes. So are unmet needs.

- *Self-centered behavior.* The person cares only about his or her own needs. The needs of others are ignored. The person demands the time and attention of others. The person becomes impatient if needs are not met.

- *Aggressive behavior.* The person may swear, bite, hit, pinch, scratch, or kick. Fear, anger, pain, and dementia (Chapter 49) are causes. Protect the person, others, and yourself from harm (Chapter 13).

- *Withdrawal.* The person has little or no contact with family, friends, and staff. He or she spends time alone and does not take part in social or group events. This may signal physical illness or depression. Some people are not social. They prefer to be alone.

- *Inappropriate sexual behavior.* Some people make inappropriate sexual remarks. Or they touch others in the wrong way. Some disrobe or masturbate in public. These behaviors may be on purpose. Or they are caused by disease, confusion, dementia, or drug side effects.

You cannot avoid the person or lose control. Good communication is needed. Behaviors are addressed in the care plan. The care plan may include some of the guidelines in Box 9-2.

See *Focus on Communication: Behavior Issues.*

See *Teamwork and Time Management: Behavior Issues.*

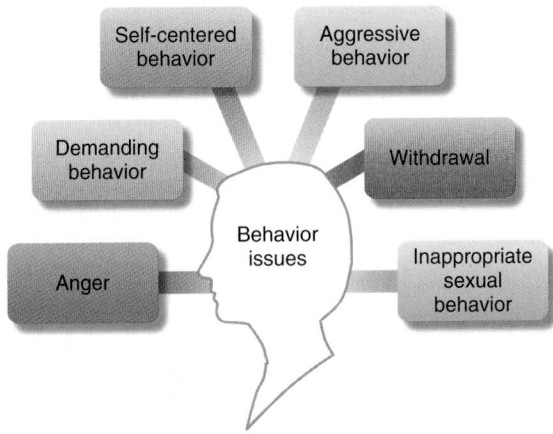

FIGURE 9-9 Behavior issues are a response to illness, injury, or disability, or they are life-long.

BOX 9-2	Dealing With Behavior Issues

- Recognize frustrating and frightening situations. Put yourself in the person's situation. How would you feel? How would you want to be treated?
- Treat the person with dignity and respect.
- Answer questions clearly and thoroughly. Ask the nurse to answer questions you cannot answer.
- Keep the person informed. Tell the person what you are going to do and when.
- Do not keep the person waiting. Answer call lights promptly. If you tell the person that you will do something for him or her, do it promptly.
- Explain the reason for long waits. Ask if you can get or do something to increase the person's comfort.
- Stay calm and professional, especially if the person is angry or hostile. Often the person is not angry at you. He or she is angry at another person or situation.
- Do not argue with the person.
- Listen and use silence. The person may feel better if able to express his or her feelings.
- Protect yourself from violent behaviors (Chapter 13).
- Report the person's behavior to the nurse. Discuss how to deal with the person.

FOCUS ON COMMUNICATION

Behavior Issues

Anger is a common response to illness and disability. Patients and residents may be angry with their situation. Anger may be directed at you. You might have problems dealing with the person's anger. You must act professionally. Stay calm. Do not yell at or insult the person. Listen to his or her concerns. Give needed care. Try not to take angry statements personally. If a person says hurtful things, you can kindly say: "Please don't say those things. I'm trying to help you." Tell the nurse about the person's behavior.

Caring for demanding or angry persons can be hard. Ask the nurse or co-workers to help if needed.

TEAMWORK AND TIME MANAGEMENT

Behavior Issues

Persons who are demanding can take a lot of time. A simple task, such as filling a water mug, can take several minutes. The mug may be too full or not full enough. The water may be too warm or too cold. Or the person may have a list of other care needs.

This may happen to you or to co-workers. Learn to recognize these situations. Offer to help co-workers with the person or other tasks. Hopefully they also will help you.

FOCUS ON **PRIDE**

The Person, Family, and Yourself

P ersonal and Professional Responsibility

Improving communication is an on-going process. You may be uncomfortable with patient or resident interactions at first. You will have many chances to develop communication skills. You are responsible for taking advantage of these opportunities. To improve your communication:

- Use methods such as listening and clarifying.
- Pay attention to the nonverbal messages you may be sending.
- Avoid the communication barriers.
- Know where your agency keeps resources to aid with communication. These may include devices like those shown in Figure 9-6 or translation lists with useful words or phrases (see *Evolve Student Learning Resources*).
- Learn from your mistakes.

With practice, you will communicate more effectively. This is a valuable skill.

R ights and Respect

You may care for young and old persons, ill and disabled persons, persons who are obese, those with mental health disorders, and persons from other cultures. Each person is different. Each has his or her own needs and concerns.

Avoid labeling the person or making assumptions. For example, a person is obese. That does not mean the person is lazy or lacks control. Or a person has a mental health disorder. That does not mean the person is unstable or "crazy." Or a person is elderly. Myths about older persons are common. See Chapter 12.

Each person is unique and has value. Try to understand the person. Listen and use good communication. Treat the person with dignity and respect.

I ndependence and Social Interaction

Fear and anxiety are common emotions for persons in nursing centers and hospitals. Nursing center residents may feel lonely or abandoned by their families and friends. Patients may fear loss of function that will have social effects. For example, a stroke can cause a person to lose function on 1 side of the body. The person may lose the ability to work, live at home, perform daily activities, walk, drive, and so on. Feeling abandoned or worthless affects self-esteem and health.

To provide a sense of identity, worth, and belonging:

- Greet each person by name.
- Talk to the person while providing care.
- Take an extra minute to talk or just listen.
- Treat each person with dignity and respect.
- Encourage as much independence as possible.
- Focus on the person's abilities, not his or her disabilities.
- Allow private time with visitors.

D elegation and Teamwork

Caring for persons with behavior issues requires great teamwork. Staff members may become frustrated. But the person's quality of care must not be lowered. The health team must work together to manage such persons. Care assignments may rotate to allow breaks.

When not assigned to such a person, assist your co-worker with the person or other tasks. When you interact with the person, be respectful. Treat the person as nicely as you treat others. Often when treated kindly, the person's behavior will improve. A supportive and encouraging team makes caring for persons with behavior issues easier.

E thics and Laws

You will care for persons with different ideas, values, and life-styles. These shape the person's character and identity. It is not ethical to:

- Force your views and beliefs on another person.
- Make negative comments or insult the person's customs.
- Argue with a person about health care or religious beliefs.

Respect the person as a whole. This includes his or her cultural and religious practices.

FOCUS ON **PRIDE**: *Application*

Imagine yourself as a patient or resident. What would you want the staff to know about you? Ask 1 or 2 others what would be important to them. How does understanding the person allow you to give better care?

REVIEW QUESTIONS

Circle the BEST answer.

1 You work in a health care agency. You focus on
   a The person's care plan
   b The person's physical, safety and security, and self-esteem needs
   c The person as a physical, psychological, social, and spiritual being
   d The person's cultural and spiritual needs

2 Which basic need is the *most* essential?
   a The need to feel safe
   b The need to feel valued
   c The need for affection
   d The need for food

3 A person says: "I'm falling!" Which needs are *most* important at the time?
   a Self-actualization needs
   b Safety and security needs
   c Love and belonging needs
   d Self-esteem needs

4 A person has a garden behind the nursing center. This relates to
   a Self-actualization
   b Self-esteem
   c Love and belonging
   d Safety and security

Continued

REVIEW QUESTIONS—cont'd

5 Which statement about culture and religion is *true?*
  a Cultural and religious practices are not allowed in nursing centers.
  b A person must follow all beliefs and practices of his or her culture or religion.
  c Culture and religion influence health and illness practices.
  d Culture and religion do not influence food choices.

6 Which is *true?*
  a Mental health disorders are the focus of pediatrics.
  b Sick children are the focus of obstetrics.
  c The diseases of aging are the focus of geriatrics.
  d Childbirth is the focus of pediatrics.

7 These statements are about illness and disability. Which is *true?*
  a They are matters of personal choice.
  b Normal activities are not affected.
  c Only physical effects occur.
  d Maintaining optimal function is a goal.

8 Alert and oriented residents need nursing center care because they
  a Are very disabled and confused
  b Have trouble remembering things
  c Have physical problems
  d Need surgery

9 Which is *true?*
  a Nonverbal communication uses the written or spoken word.
  b Verbal communication is the truest reflection of a person's feelings.
  c Body language cannot be controlled.
  d Touch means different things to different people.

10 To communicate with the person you should
  a Use medical words and phrases
  b Change the subject often
  c Give your opinions
  d Be quiet when the person is silent

11 Which shows that you are listening?
  a You sit with your arms crossed.
  b You have eye contact with the person.
  c You avoid asking questions.
  d You use communication barriers.

12 Which is an open-ended question?
  a "What hobbies do you enjoy?"
  b "Do you want to wear your red sweater?"
  c "Would you like eggs and toast for breakfast?"
  d "Do you want to sit in your chair?"

13 You ask: "What is your name?" This is
  a A communication barrier
  b A direct question
  c Paraphrasing
  d An open-ended question

14 Focusing is useful when
  a A person is rambling
  b You want to make sure you understand the message
  c You want the person to share thoughts and feelings
  d A person is silent

15 Which promotes communication?
  a "Don't worry."
  b "Everything will be fine."
  c "This is a good nursing center."
  d "Why are you crying?"

16 Which is a barrier to communication?
  a Focusing
  b Asking questions
  c Pretending to listen
  d Using familiar language

17 A person uses a wheelchair. For effective communication, you should
  a Lean on the wheelchair
  b Pat the person on the head
  c Direct questions to the companion
  d Sit or squat next to the person

18 A person is comatose. Which action is correct?
  a You assume that the person cannot hear.
  b You explain what you are going to do.
  c You use listening and silence to communicate.
  d You enter the room without knocking.

19 A person has many visitors. Which is *true?*
  a They can help meet basic needs.
  b You can discuss the person's condition with them.
  c You can answer their questions about the person's care.
  d You decide who stays in the room when care is given.

20 A visitor seems to tire a person. What should you do?
  a Ask the person to leave.
  b Tell the nurse.
  c Stay in the room to observe the person and visitor.
  d Find out the visitor's relationship to the person.

21 A person wants care given at a certain time and in a certain way. Nothing seems to please the person. The person is most likely demonstrating
  a Angry behavior
  b Withdrawn behavior
  c Demanding behavior
  d Aggressive behavior

22 A person is demonstrating problem behavior. You should
  a Put yourself in the person's situation
  b Ignore the behavior
  c Ask the person to be nicer
  d Avoid the person

Answers to Chapter 9 questions are on p. 870.

FOCUS ON **PRACTICE**

Problem Solving

Mr. Hawn is a new resident. He was admitted to the center last month after his wife died. He could not care for himself at home. Mr. Hawn is withdrawn and angry toward the staff. He is impatient and agitated when his needs are not met right away. Explain possible reasons for his behaviors. How will you manage his behaviors and provide quality care?

Body Structure and Function

OBJECTIVES

- Define the key terms and key abbreviations in this chapter.
- Identify the basic structures of the cell.
- Explain how cells divide.
- Describe 4 types of tissues.

- Identify the structures and functions of each body system.
- Explain how to promote PRIDE in the person, the family, and yourself.

KEY TERMS

artery A blood vessel that carries blood away from the heart
capillary A very tiny blood vessel; food, oxygen, and other substances pass from the capillaries into the cells
cell The basic unit of body structure
digestion The process that breaks down food physically and chemically so it can be absorbed for use by the cells
hemoglobin The substance in red blood cells that carries oxygen and gives blood its red color
hormone A chemical substance secreted by the endocrine glands into the bloodstream
immunity Protection against a disease or condition; the person will not get or be affected by the disease
joint The point at which 2 or more bones meet to allow movement

menstruation The process in which the lining of the uterus *(endometrium)* breaks up and is discharged from the body through the vagina
metabolism The burning of food for heat and energy by the cells
organ Groups of tissue with the same function
peristalsis Involuntary muscle contractions in the digestive system that move food down the esophagus through the alimentary canal
respiration The process of supplying the cells with oxygen and removing carbon dioxide from them
system Organs that work together to perform special functions
tissue A group of cells with similar functions
vein A blood vessel that returns blood to the heart

KEY ABBREVIATIONS

CNS	Central nervous system	**RBC**	Red blood cell
GI	Gastro-intestinal	**WBC**	White blood cell
mL	Milliliter		

Ideally, the human body is in a steady state called *homeostasis. (Homeo* means *sameness. Stasis* means *standing still.)* Various body functions and processes work to promote health and survival. Homeostasis is affected by illness, disease, and injury.

You help patients and residents meet their basic needs. Your care promotes comfort, healing, and recovery. Therefore you need to know the body's normal structure *(anatomy)* and function *(physiology)*. They will help you understand signs, symptoms, and the reasons for care and procedures. You will give safe and more effective care.

See Chapter 12 for the changes in body structure and function that occur with aging.

CELLS, TISSUES, AND ORGANS

The basic unit of body structure is the **cell.** Cells have the same basic structure. Function, size, and shape may differ. Cells are very small. You need a microscope to see them. Cells need food, water, and oxygen to live and function.

Figure 10-1 shows the cell and its structures. The *cell membrane* is the outer covering. It encloses the cell and helps hold the cell's shape. The *nucleus* is the control center of the cell. It directs the cell's activities. The nucleus is in the center of the cell. The *cytoplasm* surrounds the nucleus. Cytoplasm contains smaller structures that perform cell functions. *Protoplasm* means "living substance." It refers to all structures, substances, and water within the cell. Protoplasm is a semi-liquid substance much like an egg white.

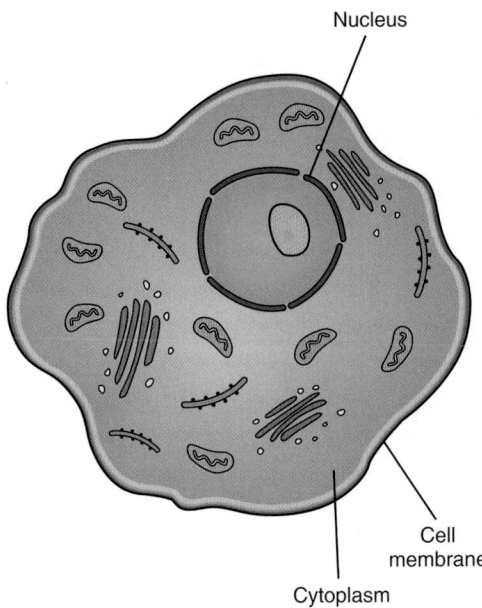

FIGURE 10-1 Parts of a cell.

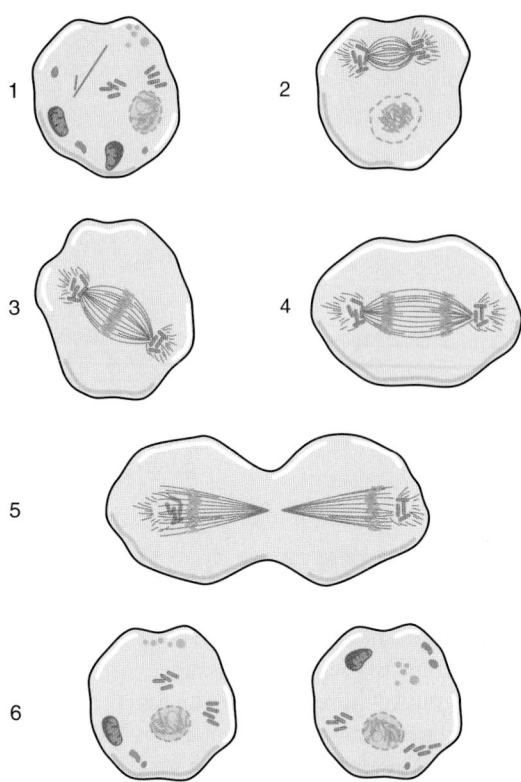

FIGURE 10-2 Cell division.

Chromosomes are thread-like structures in the nucleus. Each cell has 46 chromosomes. Chromosomes contain *genes*. Genes control the traits children inherit from their parents. Height, eye color, and skin color are examples.

The nucleus controls cell reproduction. Cells reproduce by dividing in half. The process of cell division is called *mitosis*. It is needed for tissue growth and repair. During mitosis, the 46 chromosomes arrange themselves in 23 pairs. As the cell divides, the 23 pairs are pulled in half. The 2 new cells are identical. Each has 46 chromosomes (Fig. 10-2).

Cells are the body's building blocks. *Groups of cells with similar functions combine to form* **tissues.**

- *Epithelial tissue* covers internal and external body surfaces. Tissue lining the nose, mouth, respiratory tract, stomach, and intestines is epithelial tissue. So are the skin, hair, nails, and glands.
- *Connective tissue* anchors, connects, and supports other tissues. It is in every part of the body. Bones, tendons, ligaments, and cartilage are connective tissue. Blood is a form of connective tissue.
- *Muscle tissue* stretches and contracts to let the body move.
- *Nerve tissue* receives and carries impulses to the brain and back to body parts.

Groups of tissue with the same function form **organs.** An organ has 1 or more functions. Examples of organs are the heart, brain, liver, lungs, and kidneys. **Systems** *are formed by organs that work together to perform special functions* (Fig. 10-3).

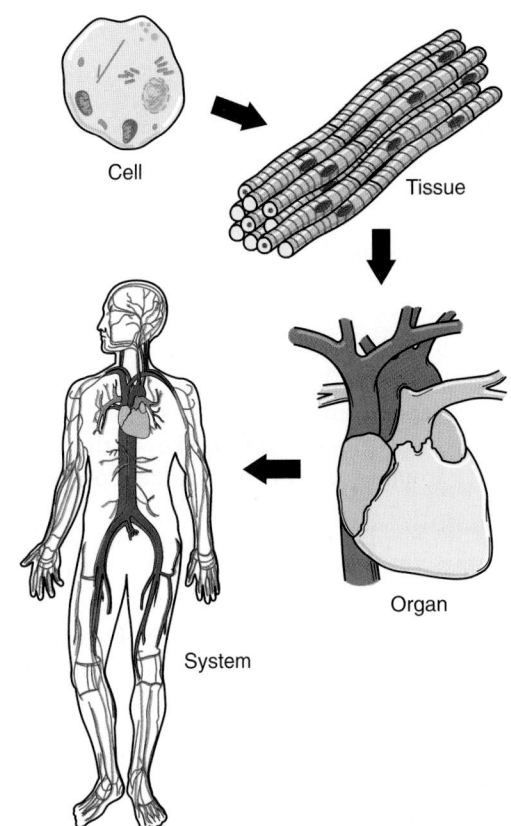

FIGURE 10-3 Organization of the body.

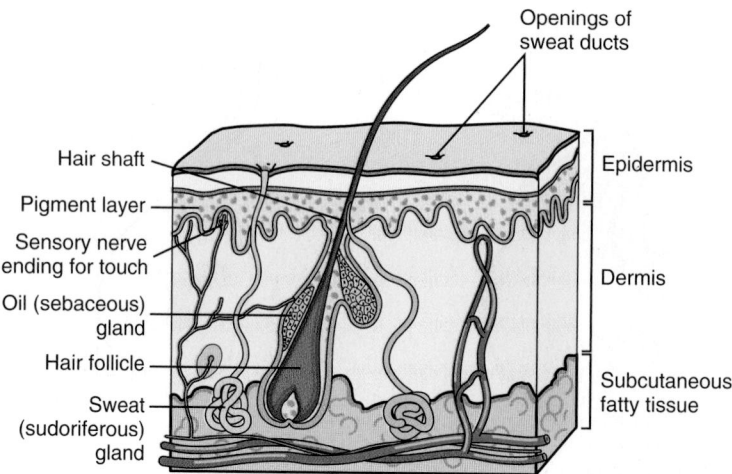

FIGURE 10-4 Layers of the skin.

THE INTEGUMENTARY SYSTEM

The *integumentary system*, or *skin*, is the largest system. *Integument* means *covering*. The skin covers the body. It has epithelial, connective, and nerve tissue. It also has oil glands and sweat glands. There are 2 skin layers (Fig. 10-4).

- The *epidermis* is the outer layer. It has living cells and dead cells. The dead cells were once deeper in the epidermis. They were pushed upward as the cells divided. Dead cells constantly flake off. They are replaced by living cells. Living cells die and flake off. Living cells of the epidermis contain *pigment*. Pigment gives skin its color. The epidermis has no blood vessels and few nerve endings.
- The *dermis* is the inner layer. It is made up of connective tissue. Blood vessels, nerves, sweat glands, and oil glands are found in the dermis. So are hair roots.

The epidermis and dermis are supported by *subcutaneous tissue*. The subcutaneous tissue is a thick layer of fat and connective tissue.

Oil glands and *sweat glands*, *hair*, and *nails* are skin appendages.

- Hair—covers the entire body, except the palms of the hands and the soles of the feet. Hair in the nose and ears and around the eyes protects these organs from dust, insects, and other foreign objects.
- Nails—protect the tips of the fingers and toes. Nails help fingers pick up and handle small objects.
- Sweat glands (*sudoriferous glands*)—help the body regulate temperature. Sweat consists of water, salt, and a small amount of wastes. Sweat is secreted through pores in the skin. The body is cooled as sweat evaporates.
- Oil glands (*sebaceous glands*)—lie near the hair shafts. They secrete an oily substance into the space near the hair shaft. Oil travels to the skin surface. This helps keep the hair and skin soft and shiny.

The skin has many functions.

- It is the body's protective covering.
- It prevents microorganisms and other substances from entering the body.
- It prevents excess amounts of water from leaving the body.
- It protects organs from injury.
- Nerve endings in the skin sense both pleasant and unpleasant stimulation. Nerve endings are over the entire body. They sense cold, pain, touch, and pressure to protect the body from injury.
- It helps regulate body temperature. Blood vessels *dilate* (widen) when temperature outside the body is high. More blood is brought to the body surface for cooling during evaporation. When blood vessels *constrict* (narrow), the body retains heat. This is because less blood reaches the skin.
- It stores fat and water.

THE MUSCULO-SKELETAL SYSTEM

The *musculo-skeletal system* provides the framework for the body. It lets the body move. This system also protects internal organs and gives the body shape.

Bones

The human body has 206 *bones* (Fig. 10-5). There are 4 types of bones.

- *Long bones* bear the body's weight. Leg bones are long bones.
- *Short bones* allow skill and ease in movement. Bones in the wrists, fingers, ankles, and toes are short bones.
- *Flat bones* protect the organs. They include the ribs, skull, pelvic bones, and shoulder blades.
- *Irregular bones* are the vertebrae in the spinal column. They allow various degrees of movement and flexibility.

Bones are hard, rigid structures. They are made up of living cells. Calcium and phosphorus are needed for bone formation and strength. Bones store these minerals for use by the body.

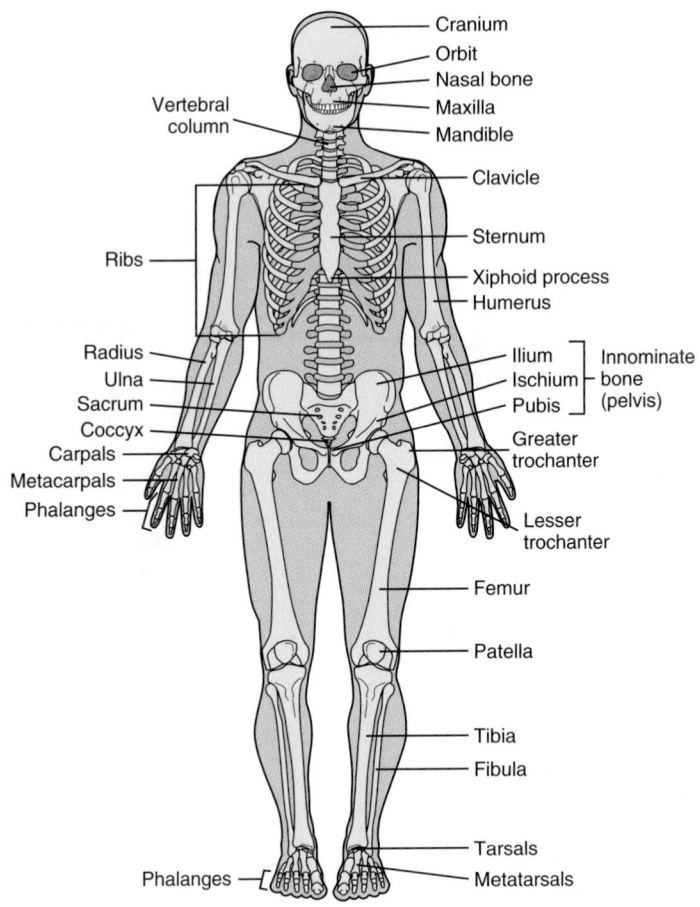

FIGURE 10-5 Bones of the body.

Bones are covered by a membrane called *periosteum*. Periosteum contains blood vessels that supply bone cells with oxygen and food. Inside the hollow centers of the bones is a substance called *bone marrow*. Blood cells are formed in the bone marrow.

Joints

A *joint* is the point at which 2 or more bones meet. Joints allow movement (Chapter 30). *Cartilage* is connective tissue at the end of the long bones. It cushions the joint so that the bone ends do not rub together. The *synovial membrane* lines the joints. It secretes *synovial fluid*. Synovial fluid acts as a lubricant so the joint can move smoothly. Bones are held together at the joint by strong bands of connective tissue called *ligaments*.

There are 3 major types of joints (Fig. 10-6).

* A *ball-and-socket joint* allows movement in all directions. It is made of the rounded end of 1 bone and the hollow end of another bone. The rounded end of 1 fits into the hollow end of the other. The joints of the hips and shoulders are ball-and-socket joints.
* A *hinge joint* allows movement in 1 direction. The elbow is a hinge joint.
* A *pivot joint* allows turning from side to side. A pivot joint connects the skull to the spine.

Some joints cannot move. They connect the bones of the skull.

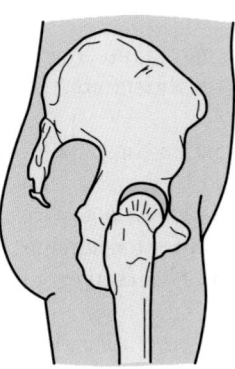

Ball-and-socket

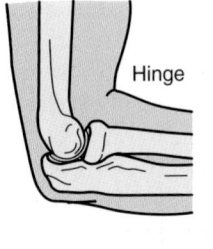

Hinge

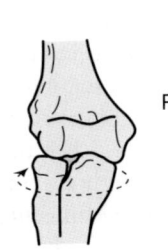

Pivot

FIGURE 10-6 Types of joints.

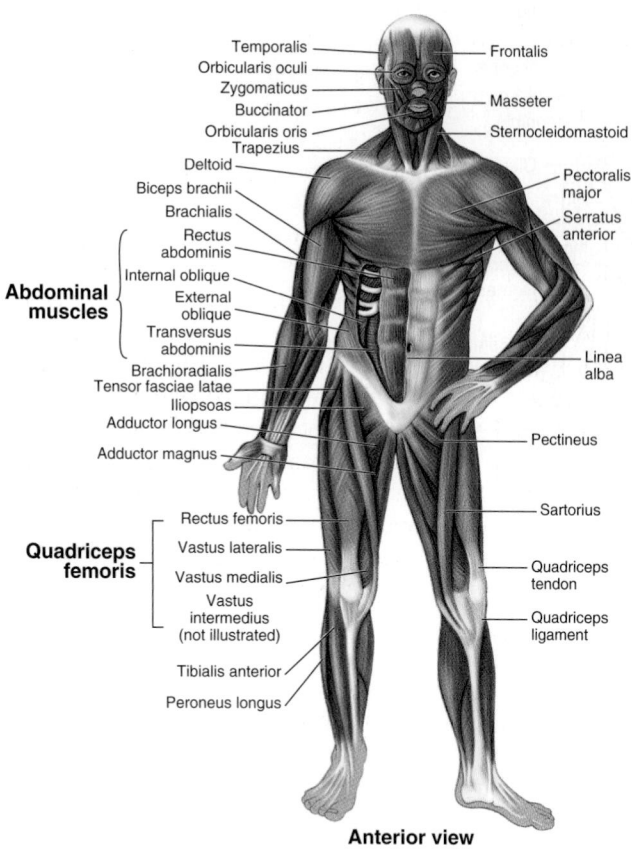

Anterior view

FIGURE 10-7 Anterior view of the muscles of the body. (From Herlihy B, Maebius NK: *The human body in health and illness,* ed 4, St Louis, 2011, Elsevier.)

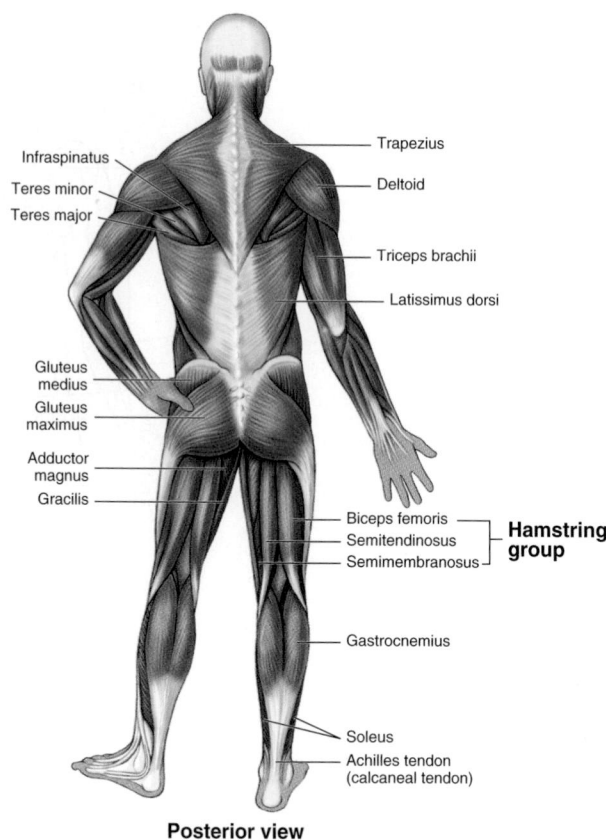

Posterior view

FIGURE 10-8 Posterior view of the muscles of the body. (From Herlihy B, Maebius NK: *The human body in health and illness,* ed 4, St Louis, 2011, Elsevier.)

Muscles

The human body has more than 500 *muscles*. See Figures 10-7 and 10-8. Some are voluntary. Others are involuntary.

- *Voluntary muscles* can be consciously controlled. Muscles attached to bones *(skeletal muscles)* are voluntary. Arm muscles do not work unless you move your arm; likewise for leg muscles. Skeletal muscles are *striated.* That is, they look striped or streaked.
- *Involuntary muscles* work automatically. You cannot control them. They control the action of the stomach, intestines, blood vessels, and other body organs. Involuntary muscles also are called *smooth muscles.* They look smooth, not streaked or striped.
- *Cardiac muscle* is in the heart. It is an involuntary muscle. However, it appears striated like skeletal muscle.

Muscles have 3 functions.

- Movement of body parts
- Maintenance of posture or muscle tone
- Production of body heat

Strong, tough connective tissues called *tendons* connect muscles to bones. When muscles *contract* (shorten), tendons at each end of the muscle cause the bone to move. The body has many tendons. See the Achilles tendon in Figure 10-8. Some muscles constantly contract to maintain the body's posture. When muscles contract, they burn food for energy. Heat is produced. The more muscle activity, the greater the amount of heat produced. Shivering is how the body produces heat when exposed to cold. Shivering is from rapid, general muscle contractions.

Sphincters are circular bands of muscle fibers. They *constrict* (narrow) a passage. Or they close a natural body opening. For example:

- The *pyloric sphincter* (Fig. 10-9) is an opening from the stomach into the small intestine. Closed, it holds food in the stomach for partial digestion. It opens to allow partially digested food to enter the small intestine.
- The *anal sphincter* keeps the anus closed. It opens for a bowel movement.
- *Urethral sphincters* seal off the bladder. This allows urine to collect in the bladder. The sphincters open for urination.

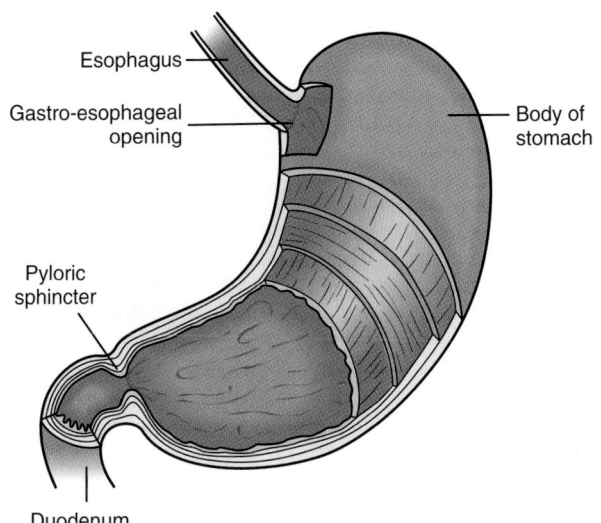

FIGURE 10-9 Pyloric sphincter. (Redrawn from Thibodeau GA, Patton KT: *The human body in health and disease*, ed 6, St Louis, 2014, Mosby.)

THE NERVOUS SYSTEM

The *nervous system* controls, directs, and coordinates body functions. Its 2 main divisions are:

- The *central nervous system* (CNS). It consists of the brain and spinal cord (Fig. 10-10).
- The *peripheral nervous system*. It involves the nerves throughout the body (Fig. 10-11).

Nerves connect to the spinal cord. Nerves carry messages or impulses to and from the brain. A *stimulus* causes a nerve impulse. A stimulus is anything that excites or causes a body part to function, become active, or respond. A *reflex* is the body's response (functioning or movement) to a stimulus. Reflexes are involuntary, unconscious, and immediate. The person cannot control reflexes.

Nerves are easily damaged and take a long time to heal. Some nerve fibers have a protective covering called a *myelin sheath*. The myelin sheath also insulates the nerve fiber. Nerve fibers covered with myelin conduct impulses faster than those fibers without it.

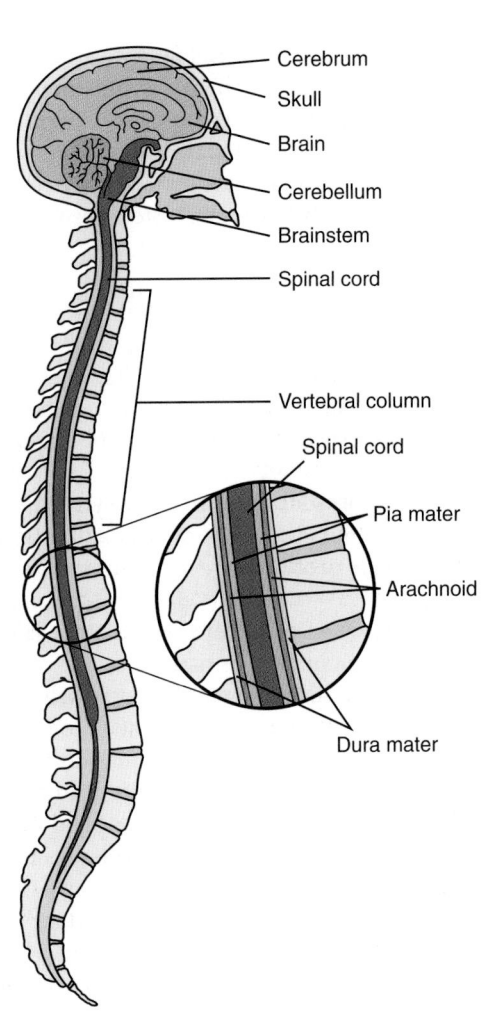

FIGURE 10-10 Central nervous system.

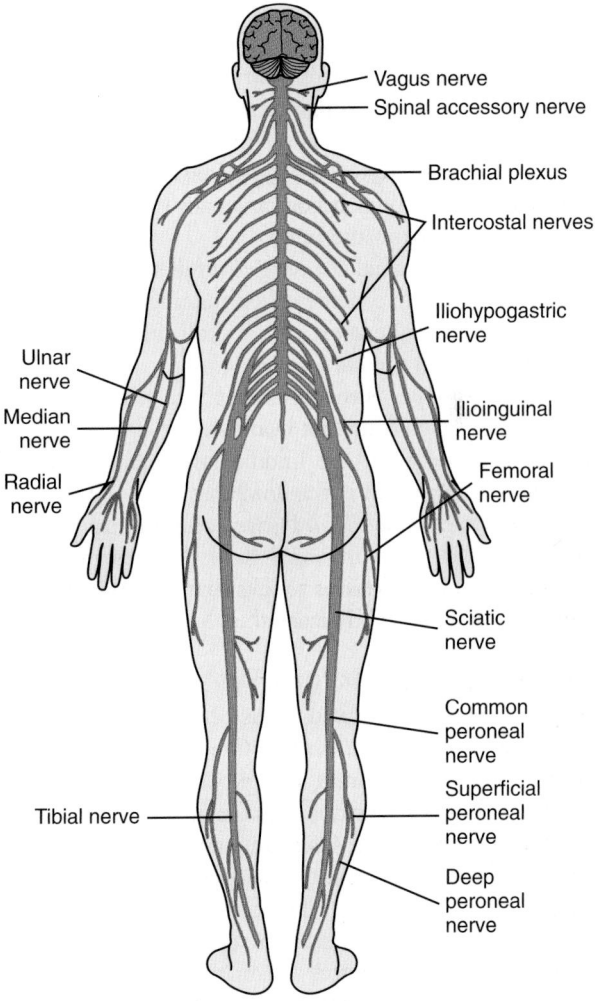

FIGURE 10-11 Peripheral nervous system.

The Central Nervous System

The *brain* and *spinal cord* make up the central nervous system. The brain is covered by the skull. The 3 main parts of the brain are the *cerebrum*, the *cerebellum*, and the *brainstem* (Fig. 10-12).

The cerebrum is the largest part of the brain. It is the center of thought and intelligence. The cerebrum is divided into 2 halves called *right* and *left hemispheres*. The right hemisphere controls movement and activities on the body's left side. The left hemisphere controls the right side.

The outside of the cerebrum is called the *cerebral cortex*. It controls the highest functions of the brain. These include reasoning, memory, consciousness, speech, voluntary muscle movement, vision, hearing, sensation, and other activities.

The cerebellum regulates and coordinates body movements. It controls balance and the smooth movements of voluntary muscles. Injury to the cerebellum results in jerky movements, loss of coordination, and muscle weakness.

The brainstem connects the cerebrum to the spinal cord. The brainstem contains the *midbrain, pons,* and *medulla*. The midbrain and pons relay messages between the medulla and the cerebrum. The medulla is below the pons. The medulla controls heart rate, breathing, blood vessel size, swallowing, coughing, and vomiting. The brain connects to the spinal cord at the lower end of the medulla.

The spinal cord lies within the spinal column. The cord is 17 to 18 inches long. It contains pathways that conduct messages to and from the brain.

The brain and spinal cord are covered and protected by 3 layers of connective tissue called meninges.
- The outer layer lies next to the skull. It is a tough covering called the *dura mater*.
- The middle layer is the *arachnoid*.
- The inner layer is the *pia mater*.

The space between the middle layer (arachnoid) and inner layer (pia mater) is the *arachnoid space*. The space is filled with *cerebrospinal fluid*. It circulates around the brain and spinal cord. Cerebrospinal fluid protects the central nervous system. It cushions shocks that could easily injure brain and spinal cord structures.

The Peripheral Nervous System

The peripheral nervous system has 12 pairs of *cranial nerves* and 31 pairs of *spinal nerves*. Cranial nerves conduct impulses between the brain and the head, neck, chest, and abdomen. They conduct impulses for smell, vision, hearing, pain, touch, temperature, and pressure. They also conduct impulses for voluntary and involuntary muscles. Spinal nerves carry impulses from the skin, extremities, and internal structures not supplied by the cranial nerves.

Some peripheral nerves form the *autonomic nervous system*. This system controls involuntary muscles and certain body functions. The functions include the heartbeat, blood pressure, intestinal contractions, and glandular secretions. These functions occur automatically.

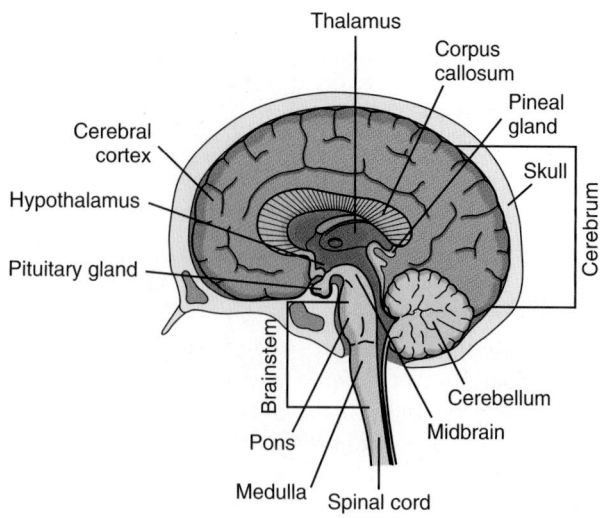

FIGURE 10-12 The brain.

The autonomic nervous system is divided into the *sympathetic nervous system* and the *parasympathetic nervous system*. They balance each other. The sympathetic nervous system speeds up functions. The parasympathetic nervous system slows functions. When you are angry, scared, excited, or exercising, the sympathetic nervous system is stimulated. The parasympathetic system is activated when you relax or when the sympathetic system is stimulated for too long.

The Sense Organs

The 5 senses are *sight, hearing, taste, smell,* and *touch*. Receptors for taste are in the tongue. They are called *taste buds*. Receptors for smell are in the nose. Touch receptors are in the dermis, especially in the toes and fingertips.

The Eye. Receptors for vision are in the eyes (Fig. 10-13). The eye is easily injured. Bones of the skull, eyelids and eyelashes, and tears protect the eyes from injury. The eye has 3 layers.
- The *sclera*, the white of the eye, is the outer layer. It is made of tough connective tissue.
- The *choroid* is the second layer. Blood vessels, the *ciliary muscle*, and the *iris* make up the choroid. The iris gives the eye its color. The opening in the middle of the iris is the *pupil*. Pupil size varies with the amount of light entering the eye. The pupil constricts (narrows) in bright light. It dilates (widens) in dim or dark places.
- The *retina* is the inner layer. It has receptors for vision and the nerve fibers of the *optic nerve*.

Light enters the eye through the *cornea*. It is the transparent part of the outer layer that lies over the eye. Light rays pass to the *lens*, which lies behind the pupil. The light is then reflected to the retina. Light is carried to the brain by the optic nerve.

The *aqueous chamber* separates the cornea from the lens. The chamber is filled with a fluid called *aqueous humor.* The fluid helps the cornea keep its shape and position. The *vitreous humor* is behind the lens. It is a gelatin-like substance that supports the retina and maintains the eye's shape.

The Ear. The *ear* is a sense organ (Fig. 10-14). It functions in hearing and balance. The ear has 3 parts: the *external ear, middle ear,* and *inner ear.*

The external ear (outer part) is called the *pinna* or *auricle.* Sound waves are guided through the external ear into the *auditory canal.* Glands in the auditory canal secrete a waxy substance called *cerumen.* The auditory canal extends about 1 inch into the *eardrum.* The eardrum *(tympanic membrane)* separates the external and middle ear.

The middle ear is a small space. It contains the *eustachian tube* and 3 small bones called *ossicles.* The eustachian tube connects the middle ear and the throat. Air enters the eustachian tube so there is equal pressure on both sides of the eardrum. The ossicles amplify sound received from the eardrum and transmit the sound to the inner ear. The 3 ossicles are:

* The *malleus.* It look like a hammer.
* The *incus.* It looks like an anvil.
* The *stapes.* It is shaped like a stirrup.

The inner ear consists of *semicircular canals* and the *cochlea.* The cochlea looks like a snail shell. It contains fluid. The fluid carries sound waves from the middle ear to the *acoustic nerve.* The acoustic nerve then carries messages to the brain.

The 3 semicircular canals are involved with balance. They sense the head's position and changes in position. They send messages to the brain.

THE CIRCULATORY SYSTEM

The *circulatory system (cardiovascular system)* is made up of the *blood, heart,* and *blood vessels.* The heart pumps blood through the blood vessels. The circulatory system has many functions.

* Blood carries food, hormones, and other substances to the cells.
* Blood transports (carries) the gases of respiration (p. 118). It brings oxygen to the cells.
* Blood removes waste products from cells.
* Blood plays a role in maintaining the body's fluid balance.
* Blood and blood vessels help regulate body temperature. The blood carries heat from muscle activity to other body parts. Blood vessels in the skin dilate to cool the body. They constrict to retain heat.
* The system produces and carries cells that defend the body from microbes that cause disease.

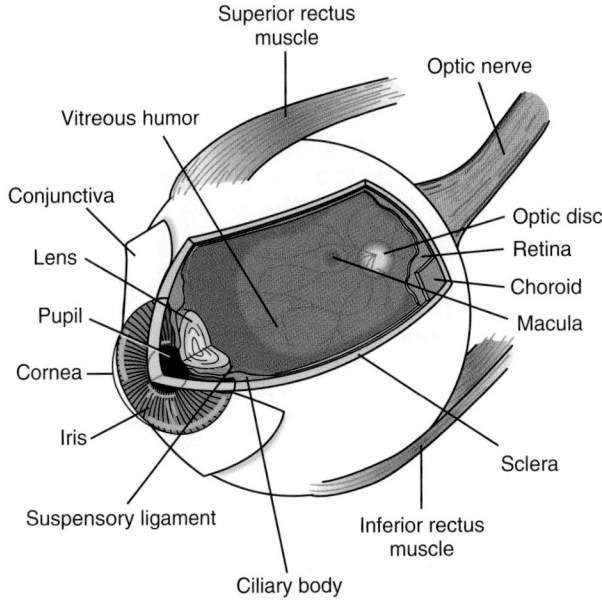

FIGURE 10-13 The eye.

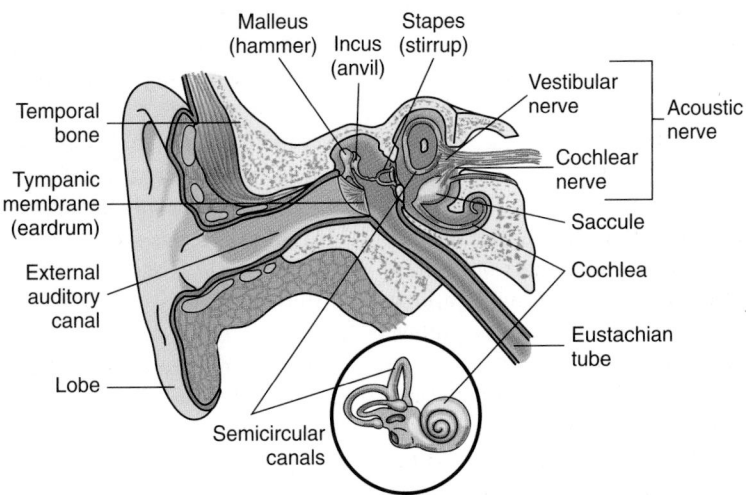

FIGURE 10-14 The ear.

The Blood

The *blood* consists of blood cells and *plasma*. Plasma is mostly water. It carries blood to other body cells. Plasma also carries substances that cells need to function. This includes food (proteins, fats, and carbohydrates), hormones (p. 122), and chemicals.

Red blood cells (RBCs) are called *erythrocytes*. **Hemoglobin** is a substance in RBCs that carries oxygen and gives blood its red color. As RBCs circulate through the lungs, hemoglobin picks up oxygen. Hemoglobin carries oxygen to the cells. When blood is bright red, hemoglobin in the RBCs is filled with oxygen. As blood circulates through the body, oxygen is given to the cells. Cells release carbon dioxide (a waste product). It is picked up by the hemoglobin. RBCs filled with carbon dioxide make the blood look dark red.

The body has about 25 trillion (25,000,000,000,000) RBCs. About 4½ to 5 million cells are in a cubic millimeter of blood (the size of a tiny drop). RBCs live for 3 to 4 months. They are destroyed by the liver and spleen as they wear out. New RBCs are formed in the bone marrow. About 1 million RBCs are produced every second.

White blood cells (WBCs) are called *leukocytes*. They have no color. They protect the body against infection. There are about 5000 to 10,000 WBCs in a cubic millimeter of blood. At the first sign of infection, WBCs rush to the infection site. There they multiply rapidly. The number of WBCs increases when there is an infection. WBCs are formed by the bone marrow. They live about 9 days.

Platelets (thrombocytes) are needed for blood clotting. They are formed by the bone marrow. There are about 200,000 to 400,000 platelets in a cubic millimeter of blood. A platelet lives about 4 days.

The Heart

The *heart* is a muscle. It pumps blood through the blood vessels to the tissues and cells. The heart lies in the middle to lower part of the chest cavity toward the left side (Fig. 10-15). The heart is hollow and has 3 layers (Fig. 10-16).

- The *pericardium* is the outer layer. It is a thin sac covering the heart.
- The *myocardium* is the second layer. It is the thick, muscular part of the heart.
- The *endocardium* is the inner layer. A membrane, it lines the inner surface of the heart.

The heart has 4 chambers (see Fig. 10-16). Upper chambers receive blood and are called *atria*. The *right atrium* receives blood from body tissues. The *left atrium* receives blood from the lungs. Lower chambers are called *ventricles*. Ventricles pump blood. The *right ventricle* pumps blood to the lungs for oxygen. The *left ventricle* pumps blood to all parts of the body.

Valves are between the atria and ventricles. The valves allow blood flow in 1 direction. They prevent blood from flowing back into the atria from the ventricles. The *tricuspid valve* is between the right atrium and the right ventricle. The *mitral valve (bicuspid valve)* is between the left atrium and left ventricle.

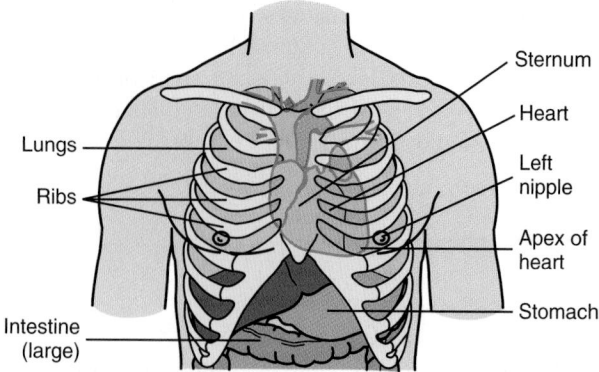

FIGURE 10-15 Location of the heart in the chest cavity.

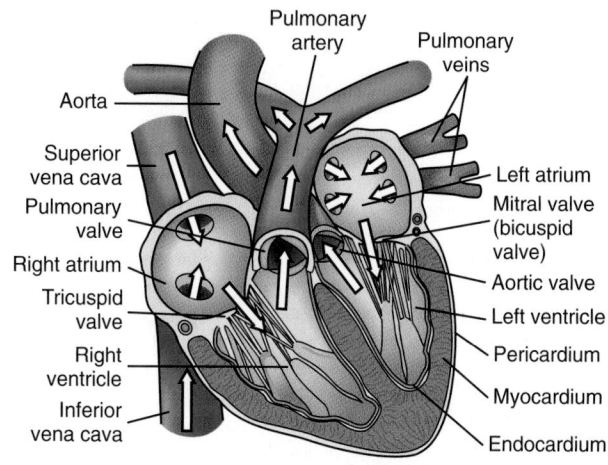

FIGURE 10-16 Structures of the heart.

Heart action has 2 phases.
- *Diastole.* It is the resting phase. Heart chambers fill with blood.
- *Systole.* It is the working phase. The heart contracts. Blood is pumped through the blood vessels when the heart contracts.

The Blood Vessels

Blood flows to body tissues and cells through the blood vessels. There are 3 groups of blood vessels: arteries, capillaries, and veins.

Arteries carry blood away from the heart. Arterial blood is rich in oxygen. The *aorta* is the largest artery. It receives blood directly from the left ventricle. The aorta branches into other arteries that carry blood to all parts of the body (Fig. 10-17). These arteries branch into smaller parts within the tissues. The smallest branch of an artery is an *arteriole.*

Arterioles connect to capillaries. *Capillaries* are very tiny blood vessels. Food, oxygen, and other substances pass from capillaries into the cells. The capillaries pick up waste products (including carbon dioxide) from the cells. Veins carry waste products back to the heart.

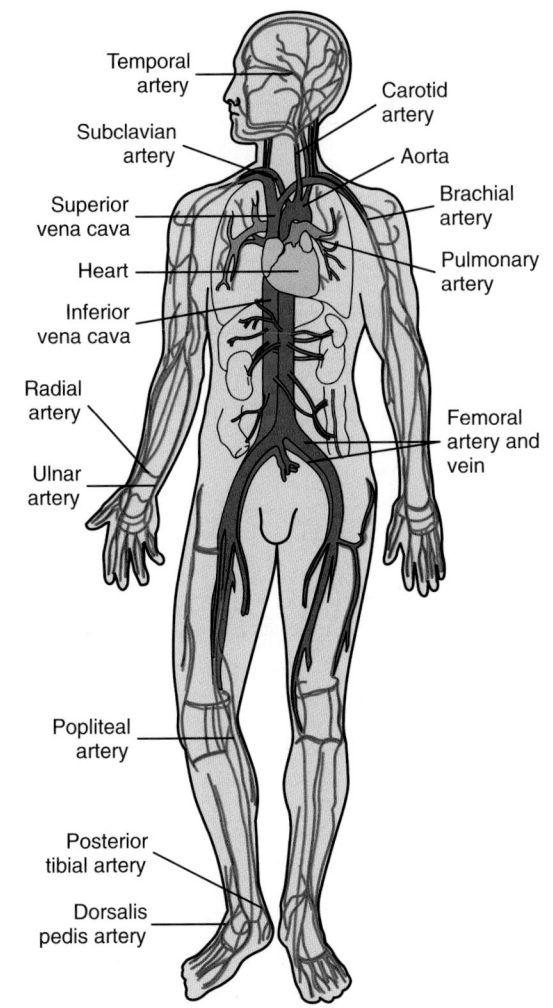

FIGURE 10-17 Arterial (red) and venous (blue) systems.

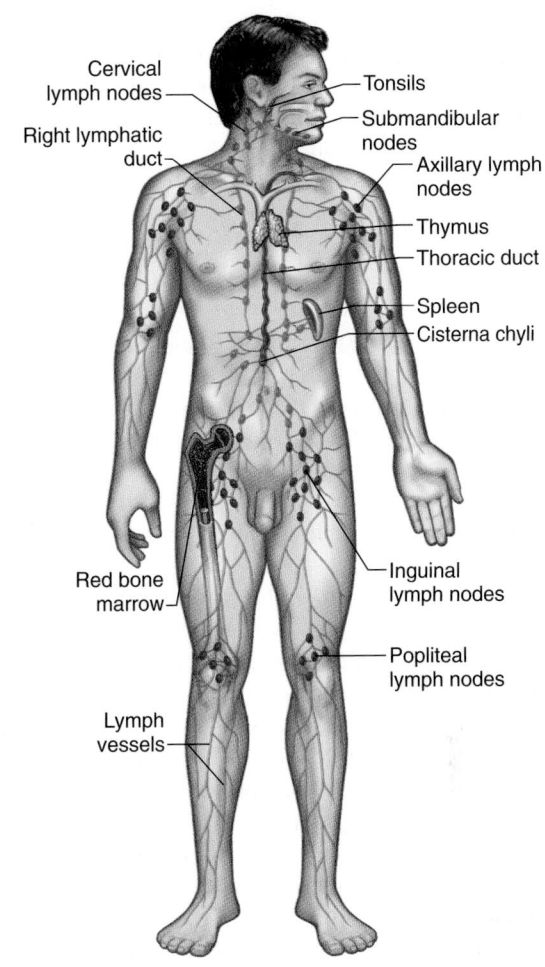

FIGURE 10-18 Lymphatic system. (From Patton KT, Thibodeau GA: *The human body in health and disease,* ed 6, St Louis, 2014, Mosby.)

Veins *return blood to the heart.* They connect to the capillaries by *venules.* Venules are small veins. Venules branch together to form veins. The many veins also branch together as they near the heart to form 2 main veins (see Fig. 10-17). The 2 main veins are the *inferior vena cava* and the *superior vena cava.* Both empty into the right atrium. The inferior vena cava carries blood from the legs and trunk. The superior vena cava carries blood from the head and arms. Venous blood is dark red. It has little oxygen and a lot of carbon dioxide.

Blood flow through the circulatory system is shown in Figure 10-16. The path of blood flow is as follows.

- Venous blood, poor in oxygen, empties into the right atrium.
- Blood flows through the tricuspid valve into the right ventricle.
- The right ventricle pumps blood into the lungs to pick up oxygen.
- Oxygen-rich blood from the lungs enters the left atrium.
- Blood from the left atrium passes through the mitral valve into the left ventricle.
- The left ventricle pumps the blood into the aorta. It branches off to form other arteries.
- Arterial blood is carried to the tissues by arterioles and to the cells by capillaries.

- Cells and capillaries exchange oxygen and nutrients for carbon dioxide and waste products.
- Capillaries connect with venules. Venules carry blood that has carbon dioxide and waste products.
- Venules form veins.
- Veins return blood to the heart.

THE LYMPHATIC SYSTEM

The lymphatic (lymph) system is a complex network that transports lymph throughout the body (Fig. 10-18). *Lymph* is a clear, thin, watery fluid. Lymph contains proteins and fats from the intestines. Lymph also contains white blood cells (WBCs). The lymphatic system:

- Collects extra lymph from the tissues and returns it to the blood. This helps maintain fluid balance. Water, proteins, and other substances normally leak out of the capillaries. The lymphatic system drains the extra fluid from the tissues. Otherwise, the tissues swell.
- Defends the body against infection by producing lymphocytes. *Lymphocytes* are a type of WBC that defends the body against microorganisms that cause infection (Chapter 16).
- Absorbs fats from the intestines and transports them to the blood.

Lymph is formed in the tissues. Lymph is transported by *lymphatic vessels*—lymphatic capillaries to lymphatic venules to the right lymphatic duct and the thoracic duct. Lymph then enters the blood in veins near the neck.

- The *right lymphatic duct* collects lymph from the right arm and from the right side of the head, neck, and chest. It empties into a vein on the right side of the neck.
- The *thoracic duct (left lymphatic duct)* collects lymph from the pelvis, abdomen, lower chest, and rest of the body. It empties into a vein on the left side of the neck.

Lymph nodes are shaped like beans. They range from the size of a pinhead to as large as a lima bean. They are found in the neck, underarm, groin area, chest, abdomen, and pelvis. Usually, you cannot see or feel lymph nodes. They swell when producing more lymphocytes to fight infection.

Lymph enters lymph nodes through the lymphatic vessels. The lymph nodes filter bacteria, cancer cells, and damaged cells from the lymph. This prevents such substances from entering and circulating throughout the body.

See Figure 10-18 for the location of the *thymus (thymus gland)*. Certain lymphocytes—T lymphocytes (T cells)—develop in the thymus. Such lymphocytes are important for immune system function (p. 123). The thymus reaches full growth at puberty. Then thymus tissue is slowly replaced by fat and connective tissue. By age 80, it is usually gone.

The *tonsils* are in the back of the throat. *Adenoids* are behind the nose. These structures trap microorganisms in the mouth and nose to help prevent infection.

The *spleen* is the largest structure in the lymphatic system. It is about the size of a fist. The spleen has a rich blood supply—about 500 milliliters (mL) (1 pint) of blood. The spleen:

- Filters and removes bacteria and other substances.
- Destroys old RBCs.
- Saves the iron found in hemoglobin when RBCs are destroyed.
- Stores blood. When needed, the blood is returned to the circulatory system.

THE RESPIRATORY SYSTEM

Oxygen is needed to live. Every cell needs oxygen. Air contains about 21% oxygen. This meets the body's needs under normal conditions. The respiratory system (Fig. 10-19) brings oxygen into the lungs and removes carbon dioxide. **Respiration** *is the process of supplying the cells with oxygen and removing carbon dioxide from them.* Respiration involves *inhalation* (breathing in) and *exhalation* (breathing out). The terms *inspiration* (breathing in) and *expiration* (breathing out) also are used.

Air enters the body through the *nose*. The air then passes into the *pharynx* (throat). It is a tube-shaped passageway for air and food. Air passes from the pharynx into the *larynx* (voice box). A piece of cartilage, the *epiglottis*, acts

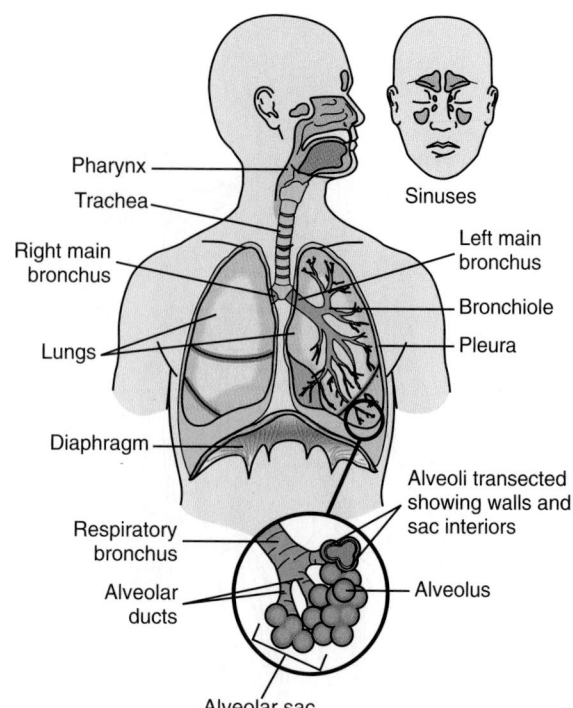

FIGURE 10-19 Respiratory system.

like a lid over the larynx. The epiglottis prevents food from entering the airway during swallowing. During inhalation the epiglottis lifts up to let air pass over the larynx. Air passes from the larynx into the *trachea* (windpipe).

The trachea divides at its lower end into the *right bronchus* and the *left bronchus*. Each bronchus enters a lung. Upon entering the lungs, the bronchi divide many times into smaller branches called *bronchioles*. Eventually the bronchioles subdivide. They end up in tiny 1-celled air sacs called *alveoli*.

Alveoli look like small clusters of grapes. They are supplied by capillaries. Oxygen and carbon dioxide are exchanged between the alveoli and capillaries. Blood in the capillaries picks up oxygen from the alveoli. Then the blood is returned to the left side of the heart and pumped to the rest of the body. Alveoli pick up carbon dioxide from the capillaries for exhalation.

The lungs are spongy tissues. They are filled with alveoli, blood vessels, and nerves. Each lung is divided into lobes. The right lung has 3 lobes; the left lung has 2. The lungs are separated from the abdominal cavity by a muscle called the *diaphragm*.

Each lung is covered by a 2-layered sac called the *pleura*. One layer is attached to the lung and the other to the chest wall. The pleura secretes a very thin fluid that fills the space between the layers. The fluid prevents the layers from rubbing together during inhalation and exhalation. A bony framework made up of the ribs, sternum, and vertebrae protects the lungs.

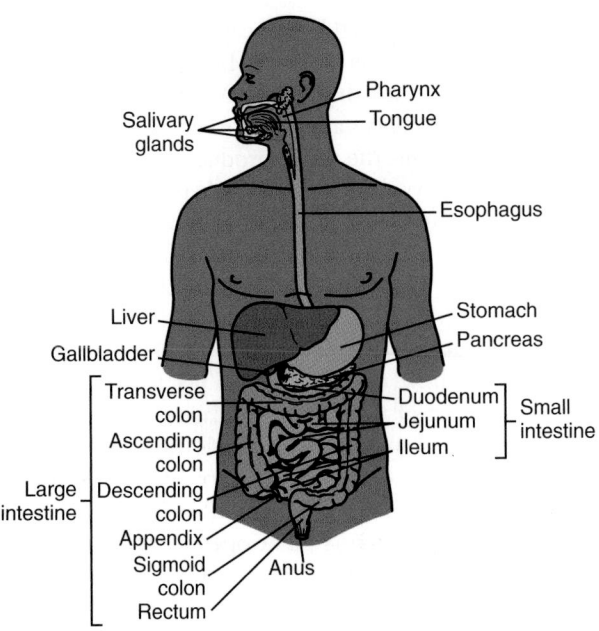

FIGURE 10-20 Digestive system.

THE DIGESTIVE SYSTEM

Digestion is the process that breaks down food physically and chemically so it can be absorbed for use by the cells. The digestive system is also called the gastro-intestinal (GI) system. The system also removes solid wastes from the body.

The digestive system involves the *alimentary canal (GI tract)* and the accessory organs of digestion (Fig. 10-20). The alimentary canal is a long tube. It extends from the mouth to the anus. Its major parts are the mouth, pharynx, esophagus, stomach, small intestine, and large intestine. Accessory organs are the teeth, tongue, salivary glands, liver, gallbladder, and pancreas.

Digestion begins in the *mouth (oral cavity).* It receives food and prepares it for digestion. Using chewing motions, the *teeth* cut, chop, and grind food into small particles for digestion and swallowing. The *tongue* aids in chewing and swallowing. *Taste buds* on the tongue's surface contain nerve endings. Taste buds allow sweet, sour, bitter, and salty tastes to be sensed. *Salivary glands* in the mouth secrete *saliva.* Saliva moistens food particles to ease swallowing and begin digestion. During swallowing, the tongue pushes food into the *pharynx.*

The pharynx (throat) is a muscular tube. Swallowing continues as the pharynx contracts. Contraction of the pharynx pushes food into the *esophagus.* The esophagus is a muscular tube about 10 inches long. It extends from the pharynx to the *stomach. Involuntary muscle contractions move food down the esophagus through the alimentary canal (peristalsis).*

The stomach is a muscular, pouch-like sac. It is in the upper left part of the abdominal cavity. Strong stomach muscles stir and churn food to break it up into even smaller particles. A mucous membrane lines the stomach. It contains glands that secrete *gastric juices.* Food is mixed and churned with the gastric juices to form a semi-liquid substance called *chyme.* Through peristalsis, the chyme is pushed from the stomach into the small intestine.

The *small intestine* is about 20 feet long. It has 3 parts. The first part is the *duodenum.* There more digestive juices are added to the chyme. One is called *bile.* Bile is a greenish liquid made in the *liver.* Bile is stored in the *gallbladder.* Juices from the *pancreas* and small intestine are added to the chyme. Digestive juices chemically break down food so it can be absorbed.

Peristalsis moves the chyme through the 2 other parts of the small intestine: the *jejunum* and the *ileum.* Tiny projections called *villi* line the small intestine. Villi absorb the digested food into the capillaries. Most food absorption takes place in the jejunum and the ileum.

Some chyme is not digested. Undigested chyme passes from the small intestine into the large *intestine (large bowel or colon).* The colon absorbs most of the water from the chyme. The remaining semi-solid material is called *feces.* Feces contain a small amount of water, solid wastes, and some mucus and germs. These are the waste products of digestion. Feces pass through the colon into the *rectum* by peristalsis. Feces pass out of the body through the *anus.*

THE URINARY SYSTEM

The digestive system rids the body of solid wastes. The lungs rid the body of carbon dioxide. Water and other substances leave the body through sweat. There are other waste products in the blood from cells burning food for energy. The urinary system (Fig. 10-21, p. 120):

- Removes waste products from the blood.
- Maintains water balance within the body.
- Maintains electrolyte balance. *Electrolytes* are substances that dissolve in water—sodium, potassium, and calcium.
  - Sodium is needed for fluid balance. The body retains water if sodium levels are high. Loss of sodium (through vomiting, diarrhea, some drugs, and so on) can result in dehydration.
  - Potassium and calcium are needed for the proper function of skeletal and cardiac muscles.
- Maintains acid-base balance. A pH scale measures if a substance is acidic, neutral, or basic. A pH of 7 is neutral. Anything below 7 is acidic. Anything above 7 is basic. The blood must remain within a certain pH range (7.35–7.45) for the body to function normally.

The *kidneys* are 2 bean-shaped organs in the upper abdomen. They lie against the back muscles on each side of the spine. They are protected by the lower edge of the rib cage.

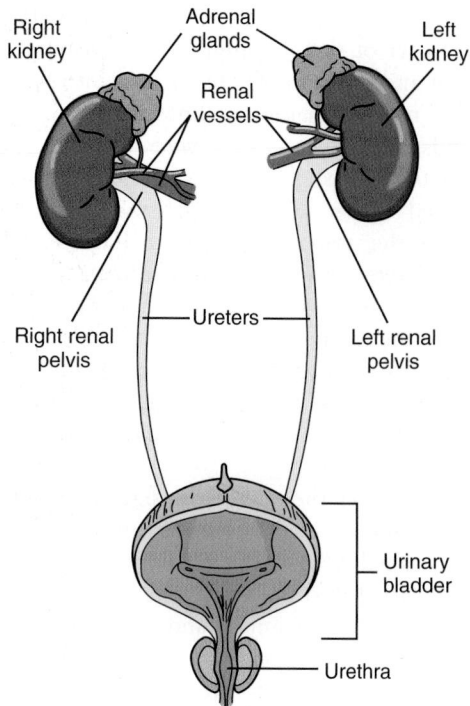

FIGURE 10-21 Urinary system.

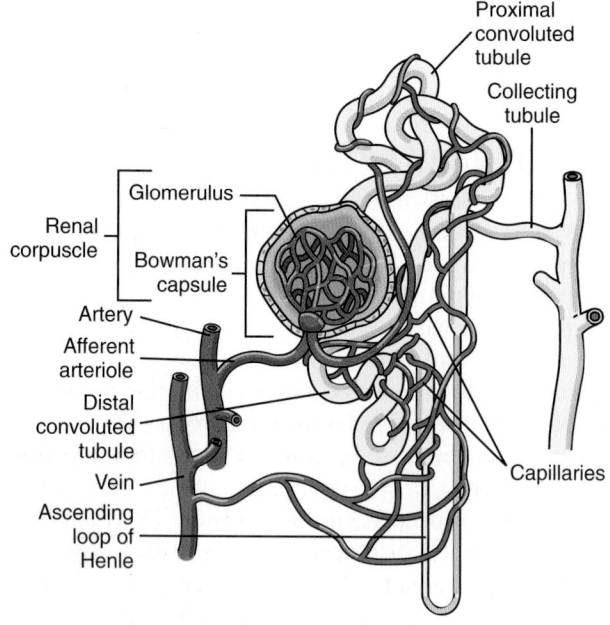

FIGURE 10-22 A nephron.

Each kidney has over a million tiny *nephrons* (Fig. 10-22). Each nephron is the basic working unit of the kidney. Each nephron has a *convoluted tubule*, which is a tiny coiled tubule. Each convoluted tubule has a *Bowman's capsule* at 1 end. The capsule partly surrounds a cluster of capillaries called a *glomerulus*. Blood passes through the glomerulus and is filtered by the capillaries. The fluid part of the blood is squeezed into the Bowman's capsule. The fluid then passes into the tubule. Most of the water and other needed substances are re-absorbed by the blood. The rest of the fluid and the waste products form *urine* in the tubule. Urine flows through the tubule to a *collecting tubule*. All collecting tubules drain into the *renal pelvis* in the kidney.

A tube called the *ureter* is attached to the renal pelvis of the kidney. Each ureter is about 10 to 12 inches long. The ureters carry urine from the kidneys to the *bladder*. The bladder is a hollow, muscular sac. It lies toward the front in the lower part of the abdominal cavity.

Urine is stored in the bladder until the need to urinate is felt. This usually occurs when there is about a half pint (250 mL) of urine in the bladder. Urine passes from the bladder through the *urethra*. The opening at the end of the urethra is called the *meatus*. Urine passes from the body through the meatus. Urine is a clear, yellowish fluid.

THE REPRODUCTIVE SYSTEM

Human reproduction results from the union of a male sex cell and a female sex cell. The male and female reproductive systems are different. This allows for the process of reproduction.

The Male Reproductive System

The male reproductive system is shown in Figure 10-23. The *testes (testicles)* are the male sex glands. Sex glands also are called *gonads*. The 2 testes are oval or almond-shaped glands. Male sex cells are produced in the testes. Male sex cells are called *sperm* cells.

Testosterone, the male hormone, is produced in the testes. This hormone is needed for reproductive organ function. It also is needed for the development of the male secondary sex characteristics. There is facial hair; pubic and axillary (underarm) hair; and hair on the arms, chest, and legs. Neck and shoulder sizes increase.

The testes are suspended between the thighs in a sac called the *scrotum*. The scrotum is made of skin and muscle.

Sperm travel from the testis to the *epididymis*. The epididymis is a coiled tube on top and to the side of the testis. From the epididymis, sperm travel through a tube called the *vas deferens*. Each vas deferens joins a *seminal vesicle*. The 2 seminal vesicles store sperm and produce *semen*. Semen is a fluid that carries sperm from the male reproductive tract. The ducts of the seminal vesicles unite to form the *ejaculatory duct*. It passes through the *prostate gland*.

The prostate gland lies just below the bladder. It is shaped like a donut. The gland secretes fluid into the semen. As the ejaculatory ducts leave the prostate, they join the *urethra*. The urethra runs through the prostate gland. The urethra is the outlet for urine and semen. The urethra is contained within the *penis*.

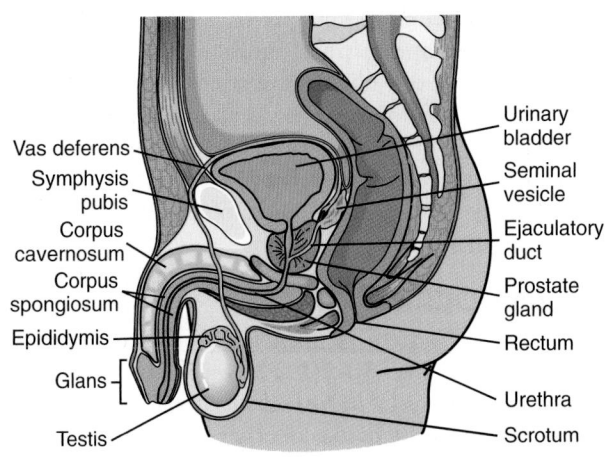

FIGURE 10-23 Male reproductive system.

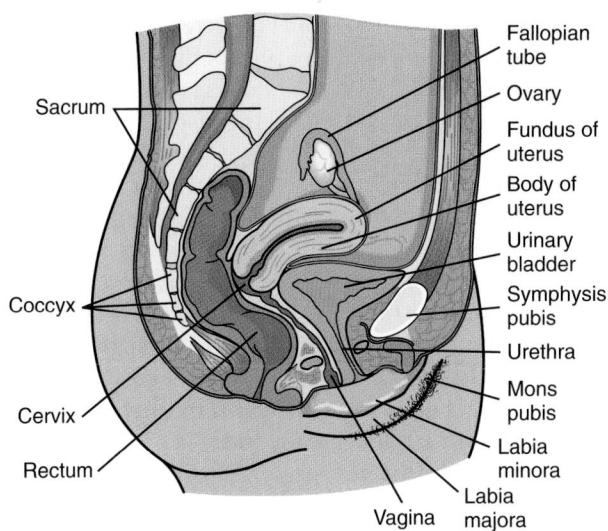

FIGURE 10-24 Female reproductive system.

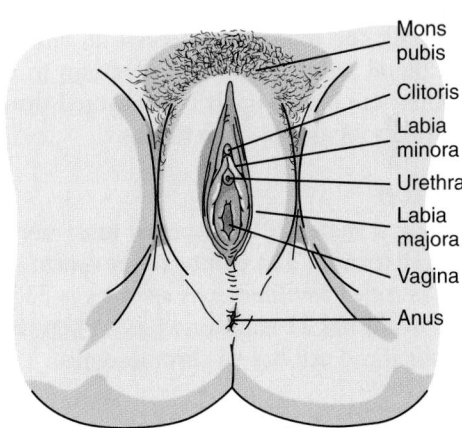

FIGURE 10-25 External female genitalia.

The penis is outside of the body. The *glans* is at the end of the penis. The urethra opens at the end of the glans. A fold of skin (*prepuce* or *foreskin*) is at the end of the penis (Chapters 22 and 25).

The penis has *erectile* tissue. When a man is sexually excited, blood fills the erectile tissue. The penis enlarges and becomes hard and erect. The erect penis can enter a female's vagina. *Cowper's glands* are 2 pea-sized glands under the prostate. They produce a clear, colorless fluid before ejaculation (release of semen). The fluid cleanses the urethra, protects sperm from damage, and provides some lubrication for intercourse. With ejaculation, semen—containing sperm—is released into the vagina.

The Female Reproductive System

Figure 10-24 shows the female reproductive system. The female gonads are 2 almond-shaped glands called *ovaries*. An ovary is on each side of the uterus in the abdominal cavity.

The ovaries contain *ova* or eggs. Ova are the female sex cells. One ovum (egg) is released monthly during the woman's reproductive years. Release of an ovum is called *ovulation.*

The ovaries secrete the female hormones *estrogen* and *progesterone*. These hormones are needed for reproductive system function. They also are needed for the development of secondary sex characteristics in the female. These include increased breast size, pubic and axillary (underarm) hair, slight deepening of the voice, and widening and rounding of the hips.

When an ovum is released from an ovary, it travels through a *fallopian tube*. There are 2 fallopian tubes, 1 on each side. The tubes are attached at 1 end to the *uterus.* The ovum travels through the fallopian tube to the uterus.

The uterus is a hollow, muscular organ shaped like a pear. It is in the center of the pelvic cavity behind the bladder and in front of the rectum. The main part of the uterus is the *fundus.* The neck or narrow section of the uterus is the *cervix.* Tissue lining the uterus is the *endometrium.* The endometrium has many blood vessels. If sex cells from the male and female unite into 1 cell, that cell implants into the endometrium. There the cell grows into a *fetus* (unborn baby) and receives nourishment.

The cervix of the uterus projects into a muscular canal called the *vagina.* The vagina opens to the outside of the body. It is just behind the urethra. The vagina receives the penis during intercourse. It also is part of the birth canal. Glands in the vaginal wall keep it moistened with secretions. The Bartholin's glands are examples. In young girls, the external vaginal opening is partially closed by a membrane called the *hymen.* The hymen ruptures when the female has intercourse for the first time.

The external female genitalia are called the *vulva* (Fig. 10-25).

- The *mons pubis* is a rounded, fatty pad over a bone called the *symphysis pubis*. The mons pubis is covered with hair in the adult female.
- The *labia majora* and *labia minora* are 2 folds of tissue on each side of the vaginal opening.
- The *clitoris* is a small organ composed of erectile tissue. It becomes hard when sexually stimulated.

The *mammary glands (breasts)* secrete milk after childbirth. The glands are on the outside of the chest. They are made up of glandular tissue and fat (Fig. 10-26). The milk drains into ducts that open onto the *nipple.*

Menstruation. The endometrium is rich in blood to nourish the cell that grows into a fetus. If pregnancy does not occur, menstruation begins. *Menstruation is the process in which the lining of the uterus (endometrium) breaks up and is discharged from the body through the vagina.* It occurs about every 28 days. Therefore it is called the *menstrual cycle.*

The first day of the menstrual cycle begins with menstruation. Blood flows from the uterus through the vaginal opening. Menstrual flow usually lasts 3 to 7 days. Ovulation occurs during the next phase. An ovum matures in an ovary and is released. Ovulation usually occurs on or about day 14 of the cycle.

Meanwhile, estrogen and progesterone (the female hormones) are secreted by the ovaries. These hormones cause the endometrium to thicken for pregnancy. If pregnancy does not occur, the hormones decrease in amount. This causes the blood supply to the endometrium to decrease. The endometrium breaks up. It is discharged through the vagina. Another menstrual cycle begins.

Fertilization

To reproduce, a male sex cell (sperm) must unite with a female sex cell (ovum). The uniting of the sperm and ovum into 1 cell is called *fertilization.* A sperm has 23 chromosomes. An ovum has 23 chromosomes. When the 2 cells unite, the fertilized cell has 46 chromosomes.

During intercourse, millions of sperm are deposited into the vagina. Sperm travel up the cervix, through the uterus, and into the fallopian tubes. If a sperm and an ovum unite in a fallopian tube, fertilization results. Pregnancy occurs. The fertilized cell travels down the fallopian tube to the uterus. After a short time, the fertilized cell implants into the thick endometrium and grows during pregnancy.

THE ENDOCRINE SYSTEM

The endocrine system is made up of glands called the *endocrine glands* (Fig. 10-27). *The endocrine glands secrete chemical substances called* **hormones** *into the bloodstream.* Hormones regulate the activities of other organs and glands in the body.

The *pituitary gland* is called the *master gland.* About the size of a cherry, it is at the base of the brain behind the eyes. The pituitary gland is divided into the *anterior pituitary lobe* and the *posterior pituitary lobe.* The anterior pituitary lobe secretes:

- *Growth hormone (GH)*—needed for growth of muscles, bones, and other organs. It is needed throughout life to maintain normal-sized bones and muscles. Growth is stunted if a baby is born with deficient amounts of growth hormones. Too much of the hormone causes excessive growth.
- *Thyroid-stimulating hormone (TSH)*—needed for thyroid gland function.
- *Adrenocorticotropic hormone (ACTH)*—stimulates the adrenal glands.

The anterior lobe also secretes hormones that regulate growth, development, and function of the male and female reproductive systems.

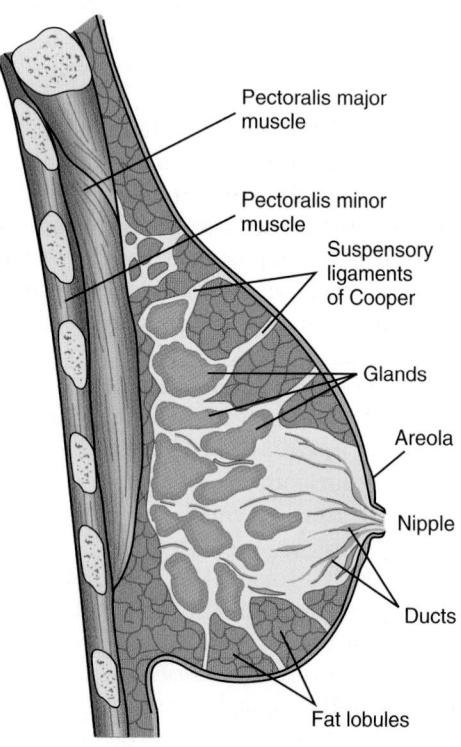

Pectoralis major muscle

Pectoralis minor muscle

Suspensory ligaments of Cooper

Glands

Areola

Nipple

Ducts

Fat lobules

FIGURE 10-26 The female breast.

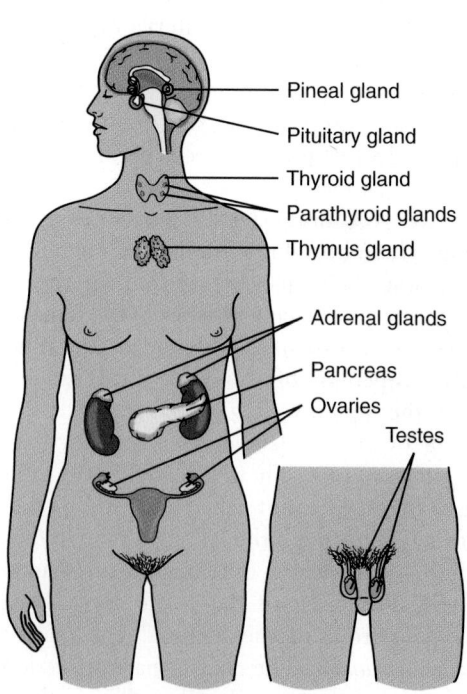

Pineal gland

Pituitary gland

Thyroid gland

Parathyroid glands

Thymus gland

Adrenal glands

Pancreas

Ovaries

Testes

FIGURE 10-27 Endocrine system.

The posterior pituitary lobe secretes *antidiuretic hormone (ADH)* and *oxytocin*. ADH prevents the kidneys from excreting excessive amounts of water. Oxytocin causes uterine muscles to contract during childbirth.

The *thyroid gland*, shaped like a butterfly, is in the neck in front of the larynx. *Thyroid hormone (TH, thyroxine)* is secreted by the thyroid gland. It regulates metabolism. *Metabolism is the burning of food for heat and energy by the cells.* Too little TH results in slowed body processes, slowed movements, and weight gain. Too much TH causes increased metabolism, excess energy, and weight loss. Some babies are born with deficient amounts of TH. Their physical growth and mental growth are stunted.

The 4 *parathyroid glands* secrete *parathormone*. Two lie on each side of the thyroid gland. Parathormone regulates calcium use. Calcium is needed for nerve and muscle function. Insufficient amounts of calcium cause *tetany*. Tetany is a state of severe muscle contraction and spasm. If untreated, tetany can cause death.

The *thymus* secretes the hormone *thymosin*. This hormone is important for the development and function of the immune system.

The *pancreas* secretes *insulin*. Insulin regulates the amount of sugar in the blood available for use by the cells. Insulin is needed for sugar to enter the cells. If there is too little insulin, sugar cannot enter the cells. If sugar cannot enter the cells, excess amounts build up in the blood. This condition is called *diabetes*.

There are 2 *adrenal glands*. An adrenal gland is on the top of each kidney. The adrenal gland has 2 parts: the *adrenal medulla* and the *adrenal cortex*. The adrenal medulla secretes *epinephrine* and *norepinephrine*. These hormones stimulate the body to quickly produce energy during emergencies. Heart rate, blood pressure, muscle power, and energy all increase.

The adrenal cortex secretes 3 groups of hormones needed for life.
- *Glucocorticoids*—regulate metabolism of carbohydrates. They also control the body's response to stress and inflammation.
- *Mineralocorticoids*—regulate the amount of salt and water that is absorbed and lost by the kidneys.
- Small amounts of male and female sex hormones are secreted.

The *gonads* are the glands of human reproduction. Male sex glands (testes) secrete *testosterone*. Female sex glands (ovaries) secrete *estrogen* and *progesterone*.

THE IMMUNE SYSTEM

The immune system protects the body from disease and infection. Abnormal body cells can grow into tumors. Sometimes the body produces substances that cause the body to attack itself. Microorganisms (bacteria, viruses, and other germs) can cause an infection. The immune system defends against threats inside and outside the body.

The immune system gives the body immunity. *Immunity means that a person has protection against a disease or condition. The person will not get or be affected by the disease.*
- *Specific immunity* is the body's reaction to a certain threat.
- *Non-specific immunity* is the body's reaction to anything it does not recognize as a normal body substance.

Special cells and substances function to produce immunity.
- *Antibodies*—normal body substances that recognize other substances. They are involved in destroying abnormal or unwanted substances.
- *Antigens*—substances that cause an immune response. Antibodies recognize and bind with unwanted antigens. This leads to the destruction of unwanted substances and the production of more antibodies.
- *Phagocytes*—white blood cells (WBCs) that digest and destroy microorganisms and other unwanted substances (Fig. 10-28).
- *Lymphocytes*—WBCs that produce antibodies. Lymphocyte production increases as the body responds to an infection.
  - *B lymphocytes (B cells)*—cause the production of antibodies that circulate in the plasma. The antibodies react to specific antigens.
  - *T lymphocytes (T cells)*—destroy invading cells. *Killer T cells* produce poisons near the invading cells. Some T cells attract other cells. The other cells destroy the invaders.

When the body senses an antigen from an unwanted substance, the immune system acts. Phagocyte and lymphocyte production increases. Phagocytes destroy the invaders through digestion. The lymphocytes produce antibodies that identify and destroy the unwanted substances.

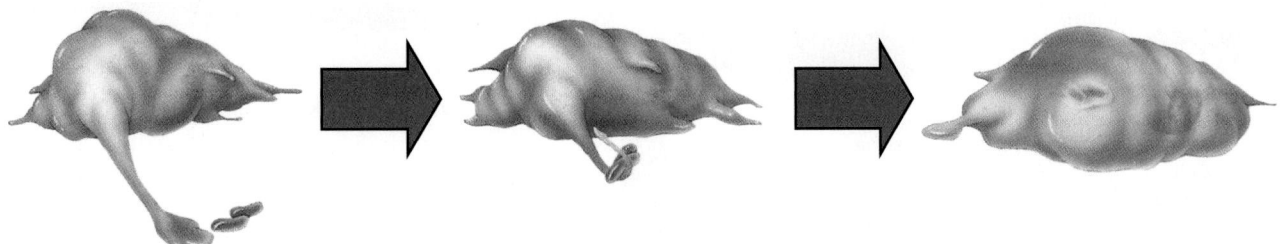

FIGURE 10-28 A phagocyte digests and destroys a microorganism. (From Thibodeau GA, Patton KT: *Structure and function of the body*, ed 11, St Louis, 2000, Mosby.)

FOCUS ON PRIDE

The Person, Family, and Yourself

Personal and Professional Responsibility

Taking care of yourself is a personal and professional responsibility. To care for others you need a strong and healthy body.

- Eat a healthy diet (Chapter 27), exercise, and get enough rest.
- See your doctor for a check-up at least once a year. Or do so sooner if you have a concern.
- Take prescription or over-the-counter drugs only as instructed.
- Keep your immunizations up to date. For example, get a tetanus booster every 10 years.
- Protect your bones and muscles from injury by using good body mechanics (Chapter 17).
- Protect yourself from infection. Follow Standard Precautions and practice good hand hygiene (Chapter 16).

Rights and Respect

Patients and residents have the right to make decisions about their bodies. You may not agree with those decisions. But you must respect the person's choices. If the decision will cause no harm, comply with the request. For example, Mr. Ferris does not want to wear his hearing aid today. He says: "I don't need that thing." His request will not harm him. Respect his choice. Tell the nurse.

If the person's decision may cause harm, tell the nurse at once. For example, Ms. Lane's kidneys do not function. She goes to dialysis 3 times a week. (*Dialysis* is the process of artificially removing wastes from the blood when the kidneys do not function.) Ms. Lane does not want to go today. She says: "I just can't sit there for that long." You know the importance of the urinary system. Without dialysis, she will become very sick. You tell the nurse. Ms. Lane cannot be forced to go to dialysis. But the nurse can talk with Ms. Lane about her decision, the consequences, and possible solutions.

Independence and Social Interaction

The body does not always work right. People become ill or injured. Some illnesses cannot be cured. Sometimes the health team cannot prevent loss of function. To help maintain the person's optimal level of function:

- Do not treat the person as a sick, dependent person.
- Encourage the person to be as independent as possible.
- Always focus on the person's abilities, not disabilities.
- Tell the person when you notice progress.
- Promote social interaction. This improves mental performance.

Take pride in helping each person regain or maintain the highest level of functioning possible.

Delegation and Teamwork

The body works like a team. Each system has independent functions. But all systems interact and depend on each other. They work together to keep the body functioning. When a person has a problem with 1 body system, other systems are affected. Understanding each system and how the systems interact helps you provide better care.

Ethics and Laws

Sometimes a person is not able to make decisions about his or her own body. For example, the person has dementia. Or the person is unconscious or affected by drugs or alcohol. Maybe the person thinks about harming himself or herself. Or the person is a child. Ethical issues may arise over who makes decisions for such persons.

Spouses, parents, family members, or legal representatives may make decisions. Some persons have an advance directive (Chapter 55). Sometimes the court appoints a guardian for a short time. Finally, the agency's ethics committee may address complex issues. The person's safety and best interests must guide the care given.

FOCUS ON PRIDE: *Application*

Body systems interact for normal function. Explain how the body systems below interact with other systems. How might a problem in 1 system affect another?

- Nervous system
- Circulatory system
- Respiratory system
- Endocrine system

REVIEW QUESTIONS

Circle the BEST answer.

1 The basic unit of body structure is the
   a Cell
   b Neuron
   c Nephron
   d Ovum

2 The outer layer of the skin is called the
   a Dermis
   b Epidermis
   c Integument
   d Myelin

Continued

REVIEW QUESTIONS—cont'd

3 Which is a function of the skin?
a Provides the protective covering for the body
b Transports lymph
c Forms blood cells
d Provides the shape and framework for the body

4 Which allows movement?
a Bone marrow
b Synovial membrane
c Joints
d Ligaments

5 Skeletal muscles
a Are under involuntary control
b Appear smooth
c Are under voluntary control
d Appear striped and smooth

6 The highest functions in the brain take place in the
a Cerebral cortex
b Medulla
c Brainstem
d Spinal nerves

7 The ear is involved with
a Regulating body movements
b Balance
c Smoothness of body movements
d Controlling involuntary muscles

8 The liquid part of blood is the
a Hemoglobin
b Red blood cell
c Plasma
d White blood cell

9 Which part of the heart pumps blood to the body?
a Right atrium
b Left atrium
c Right ventricle
d Left ventricle

10 Which carry blood away from the heart?
a Capillaries
b Veins
c Venules
d Arteries

11 Which statement about the lymphatic system is *true*?
a The tonsils are the largest structures in the lymphatic system.
b Lymph transports oxygen and nutrients to cells.
c The spleen filters bacteria and damaged cells.
d Extra lymph from the blood is moved to the tissues.

12 Oxygen and carbon dioxide are exchanged
a In the bronchi
b Between the alveoli and capillaries
c Between the lungs and pleura
d In the trachea

13 Digestion begins in the
a Mouth
b Stomach
c Small intestine
d Colon

14 Most food absorption takes place in the
a Stomach
b Small intestine
c Colon
d Large intestine

15 Urine is formed by the
a Jejunum
b Kidneys
c Bladder
d Liver

16 Urine passes from the body through the
a Ureters
b Urethra
c Anus
d Nephrons

17 The male sex gland is called the
a Penis
b Semen
c Testis
d Scrotum

18 The male sex cell is the
a Semen
b Ovum
c Gonad
d Sperm

19 The female sex gland is the
a Ovary
b Cervix
c Uterus
d Vagina

20 The discharge of the lining of the uterus is called
a The endometrium
b Ovulation
c Fertilization
d Menstruation

21 The endocrine glands secrete
a Hormones
b Mucus
c Semen
d Antibodies

22 The immune system protects the body from
a Low blood sugar
b Disease and infection
c Loss of fluid
d Stunted growth

Answers to Chapter 10 questions are on p. 870.

FOCUS ON **PRACTICE**

Problem Solving

A patient has a disorder that affects the immune system. How does this affect body function? How will you provide care in a way that protects the person?

Growth and Development

KEY TERMS

adolescence The time between puberty and adulthood; a time of rapid growth and physical, sexual, emotional, and social changes

development Changes in mental, emotional, and social function

developmental task A skill that must be completed during a stage of development

ejaculation The release of semen

growth The physical changes that are measured and that occur in a steady, orderly manner

infancy The first year of life

menarche The first menstruation and the start of menstrual cycles

menopause The time when menstruation stops and menstrual cycles end

peer A person of the same age-group and background

primary caregiver The person mainly responsible for providing or assisting with the child's basic needs

puberty The period when reproductive organs begin to function and secondary sex characteristics appear

reflex An involuntary movement

sexual orientation Sexual arousal or romantic attraction to persons of the other gender (heterosexual), the same gender (homosexual), or both genders (bisexual)

teen dating violence The physical, sexual, psychological, or emotional violence within a dating relationship as well as stalking

KEY ABBREVIATIONS

CDC Centers for Disease Control and Prevention
CNS Central nervous system

IPV Intimate partner violence

---

*G*rowth *is the physical changes that are measured and that occur in a steady and orderly manner.* Growth is measured in weight, height, and changes in appearance and body functions (Fig. 11-1). *Development relates to changes in mental, emotional, and social function.* A person behaves and thinks in certain ways in each stage of development. For example, babies depend on adults for basic needs. Adults can meet most of their basic needs without help.

This chapter presents the basic stages of growth and development that occur in normal, healthy persons from birth until death. The stages overlap. It is hard to see the start and end of each stage. Also, the rate of growth and development varies with each person.

Growth and development theories usually involve the 2-parent family. Single-parent households are common. Sometimes relatives care for children. In this chapter, *primary caregiver* is used in place of *mother, father, or parent.* The **primary caregiver** *is the person mainly responsible for providing or assisting with the child's basic needs.* A mother, father, grandparent, sister, brother, aunt, uncle, or court-appointed guardian may have this role. *Parent* and *parents* are used in this chapter. However, another primary caregiver may have the parent role.

Growth and development stages vary among experts. The groups and content in this chapter are broad and general.

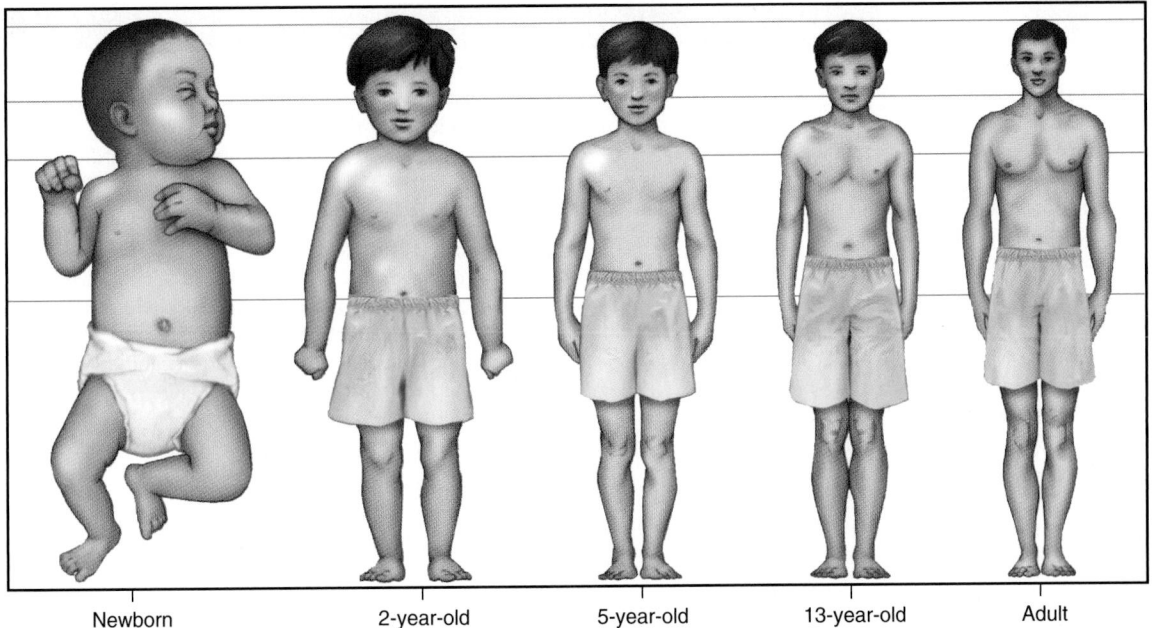

FIGURE 11-1 Changes in appearance from birth to maturity. (From Patton KT, Thibodeau GA: *The human body in health and disease*, ed 6, St Louis, 2014, Mosby.)

PRINCIPLES

Growth and development is a process affecting the whole person. Although they differ, growth and development:

- Overlap.
- Depend on each other.
- Occur at the same time.

For example, an infant coos or babbles (development) when the physical structures for speech are strong enough (growth). Basic principles of growth and development are:

- The process starts at fertilization and continues until death.
- The process proceeds from the simple to the complex. A baby sits before standing, stands before walking, and walks before running.
- The process occurs in certain directions.
  - From head to foot. Babies hold their heads up before sitting. They sit before standing.
  - From the center of the body outward. Babies control shoulder movements before controlling hand movements.
- The process occurs in a sequence, order, and pattern. Certain skills are completed during each stage. A *developmental task is a skill that must be completed during a stage of development.* A stage cannot be skipped. Each stage is the basis for the next stage. See Box 11-1, p. 128.
- The rate of the process is uneven. It is not at a set pace. Growth is rapid during infancy. Children have growth spurts. Some children develop fast. Others develop slowly.
- Each stage has its own characteristics and developmental tasks.

INFANCY (BIRTH TO 1 YEAR)

Infancy is the first year of life. Growth and development are rapid during this time. During this stage infants:

- Learn to walk.
- Learn to eat solid foods.
- Begin to talk and communicate with others.
- Learn to trust.
- Begin to have emotional relationships with parents, brothers, and sisters.
- Develop stable sleep and feeding patterns.

The Newborn (Birth to 1 Month)

The *neonatal* period of infancy is from birth to 1 month. A baby is called a *neonate* or *newborn* at this time. *(Neo* means *new; natal* and *nate* mean *born.)* The average newborn weighs 6 to 9 pounds. Birth weight doubles by 5 to 6 months of age. Birth weight triples by 1 year of age. The average 1-year-old weighs 21½ pounds.

The average newborn is about 20 inches long. Length increases in spurts. At 6 months, the average length is 25½ inches. At 1 year the infant is about 29 inches.

The newborn's head is larger than the chest. The trunk is long. The abdomen is large, round, and soft. The newborn has fat, pudgy cheeks, a flat nose, and a receding chin (Fig. 11-2, p. 128). At 1 year, the chest is larger than the head.

The skin is smooth. Light-skinned babies are reddish at birth but turn pink a few days later. Dark-skinned newborns may appear pinkish to yellowish brown. The skin turns to its natural color in a few days. Eyes are dark gray or deep blue in light-skinned babies. Dark-skinned babies have brown eyes.

BOX 11-1   Growth and Development—Developmental Tasks

Infancy (Birth to 1 Year)
- Learning to walk
- Learning to eat solid foods
- Beginning to talk and communicate with others
- Learning to trust
- Beginning to have emotional relationships with parents, brothers, and sisters
- Developing stable sleep and feeding patterns

Toddlerhood (1 to 3 Years)
- Tolerating separation from the primary caregiver
- Gaining control of bowel and bladder function
- Using words to communicate
- Becoming less dependent on the primary caregiver

Preschool (3 to 6 Years)
- Increasing the ability to communicate and understand others
- Performing self-care
- Learning gender differences and developing sexual modesty
- Learning right from wrong and good from bad
- Learning to play with others
- Developing family relationships

School Age (6 to 9 or 10 Years)
- Developing the social and physical skills needed for playing games
- Learning to get along with *persons of the same age-group and background* **(peers)**
- Learning gender-appropriate behaviors and attitudes
- Learning basic reading, writing, and math skills
- Developing a conscience and morals
- Developing a good feeling and attitude about oneself

Late Childhood (9 or 10 to 12 Years)
- Becoming independent of adults and learning to depend on oneself
- Developing and keeping friendships with peers

Late Childhood (9 or 10 to 12 Years)—cont'd
- Understanding physical, psychological, and social changes
- Developing moral and ethical behavior
- Developing greater muscular strength, coordination, and balance
- Learning how to study

Adolescence (12 to 18 Years)
- Accepting changes in the body and appearance
- Developing appropriate relationships with others and beginning to attract partners
- Becoming independent from parents and adults
- Preparing for marriage and family life
- Preparing for a career
- Developing morals, attitudes, and values needed to function in society

Young Adulthood (18 to 40 Years)
- Choosing education and a career
- Selecting a partner
- Learning to live with a partner
- Becoming a parent and raising children
- Developing a satisfactory sex life

Middle Adulthood (40 to 65 Years)
- Adjusting to physical changes
- Having grown children
- Developing leisure-time activities
- Adjusting to aging parents

Late Adulthood (65 Years and Older)
- Adjusting to decreased strength and loss of health
- Adjusting to retirement and reduced income
- Coping with a partner's death
- Developing new friends and relationships
- Preparing for one's own death

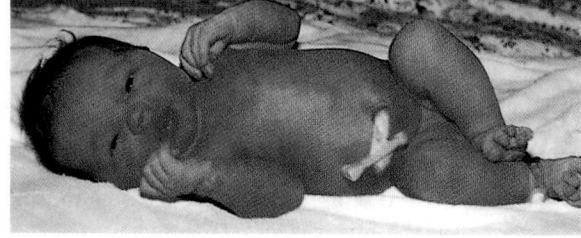

FIGURE 11-2 A newborn. (Courtesy Marjori M. Pyle for LifeCircle, Costa Mesa, Calif.)

The newborn's central nervous system (CNS) is not well-developed. Movements lack purpose and are uncoordinated. Newborns can see from about 8 to 12 inches and can follow large objects. They like faces and bright colors. Newborns hear well. Loud sounds startle them. Soft sounds soothe them. They know the mother's voice. They react to touch and pain. They can taste and smell.

Newborns have certain **reflexes** *(involuntary movements).* These reflexes decline and then disappear as the CNS develops.

- *Moro reflex (startle reflex)*—occurs when the baby is startled by a loud noise, a sudden movement, or the head falling back. The arms are thrown apart. The legs extend and then flex. A brief cry is common. See Figure 11-3.
- *Rooting reflex*—occurs when the cheek is touched near the mouth (Fig. 11-4). The mouth opens and the head turns toward the touch. This reflex is needed for feeding. It guides the baby's mouth to the nipple.
- *Sucking reflex*—occurs when the lips are touched.
- *Palmar grasp reflex*—occurs when the palm is stroked. The fingers close firmly around the object (Fig. 11-5).
- *Step (dance) reflex*—occurs when the baby is held upright and the feet touch a surface. The feet move up and down and in stepping motions (Fig. 11-6).

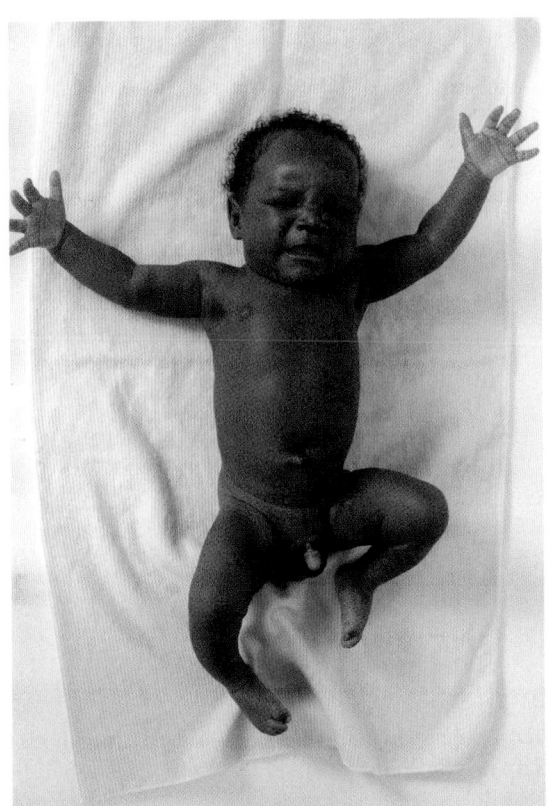

FIGURE 11-3 Moro reflex. (Courtesy Paul Vincent Kuntz, Texas Children's Hospital, as found in Hockenberry MJ, Wilson D: *Wong's nursing care of infants and children,* ed 10, St Louis, 2015, Mosby.)

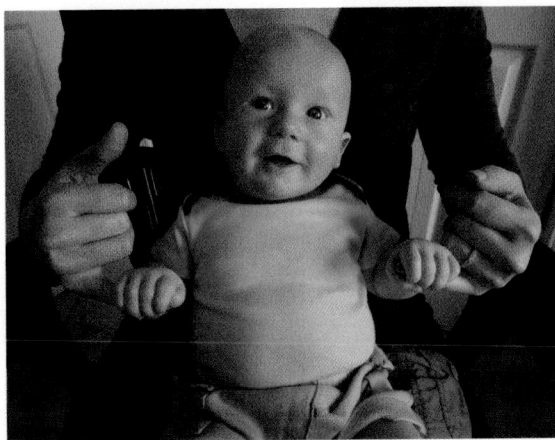

FIGURE 11-5 The grasp reflex. (Courtesy Anne Skowronski, Mount Juliet, Tennessee.)

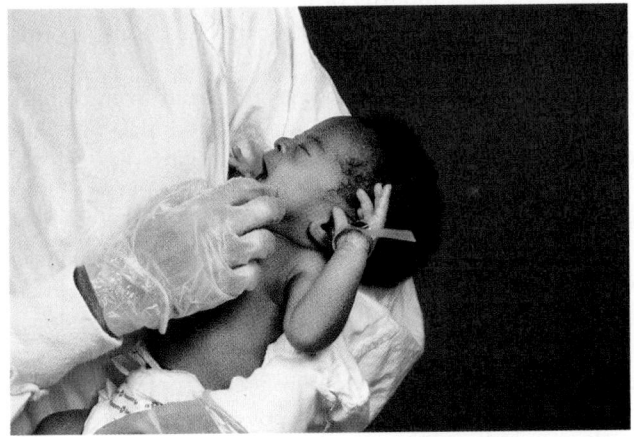

FIGURE 11-4 Rooting reflex. (From Seidel HM and others: *Mosby's guide to physical examination,* ed 3, St Louis, 1995, Mosby.)

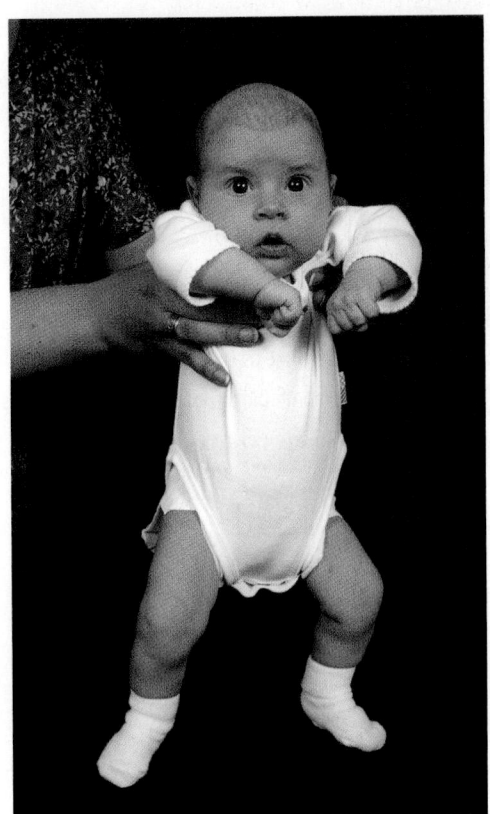

FIGURE 11-6 Step (dance) reflex.

Specific, voluntary, and coordinated movements occur as the nervous and muscular systems develop. Newborns cannot hold their heads up. They turn their heads from side to side.

Newborns sleep 16 to 18 hours a day. They awaken when hungry and fall asleep after a feeding. Bottle-fed infants feed every 2½ to 4 hours. Breast-fed infants are hungry more often—every 2 to 3 hours. The time between feedings lengthens as infants grow and develop. They also stay awake more and sleep less.

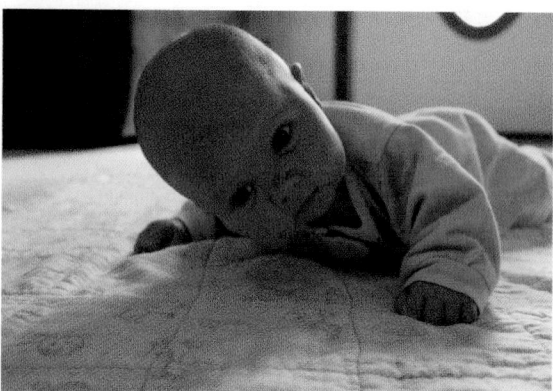

FIGURE 11-7 The 1-month-old can briefly lift the head when lying on the stomach.

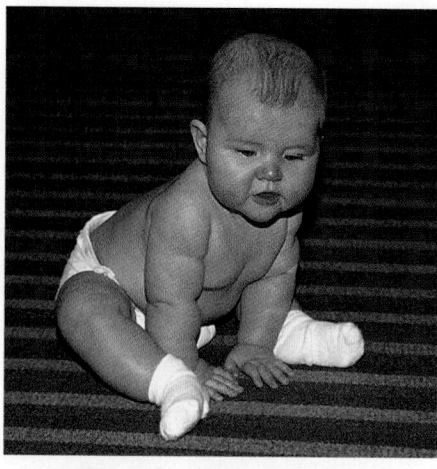

FIGURE 11-10 A 6-month-old sits forward leaning on the hands. (From James SR, Ashwill JW, Droske SC: *Nursing care of children: principles and practices,* ed 3, Philadelphia, 2007, Saunders.)

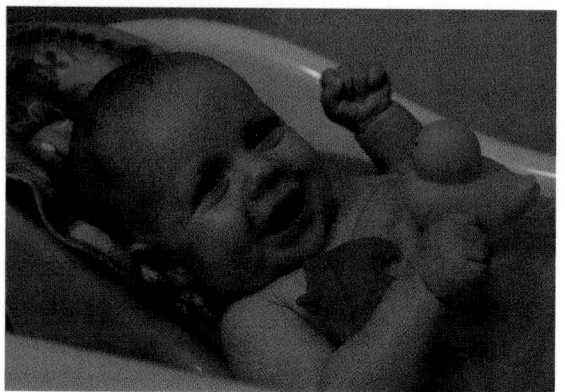

FIGURE 11-8 A 2-month-old smiles in response to others.

Infants (1 Month to 1 Year)

When on their stomachs, 1-month-old infants can lift their heads up briefly (Fig. 11-7). They also can turn their heads. They smile.

Two-month-old infants can hold their heads up when held straight. When on their stomachs, they can turn their heads from side to side. They need support to sit in an angled position. They smile in response to others (Fig. 11-8).

Infants 3 to 4 months of age can hold their heads up (Fig. 11-9). They reach for objects. The Moro, rooting, and grasp reflexes disappear.

By 4 to 5 months, infants can roll from front to back. They roll from back to front by 5 to 6 months. They also can sit by leaning forward on their hands (Fig. 11-10). Teething may begin with the bottom front teeth. They sleep all night. They can play "peek-a-boo."

Solid foods are given at 4 to 6 months. Rice cereal mixed with breast-milk or formula is given first with an infant spoon. Fruits, vegetables, and meats are introduced slowly. These foods are pureed and thin at first. Thicker and chunkier foods are given as more teeth erupt and chewing and swallowing skills increase.

At 6 months, infants can bear weight when pulled to a standing position. They sit with support and move around by rolling. Some start to drink from a cup. They smile at themselves in a mirror. They respond to their names.

Crawling may start at 7 months. Infants can stand while holding on for support. They make sounds in response to caregivers.

At 8 months, infants can sit for long periods. They can change from lying to sitting and from sitting to lying positions. The pincer grasp develops—holding small objects with the thumb and index finger (Fig. 11-11). Infants can pick up small finger foods. They drink from a cup with handles.

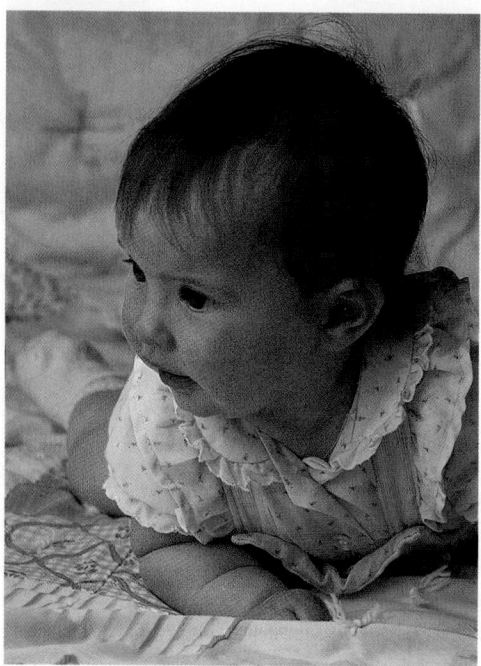

FIGURE 11-9 The 3-month-old child can raise the head and shoulders.

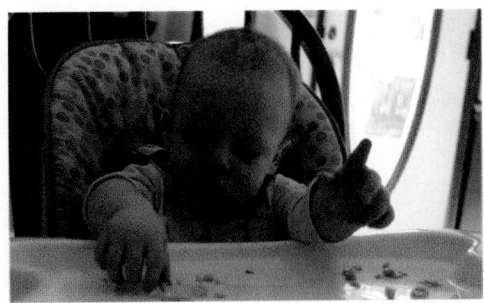

FIGURE 11-11 An 8-month-old uses a pincer grasp to pick up small objects.

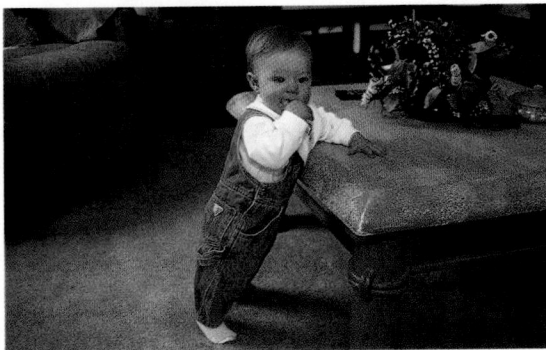

FIGURE 11-12 A 10-month-old infant can walk while holding on to furniture.

BOX 11-2	Language Development in Infants

By the End of 3 Months
- Smiles when the parent appears.
- Startles at loud sounds.
- Makes "cooing" sounds.
- Becomes quiet or smiles when spoken to.
- Seems to know the parent's voice.
- Has different cries for different needs.

By the End of 6 Months
- Makes gurgling sounds when playing alone or with others.
- Babbles and makes other sounds.
- Makes sounds to voice pleasure or displeasure.
- Moves the eyes toward sounds.
- Responds to changes in the parent's voice.
- Notices toy sounds.
- Pays attention to music.

By the End of 12 Months
- Tries to imitate a few words.
- Says some words. "Mama," "dada," and "uh-oh" are examples.
- Understands simple instructions. "Come here" is an example.
- Knows words for common items. "Shoe" and "book" are examples.
- Turns and looks toward sounds.
- Responds to "no."

Modified from Mayo Foundation for Medical Education and Research: Language development: speech milestones for babies, *Mayo Clinic.*

When holding on to something, 9-month-olds can pull up into a standing position. They can hold a bottle, play "pat-a-cake," and drink from a cup or glass. They understand their names and "no." They point and use gestures to communicate.

At 10 months, infants can stand alone. They may walk with help or while holding on to something (Fig. 11-12). They also may crawl up stairs. At 11 months, they may walk alone and use push toys.

At 12 months, walking skills increase. They can climb onto furniture. They can turn book pages and put objects into a container. Weaning (stopping bottle or breast-feeding) may begin.

The infant must develop a sense of trust. If successful, the infant trusts himself or herself and others. Trust develops with consistent care. The infant's physical and safety needs are met—feeding, comfort, warmth, touch, stimulation, and caring.

See *Promoting Safety and Comfort: Infants (1 Month to 1 Year).*

PROMOTING SAFETY AND COMFORT

Infants (1 Month to 1 Year)

Safety
Infants cannot protect themselves. Safety measures for infants are presented in Chapters 13 and 52. Also see *Focus on Children and Older Persons* boxes throughout this book.

Language Development. The rate of speech development varies among infants. Some will say "ma ma" and "da da" around 6 months. Others may not do so until 8 months. The health team has guidelines for normal speech and language development in infants. An example is given in Box 11-2.

TODDLERHOOD (1 TO 3 YEARS)

The growth rate is slower than during infancy. Toddlers learn to:
- Tolerate separation from the primary caregiver.
- Gain control of bowel and bladder function.
- Use words to communicate.
- Become less dependent on the primary caregiver.

Toddlers learn to walk well. They are curious and get into everything and anything. They touch, smell, and taste everything within reach. They climb onto tables, chairs, counters, and other high places. These skills allow toddlers to explore their settings. They go farther away from primary caregivers. They learn to do some things without a primary caregiver. By the age of 3, they can run, jump, climb, ride a tricycle, and walk up and down stairs.

Hand coordination increases. They learn to feed themselves—from eating with fingers to using a spoon (Fig. 11-13, p. 132). They can scribble, build towers with blocks, and string beads. Right- or left-handedness is seen during year 2.

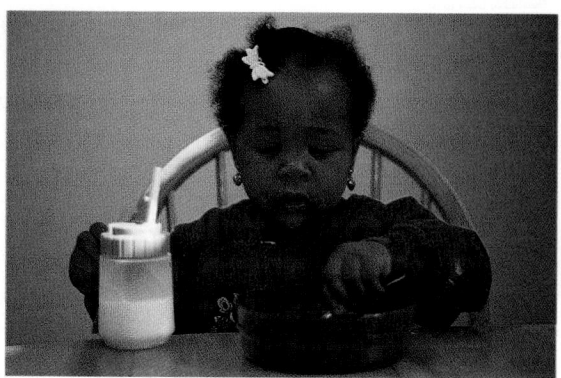

FIGURE 11-13 A toddler uses a spoon.

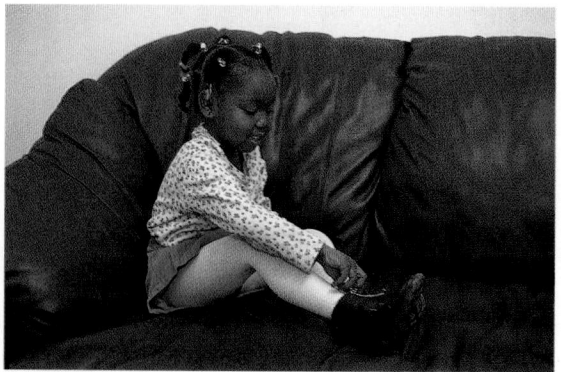

FIGURE 11-14 A 3-year-old has increased coordination.

Computer use often begins in toddlerhood. Toddlers like to push keys, move a mouse, and play with levers and buttons common on computer toys. Such actions help develop fine motor skills and hand-eye coordination.

Toilet training is a major developmental task. Bowel and bladder control is related to CNS development. Children must be mentally and physically ready for toilet training. Some are ready at 2 years. Others are ready at 2½ to 3 years of age. The process starts with bowel control. Bladder control during the day occurs before bladder control at night.

Speech and language skills increase. Speech is clearer. Toddlers imitate others to learn words. They understand more words than they say. "Me" and "mine" are used often.

Play skills increase. The child plays alongside other children but not with them. Toddlers do not share toys. They are possessive and do not understand sharing.

Temper tantrums and saying "no" are common. Toddlers kick and scream to express anger and frustration. That is how they object when independence is challenged. Using "no" can frustrate primary caregivers. Almost every request may be answered "no," even if the child follows the request.

Toddlers learn to tolerate separation from the primary caregiver. As toddlers start to explore, they move away from the primary caregiver. With discomfort, frustration, fear, or injury, they quickly return to primary caregivers or cry for attention. If primary caregivers are consistently present when needed, children learn to feel secure. They learn to tolerate brief periods of separation.

PRESCHOOL (3 TO 6 YEARS)

Preschool children grow 2 to 3 inches per year. They gain about 5 pounds a year. Preschoolers are thinner, more coordinated, and more graceful than toddlers. Preschoolers:

* Increase their ability to communicate and understand others.
* Perform self-care.
* Learn gender differences and develop sexual modesty.
* Learn right from wrong and good from bad.
* Learn to play with others.
* Develop family relationships.

The 3-Year-Old

More coordinated, 3-year-olds can walk on tiptoe and balance on 1 foot for a few seconds. They run, jump, kick a ball, and climb with ease.

Personal care skills increase. They put on clothes and shoes, manage buttons, wash their hands, and brush their teeth (Fig. 11-14). They feed themselves, pour from a bottle, and help set the table without breaking dishes. They can draw circles and crosses.

Language skills increase. Three-year-olds talk and ask questions ("how" and "why") constantly. They can name body parts, family members, and friends. They like talking and musical toys.

Play is important. They play with 2 or 3 other children and can share. They play simple games and learn simple rules. Imaginary friends and imitating adults are common. They enjoy crayons, cutting paper, pasting, painting, computer games, and playing "house" and "dress-up" (Fig. 11-15). They like wagons, tricycles, and other riding toys.

Three-year-olds know that there are 2 sexes. They also know their own sex. Little girls may wonder how the penis works and why they do not have one. Little boys may wonder how girls can urinate without a penis.

The concept of time develops. Three-year-olds may speak of the past, present, and future. "Yesterday" and "tomorrow" are confusing. Children may fear the dark and need bedroom night-lights. Nightmares are common.

Three-year-olds are less fearful of strangers. They can be away from primary caregivers for short periods. They are less jealous than toddlers of a new baby. They try to please primary caregivers.

The 4-Year-Old

Four-year-olds can hop, skip, and throw and catch a ball. They can lace shoes, draw faces, and copy a square. They try to print letters. With help, they can bathe and tend to toileting needs.

They know more words. They ask many questions and exaggerate stories. They can sing simple songs, repeat 4 numbers, count to 5, and name a few colors.

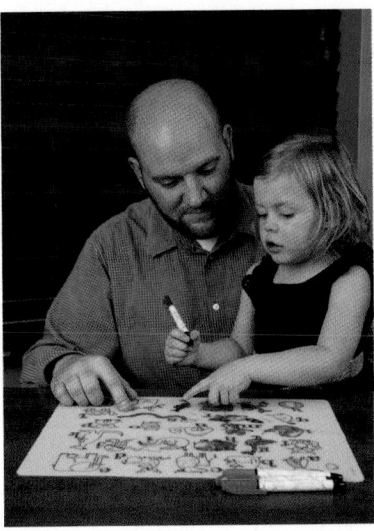

FIGURE 11-15 This 3-year-old enjoys coloring.

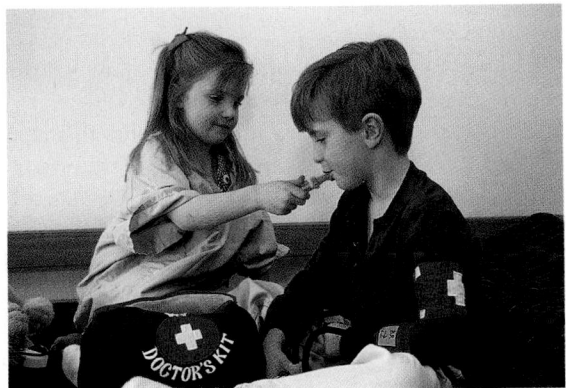

FIGURE 11-16 Four-year-olds play "doctor and nurse."

Four-year-olds tend to tease, tattle, and tell fibs. When bad, they may blame an imaginary friend. Bragging, telling tales about family, and showing off are common. They can play with other children. They are proud of achievements but have mood swings.

These children enjoy playing "dress-up," wearing costumes, and telling and hearing stories. They like to draw and make things. Imagination, drama, and imitating adults are part of play. Interest in computer games continues. They play in groups of 2 or 3 and tend to be bossy. Playing "doctor and nurse" is common as curiosity about the other sex continues (Fig. 11-16).

The primary caregiver of the other sex is preferred. Rivalries with brothers and sisters are seen, especially when a younger child takes the 4-year-old's things. Rivalries also occur when older children have more and different privileges. The family is often the focus of the child's frustrations and aggressive behavior. A 4-year-old may try to run away from home.

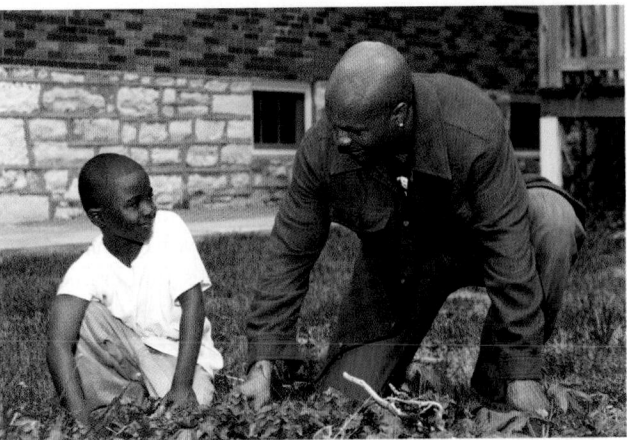

FIGURE 11-17 This 5-year-old does yard work with his father.

The 5-Year-Old

Coordination increases. Five-year-olds can jump rope, skate, tie shoelaces, dress, and bathe. They can use a pencil well and copy diamond and triangle shapes. They can print a few letters, numbers, and their first names. Drawings of people include body parts.

Communication skills increase. They speak in full sentences. Questions have more meaning. They want words defined and take part in conversations. They can name colors, coins, days, and the months. They specify and describe drawings.

Five-year-olds are more responsible and truthful. They quarrel less. They are more aware of rules and are eager to do things right. They have manners, are independent, and can be trusted within limits. Fears are fewer but nightmares and dreams are common. They are proud of achievements.

These children like books about animals and other children. They like computer and board games and try to follow rules. They imitate adults during play and are interested in TV. They also enjoy doing things with the primary caregiver of the same sex (Fig. 11-17). These include cooking, housekeeping, shopping, yard work, and sports.

Younger children are considered a nuisance. However, 5-year-olds usually protect them. They tolerate brothers and sisters well.

SCHOOL AGE (6 TO 9 OR 10 YEARS)

School-age children enter the world of peer groups, games, and learning. They grow 2 to 3 inches a year. They gain 4½ to 6½ pounds a year. They need to:
- Develop the social and physical skills needed for playing games.
- Learn to get along with persons of the same age-group and background (peers).
- Learn gender-appropriate behaviors and attitudes.
- Learn basic reading, writing, and math skills.
- Develop a conscience and morals.
- Develop a good feeling and attitude about oneself.

Baby teeth are lost and permanent teeth erupt. This starts around age 6.

These children can run, jump, skip, hop, and ride a 2-wheeled bike. They can swim, skate, dance, and jump rope. Learning to play in groups, they can take part in team sports. Soccer, T-ball, baseball, football, and volleyball are examples (Fig. 11-18). They learn teamwork and sportsmanship and follow rules. Quiet play involves collections, board games, computer and video games, and crafts.

Reading, writing, grammar, and math skills develop. They learn print and then cursive writing. Sentences are longer and more complex. As reading skills increase, so do language skills. Children like to read and be read to.

Play activities have purpose and involve "work." School-age children like household tasks—cleaning, cooking, yard work. They also like crafts, building things, and scout groups. Rewards are important—good grades, trophies, payment for chores, scouting badges.

At about age 7, boys prefer playing with boys. Girls prefer playing with girls. From 8 to 9 years, some play involves boys and girls. Interest in boy-girl relationships starts at about 8 to 9 years. However, children may deny such interest.

School-age children want to be well-liked. Peer groups are important for love, belonging, and self-esteem needs. These children get along well with and need adults. However, they prefer peer group fads, opinions, and activities (Fig. 11-19).

LATE CHILDHOOD (9 OR 10 TO 12 YEARS)

Late childhood (*pre-adolescence*) is the time between childhood and adolescence. Developmental tasks are like those for school-age children. In addition, pre-adolescents are expected to:

- Become independent of adults and learn to depend on oneself.
- Develop and keep friendships with peers.
- Understand physical, psychological, and social changes.
- Develop moral and ethical behavior.
- Develop greater muscular strength, coordination, and balance.
- Learn how to study.

Many permanent teeth erupt. Girls have a growth spurt. By age 12 years, they are taller and heavier than boys. Both boys and girls are more graceful and coordinated (Fig. 11-20). Muscle strength and physical skills increase. Skill in team sports is important.

Math and language skills increase. These children read for information and pleasure. They read the news. They enjoy books and stories about romance, mystery, adventure, and science fiction.

The onset of puberty nears. *Puberty is the period when reproductive organs begin to function and secondary sex characteristics appear.* In girls, the hips widen and breast buds appear. Some 9-, 10-, and 11-year-old girls begin puberty. Boys show fewer signs of maturing sexually. Genital organs begin to grow. There is concern about body image.

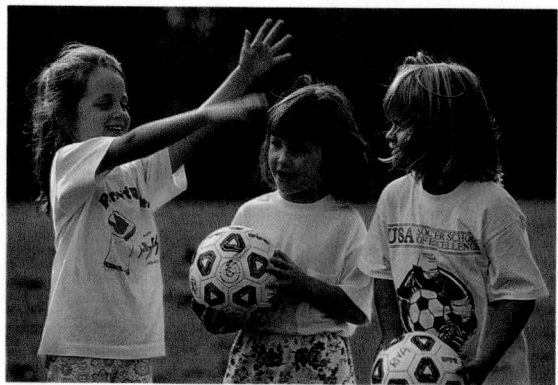

FIGURE 11-18 These 6-year-old girls enjoy soccer.

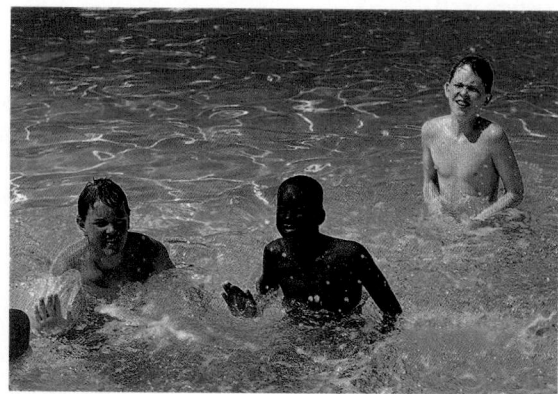

FIGURE 11-19 Belonging to a peer group is important to school-age children.

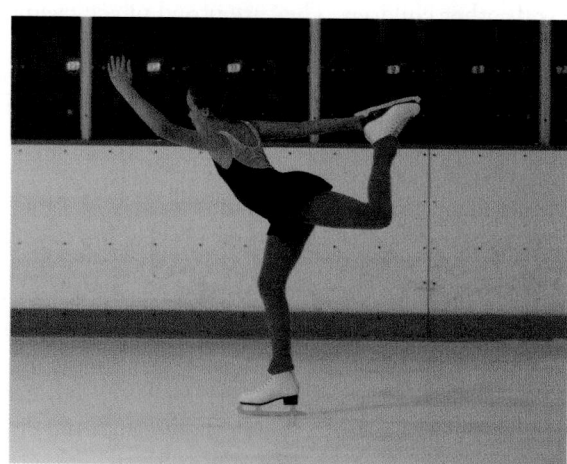

FIGURE 11-20 Movements are smooth and graceful in late childhood. (Courtesy Kevin Devine Photography, Kansas City, Missouri.)

Factual sex information is important. Information shared by friends is often not complete and not accurate. Parents and children may not want to discuss sex with each other. They may avoid the subject. When children ask questions, answers must be honest, complete, and in terms that children understand.

Peer groups are the center of activities. The group affects attitudes and behavior. Friends of the same sex are preferred. Friends are loyal and share problems. A "best friend" is common. Interest in and feeling attraction to others begins.

These children are aware of the mistakes and faults of adults. Adult rules and standards are questioned. It is common to rebel against adults and test limits. Parents and children disagree. However, parents are needed for the child's development.

ADOLESCENCE (12 TO 18 YEARS)

Adolescence is the time between puberty and adulthood. There is rapid growth and physical, sexual, emotional, and social changes. The stage begins with puberty. Girls reach puberty between 9 and 16 years. Boys reach puberty between 13 and 15 years. Adolescents need to:

- Accept changes in the body and appearance.
- Develop appropriate relationships with others and begin to attract partners.
- Become independent from parents and adults.
- Prepare for marriage and family life.
- Prepare for a career.
- Develop the morals, attitudes, and values needed to function in society.

Boys and girls have a growth spurt. Both gain height and weight. They need about $9\frac{1}{2}$ hours of sleep because of such rapid growth. Girls usually complete physical development by age 17. Boys usually stop growing between 18 and 21 years.

Active oil glands lead to acne. Sweat glands are more active. Good hygiene is needed. Deodorants or antiperspirants prevent body odors.

Menarche marks the onset of puberty in girls. *Menarche is the first menstruation and the start of menstrual cycles* (Chapter 10). *Pregnancy can now occur.* Secondary sex characteristics appear. They include:

- Increase in breast size
- Pubic, axillary (underarm), and leg hair
- Slight deepening of the voice
- Widening and rounding of the hips

Ejaculation (the release of semen) signals the onset of puberty in boys. *Nocturnal emissions* ("wet dreams") occur. During sleep *(nocturnal)* the penis becomes erect. Semen is released *(emission)*. *The male can father children.* Other secondary sex characteristics include:

- Facial, pubic, and axillary (underarm) hair
- Hair on the chest, arms, and legs
- Deepening of the voice
- Increases in neck and shoulder sizes

Movements seem awkward and clumsy. Muscle and bone growth is uneven. Coordination and graceful movements develop as muscle and bone growth even out.

Accepting body changes and appearance occurs over time. Girls worry about weight gain. Breast development can embarrass girls, especially if breasts are large or small. Some do not like wearing a bra. Others wear clothes that show off the breasts. Boys may worry about genital size. Height is a concern for both genders. Being small limits play in some sports. Boys do not like being shorter than their peers. Tall girls may be embarrassed about being taller than other girls and boys.

Mood swings occur. Emotional reactions vary from high to low. They can be happy one moment and sad the next. Reactions to comments or events are hard to predict. They control emotions better later in this stage. Sometimes 14- to 18-year-olds are sad and depressed. However, they have more control over the time and place of emotional reactions.

Adolescents need to become independent of parents and other adults. They must learn to function, make decisions, and act responsibly without adult supervision. Many teenagers have part-time jobs or babysit (Fig. 11-21). They go to dances and parties, shop without an adult, and stay home alone. Many take part in school clubs and organizations.

Judgment and reasoning are not always sound. They still need guidance, discipline, and emotional and financial support from parents. The child and parents often disagree about behavior and activity restrictions and limits. Teens prefer doing things with their peers rather than with family. They tend to confide in and seek advice from adults other than their parents.

Interests and activities also reflect the need to develop intimate relationships. Adolescents may begin to feel or show a sexual orientation (Chapter 51). *Sexual orientation is sexual arousal or romantic attraction to persons of the other gender (heterosexual), the same gender (homosexual), or both genders (bisexual).*

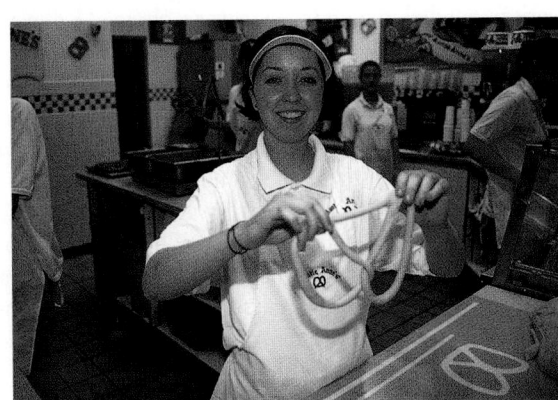

FIGURE 11-21 This teenager has a part-time job.

Teens like parties, dances, and other social events. Appearance is important (clothing, hairstyles). Teens experiment with make-up and hairstyles. They spend time talking to friends on the phone, texting, on social media sites, listening to music, and reading teen magazines.

Thoughts about careers and what to do after high school become a focus. Interests, skills, talents, and money are some factors that influence college or job choices.

Teens need to develop morals, values, and attitudes for living in society. They need to develop a sense about good and bad, right and wrong, and the important and unimportant. Parents, peers, culture, religion, the media, and school are influencing factors. Substance abuse, unwanted pregnancy, criminal acts, and suicide are risks for troubled teens.

Teen Dating

The age for dating varies. At first, dating involves school events, such as dances or football games. Group dating is common. The same group of girls is with the same group of boys. Pairing off as a couple replaces group dating. Couples may be sexual partners.

Parents and teens often disagree about dating. Parents worry about sexual activities, pregnancy, and sexually transmitted diseases. Teens usually do not understand or appreciate these concerns. Dating helps meet security, love and belonging, and self-esteem needs. Teens may have problems controlling sexual urges and considering the results of sexual activity.

See *Promoting Safety and Comfort: Teen Dating.*

YOUNG ADULTHOOD (18 TO 40 YEARS)

Mental and social development continue during young adulthood. There is little physical growth. Adult height has been reached. Body systems are fully developed. Young adulthood involves:
- Choosing education and a career.
- Selecting a partner.
- Learning to live with a partner.
- Becoming a parent and raising children.
- Developing a satisfactory sex life.

Most jobs require certain knowledge and skills. The education needed depends on career choice. Education usually increases job choices. Employment is needed for economic independence and to support a family.

Most adults marry at least once (Fig. 11-22). Others choose to remain single. They may live alone or with friends of the same or other gender. Gay and lesbian persons may commit to a partner or get married.

People marry for many reasons. They include love, emotional security, wanting a family, and sex. Some leave an unhappy home life. Some marry for social status, money, and companionship. Some marry to feel wanted, needed, and desirable.

PROMOTING SAFETY AND COMFORT

Teen Dating

Safety

Intimate partner violence (IPV) (Chapter 5) can start with teen dating. The Centers for Disease Control and Prevention (CDC) defines *teen dating violence as the physical, sexual, psychological, or emotional violence within a dating relationship as well as stalking.*

Teen dating violence often begins with teasing and name calling. Such behaviors can lead to serious violence such as assault and rape. In a CDC survey, almost 10 percent of high school students reported being hit, slapped, or physically hurt by a dating partner. According to the CDC, 25 percent of adolescents reported verbal, emotional, physical, or sexual dating violence. Victims of teen dating violence are at risk for:
- Doing poorly in school
- Using alcohol, drugs, and tobacco
- Suicide attempts
- Fighting
- Violence in future relationships

Adult behaviors, TV, and movies may suggest that IPV and teen dating violence are okay. Violence is never okay. According to the CDC, teens at risk include those who:
- Approve of using threats or violence to get their way or to express anger or frustration.
- Use alcohol or drugs.
- Cannot manage anger or frustration.
- Have violent peers.
- Have conflict with a partner.
- Have multiple sexual partners.
- Have a friend involved in dating violence.
- Are depressed or anxious.
- Witness violence at home or in the community.
- Have a history of aggressive behavior or bullying.

See Chapter 5 for IPV. Teen dating violence can occur in person, electronically, and with a current or former dating partner. Helpful resources include:
- National Teen Dating Abuse Helpline
- National Sexual Assault Hotline
- National Sexual Assault Online Hotline
- National Domestic Violence Hotline

Many factors affect partner selection. They include age, religion, interests, education, race, personality, and love. Some marriages or partnerships are happy and successful. Others are not. Partners must work together to build a relationship based on trust, respect, caring, and friendship.

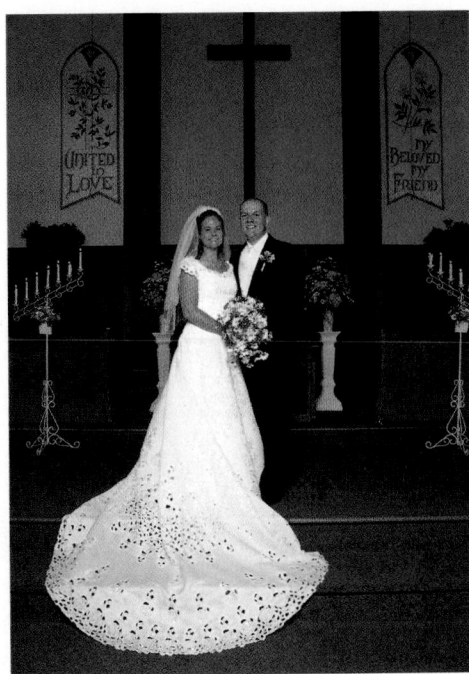

FIGURE 11-22 A wedding celebrates a couple's marriage. (Courtesy Dean Williams Photography, Springfield, Illinois.)

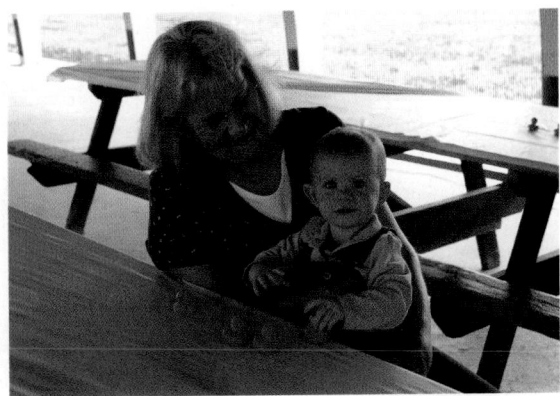

FIGURE 11-23 This woman enjoys time with her grandchild.

Partners must learn to live together. Habits, routines, meals, and pastimes are changed or adjusted to "fit" the other person's needs. They learn to solve problems and make decisions together. They need to work toward the same goals. Open and honest communication is needed.

Sexual frequency, desires, practices, and preferences vary. For a satisfying and intimate relationship, partners must understand and accept the other's needs.

Birth control methods allow couples to plan when to have children and how many to have. Some pregnancies are not planned. Some couples choose not to have children. Physical problems in the man or woman can interfere with or prevent pregnancy.

Parents must agree on child-rearing practices and discipline methods. They need to adjust to the child and to the child's needs for parental time, energy, and attention.

MIDDLE ADULTHOOD (40 TO 65 YEARS)

This stage is more stable and comfortable. Children are usually grown and have moved away. Partners have time together. Worries about children and money are fewer.

Middle-age adults:
* Adjust to physical changes.
* Adjust to having grown children.
* Develop leisure-time activities.
* Adjust to aging parents.

Physical changes occur. Many are gradual and are not noticed. Others are seen early. Energy and endurance begin to slow down. So do metabolism and physical activities. Therefore weight control becomes a problem. Facial wrinkles and gray hair appear. Needing eyeglasses is common. Hair loss may begin. *Menstruation stops and menstrual cycles end (menopause).* It occurs between the ages of 45 and 55 years. Ovaries stop secreting hormones. The woman cannot have children.

Many diseases and illnesses can develop. The disorders become chronic and threaten life.

Children leave home for college, marry, move to their own homes, and start families. Adults have to let children go and adjust to being in-laws and grandparents (Fig. 11-23). Parents must let children lead their own lives. However, they provide emotional support when needed.

Spare time increases as parenting demands decrease. Hobbies and pastimes bring pleasure. They include gardening, fishing, painting, golfing, volunteer work, and being part of clubs and organizations (Fig. 11-24, p. 138). These activities are even more important after retirement and during late adulthood.

Some middle-age adults have aging parents in poor health. Responsibility for aging parents may begin during this stage. Many middle-age adults deal with the death of parents.

LATE ADULTHOOD (65 YEARS AND OLDER)

Chapter 12 describes the many changes that occur in older persons. Older persons:
* Adjust to decreased strength and loss of health.
* Adjust to retirement and reduced income.
* Cope with a partner's death.
* Develop new friends and relationships.
* Prepare for one's own death.

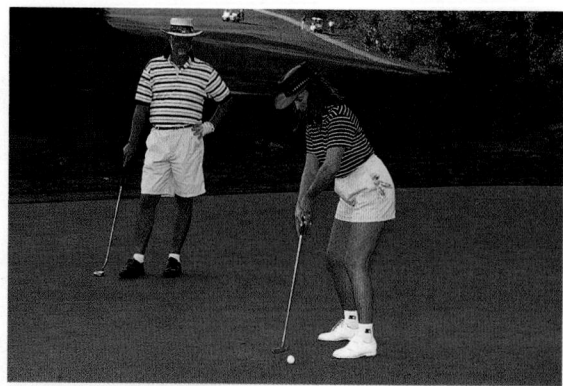

FIGURE 11-24 Middle-age adults usually have more time for leisure activities.

FOCUS ON **PRIDE**

The Person, Family, and Yourself

Personal and Professional Responsibility

Development affects the care you give. Care measures and procedures change. Safety concerns differ. The person's level of trust and fears vary. These affect your interactions. For example, you are caring for a 1-year-old. You need to use your stethoscope to check an apical pulse (Chapter 29). You know 1-year-olds are learning to trust. The child may be afraid of you and your stethoscope. To gain the child's trust:

• Ask the parent to hold the child.
• Show the child the procedure on the parent.
• Let the child play with the stethoscope.
• Talk in a kind, playful voice.

You are responsible for knowing how development affects the care you give. Throughout this book, read the *Focus on Children and Older Persons* boxes. They explain how to adjust your care for the different stages of development.

Rights and Respect

Family situations may conflict with your values. Show respect to all persons. Do not gossip. Be kind. Take pride in not letting your personal opinions affect the care you give.

Independence and Social Interaction

Developmental monitoring and screening are used to determine if a child is developing normally. For example, does the child move, play, learn, and behave as expected? Is the child learning independence? Does the child communicate and interact normally?

The health team uses a screening tool to see if milestones are being met. Milestones are guides for what a child should be able to do at a certain age. Developmental delays may indicate a disability (Chapter 50).

Delegation and Teamwork

For children, the primary caregiver is an important part of the health team. The nurse teaches the caregiver how to help with care. For example, an infant is bottle-fed. The mother is taught her role in measuring intake and output (Chapter 27). The nurse instructs her to save the bottles and report intake to the nursing staff. She is also taught to save the diapers to be weighed for output.

When interacting with caregivers:

• Be polite. Treat them with kindness and respect.
• Thank them for helping with the child's care.
• Praise actions that are done well.
• Remind them of care measures taught by the nurse.
• Tell the nurse about any questions or concerns.
• Tell the nurse if you notice that they need more teaching.

Ethics and Laws

Development affects a person's ability to make health care decisions. A child does not have the reasoning and judgment to make decisions. As one develops, he or she gains independence and the ability to function in society.

State laws determine the age of adulthood for making legal and health care decisions. This age varies but age 18 is common. *Minors* are under the age to legally make decisions. A parent or legal guardian makes decisions for a minor.

An *emancipated minor* is under the legal age but is able to make his or her own decisions. This can occur by marriage, by joining the armed forces, or by a court ruling. In some states, pregnancy and having children are other ways. Agencies often have individuals or groups responsible for handling questions of emancipation. Risk management nurses and ethics committees are examples.

FOCUS ON **PRIDE**: *Application*

Choose 3 age-groups. Describe normal development for each group. Explain how the person's developmental level affects your approach to care.

REVIEW QUESTIONS

Circle the BEST answer.

1 Changes in mental, emotional, and social function are called
   a Growth
   b Development
   c A reflex
   d A stage

2 These statements are about growth and development. Which is *true?*
   a They occur from complex to simple.
   b They occur at a set pace.
   c There is no order or pattern.
   d Each stage has its own characteristics.

3 Which reflexes does the infant need for feeding?
   a The Moro and startle reflexes
   b The rooting and sucking reflexes
   c The grasping and Moro reflexes
   d The rooting and grasping reflexes

4 Which occurs first in infants?
   a Holding the head up
   b Rolling from front to back
   c Rolling from back to front
   d The pincer grasp

5 An infant can stand alone at about
   a 8 months
   b 10 months
   c 11 months
   d 12 months

6 A 6-month-old can
   a Say 3 to 5 words
   b Understand simple instructions
   c Babble and make gurgling sounds
   d Respond to "no"

7 Toilet training begins
   a During infancy
   b During the toddler years
   c When the primary caregiver is ready
   d At the age of 3 years

8 The toddler can
   a Use a spoon and cup
   b Ride a bike
   c Help set the table
   d Put on clothes and shoes

9 Playing with other children begins during
   a Infancy
   b The toddler years
   c The preschool years
   d The school-age years

10 Losing baby teeth usually begins at the age of
   a 4 years
   b 5 years
   c 6 years
   d 7 years

11 Peer groups become important to
   a Toddlers
   b Preschool children
   c School-age children
   d Young adults

12 Reproductive organs begin to function. Secondary sex characteristics appear. This is called
   a Late childhood
   b Puberty
   c Adolescence
   d Adulthood

13 Which is *true?*
   a Boys begin puberty earlier than girls.
   b Boys begin puberty between the ages of 9 and 11.
   c Little growth occurs during adolescence.
   d Menarche marks the onset of puberty in girls.

14 Dating usually begins
   a During late childhood
   b Before puberty
   c With "pairing off"
   d During adolescence

15 Dating violence
   a Can occur electronically or in person
   b Does not include stalking
   c Rarely occurs with teenagers
   d Often begins with physical violence

16 Adolescence is a time when parents and children
   a Talk openly about sex
   b Express love and affection
   c Disagree
   d Do things as a family

17 Young adulthood involves
   a Caring for aging parents
   b Making career choices
   c Physical growth and changes in body appearance
   d Adjusting to grown children

18 Middle adulthood ranges from
   a 20 to 35 years
   b 30 to 40 years
   c 35 to 45 years
   d 40 to 65 years

19 Middle adulthood is a time when
   a Families are started
   b Physical energy and free time increase
   c Children are grown and leave home
   d People need to prepare for death

20 Late adulthood involves
   a Retirement
   b Menopause
   c Stable health
   d Few changes

Answers to Chapter 11 questions are on p. 870.

FOCUS ON **PRACTICE**

Problem Solving

You are caring for a 2-year-old boy. You take the child to another room to weigh him. The child's mother stays in his room with her child. You ask the child to stand on the scale. He says: "No." You reach for him to place him on the scale. He cries and runs from you. Is this response normal? What could have been done to avoid this?

OBJECTIVES

- Define the key terms and key abbreviations in this chapter.
- Identify the psychological and social changes common in older adulthood.
- Describe the physical changes from aging and the care required.
- Describe housing options for older persons.
- Describe the personal gains and losses related to long-term care.
- Explain how to promote PRIDE in the person, the family, and yourself.

KEY TERMS

atrophy Shrink
geriatrics The care of aging people

gerontology The study of the aging process

KEY ABBREVIATIONS

ADU Accessory dwelling unit
CCRC Continuing care retirement community

CMS Centers for Medicare & Medicaid Services
ECHO Elder Cottage Housing Opportunity

People live longer than ever before. They are healthier and more active. Late adulthood ranges from 65 years of age and older. The oldest-old are 85 years of age and older. Chronic illness is common in older persons. Disability often results. Many older persons have at least 1 disability. Disabilities increase and become more severe with aging. They can interfere with:

- Self-care—bathing, dressing, eating, elimination
- Mobility and getting around one's home and other settings
- Fixing meals
- Shopping
- Managing money
- Using a phone
- Doing housework
- Taking drugs
- Leisure and recreational activities

Most older people live in a family setting. They live with a spouse, partner, children, brothers or sisters, or other family. Some live alone or with friends. Still others live in assisted living residences or nursing centers. The need for nursing center care increases with aging.

Gerontology is the study of the aging process. Geriatrics is the care of aging people. Aging is normal. It is not a disease. Normal changes occur in body structure and function. The risk for illness, injury, and disability increases. Psychological

and social changes also occur. Often changes are slow. Most people adjust well and lead happy, meaningful lives.

There are many myths about aging and older persons. A *myth* is a widely believed story that is not true. To provide good care, you need to know the facts about older persons and aging. See Box 12-1 for some common myths and facts.

PSYCHOLOGICAL AND SOCIAL CHANGES

Graying hair, wrinkles, and slow movements are physical reminders of aging. These changes threaten self-esteem, self-image, and feelings of self-worth. They also threaten independence.

Social roles change. A parent may rely on an adult child for care. Retirees need activities to replace the work role. Adjusting to the deaths of parents, family members, and friends is common. The person faces his or her own death.

People cope with aging in their own way. How they cope depends on:

- Health status
- Life experiences
- Finances
- Education
- Social support systems

BOX 12-1	Myths and Facts About Aging
Myth	**Fact**
Aging means disability and death.	Most older adults are healthy. Good nutrition, exercise, and not smoking can reverse or slow many changes blamed on aging.
Older persons cannot or should not have sex.	Many older people enjoy a fulfilling sex life. Sexuality remains important. Intimacy, love, and companionship are needed.
Older people are lonely.	Frequent contact with children is common. So is taking part in family activities. Brothers and sisters can provide support and companionship. Many older persons have jobs, are volunteers, and enjoy hobbies.
Mental function declines with age.	People may receive and process information more slowly with aging. However, people learn until very late in life. Heredity, exercise, diet, and social interaction are some factors affecting mental function.
Most older people live in nursing centers.	According to the 2010 census, only about 1,600,000 (4.1%) of the people 65 years and older lived in nursing centers or other care settings.
Older people are crabby and rude.	Older persons who are crabby and rude were probably crabby and rude when younger.

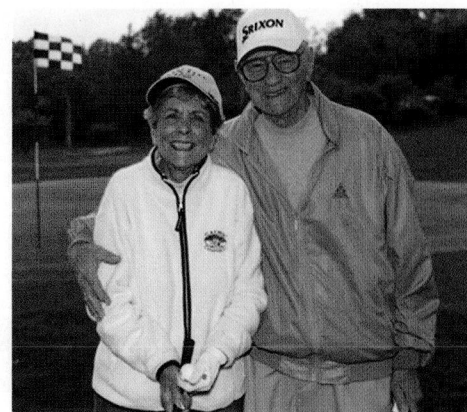

FIGURE 12-1 A retired couple enjoys golf as a leisure-time activity.

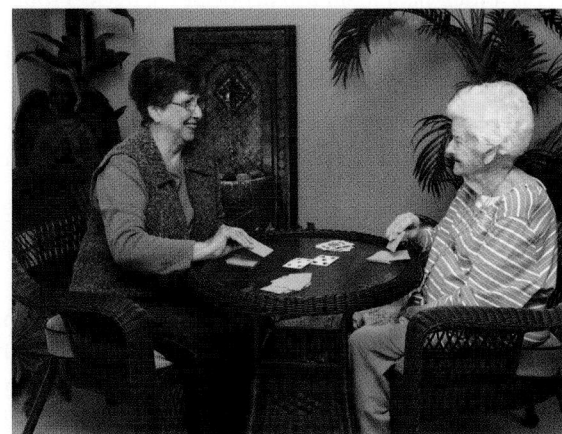

FIGURE 12-2 This retired woman is a nursing center volunteer.

Retirement

Age 65 is the common retirement age. Some retire earlier. Others work longer. Retirement allows the person to relax and enjoy life (Fig. 12-1). Travel, leisure, and doing what one wants are retirement "benefits." Many people enjoy retirement. For others, poor health, disability, and medical bills can make retirement very hard.

Work meets love, belonging, and self-esteem needs. The person feels fulfilled and useful. Friendships form. Co-workers share daily events. Leisure time, recreation, and companionship often involve co-workers. Some retired people have part-time jobs or do volunteer work (Fig. 12-2).

Reduced Income. Retirement often means reduced income. Social Security may provide the only income.

The retired person still has expenses. House or rent payments continue. Food, clothing, utility bills, and taxes are other expenses. Car expenses, home repairs, drugs, and health care are other costs. So are entertainment and gifts.

Reduced income may force life-style changes. Examples include:

- Limiting social and leisure events
- Buying cheaper food, clothes, and household items
- Moving to cheaper housing
- Living with children or other family
- Avoiding health care or needed drugs
- Relying on children or other family for money or needed items

Severe money problems can result. Some people plan for retirement with savings, investments, retirement plans, and insurance. They are financially comfortable during retirement.

CARING ABOUT CULTURE
Foreign-Born Persons

Some older persons speak and understand a foreign language. They communicate with family and friends who speak the same language. They also share cultural values and practices. Family and friends may move away or die. The person may not have anyone to talk to. He or she may not be understood by others. The person feels greater loneliness and isolation.

Social Relationships

Social relationships change throughout life. (See *Caring About Culture: Foreign-Born Persons.*) Children grow up, leave home, and have families. Some live far away from parents. Older family members and friends die, move away, or are disabled. Yet most older people have regular contact with children, grandchildren, family, and friends. Others are lonely. Separation from children is a common cause. So is lack of companionship with people their own age (Fig. 12-3, p. 142).

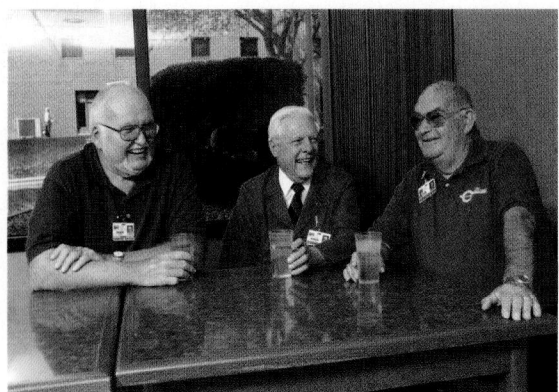

FIGURE 12-3 Older people enjoy being with others of their own age.

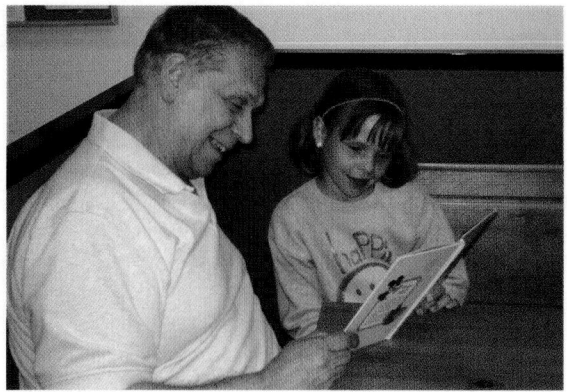

FIGURE 12-4 An older man reads to his grandchild.

Many older people adjust to social changes. Hobbies, religious and community events, and new friends help prevent loneliness. Some community groups sponsor bus trips to ball games, shopping, plays, and concerts.

Grandchildren can bring great love and joy (Fig. 12-4). Family times help prevent loneliness. They help the older person feel useful and wanted.

See *Focus on Communication: Social Relationships.*

Children as Caregivers

Sometimes parents and children change roles. The child cares for the parent. Some older persons feel more secure. Others feel unwanted, in the way, and useless. Some lose dignity and self-respect. Tensions may occur among the child, parent, and other household members. Lack of privacy is a cause. So are disagreements and criticisms about housekeeping, raising children, cooking, and friends.

Death and Grieving

As couples age, chances increase that a partner will die. A person may try to prepare for a partner's death. When death occurs, the loss is crushing. No amount of preparation is ever enough for the emptiness and changes that result. The person loses a lover, friend, companion, and confidant. Grief may be very great. The person's life will likely change. Serious physical and mental health problems result. Some lose the will to live. Some attempt suicide.

The surviving spouse may live alone. Others need to decide on housing options. (See "Housing Options," p. 147.) Some people re-marry or have live-in arrangements with new partners.

Death of a Child. Sadly, children die. They may be newborns, infants, toddlers, school-age, or older. Death of a child at any age seems to be against the natural order of things. That is, parents should die before their children.

FOCUS ON COMMUNICATION

Social Relationships

The social changes of aging can cause loneliness. With nursing center care, the loneliness can seem greater. Staff and other residents do not replace family and friends. To help the person feel less lonely, you can:
- Suggest that the person call a family member or friend. Offer to help with phone numbers and dialing. Many residents have wireless phones.
- Keep the phone within the person's reach. Calls can be placed or answered with greater ease.
- Suggest that the person read cards and letters. Offer to assist.
- Visit with the person a few times during your shift.
- Introduce new residents to other residents and staff. Often new friendships develop.
- Encourage the person to e-mail or have video calls with family and friends. Some residents have their own computers with the center providing Internet access.

Parents of any age experience great grief when a child dies. As people live longer, some out-live their adult children. Their emotional needs are great. Sadly, often few family and friends are left to provide support and comfort.

PHYSICAL CHANGES

Physical changes of aging happen to everyone (Box 12-2). Body processes slow. Energy level and body efficiency decline. The rate and degree of changes vary with each person. They depend on diet, health, exercise, stress, environment, heredity, and other factors. Changes are slow over many years. Often they are not seen for a long time.

Normal aging does not mean loss of health. Quality of life does not have to decline. The person can adjust to many of the changes.

BOX 12-2	**Common Physical Changes During the Aging Process**

Integumentary System
- Skin becomes less elastic
- Skin loses strength
- Brown spots ("age spots" or "liver spots") on the wrists and hands
- Fewer nerve endings
- Fewer blood vessels
- Fatty tissue layer is lost
- Skin thins and sags
- Skin is fragile and easily injured
- Folds, lines, and wrinkles appear
- Blood vessels become more fragile
- Decreased secretion of oil and sweat glands
- Dry, itchy skin
- More sensitive to cold
- Decreased sensitivity to pain
- Nails become thick and tough
- Whitening or graying hair
- Facial hair in some women
- Loss or thinning of hair
- Drier hair

Musculo-Skeletal System
- Muscles *atrophy (shrink)*
- Muscle strength, tone, and contractility decrease
- Bone mass decreases
- Bones become weaker
- Bones become brittle; can break easily
- Vertebrae shorten
- Joints become stiff and painful
- Hip and knee joints become flexed
- Gradual loss of height; trunk becomes shorter
- Decreased mobility

Nervous System
- Brain and spinal cord lose nerve cells
- Nerve cells send messages at a slower rate
- Reflexes slow
- Reduced blood flow to the brain
- Abnormal structures can form in the brain
- Brain tissue may atrophy
- Changes in brain cells
- Shorter memory
- Forgetfulness
- Slower ability to respond
- Confusion
- Dizziness
- Sleep patterns change
- Reduced sensitivity to pain and touch
- Smell and taste decrease
- Eyelids thin and wrinkle
- Less tear secretion
- Pupils less responsive to light
- Decreased vision at night or in dark rooms
- Problems seeing green and blue colors
- Poor vision
- Changes in acoustic nerve
- Eardrums atrophy
- High-pitched sounds are not heard
- Decreased earwax secretion
- Hearing loss

Circulatory System
- Heart pumps with less force
- Heart valves thicken and become stiff
- Heart rate may slow
- Abnormal heart rhythms may occur
- Heart may enlarge slightly
- Heart walls thicken
- Arteries narrow and become stiffer
- Less blood flows through narrowed arteries
- Weakened heart works harder to pump blood through narrowed vessels
- Number of red blood cells decreases

Respiratory System
- Respiratory muscles weaken
- Some lung tissue is lost
- Lung tissue becomes less elastic
- Chest is less able to stretch to breathe
- Difficulty breathing *(dyspnea)*
- Decreased strength for coughing and clearing the airway

Digestive System
- Decreased saliva production
- Difficulty swallowing *(dysphagia)*
- Decreased appetite
- Decreased secretion of digestive juices
- Difficulty digesting fried and fatty foods
- Indigestion
- Loss of teeth
- Decreased peristalsis causing flatulence and constipation

Urinary System
- Kidney function decreases
- Reduced blood supply to kidneys
- Kidneys atrophy
- Bladder tissues less able to stretch
- Bladder muscles weaken
- Bladder may not empty completely
- Urinary frequency
- Urinary urgency may occur
- Urinary incontinence may occur
- Night-time urination may occur

Reproductive System
- Men
  - Testosterone decreases slightly
  - Erections take longer
  - Longer phase between erection and orgasm
  - Less forceful orgasms
  - Erections lost quickly
  - Longer time between erections
- Women
  - Menopause
  - Estrogen and progesterone decrease
  - Uterus, vagina, and genitalia atrophy
  - Thinning of vaginal walls
  - Vaginal dryness
  - Arousal takes longer
  - Less intense orgasms
  - Quicker return to pre-excitement state

The Integumentary System

The skin loses elasticity, strength, and the fatty tissue layer. The skin thins and sags. Wrinkles appear. Oil and sweat gland secretions decrease. The skin is dry, itchy, fragile, and easily injured. Brown spots ("age spots," "liver spots") are common on the wrists and hands. The skin's blood vessels are fragile, increasing the risk for:

- Skin breakdown
- Skin tears (Chapter 36)
- Pressure ulcers (Chapter 37)
- Bruising
- Delayed healing

Loss of the fatty tissue layer affects body temperature. More sensitive to cold, protect the person from drafts and cold. Sweaters, lap blankets, socks, and extra blankets are helpful. So are higher thermostat settings.

Dry, itchy skin is easily damaged. A shower or bath twice a week is enough for hygiene. Partial baths are taken at other times. Mild soaps or soap substitutes clean the underarms, genitals, and under the breasts. Often soap is not used on the arms, legs, back, chest, and abdomen. Lotions and creams prevent drying and itching. Decreased sweat gland secretion may lessen the need for deodorants. See Chapter 22 for hygiene.

Nails become thick and tough. Feet usually have poor circulation. A nick or cut can lead to a serious infection. See Chapter 22 for nail and foot care.

The skin has fewer nerve endings. This affects sensing heat, cold, pressure, and pain. Burns are great risks because of fragile skin, poor circulation, and decreased sensing of heat and cold. Provide socks for cold feet. Do not use hot water bottles and heating pads on feet because of the burn risk.

White or gray hair is common. Hair loss occurs in men. Hair thins on men and women—head, pubic area, and underarms. Women and men may choose to wear wigs. Some color hair to cover graying. Facial hair (lip and chin) may occur in women.

Decreases in scalp oils make hair dryer. Brushing promotes circulation and oil production. Shampoo frequency usually decreases with age. It is done as needed for hygiene and comfort.

Skin disorders and skin cancer increase with age. They rarely cause death if treated early. Prolonged sun exposure is a cause of skin cancer.

Changes to the integumentary system can be seen. Gray hair, hair loss, brown spots, wrinkles, and sagging skin are some examples. These changes can affect self-esteem and body image.

The Musculo-Skeletal System

Muscle cells decrease in number. Muscles *atrophy (shrink).* They decrease in strength.

Bones lose minerals, especially calcium. Bones lose strength, become brittle, and break easily. Sometimes just turning in bed can cause fractures (broken bones).

Vertebrae shorten. Joints become stiff and painful. Hip and knee joints flex (bend) slightly. These changes cause gradual loss of height and strength. Mobility also decreases.

Activity, exercise, and diet help prevent bone loss and loss of muscle strength. Walking is good exercise. Exercise groups and range-of-motion exercises are helpful (Chapter 30). A diet high in protein, calcium, and vitamins is needed.

Bones can break easily. Protect the person from injury and falls (Chapters 13 and 14). Turn and move the person gently and carefully (Chapters 18 and 19). Some persons need help and support getting out of bed. Some need help walking.

The Nervous System

Nerve cells are lost in the brain and spinal cord. Nerve conduction and reflexes slow. Responses are slower. For example, an older person slips. The message telling the brain of the slip travels slowly. The message from the brain to prevent the fall also travels slowly. The person falls.

Blood flow to the brain is reduced. Dizziness may occur, increasing the risk for falls. Practice measures to prevent falls (Chapter 14). Remind the person to get up slowly from bed to chair or standing. This helps prevent dizziness (Chapter 30).

Changes occur in the brain. This affects personality and mental function. So does the reduced blood flow to the brain. Memory is shorter. Forgetfulness increases. Responses slow. Confusion, dizziness, and fatigue may occur. Older persons often remember events from long ago better than recent ones. When mentally active and involved in current events, older people show fewer personality and mental changes. (See Chapter 49.)

Sleep patterns change. Falling asleep is harder. Sleep periods are shorter. Older persons wake often at night and have less deep sleep. Less sleep is needed. Loss of energy and decreased blood flow may cause fatigue. They may rest or nap during the day. They may go to bed early and get up early.

The Senses. Aging affects touch, smell, taste, sight, and hearing.

Touch. Touch and sensitivity to pain and pressure are often reduced. So is sensing heat and cold. These changes increase the risk for injury. The person may not notice painful injuries or diseases. Or the person feels minor pain. You need to:

- Protect older persons from injury (Chapters 13 and 14).
- Follow safety measures for heat and cold (Chapter 38).
- Check for signs of skin breakdown (Chapters 22, 36, and 37).
- Give good skin care (Chapter 22).
- Prevent skin tears (Chapter 36) and pressure ulcers (Chapter 37).

Taste and Smell. Taste and smell dull. Appetite decreases. Taste buds decrease in number. The tongue senses sweet, salty, bitter, and sour tastes. Sweet and salty tastes are lost first. Older people often complain that food has no taste or tastes bitter. They like more salt and sugar on food.

The Eye. Eyelids thin and wrinkle. Tear secretion is less. Dust and pollution can irritate the eye.

The pupil becomes smaller and responds less to light. Vision is poor at night or in dark rooms. The eye takes longer adjusting to lighting changes, causing vision problems when:

• Going from a dark to a bright room
• Going from a bright to a dark room

Clear vision is reduced. Eyeglasses are often needed. The lens of the eye yellows, making greens and blues harder to see.

Gradually the eyes lose the ability to focus on near objects. Older persons become more farsighted. That is, the person sees objects at a distance more clearly than close objects. The lens becomes more rigid with age. It is harder for the eye to shift from far to near vision and from near to far vision. Falls and accidents are risks. The risk is greater on stairs and where lighting is poor. Eyeglasses are worn as needed. Keep rooms well-lit. Night-lights are helpful.

The Ear. Changes occur in the acoustic nerve. Eardrums atrophy. High-pitched sounds are hard to hear. Severe hearing loss occurs as changes progress. A hearing aid may be needed (Chapter 42).

Wax secretion decreases. Wax becomes harder and thicker. It is easily impacted (wedged in the ear). This can cause hearing loss. A doctor or nurse removes the wax.

The Circulatory System

The number of red blood cells decreases. This can cause fatigue.

The heart muscle weakens. It pumps blood with less force. Activity, exercise, excitement, and illness increase the body's need for oxygen and nutrients. A damaged or weak heart cannot meet these needs.

Arteries narrow and are less elastic. Less blood flows through them. Poor circulation occurs in many body parts. A weak heart works harder to pump blood through narrowed vessels.

Exercise helps maintain health and well-being (Fig. 12-5). Many older persons exercise daily. They walk, jog, golf, and bicycle. They also hike, ski, play tennis, swim, and play other sports. Older persons need to be as active as possible.

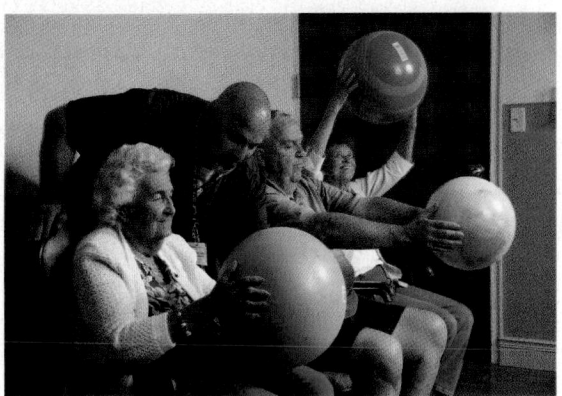

FIGURE 12-5 These residents take part in an exercise program.

Sometimes circulatory changes are severe. Rest is needed during the day. Over-exertion is avoided. The person should not walk far, climb many stairs, or carry heavy things. Personal care items, TV, phone, and other needed items are kept nearby. Some exercise helps circulation. It also prevents blood clots in leg veins. Some persons need to stay in bed. They need range-of-motion exercises (Chapter 30). Doctors may order certain exercise and activity limits.

The Respiratory System

Respiratory muscles weaken. Lung tissue becomes less elastic. Difficult, labored, or painful breathing *(dyspnea)* may occur with activity. *(Dys* means *difficult. Pnea* means *breathing.)* The person may lack strength to cough and clear the airway of secretions. Respiratory infections and diseases may develop. These can threaten life.

Normal breathing is promoted. Avoid heavy bed linens over the chest. They prevent normal chest expansion. Turning, re-positioning, and deep breathing are important. Breathing usually is easier in semi-Fowler's position (Chapter 20). The person should be as active as possible.

The Digestive System

Salivary glands produce less saliva. This can cause difficulty swallowing *(dysphagia)*. *(Dys* means *difficult. Phagia* means *swallowing.)* Dry foods may be hard to swallow. Taste and smell dull. This decreases appetite. Oral hygiene and denture care improve taste.

Secretion of digestive juices decreases. Fried and fatty foods are hard to digest. They may cause indigestion. Dry, fried, and fatty foods are avoided. This helps swallowing and digestion problems. Some people do not have teeth or dentures. Their food is pureed or ground.

Loss of teeth and ill-fitting dentures cause chewing problems. This causes digestion problems. Hard-to-chew foods are avoided. Ground or chopped meat is easier to chew and swallow.

Peristalsis decreases. The stomach and colon empty slower. Flatulence and constipation can occur (Chapter 26). High-fiber foods help prevent constipation. However, they are hard to chew and can irritate the intestines. They include apricots, celery, and fruits and vegetables with skins and seeds. Persons with chewing problems or constipation often need foods that provide soft bulk. They include whole-grain cereals and cooked fruits and vegetables.

Fewer calories are needed because energy and activity levels decline. More fluids are needed for chewing, swallowing, digestion, and kidney function. Foods are needed to prevent constipation and bone changes. High-protein foods are needed for tissue growth and repair. However, some older persons lack protein in their diets. High-protein foods (meat and fish) are costly.

The Urinary System

Kidney function decreases. The kidneys shrink. Blood flow to the kidneys is reduced. Waste removal is less efficient.

The ureters, bladder, and urethra lose tone and elasticity. Bladder muscles weaken. Bladder size decreases, storing less urine. Urinary frequency or urgency may occur. Many older persons have to urinate (void) during the night. Urinary incontinence (the loss of bladder control) may occur (Chapter 24).

In men, the prostate gland enlarges. This puts pressure on the urethra. Difficulty voiding or frequent urination occurs.

Urinary tract infections are risks. Adequate fluids are needed—water, juices, milk, gelatin. Follow the care plan. Remind the person to drink. Offer fluids often to those needing help. Most fluids should be taken before 1700 (5:00 PM). This reduces the need to void during the night.

Persons with incontinence may need bladder training programs. Sometimes catheters are needed (Chapter 25).

The Reproductive System

Reproductive organs change with aging. For the effects of aging on sexuality, see Chapter 51.

- *Men.* The hormone *testosterone* decreases slightly. It affects strength, sperm production, and reproductive tissues. These changes affect sexual activity. An erection takes longer. The phase between erection and orgasm also is longer. Orgasm is less forceful than when younger. Erections are lost quickly. The time between erections also is longer. Older men may need the penis stimulated for arousal. Fatigue, over-eating, and too much alcohol affect erections. Some men fear performance problems. They may avoid closeness.

BOX 12-3   In-Home and Community-Based Services

- *Adult day care.* Provides a safe setting for those who cannot be alone during the day. Services may include personal care, social and recreational activities, meals, drug reminders, counseling, and home health aide services.
- *Caregiver programs.* These programs are for those who care for older adults and for grandparents raising grandchildren.
- *Case management.* A case manager assesses the needs of the older person and family. Arrangements are made for needed services.
- *Companionship services.* A volunteer visits the older person at home. Supervision and support services are provided as needed.
- *Elder abuse prevention programs.* Cases of suspected abuse and neglect are investigated. Help is given as needed.
- *Emergency response systems.* In-home 24-hour alarm systems allow the person to call for emergency help. For example, the person wears a necklace or bracelet with a button to push if help is needed. The person pushes the button in case of a fall or an emergency. He or she is connected to an operator who will send help.
- *Financial counseling.* Help is given with checking accounts, paying bills, taxes, and insurance claims and forms. Counseling is available about Social Security benefits, prescription drug programs, food stamps, and other programs.
- *Home health care.* Nursing and physical, occupational, and speech therapies are provided. The person may need help with such things as taking drugs, changing dressings, or catheter care.
- *Homemaker services.* Help is given with household tasks. Cleaning, laundry, shopping, and preparing meals are examples. Some people need help with personal care.
- *Home repair and modification.* Programs are available to keep the house in good repair. Roofing and plumbing are examples. See *Focus on Long-Term Care and Home Care: Housing Options* for home changes.
- *Hospice care.* See Chapters 1 and 55. Nursing, comfort, and homemaker services are provided.
- *Legal assistance.* Advice is given for some legal matters. Wills, renters' rights, and consumer problems are examples. A lawyer may represent the person in court.
- *Meal programs.* Meals are provided in-home or in a senior center.
- *Personal care.* Help is given with eating, bathing, oral care, grooming, and dressing.
- *Rehabilitation.* Therapies are given to assist the person to regain or maintain his or her highest level of functioning.
- *Respite care.* This service relieves caregivers of daily care for a short time.
- *Senior centers.* These centers offer many social and recreational activities. Classes, day trips, travel groups, performing arts, and nature activities are examples. Services also include meals, counseling, legal help, health screenings, and transportation.
- *Phone reassurance.* Regular phone contact is provided. The person is called at various times. If the person does not answer, someone is sent to the person's home. Also, the older person can call the service when help is needed.
- *Transportation.* Older persons are given rides to and from doctor visits, appointments, shopping, religious services, and other places.
- *Wellness programs.* Blood pressure, blood sugar, and other tests are done to promote health. Sessions are held about fitness, nutrition, and other health topics.

- *Women. Menopause* is when menstruation stops and there has been at least 1 year without a menstrual period. Women can no longer have children. This occurs between 45 and 55 years of age. Female hormones (*estrogen* and *progesterone*) decrease. The uterus, vagina, and genitalia atrophy. Thin vaginal walls and dryness make intercourse uncomfortable or painful. Arousal takes longer. Orgasm is less intense. The pre-excitement state returns more quickly.

HOUSING OPTIONS

A person's home is more than a place to live. A home has family memories. It is a link to neighbors and the community. It brings pride and self-esteem. Aging can lead to changes in a person's home setting.

Most older people live in their own homes. Many function without help. Others need help from family, home care, or community-based services for daily living and safety (Box 12-3). Bathing, dressing, meals, housekeeping, shopping, and transportation are examples. Many services also provide social contact.

Some older persons choose smaller homes when children are gone. Others retire to warmer climates or move closer to children and family. Some choose other housing. Reduced income, taxes, home repairs, and yard work are factors. Some people cannot care for themselves.

Many housing options meet the needs of older people. A new home setting could maintain or improve the person's quality of life.

See *Focus on Long-Term Care and Home Care: Housing Options.*

FOCUS ON LONG-TERM CARE AND HOME CARE

Housing Options

Home Care
Simple changes can make a home safe, easy to use, and promote independence. The nurse discusses needed changes with the patient and family.

The Bathroom
- Non-slick flooring
- Grab bars by showers, tubs, and toilets
- Non-skid surfaces in showers and tubs (bath mats, non-skid bath decals)
- Rugs with non-slip backing outside the tub and shower and in front of the toilet
- Hand-held shower nozzle or adjustable shower head
- Shower chair for shower or bathtub
- Transfer bench
- Lever-handle faucets
- Water controls close to the shower or tub entrance
- Anti-scald devices on faucets and shower heads
- Towel bars or hooks raised or lowered for the person's reach
- Comfort-height toilet, raised toilet seat, or a toilet seat riser
- Chair placed in front of the sink for sitting
- Knee space under the sink for the person who sits
- Bright, non-glare lighting

The Bedroom
- Closet rods that adjust for height
- Lowered shelves or pull-down shelves
- Pull-out drawers, bins, and baskets in closets
- A commode chair near the bed for night-time use (Chapter 24)

The Kitchen
- Appliances within reach—side-by-side refrigerator/freezer, cook-top range, wall-mounted oven, dishwasher raised off the floor
- Stove controls on the front of the stove
- Stove controls clearly marked and easy to see
- Lowered shelves or pull-down shelves
- Height of sink and countertops adjusted for the person's needs (lowered for wheelchair use; raised for the person who cannot bend easily)

The Kitchen—cont'd
- Anti-scald devices on faucets
- Lever-handle faucets
- Spray attachment to the sink—pots can be filled after placing them on the stove

Other
- Lever door handles on all doors
- Easy-to-grasp cabinet and drawer handles
- Hand rails on both sides of stairways and outside steps
- Keyless locking system
- Security system
- Shelves near outside doors—items can be set down to open the door
- Bright lights inside and outside entry-ways
- Motion-activated entrance lights
- Slip-free walk-ways and entry-ways
- House numbers that are easy to see from the street
- Automatic garage door opener
- Rocker light switches that turn on and off with a push
- Electrical outlets 18 inches above the floor
- Peepholes or view panels in doors at the correct height for the person
- Washer and dryer on the main floor
- Wall-mounted, fold-down ironing board
- Stair or platform lifts
- No scatter or throw rugs
- Thick carpeting replaced with low pile carpeting
- Furniture arranged for wheelchair use
- Phones in all rooms, including the bathroom
- Cordless phone or wireless phone
- Chairs throughout the home so the person can sit when tired, weak, dizzy, and so on
- Smoke detectors as required by local fire code
- Carbon monoxide detectors
- For poor eyesight—see Chapter 42
- For hearing loss—see Chapter 42

Living With Family

Sometimes older brothers, sisters, and cousins live together. They:

- Provide companionship.
- Share living expenses.
- Provide care during illness or disability.

Living with children is an option. The older parent (parents) moves in with the child. Or the child moves to the parent's home. The parent may be healthy, may need some help, or may be ill or disabled. Some adult children give care to avoid nursing center care.

Living with an adult child is a social change. Everyone in the home must adjust. If no spare bedroom, sleeping plans may change. The parent may need a hospital bed. It can go in a family or living room, dining room, den, or bedroom.

The adult child's family needs time alone. Other family members may help give care. Respite care is an option. (*Respite* means *a short period of rest or relief.*) The person goes to a nursing center for a short time. This gives the family relief from the person's care. Home care agencies can provide nurses or home health aides. Many community and church groups have volunteers who help give care.

Adult Day Care. Many children work even though the parent cannot stay alone. Adult day-care centers provide meals, supervision, and activities. Some give rides to and from the center. Some have rehabilitation services (Chapter 41) and serve persons with dementia (Chapter 49).

Requirements vary. Some require the ability to walk. A cane or walker is used as needed. Others allow wheelchairs. Most require some self-care abilities.

Cards, board games, movies, crafts, dancing, walks, exercise groups, and lectures are common activities (Fig. 12-6). Some provide bowling and swimming. All activities are supervised. Needed help is given.

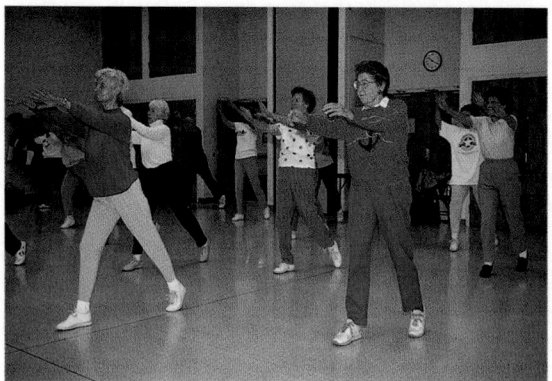

FIGURE 12-6 An adult day-care center activity.

Some areas have inter-generational day-care centers. Children and older persons are in the same center. They work together on some activities. They eat and play together. Young children bring much joy to older persons. They give older persons purpose, love, and affection. In turn, children learn about aging. They also receive love and affection.

Elder Cottage Housing Opportunity and Accessory Dwelling Units

Elder Cottage Housing Opportunity (ECHO) homes are small homes designed for older and disabled persons. The portable home is placed in the yard of a single-family home. Some ECHO homes attach to a house as a home addition.

An *accessory dwelling unit (ADU)* is a separate living area in a home. It can be over a garage, in the basement, or an addition to the house. It has a kitchen, bedroom, and bathroom. Some have a small living room. Some children have these apartments for their parents. Or the older person's home may have an apartment.

ADUs are also called "in-law apartments," "granny flats," "accessory apartments," "second units," and other names. ECHO homes and ADUs allow older persons to live independently but near family and friends.

Rental Options

Instead of owning a home, many older persons choose to rent. Rental options include a single-family home, an apartment, a condo, a mobile home, or a room in a house.

The renter pays rent and utility bills. The benefits of renting include:

- The renter is free from the responsibilities of home ownership.
- The owner (landlord) provides maintenance, yard work, snow removal, and repairs.
- The older person remains independent.
- The older person can keep personal items.
  Downsides to renting include:
- Restrictions about having pets
- Relying on the landlord for repairs and maintenance
- Rent increases
- Ending rental agreements before the person wants to move
- Lack of gardening or yard work opportunities

Senior Citizen Housing. In many areas, state and federal funds support apartment complexes for older and disabled persons. Such persons have low to moderate incomes. Monthly rents are lower. The rent depends on the person's monthly income.

Residential Hotels. Some cities have residential hotels. Private rooms or small apartments are rented. Food services may include a dining room, cafeteria, or room service. Some provide recreational activities and emergency medical services. Most hotels are close to shopping, places of worship, and other civic services.

Home-Sharing

Two or more people share a house or apartment. Each person has a bedroom. They share other living spaces—kitchen, bathroom, living room. They share household chores and expenses. Or cooking, cleaning, and yard work are exchanged for rent.

Shared housing is a way to avoid living alone. It provides companionship. Some people feel safer when living with another person.

Group Settings

Group settings provide housing, in-home support services, and social activities. Services provided relate to personal care and independent living.
- Personal hygiene and grooming
- Eating
- Getting in and out of bed or chairs
- Using the bathroom
- Using the phone
- Housework
- Preparing meals
- Shopping
- Managing money

Assisted Living Residences. Assisted living residences are for persons who need help with daily living (Chapters 1 and 53). Residents have social contact with others in a home-like setting. Staff are available to assist 24 hours a day.

Board and Care Homes. Board and care homes (group homes) are often private, single-family homes. The homes have been adapted for group living. Residents have roommates or their own rooms.

Some homes are for older persons. Others are for people with certain problems. Dementia, mental health disorders, and intellectual and developmental disabilities are examples.

Homes house 4 to 10 people or more. The care provided and rules vary from state to state. The person pays monthly rent. Some board and care homes receive government funds.

Adult Foster Care. Adult foster care can take 2 forms.
- An older person lives with a family.
- A single family home serves 4 to 5 persons with special needs. They may be older, disabled, or have mental health disorders.

The person receives help with personal care and independent living. The person receives needed health care.

Adult Care Facilities. Adult care facilities are also called *congregate housing*. *Congregate* means *a group, gathering, or cluster*. In this group setting, private apartments are designed for older people. Buildings have wheelchair access, hand rails, elevators, and other safety features.

Services are many. A doctor or nurse is on call. Someone checks on the person daily. A dining room is common. Rides are provided to places of worship, the doctor, or shopping areas. Tenants pay monthly rent.

Continuing Care Retirement Communities. Continuing care retirement communities (CCRCs) offer many services. They range from independent living units to 24-hour nursing care. CCRCs have housing, activity, and health care services. They meet the changing needs of older persons living alone or with a partner.

Independent living units are small apartments. Residents perform self-care and take their own drugs. Food service is provided. Help is nearby if needed. Many people travel or drive about in their own cars. Rides are provided for those who need them.

Services are added as the person's needs change. Over time, some persons need nursing center care. They move into the nursing center within the CCRC. Many older couples find comfort in this plan. One partner needs nursing care. The other is close by and can visit often.

The person signs a contract with the CCRC. The contract is for a certain time or for the person's life-time. The contract lists services provided and the required fees.

Nursing Centers

Some older persons cannot care for themselves. Nursing centers are options for them (Chapter 1). Some people stay in nursing centers until death. Others return home when able. The nursing center is the person's temporary or permanent home. The setting is as home-like as possible (Fig. 12-7).

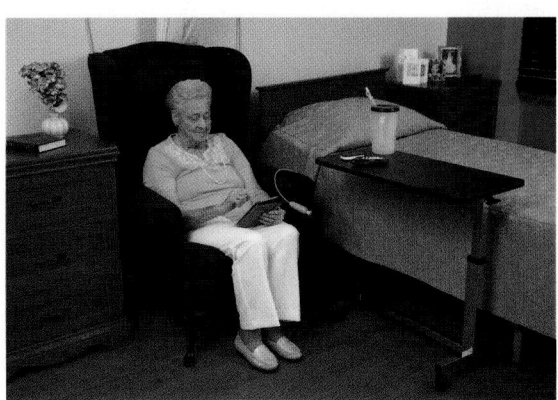

FIGURE 12-7 A nursing center is as home-like as possible. Some centers allow residents to bring their own bed and furniture from home.

The person needing nursing center care may suffer some or all of these losses.

- Loss of identity as a productive member of a family and community
- Loss of possessions—home, household items, care, and so on
- Loss of independence
- Loss of real-world experiences—shopping, traveling, cooking, driving, hobbies, and so on
- Loss of health and mobility

The person may feel useless, powerless, and hopeless. The health team helps the person cope with loss and improve quality of life. Treat the person with dignity and respect. Also practice good communication skills. Follow the care plan.

Most nursing centers receive Medicare or Medicaid funds. They must meet requirements of the *Omnibus Budget Reconciliation Act of 1987 (OBRA)*. OBRA protects the person's rights and promotes quality of life. The Centers for Medicare & Medicaid Services (CMS) has rules and regulations for OBRA. See Box 12-4.

Nursing centers serve to meet the needs of older and disabled persons. Physical changes of aging are considered in the design. So are safety needs. Programs and services meet the person's basic needs. Box 12-5 lists the features of a quality nursing center.

BOX 12-4	Environment Requirements

- The center provides a clean, comfortable, and home-like setting. Residents are allowed to use personal belongings.
- The person's care equipment is clean and properly stored. This includes toothbrushes, dentures, denture cups, water mugs, emesis (kidney) basins, hair brushes and combs, bedpans, urinals, feeding tubes, leg bags and catheter bags, waterproof under-pads, and positioning devices.
- The call system functions properly. Residents have call lights within reach.
- Bed linens are clean and in good condition.
- There are clean towels and washcloths for each person.
- The person has closet space with shelves. The person can reach the shelves.
- Lighting levels are comfortable and adequate.
- Temperature levels are comfortable and safe. The temperature is between 71°F and 81°F (Fahrenheit).
- Sound levels are comfortable. Sound levels allow for hearing, privacy, and social interaction.

- Safety measures are followed for persons who smoke. See Chapter 13.
- Hand rails, assistive devices, and other surfaces are in good repair. They are free from sharp edges or other hazards.
- Furniture is appropriate for the residents.
- The person's setting is as free from accident hazards as possible.
  - Resident care equipment is used following the manufacturer's instructions.
  - Safety measures are practiced for hazardous substances (Chapter 13).
  - Safety measures are practiced to prevent equipment accidents (Chapter 13). This includes electrical safety.
  - Safety measures are practiced to prevent accidents from assistive (adaptive) devices and equipment. This includes canes, walkers, wheelchairs, mechanical lifts, restraints, bed rails, mattresses, and so on.

Modified from Centers for Medicare & Medicaid Services: Environment observations—FORM CMS-20061 Baltimore, March 2013, U.S. Department of Health and Human Services.

BOX 12-5   Features of a Quality Nursing Center

Basic Information

- The center is Medicare-certified.
- The center is Medicaid-certified.
- The center is a skilled nursing facility.
- The administrator is licensed by the state.
- The center conducts background checks on all staff.
- The center provides training on preventing abuse and neglect.
- The center provides the level of care needed. Rehabilitation, dementia, ventilator, and hospice services are examples.
- The center is located close enough for family and friends to visit.
- The center has policies and procedures to protect resident belongings.

Resident Appearance

- Residents are clean and well-groomed.
- Residents are dressed correctly for the season or time of day.

Living Spaces

- The center is free from strong, unpleasant odors.
- The center appears clean and well-kept.
- The temperature is comfortable for the residents.
- The center has good lighting.
- Noise levels in the dining room and in common areas are comfortable.
- Smoking is not allowed. If allowed, it is restricted to certain areas.
- Furnishings in rooms and lounges are sturdy, comfortable, and attractive.

Staff

- The relationship between the staff and residents appears to be warm, polite, and respectful.
- Staff are respectful to each other.
- All staff wear name tags.
- Staff knock on the person's door before entering the room.
- Staff refer to residents by name.
- The center offers a training and continuing education program for all staff.
- The center has licensed nurses 24 hours a day. An RN (registered nurse) is present at least 8 hours a day, 7 days a week.
- Nurses and nursing assistants work as a team to meet resident needs.
- Residents have the same caregivers on a daily basis.
- The center is adequately staffed on weekends and holidays.
- Nursing assistants take part in care planning meetings.
- The center has a full-time social worker on staff.
- A licensed doctor is on staff. He or she is there daily and can be reached at all times.
- The center's management team has worked together for at least 1 year. This includes the administrator and director of nursing.

Residents' Rooms

- Residents may have personal belongings and furniture in their rooms.
- Each resident has a storage space (closet and drawers) in his or her room.
- Each resident has a window in his or her room.
- Residents have access to a personal phone.
- Residents have access to a personal TV.
- Residents have a choice of roommates.
- The resident can reach his or her water mug.

Hallways, Stairs, Lounges, and Bathrooms

- Exits are clearly marked.
- The center has quiet areas where residents can visit with family and friends.
- All common areas, resident rooms, and doorways are designed for wheelchair use.
- The center has hand rails in the hallways.
- The center has grab bars in bathrooms.
- Spills are cleaned up quickly.
- Hallways are free of clutter.
- Hallways have good lighting.

Food and Fluids

- Residents have food choices at meal times.
- The person's favorite foods are served.
- Food smells good and looks good.
- Food is served at the correct temperature.
- Nutritious snacks are available upon request.
- Each resident has a filled water mug.
- Staff help residents eat and drink if help is needed.
- Dining rooms allow residents to relax, socialize, and enjoy their food.
- Residents are weighed regularly.

Activities

- Residents may choose a variety of activities. This includes residents who cannot leave their rooms.
- The center has outdoor areas for resident use. Staff help residents to go outside.
- The center has an active volunteer program.

Safety and Care

- The center has smoke alarms and sprinklers.
- The center has an emergency evacuation plan.
- Regular fire drills are held. Residents, including bed-bound residents, are moved to safety.
- There are enough staff to move residents quickly in an emergency.
- Staff respond quickly to call lights and requests for help.
- Residents receive preventive care to stay healthy. Yearly flu shots are an example.
- Residents may see their personal doctors.
- The center has an arrangement with a nearby hospital for emergencies.
- Care plan meetings are held with residents and family members.
- The center has corrected all problems on its last state inspection report.

Modified from Centers for Medicare & Medicaid Services: Your guide to choosing a nursing home or other long-term care, *Baltimore, revised December 2013, U.S. Department of Health and Human Services.*

FOCUS ON PRIDE
The Person, Family and Yourself

Personal and Professional Responsibility
Myths about aging are common. Some believe that all older persons have decreased mental and physical function. For example, they are hard-of-hearing, confused, or move slowly. Others think the elderly cannot care for themselves. Or they lose interest in activities.

Your beliefs affect the care you give. You may struggle with a myth. Review the facts about aging in Box 12-1. Each person is unique. Treat each person as an individual.

Rights and Respect
A nursing center provides a temporary or permanent residence for some persons. The setting must promote quality of life. It must be clean, safe, comfortable, and as home-like as possible. Give care that reflects these principles. To do so:
- Knock before entering the person's room.
- Make sure the person, clothes, and linens are clean and dry.
- Keep the person's room clean and orderly.
- Place soiled linens in the correct containers. Empty the containers often. Do not let them over-flow.
- Clean up your work area and the bathroom after giving care.
- Help the person display belongings if asked. Do not touch the person's items without permission.
- Treat the person as if you were in his or her home.
- Respect the person and his or her setting.

Independence and Social Interaction
Older persons may feel lonely and isolated. Loss of friends and loved ones, a new home setting, reduced income, and physical changes are causes. To promote social interaction:
- Encourage the person to talk about friends and family.
- Ask about the person's hobbies and interests.
- Use touch to show caring. For example, gently place your hand on the person's shoulder or arm. Remember to maintain professional boundaries.
- Take time to listen. Avoid seeming rushed.

Some persons prefer quiet and privacy. They may avoid social contacts. Respect their wishes for privacy. Take pride in considering their social needs.

Delegation and Teamwork
Team members often work together to assist older persons. For example, 2 nursing assistants help an older woman to the bathroom. Or team members work close by with groups of older persons. For example, 2 Russian-speaking nursing assistants sit near each other when feeding residents. When working this way, they may be tempted to talk to each other in their native language.

Co-workers may be closer to your age, share your interests, relate to your work, share your native language, and so on. You must not ignore the patient, resident, or group or speak in a foreign language. Talk with the person or group. Focus on them, not on others. This promotes a sense of belonging and self-worth.

Ethics and Laws
The CMS is a federal agency. It issues standards, rules, and regulations. Employers and employees must comply with them. Unannounced surveys are conducted for agency compliance. If requirements are not met, funding is lost. A survey team will:
- Review policies, procedures, and medical records.
- Interview staff, patients and residents, and families.
- Check for cleanliness and safety.
- Make sure staff meet state requirements.
- Observe how care is given.

You may be observed or asked questions during a survey. You must provide safe, quality care and protect the person's rights. Also, you must help keep the agency clean and follow agency policies and procedures. Answer survey questions completely and honestly. Act professionally and use good work ethics (Chapter 6).

You may be tempted to act differently when surveyors are present. This is wrong. Your conduct and care must reflect a normal day. Provide the same quality care every day.

FOCUS ON PRIDE: Application
The changes of aging affect the whole person. List 5 changes that occur with aging. Describe how each affects the person. How would you modify care to meet the person's needs?

REVIEW QUESTIONS
Circle the BEST answer.

1 Late adulthood begins at age
 a 55
 b 65
 c 75
 d 85

2 The study of the aging process is called
 a Geriatrics
 b Dysphagia
 c Gerontology
 d Dyspnea

3 Retirement usually means
 a Lowered income
 b Changes from aging
 c Less free time
 d Financial security

4 Which causes loneliness in older persons?
 a Having hobbies
 b Children moving away
 c Attending community events
 d Contact with other older persons

REVIEW QUESTIONS—cont'd

5 Older persons living with their children often feel
  a Independent
  b Wanted and a part of things
  c Useless
  d Dignified

6 Which statement about a partner's death is *true*?
  a The surviving partner's life will not likely change.
  b Preparing for the event lessens grief.
  c Grief cannot cause physical problems.
  d Feelings of loss and emptiness occur.

7 Skin changes occur with aging. Care should include
  a Keeping the room cool
  b A daily bath with soap
  c Applying lotion
  d Bathing in hot water

8 An older person complains of cold feet. You should
  a Provide socks
  b Apply a hot water bottle
  c Soak the feet in hot water
  d Apply a heating pad

9 Musculo-skeletal changes occur with aging. Which is *true*?
  a Bones become firm.
  b Exercise promotes muscle atrophy.
  c Joints become stiff and painful.
  d Bedrest prevents loss of strength.

10 Changes occur in the nervous system. Which is *true*?
  a Less sleep is needed than when younger.
  b The person forgets events from long ago.
  c Sensitivity to pressure increases.
  d Confusion occurs in all older persons.

11 Changes occur in the eye with aging. Which is *true*?
  a Tear secretion increases.
  b There is no change in seeing colors.
  c There is more trouble focusing on far objects.
  d Vision is poor at night and in dark rooms.

12 Which is *true* of hearing loss in older persons?
  a Low-pitched sounds are hard to hear.
  b Acoustic nerve changes affect hearing.
  c Earwax cannot affect hearing.
  d Ear infections often cause hearing loss.

13 Arteries narrow and lose their elasticity. These changes result in
  a A slower heart rate
  b Lower blood pressure
  c Poor circulation to many body parts
  d Less blood in the body

14 An older person has circulatory changes. Which care measure would you question?
  a Keep needed items nearby
  b Get a moderate amount of daily exercise
  c Avoid exertion
  d Take long walks

15 Respiratory changes occur with aging. Which is *true*?
  a Heavy bed linens are used.
  b The person is turned often if on bedrest.
  c The side-lying position is best for breathing.
  d Deep breathing is avoided.

16 Older persons should avoid dry foods because of
  a Decreases in saliva
  b Loss of teeth or ill-fitting dentures
  c Decreased amounts of digestive juices
  d Decreased peristalsis

17 Changes occur in the digestive system. Older persons should eat
  a Fruits and vegetables with skins and seeds
  b Dry and fatty foods
  c Raw apricots and celery
  d Protein foods

18 Changes occur in the urinary system. Which is *true*?
  a Kidneys increase in size.
  b Fluids are needed for kidney function.
  c The bladder becomes larger.
  d Blood flow to the kidneys increases.

19 The doctor orders increased fluid intake for an older person. You should
  a Give most of the fluid before 1700 (5:00 PM)
  b Provide mostly water
  c Start a bladder training program
  d Insert a catheter

20 Most older people are
  a In nursing centers
  b In a family setting
  c With children
  d In senior citizen housing

21 Adult day-care centers
  a Provide meals, supervision, and activities
  b Provide housing and nursing care
  c Offer help for persons who cannot perform self-care
  d Provide personal care

22 A husband needs 24-hour nursing care. His wife needs an independent living unit. Which would meet their needs?
  a Adult foster care
  b Home health care
  c A continuing care retirement community
  d An assisted living residence

23 A quality nursing center
  a Is Medicare and Medicaid certified
  b Is owned by doctors and nurses
  c Has independent living units
  d Provides adult and child day care

Answers to Chapter 12 questions are on p. 870.

FOCUS ON PRACTICE

Problem Solving

Ms. Hild has urinary incontinence and chewing and swallowing problems due to changes from aging. A co-worker uses the term "diaper" to describe her incontinence product and "bib" for her clothing protector. The co-worker wipes spilled food from Ms. Hild's face with a spoon and threatens to with-hold privileges if she does not finish meals.

Explain why it is important to treat the person as an adult and not a child. Describe ways to provide age-appropriate care. How will you respond to your co-worker's statements and actions?

OBJECTIVES

- Define the key terms and key abbreviations in this chapter.
- Describe accident risk factors.
- Explain why you identify a person before giving care.
- Explain how to correctly identify a person.
- Describe the safety measures to prevent burns, poisoning, and suffocation.
- Identify the signs and causes of choking.
- Explain how to prevent equipment accidents.
- Explain how to handle hazardous chemicals.

- Identify natural and human-made disasters.
- Describe fire prevention measures and oxygen safety.
- Explain what to do during a fire.
- Explain how to protect yourself from workplace violence.
- Describe your role in risk management.
- Perform the procedures described in this chapter.
- Explain how to promote PRIDE in the person, the family, and yourself.

KEY TERMS

coma A state of being unaware of one's setting and being unable to react or respond to people, places, or things

dementia The loss of cognitive and social function caused by changes in the brain

disaster A sudden, catastrophic event in which people are injured and killed and property is destroyed

electrical shock When electrical current passes through the body

elopement When a patient or resident leaves the agency without staff knowledge

ground That which carries leaking electricity to the earth and away from an electrical item

hazard Any thing in the person's setting that could cause injury or illness

hazardous chemical Any chemical that is a health hazard or a physical hazard

hemiplegia Paralysis *(plegia)* on 1 side *(hemi)* of the body

incident Any event that has harmed or could harm a patient, resident, visitor, or staff member

paralysis Loss of muscle function, sensation, or both

paraplegia Paralysis in the legs and lower trunk *(para* means *beyond; plegia* means *paralysis)*

poison Any substance harmful to the body when ingested, inhaled, injected, or absorbed through the skin

quadriplegia Paralysis in the arms, legs, and trunk *(quad* means *4; plegia* means *paralysis);* tetraplegia

suffocation When breathing stops from the lack of oxygen

tetraplegia See "quadriplegia" *(tetra* means *4; plegia* means *paralysis)*

workplace violence Violent acts (including assault or threat of assault) directed toward persons at work or while on duty

KEY ABBREVIATIONS

AED	Automated external defibrillator	**HCS**	Hazard Communication Standard
C	Centigrade	**ID**	Identification
CDC	Centers for Disease Control and Prevention	**MET**	Medical Emergency Team
CMS	Centers for Medicare & Medicaid Services	**OSHA**	Occupational Safety and Health Administration
CO	Carbon monoxide	**PASS**	*Pull* the safety pin, *aim* low, *squeeze* the lever, *sweep* back and forth
CPR	Cardiopulmonary resuscitation		
EMS	Emergency Medical Services	**RACE**	Rescue, alarm, confine, extinguish
F	Fahrenheit	**RRT**	Rapid Response Team
FBAO	Foreign-body airway obstruction	**SDS**	Safety data sheet

Safety is a basic need. Patients and residents are at great risk for accidents and falls. (See Chapter 14 for falls.) Some accidents and injuries cause death.

The health team must provide for safety. This includes you. Common sense and simple safety measures can prevent most accidents. Sometimes extraordinary measures are needed. You must protect patients, residents, visitors, co-workers, and yourself. The safety measures in this chapter apply to all health care settings and everyday life.

The goal is to decrease the person's risk of accidents and injuries without limiting mobility and independence. The care plan lists other safety measures for the person. Measures to promote safety must not interfere with the person's rights (Chapter 2).

See *Focus on Surveys: Safety.*

A SAFE SETTING

In a safe setting, a person has little risk of illness or injury. The person's setting is free of hazards to the extent possible. The person feels safe and secure physically and mentally. The risk for infection, falls, burns, poisoning, and other injuries is low. Temperature and noise levels are comfortable. Smells are pleasant. There is enough room and light to move about safely. The person and the person's property are safe from fire and intruders. The person is not afraid and has few worries and concerns.

The person must receive the right care and treatment. To protect the person from harm, follow the person's care plan. Also practice the safety measures in this chapter.

See *Teamwork and Time Management: A Safe Setting.*

FOCUS ON **SURVEYS**

Safety

A survey team will observe the agency setting and patient or resident rooms.

- For potential or actual hazards. A *hazard* is any thing in the person's setting that could cause injury or illness. Examples include spills, loose hand rails, unanswered call lights, burnt-out bulbs, unsafe equipment, and other safety issues described in this chapter.
- For how staff respond to potential or actual hazards.
- If the care plan was followed on each shift for persons at risk.
- How staff supervise persons at risk.
- If the staff have removed or changed a hazard.
  The survey team will interview staff. A surveyor may ask you:
- About measures in the person's care plan to reduce the risk for an accident.
- When and how you report risks and hazards.
- When and how you correct an immediate hazard. A spill is an example.
- The agency's procedures for removing or reducing a hazard.
  You must provide for safety at all times. And you must know what to do if you find a hazard. Remember to give surveyors complete and honest answers. Surveys protect patients and residents.

TEAMWORK AND TIME MANAGEMENT

A Safe Setting

You may see something unsafe. Correct the matter right away if it is something you can do. For example:

- Wipe up spills right away. Do so even if you did not cause the spill.
- A person is sliding out of a wheelchair. Position the person correctly in the chair. Do so even if a co-worker is responsible for the person's care.
- A person has problems holding a coffee cup. Offer to help the person.
- Food is left unattended in an oven. Turn off the oven. Then tell your co-worker the reason for your action.
  You cannot correct some safety issues. Follow agency policy to report such problems. They include:
- Electrical outlets or switches coming out of the wall
- Electrical outlets that do not work
- Water leaks from windows, doors, ceilings, pipes, faucets, tubs, showers, toilets, water heaters, and other sources
- Toilets that do not work properly
- Water from faucets that does not warm up or that is very hot
- Broken or damaged windows or furniture
- Windows and doors that do not work properly
- Knobs and handles that are broken or do not work properly
- Hand rails and grab bars that are loose or need repair
- Odd smells, odors, and sounds
- Signs of rodents, flies, ants, or other pests
- Lights and lamps that do not work or have burnt-out bulbs
- Flooring (carpeting, tiles) needing repair

ACCIDENT RISK FACTORS

Some people cannot protect themselves. They present dangers to themselves and others. They rely on others for safety. Certain factors increase the risk of accidents and injuries. Follow the person's care plan.

- *Age.* Children and older persons are at risk for injuries. See *Focus on Children and Older Persons: Accident Risk Factors (Age).*
- *Awareness of surroundings.* People need to know their surroundings to protect themselves from injury. Confused and disoriented persons may not understand what is happening to and around them. A coma can occur from illness or injury. *Coma is a state of being unaware of one's setting and being unable to react or respond to people, places, or things.*
- *Agitated and aggressive behaviors.* Pain can cause these behaviors. So can confusion, decreased awareness of surroundings, and fear of what may happen.
- *Vision loss.* Persons with poor vision can fall or trip over toys, rugs, equipment, furniture, and cords. Some cannot read container labels. Poisoning can result. Harm can result from taking the wrong drug or the wrong dose.

FOCUS ON CHILDREN AND OLDER PERSONS

Accident Risk Factors (Age)

Children

Infants are helpless. Young children have not learned safety and danger. They explore their settings, put objects in their mouths, and touch and feel new things. Falls, poisoning, choking, burns, and other accidents are risks. Practice the safety measures in Chapter 52 and Appendix D, p. 877.

Older Persons

Changes from aging increase the risk for falls and other injuries. Many older persons have decreased strength and move slowly. Some are unsteady. Often balance is affected. These changes prevent quick and sudden movements to avoid dangers and falls. Older persons also are less sensitive to heat and cold. They have poor vision, hearing problems, and a dulled sense of smell. Confusion, poor judgment, memory problems, and disorientation may occur (Chapter 49).

Some persons have dementia. *Dementia is the loss of cognitive and social function caused by changes in the brain* (Chapter 49). *(Cognitive relates to knowledge.)* Memory and the ability to think and reason are lost.

Persons with dementia are confused and disoriented. Their awareness of surroundings is reduced. They may not understand what is happening to and around them. Judgment is poor. They no longer know what is safe and what are dangers. They may access closets, cupboards, or other unsafe and unlocked areas. They may eat or drink cleaning products, drugs, or poisons. Accidents and injuries are great risks.

- *Hearing loss.* Persons with hearing loss have problems hearing the spoken word. They may not hear warning signals or fire alarms. Some cannot hear approaching meal carts, drug carts, stretchers, or wheelchairs. They do not know to move to safety.
- *Impaired smell and touch.* Illness and aging affect smell and touch. The person may not detect smoke or gas odors. Burns are a risk from impaired touch. The person has problems sensing heat and cold. Some people have a decreased sense of pain. They may be unaware of injury. For example, Mrs. Parks does not feel a blister from her shoes. She has poor circulation in her legs and feet. The blister can become a serious wound.
- *Impaired mobility.* Some diseases and injuries affect mobility. A person may know there is danger but cannot move to safety. Some persons cannot walk or propel wheelchairs. Some persons are paralyzed.
  - *Paralysis means loss of muscle function, sensation, or both.*
  - *Paraplegia is paralysis in the legs and lower trunk.* (Para *means* beyond. Plegia *means* paralysis.)
  - *Quadriplegia (tetraplegia) is paralysis in the arms, legs, and trunk.* (Quad *and* tetra *mean* 4. Plegia *means* paralysis.)
  - *Hemiplegia is paralysis* (plegia) *on 1 side* (hemi) *of the body.*
- *Drugs.* Drug side effects may include loss of balance, drowsiness, and lack of coordination. Reduced awareness, confusion, and disorientation may occur. The person may be fearful and uncooperative. Report behavior changes and the person's complaints to the nurse.

IDENTIFYING THE PERSON

Each person has different treatments, therapies, and activity limits. Life and health are threatened from the wrong care.

The person may receive an identification (ID) bracelet when admitted to the agency (Fig. 13-1). The bracelet has the person's name, room and bed number, birth date, age, doctor, and other identifying information.

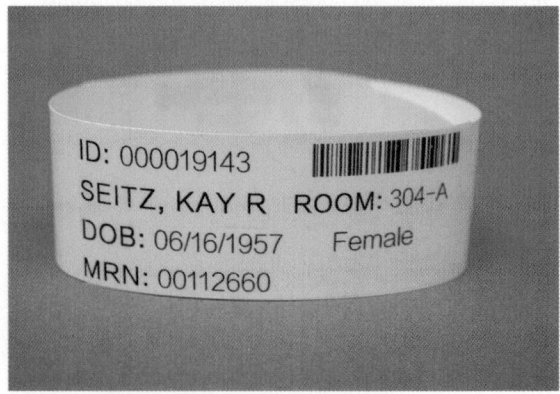

FIGURE 13-1 ID bracelet.

You use the bracelet to identify the person before giving care. Your assignment sheet states what care to give. To identify the person:

- Compare identifying information on the assignment sheet with that on the ID bracelet (Fig. 13-2). Carefully check the information. Some people have the same first and last names. For example, John Smith is a very common name.
- Use at least 2 identifiers. An identifier cannot be the person's room or bed number. Some agencies require the person to state and spell his or her name and give his or her birth date. Others require using the person's ID number. Always follow agency policy.
- Call the person by name when checking the ID bracelet. This is a courtesy given as you touch the person and before giving care. Just calling the person by name is not enough for identification. Confused, disoriented, drowsy, hard-of-hearing, or distracted persons may answer to any name.

See *Focus on Communication: Identifying the Person.*

See *Focus on Long-Term Care and Home Care: Identifying the Person.*

See *Promoting Safety and Comfort: Identifying the Person.*

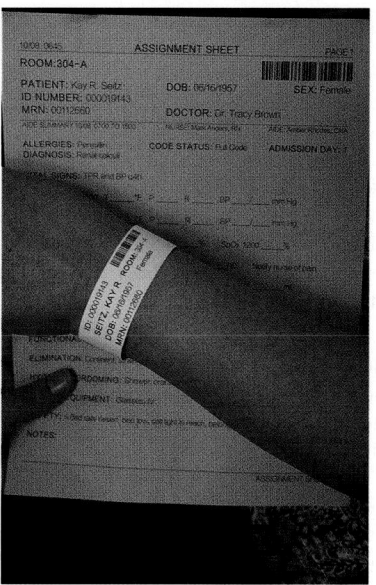

FIGURE 13-2 The ID bracelet is checked against the assignment sheet to accurately identify the person.

FOCUS ON **COMMUNICATION**

Identifying the Person

To identify the person, call the person by name. Ask to see the ID bracelet. For example: "Hello, Mr. Hall. May I see your ID bracelet?" Then ask for 2 identifiers. You can say: "Please tell me your full name and birth date." Compare the identifiers with the information on the ID bracelet and your assignment sheet.

For some persons, identifying themselves is annoying. The person may say: "Do I have to say it again? You know who I am." Be polite. Explain why you check the person's identity. You can say: "It is important to check so I give care to the right person. It is for your safety." Thank the person. Use his or her title and name. For example: "Thank you, Mr. Green."

PROMOTING SAFETY AND COMFORT

Identifying the Person

Safety
Always identify the person before starting a task or procedure. Do not identify the person and then leave the room for supplies and equipment. You could go to the wrong room and give care to the wrong person. And the person for whom the care was intended would not receive it. This too could cause harm.

Sometimes ID bracelets are damaged from water, spilled food and fluids, and everyday wear and tear. If you cannot read the information on the ID bracelet, tell the nurse. The nurse can have a new bracelet made.

Comfort
Make sure ID bracelets are not too loose or too tight. You should be able to slide 1 or 2 fingers under a bracelet. If it is too loose or too tight, tell the nurse.

FOCUS ON **LONG-TERM CARE AND HOME CARE**

Identifying the Person

Long-Term Care
Alert and oriented residents may choose not to wear ID bracelets. This is noted on the person's care plan. Follow center policy and the care plan to identify the person.

Some nursing centers have photo ID systems (Fig. 13-3). The person's photo is taken on admission. Then it is placed in the person's medical record. If your center uses such a system, learn to use it safely.

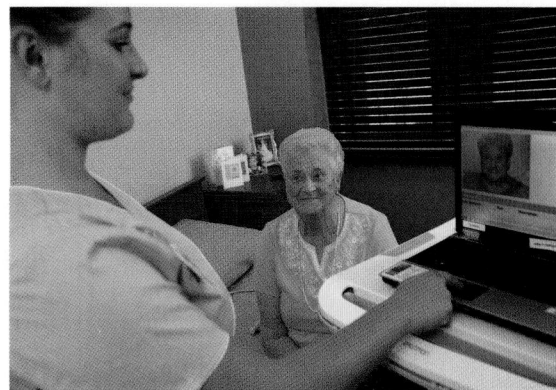

FIGURE 13-3 The nursing assistant uses the photo to identify the person.

BOX 13-1	Preventing Burns

Smoke Alarms
- Have working smoke alarms.
  - Have smoke alarms on every level of the home, in each bedroom, and outside each bedroom or sleeping area.
  - Test alarms every month.
  - Replace batteries when Daylight Savings Time changes in the spring and fall. Replace batteries even if alarms are hard-wired.
  - Use alarms with flashing strobe lights if hard-of-hearing.

Children
- Do not leave children home alone.
- Supervise young children at all times.
- Do not leave children alone in the kitchen, bathroom, or a room with a fireplace.
- Secure fireplaces with door guards or heat-resistant gates.
- Install barriers around fireplaces, ovens, and furnaces. Avoid using glass screens that can become very hot and take a long time to cool down.
- Store matches, lighters, lamp oils, or other flammable materials in locked cabinets. Or store them out of the reach of children.
- Do not let children near stoves, space heaters, fireplaces, barbecue grills, radiators, registers, oil lamps, candles, curling irons, and other heat sources.
- Do not carry or hold a child while cooking.
- Keep space heaters and materials that can catch fire away from children.
- Teach children fire safety and fire prevention measures. Also teach the dangers of fire.
- Check metal playground equipment. Metal surfaces exposed to sunlight can heat to high temperatures. They can burn a child's face, hands, arms, legs, and buttocks.
- Check car seats, seat belts, and seat-belt buckles. If hot, they can burn children.
- Cover car seats with towels if you park in the sun. Also use a sun visor for the windshield.
- Protect children from sun exposure.
  - Use a sunscreen.
  - Cover exposed areas.
  - Limit time in the sun.

Kitchen and Cooking
- Do not let children help you cook at the stove, in a microwave oven, or on a barbecue grill.
- Use the back burners of stoves when cooking.
- Point pot and pan handles inward, toward the back. They point away from where people stand and walk.
- Do not leave cooking utensils in pots and pans.
- Do not wear clothes with long sleeves or that are loose-fitting when cooking.
- Keep things that can catch fire away from stoves. This includes paper towels, oven mitts, pot-holders, curtains, and so on.
- Do not put wet food into frying pans or deep-fryers. The water causes the oil to splatter.

Kitchen and Cooking—cont'd
- Use dry oven mitts and pot-holders. Water conducts heat.
- Stay near the stove, oven, microwave oven, and barbecue grill when cooking. Do not leave cooking unattended.
- Open or uncover microwaved foods slowly. Steam can burn your fingers, hands, or face.
- Keep hot food and liquids away from counter and table edges. Use the center of the counter or table.
- Turn the oven and stove burners off when not in use.

Eating and Drinking
- Assist with eating and drinking as needed. Spilled hot food or fluids can cause burns.
- Be careful when carrying hot foods and fluids, especially when near children and older persons.
- Do not pour hot liquids near a child or older person.

Water
- Set the hot water heater temperature no higher than 120°F.
- Have anti-scald devices installed on faucets and shower-heads.
- Turn on cold water first, then hot water. Turn off hot water first, then cold water.
- Measure bath or shower water temperature (Chapter 22). Check it before bathing a baby or before a person gets into the tub or shower.
- Check for "hot spots" in bath water. Move your hand back and forth.

Appliances and Other Electrical Equipment
- See "Preventing Equipment Accidents" (p. 169).
- Do not allow the use of space heaters. If used, they must be at least 3 feet away from items that can burn. Turn off the heater before leaving the room.
- Do not let the person sleep with a heating pad.
- Do not let the person use an electric blanket.
- Turn off and unplug irons, curling irons, electric rollers, and hair dryers when not in use.

Smoking
- Be sure patients and residents smoke only in smoking areas.
- Do not leave smoking materials at the bedside. They are left at the beside only if the person is trusted to smoke alone in smoking areas. Follow the care plan.
- Supervise the smoking of persons who cannot protect themselves.
- Do not allow smoking in bed.
- Do not allow smoking where oxygen is used or stored (Chapter 39).
- Be alert to ashes that may fall onto a person.

Other
- See "Preventing Fires" (p. 175).
- Follow safety guidelines when applying heat and cold (Chapter 38).

PREVENTING BURNS

Burns are a leading cause of death among children and older persons. Smoking, spilled hot liquids, children playing with matches, barbecue grills, fireplaces, and stoves are common causes. So are electrical items and very hot water (sinks, tubs, showers). The safety measures in Box 13-1 can prevent burns.

Burn severity (Chapter 54) depends on water temperature and length of exposure (Table 13-1). The person's condition is also a factor.

- *Superficial (first degree) burn*—involves the epidermis (top layer of skin). Sunburn is an example. The skin is red and painful to touch. There may be mild swelling.
- *Partial-thickness (second degree) burn*—involves the epidermis and dermis. The skin appears deep red. The person has pain and blisters. The skin may appear glossy from leaking fluid.
- *Full-thickness (third degree) burn*—the epidermis and dermis, fat, muscle, and bone may be injured or destroyed. These burns are not painful. Nerve endings are destroyed. The skin appears charred or has white, brown, or black patches.

See *Focus on Children and Older Persons: Preventing Burns.*

TABLE 13-1	Temperature and Time for a Third Degree Burn	
Fahrenheit (F)	**Centigrade (C)**	**Time Required for a Third Degree Burn to Occur**
155°F	68°C	1 second
148°F	64°C	2 seconds
140°F	60°C	5 seconds
133°F	56°C	15 seconds
127°F	52°C	1 minute
124°F	51°C	3 minutes
120°F	48°C	5 minutes
100°F	37°C	Usually a safe temperature for bathing

Modified from Centers for Medicare & Medicaid Services: State operations manual, Baltimore, 2015, U.S. Department of Health and Human Services.

FOCUS ON CHILDREN AND OLDER PERSONS

Preventing Burns

Older Persons

Older persons are at risk for burns. Risk factors include decreased skin thickness, decreased sensitivity to heat, reduced reaction time, decreased mobility, communication problems, confusion, and dementia. Many of the measures in Box 13-1 for children apply to persons who are confused or have dementia.

PREVENTING POISONING

A *poison is any substance harmful to the body when ingested, inhaled, injected, or absorbed through the skin.* If too much is taken, any substance can be poisonous. Poisonings are intentional or unintentional.

- *Unintentional*—the person takes or gives a substance without intending to cause harm. This includes drugs or chemicals used in excess amounts—an "over-dose."
- *Intentional*—the person takes (suicide) or gives (assault or homicide) a substance intending to cause harm.

Poisoning can cause illness, brain damage, coma, and death. Children and older persons are at risk. Drugs and household products are common poisons. Poisoning in adults may be from carelessness, confusion, or poor vision when reading labels. As a result, a person may take too much of a drug.

Common poisons include:

- Drugs (legal and illegal) and vitamins
- Household products—detergents, soaps, sprays, furniture polish, window cleaners, bleach, paint, paint thinner, toilet bowl and other cleaners, gasoline, kerosene, glue, and so on
- Personal care products—soaps, shampoos, hair conditioners, bath oils, powders, lotions, nail polish removers, sprays, make-up, perfumes, after-shave lotions, deodorants, mouthwashes, and so on
- Fertilizers, insecticides, bug sprays, and so on
- Lead (p. 161)
- House plants
- Wild mushrooms
- Alcohol
- Carbon monoxide (p. 161)

The measures in Box 13-2 (p. 160) can prevent poisoning.

See *Focus on Long-Term Care and Home Care: Preventing Poisoning.*

See *Promoting Safety and Comfort: Preventing Poisoning,* p. 161.

FOCUS ON LONG-TERM CARE AND HOME CARE

Preventing Poisoning

Home Care

Provide good lighting when patients are taking their drugs. Make sure they read prescription labels correctly and are taking the correct drug and dosage (Chapter 53).

Bathroom medicine cabinets, drawers, and counters are checked for out-dated products and drugs. Also check for such items in kitchens and bedrooms. To safely dispose of out-dated items:

- Obtain permission from the person and the nurse.
- Follow agency policy for disposal.

BOX 13-2	Preventing Poisoning

All Ages

- Keep harmful products in high, locked areas (Fig. 13-4). Children and confused persons cannot see or reach them.
- Use prescription drugs correctly.
  - Only take prescription drugs prescribed by a licensed health care professional.
  - Take drugs as prescribed. Do not take larger or more frequent doses. This is especially important for pain-relief drugs.
  - Do not share or sell prescription drugs.
  - Keep all drugs in a safe place. Keep them where children cannot reach them.
  - Read all directions and warning labels. Have good lighting.
  - Follow all directions.
  - Keep drugs in their original bottles or containers.
  - Dispose of unused, no longer needed, and out-dated drugs.
- Buy products with child-resistant packaging.
- Keep child-resistant caps on all harmful products.
- Keep harmful products in their original containers. Do not store them in food containers.
- Leave the original label on harmful products (p. 171).
- Store personal care items according to agency policy. Soap, mouthwash, lotion, deodorant, and shampoo are examples. These items could cause harm when swallowed.
- Use and store harmful products according to the manufacturer's instructions (p. 171).
- Do not sniff chemical containers.
- Read all labels carefully before using the product. Have good lighting.
- Do not leave harmful products unattended when in use.
- Do not mix cleaners or other household products together.
- Turn on fans and open windows when using cleaners and other household products.
- Point spray nozzles away from your face and other people.
- Do not store harmful products near food.
- Discard harmful products that are out-dated.

All Ages—cont'd

- Use safety latches on kitchen, bathroom, utility, garage, basement, and workshop cabinets and drawers.
- Discard poisonous household plants. Or place them where persons at risk cannot reach them.
- Keep emergency numbers by the phone: Poison Control Center (1-800-222-1222), police, ambulance, hospital, and doctor.
- Prevent carbon monoxide poisoning.

Children

- Keep children in your sight when using a harmful product.
- Teach children not to eat plants and unknown foods. Teach them not to eat leaves, stems, seeds, berries, nuts, or bark.
- Do not leave lamp oil, lamps with lamp oil, or candles containing lamp oil where children can reach them. Lamp oil is harmful if ingested.
- Practice safe drug use.
  - Do not call drugs or vitamins "candy."
  - Do not take drugs in front of children.
  - Do not put a dose on a counter or table where a child can reach it.
  - Do not leave drugs unattended if you need to do something else when taking drugs. Take children with you.
  - Secure child-safety caps on every drug.
  - Put drugs away after taking them. Put them out of the sight and reach of children.
  - Be aware that guests (including family and friends) may bring legal or illegal drugs into your home. Do not let children have access to purses, handbags, briefcases, backpacks, coat pockets, or similar items.
- Place warning stickers ("Mr. Yuk") on harmful substances (Fig. 13-5).
- Supervise children when visiting family and friends. Look for harmful products in and on counters, tables, bathrooms, and other areas and surfaces.
- Prevent lead poisoning.

PROMOTING SAFETY AND COMFORT

Preventing Poisoning

Safety

The Poison Control Center number is 1-800-222-1222. If you need to call the Poison Control Center, give the following information.

- The person's age
- The person's weight
- The person's condition and health problems
- The substance, containers, or bottles involved

- How the substance entered the body
  - Swallowed
  - Inhaled or smelled
  - Injected
  - Skin contact
  - Splashed into the eyes
- When the substance entered the body
- First aid given (Chapter 54)
- If the person has vomited
- Your location, name, and phone number
- Distance to the nearest hospital

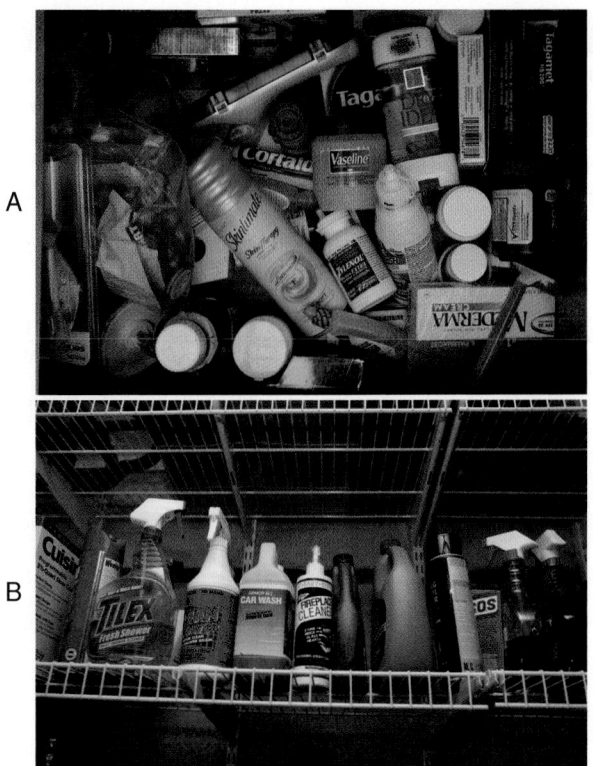

FIGURE 13-4 Harmful products must be kept in locked areas and out of the reach of children. **A,** Bathroom drawers and cabinets hold many harmful products. **B,** Household cleaners must be kept out of reach.

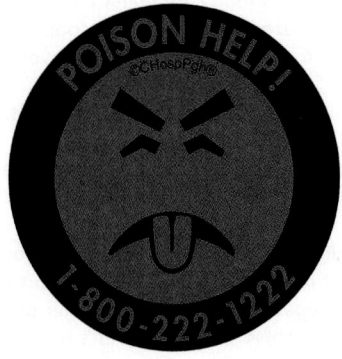

FIGURE 13-5 The "Mr. Yuk" warning sticker is placed on harmful products. (Courtesy Children's Hospital, Pittsburgh Poison Center, Pittsburgh, Pa.).

Lead Poisoning

Lead is a metal. When in the body, it affects normal body functions. A very strong poison, it can injure the brain, nervous system, red blood cells, kidneys, liver, teeth, and bones. It can lower intelligence and cause learning and behavior problems. See Box 13-3, p. 162, for the sources of lead poisoning.

Lead enters the body through:
- *Inhaling dust.* Windows may have lead-based paint. When windows are opened and closed, dust is created. Dust from soil may contain lead.
- *Ingestion.* Young children can eat, chew, and suck on non-food items containing lead. Toys and lead-painted surfaces—window sills and railings—are examples. They may eat paint chips. Water is a source of lead if plumbing materials contain lead.

Children between the ages of 6 months and 6 years are at risk for lead poisoning. Lead can affect almost every body system. Signs and symptoms are usually gradual in onset. They are not always obvious. See Box 13-3 for signs, symptoms, and safety measures.

See *Focus on Long-Term Care and Home Care: Lead Poisoning.*

Carbon Monoxide Poisoning

Carbon monoxide (CO) is a deadly colorless, odorless, and tasteless gas. It is produced by the burning of fuel—gas, oil, kerosene, wood, charcoal (Box 13-4, p. 163). Fuel-burning devices must work properly and must be used correctly. Otherwise, dangerous levels of CO can build up in closed or semi-closed areas. Instead of breathing in oxygen, the person breathes in air filled with CO. Red blood cells pick up CO faster than oxygen. Oxygen does not get into the body. CO can quickly or slowly kill. If not fatal, brain and nervous system damage can result.

People and animals are at risk for CO poisoning. Sleeping or intoxicated persons can die before having symptoms. CO poisoning may be unintentional or intentional as a suicide attempt. See Box 13-4 for the signs and symptoms of CO poisoning and safety measures.

BOX 13-3   Lead Poisoning

Sources of Lead Poisoning

- House paint before 1978. Children can swallow peeling paint and paint chips. When paint is stripped or sanded, lead dust is released into the air.
- Toys and furniture painted before 1976.
- Painted toys and decorations made outside of the United States.
- Lead bullets.
- Fishing sinkers.
- Curtain weights.
- Plumbing, pipes, and faucets. Lead can be found in drinking water if these devices contain lead.
- The soil near highways and houses. The soil may be contaminated with car exhaust and paint scrapings from houses.
- Hobbies that involve soldering, stained glass, making jewelry, pottery, and lead figures.
- Children's paint sets and art supplies.
- Pewter pitchers and dinnerware.
- Storage batteries.

Lead Poisoning in Children: Signs and Symptoms

- Abdominal pain; cramping
- Activity: decreased
- Anemia
- Appetite: poor
- Attention and learning problems
- Behavior problems; aggressive behavior
- Bowel problems: constipation and diarrhea
- Coma
- Coordination: poor
- Fatigue
- Growth: slowed
- Headaches
- Hearing loss
- Hyperactivity
- Irritability
- Kidney damage
- Language and speech problems
- Memory problems
- Muscle weakness
- *Pallor* (paleness)
- Reflexes: slow
- Seizures
- Sensations: reduced
- Sleep problems
- Sluggishness
- Vomiting
- Walking problems; staggering
- Weight loss

Safety Measures to Prevent Lead Poisoning

- Prevent or discourage children from eating, chewing, or sucking on non-food items. They include:
  - Toys and furniture painted before 1976
  - Painted toys and decorations made outside the United States
  - Paint chips
  - Dirt
  - Keys
  - Pewter and lead-based figurines
  - Fishing sinkers
  - Other sources of lead as listed in this box

Safety Measures to Prevent Lead Poisoning—cont'd

- Do not let children play in dirt. Have them play in grassy or sandy areas.
- Assist the child with hand-washing before eating, after playing outside, and before going to bed.
- Wash toys often.
- Rinse pacifiers, baby bottles, and other items that fall to the floor.
- Prevent exposure to lead-based plumbing.
  - Do not use hot tap water for cooking or drinking. Let cold water run for 1 to 2 minutes before drinking water or using it for coffee or cooking. This helps flush the lead out of the plumbing.
  - Do not use hot tap water to make baby formula.
- Prevent exposure to lead-based paint.
  - Keep children away from paint chips.
  - Keep children away from dust contaminated with lead paint.
  - Do not sweep or vacuum lead-based paint dust or paint chips.
  - Use a wet mop and wet cloths to clean up dust and paint chips.
  - Use a wet mop and wet cloths to clean furniture, window sills, and dusty surfaces.
  - Use duct tape to cover peeling or chipping paint. This is only a temporary measure. Peeling and chipping paint must be removed.
  - Do not bump into walls or furniture that may contain lead-based paint. This prevents dust and paint chips.
  - Do not open and close windows that have lead-based paint. This prevents dust and paint chips.
  - Keep the home as dust-free as possible.
- Prevent exposure to food contaminated with lead.
  - Do not use glazed pottery to cook food.
  - Do not eat foods that are stored or served in glazed pottery.
  - Do not eat foods that are canned outside the United States.
- Do not store wine, alcohol, or vinegar-based salad dressings in lead crystal decanters for long periods. Lead can get into the liquid.
- Prevent children from having contact with work or hobby materials that may contain lead. Welding, pottery, home building and repair, and automotive repair products and supplies are examples. So are children's paint sets and art supplies.
  - Store lead-based products where children cannot see or reach them.
  - Take shoes off before entering the home.
  - Shower and change clothes before contact with children.
  - Wash and store clothes contaminated with lead separately from others.
- Do not let children handle or play with old newspapers, magazines, or comic books. The ink may contain lead.

BOX 13-4	Carbon Monoxide Poisoning

Sources of Carbon Monoxide: Examples
- Fireplaces: wood and gas
- Furnaces
- Gas clothes dryers
- Gas stove and ovens
- Gas water heaters
- Generators: portable
- Grills and camp stoves used indoors: gas, charcoal
- Lanterns
- Lawn mowers
- Motor vehicles
- Snow blowers
- Space heaters: gas, kerosene
- Weed trimmers
- Wood-burning stoves

Signs and Symptoms
- Breathing problems
- Cherry-pink skin
- Chest pain
- Confusion
- Dizziness
- Fainting
- Headache
- Nausea
- Sleepiness
- Slurred speech
- Vomiting
- Weakness

Safety Measures to Prevent Carbon Monoxide Poisoning
- Have CO alarms installed in each sleeping area and in rooms with fireplaces. Also install them near furnaces and gas appliances (outside of kitchens, laundry rooms, and so on).
- Have vehicle exhaust systems checked regularly.
- Have the furnace inspected and repaired before every heating season.
- Have chimneys and flues inspected and repaired.
- Have fuel-burning appliances checked regularly. See "Sources of Carbon Monoxide: Examples" in this box.
- Follow the manufacturer's instructions when using fuel-burning devices.
- Use the correct fuel for fuel-burning devices.
- Do not idle a vehicle, lawn mower, snow blower, weed trimmer, or other device in an open or closed area or garage. Fumes can leak into the house.
- Have fuel-burning devices, chimneys, and flues checked when people in the same building show signs and symptoms.
- Ventilate the room when using a space heater.
- If you or others have signs and symptoms:
  - Open doors and windows.
  - Turn off appliances.
  - Leave the home.
  - Go to an emergency room.
- Open doors and windows if you notice gas odors. Turn off appliances and leave the home.
- Have gas odors checked by trained professionals.
- Do not use a gas stove or oven to heat a home or room. Do not use a gas stove or oven to dry clothing or other items.
- Do not use charcoal grills, barbecue grills, and gas camp stoves indoors or in a garage.
- Never burn charcoal indoors.
- Do not use a generator indoors, in a basement, in a garage, or by a window, door, or vent.

PREVENTING SUFFOCATION

Suffocation is when breathing stops from the lack of oxygen. Death occurs if the person does not start breathing. Common causes include choking, drowning, inhaling gas or smoke, strangulation, and electrical shock (p. 169).

Measures to prevent suffocation are listed in Box 13-5, p. 164. Clear the airway if the person is choking.

Choking

Foreign bodies can obstruct the airway. This is called *choking* or *foreign-body airway obstruction (FBAO)*. Air cannot pass through the airways into the lungs. The body does not get enough oxygen. Death can result.

Choking often occurs during eating. A large, poorly chewed piece of meat is the most common cause. Laughing and talking while eating also are common causes. So is excessive alcohol intake.

Unconscious persons can choke. Common causes are aspiration of vomitus and the tongue falling back into the airway.

Foreign bodies can cause mild or severe airway obstruction. With *mild airway obstruction*, some air moves in and out of the lungs. The person is conscious and usually can speak. Often forceful coughing can remove the object. Breathing may sound like wheezing between coughs. For mild airway obstruction:
- Stay with the person.
- Encourage the person to keep coughing to expel the object.
- Do not interrupt the person's efforts to clear the airway. If the person is breathing and coughing, abdominal thrusts (p. 165) are not needed.
- If the obstruction persists, call for help.

A person with *severe airway obstruction* has difficulty breathing. Air does not move in and out of the lungs. The person may not be able to breathe, speak, or cough. If able to cough, the cough is of poor quality. When the person tries to inhale, there is no noise or a high-pitched noise. The person may appear pale and cyanotic (bluish color).

BOX 13-5   Preventing Suffocation

All Age-Groups
- Cut foods into small, bite-sized pieces for persons who cannot do so themselves.
- Make sure dentures fit properly and are in place.
- Make sure the person can chew and swallow the food served.
- Report loose teeth or dentures.
- Check the care plan for swallowing problems before serving food (including snacks) or fluids. The person may ask for something that he or she cannot swallow.
- Tell the nurse at once if the person has swallowing problems.
- Do not give oral foods or fluids to persons with feeding tubes (Chapter 28).
- Follow aspiration precautions (Chapter 27).
- Do not leave a person unattended in a bathtub or shower.
- Remove the key for a gas fireplace. Store it out of reach.
- Move all persons from the area if you smell smoke.
- Position the person in bed properly (Chapter 17).
- Use bed rails correctly (Chapter 20).
- Use restraints correctly (Chapter 15).
- Prevent entrapment in the bed system (Chapter 20).
- Do not use power strips for care equipment.
- See "Preventing Equipment Accidents," p. 169.

Children
- Practice crib safety measures (Chapter 52).
- Plastics safety:
  - Keep plastic bags, covers, and dry-cleaning bags away from children.
  - Tie large plastic bags and garment bags in knots. Then discard them.
- Electrical safety:
  - Use safety plugs in outlets with caution. Children can remove and choke on them. And they can be misplaced when removed to use the outlet.
  - Keep electrical cords and electrical items out of the reach of children.
  - See "Preventing Equipment Accidents," p. 169.
- Sleep and position safety:
  - Position infants on their backs for sleep. (See Chapter 52.) This reduces the risk for sudden infant death syndrome (SIDS) (Chapter 52).
  - Do not use pillows to position infants.
  - Do not use pillows to prevent infants from falling off of beds and furniture.
  - Remove pillows, loose sheets or blankets, comforters, quilts, sheepskin, stuffed toys, crib bumpers, sleep positioners, and other soft items from the crib when the baby is sleeping.
  - Have babies wear sleep sacks for warmth when sleeping. A sleep sack is a wearable blanket.
  - Do not let babies sleep on soft surfaces (beds, sofas, chairs), recliners, bouncy chairs, or swings.

Children—cont'd
- Food safety:
  - Do not feed an infant while he or she is lying down.
  - Do not leave a baby alone when drinking from a bottle. The baby could aspirate milk and choke.
  - Have children sit when they eat. They should not eat or suck on anything while lying down or playing.
  - Do not give infants and young children small, round, or hard foods. This includes hot dogs, peanuts, peanut butter, popcorn, nuts, grapes, raisins, hard candy, jellybeans, gum, raw vegetables, raw and unpeeled fruit slices, dried fruits, and chunks of meat.
  - Remove small bones from fish and chicken.
  - Cut foods into small pieces.
  - Give infants soft foods that do not require chewing.
  - Do not let children play with dried beans or dried peas.
- Balloon safety:
  - Use Mylar balloons instead of latex ones.
  - Store latex balloons where children cannot see or reach them.
  - Do not let children inflate or deflate latex balloons.
  - Deflate and discard latex balloons after use.
  - Pick up and discard broken balloon pieces at once. Do not let children near them.
- Small object and toy safety:
  - Check floors for small objects—buttons, coins, beads, marbles, pins, tacks, nails, screws, jewelry, and so on. Keep them out of a child's reach. Pick up and store or discard such objects. Children can choke on them. When checking floors, it is best to get on the floor on your hands and knees—the child's eye level.
  - Remove rubber knobs or tips from door stops.
  - Check toys for removable parts.
  - Do not let babies play with small toys or toys with small parts.
- Cord and ribbon safety:
  - Do not string or hang any object on or near a crib. This includes a mobile, toy, or diaper bag. The child can get caught in it and strangle.
  - Never tie pacifiers or teethers around a child's neck.
  - Do not use bibs, clothes with ribbons or cords, or necklaces whenever the child is put in a crib or playpen.
  - Make sure dangling cords are not within a baby's reach. This includes cords from venetian blinds.
- Other:
  - Keep appliance doors closed—ovens, refrigerators, clothes dryers, washing machines, freezers, dishwashers, coolers, and so on.
- See Chapter 52 for other child safety measures.

Older Persons
- Report signs & symptoms of weakness.
- Report dentures that fit poorly.
- Report signs or symptoms of difficulty swallowing (dysphagia).
- Be aware of chronic illnesses.

The conscious person clutches at the throat (Fig. 13-6). Clutching at the throat is often called the "universal sign of choking." The conscious person is very frightened. If the obstruction is not removed, the person will die. Severe airway obstruction is an emergency.

Relieving Choking. *Abdominal thrusts* are used to relieve severe airway obstruction. Abdominal thrusts are quick, upward thrusts to the abdomen. This is also known as the *Heimlich maneuver*. The thrusts force air out of the lungs and create an artificial cough. They are done to try to expel the foreign body from the airway.

You may observe a person choking. And you may perform emergency measures to relieve choking. Relief of choking occurs when the foreign body is removed. Or it occurs when you feel air move and see the chest rise and fall when giving rescue breaths. The person may still be unresponsive.

If you assist a choking person, report and record what happened. Include what you did and the person's response.

Chest thrusts are used for obese or pregnant persons (Fig. 13-7). If you are alone and choking, perform self-administered abdominal thrusts. See Box 13-6.

See *Focus on Children and Older Persons: Relieving Choking*, p. 166.

See procedure: *Relieving Choking—Adult or Child (Over 1 Year of Age)*, p. 166.

See procedure: *Relieving Choking—In the Infant (Less Than 1 Year of Age)*, p. 168.

Text continued on p. 169.

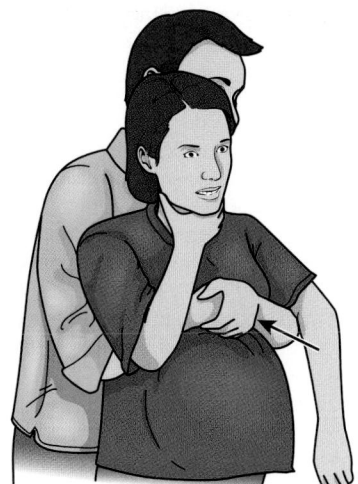
FIGURE 13-7 Chest thrusts to relieve choking in a pregnant woman.

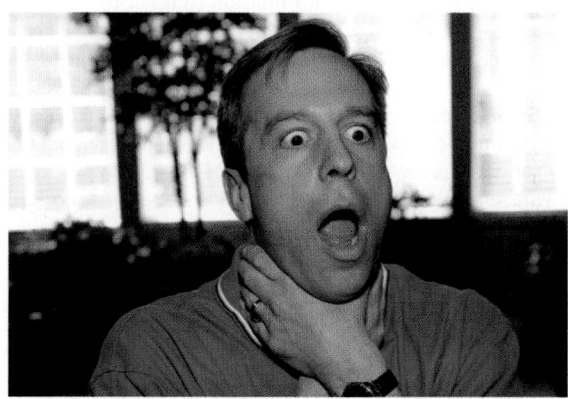
FIGURE 13-6 A choking person clutches at the throat.

BOX 13-6   Relieving Choking

Chest Thrusts for Obese or Pregnant Persons
1. Stand behind the person.
2. Place your arms under the person's underarms. Wrap your arms around the person's chest.
3. Make a fist. Place the thumb side of the fist on the middle of the sternum (breastbone).
4. Grasp the fist with your other hand.
5. Give chest thrusts until the object is expelled or the person becomes unresponsive.
6. If the person becomes unresponsive, have someone activate the Emergency Medical Services (EMS) system or the agency's Rapid Response Team (RRT) or Medical Emergency Team (MET) if not already done. This team quickly responds to give care in life-threatening situations. Start cardiopulmonary resuscitation (CPR). See Chapter 54.

Self-Administered Abdominal Thrusts
1. Make a fist with 1 hand.
2. Place the thumb side of the fist above your navel and below the lower end of the sternum.
3. Grasp your fist with your other hand.
4. Press inward and upward quickly.
5. Press the upper abdomen against a hard surface if the thrust did not relieve the obstruction. Use the back of a chair, a table, or a railing.
6. Use as many thrusts as needed.

FOCUS ON CHILDREN AND OLDER PERSONS

Relieving Choking

Children

Respiratory infections can cause airway obstruction in infants and children. Airway structures become swollen. The airway narrows or becomes completely obstructed. Air cannot enter the airway. The child needs emergency care at once.

The procedures that follow will not relieve airway obstruction caused by an infection. Do not try them if the child has a fever, rash, congestion, hoarseness, or other signs and symptoms of respiratory infection. You will waste precious time. Activate the EMS system or the agency's RRT. Give rescue breaths if the child is not breathing but has a pulse. Start CPR if the child is not responding, not breathing or not breathing normally (gasping), and has no pulse. See Chapter 54.

Abdominal thrusts are not given to infants. They can damage the liver and other organs. Back slaps (back blows) and chest thrusts are used for infants.

Basic Life Support guidelines are updated as new information becomes available. You are responsible for following current guidelines. Updates can be found on-line at ECCguidelines.heart.org.

Relieving Choking—Adult or Child (Over 1 Year of Age)

PROCEDURE

1 Ask the person if he or she is choking. Help the person if he or she nods "yes" and cannot talk.
2 Have someone call for help.
  a *In a public area,* have someone activate the EMS system by calling 911. Send someone to get an automated external defibrillator (AED) (Chapter 54).
  b *In an agency,* have someone call the agency's RRT (MET) and get a defibrillator (AED).
3 Give abdominal thrusts.
  a *If the person is standing or sitting:*
    1) Stand or kneel behind the person.
    2) Wrap your arms around the person's waist.
    3) Make a fist with 1 hand.
    4) Place the thumb side of the fist against the abdomen. The fist is slightly above the navel in the middle of the abdomen and well below the end of the sternum (breastbone). See Figure 13-8, *A.*
    5) Grasp the fist with your other hand (Fig. 13-8, *B*).
    6) Press your fist into the person's abdomen with a quick, upward thrust (Fig. 13-9).
  b *If the person is lying down but responsive* (Fig. 13-10):
    1) Straddle the person's thighs.
    2) Place the heel of 1 hand against the abdomen. It is in the middle slightly above the navel and well below the end of the sternum (breastbone).
    3) Place your second hand on top of your first hand.
    4) Press both hands into the abdomen with a quick, upward thrust.
4 Repeat thrusts until the object is expelled or the person becomes unresponsive.
5 *If the object is dislodged,* encourage hospital care. Injuries can occur from abdominal thrusts.

6 *If the person becomes unresponsive,* lower the person to the floor or ground. Position the person supine (lying flat on the back). Make sure the EMS or RRT (MET) was called.
  a *If alone with a wireless phone,* use it while continuing to give care.
  b *If alone without a wireless phone,* give about 2 minutes of CPR first. Then call the EMS or RRT (MET) and get an AED.
7 Start CPR. See Chapter 54. Do not check for a pulse.
  a Begin with compressions. Give 30 compressions.
  b Use the head tilt–chin lift method to open the airway (Fig. 13-11). Open wide the person's mouth. Look for an object. Remove the object if you can see it and can remove it easily.
  c Give 2 breaths.
  d Continue cycles of 30 compressions and 2 breaths. Look for an object every time you open the airway.
8 *If you relieve choking in an unresponsive person,* check for a response, breathing, and a pulse.
  a *If no response, no normal breathing, and no pulse—* continue CPR. Use the AED as soon as possible (Chapter 54).
  b *If no response and no normal breathing but there is a pulse—*give rescue breaths. For an adult, give 1 breath every 5 to 6 seconds. For a child, give 1 breath every 3 to 5 seconds. Check for a pulse about every 2 minutes. If no pulse, begin CPR.
  c *If the person has normal breathing and a pulse—*place the person in the recovery position if there is no response (Chapter 54). Continue to check the person until help arrives. Encourage hospital care.

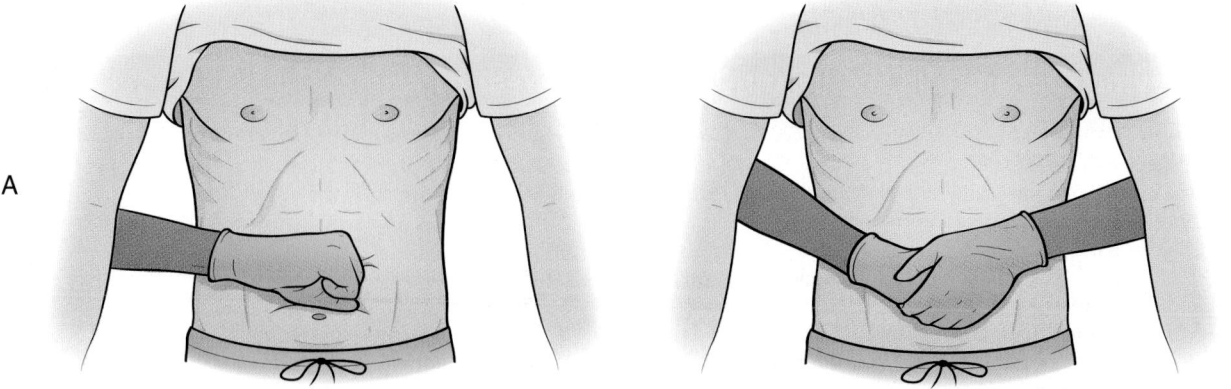

FIGURE 13-8 **Hand positioning for abdominal thrusts. A,** The fist is slightly above the navel in the mid-line of the abdomen. **B,** The other hand clasps the first.

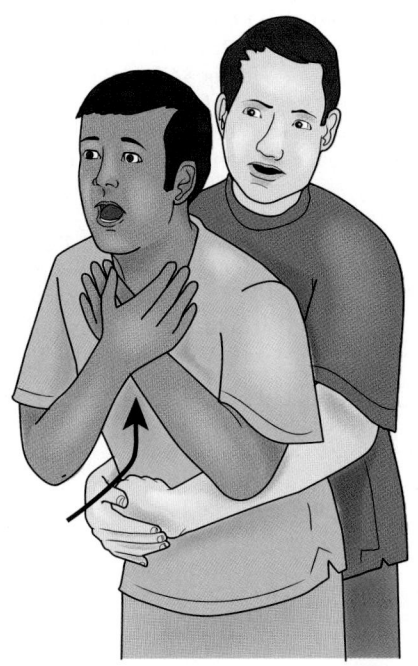

FIGURE 13-9 Abdominal thrusts with the person standing.

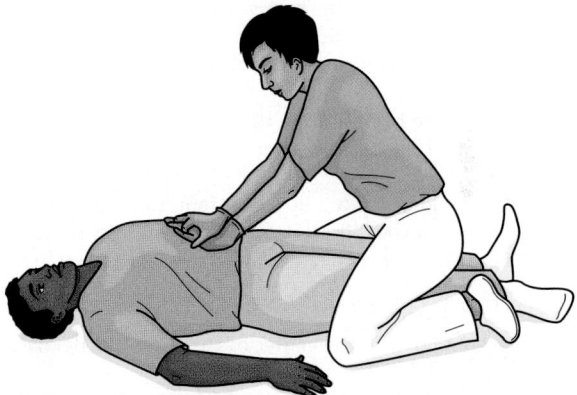

FIGURE 13-10 Abdominal thrusts with the person lying down.

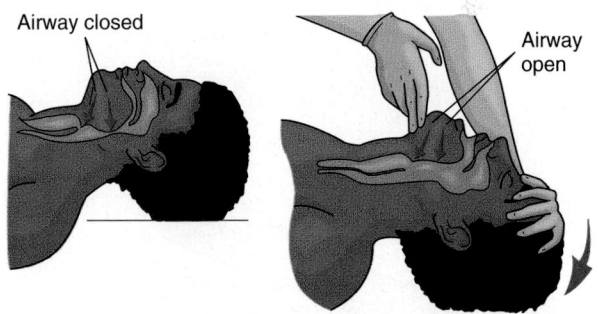

Airway closed

Airway open

FIGURE 13-11 The head tilt–chin lift method opens the airway. One hand is on the person's forehead. Pressure is applied to lift the head back. The chin is lifted with the fingers of the other hand.

Basic Life Support guidelines are updated as new information becomes available. You are responsible for following current guidelines. Updates can be found on-line at ECCguidelines.heart.org.

Relieving Choking—In the Infant (Less Than 1 Year of Age)

PROCEDURE

1 Have someone call for help.
 a *In a public area,* have someone activate the EMS system by calling 911. Send someone to get an AED. See Chapter 54.
 b *In an agency,* have someone call the agency's RRT (MET) and get a defibrillator (AED).
2 Kneel next to the infant. Or sit with the infant in your lap.
3 Expose the infant's chest and back. Perform this step only if it can be done easily.
4 Hold the infant face down over your forearm. (Support your arm on your thigh or lap.) The infant's head is lower than the chest. Support the head and jaw with your hand.
5 Give up to 5 forceful back slaps (back blows) (Fig. 13-12). Use the heel of your hand. Give the back slaps between the shoulder blades. (Stop the back slaps if the object is expelled.)
6 Turn the infant as a unit.
 a Continue to support the infant's face, jaw, head, neck, and chest with 1 hand.
 b Support the back and the back of the infant's head with your other hand. Your palm supports the back of the head.
 c Turn the infant as a unit. The infant is in a back-lying position on your forearm. Your forearm rests on your thigh. The infant's head is lower than the chest.
7 Give up to 5 chest thrusts (Fig. 13-13). The chest thrusts are quick and downward.
 a Place 2 fingers in the center of the chest just below the nipple line.

 b Give chest thrusts at a rate of about 1 every second.
 c Stop chest thrusts if the object is expelled.
8 Continue giving 5 back slaps followed by 5 chest thrusts until:
 a The object is expelled.
 b The infant becomes unresponsive.
9 *If the infant becomes unresponsive:*
 a Send someone to activate the EMS system or RRT (MET) if not already done (step 1). If alone, do the following.
  1) *If alone with a wireless phone,* use it while continuing to give care.
  2) *If alone without a wireless phone,* give about 2 minutes of CPR first. Then call the EMS or RRT (MET) and get an AED.
 b Place the infant on a firm, flat surface.
 c Start CPR (Chapter 54). Begin with compressions. Give 30 compressions. (See Chapter 54 for infant CPR.)
 d Open the airway. Use the head tilt–chin lift method. Open the infant's mouth. Look for an object. Remove the object if you see it and can remove it easily. Use your fingers.
 e Give 2 breaths.
 f Continue cycles of 30 compressions and 2 breaths. Look for an object if you see it and can remove it easily. Use your fingers.
 g Continue CPR until help takes over or until choking is relieved.

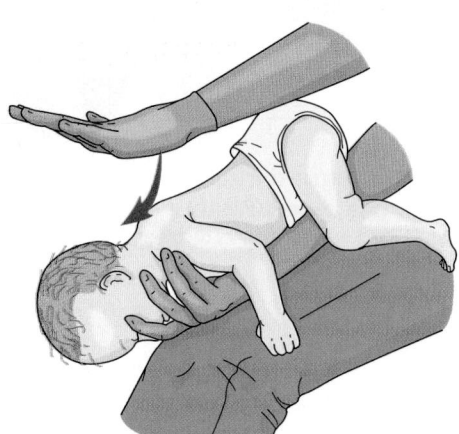

FIGURE 13-12 Back slaps (back blows). The infant is held face down and supported with 1 hand. The rescuer's forearm is supported on his or her thigh. Back slaps are given between the shoulder blades with the heel of 1 hand.

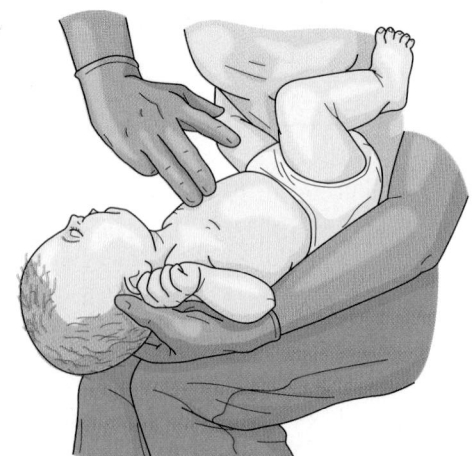

FIGURE 13-13 Chest thrusts. The infant is in the back-lying position. The rescuer uses 2 fingers to compress the center of the chest just below the nipple line.

PREVENTING EQUIPMENT ACCIDENTS

All equipment is unsafe if broken, not used correctly, or not working properly. This includes hospital beds. Inspect all equipment before use. Check all items for cracks, chips, and sharp or rough edges. They can cause cuts, stabs, or scratches. Follow the Bloodborne Pathogen Standard (Chapter 16).

Electrical Equipment

Electrical items must work properly and be in good repair. Frayed cords (Fig. 13-14, *A*) and over-loaded electrical outlets (Fig. 13-14, *B*) can cause fires, burns, and electrical shocks. *Electrical shock is when electrical current passes through the body.* It can burn the skin, muscles, nerves, and other tissues. It can affect the heart and cause death.

Three-pronged plugs (Fig. 13-15) are used on all electrical items. Two prongs carry electrical current. The third prong is the ground. A *ground carries leaking electricity to the earth and away from an electrical item.* Without a ground, leaking electricity can be conducted to the person. It can cause electrical shocks and possible death. If you receive a shock, report it at once. Do not use the item.

Warning signs of a faulty electrical item include:
- Shocks
- Loss of power or a power surge
- Dimming or flickering lights
- Sparks
- Sizzling or buzzing sounds
- Burning odor
- Loose plugs

Do not use or give damaged items to patients or residents. Take the item to the nurse. The nurse will have you do 1 of the following.
- Discard the item. Follow agency policy.
- Tag the item and send it for repair. Follow agency policy.

Practice the safety measures in Box 13-7, p. 170. Complete an incident report (p. 182) for an equipment-related accident. The *Safe Medical Devices Act* requires that agencies report equipment-related illnesses, injuries, and deaths.

Bariatric-Safe Equipment

Beds, chairs, wheelchairs, stretchers, toilets, commodes, and other equipment usually have a weight capacity of 250 to 350 pounds. Bariatric patients and residents can weigh from 250 pounds to over 1000 pounds. Equipment must support the person's weight.

Bariatric equipment is labeled with:
- "EC" for "expanded capacity"
- The weight limit suggested by the manufacturer

You must know the equipment's weight capacity and the person's weight. Do not use the item if the person's weight is greater than the weight capacity. Follow the nurse's directions and the care plan.

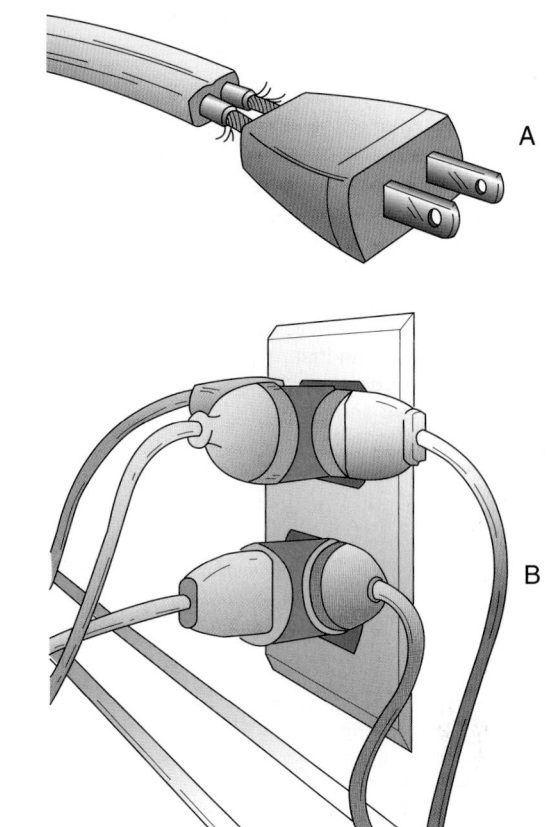

FIGURE 13-14 A, A frayed electrical cord. **B,** An over-loaded electrical outlet.

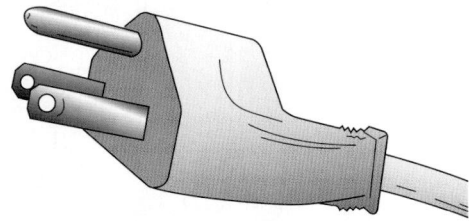

FIGURE 13-15 A three-pronged plug.

BOX 13-7	Preventing Equipment Accidents

General Safety

- Follow agency policies and procedures.
- Follow the manufacturer's instructions. Use equipment correctly.
- Read all caution and warning labels.
- Do not use an unfamiliar item. Ask for training. Also ask a nurse to supervise you the first time you use the item.
- Use an item only for its intended purpose.
- Make sure the item works before you begin.
- Make sure you have all needed equipment. For example, you need to plug in an item. There must be an outlet.
- Show a broken or damaged item to the nurse. Follow the nurse's instructions and agency policies for discarding items or sending them for repair.
- Do not try to repair broken or damaged items.
- Do not use broken or damaged items.

Electrical Safety

- Check cords and equipment for damage. Make sure they are in good repair.
- Use 3-pronged plugs on all electrical devices (see Fig. 13-15).
- Avoid using extension cords. If you need one, use it for only 1 device. This prevents over-loading a circuit.
- Do not use power strips for care equipment.
- Do not cover any electrical cord with rugs, carpets, linens, or other materials. Do not run power cords under rugs.
- Connect a bed power cord directly to a wall outlet. Do not connect a bed power cord to an extension cord or outlet strip.

Electrical Safety—cont'd

- Do not use electrical items owned by the person until they are safety checked. The maintenance staff does this.
- Keep electrical items away from water.
- Keep work areas clean and dry. Wipe up spills right away.
- Do not touch electrical items if you are wet, if your hands are wet, or if you are standing in water.
- Do not put a finger or any item into an outlet.
- Use tamper-resistant outlets. If necessary, use outlet safety covers or plates over standard electrical outlets (Fig. 13-16, A). Use safety plugs with caution (Fig. 13-16, B). Children can remove and choke on outlet plugs or stick their fingers or small objects into outlet openings. Use power strip covers for power strips and attached cords.
- Turn off equipment before unplugging it. Sparks occur when electrical items are unplugged while turned on.
- Hold on to the plug (not the cord) when removing it from an outlet (Fig. 13-17).
- Do not give showers or tub baths during electrical storms. Lightning can travel through pipes.
- Do not use electrical items or phones during storms.
- Do not use water to put out an electrical fire. If possible, turn off or unplug the item.
- Do not touch a person who is having an electrical shock. If possible, turn off or unplug the item. Call for help at once.
- Keep electrical cords away from heating vents and other heat sources.
- Turn off the device when done using the item.
- Unplug all devices when not in use.

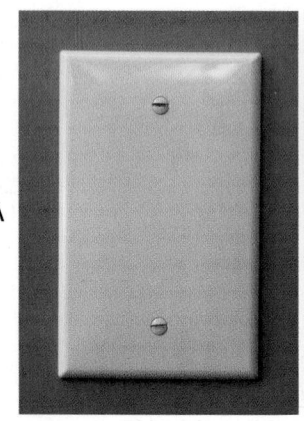 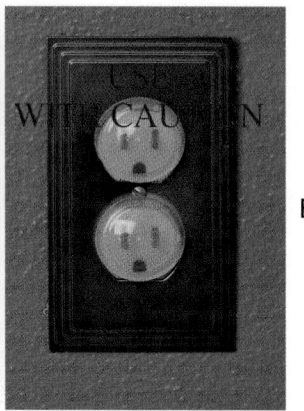

A   B

FIGURE 13-16 Outlet safety. A, Outlet safety cover. **B,** Outlet plugs. Use plugs with caution.

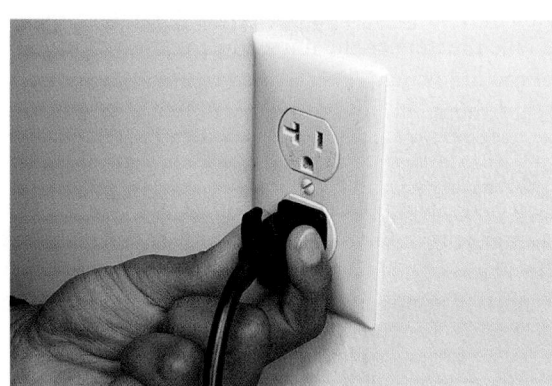

FIGURE 13-17 Hold on to the plug to remove it from the outlet.

Wheelchair and Stretcher Safety

Wheelchairs are useful for people who cannot walk or who have severe problems walking. Stretchers are used to transport persons who cannot use wheelchairs. They cannot sit up or must lie down.

The person can fall from the wheelchair or stretcher. Or the person can fall during transfers to and from the wheelchair or stretcher. See Chapter 19 for wheelchair and stretcher safety.

HAZARDOUS CHEMICALS

A *hazardous chemical* is any chemical that is a health hazard or a physical hazard. Physical hazards can cause fires or explosions. Health hazards can cause acute or chronic health problems. Health hazards can:

- Cause cancer.
- Affect blood cell formation and function.
- Damage the kidneys, nervous system, lungs, skin, eyes, or mucous membranes.
- Cause birth defects, miscarriages, and fertility problems.

Exposure to hazardous chemicals can occur under normal working conditions or during certain emergencies. Examples include equipment failures, container ruptures, or the uncontrolled release of a hazard into the workplace. Workplace hazards include:

- Latex gloves (Chapter 16)
- Thermometers and blood pressure equipment containing mercury (Chapter 29)
- Cleaners and disinfectants (Chapter 16)

The *Hazard Communication Standard (HCS)* is a policy of the Occupational Safety and Health Administration (OSHA). It requires container labeling (Fig. 13-18), safety data sheets (SDSs), and employee training. The standard also requires eyewash and total body wash stations where hazardous substances are used.

Labeling

Hazardous chemical containers have warning labels. The HCS requires the following.

- Name, address, and phone number of the manufacturer, importer, or responsible party.
- Product identifier. This is the chemical name, code number, or batch number.
- Signal word. This is a word used to communicate the severity of a potential hazard.
  - Danger—used for severe hazards.
  - Warning—used for less severe hazards.
- Hazard statements. These describe the nature of the hazard. Examples include:
  - "Causes severe skin burns and eye damage"
  - "Harmful if swallowed"

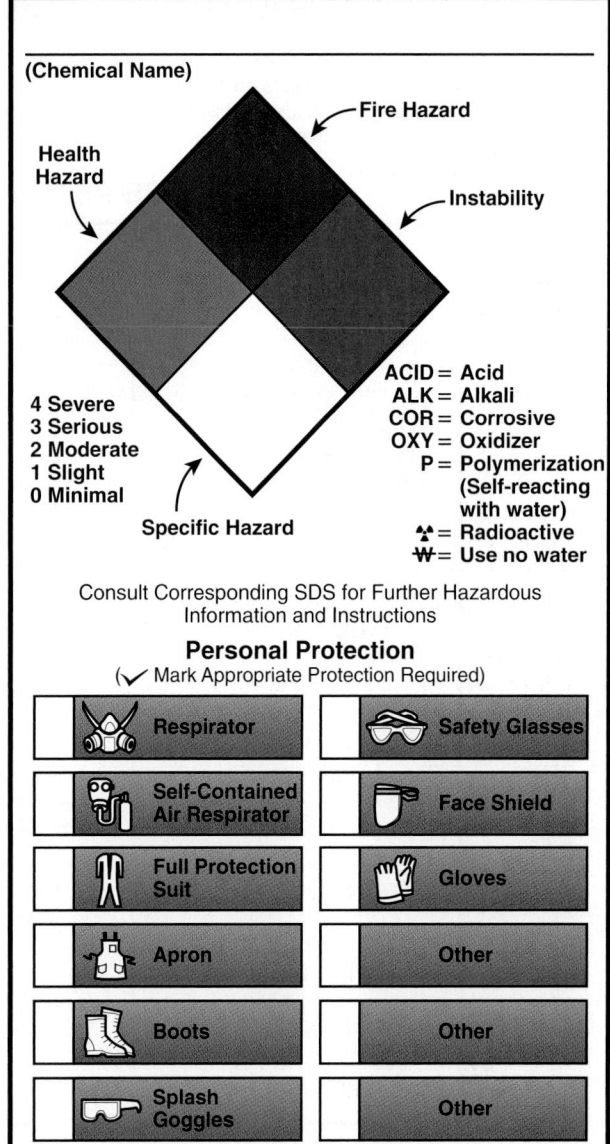

FIGURE 13-18 Sample warning label. (Redrawn and modified from Chemical Hazard Warning Labels, Seton, Branford, Conn.)

- Precautionary statements. These describe the measures to take if exposed to a hazardous chemical. The 4 types of precautionary statements are:
  - Prevention—how to minimize exposure
  - Response—emergency response and first aid
  - Storage—how to store the chemical
  - Disposal—how to dispose of the chemical
- Pictograms. A *pictogram* is a symbol used to communicate specific information about a chemical hazard (Fig. 13-19, p. 172).

If a warning label is removed or damaged, do not use the substance. Show the container to the nurse and explain the problem. Do not leave the container unattended.

Hazard Communication Standard Pictogram

As of June 1, 2015, the Hazard Communication Standard (HCS) will require pictograms on labels to alert users of the chemical hazards to which they may be exposed. Each pictogram consists of a symbol on a white background framed within a red border and represents a distinct hazard(s). The pictogram on the label is determined by the chemical hazard classification.

HCS Pictograms and Hazards

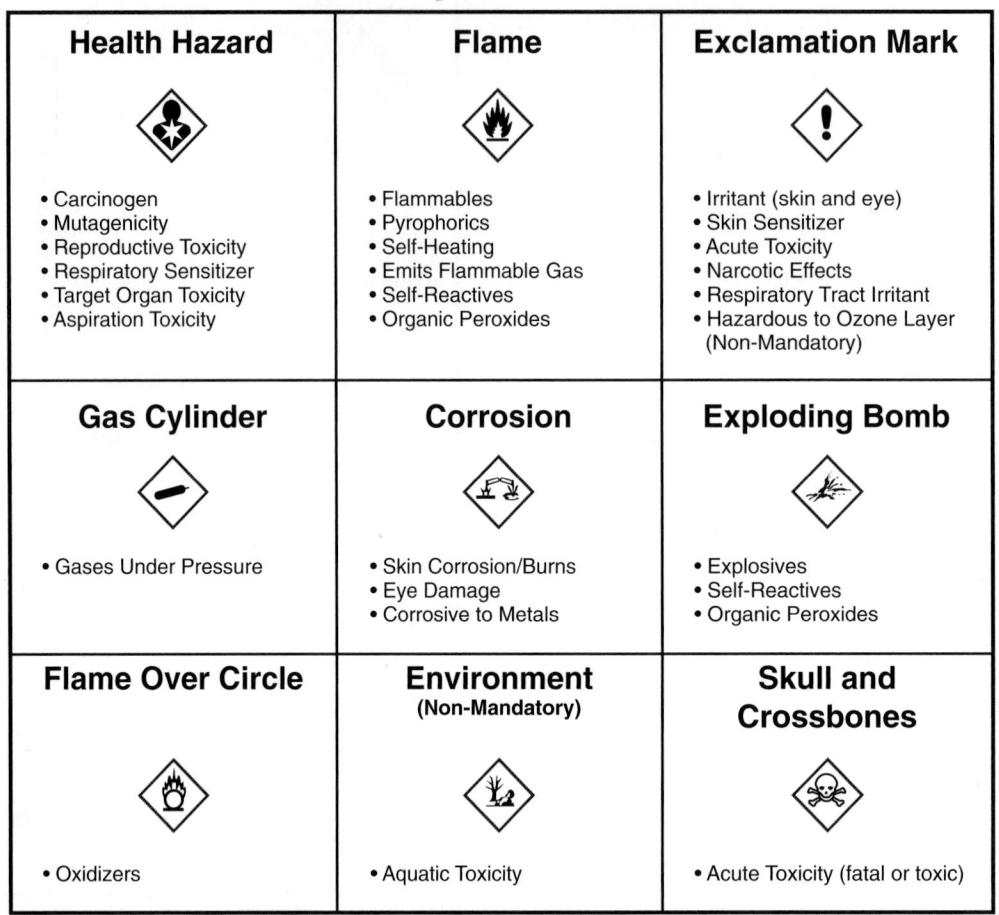

Health Hazard	Flame	Exclamation Mark
• Carcinogen • Mutagenicity • Reproductive Toxicity • Respiratory Sensitizer • Target Organ Toxicity • Aspiration Toxicity	• Flammables • Pyrophorics • Self-Heating • Emits Flammable Gas • Self-Reactives • Organic Peroxides	• Irritant (skin and eye) • Skin Sensitizer • Acute Toxicity • Narcotic Effects • Respiratory Tract Irritant • Hazardous to Ozone Layer (Non-Mandatory)
Gas Cylinder	**Corrosion**	**Exploding Bomb**
• Gases Under Pressure	• Skin Corrosion/Burns • Eye Damage • Corrosive to Metals	• Explosives • Self-Reactives • Organic Peroxides
Flame Over Circle	**Environment** (Non-Mandatory)	**Skull and Crossbones**
• Oxidizers	• Aquatic Toxicity	• Acute Toxicity (fatal or toxic)

FIGURE 13-19 Hazard Communication Standard pictograms. (Redrawn from OSHA Quick Card™, OSHA® Occupational Safety and Health Administration. U.S. Department of Labor, Washington, D.C.)

Safety Data Sheets

Every hazardous substance has an SDS (called material safety data sheet [MSDS] in some agencies). Information provided includes:
• Name and common names
• All hazards about the chemical
• Chemical ingredients
• First aid measures
• Fire-fighting measures
• Accidental release measures
• Safe handling and storage measures
• Exposure controls and personal protection measures
  Know where to find SDSs on your nursing unit. Check the SDS before using a hazardous chemical, cleaning up a leak or spill, or disposing of the substance. Call for the nurse about a leak or spill right away. Do not leave a leak or spill unattended.

Employee Training

Your employer provides hazardous chemical training. You learn about hazards, exposure risks, and protection measures. You learn to read and use warning labels and the SDS.

Each hazardous chemical requires certain protection measures. Box 13-8 lists general rules to safely handle hazardous chemicals.

BOX 13-8	**Hazardous Chemical Safety Measures**

- Read all warning labels.
- Follow the safety measures on the warning label and SDS.
- Make sure each container has a warning label that is not damaged.
- Use a leak-proof container to carry or transport a hazardous chemical.
- Wear personal protective equipment (PPE) to clean up spills and leaks. The warning label or SDS tells you what to wear (mask, gown, gloves, eye protection, safety boots).
- Clean up spills at once. Work from clean areas to dirty areas with circular motions.
- Dispose of hazardous chemicals in sealed bags or containers.
- Stand behind a lead shield during x-ray or radiation therapy procedures. Follow agency procedures to prevent radiation exposure.
- Do not enter a room while a person is having x-rays or radiation therapy.
- Wash your hands after handling hazardous chemicals.
- Work in well-ventilated areas to avoid inhaling gases.
- Use cleaning products safely.
  - Read and follow warnings and label directions.
  - Keep all products in their original containers.
  - Make sure the area is well-ventilated.
  - Do not mix products. Mixing products can cause dangerous gases. For example, do not mix ammonia and bleach.
  - Close containers properly.
  - Put cleaning products away after use.
  - Do not store cleaning products near food.
  - Empty buckets, pails, basins, and other containers with cleaning solutions.
  - Do not use an empty container for other purposes or things.
- Store a hazardous substance according to the SDS.

DISASTERS

A *disaster is a sudden catastrophic event. People are injured and killed. Property is destroyed.* Natural disasters include tornadoes, hurricanes, blizzards, earthquakes, volcano eruptions, floods, and some fires. Human-made disasters include auto, bus, train, and airplane accidents. They also include fires, bombings, nuclear power plant accidents, gas or chemical leaks, explosions, and wars.

Communities, fire and police departments, and health care agencies have disaster plans. They include how to deal with people needing treatment. The disaster plan includes evacuation procedures if the agency is damaged. The plan generally provides for:

- Discharging persons who can go home
- Assigning staff and equipment to an emergency area
- Assigning staff to transport persons from treatment areas
- Calling off-duty staff to work
- Evacuation procedures if the agency is damaged
  See *Focus on Long-Term Care and Home Care: Disasters.*
  See *Focus on Surveys: Disasters.*

FOCUS ON **LONG-TERM CARE AND HOME CARE**

Disasters

Home Care
A severe storm may occur when you are in a patient's home. For safety:
- Stay informed through local TV and radio stations. Satellite TV service may not have a signal with heavy storm clouds.
- Keep a flashlight with you for power outages.
- Move the patient, family, and yourself to a "safe room."
  - Basement
  - Room on the ground floor
  - Interior room away from outside walls, windows, and doors
  - Center hallway
  - Bathroom
  - Closet

FOCUS ON **SURVEYS**

Disasters

The Centers for Medicare & Medicaid Services (CMS) requires staff training in emergency procedures. There may be unannounced disaster drills during a survey. They are done to test staff efficiency, knowledge, and response if a disaster occurs.

A surveyor may ask you:
- About fire safety. See "Fire Safety" on p. 174. This includes:
  - What to do if a fire alarm goes off.
  - What to do if you find a fire in a person's room.
  - Where to find fire alarms and fire extinguishers.
  - How to use a fire extinguisher.
- What to do if a patient or resident is missing. See "Elopement" on p. 176.

Bomb Threats

Follow agency procedures for a bomb threat or if you find an item that looks or sounds strange. Bomb threats can be sent by phone, mail, e-mail, messenger, or other means. Or the person can leave a bomb in the agency. If you see a stranger in the agency, tell the nurse at once. You cannot be too safe.

Fire Safety

Faulty electrical equipment and wiring, over-loaded electrical circuits, and smoking are major causes of fires. The health team must prevent fires and act quickly during a fire. See Box 13-9.

See *Focus on Long-Term Care and Home Care: Fire Safety.*

BOX 13-9   **Fire Prevention Measures**

- Follow the safety measures:
  - For oxygen use
  - To prevent equipment accidents (p. 169)
  - To prevent burns (p. 159)
- Practice smoking and ashtray safety.
  - Supervise persons who smoke. This is very important for persons who are confused, disoriented, or sedated.
  - Provide ashtrays for persons who are allowed to smoke. Deep, wide ashtrays on a sturdy table are best.
  - Empty ashtrays only when sure that all ashes, cigars, cigarettes, and other smoking materials are out.
  - Empty ashtrays into a metal container partially filled with sand or water. Do not empty ashtrays into plastic containers or wastebaskets lined with paper or plastic bags.
  - Smoke only where allowed to do so. Do not smoke in patients' homes.
- Keep matches, lighters, flammable liquids and materials away from children and confused or disoriented persons.
- Light matches carefully.
  - Be alert for sparks when lighting a match. The sparks can ignite materials that can burn.
  - Keep your hair, clothing, and anything that will burn away from the match and flame.
- Do not leave cooking unattended on stoves, in ovens, in microwave ovens, or on grills.
- Practice safety measures for candles.
  - Avoid using candles in bedrooms or other sleeping areas.
  - Use sturdy candle holders.
  - Place candle holders on a sturdy, clutter-free surface. Do not leave candles unattended.
  - Keep candles at least 12 inches away from anything that can burn.
  - Blow out candles when you leave the room or go to bed.
  - Do not use candles during power outages. Use flashlights and battery-operated lighting.
  - Keep candles and incense away from flammable liquids and materials.
- Store flammable liquids outside in their original containers. Keep containers where children and confused or disoriented persons cannot reach them.
- Keep materials that will burn away from space heaters, fireplaces, radiators, registers, candles, incense, oil lamps, and other heat sources. Stacked newspapers, magazines, books, and paint rags are examples.
- Do not smoke or light matches or lighters around flammable liquids or materials.
- Use clothes dryers safely.
  - Clean the lint filter before and after each use.
  - Use the correct plug and outlet.
  - Turn the dryer off when you leave the home.
  - Do not run clothes dryers when people are sleeping.

FOCUS ON LONG-TERM CARE AND HOME CARE

Fire Safety

Home Care
Fire and the Use of Oxygen
Home care patients may need oxygen therapy. Remind the patient, family, and visitors about safety measures. See Chapter 39.

Preventing Fires
Smoke alarms save lives, prevent injuries, and lessen property damage. Always locate them in a patient's home. They should be outside every sleeping area, in every bedroom, and on every floor. Make sure they are working. Tell the nurse, patient, and family if a smoke alarm does not work.

Cooking equipment is the leading cause of home fires. Practice safety measures to prevent burns (p. 159).

Space heaters present fire hazards. Electric and fuel-burning heaters are common. Practice these safety measures.
- Follow the manufacturer's instructions. Use the correct fuel.
- Light a gas space heater correctly.
  - Strike the match first.
  - Then turn on the gas.
- Do not use extension cords with space heaters.
- Keep heaters at least 3 feet away from any person, window coverings, furniture, and anything that will burn.
- Do not place heaters on stairs, in doorways, or where people walk.
- Protect yourself and others from burns. Heaters are hot. Do not touch them. Keep them away from children and persons who cannot protect themselves.
- Prevent electrocution (being injured or killed by electrical shock). Keep electric heaters away from water. (Water conducts electricity.) Make sure the cord is in good repair.
- Do not leave heaters unattended.
- Store fuel in the original container. Keep the fuel container outside.
- Refill the fuel container outside.
- Do not add fuel while the heater is running or hot. Do not over-fill the heater.

What To Do During a Fire
Know 2 exits from each room and 2 exits from the building. Keep exits clear. Keep furniture and heavy items away from doors and windows.

If a fire occurs, get the patient, family, and yourself out as fast as possible. Do not use elevators. In an apartment building, alert others to the fire. Use the fire alarm system and yell "FIRE" in the hallways. Call 911 or the fire department when out of the building. Do not go back into the building.

Using a Fire Extinguisher
Locate fire extinguishers in the patient's home. Read the manufacturer's instructions. Make sure the device works. Tell the nurse, patient, and family if a fire extinguisher does not work.

Fire and Oxygen. Three things are needed for a fire.
- A spark or flame
- A material that will burn
- Oxygen

Air has some oxygen. However, some people need extra oxygen (Chapter 39). Safety measures are needed where oxygen is used and stored.

- NO SMOKING signs are placed on the door and near the bed.
- The person and visitors cannot smoke in the room.
- Smoking materials (cigarettes, cigars, and pipes), matches, and lighters are removed from the room.
- Safety measures to prevent equipment accidents are followed (see Box 13-7).
- Wool blankets and synthetic fabrics that cause static electricity are removed from the person's room.
- The person wears a cotton gown or pajamas.
- Lit candles, incense, and other open flames are not allowed.
- Materials that ignite easily are removed from the room. They include oil, grease, nail polish remover, and so on.

Agencies have no-smoking policies and smoke-free areas. No smoking is allowed inside the buildings. Signs are posted on all entry doors. Some people ignore such rules. Remind them about the no-smoking rules.

See *Focus on Communication: Fire and Oxygen.*

FOCUS ON COMMUNICATION

Fire and Oxygen

You may have to remind a patient, resident, or visitor not to smoke inside the agency. You can simply say:
- "Mrs. Murphy, this is a smoke-free area. Here is an ashtray to put out your cigarette. If you want to smoke, I'll show you the smoking area outside."
- "Mr. Garcia, please don't smoke inside the center. We have a smoking area outside the back entrance on hallway 2. I can show you the way."

Tell the nurse what happened and what you said and did. The nurse may need to speak with the person about not smoking.

Preventing Fires. Fire prevention measures were described in relation to burns, equipment accidents, and oxygen use. Other fire safety measures are listed in Box 13-9.

What To Do During a Fire. Know your agency's procedures for fire emergencies. This includes evacuation procedures. Know where to find fire alarms, fire extinguishers, and emergency exits. Fire drills are held to practice emergency fire procedures. Remember the word *RACE* (Fig. 13-20).

- *R*—for *rescue*. Rescue persons in immediate danger. Move them to a safe place.
- *A*—for *alarm*. Sound the nearest fire alarm. Call the operator.
- *C*—for *confine*. Close doors and windows to confine the fire. Turn off oxygen or electrical items used in the general area of the fire.
- *E*—for *extinguish*. Use a fire extinguisher on a small fire that has not spread to a larger area.

Clear equipment from all normal and emergency exits. *Do not use elevators if there is a fire.*

See *Promoting Safety and Comfort: What To Do During a Fire*, p. 176.

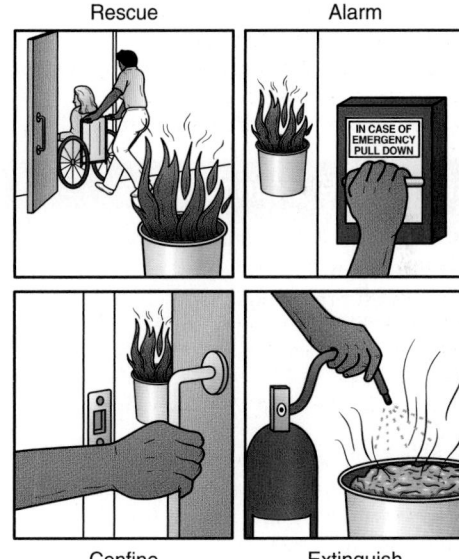

FIGURE 13-20 During a fire, remember *RACE: Rescue, Alarm, Confine, Extinguish.*

PROMOTING SAFETY AND COMFORT

What To Do During a Fire

Safety

Touch doors before opening them. Do not open a hot door. Use another way out of the room or building. If your clothing is on fire, do not run. Drop to the floor or ground. Cover your face. Roll to smother flames. If another person's clothing is on fire, get the person to the floor or ground. Roll the person or cover the person with a blanket, bedspread, or coat. This smothers the flames.

If smoke is present, cover your nose and mouth with a damp cloth. Do the same for patients, residents, visitors, and other staff. Have everyone crawl to the nearest exit.

Do the following if you cannot get out of the building because of flames or smoke.

- Call 911 or the fire department. Tell the operator where you are. Give exact information: agency name or the home care patient's name, address, phone number, and where you are in the building or home.
- Cover your nose and mouth with a damp cloth. Do the same for patients, residents, visitors, and other staff.
- Move away from the fire. Go to a room with a window. Close the room door. Stuff wet towels, blankets, sheets, or bedspreads at the bottom of the door.
- Open the window.
- Hang something from the window (towel, sheet, blanket, clothing). This helps firefighters find you.

Using a Fire Extinguisher. Different extinguishers are used for different kinds of fires.

- Oil and grease fires
- Electrical fires
- Paper and wood fires

A general procedure for using a fire extinguisher follows. See procedure: *Using a Fire Extinguisher*.

Evacuating. Agencies have evacuation procedures. If evacuation is necessary, patients and residents closest to the fire go out first. Those who can walk are given blankets to wrap around themselves. A staff member takes them to a safe place. Figures 13-22 and 13-23 (p. 178) show how to rescue persons who cannot walk. Once firefighters arrive, they direct rescue efforts.

Elopement

The CMS requires that an agency's disaster plan address elopement. *Elopement is when a patient or resident leaves the agency without staff knowledge.* The person who leaves a safe setting is at risk for many dangers. Heat or cold exposure, dehydration, drowning, and being struck by a vehicle are examples.

The agency must:

- Identify persons at risk for elopement.
- Monitor and supervise persons at risk.
- Address elopement in the person's care plan.
- Have a plan to find a missing patient or resident.

Using a Fire Extinguisher

PROCEDURE

1 Pull the fire alarm.
2 Get the nearest fire extinguisher.
3 Carry it upright.
4 Take it to the fire.

5 Follow the word *PASS*.
  a *P*—for *pull the safety pin* (Fig. 13-21, *A*). This unlocks the handle.
  b *A*—for *aim low* (Fig. 13-21, *B*). Direct the hose or nozzle at the base of the fire. Do not try to spray the tops of the flames.
  c *S*—for *squeeze the lever* (Fig. 13-21, *C*). Squeeze or push down on the lever, handle, or button to start the stream. Release the lever, handle, or button to stop the stream.
  d *S*—for *sweep back and forth* (Fig. 13-21, *D*). Sweep the stream back and forth (side to side) at the base of the fire.

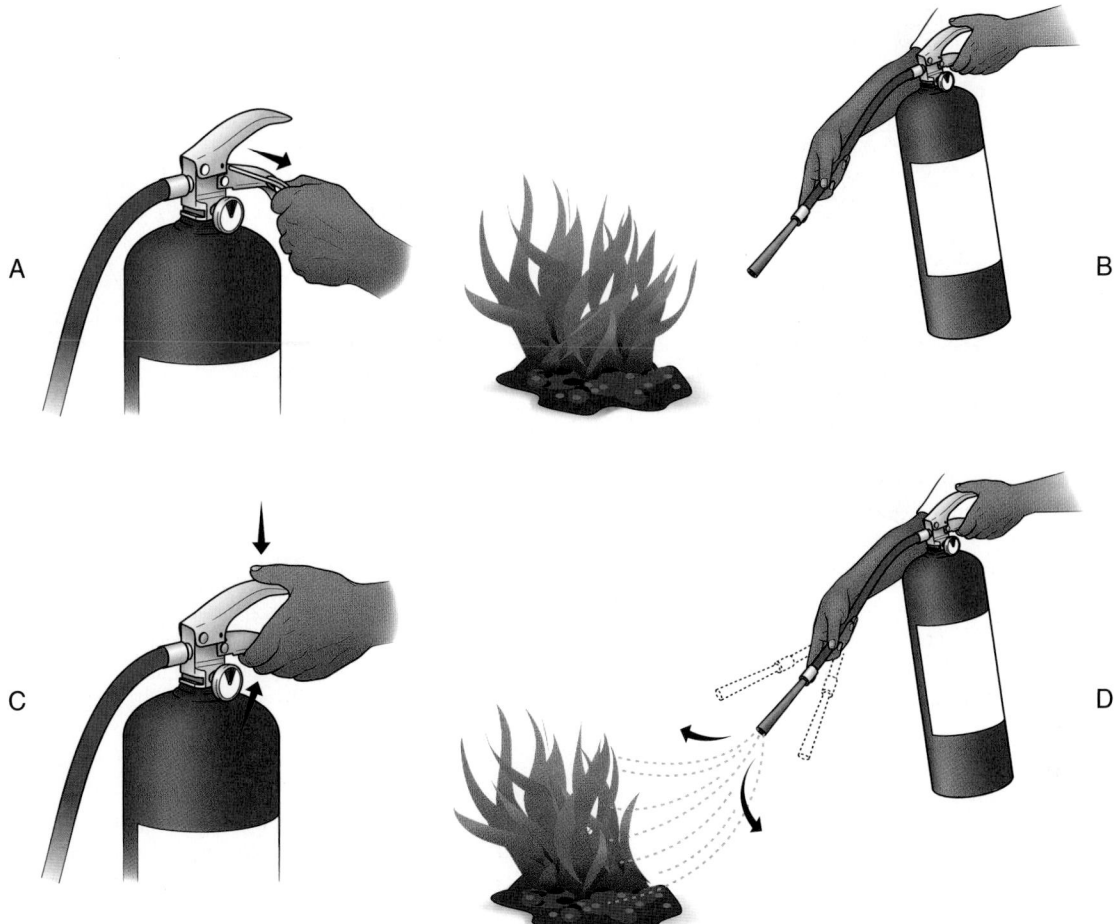

FIGURE 13-21 Using a fire extinguisher. A, *Pull* the safety pin. **B,** *Aim* the hose at the base of the fire. **C,** *Squeeze* the top handle down. **D,** *Sweep* back and forth.

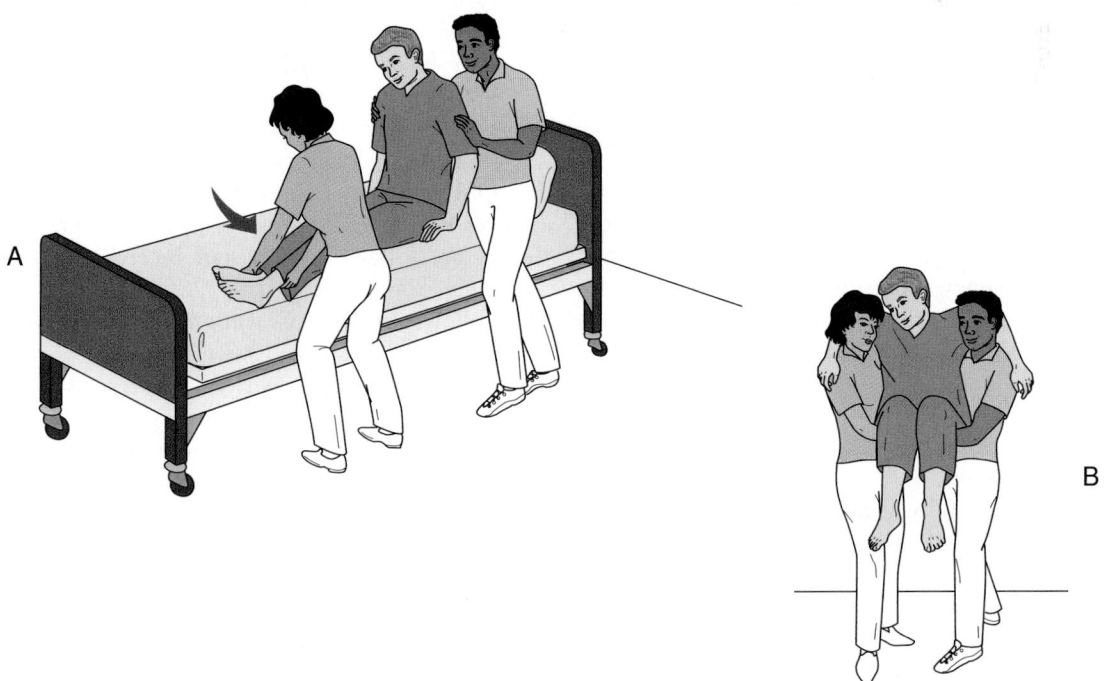

FIGURE 13-22 Swing-carry technique. A, Assist the person to a sitting position. A co-worker grasps the person's ankles as you both turn the person so he sits on the side of the bed. **B,** Pull the person's arm over your shoulder. With 1 arm, reach across the person's back to your co-worker's shoulder. Reach under the person's knees and grasp your co-worker's arm. Your co-worker does the same.

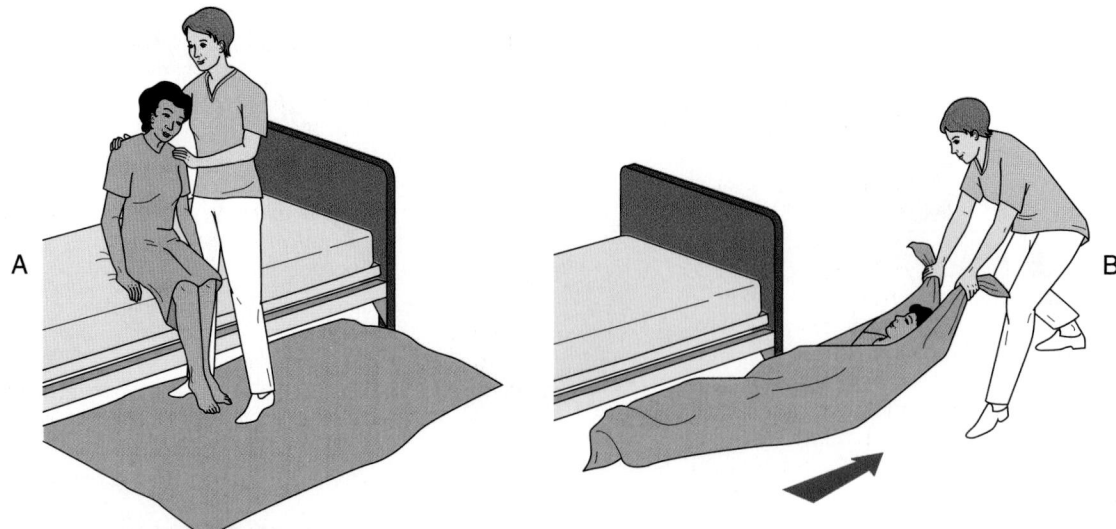

FIGURE 13-23 One-rescuer carry. **A,** Spread a blanket on the floor. Make sure the blanket will extend beyond the person's head. Assist the person to sit on the side of the bed. Grasp the person under the arms and cross your hands over her chest. Lower the person to the floor by sliding her down 1 of your legs. **B,** Wrap the blanket around the person. Grasp the blanket over the head area. Pull the person to a safe area.

WORKPLACE VIOLENCE

Workplace violence is violent acts (including assault or threat of assault) directed toward persons at work or while on duty. It includes:
- Murders
- Beatings, stabbings, and shootings
- Rapes and sexual assaults
- Use of weapons—firearms, bombs, knives, and so on
- Kidnapping
- Robbery
- Threats—obscene phone calls; threatening oral, written, or body language; and harassment of any nature (being followed, sworn at, or shouted at)
- Terrorism

Violence occurs in health care settings. It can occur anywhere in the agency. Common settings are mental health units, emergency rooms, waiting rooms, and geriatric units. Nurses and nursing assistants are at risk. They have the most contact with patients, residents, and visitors.

Assaults are a serious safety hazard in health care. Risk factors include:
- People with weapons.
- Police holds—persons arrested or convicted of crimes.
- Acutely disturbed and violent persons seeking health care.
- Alcohol and drug abuse.
- Persons with mental health disorders who do not take needed drugs, do not have follow-up care, and are not in hospitals unless they are an immediate threat to themselves or others.
- Agencies have drugs and are a target for robberies.
- Gang members and substance abusers are patients, residents, or visitors.
- Upset, agitated, and disturbed family and visitors.
- Long waits for emergency care or other services.
- Being alone with the person during care or transport to areas.
- Low staff levels during meals, emergencies, and at night.
- Poor lighting in hallways, rooms, parking lots, and other areas.
- Lack of training in recognizing and managing potentially violent situations.

OSHA has guidelines for preventing workplace violence. Work-site hazards are identified. Prevention measures are followed. Also, staff receive safety and health training. You need to:
- Follow your agency's workplace violence prevention programs.
- Follow safety and security measures.
- Voice safety and security concerns.
- Report suspicious persons right away.
- Report violent incidents promptly and accurately.
- Serve on health and safety committees that review workplace violence.
- Attend training programs that help you recognize and manage agitation, assaultive behavior, and criminal intent.

BOX 13-10 Workplace Violence—Safety Measures

Agitated or Aggressive Persons

- Stand away from the person. Judge the length of the person's arms and legs. Stand far enough away that the person cannot hit or kick you.
- Stand close to the door. Do not become trapped in the room.
- Identify items in the room that can be used as weapons. Move away from such objects. Vases, phones, radios, letter openers, paper weights, and belts are examples.
- Know where to find panic buttons, call lights, alarms, closed-circuit monitors, and other security devices.
- Keep your hands free.
- Stay calm. Talk to the person in a calm manner. Do not raise your voice or argue, scold, or interrupt the person.
- Be aware of your body language. Do not point a finger or glare at the person. Do not put your hands on your hips.
- Do not touch the person.
- Tell the person that you will get the nurse to speak to him or her.
- Leave the room as soon as you can. Make sure the person is safe.
- Tell the nurse or security officer about the matter at once. Report items in the room that can be used as weapons.

Safety Devices

- Alarm systems, closed-circuit video monitors, panic buttons, hand-held alarms, wireless phones, 2-way radios, and phone systems are installed (Fig. 13-24). These systems have a direct line to security staff or the police.
- Metal detectors are at entrances to identify guns, knives, or other weapons.
- Curved mirrors are at hallway intersections and hard-to-see areas.
- Bullet-resistant, shatter-proof glass is at nurses' stations.
- Door alarms remain on.
- Staff do not share security codes with anyone.

Weapons

- Jewelry and scarves are not worn. They can be used as weapons. For example, a person can grab earrings and bracelets. Or a person can strangle someone with a necklace or scarf.
- Long hair is worn up and off the collar (Chapter 6). A person can pull long hair and cause head injuries.

Weapons—cont'd

- Keys, scissors, pens, or other items that can serve as weapons are not visible.
- Pictures, vases, and other items that can serve as weapons are few in number.
- Tools or items left by maintenance staff or visitors are removed if they can serve as weapons.

Family and Visitors

- Visitors sign in and receive a pass to access patient and resident areas.
- Visiting hours and policies are enforced.
- A list of "restricted visitors" is made for patients and residents with a history of violence or who are victims of violence.
- Waiting rooms and lounges are comfortable and reduce stress.
- Family and visitors are informed in a timely manner.

Building Safety and Security

- Unused doors are locked.
- Bright lights are inside and outside buildings.
- Broken lights, windows, and door locks are replaced or repaired.
- Staff restrooms lock and prevent access to visitors.
- Access to the pharmacy and drug storage areas is controlled.
- Furniture is placed to prevent entrapment. This includes furniture in patient and resident rooms and in therapy areas, dining rooms, and lounges.
- Keys are always attended and secure.

Staff Safety Measures

- Staff are not alone when caring for persons with agitated or aggressive behaviors.
- Staff wear ID badges that prove employment.
- Staff use a "buddy system" when using elevators, stairways, restrooms, and low traffic areas.
- Uniforms fit well. Tight uniforms limit running. An attacker can grab loose uniforms.
- Shoes have good soles. Shoes that cause slipping limit running.
- Vehicles are locked and in good repair.
- Security escort services are used for walking to vehicles, bus stops, or train stations.

Box 13-10 has some safety measures to prevent or control workplace violence. Box 13-11 (p. 180) lists personal safety practices. Follow them all the time. Complete an incident report for workplace violence.

Restraints may be ordered if persons are a threat to themselves or others (Chapter 15). Persons with mental health disorders are supervised as they move about in the agency. Aggressive and agitated persons are treated in open areas. Privacy and confidentiality are maintained. Security officers deal with agitated, aggressive, or disruptive persons.

See *Focus on Long-Term Care and Home Care: Workplace Violence*, p. 181.

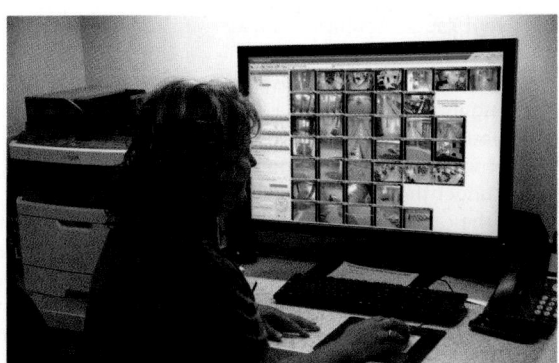

FIGURE 13-24 People entering and leaving the agency are monitored on a closed-circuit TV.

BOX 13-11   Personal Safety

General Measures

- Know the area where you are going. Ask questions about the area.
- Make a "dry run" of the area. Know the way in advance. The shortest way is not always the safest.
- Let someone know where you are at all times. Tell someone when you leave and when you arrive at your destination. If you do not call when expected, the person knows something is wrong.
- Make it known that you do not carry drugs, needles, or syringes.
- Do not carry large amounts of money or valuables. Leave them at home or in the locked car trunk. If someone wants what you have, give it. The only thing of value is you.
- Carry wallets, purses, and backpacks safely.
  - Men—Carry wallets in an inside coat pocket or side pant pocket. Never carry wallets in the rear pocket.
  - Women—Keep a firm grip on a purse. Keep it close to your body.
- Do not display money or other targets of theft. Wireless phones and other hand-held electronic devices are examples.
- Keep your wireless phone in your hand but not visible to others. Clutch it in your closed hand.
- Keep your wireless phone charged.
- Carry a whistle or shriek alarm.
- Avoid ATMs (automated teller machines) at night.
- Be careful when getting on elevators and when entering stairways.
- Do not approach a stranger or someone acting in a strange way. Report the matter at once.

Home Settings

- Keep doors and windows to the home locked at all times.
- Do not open doors to strangers. Ask for identification.
- Do not let a stranger into the home to use a phone or bathroom. Offer to call the police if the person needs help.
- Do not give personal information to callers or people at the door.

Car Safety

- Have plenty of gas in your car.
- Keep your car in good working order.
- Keep these in your car—local map, flashlight with working batteries, flares, a fire extinguisher, first aid kit.
- Raise the hood and use the flares if the car breaks down. Stay in the car. Call the police if you have a wireless phone. If someone stops by to help, ask the person to call the police.
- Lock your car. Sometimes you may want to leave it unlocked. If you need to get in the car fast, you do not want to fumble with keys. Use your judgment. Do not leave anything in the car if you leave it unlocked.
- Have your car key ready so you can get into the car quickly. Do not fumble for keys on the way to or at the car.
- Check under the car as you approach it. A person hiding under the car can grab your ankle or leg. Leave at once if someone is under the car. The person under the car may be working with someone who is waiting to attack you while you are being held or injured at the leg or ankle.
- Check the back seat before getting into the car. Make sure no one is in the car. Leave at once if someone is in the car.
- Lock car doors when you get in the car. Keep windows rolled up.

Car Safety—cont'd

- Do not open the car door or window to talk to a person approaching your car.
- Do not get out of the car to remove something from the windshield.
- Keep purses, backpacks, and other valuables under the seat or near your side. Do not leave them on the seat. They are easy targets for smash-and-grab robbers.
- Do not hitchhike or pick up hitchhikers.
- Practice safety at a gas pump.
  - Take your wallet or purse with you to the pump. If you must keep your wallet, purse, or backpack in the car, keep all windows up and lock all doors. Keep your wallet, purse, and belongings out-of-sight. Called "sliders" by police, thieves can open the car door (or reach in a window) away from where you are standing and grab purses and other valuables.
  - Keep the car key in your hand. Newer cars with "smart keys" only need to sense that the key is in the car. The car can simply be started with a foot on the brake and pushing the "start" button.
  - Protect children in the car. Lock all doors and keep the door closest to you open.

Parking Your Car

- Check for places to park. Choose a well-lit area. In a parking garage, park near entrances, exits, and on the lower level. Try to get close to the attendant if possible. The closest space to your destination is not always the safest for parking.
- Park so you can leave quickly and easily. Park at street corners so no one can park in front of you. In parking lots, back in. You see more from the front windshield than from the back window.

Walking

- Do not wear headphones or earbuds. You cannot hear cars, buses, trains, and people around you.
- Use well-lit and busy streets. Avoid vacant lots, alleys, wooded areas, and construction sites. The shortest way is not always the safest.
- Walk near the curb. Stay away from doorways, shrubs, and bushes.
- Carry a wireless phone. Know your location, and keep phone calls simple.
- Switch directions or cross the street if you think someone is following you. If the person follows you, move quickly to an open store, restaurant, or other public place. Ask for help. If nearby, go to a police or fire station.

Public Transportation

- Carry money for bus, train, or taxi fares. Have money in your pocket to avoid fumbling with a purse or wallet.
- Stand with others and near the ticket booth.
- Sit near the driver or conductor.
- Keep your wireless phone in your hand.

BOX 13-11	Personal Safety—cont'd

If You Are Threatened or Attacked

- Scream as loud and as long as you can. Keep screaming. Men and women should scream.
- Yell "FIRE," not "help." Most people will respond to "FIRE."
- Use your car keys or house key as a weapon. Hold them in your strong hand. Have 1 key extended (Fig. 13-25). Hold the key firmly. If you are attacked, go for the person's face. Slash the person's face with the key. Do not use poking motions. Do not try for a certain target because you might miss. Do not be shy—your attacker will not be.

If You Are Threatened or Attacked—cont'd

- Remember, you have 2 arms, 2 hands, 2 feet, and 2 knees. You can attack from more than 1 direction at once. Do not be shy—your attacker will not be. Push, pull, yank, and so on. You can attack a man's or woman's genitals.
- Use your thumbs as weapons. Go for the eyes and push hard.
- Carry a travel size can of aerosol hair spray. Go for the face.

FOCUS ON LONG-TERM CARE AND HOME CARE

Workplace Violence

Home Care

More measures are needed for home safety.

- Always keep doors locked.
- Do not let strangers into the home or building.
- Do not give information over the phone (Chapter 7).
- Do not let any stranger know that you are with a child or an older, ill, or disabled person.

Child abuse, elder abuse, intimate partner violence, and workplace violence can occur in home settings. If you feel uncomfortable or threatened in any way, tell the nurse. Give as much information as you can. Failing to report the matter does not help you or the patient. Follow agency policy for what to do if you are threatened or feel threatened.

The following can threaten your safety. Report these and other threats to the nurse.

- Sexual abuse or harassment by the patient or any person in the home—husband, wife, sister, brother, boyfriend, girlfriend, son, daughter, family, friends. See Chapter 5.
- Hitting, kicking, slapping, spitting, biting, scratching, pinching, pushing, or other attacks by the patient or anyone in the home.
- Attacks or threatened attacks with a weapon—knife, gun, bat, rope, tool (hammer, screwdriver, and so on), razor, scissors, spray, pot, pan, cane, chair, and so on.
- Denial of meal breaks, water, bathroom use, toilet paper, or hand-washing facilities.
- Denial of adequate sleeping conditions for a live-in situation.
- Inadequate heating or ventilation.
- Name calling, obscene language, or racial or cultural slurs.
- Exposure to unsafe conditions—blocked fire escapes, broken stairways, pest infestations, and so on.

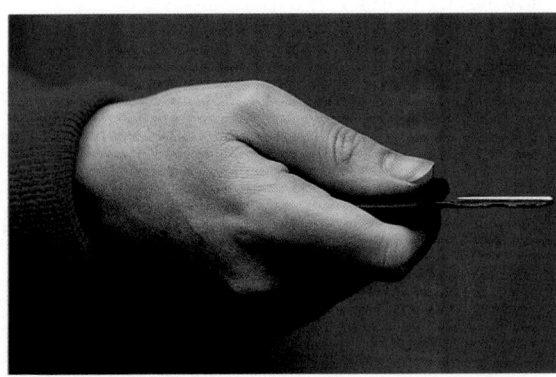

FIGURE 13-25 A key can be used as a weapon.

RISK MANAGEMENT

Risk management involves identifying and controlling risks and safety hazards affecting the agency. The intent is to:

- Protect everyone in the agency—patients, residents, visitors, and staff.
- Protect agency property from harm or danger.
- Protect the person's valuables.
- Prevent accidents and injuries.

Risk management deals with these and other safety issues.

- Accident and fire prevention
- Negligence and malpractice
- Abuse
- Workplace violence
- Federal and state requirements

Risk managers look for patterns and trends in incidents, complaints (patients, residents, staff), and accident and injury investigations. Unsafe situations are corrected. Procedure changes and training recommendations are made as needed.

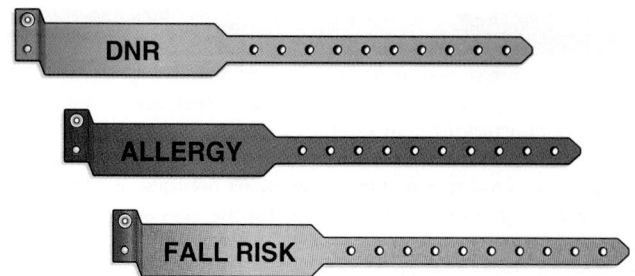

FIGURE 13-26 Color-coded wristbands. The alert is printed on the band.

Color-Coded Wristbands

Color-coded wristbands promote the person's safety and prevent harm. They quickly communicate an alert or warning (Fig. 13-26). The type of alert is printed on the band. The printing is useful in dim lighting and for persons who are color blind. These colors are common.

- Red—for an "allergy alert." Red is a warning to "stop." A red wristband warns of allergies to food, drugs, treatment supplies such as tape or latex gloves, dust, plants, grass, and so on. Allergies are not listed on the wristband.
- Yellow—for a "fall risk." Yellow implies "caution." Yellow wristbands are used for persons with a history of falls. Or they are used for persons at risk for falls because of dizziness, balance problems, confusion, and so on.
- Purple—for a "Do Not Resuscitate" (DNR) order. See Chapter 55.

Some agencies have colors for other alerts. For example, pink is for a "limb alert." This means that an arm or leg is not used for blood pressure measurements, blood draws, or intravenous infusions. To safely use color-coded wristbands:

- Know the wristband colors used in your agency. Colors may vary among agencies.
- Check the care plan and your assignment sheet when you see a color-coded wristband. You need to know the reason for the wristband and the care measures needed. Ask the nurse if you have questions.
- Do not confuse "social cause" bands with your agency's color-coded wristbands. "Live Strong" is an example.
- Check for wristbands on persons transferred from another agency. That agency may use different colors. Or the meanings may differ from those in your agency. The nurse needs to remove wristbands from another agency.
- Tell the nurse if you think a person needs a color-coded wristband.

Personal Belongings

The person's belongings must be kept safe. Often they are sent home with the family. A personal belongings list is completed. Each item is listed and described. The staff member and the person sign the completed list.

A valuables envelope is used for jewelry and money. Each jewelry item is listed and described on the envelope. Describe what you see. For example, describe a ring as having a white stone with 6 prongs in a yellow setting. Do not assume the stone is a diamond in a gold setting. For valuables:

- Count money with the person.
- Put money and each jewelry item in the envelope. Have the person watch. Seal and sign the envelope like a personal belongings list.
- Give the envelope to the nurse. The nurse takes it to the safe or sends it home with the family.

Dentures, eyeglasses, hearing aids, watches, some jewelry, radios, computers, and other electronic devices are kept at the bedside. Items kept at the bedside are listed in the person's record. Some people keep money for newspapers and personal items. The amount kept is noted in the person's record.

See *Focus on Long-Term Care and Home Care: Personal Belongings.*

Reporting Incidents

An *incident is any event that has harmed or could harm a patient, resident, visitor, or staff member.* This includes:

- Accidents involving patients, residents, visitors, or staff.
- Errors in care—giving the wrong care, giving care to the wrong person, not giving care.
- Broken or lost items owned by the person. Dentures, hearing aids, and eyeglasses are examples.
- Lost money or clothing.
- Hazardous chemical incidents.
- Workplace violence incidents.

Report accidents and errors at once. An *incident report* is completed as soon as possible. Incident reports are reviewed by risk management and a health care committee. They look for patterns and trends in accidents or errors. For example, are falls occurring on the same shift and on the same unit? Are lost or missing items being reported on the same shift or same unit? Are residents being injured on the same shift or same unit? There may be new policies and procedures to prevent future incidents.

FOCUS ON **PRIDE**

The Person, Family, and Yourself

P ersonal and Professional Responsibility

Accidents happen. Errors occur. No matter how much you try, mistakes are made. Do not lie or try to hide the incident. You must:

- Be honest.
- Tell the nurse.
- Fill out an incident report.

Incident reports are used to improve systems and promote safety, not for punishment. Information gained signals areas for improvement. Processes may be changed to make mistakes more difficult. Or they are changed to make it easier to do the right thing.

Always do your best to give safe care. When errors or accidents happen, take responsibility. Be accountable. Take pride in doing the right thing by honest reporting.

R ights and Respect

Having respect for others' well-being motivates your actions. If you value the person's safety, you will perform safety measures. For example, you will:

- Identify the person before giving care.
- Check water temperature before bathing.
- Use and store harmful products safely.
- Cut food into small pieces.
- Monitor closely for swallowing problems and signs of choking.
- Use the agency's and person's equipment correctly.
- Know what to do during a fire or disaster.
- Report concerns and incidents.

Show respect for the person in how you give care. Take pride in providing safe care.

I ndependence and Social Interaction

Children and older persons are at increased risk for injury. Children often try to show independence before they are able to judge safety. Older persons often cannot do things they used to do. They still may try. To promote safety:

- Know who you need to protect.
- Know common safety hazards and the causes of accidents.
- Practice safety measures to prevent accidents and injuries.
- Respect the desire of older persons to maintain independence. Listen to them. Discuss letting them try a task with help. Let them do as much as they safely can. Kindly communicate safety limits.

D elegation and Teamwork

Personal safety practices protect yourself and co-workers. Work as a team to ensure the safety of all staff arriving and leaving the agency.

- Wait for a person finishing work a few minutes late. Ask if you can help the person.
- Walk with others to and from the parking area.
- Walk in well-lit areas at night.
- Do not leave the parking area until all of your co-workers are safely in their vehicles.
- Offer to call security escort services for a co-worker going to a different location. For example, a person is walking to a bus stop.

Take pride in caring about the safety of all team members.

E thics and Laws

Some persons are at risk for choking. Persons with developmental disabilities (Chapter 50), young children, and older persons are examples. Safety measures must be taken to avoid harm. The following case shows what can occur when safety measures are neglected.

A 32-year-old man was a patient at a developmental center. He had an intellectual disability and epilepsy (a seizure disorder). He was a patient at the center since the age of 25.

According to the facts reported in the court case, the following occurred.

- *He had a dinner of braised beef and noodles. The pieces of beef were about ½ inch wide and ¾ inch long.*
- *While eating, he stood up, coughed out his milk, reached for his throat, and collapsed.*
- *Efforts were made to revive him.*
- *He was transported to the hospital where he died a short while later.*
- *His death was caused by "meat mass inhalation... associated with mental retardation with chronic seizure disorder..."*

The lawsuit claimed negligence because:

- *His swallowing was affected by the dosage of a drug.*
- *He was not given a soft diet.*
- *He was not properly supervised at meal time.*

In the Court's opinion, negligent care resulted in the patient's death.

(B. Szydelko v The Department of Mental Health of the State of Illinois, 1984.)

You can help prevent such incidents. Know which persons are at risk for choking. Ask the nurse or check the care plan. Monitor those persons closely. Check that they have the right diet. See Chapter 27 for more precautions.

FOCUS ON **PRIDE**: *Application*

As a student or new nursing assistant, it is normal to have fears of causing harm. This stress can have positive effects. For example, it motivates you to perform safety measures. Or it can have negative effects. You are hesitant to interact with patients or residents. What concerns do you have? How will you overcome your fears?

REVIEW QUESTIONS

Circle the BEST answer.

1 Who provides a safe setting for the person?
   a The health team
   b The family
   c The administrator
   d The risk manager

2 Which is safe?
   a Not wearing needed eyeglasses
   b Hearing problems
   c Memory problems
   d Oriented to person, time, and place

3 A person in a coma
   a Has suffered an electrical shock
   b Has dementia
   c Is unaware of surroundings
   d Has stopped breathing

4 A person with dementia
   a Has problems with thinking and reasoning
   b Is not aware of his or her surroundings
   c Is paralyzed
   d Has suffered an electrical shock

5 A person with quadriplegia is paralyzed
   a From the waist down
   b From the neck down
   c On the right side of the body
   d On the left side of the body

6 To identify a person, you
   a Call the person by name
   b Ask the person his or her name
   c Compare information on the ID bracelet against your assignment sheet
   d Ask both roommates their names

7 To prevent burns
   a Keep smoking materials at the person's bedside
   b Pour hot liquids near a person
   c Turn on hot water first
   d Check water temperature before the person enters the shower

8 Which prevents poisoning?
   a Keeping harmful products in low storage areas
   b Keeping child-resistant caps on harmful products
   c Removing product labels
   d Storing harmful products near food

9 Which signals a poison?
   a The "Mr. Yuk" sticker
   b OSHA
   c RACE
   d PASS

10 Who has the greatest risk of lead poisoning?
   a Newborns
   b Infants between the ages of 1 and 6 months
   c Children between the ages of 6 months and 6 years
   d Older persons

11 A home has lead-based plumbing. You should
   a Use hot tap water for cooking and drinking
   b Use hot tap water to make baby formula
   c Let cold water run for 1 to 2 minutes before using it for cooking
   d Be alert for signs of carbon monoxide poisoning

12 Which can cause suffocation?
   a Reporting loose teeth or dentures
   b Using electrical items that are in good repair
   c Cutting food into small, bite-sized pieces
   d Restraints

13 The most common cause of choking in adults is
   a A loose denture
   b Meat
   c Marbles
   d Candy

14 If severe airway obstruction occurs, the person usually
   a Clutches at the throat
   b Can speak, cough, and breathe
   c Is calm
   d Has a seizure

15 These statements are about FBAO. Which is *true?*
   a A person is coughing forcefully. Give abdominal thrusts.
   b A person is pregnant. Give abdominal thrusts.
   c Injuries can occur from abdominal or chest thrusts.
   d Unconscious persons cannot choke.

16 You need to shave a new resident with his electric shaver. *First,*
   a Fill the sink with water
   b The maintenance staff must check the device
   c Check the SDS
   d Get an extension cord

17 You are using electrical equipment. Which measure is unsafe?
   a Following the manufacturer's instructions
   b Keeping electrical items away from water and spills
   c Pulling on the cord to remove a plug from an outlet
   d Turning off electrical items after using them

18 Which is unsafe?
   a A chair's weight capacity exceeds the person's weight.
   b A person's weight exceeds a wheelchair's weight capacity.
   c A person who cannot walk uses a wheelchair.
   d A person who cannot sit up is transported by stretcher.

19 You spilled a hazardous substance. You should
   a Follow the instructions on the safety data sheet
   b Cover the spill and go tell the nurse
   c Wipe up the spill with paper towels
   d Leave the spill for housekeeping

20 The fire alarm sounds. Which action is correct?
   a Leave oxygen on.
   b Use elevators.
   c Open doors and windows.
   d Move residents to a safe place.

REVIEW QUESTIONS—cont'd

21 Your clothing is on fire. What should you do *first*?
a Run to get help.
b Call 911.
c Use a fire extinguisher.
d Drop to the floor and roll to smother the flames.

22 You work in a nursing center. In a severe weather alert, you should
a Take cover
b Follow the center's disaster plan
c Make sure your family is safe
d Pull the fire alarm

23 A person is agitated and aggressive. Which is unsafe?
a Standing away from the person
b Standing close to the door
c Using touch to show you care
d Talking to the person without raising your voice

24 A person has a yellow wristband. You should
a Monitor the person closely for falls
b Avoid wearing latex gloves
c Use the person's right arm for checking blood pressure
d Not perform CPR on the person

25 You see a color-coded wristband. You should
a Read the wristband for special instructions or care measures
b Ask the person what it means
c Check your assignment sheet and the person's care plan
d Remove the wristband when the risk is no longer present

26 You work the night shift. Which is safe?
a Parking in a dimly-lit area
b Walking to your car alone
c Finding your keys after getting to the car
d Checking under the car and in your back seat

27 A resident brought a radio from home. To prevent property loss
a Send the item home with the family
b Label the item with the person's name
c Put the item in a safe
d Use a wheelchair pouch for the item

28 You gave a person the wrong treatment. Which is *true*?
a Report the error at the end of the shift.
b Take action only if the person was injured.
c You are guilty of negligence.
d You must complete an incident report.

Answers to Chapter 13 questions are on p. 870.

FOCUS ON **PRACTICE**

Problem Solving

You are assisting Mr. Park with feeding. He begins to cough loudly. He can speak a few words. You hear wheezing between breaths. What do you do? Mr. Park is suddenly unable to cough, speak, or breathe. What do you do?

OBJECTIVES

- Define the key terms and key abbreviations in this chapter.
- Identify the causes and risk factors for falls.
- Describe the safety measures that prevent falls.
- Explain how to use bed and chair alarms safely.
- Explain how to use bed rails safely.
- Explain the purpose of hand rails and grab bars.

- Explain how to use wheel locks safely.
- Describe how to use transfer/gait belts.
- Explain how to help the person who is falling.
- Perform the procedures described in this chapter.
- Explain how to promote PRIDE in the person, the family, and yourself.

KEY TERMS

bed rail A device that serves as a guard or barrier along the side of the bed; side rail
gait belt See "transfer belt"

transfer belt A device applied around the waist used to support a person who is unsteady or disabled; gait belt

KEY ABBREVIATIONS

CDC Centers for Disease Control and Prevention

CMS Centers for Medicare & Medicaid Services

The risk of falling increases with age. Persons older than 65 years are at risk. A history of falls increases the risk of falling again. Falls are the most common accidents in nursing centers.

According to the Centers for Disease Control and Prevention (CDC):

- Each year, ⅓ of adults age 65 and older fall.
- Falls are the main cause of injuries and injury-related deaths in older adults.
- About 1800 nursing center residents die each year from falls.
- Falls can cause serious injury, including fractures. Fractures of the spine, hip, forearm, leg, ankle, pelvis, upper arm, and hand are the most common. Hip fractures and head trauma increase the risk of death.
- Falls result in disability, decline in function, and reduced quality of life.
- Fear of falling can cause further loss of function, depression, feelings of helplessness, and social isolation. This may increase the person's risk of falling again.

See *Focus on Surveys: Fall Prevention.*

FOCUS ON **SURVEYS**

Fall Prevention

The Centers for Medicare & Medicaid Services (CMS) defines a fall as:

- Unintentionally coming to rest on the ground, floor, or other lower level. Force, such as being pushed, was not involved.
- When a person loses his or her balance and would have fallen if staff did not act to prevent the fall.
- When a person is found on the floor unless matters suggest otherwise.
  The survey team will observe:
- For the fall risk factors described in this chapter.
- For hazards described in this chapter and in Chapter 13.
- For safety measures to prevent falls.
- For the safe repair and use of bed rails, hand rails and grab bars, and wheel locks.
- For the use of assistive (adaptive) devices. Canes, walkers, and transfer/gait belts are examples.
- For safe transfer (Chapter 19) and ambulation (Chapter 30) procedures.
- If call lights are answered promptly.
- If the person's care needs are addressed.
- If the person's care plan is followed.
  The survey team may interview you about identifying hazards (Chapter 13) and preventing falls.

CAUSES AND RISK FACTORS FOR FALLS

Most falls are caused by multiple risk factors. The more risk factors present, the greater the risk of falling. Most falls occur in patient and resident rooms. Poor lighting, cluttered floors, throw rugs, and out-of-place furniture are causes. So are wet and slippery floors, bathtubs, and showers. Weakness, walking problems, and needing to use the bathroom are major causes. For example, Mrs. Hines is weak and has an urgent need to urinate. She falls trying to get to the bathroom.

BOX 14-1   Fall Risk Factors

Care Setting
- Bed height: too low or too high
- Care equipment: IV (intravenous) poles, drainage tubes and bags, and others
- Floors: cluttered, wet, slippery, or uneven
- Furniture out-of-place
- Lacks hand rails or grab bars
- Lighting: poor or glares
- Restraint use
- Setting: new, strange, and unfamiliar
- Throw rugs or other tripping hazards
- Wet and slippery bathtubs and showers
- Wheelchairs, walkers, canes, and crutches: improper use or fit

The Person
- Age: over 65 years
- Alcohol: over-use
- Balance problems
- Blood pressure: low or high
- Confusion
- Depression
- Disorientation
- Dizziness; dizziness on standing
- Drug side effects
  - Low blood pressure when standing or sitting
  - Drowsiness
  - Fainting
  - Dizziness
  - Coordination: poor
  - Unsteadiness
  - Urination: frequent
  - Diarrhea
  - Confusion and disorientation
- Elimination: incontinence, frequency, urgency, urinating at night (nocturia)
- Falls: history of
- Fear of falling
- Foot problems
- Gait: unsteady
- Incontinence: urinary or fecal
- Joint pain and stiffness
- Judgment: poor
- Light-headedness
- Memory problems
- Mobility: impaired
- Muscle weakness
- Reaction time: slow
- Shoes that fit poorly
- Sleep problems
- Vision problems
- Weakness

The accident risk factors described in Chapter 13 can lead to falls. The problems listed in Box 14-1 increase a person's risk of falling.

See *Focus on Long-Term Care and Home Care: Causes and Risk Factors for Falls.*

See *Teamwork and Time Management: Causes and Risk Factors for Falls.*

FOCUS ON LONG-TERM CARE AND HOME CARE

Causes and Risk Factors for Falls

Long-Term Care
Nursing center residents are at increased risk for falls. Reasons given by the CDC include:
- Residents are often older and more frail than older adults in the community.
- Residents tend to have more problems with their health, thinking and memory, and ability to perform activities of daily living (ADL).
- Many residents have trouble walking and need help with mobility (ability to move about).

Weakness and walking problems are the most common causes of falls in nursing centers. Care setting hazards are other causes—poor lighting, wet floors, incorrect bed height. Other risk factors are transfer problems (Chapter 19), shoes that fit poorly, and improper use or fit of wheelchairs, walkers, canes, and other devices.

Home Care
In the home, many factors increase the risk for falls. Hazards include:
- Cluttered rooms, stairways, and hallways
- Objects on the floor and stairways—wires, cords, shoes, books, magazines, blankets, and so on
- Throw rugs
- Pets
- Flooring problems—loose tiles and floor boards, raised linoleum, frayed carpet
- Wet floors and slippery bathtub or shower floors
- Ice or snow on driveways, steps, and sidewalks
- Loose or missing hand rails and grab bars (p. 192)
- Poor lighting
- No footwear or unsafe footwear—slippers, shoes without non-skid surfaces, and shoes with long shoelaces
- Assistive (adaptive) devices that need repair—walkers, canes, wheelchairs
- Having to climb or reach for objects

TEAMWORK AND TIME MANAGEMENT

Causes and Risk Factors for Falls

The entire health team must protect the person. If you see something unsafe, tell the nurse at once. Do not assume the nurse knows or that someone is handling the matter.

Answer call lights promptly. This includes the call lights of patients and residents assigned to co-workers.

During shift changes, staff are busy going off and coming on duty. Confusion can occur about who gives care and answers call lights. Falls can result. Know your role during shift changes. Nursing staff must work together to prevent falls.

FALL PREVENTION PROGRAMS

Agencies have fall prevention programs. The measures listed in Box 14-2 are part of the program and the person's care plan. Many measures also apply to home settings. The care plan also lists measures for the person's risk factors.

Common sense and simple safety measures can prevent many falls. The health team works with the person and family to reduce the fall risk. The goal is to prevent falls without decreasing quality of life.

See *Focus on Communication: Fall Prevention Programs*.

See *Focus on Long-Term Care and Home Care: Fall Prevention Programs*.

See *Promoting Safety and Comfort: Fall Prevention Programs*.

BOX 14-2	Safety Measures to Prevent Falls

Basic Needs
- Fluid needs are met.
- Eyeglasses and hearing aids are worn as needed. Reading glasses are not worn when up and about.
- Tasks are explained before and while performing them.
- Help is given with elimination needs. Assist the person to the bathroom. Or provide the bedpan, urinal, or commode.
- The bedpan, urinal, or commode is kept within easy reach if the person can use the device without help.
- A warm drink, soft lights, or a back massage is used to calm the person who is agitated.
- Barriers are used to prevent wandering (Fig. 14-1).
- The person is properly positioned when in bed, a chair, or a wheelchair. Use pillows, wedge pads, seats, or other positioning devices as the nurse and care plan direct (Chapter 17).
- Correct procedures and equipment are used for transfers (Chapter 19). Follow the care plan.
- The person is involved in meaningful activities.
- Exercise programs are followed. They help improve balance, strength, walking, and physical function.

Bathrooms and Shower/Tub Rooms
- Tubs and showers have non-slip surfaces or non-slip bath mats.
- Grab bars (safety bars) are in showers (p. 192). They also are by tubs and toilets.
- The person uses grab bars in bathrooms and shower/tub rooms.
- Shower chairs are used (Chapter 22).
- Safety measures for tub baths and showers are followed (Chapter 22).

Floors
- Carpeting (if used) is wall-to-wall or tacked down.
- Scatter, area, and throw rugs are not used.
- Floor covers are 1 color. Bold designs can cause dizziness in older persons.
- Floors have non-glare, non-slip surfaces.
- Non-skid wax is used on hardwood, tiled, or linoleum floors.
- Loose floor boards and tiles are reported. So are frayed rugs and carpets.
- Floors and stairs are free of clutter, cords, and other items that can cause tripping.
- Floors are free of spills. Wipe up spills at once. Put a WET FLOOR sign by the wet area.
- Floors are free of excess furniture and equipment.
- Electrical and extension cords are out of the way. This includes power strips.
- Equipment and supplies are kept on 1 side of the hallway.

Furniture
- Furniture is placed for easy movement.
- Furniture is kept in place. It is not re-arranged.
- Chairs have armrests. Armrests give support when standing or sitting.
- A phone, lamp, and personal belongings are within reach.

Beds and Other Equipment
- The bed is at the correct height for the person. Follow the care plan. The bed is raised to give bedside care. Then it is lowered to a safe and comfortable level appropriate for the person. The distance from the bed to the floor is reduced if the person falls or gets out of bed.
- Bed rails (p. 190) are used according to the care plan.
- A mattress, special mat, or floor cushion is placed on the floor beside the bed (Fig. 14-2, p. 190). This reduces the chance of injury if the person falls or gets out of bed.
- Wheelchairs, walkers, canes, and crutches fit properly. They are in good repair. Another person's equipment is not used.
- Crutches, canes, and walkers have non-skid tips.
- Wheelchair and stretcher safety is followed (Chapter 19).
- Wheel locks on beds (p. 192), wheelchairs, and stretchers are in working order.
- Bed and wheelchair or stretcher wheels are locked for transfers.
- Linens are checked for sharp objects and for the person's property (dentures, eyeglasses, hearing aids, and so on).

Lighting
- Rooms, hallways, and stairways have good lighting. So do bathrooms and shower/tub rooms.
- Light switches (including those in bathrooms) are within reach and easy to find.
- Night-lights are in bedrooms, hallways, and bathrooms.

Shoes and Clothing
- Non-skid footwear is worn. Socks, bedroom slippers, and long shoelaces are avoided.
- Shoes fit well. They should not slip up and down on the feet. All shoelaces and straps are fastened.
- Clothing fits properly. Clothing is not loose. It does not drag on the floor.
- Belts are tied or secured in place.

BOX 14-2	Safety Measures to Prevent Falls—cont'd

Call Lights and Alarms

- The person is taught how to use the call light (Chapter 20).
- The call light is always within the person's reach. This includes when sitting in the chair, on the commode, and in the bathroom and shower/tub room.
- The person is asked to call for assistance when help is needed.
  - To get out of bed or a chair
  - To walk
  - To get to or from the bathroom or commode
  - To get on or off the bedpan
- Call lights are answered promptly. The person may need help right away. He or she may not wait for help.
- Bed, chair, door, floor mat, and belt alarms are used. They sense when the person tries to get up, get out of bed, or open a door.
- Alarms are responded to at once.

Other

- Color-coded alerts are used to warn of a fall risk. Yellow is the common color for a fall alert. Besides wristbands (Chapter 13), some agencies also use color-coded blankets, non-skid footwear, socks, and magnets or stickers to place on room doors.
- The person is checked often. This may be every 15 minutes or as required by the care plan. Careful and frequent observation is important.

Other—cont'd

- Frequent checks are made on persons with poor judgment or memory. This may be every 15 minutes or as required by the care plan.
- Persons at risk for falls are close to the nurses' station.
- Hand rails (p. 192) are on both sides of stairs and hallways.
- The person uses hand rails when walking or using stairs.
- Family and friends are asked to visit during busy times. Meal times and shift changes are examples. They are also asked to visit during the evening and night shifts.
- Companions are provided. Sitters, companions, or volunteers are with the person.
- Non-slip strips are on the floor next to the bed and in the bathroom. They are intact.
- Caution is used when turning corners, entering corridor intersections, and going through doors. You could injure a person coming from the other direction.
- Pull (do not push) wheelchairs, stretchers, carts, and other wheeled equipment through doorways. This allows you to lead the way and to see where you are going.
- A safety check is made of the room after visitors leave. (See the inside of the front cover.) They may have lowered a bed rail, moved a call light, or moved a walker out of reach. Or they may have brought an item that could harm the person.

FOCUS ON COMMUNICATION

Fall Prevention Programs

Often falls occur when the person tries to get needed items. The person has to reach too far and falls. Or the person tries to get up without help. Prevent falls by asking the person these questions.

- "What things would you like near you?"
- "Can I move this closer to you?"
- "Can you reach the call light?"
- "Can you reach your cane?" (Walker and wheelchair are other examples.)
- "Do you need to use the bathroom?"
- "Is there anything else you need before I leave the room?"

FOCUS ON LONG-TERM CARE AND HOME CARE

Fall Prevention Programs

Home Care

People of all ages fall in home settings. Older persons are at risk. Simple changes can prevent falls (Chapter 12). So can some of the measures in Box 14-2. For example:

- Place furniture to allow a clear path for walking.
- Remove throw rugs.
- Keep objects off the floor and stairs.
- Use night-lights in bedrooms, hallways, and bathrooms.
- Place a lamp near the bed if bedroom lights are hard to reach.
- Keep often-used items within easy reach. In kitchens, move items to lower shelves.
- Place non-slip bath mats or self-stick strips in showers and tubs.

PROMOTING SAFETY AND COMFORT

Fall Prevention Programs

Safety

Some people are visually impaired. Besides the measures in Box 14-2, other safety measures are needed to prevent falls. See Chapter 42.

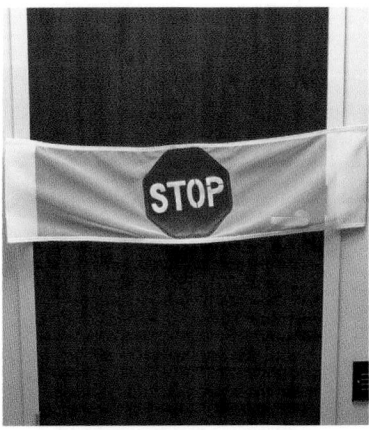

FIGURE 14-1 Barriers are used to prevent wandering.

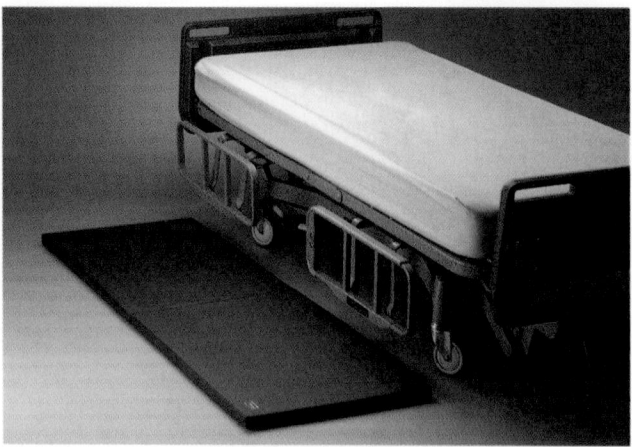

FIGURE 14-2 Floor cushion. (Image courtesy Posey Co., Arcadia, Calif.)

Bed and Chair Alarms

Bed and chair alarms alert the staff that a person is moving from the bed or chair. See Figure 14-3. The device attaches to the person's clothing. Or the person sits or lies on a flat sensor. To alert staff, the device makes a sound—alarm, beep, chime, music, and so on. Or a recorded message is played. For example: "Please do not get up. Sit down and use your call light for help."

To use bed and chair alarms safely:
- Follow the manufacturer's instructions.
- Test the alarm before leaving the person alone. If the device does not work, stay with the person. Call for the nurse.
- Respond to alarms at once.

For alarms that attach to clothing:
- Mount the alarm securely out of the person's reach.
- Place the alarm at least 2 feet away from the person's ear. Alarms close to the ear may cause hearing loss or injury.
- Attach the clip securely out of the person's reach. The clip is near the shoulder. Check that clothing is not frayed or torn.
- Check the cord. The cord should allow enough movement for comfort but be short enough to activate the alarm if the person moves from the safe area. The cord must not be tangled in bed rails, linen, chair parts, and so on.

Alarms are not a substitute for close observation. Persons at risk for falls are checked often. Careful and frequent observation is important.

Bed Rails

A ***bed rail*** *(side rail) is a device that serves as a guard or barrier along the side of the bed.* Bed rails are raised and lowered (Fig. 14-4). They lock in place with levers, latches, or buttons. Bed rails are half, three quarters (¾), or the full length of the bed. When half-length rails are used, each side may have 2 rails. One is for the upper part of the bed, the other for the lower part.

The nurse and the care plan tell you when to raise bed rails. They are needed by persons who are unconscious or sedated with drugs. Some confused or disoriented people need them. If a person needs bed rails, keep them up at all times except when giving bedside care.

Bed rails present hazards. The person can fall when trying to climb over them or the person cannot get out of bed to use the bathroom. *Entrapment* is a risk (Chapter 20). That is, the person can get caught, trapped, entangled, or strangled.

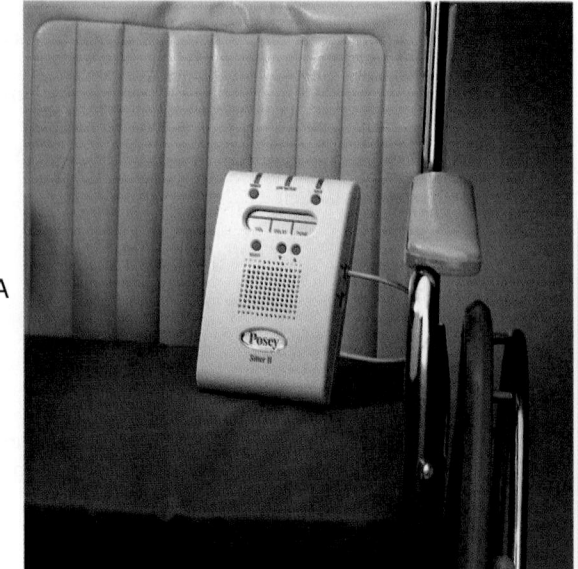
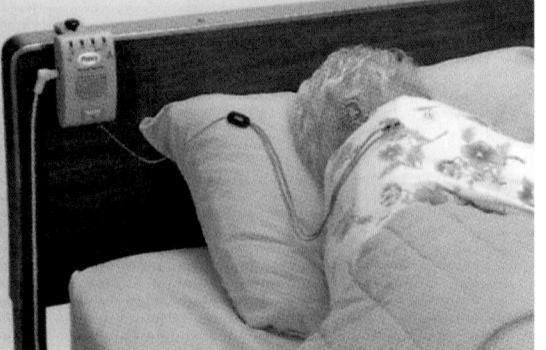

FIGURE 14-3 Alarms. A, Chair alarm. **B,** Bed alarm. (Images courtesy Posey Co., Arcadia, Calif.)

The CMS considers bed rails restraints (Chapter 15) if:
• The person cannot get out of bed.
• The person cannot lower them without help.

Accrediting agency standards and federal and state laws affect bed rail use. They are allowed when the person's condition requires them. Bed rails must be in the person's best interests. Some people feel safer with bed rails up. Others use them for position changes in bed. The person or legal representative must give written consent for raised bed rails. The need for bed rails is carefully noted in the person's medical record and care plan.

The procedures in this book include using bed rails. This helps you learn to use them correctly. The nurse, the care plan, and your assignment sheet tell you who uses bed rails. If a person does not use them, omit the "raise bed rails" and "lower bed rails" steps.

Check the person often. Report to the nurse that you checked the person. If allowed to chart, record when you checked the person and your observations (Fig. 14-5).

See *Focus on Children and Older Persons: Bed Rails.*

See *Focus on Long-Term Care and Home Care: Bed Rails,* p. 192.

See *Promoting Safety and Comfort: Bed Rails,* p. 192.

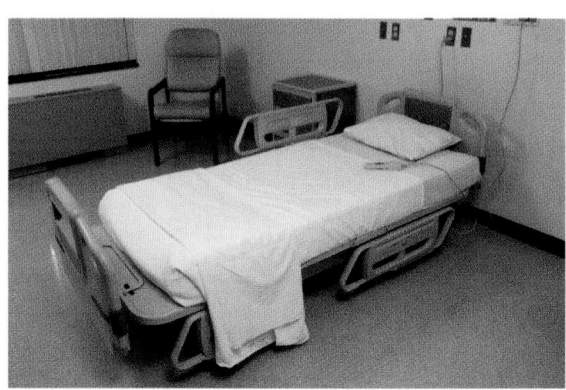

FIGURE 14-4 Bed rails. The far bed rail is raised. The near bed rail is lowered.

FOCUS ON CHILDREN AND OLDER PERSONS

Bed Rails

Children

Cribs must meet federal safety standards. In 2010, the United States government set new safety standards for consumer cribs. Drop-side cribs do not meet current safety standards. If a drop-side crib cannot be replaced, keep the rail up and locked. Some crib manufacturers make immobilizers to secure the drop side. Check the crib often to make sure all parts are secure. Medical cribs with drop sides are allowed in hospitals.

Crib rails must be safe. Slats must not be missing, loose, or cracked. The space between crib rail slats must be no more than $2\frac{3}{8}$ inches. If the space is larger, the baby's head can get caught between the slats. The baby can suffocate.

For toddlers and older children, rails may be placed on beds. Entrapment is a risk (Chapter 20). Rails must fit the child's bed and be installed according to the manufacturer's instructions.

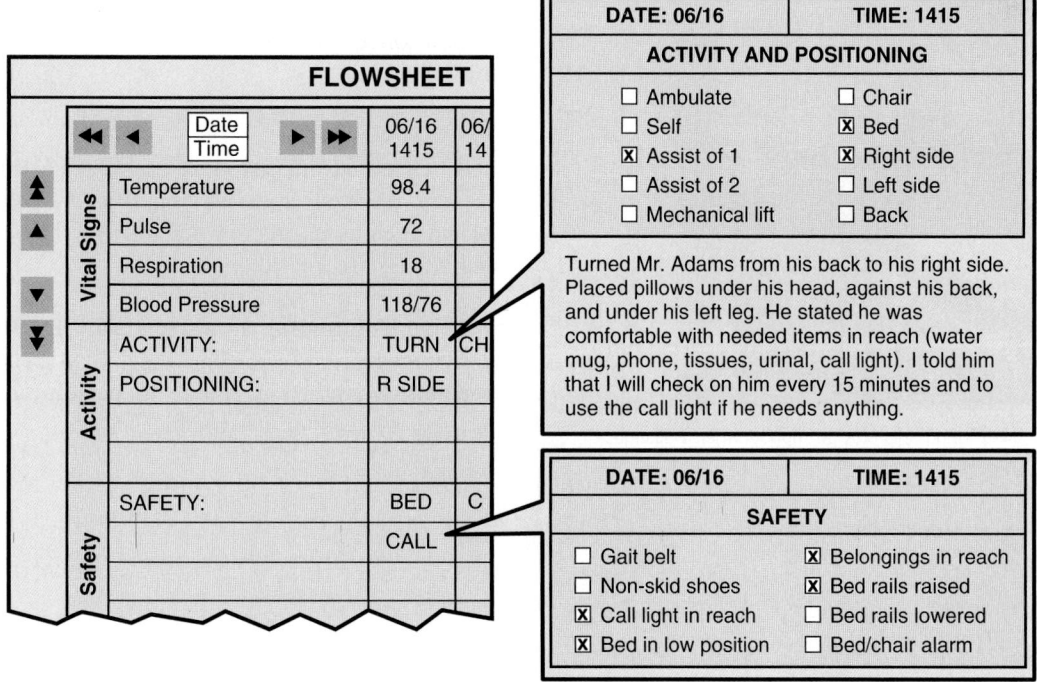

FIGURE 14-5 Charting sample.

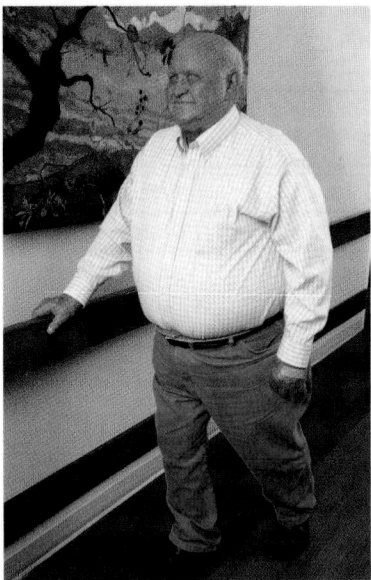

FIGURE 14-6 Hand rails provide support when walking.

Hand Rails and Grab Bars
Hand rails are in hallways and stairways (Fig. 14-6). They give support to persons who are weak or unsteady when walking.

Grab bars are in bathrooms and in shower/tub rooms (Fig. 14-7). They provide support to sit down or get up from a toilet. They also are used to get in and out of the shower or tub.

Wheel Locks
Beds wheels let the bed move easily. Wheels have locks to prevent the bed from moving (Fig. 14-8). Wheels are locked at all times except when moving the bed. Make sure bed wheels are locked:
- When giving bedside care
- When you transfer a person to and from bed

Wheelchair and stretcher wheels also are locked during transfers (Chapter 19). You or the person can be injured if the bed, wheelchair, or stretcher moves.

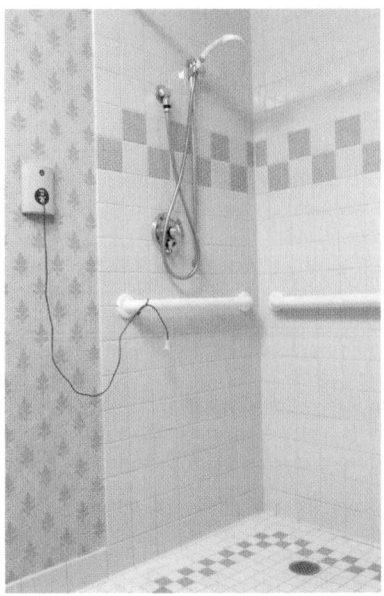

FIGURE 14-7 Grab bars in a shower.

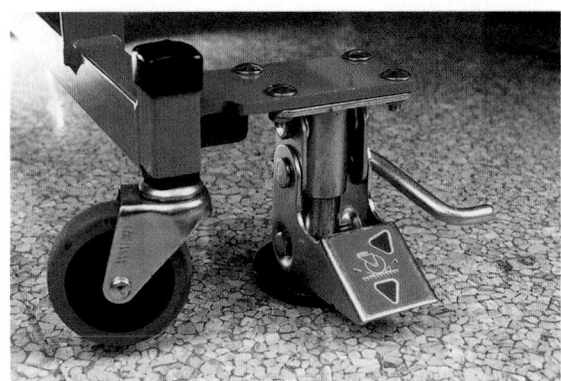

FIGURE 14-8 Bed wheel lock.

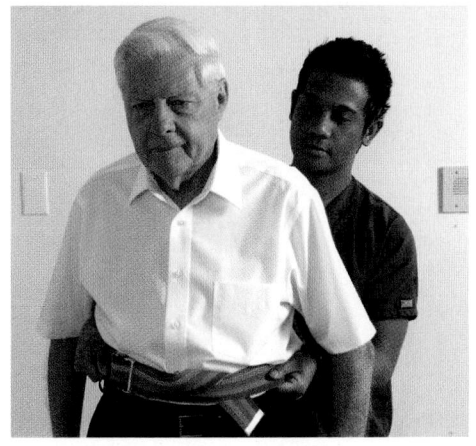

FIGURE 14-9 Transfer/gait belt. The buckle is off-center and not over the spine. Excess strap is tucked into the belt. The nursing assistant grasps the belt from underneath.

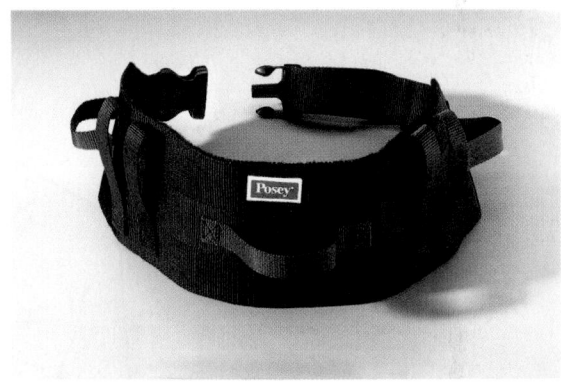

FIGURE 14-10 A transfer/gait belt with handles. (Image courtesy Posey Co., Arcadia, Calif.)

TRANSFER/GAIT BELTS

A ***transfer belt (gait belt)*** *is a device applied around the waist used to support a person who is unsteady or disabled* (Fig. 14-9). It helps prevent falls and injuries. When used to transfer a person (Chapter 19), it is called a *transfer belt*. When used to help a person walk, it is called a *gait belt*.

The belt goes around the waist. Grasp the belt from underneath to support the person during the transfer or when assisting the person to walk. If the belt has handles, grasp the belt by the handles (Fig. 14-10).

The standard-sized transfer/gait belt fits waist sizes up to 51 inches. Bariatric-sized belts fit waist sizes up to 71 inches. The nurse and care plan tell you what size to use. If the person's waist size is greater than 71 inches, follow the nurse's directions and the care plan.

See *Focus on Communication: Transfer/Gait Belts.*

See *Promoting Safety and Comfort: Transfer/Gait Belts,* p. 194.

See procedure: *Using a Transfer/Gait Belt,* p. 195.

FOCUS ON **COMMUNICATION**

Transfer/Gait Belts

When applying a transfer/gait belt, ask about the person's comfort. You can say: "How does that feel? Is the belt too loose? Is it too tight?" Adjust the belt as needed for the person's comfort and safety.

PROMOTING SAFETY AND COMFORT
Transfer/Gait Belts

Safety

Transfer/gait belts are routinely used in nursing centers. If the person needs help, a belt is required. For safe use, always follow the manufacturer's instructions.

Some transfer/gait belts have a quick-release buckle (Fig. 14-11). Position the quick-release buckle at the person's back where he or she cannot reach it. The person cannot release the buckle during the procedure. Injury could result if the buckle is released.

Do not leave excess strap dangling. Tuck the excess strap into the belt (see Fig. 14-9).

Remove the belt after the procedure. Do not leave the person alone while he or she is wearing a transfer/gait belt.

Using a transfer/gait belt is unsafe for some persons. The belt could cause pressure or rub against care equipment.

Safety—cont'd

Check with the nurse and the care plan before using a transfer/gait belt if the person has:

- An ostomy—colostomy, ileostomy, urostomy (Chapters 26 and 47)
- A gastrostomy tube (Chapter 28)
- Chronic obstructive pulmonary disease (Chapter 45)
- An abdominal or chest wound, incision, or drainage tube
- Monitoring equipment
- A hernia (part of an organ protrudes or projects through an opening in a muscle wall. Hernias often involve a loop of bowel or the stomach.)
- Other conditions or care equipment involving the chest or abdomen

Comfort

A transfer/gait belt is always applied over clothing. It is never applied over bare skin. Also, it is applied around the waist and under the breasts. Breasts must not be caught under the belt. The belt buckle is never positioned over the person's spine.

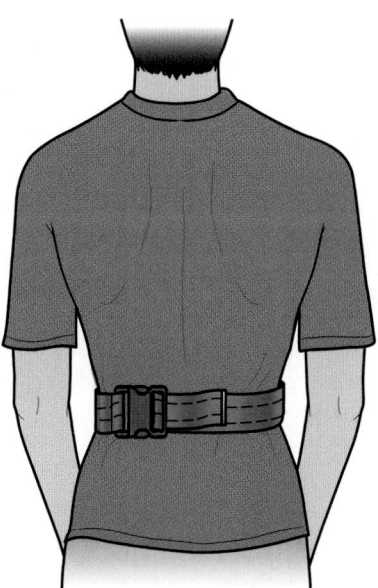

FIGURE 14-11 A transfer/gait belt with a quick-release buckle. The buckle is positioned off-center at the back.

Using a Transfer/Gait Belt

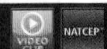

QUALITY OF LIFE

- Knock before entering the person's room.
- Address the person by name.
- Introduce yourself by name and title.

- Explain the procedure before starting and during the procedure.
- Protect the person's rights during the procedure.
- Handle the person gently during the procedure.

PRE-PROCEDURE

1 See *Promoting Safety and Comfort: Transfer/Gait Belts.*
2 Practice hand hygiene.
3 Obtain a transfer/gait belt of the correct type and size.

4 Identify the person. Check the identification (ID) bracelet against the assignment sheet. Use 2 identifiers (Chapter 13). Also call the person by name.
5 Provide for privacy.

PROCEDURE

6 Assist the person to a sitting position.
7 Apply the belt. Hold the belt by the buckle. Wrap the belt around the person's waist. Apply the belt over clothing. Do not apply it over bare skin.
   a For a belt with a metal buckle:
      1) Insert the belt's metal tip into the buckle. Pass the belt through the side with the teeth first (Fig. 14-12, *A*).
      2) Bring the belt tip across the front of the buckle. Insert the tip through the buckle's smooth side (Fig. 14-12, *B*).
   b For a belt with a quick-release buckle, push the belt ends together to secure the buckle.
8 Tighten the belt so it is snug. It should not cause discomfort or impair breathing. You should be able to slide your open, flat hand under the belt. Ask the person about his or her comfort.

9 Make sure that a woman's breasts are not caught under the belt.
10 Place the buckle off-center in the front or off-center in the back for the person's comfort (Fig. 14-12, *C*). A quick-release buckle is turned around to the person's back out of his or her reach. The buckle is not over the spine.
11 Tuck any excess strap into the belt (see Fig. 14-12, *C*).
12 Complete the transfer (Chapter 19) or ambulation procedure (Chapter 30). Grasp the belt from underneath with 2 hands. See Figure 14-9. Or grasp the belt by the handles.

POST-PROCEDURE

13 Remove the belt after the procedure in step 12. The person is not left alone wearing the belt.
   a For a belt with a metal buckle:
      1) Bring the belt strap back through the buckle's smooth side.
      2) Pull the belt through the side with the teeth.
   b For a belt with a quick-release buckle, push inward on the quick-release buttons.
   c Remove the belt from the person's waist. Avoid dragging the belt across the waist.

14 Provide for comfort. (See the inside of the front cover.)
15 Place the call light and other needed items within reach.
16 Unscreen the person.
17 Complete a safety check of the room. (See the inside of the front cover.)
18 Return the transfer/gait belt to its proper place.
19 Practice hand hygiene.
20 Report and record your observations.

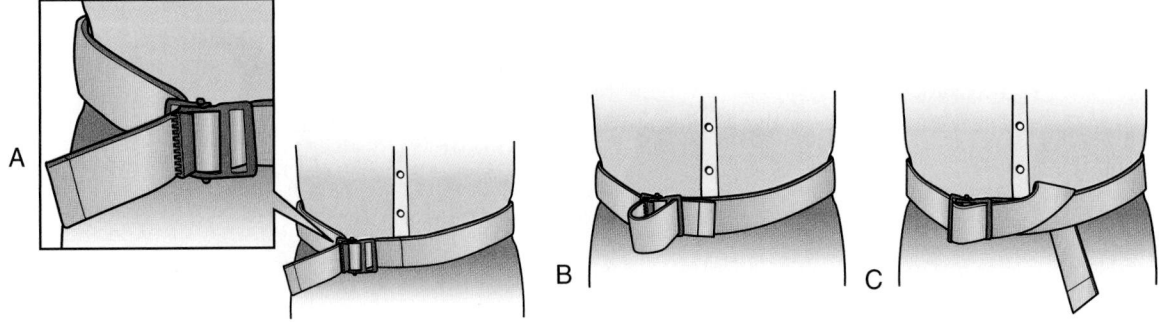

FIGURE 14-12 Applying a transfer/gait belt at the waist. **A,** The belt is inserted into the buckle. The belt goes through the side with the teeth first. **B,** The belt is inserted into the buckle's smooth side. **C,** The buckle is in the front. Excess strap is tucked into the belt.

THE FALLING PERSON

A person may start to fall when standing or walking. The person may be weak, light-headed, or dizzy. Fainting may occur. Falling may be caused by slipping or sliding on spills, waxed floors, throw rugs, or improper shoes. See p. 187 for the causes and risk factors for falls.

Do not try to prevent the fall. You could injure yourself and the person while twisting and straining to prevent the fall. Balance is lost as the person falls. If you try to prevent the fall, you could lose your balance. You both could fall. Head, wrist, arm, hip, knee, and back injuries could occur.

If a person starts to fall, ease him or her to the floor. This lets you control the direction of the fall. You can also protect the person's head. Do not let the person move or get up before the nurse checks for injuries. Calmly explain that the nurse will check for injuries such as broken bones.

If you find a person on the floor, do not move the person. Stay with the person and call for the nurse.

An incident report is completed after all falls (Chapter 13). The nurse may ask you to help with the report.

See *Focus on Children and Older Persons: The Falling Person.*

See *Promoting Safety and Comfort: The Falling Person.*

See procedure: *Helping the Falling Person.*

FOCUS ON CHILDREN AND OLDER PERSONS

The Falling Person

Older Persons

Some older persons are confused. A confused person may not understand why you do not want him or her to move or get up after a fall. Forcing a person not to move may injure the person and you. You may need to let the person move for his or her safety and your own. Never use force to hold a person down. Stay calm and protect the person from injury. Talk to the person in a quiet, soothing voice. Call for help.

PROMOTING SAFETY AND COMFORT

The Falling Person

Safety

If a bariatric person starts to fall, there is little that you can do. For the person's safety and yours:

- Do *not* use the procedure: *Helping the Falling Person.*
- Move items out of the way that could cause injury. Do so as fast as possible.
- Try to protect the person's head. Protect the person's head from striking the floor, equipment, or other objects.
- Call for the nurse at once. Stay with the person.
- Assist the health team as needed to return the person to bed.

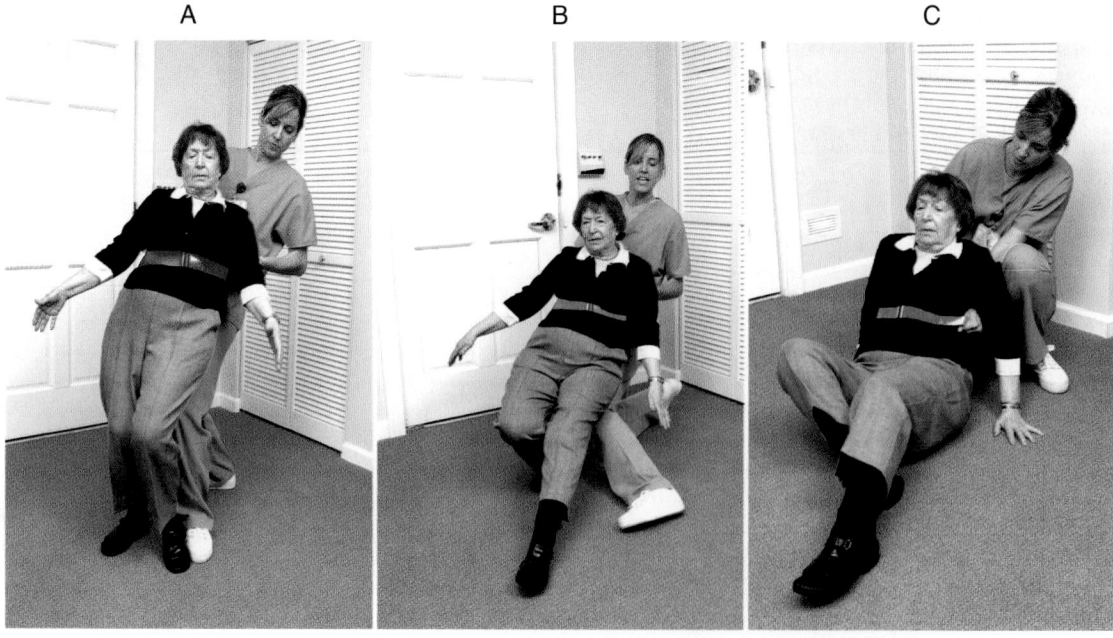

FIGURE 14-13 The falling person. A, The falling person is supported with the gait belt. **B,** The person's buttocks rest on the nursing assistant's leg. **C,** The person is eased to the floor on the nursing assistant's leg.

Helping the Falling Person

PROCEDURE

1 Stand behind the person with your feet apart. Keep your back straight.
2 Bring the person close to your body as fast as possible (Fig. 14-13, *A*). Use the transfer/gait belt. Or wrap your arms around the person's waist. If necessary, you can also hold the person under the arms.
3 Move your leg so the person's buttocks rest on it (Fig. 14-13, *B*). Move your leg that is near the person.

4 Lower the person to the floor. The person slides down your leg to the floor (Fig. 14-13, *C*). Bend at your hips and knees as you lower the person.
5 Call a nurse to check the person. Stay with the person.
6 Help the nurse return the person to bed. Ask other staff to help if needed.

POST-PROCEDURE

7 Provide for comfort. (See the inside of the front cover.)
8 Place the call light and other needed items within reach.
9 Raise or lower bed rails. Follow the care plan.
10 Complete a safety check of the room. (See the inside of the front cover.)
11 Practice hand hygiene.

12 Report and record the following.
  * How the fall occurred
  * How far the person walked
  * How activity was tolerated before the fall
  * Complaints before the fall
  * How much help the person needed while walking
13 Complete an incident report (Chapter 13).

MOVING THE PERSON FROM THE FLOOR

After a fall, wait for the nurse before moving the person. The nurse will assess the person for injuries. Special procedures are used for persons with severe injuries. Assist as the nurse directs.

For a person with no injuries or minor injuries, follow the nurse's directions to help move the person from the floor. The Occupational Safety and Health Administration (OSHA) recommends minimal manual lifting and eliminating it when possible. Often a mechanical lift (Chapter 19) is used to move the person (Fig. 14-14). The lift must reach the floor.

If the person can stand alone, the nurse has staff stand by as the person stands up. Or a transfer/gait belt is used to assist the person.

If a manual lift is required, protect yourself from injury.
* Use good body mechanics (Chapter 17).
* Roll the person onto his or her side and position an assist device. A blanket or drawsheet (Chapter 21) are examples. Avoid reaching across the person.
* Have at least 2 staff members on each side of the person. The larger the person, the more staff needed.
* Bend your knees, not your back. Do not twist.
* For the lift:
  1. Kneel on 1 knee.
  2. Grasp the blanket, drawsheet, or other device.
  3. Lift smoothly with your legs as you stand. Stand together on the "count of 3." Do not bend your back.

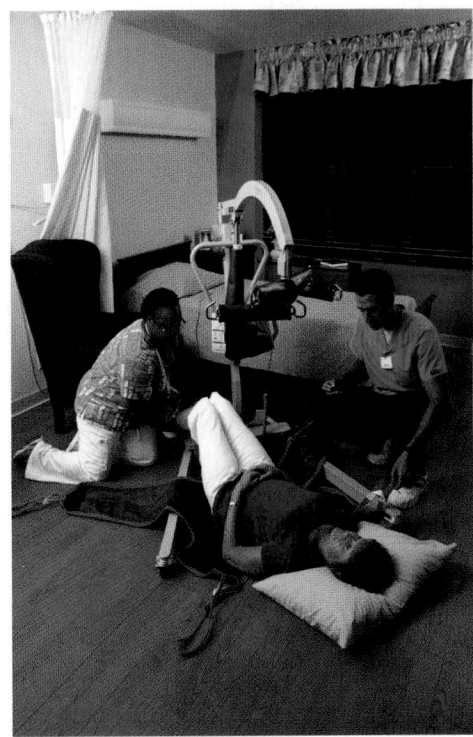

FIGURE 14-14 Moving the person from the floor using a mechanical lift.

FOCUS ON PRIDE

The Person, Family, and Yourself

Personal and Professional Responsibility

Safety measures can take time. Maybe you need to get a transfer/gait belt or walker. Or you must put on the person's shoes. Resist the urge to take short cuts. Take the time to:

- Find and use assistive devices.
- Put proper footwear on the person.
- Raise or lower the bed and bed rails as appropriate.
- Lock wheels on beds, stretchers, and wheelchairs.
- Ask for help if needed.

Safe care includes taking measures to prevent falls. See Box 14-2. Take time for safety. Take pride in doing the right thing.

Rights and Respect

Safety and security are not only rights, but basic needs (Chapter 9). Fear of falling does not make a person feel safe. Before moving a person, explain what you are going to do and what he or she needs to do. Also give step-by-step instructions as you progress. Do not move the person without telling him or her first. Good communication promotes comfort. It supports the person's right to safety and security. See Chapters 18 and 19 for how to safely move and transfer the person.

Independence and Social Interaction

Some people feel that safety devices limit independence. For example, Ms. Mills does not like having bed rails up. She says: "I feel trapped. Do these have to be up?" Ms. Mills has fallen out of bed at night. The care plan includes having bed rails up while she is in bed.

Listen to the person's concerns. Kindly explain the reason for the safety device. If the person still refuses, tell the nurse. Do not let the person talk you out of a safety measure or using a safety device. Safety is always a priority.

Delegation and Teamwork

Helping co-workers is an important part of teamwork. However, you may not be familiar with a person and his or her care plan. You must promote safety. Communication is essential. When assisting with the transfer of a co-worker's patient or resident, you must have certain information. Ask the nurse or co-worker:

- Is the person at risk for falls?
- Is the person weak? Can he or she bear weight?
- Are there activity limits?
- How many staff are needed for the transfer?
- Are assistive devices needed? A cane, transfer belt, wheelchair, and walker are examples.
- Is other equipment needed? Oxygen and braces are examples.

Ethics and Laws

Falls are a serious matter. Failing to prevent falls can result in legal action. The following is a real case in which the nursing staff neglected to use safety measures to prevent a fall.

A hospital patient fell and injured her right shoulder 6 days after knee surgery. The patient claimed that the nursing staff did not follow orders to assist with walking to and from the bathroom. According to the patient:

- *She asked for help to raise herself from a commode to a standing position.*
- *She was not given assistance.*
- *She fell when the commode (with wheels) shifted while she tried to stand.*

According to the hospital's lawyers, the staff did not use a transfer belt. Failure to use the belt violated hospital policy. The case settled for $25,000.

(N. Martinez and M. Martinez v St. Catherine's Hospital, Sentry Insurance and Wisconsin Patient Compensation Fund, 1998, Wisconsin.)

You must prevent falls. Follow the safety measures presented in this chapter. Take pride in protecting the person, yourself, and the agency.

FOCUS ON PRIDE: Application

Mr. Stark is embarrassed about needing to use a transfer/gait belt and walker. How will you promote his safety and dignity? What if he refuses to use the devices?

REVIEW QUESTIONS

Circle the BEST answer.

1 These statements are about falls. Which is *true?*
   a Most are caused by multiple risk factors.
   b Serious injuries are unlikely.
   c Most occur outdoors.
   d Nursing center residents are at decreased risk.

2 Which person has the lowest risk of falls?
   a A 75-year-old with confusion
   b A 68-year-old with a history of falls
   c A 60-year-old with a hearing aid
   d An 80-year-old with urinary incontinence

3 A person's care plan includes fall prevention measures. Which should you question?
   a Assist with elimination needs.
   b Keep phone, lamp, and TV controls within reach.
   c Check the person every 2 hours.
   d Complete a safety check after visitors leave the room.

4 You observe the following in the person's room. Which is unsafe?
   a The lamp cord is by the chair.
   b The chair has armrests.
   c The night-light is on.
   d The bed is in a low position.

5 You note the following after a person got dressed. Which is safe?
   a Pant cuffs are dragging on the floor.
   b The person is wearing non-skid shoes.
   c The belt is not fastened.
   d The shirt is too big.

6 A co-worker is helping Mr. Polk today. His chair alarm goes off. What should you do?
   a Find your co-worker.
   b Tell the nurse.
   c Assist Mr. Polk.
   d Wait for someone to respond to the alarm.

7 To help prevent falls, you need to report
   a Equipment and supplies being on 1 side of the hallway
   b A floor cushion beside the bed
   c A co-worker pulling a wheelchair through a doorway
   d Clutter on stairways

8 Bed rails are used
   a When you think they are needed
   b According to the care plan
   c When the bed is raised
   d To support persons who are weak or unsteady

9 Before transferring a person to the bed, you must
   a Raise the bed rails
   b Get a grab bar
   c Lock the bed wheels
   d Remove the person's shoes

10 A transfer/gait belt is applied
   a To the skin
   b Over clothing at the waist
   c Over the breasts
   d Under the robe

11 To safely use a transfer/gait belt, you must
   a Follow the manufacturer's instructions
   b Be able to slide a closed fist under the belt
   c Leave the belt on if the person is left alone
   d Position the buckle over the person's spine

12 You apply a transfer/gait belt. What should you do with the excess strap?
   a Cut it off.
   b Wrap it around the person's waist.
   c Tuck it into the belt.
   d Let it dangle.

13 A person starts to fall. Your *first* action is to
   a Try to prevent the fall
   b Call for help
   c Bring the person close to your body as fast as possible
   d Lower the person to the floor

14 When a bariatric person falls, you should
   a Try to stop the fall
   b Try to protect the person's head
   c Quickly pull the person close to you
   d Do nothing

15 You found a person lying on the floor. What should you do?
   a Lock the bed wheels.
   b Help the person back to bed.
   c Apply a transfer belt.
   d Call for the nurse.

Answers to Chapter 14 questions are on p. 870.

FOCUS ON **PRACTICE**

Problem Solving

You are assisting a resident in the bathroom. The resident is not to be left alone while in the bathroom. You hear another resident's chair alarm sound in the hallway outside the door. What will you do?

Restraint Alternatives and Safe Restraint Use

OBJECTIVES

- Define the key terms and key abbreviations in this chapter.
- Describe the purpose of restraints.
- Identify the risk factors related to restraint use.
- Identify restraint alternatives.
- Explain the legal aspects of restraint use.

- Explain how to use restraints safely.
- Perform the procedure described in this chapter.
- Explain how to promote PRIDE in the person, the family, and yourself.

KEY TERMS

chemical restraint Any drug used for discipline or convenience and not required to treat medical symptoms

convenience Any action taken to control or manage a person's behavior that requires less effort by the staff; the action is not in the person's best interest

discipline Any action taken by the agency to punish or penalize a patient or resident

enabler A device that limits freedom of movement but is used to promote independence, comfort, or safety

freedom of movement Any change in place or position of the body or any part of the body that the person is able to control

medical symptom An indication or characteristic of a physical or psychological condition

physical restraint Any manual method or physical or mechanical device, material, or equipment attached to or near the person's body that he or she cannot remove easily and that restricts freedom of movement or normal access to one's body

remove easily The manual method, device, material, or equipment used to restrain the person that can be removed intentionally by the person in the same manner it was applied by the staff

KEY ABBREVIATIONS

CMS Centers for Medicare & Medicaid Services
FDA Food and Drug Administration
OBRA Omnibus Budget Reconciliation Act of 1987

ROM Range-of-motion
TJC The Joint Commission

Chapters 13 and 14 have many safety measures. However, some persons need extra protection. They may present dangers to themselves or others (including staff).

The Centers for Medicare & Medicaid Services (CMS) has rules for using restraints. Like the *Omnibus Budget Reconciliation Act of 1987* (OBRA), CMS rules protect the person's rights and safety. This includes the right to be free from restraint. Restraints may be used only to treat a medical symptom or for the immediate physical safety of the person or others. Restraints may be used only when less restrictive measures fail to protect the person or others. They must be discontinued as soon as possible.

The CMS uses these terms.

- *Physical restraint—any manual method or physical or mechanical device, material, or equipment attached to or near the person's body that he or she cannot remove easily and that restricts freedom of movement or normal access to one's body.*

- *Chemical restraint—any drug used for discipline or convenience and not required to treat medical symptoms.* The drug or dosage is not a standard treatment for the person's condition.

- *Freedom of movement—any change in place or position of the body or any part of the body that the person is able to control.*

- *Convenience—any action taken to control or manage a person's behavior that requires less effort by the staff; the action is not in the person's best interest.*

- *Discipline—any action taken by the agency to punish or penalize a patient or resident.*

- *Remove easily—the manual method, device, material, or equipment used to restrain the person that can be removed intentionally by the person in the same manner it was applied by the staff.* For example, the person can put bed rails down, untie a knot, or unclasp a buckle.

HISTORY OF RESTRAINT USE

Restraints were once used to *prevent* falls. Research shows that restraints *cause* falls. Falls occur when persons try to get free of the restraints. Injuries are more serious from falls in restrained persons than in those not restrained.

Restraints also were used to prevent wandering or interfering with treatment. They were often used for confusion, poor judgment, or behavior problems. Older persons were restrained more often than younger persons were. Restraints were viewed as necessary devices to protect a person. However, they can cause serious harm, even death. See "Risks From Restraint Use" on p. 203.

Besides the CMS, the Food and Drug Administration (FDA), state agencies, and The Joint Commission (TJC—an accrediting agency) have guidelines for restraint use. They do not forbid restraint use. *They require considering or trying all other appropriate alternatives first.*

Every agency has policies and procedures for restraints. They include identifying persons at risk for harm, harmful behaviors, restraint alternatives, and proper restraint use. Staff training is required.

RESTRAINT ALTERNATIVES

Often there are causes and reasons for harmful behaviors. Knowing and treating the cause can prevent restraint use. This is very important for persons with speech or cognitive problems. The nurse tries to find out what the behavior means.

* Is the person in pain, ill, or injured?
* Is the person short of breath? Are cells getting enough oxygen (Chapter 39)?
* Is the person afraid in a new setting?
* Does the person need to use the bathroom?
* Is clothing or a wound dressing (Chapter 36) tight or causing other discomfort?
* Is the person's position uncomfortable?
* Are body fluids, secretions, or excretions causing skin irritation?
* Is the person too hot or too cold? Hungry or thirsty?
* What are the person's life-long habits?
* Does the person have problems communicating?
* Is the person seeing, hearing, or feeling things that are not real (Chapters 48 and 49)?
* Is the person confused or disoriented (Chapter 49)?
* Are drugs causing the behaviors?

Restraint alternatives for the person are identified in the care plan (Box 15-1). The care plan is changed as needed. Restraint alternatives may not protect the person. The doctor may need to order restraints.

BOX 15-1	**Restraint Alternatives**

Physical Needs
* Life-long habits and routines are in the care plan. For example, showers before breakfast; reads in the bathroom; walks outside before lunch; watches TV after lunch.
* Pillows, wedge cushions, and posture and positioning devices are used.
* Food, fluid, hygiene, and elimination needs are met.
* The bedpan, urinal, or commode is within the person's reach.
* Back massages are given.
* A calm, quiet setting is provided.
* Exercise programs are provided.
* Outdoor time is planned for nice weather.
* Furniture meets the person's needs (lower bed, reclining chair, rocking chair).
* Observations and visits are made at least every 15 minutes. Or as often as directed by the nurse and the care plan.
* The person is moved to a room close to the nurses' station.
* Light is adjusted to meet the person's needs and preferences.
* Staff assignments are consistent.
* Sleep is not interrupted.
* Noise levels are reduced.

Safety and Security Needs
* The call light is within reach.
* Call lights are answered promptly.
* The person wanders in safe areas.
* All staff are aware of persons tending to wander. This includes staff in housekeeping, maintenance, the business office, dietary, and so on.

Safety and Security Needs—cont'd
* Knob guards are used on doors.
* Falls and injuries from falls are prevented (Chapter 14).
    * Padded hip protectors are worn under clothing (Fig. 15-1, p. 202).
    * Floor cushions are placed next to beds (Chapter 14).
    * Roll guards are attached to the bed frame (Fig. 15-2, p. 202).
* Warning alarms are used on beds, chairs, and doors.
* Walls and furniture corners are padded.
* Procedures and care measures are explained.
* Frequent explanations are given about equipment or devices.
* Confused persons are oriented to person, time, and place. Calendars and clocks are provided. See Chapter 49.

Love, Belonging, and Self-Esteem Needs
* Diversion is provided—TV, videos, music, games, relaxation, and so on.
* Family and friends make videos of themselves for the person to watch.
* Videos are made of visits with family and friends for the person to watch.
* Time is spent in supervised areas (dining room, lounge, by the nurses' station).
* Family, friends, and volunteers visit.
* The person has companions or sitters.
* Time is spent with the person.
* Extra time is spent with a person who is restless.
* Reminiscing is done with the person.
* The person does jobs or tasks he or she consents to.

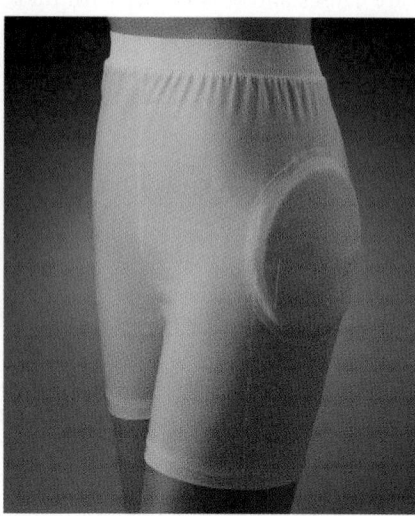

FIGURE 15-1 Hip protector. (Image courtesy Posey Company, Arcadia, Calif.)

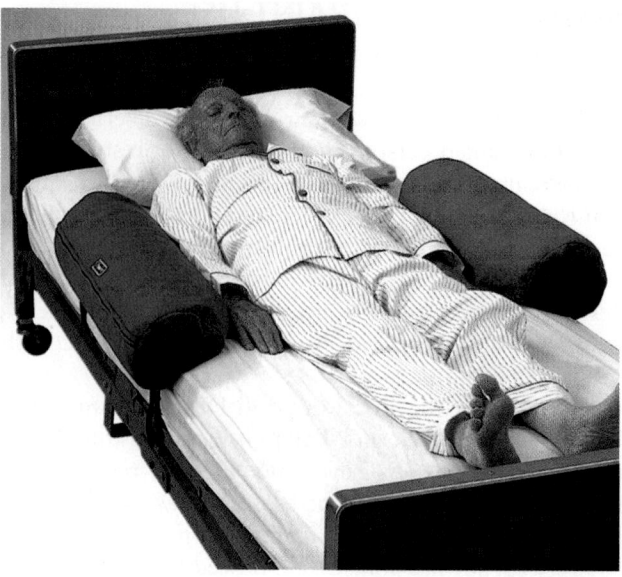

FIGURE 15-2 Roll guard. (Image courtesy Posey Company, Arcadia, Calif.)

SAFE RESTRAINT USE

Restraints can cause serious injury and even death. CMS, OBRA, FDA, and TJC rules and guidelines are followed. So are state laws. They are part of the agency's policies and procedures for restraint use.

Restraints are not used to discipline a person. They are not used for staff convenience. Restraints are used only when necessary to treat medical symptoms. A *medical symptom is an indication or characteristic of a physical or psychological condition.* Symptoms may relate to physical, emotional, or behavioral problems. Sometimes restraints are needed to protect the person or others. That is, a person may have violent or aggressive behaviors that are harmful to self or others or that are threatening to others.

See *Focus on Surveys: Safe Restraint Use.*

FOCUS ON SURVEYS

Safe Restraint Use

Agencies must have a policy about restraint use. Surveyors will try to learn if restraints were used:
- For discipline or staff convenience
- Only for a certain time for the person's well-being
Surveyors will review medical records and interview staff. Some questions will focus on:
- How staff members define "restraint."
- The medical symptoms leading to restraint use. Could they be reversed or reduced?
- The cause of the medical symptoms. Were they caused by failure to:
  - Meet the person's needs
  - Provide rehabilitation
  - Provide meaningful activities
  - Change the person's setting for safety
- If restraint alternatives were used.
- If the least restrictive restraints were used.
- If restraints were used for a short time.

Physical and Chemical Restraints

According to the CMS, a *physical restraint* includes these points.

- May be any manual method, physical or mechanical device, material, or equipment.
- Is attached to or next to the person's body.
- Cannot be removed easily by the person.
- Restricts freedom of movement or normal access to one's body.

Physical restraints are applied to the chest, waist, elbows, wrists, hands, or ankles. They confine the person to a bed or chair. Or they prevent movement of a body part. Some furniture or barriers also prevent freedom of movement.

- A device used with a chair that the person cannot remove easily. The device prevents the person from rising. Trays, tables, bars, and belts are examples (Fig. 15-3).
- Any chair that prevents the person from rising.
- Any bed or chair placed so close to the wall that the person cannot get out of the bed or chair.
- Bed rails (Chapter 14) that prevent the person from getting out of bed. For example, 4 half-length bed rails are raised. They are restraints if the person cannot lower them.
- Tucking in or using Velcro (or other device) to hold a sheet, fabric, or clothing so tightly that freedom of movement is restricted.

Drugs or drug dosages are *chemical restraints* if they:

- Control behavior or restrict movement.
- Are not standard treatment for the person's condition.

Drugs cannot be used for discipline or staff convenience. They cannot be used if they affect physical or mental function.

Sometimes drugs can help persons who are confused or disoriented. They may be anxious, agitated, or aggressive. The doctor may order drugs to control these behaviors. The drugs should not make the person sleepy and unable to function at his or her highest level.

Enablers. An *enabler is a device that limits freedom of movement but is used to promote independence, comfort, or safety.* Some devices can be restraints or enablers. When the person can easily remove the device and it helps the person function, it is an enabler. For example:

- A chair or wheelchair with a lap-top tray for meals, writing, and so on (see Fig. 15-3). The chair is an enabler. If used to limit freedom of movement, the chair is a restraint.
- A person chooses to have raised bed rails. The bed rails are used to move in bed and to prevent falling out of bed. The bed rails are enablers, not restraints.

Risks From Restraint Use

Box 15-2 lists the risks from restraints. Injuries can occur as the person tries to get free of the restraint. Injuries also occur from using the wrong restraint, applying it wrong, or keeping it on too long. Cuts, bruises, and fractures are common. *The most serious risk is death from strangulation.*

Restraints are medical devices. The *Safe Medical Devices Act* applies if a restraint causes illness, injury, or death. Also, CMS requires the reporting of any death that occurs:

- While a person is in a restraint.
- Within 24 hours after a restraint was removed.
- Within 1 week after a restraint was removed. This is done if the restraint may have contributed directly or indirectly to the person's death.

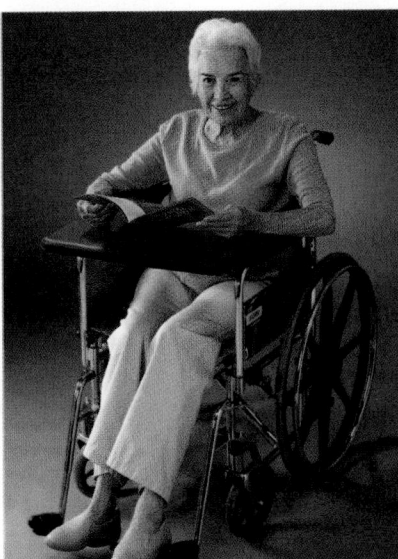

FIGURE 15-3 This lap-top tray is a restraint alternative. It is a restraint when used to prevent freedom of movement. (Image courtesy Posey Company, Arcadia, Calif.)

BOX 15-2	Risks From Restraint Use

- Constipation
- Contractures
- Cuts and bruises
- Decline in physical function (ability to walk, muscle problems)
- Dehydration
- Falls
- Fractures
- Head trauma
- Incontinence
- Infections: pneumonia and urinary tract
- Nerve injuries
- Pressure ulcers
- Social and mental health problems: agitation, anger, delirium, depression, loss of dignity, embarrassment and humiliation, mistrust, loss of self-respect, reduced social contact, withdrawal
- Strangulation

Laws, Rules, and Guidelines

Laws (federal and state) and rules (CMS, FDA) for restraint use are followed. So are accrediting agency (TJC) guidelines. Remember:

- *Restraints must protect the person.* They are not used for staff convenience or to discipline a person. Using restraints is not easier than properly supervising and observing the person. A restrained person requires more staff time for care, supervision, and observation. A restraint is used only when it is the best safety measure for the person. Restraints are not used to punish or penalize uncooperative persons.
- *A doctor's order is required.* OBRA, CMS, state laws, FDA warnings, TJC, and other accrediting agencies protect persons from unnecessary restraints. If restraints are needed for medical reasons, a doctor's order is required. The doctor gives the reason for the restraint, what body part to restrain, what to use, and how long to use it. This information is on the care plan and your assignment sheet. In an emergency, the nurse can decide to apply restraints before getting a doctor's order.
- *The least restrictive method is used.* It allows the greatest amount of movement or body access possible. Some restraints attach to the person's body and to a fixed (non-movable) object. They restrict freedom of movement or body access. Vest, jacket, ankle, wrist, hand, and some belt restraints are examples. Other restraints are near but not directly attached to the person's body (bed rails or wedge cushions). They do not totally restrict freedom of movement and are less restrictive. They allow access to certain body parts.
- *Restraints are used only after other measures fail to protect the person* (see Box 15-1). Some people can harm themselves or others. The care plan must include measures to protect the person and prevent harm to others. Many fall prevention measures are restraint alternatives (Chapter 14).
- *Unnecessary restraint is false imprisonment* (Chapter 5). You must clearly understand the reason for the restraint and its risks. If not, politely ask about its use. If you apply an unneeded restraint, you could face false imprisonment charges.
- *Informed consent is required.* The person must understand the reason for the restraint. The person is told how the restraint will help the planned medical treatment. The person is told about the risks of restraint use. If the person cannot give consent, his or her legal representative is given the information for purposes of giving consent. Consent must be given before a restraint can be used. The doctor or nurse provides needed information and obtains the consent.

Safety Guidelines

The restrained person must be kept safe. Follow the safety measures in Box 15-3. Also remember these key points.

- *Observe for increased confusion and agitation.* Restraints can increase confusion and agitation. Whether confused or alert, people are aware of restricted movements. They may try to get out of the restraint or struggle to pull at it. Some restrained persons beg others to free or to help release them. These behaviors often are viewed as signs of confusion. Some people become more confused because they do not understand what is happening to them. Restrained persons need repeated explanations and reassurance. Spending time with them has a calming effect.
- *Protect the person's quality of life.* Restraints are used for as short a time as possible. The care plan must show how to reduce restraint use. The person's needs are met with as little restraint as possible. You must meet the person's physical, emotional, and social needs. Visit with the person and explain the reason for the restraint.
- *Follow the manufacturer's instructions.* They explain how to safely apply and secure the restraint. The restraint must be snug and firm but not tight. Tight restraints affect circulation and breathing. The person must be comfortable and able to move the restrained part to a limited and safe extent. You could be negligent if you do not apply or secure a restraint properly.
- *Apply restraints with enough help to protect the person and staff from injury.* Persons in immediate danger of harming themselves or others are restrained quickly. Combative and agitated people can hurt themselves and the staff when restraints are applied. Enough staff members are needed to complete the task safely and quickly.
- *Observe the person at least every 15 minutes or as often as directed by the nurse and the care plan.* Restraints are dangerous. Injuries and deaths can result from improper restraint use and poor observation. Prevent complications. Breathing and circulation problems are examples.
- *Remove or release the restraint, re-position the person, and meet basic needs at least every 2 hours. Or do so as often as noted in the care plan.*
  - Remove or release the restraint for at least 10 minutes.
  - Provide for food, fluid, comfort, safety, hygiene, and elimination needs. Also give skin care.
  - Perform ROM exercises or help the person walk (Chapter 30). Follow the care plan.

See *Focus on Communication: Safety Guidelines,* p. 208.
See *Teamwork and Time Management: Safety Guidelines,* p. 209.

Text continued on p. 210.

BOX 15-3	Safety Measures for Using Restraints

Before Applying Restraints

- Do not use sheets, towels, tape, rope, straps, bandages, Velcro, or other items to restrain a person.
- Apply a restraint only after being instructed about its proper use.
- Demonstrate proper application of the restraint before applying it.
- Use the restraint noted in the care plan. Use the correct size. Small restraints are tight. They cause discomfort and agitation. They also restrict breathing and circulation. Strangulation is a risk from big or loose restraints.
- Use only restraints that have manufacturer's instructions and warning labels.
  - Read the warning labels. Note the front and back of the restraint.
  - Follow the instructions. Some restraints are safe for bed, chair, and wheelchair use. Others are used only with certain equipment.
- Use intact restraints.
  - Look for broken stitches, tears, cuts, or frayed fabric or straps.
  - Look for missing or loose buckles, locks, hooks, loops, or straps or other damage. The restraint must hold securely.
- Test zippers, buckles, locks, hooks, loops, and other fasteners. The device must fasten securely.
- Do not use a restraint near a fire, a flame, or smoking materials.

Applying Restraints

- Follow agency policies and procedures.
- Do not use a restraint to:
  - Position a person on a toilet.
  - Position a person on furniture that does not allow for correct application.
- Position the person in good alignment before applying the restraint (Chapter 17).
  - Semi-Fowler's position (Chapter 20) is usually preferred for a vest, jacket, or belt restraint.
  - When in a chair, position the person so the hips are well to the back of the chair.
- Pad bony areas and the skin as instructed by the nurse. This prevents pressure and injury from the restraint.
- Follow the manufacturer's instructions. A restraint applied wrong or backward may cause serious injury or death. Death may occur from suffocation or strangulation.
  - For a vest restraint, the "V" neck is in front (Fig. 15-4, p. 206).
  - For a jacket restraint, the opening is in the back.
  - For a belt restraint when in a chair—Apply the restraint at a 45-degree angle over the thighs (Fig. 15-5, p. 206).
- Do not criss-cross straps in the back unless required by the manufacturer's instructions (Fig. 15-6, p. 206). Straps may loosen when the person moves and cause serious injury.
- Secure restraints according to agency policy. The policy should follow the manufacturer's instructions and allow for quick release in an emergency. Quick-release buckles or airline-type buckles are used (Fig. 15-7, p. 206). So are quick-release ties (Fig. 15-8, p. 207).
- Secure straps out of the person's reach.
- Leave 1 to 2 inches of slack in the straps if directed to do so by the nurse. This allows some movement of the part.

Applying Restraints—cont'd

- Secure the restraint to the movable part of the bed frame (Fig. 15-9, p. 207). The restraint will not tighten or loosen when the head or foot of the bed is raised or lowered. For chairs, secure straps under the seat of the wheelchair or chair (Fig. 15-10, p. 207).
- Check for snugness after applying the restraint. The restraint should be snug but allow some movement of the restrained part. Follow the manufacturer's instructions. For example:
  - *If applied to the chest or waist*—Make sure the person can breathe easily. A flat hand should slide between the restraint and the person's body (Fig. 15-11, p. 207). Check with the nurse if you have very small or very large hands. Small or large hands could cause the restraint to be too tight or too loose.
  - *For wrist and mitt restraints*—You should be able to slide 1 finger under the restraint. Check with the nurse if you have very small or very large fingers. Small or large fingers could cause the restraint to be too tight or too loose.
- Make sure that the straps:
  - Cannot tighten, loosen, slip, or cause too much slack.
  - Will not slide in any direction. If straps slide, they change the restraint's position. The person can get suspended off the mattress or chair (Figs. 15-12 and 15-13, p. 208). Strangulation can result.
- Never secure restraints to the bed rails. The person can reach bed rails to release knots or buckles. Also, injury to the person is likely when raising or lowering bed rails.
- Use bed rail covers or gap protectors as instructed by the nurse (Fig. 15-14, p. 208). They prevent entrapment between the rails or the bed rail bars (see Fig. 15-12). Entrapment can occur between:
  - The bars of a bed rail
  - The space between half-length (split) bed rails
  - The bed rail and mattress
  - The head-board or foot-board and mattress

After Applying Restraints

- Keep full bed rails up when using a vest, jacket, or belt restraint. Also use bed rail covers or gap protectors. Otherwise the person could fall off the bed and strangle on the restraint. Or the person can get caught between half-length bed rails.
- Do not use back cushions when a person is restrained in a chair. If the cushion moves out of place, slack occurs in the straps. Strangulation is a risk if the person slides forward or down from the extra slack.
- Do not cover the person with a sheet, blanket, bedspread, or other covering. The restraint must be within plain view at all times.
- Check the person at least every 15 minutes for safety, comfort, and signs of injury. Or check the person as often as directed by the nurse and the care plan.
- Monitor persons in the supine (back-lying) position constantly. Aspiration is a great risk if vomiting occurs (Chapter 27). Call for the nurse at once.

Continued

BOX 15-3   Safety Measures for Using Restraints—cont'd

After Applying Restraints—cont'd

- Check the person's circulation at least every 15 minutes or as often as directed by the nurse and the care plan.
  - *For mitt, wrist, or ankle restraints*—You should feel a pulse at a pulse site below the restraint. Fingers or toes should be warm and pink. Tell the nurse at once if:
    - *You cannot feel a pulse.*
    - *Fingers or toes are cold, pale, or blue in color.*
    - *The person complains of pain, numbness, or tingling in the restrained part.*
    - *The skin is red or damaged.*
  - *For a belt, jacket, or vest restraint*—The person should be able to breathe easily. Also check the position of the restraint, especially in the front and back.
- Keep scissors in your pocket. In an emergency, cutting the tie may be faster than untying a knot. Never leave scissors where the person can reach them. Make sure the person cannot reach the scissors in your pocket.

After Applying Restraints—cont'd

- Remove or release the restraint and re-position the person every 2 hours or as often as noted in the care plan. The restraint is removed or released for at least 10 minutes. Meet the person's basic needs. You need to:
  - Measure vital signs.
  - Meet elimination needs.
  - Offer food and fluids.
  - Meet hygiene needs.
  - Give skin care.
  - Perform range-of-motion (ROM) exercises or help the person walk. Follow the care plan.
  - Provide for physical and emotional comfort. (See the inside of the front cover.)
- Keep the call light and other needed items within the person's reach. Chart that this was done.
- Complete a safety check before leaving the room. (See the inside of the front cover.)
- Report to the nurse every time you checked the person and removed or released the restraint. Report your observations and the care given (Fig. 15-15, p. 209). Follow agency policy for recording.

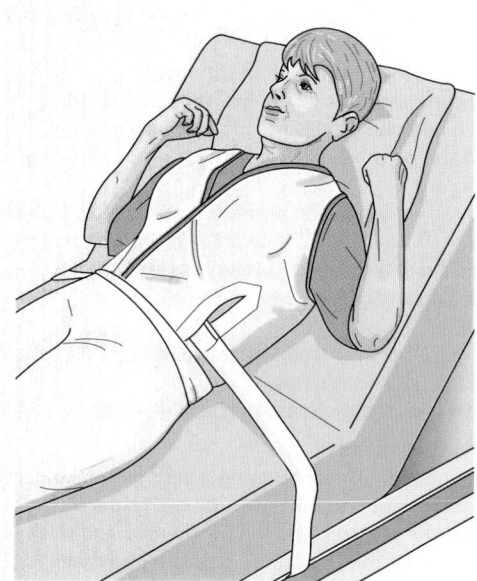

FIGURE 15-4 The vest restraint criss-crosses in front. The "V" neck is in front. (NOTE: The bed rails are raised after the restraint is applied.)

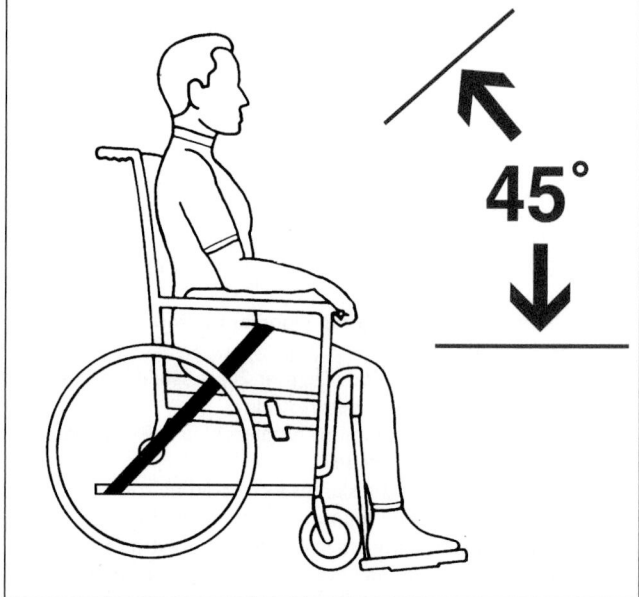

FIGURE 15-5 The belt restraint is at a 45-degree angle over the thighs. (Image courtesy Posey Company, Arcadia, Calif.)

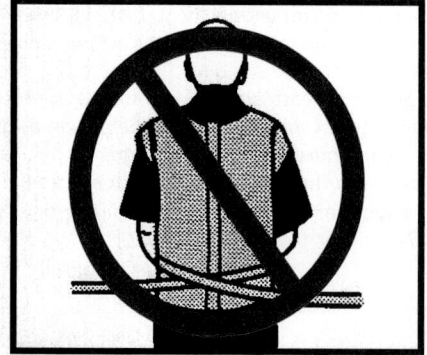

FIGURE 15-6 Never criss-cross vest or jacket straps in the back. (Image courtesy Posey Company, Arcadia, Calif.)

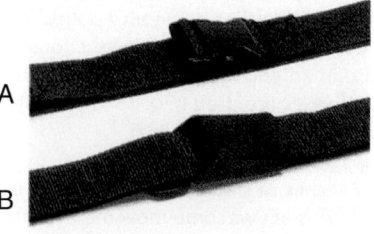

FIGURE 15-7 A, Quick-release buckle. **B,** Airline-type buckle. (Image courtesy Posey Company, Arcadia, Calif.)

How to Tie the Posey Quick-Release Tie

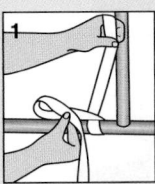 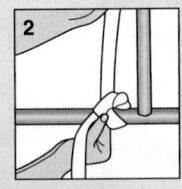 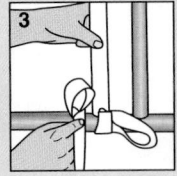 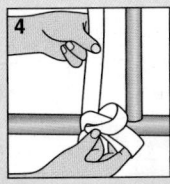 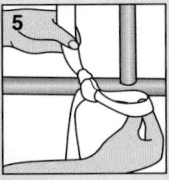

1. Wrap the strap once around a movable part of the bed frame leaving at least an 8″ (20 cm) tail. Fold the loose end in half to create a loop and cross it over the other end.
2. Insert the folded strap where the straps cross over each other, as if tying a shoelace. Pull on the loop to tighten.
3. Fold the loose end in half to create a second loop.
4. Insert the second loop into the first loop.
5. Pull on the loop to tighten. Test to make sure strap is secure and will not slide in any direction.
6. Repeat on other side. Practice quick-release ties to ensure the knot releases with one pull on the loose end of the strap.

FIGURE 15-8 The Posey quick-release tie. (Image courtesy Posey Company, Arcadia, Calif.)

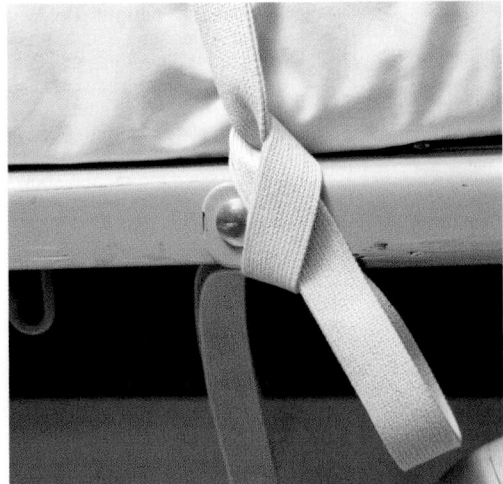

FIGURE 15-9 The restraint is secured to the movable part of the bed frame.

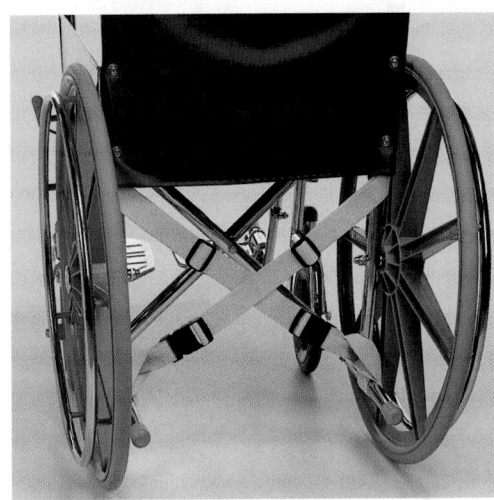

FIGURE 15-10 The restraint straps are secured to the wheelchair frame. (Image courtesy Posey Company, Arcadia, Calif.)

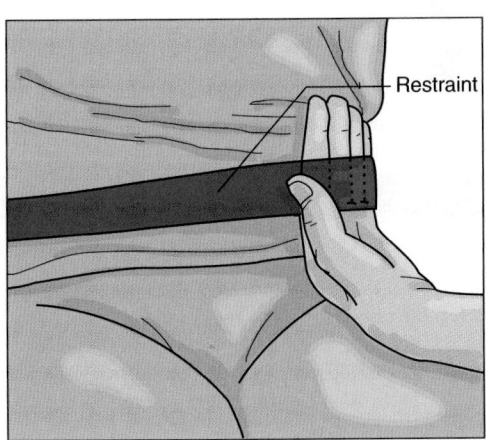

Restraint

FIGURE 15-11 A flat hand slides between the restraint and the person.

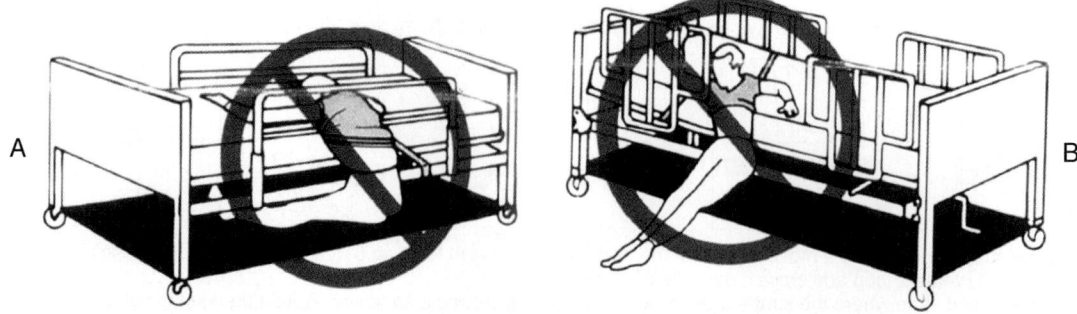

FIGURE 15-12 A, A person can get suspended and caught between bed rail bars. **B,** The person can get suspended and caught between half-length bed rails. (Images courtesy Posey Company, Arcadia, Calif.)

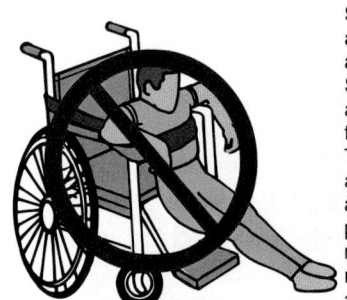

Straps to prevent sliding should always be over the thighs—NOT around the waist or chest. Straps should be at a 45° angle and secured to the chair under the seat, not behind the back. They should be snug but comfortable and not restrict breathing. If a belt or vest is too loose or applied around the waist, the person may slide partially off the seat— resulting in possible suffocation and death.

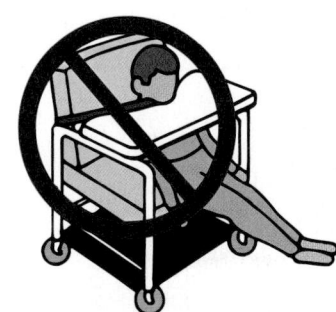

Tray tables (with or without a belt or vest) pose potential danger if the person should slide partly under the table and become caught. This could result in suffocation and death. Make sure the person's hips are positioned at the back of the chair— this may necessitate the use of an anti-slide material (Posey Grip), a pommel cushion, or a restrictive device if the person shows any tendency to slide forward.

FIGURE 15-13 Strangulation can result if the person slides forward or down because of extra slack in the restraint. (Images courtesy Posey Company, Arcadia, Calif.)

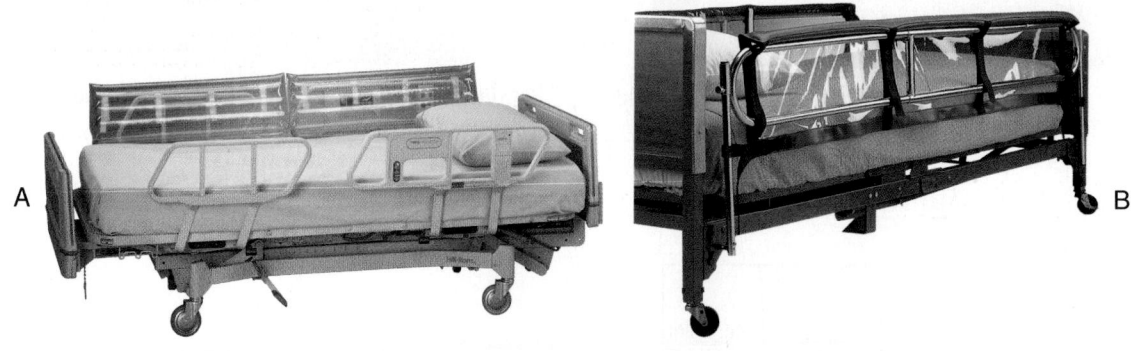

FIGURE 15-14 A, Bed rail protector. **B,** Guard rail pads. (Images courtesy Posey Company, Arcadia, Calif.)

FOCUS ON **COMMUNICATION**

Safety Guidelines

Restraints can increase confusion. Remind the person of the reason for the restraint and to call for help when it is needed. Repeat the following as often as needed.

- "Dr. Monroe ordered this restraint so you don't hurt yourself. If you need to get up, please call for help. I'll check on you every 15 minutes. Other staff will check on you too."
- "How does the restraint feel? Is it too tight? Is it too loose?"

- "Please put your call light on. I want to make sure that you can reach and use it with the restraint on."
- "Please call for help right away if the restraint is too tight."
- "Please call for help right away if you feel pain in your fingers or hands. Also call for me if you feel numbness or tingling."
- "Please call for help right away if you are having problems breathing."

RESTRAINT MONITORING

PARKER, LOUISE DOB: 7/14/1948 GENDER: Female ID# 0003788965

Room 304B DATE: Jan 04 TIME: 1430 USERNAME: Sharon Clark, CNA

Restraint Alternatives Before Restraints Applied

☒ Physical needs met	☒ Diversion	☒ Re-oriented person
☒ Safety and security needs met	☒ Increased supervision	☒ Sat quietly/talked with person
☒ Comfort measures	☐ Companion or sitter	☒ Care measures explained
☒ Pain relief measures	☒ Exercise/activity/re-positioning	☒ Fall prevention measures
☒ Calm, quiet setting	☒ Protection of IV/dressing/other	☐ Other:

Restraint Type and Location

☐ Soft limb — ☐ Right wrist ☐ Right ankle ☐ Left wrist ☐ Left ankle

☒ Mitt — ☒ Right wrist ☒ Left wrist

☐ Elbow splint — ☐ Right arm ☐ Left arm

☐ Belt ☐ Vest ☐ Jacket ☐ Other:

Care Measures

☒ Restraints released/removed Duration: 15 minutes
☒ Restraints re-applied
☐ Measures refused
Notified nurse: Evan Scott, RN

☒ Food/fluid needs met ☒ ROM/exercise/activity ☒ Urinary/bowel elimination ☒ Positioning ☒ Call light and needed items in reach

☒ Comfort measures ☒ Skin care ☒ Hygiene ☐ Other:

Vital Signs

Temp 98.4 °F Pulse 70 R 14 BP 116/72 mmHg Pain; 0 /10

Circulation Observations (Normal in blue)

Color: ☒ Pink ☐ Pale ☐ Cyanotic (bluish)
Temperature: ☐ Hot ☒ Warm ☐ Cool ☐ Cold
Sensation: ☒ Good sensation ☐ Numbness/tingling ☐ No sensation
Movement: ☒ Able to move extremities ☐ Unable to move extremities
Pulses: ☒ Pulses present in all extremities ☐ Pulse faint/absent in any extremity

Tell the nurse at once if any observations are abnormal. Notified Nurse:

Behavior Observations

☒ Alert	☐ Agitated	☐ Restless	☐ Drowsy
☒ Calm/cooperative	☐ Aggressive	☐ Confused	☐ Sleeping

FIGURE 15-15 Charting sample.

TEAMWORK AND TIME MANAGEMENT
Safety Guidelines

You may not be assigned to a restrained person. However, make sure you know who is restrained on your unit. When you walk past the person or the person's room, check if the person is safe and comfortable. Answer the person's call light promptly.

Reporting and Recording

Restraint information is recorded in the person's medical record (see Fig. 15-15). If you apply restraints or care for a restrained person, report and record:

- The type of restraint applied.
- The body part or parts restrained.
- The reason for the application.
- Safety measures taken (for example, bed rails padded and up, call light within reach).
- The time you applied the restraint.
- The time you removed or released the restraint and for how long.
- The person's vital signs.
- The care given when the restraint was removed and for how long.
- Skin color and condition.
- Condition of the limbs.
- The pulse felt in the restrained part.
- Changes in the person's behavior.
  Report the following complaints at once.
- Difficulty breathing
- Pain, numbness, or tingling in the restrained part
- Discomfort
- A tight restraint

Applying Restraints

Restraints are made of cloth or leather. Cloth restraints (soft restraints) are mitts, belts, straps, jackets, and vests. They are applied to the wrists, ankles, hands, waist, and chest. Leather restraints are applied to the wrists and ankles. Leather restraints are used for extreme agitation and combativeness.

Wrist Restraints. Wrist restraints (limb holders) limit arm movement (Fig. 15-16). They may be used when the person:

- Is at risk for pulling out tubes used for life-saving treatment (intravenous [IV] infusion, feeding tube).
- Is at risk for pulling at devices used to monitor vital signs.
- Scratches at, pulls at, or peels the skin, a wound, or a dressing. This can damage the skin or the wound.

Mitt Restraints. Hands are placed in mitt restraints. They prevent finger use. They allow hand, wrist, and arm movements. They have the same purpose as wrist restraints. Most mitts are padded (Fig. 15-17).

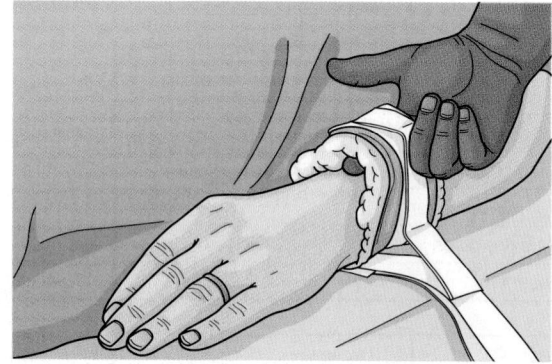

FIGURE 15-16 Wrist restraint. The soft part is toward the skin. Note that 1 finger fits between the restraint and the wrist.

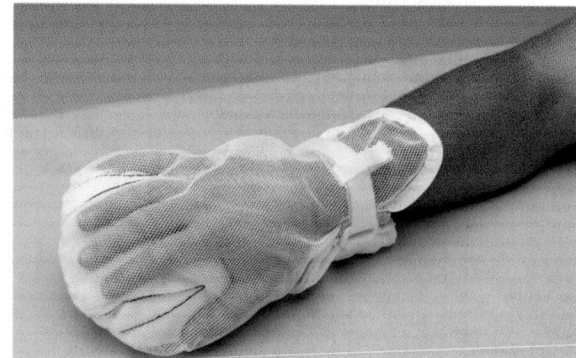

FIGURE 15-17 Mitt restraint. (Image courtesy Posey Company, Arcadia, Calif.)

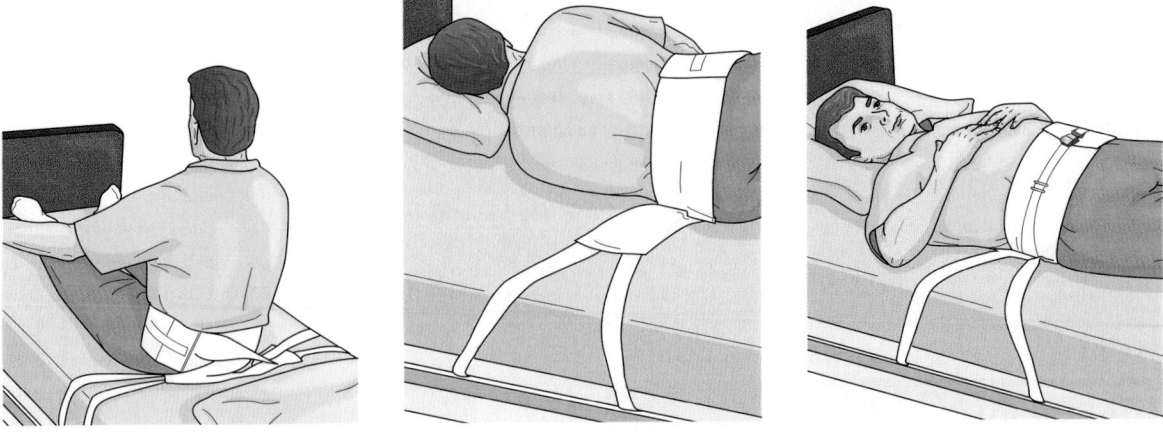

FIGURE 15-18 Belt restraint. (NOTE: The bed rails are raised after the restraint is applied.)

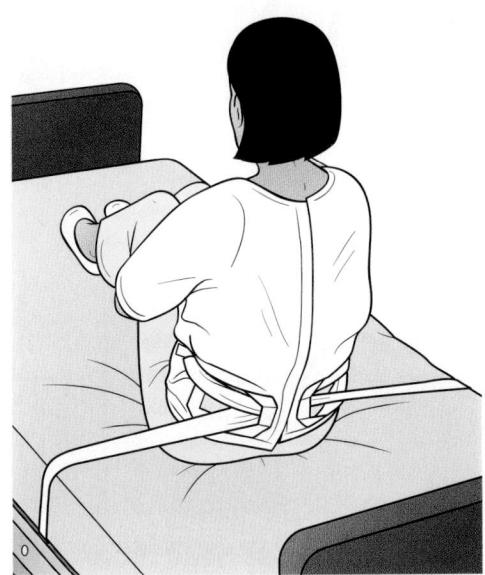

FIGURE 15-19 Jacket restraint. (NOTE: The bed rails are raised after the restraint is applied.)

FOCUS ON COMMUNICATION

Applying Restraints

If you do not know how to apply a certain restraint, do not do so. Ask the nurse to show you the correct way. You can say: "I've never applied a restraint like this before. Would you please show me how and then watch me apply it?" Thank the nurse for helping you.

When applying a restraint, explain to the person what you are going to do. Then tell the person what you are doing step-by-step. Always check for safety and comfort. You can ask: "How does the restraint feel? Is it too tight? Is it too loose?"

Make sure the person can communicate with you after leaving the room. Place the call light within reach. Make sure the person can use it with the restraint on. Remind the person to call if uncomfortable or if anything is needed.

Belt Restraints. A belt restraint (Fig. 15-18) may be used when injuries from falls are risks or for positioning during a medical treatment. The person cannot get out of bed or out of a chair. However, a roll belt allows the person to turn from side to side or to sit up in bed.

The belt is applied around the waist and secured to the bed or chair (lap belt). It is applied over a garment. The person can release the quick-release type. It is less restrictive than those that only staff can release.

Vest Restraints and Jacket Restraints. Vest and jacket restraints are applied to the chest. They have the same purpose as belt restraints. The person cannot turn in bed or get out of a chair.

A jacket restraint is applied with the opening in the back. For a vest restraint, the "V" neck is in front and the vest crosses in the front (see Fig. 15-4). Vest and jacket restraints are never worn backward. Strangulation or other injuries are risks if the person slides down in the bed or chair. The restraint is always applied over a garment. (NOTE: *The straps of vest and jacket restraints cross in the front. A vest or jacket restraint may have a positioning slot in the back* [Fig. 15-19]. *Criss-cross straps following the manufacturer's instructions.*)

Vest and jacket restraints have life-threatening risks. Death can occur from strangulation. If caught in the restraint, it can become so tight that the person's chest cannot expand to inhale air. The person quickly suffocates and dies. Correct application is critical. You are advised to only assist the nurse in applying them. The nurse should assume full responsibility for applying a vest or jacket restraint.

See *Focus on Communication: Applying Restraints.*

See *Focus on Children and Older Persons: Applying Restraints*, p. 212.

See *Delegation Guidelines: Applying Restraints*, p. 212.

See *Promoting Safety and Comfort: Applying Restraints*, p. 212.

See procedure: *Applying Restraints*, p. 213.

FOCUS ON CHILDREN AND OLDER PERSONS
Applying Restraints

Children
Elbow splints limit arm movements. They prevent infants and children from bending their elbows (Fig. 15-20). They are used to prevent scratching and touching incisions or pulling out tubes. Both arms are restrained to achieve the desired effect.

Older Persons
Restraints may increase confusion and agitation in persons with dementia. They do not understand what you are doing. They may resist your efforts to apply a restraint. They may try to get free from the restraint. Serious injury and death are risks.

Never use force to apply a restraint. If a person is confused or agitated, ask a co-worker to help apply the restraint. Report problems to the nurse at once.

DELEGATION GUIDELINES
Applying Restraints

Before applying a restraint, you need this information from the nurse and the care plan.
- Why the doctor ordered the restraint.
- What type and size to use.
- Where to apply the restraint.
- How to safely apply the restraint. Have the nurse show you how to apply it. Then show correct application back to the nurse.
- How to correctly position the person.
- What bony areas to pad and how to pad them.
- If bed rail covers or gap protectors are needed.
- If bed rails are up or down.
- What special equipment is needed.
- If the person needs to be checked more or less often than every 15 minutes. If yes, how often?
- When to apply and release the restraint.
- What observations to report and record. See "Reporting and Recording," p. 210.
- When to report observations.
- What patient or resident concerns to report at once.

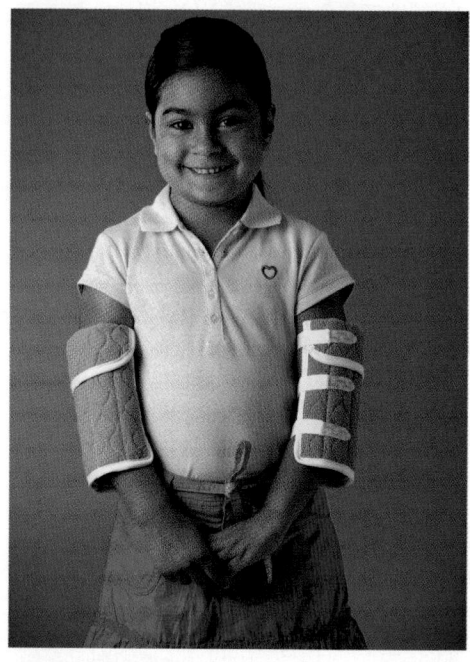

FIGURE 15-20 Elbow splints. (Image courtesy Posey Company, Arcadia, Calif.)

PROMOTING SAFETY AND COMFORT
Applying Restraints

Safety
Restraints can cause serious harm, even death. Always follow the manufacturer's instructions. The instructions for 1 restraint may not apply to another. Also, the manufacturer may have instructions for applying restraints on persons who are agitated.

Never use force. Ask a co-worker to help if a person is confused and agitated. Report problems to the nurse at once.

Check the person at least every 15 minutes or as often as directed by the nurse and the care plan. Make sure the call light is within reach. Ask the person to use the call light at the first sign of problems or discomfort.

Never use a restraint as a seat belt in a car or other vehicle.

Mitt Restraints
Mitt restraints prevent finger use. Often they are not secured to the bed or chair. Therefore the person can raise the mitt to his or her mouth. Observe the person closely to make sure that he or she does not:
- Use the teeth to remove or damage the device.
- Ingest any mitt material.

Mitt Restraints—cont'd
Persons with mitt restraints may be able to walk about. Falls are a risk. Practice safety measures to prevent falls (Chapter 14).

Belt, Vest, and Jacket Restraints
If a belt, vest, or jacket restraint is ordered, monitor the person to make sure that he or she cannot:
- Slide forward or down in the chair or bed and become suspended or entrapped.
- Fall off the chair or mattress and become suspended or entrapped.

Comfort
The person's comfort is always important when restraints are used. Restraints limit movement. This affects position changes and reaching needed items. Position the person in good alignment before applying a restraint (Chapter 17). Also make sure the person can reach needed items—call light, water mug, tissues, phone, bed controls, and so on.

Applying Restraints

QUALITY OF LIFE

- Knock before entering the person's room.
- Address the person by name.
- Introduce yourself by name and title.

- Explain the procedure before starting and during the procedure.
- Protect the person's rights during the procedure.
- Handle the person gently during the procedure.

PRE-PROCEDURE

1 Follow *Delegation Guidelines: Applying Restraints*. See *Promoting Safety and Comfort: Applying Restraints*.
2 Collect the following as instructed by the nurse.
   - Correct type and size of restraint
   - Padding for skin and bony areas
   - Bed rail pads or gap protectors (if needed)

3 Practice hand hygiene.
4 Identify the person. Check the ID (identification) bracelet against the assignment sheet. Use 2 identifiers (Chapter 13). Also call the person by name.
5 Provide for privacy.

PROCEDURE

6 Position the person for comfort and good alignment.
7 Put the bed rail pads or gap protectors (if needed) on the bed if the person is in bed. Follow the manufacturer's instructions.
8 Pad bony areas. Follow the nurse's instructions and the care plan.
9 Read the manufacturer's instructions. Note the front and back of the restraint.
10 *For wrist restraints:*
   a Apply the restraint following the manufacturer's instructions. Place the soft or foam part toward the skin.
   b Secure the restraint so it is snug but not tight. Make sure you can slide 1 finger under the restraint (see Fig. 15-16). Follow the manufacturer's instructions. Adjust the straps if the restraint is too loose or too tight. Check for snugness again.
   c Secure the straps to the movable part of the bed frame out of the person's reach. Use the buckle or a quick-release tie.
   d Repeat step 10, a–c for the other wrist.
11 *For mitt restraints:*
   a Clean and dry the person's hands.
   b Insert the person's hand into the restraint with the palm down. Follow the manufacturer's instructions.
   c Wrap the wrist strap around the smallest part of the wrist. Secure the strap with the hook-and-loop closure.
   d Secure the restraint to the bed if directed to do so. Secure the straps to the movable part of the bed frame out of the person's reach. Use the buckle or a quick-release tie.
   e Check for snugness. Slide 1 finger between the restraint and the wrist. Follow the manufacturer's instructions. Adjust the straps if the restraint is too loose or too tight. Check for snugness again.
   f Repeat step 11, b–e for the other hand.

12 *For a belt restraint:*
   a Assist the person to a sitting position.
   b Apply the restraint. Follow the manufacturer's instructions.
   c Remove wrinkles or creases from the front and back of the restraint.
   d Bring the ties through the slots in the belt.
   e Position the straps at a 45-degree angle between the wheelchair seat and sides (see Fig. 15-5). If in bed, help the person lie down.
   f Make sure the person is comfortable and in good alignment.
   g Secure the straps to the movable part of the bed frame. Use the buckle or a quick-release tie. The buckle or tie is out of the person's reach. For a wheelchair, criss-cross and secure the straps as in Figure 15-10.
   h Check for snugness. Slide an open hand between the restraint and the person. Adjust the restraint if it is too loose or too tight. Check for snugness again.
13 *For a vest restraint:*
   a Assist the person to a sitting position. If in a wheelchair:
      1) Position him or her as far back in the wheelchair as possible.
      2) Make sure the buttocks are against the chair back.
   b Apply the restraint. Follow the manufacturer's instructions. The "V" part of the vest crosses in front.
   c Bring the straps through the slots.
   d Remove wrinkles in the front and back.
   e Position the straps at a 45-degree angle between the wheelchair seat and sides. If in bed, help the person lie down.
   f Make sure the person is comfortable and in good alignment.
   g Secure the straps to the movable part of the bed frame at waist level. Use the buckle or a quick-release tie. The buckle or tie is out of the person's reach. For a wheelchair, criss-cross and secure the straps as in Figure 15-10.
   h Check for snugness. Slide an open hand between the restraint and the person. Adjust the restraint if it is too loose or too tight. Check for snugness again.

Continued

Applying Restraints—cont'd

PROCEDURE—cont'd

14 *For a jacket restraint:*
  a Assist the person to a sitting position. If in a wheelchair:
    1) Position him or her as far back in the wheelchair as possible.
    2) Make sure the buttocks are against the chair back.
  b Apply the restraint. Follow the manufacturer's instructions. The jacket opening goes in the back.
  c Close the back with the zipper, ties, or hook-and-loop closures.
  d Make sure the side seams are under the arms. Remove wrinkles in the front and back.
  e Position the straps at a 45-degree angle between the wheelchair seat and sides. If in bed, help the person lie down.
  f Make sure the person is comfortable and in good alignment.
  g Secure the straps to the movable part of the bed frame at waist level. Use the buckle or quick-release tie. The buckle or tie is out of the person's reach. For a wheelchair, criss-cross and secure the straps as in Figure 15-10.
  h Check for snugness. Slide an open hand between the restraint and the person. Adjust the restraint if it is too loose or too tight. Check for snugness again.

15 *For elbow splints:*
  a Release the adjustment straps (hook-and-loop).
  b Wrap a splint over 1 arm. The splint is centered over the elbow.
  c Secure the hook fastener to the quilted material. If necessary to hold the splint in place, use a safety pin to secure the splint to the person's clothing at the top and bottom of the splint.
  d Check for snugness. Slide 2 fingers between the splint and the person's arm. Adjust the splint if it is too loose or too tight. Check for snugness again.
  e Repeat step 15, a–d for the other arm.

POST-PROCEDURE

16 Position the person as the nurse directs.
17 Provide for comfort. (See the inside of the front cover.)
18 Place the call light and other needed items within the person's reach.
19 Raise or lower bed rails. Follow the care plan and the manufacturer's instructions for the restraint.
20 Unscreen the person.
21 Complete a safety check of the room. (See the inside of the front cover.)
22 Practice hand hygiene.
23 Check the person and the restraint at least every 15 minutes or as often as directed by the nurse and the care plan. Report and record your observations.
  a For wrist or mitt restraints or elbow splints: check the pulse, color, and temperature of the restrained parts.
  b For a vest, jacket, or belt restraint: check the person's breathing. *Call for the nurse at once if the person is not breathing or is having problems breathing.* Make sure the restraint is properly positioned in the front and back.

24 Do the following at least every 2 hours for at least 10 minutes.
  a Remove or release the restraint.
  b Measure vital signs.
  c Re-position the person.
  d Meet food, fluid, hygiene, and elimination needs.
  e Give skin care.
  f Perform ROM exercises or help the person walk. Follow the care plan.
  g Provide for physical and emotional comfort. (See the inside of the front cover.)
  h Re-apply the restraint.
25 Complete a safety check of the room. (See the inside of the front cover.)
26 Practice hand hygiene.
27 Report and record your observations and the care given.

FOCUS ON **P R I D E**

The Person, Family, and Yourself

Personal and Professional Responsibility

Restraints have many risks. See Box 15-2. Therefore restraint use brings many responsibilities. You must:

- Monitor the person for safety.
- Apply the restraint properly.
- Promote comfort.
- Observe the person closely.
- Meet basic needs.
- Report any concerns to the nurse.

If you do not know how to apply a restraint, do not do so. Ask the nurse to show you. To use restraints safely and responsibly, follow the guidelines in Box 15-3.

Rights and Respect

Every person has the right to freedom from restraint. Restraints are used only as a last resort to protect the person or others from harm. Other methods must be tried before restraints are used. You may be asked to assist with restraint alternatives (see Box 15-1). Make a genuine effort. Be honest. Do not tell the nurse you tried if you really did not. Do your best to allow the person the right to freedom from restraint.

Independence and Social Interaction

All restraints limit movement. Independence is restricted. To promote independence:

- Keep the call light within reach at all times. Make sure the person can use it. Tell the person to signal for you if anything is needed. Answer the call light and meet the person's needs promptly.
- Keep needed items within reach. This is most important with restraints that allow hand and arm use. Belt, vest, and jacket restraints and elbow splints are examples.
- Check the person at least every 15 minutes or as often as directed by the nurse and the care plan.
- Remove or release the restraint at least every 2 hours.
- Meet food, fluid, hygiene, and elimination needs.
- Assist the person with walks or ROM exercises.
- Allow choice. For example, let the person choose where to walk or what to eat and drink.
- Let the person do as much for himself or herself as safely possible.

Personal choice and freedom of movement promote independence, dignity, and self-esteem. Provide care that gives restrained persons the independence they deserve.

Delegation and Teamwork

Care conferences are held to meet the person's safety needs. The health team reviews and updates the person's care plan. Every attempt is made to protect the person without restraints.

You are an important member of the health team. Your input has value. Share your observations and ideas. For example, Mrs. Garner does not try to get out of her chair when she looks through her photo albums or reads a book. You share this with the team. They include diversion activities in her care plan.

Ethics and Laws

Imagine the following.

- Your nose itches. But your wrists are restrained. You cannot scratch your nose.
- You need to use the bathroom. Your arms are restrained with wrist restraints. You cannot get up. You cannot reach your call light. You soil yourself with urine or a bowel movement.
- Your phone is ringing. You cannot answer it.
- You are wearing mitt restraints. You cannot reach your eyeglasses or put them on. You cannot see who is coming into and going out of your room. And you cannot speak because of a stroke.
- You are uncomfortable. You have a vest restraint. You cannot move or turn in bed.
- You are thirsty. Your wrists are restrained. You cannot reach the water mug.
- You hear the fire alarm. You have on a restraint. You cannot get up to move to a safe place. You must wait until someone rescues you.

What would you do? Would you calmly lie or sit there? Would you try to get free from the restraint? Would you yell for help? Would the staff think that you are uncomfortable? Or would they think that you are agitated and uncooperative? Would you feel angry, embarrassed, or humiliated?

Ethics deals with how others are treated. Restraints lessen the person's dignity and freedom. A person should not be treated in this way. That is why restraints are a last resort. Put yourself in the person's situation. Then you can better understand how the person feels. Treat the person like you would want to be treated—with kindness, caring, respect, and dignity.

FOCUS ON **PRIDE**: *Application*

Your input has value. Do not be afraid to share your thoughts, observations, and ideas with the nurse. Describe 3 scenarios involving behavior that is dangerous or that interferes with treatment. List ideas for managing the behavior without using restraints.

REVIEW QUESTIONS

*Circle **T** if the statement is TRUE or **F** if it is FALSE.*

1 **T F** Restraint alternatives fail to protect a person. You can apply a restraint.

2 **T F** A restraint restricts a person's freedom of movement.

3 **T F** Some drugs are restraints.

4 **T F** Restraints can be used for staff convenience.

5 **T F** A device is a restraint only if it is attached to the person's body.

6 **T F** Bed rails are restraints if the person cannot lower them.

7 **T F** Restraints are used only for a person's specific medical symptom.

8 **T F** Unnecessary restraint is false imprisonment.

9 **T F** You can apply restraints when you think they are needed.

10 **T F** You can use a vest restraint to position a person on the toilet.

11 **T F** Restraints are removed or released at least every 2 hours.

12 **T F** Restraints are tied to bed rails.

13 **T F** Wrist restraints are used to prevent falls.

14 **T F** A vest restraint crosses in front.

15 **T F** Bed rails are left down when a vest restraint is used.

Circle the BEST answer.

16 Which is a restraint alternative?
  a Positioning the person's chair close to the wall
  b Raising all bed rails
  c Giving a drug that restricts movement
  d Padding walls and corners of furniture

17 Physical restraints
  a Can be removed easily by the person
  b Are not allowed by OBRA
  c Require a doctor's order
  d Are safer than chemical restraints

18 The following can occur because of restraints. Which is the *most* serious?
  a Fractures
  b Strangulation
  c Pressure ulcers
  d Urinary tract infections

19 A belt restraint is applied to a person in bed. Where should you secure the straps?
  a To the bed rails
  b To the head-board
  c To the movable part of the bed frame
  d To the foot-board

20 A person has a restraint. You should check the person and the position of the restraint at least every
  a 15 minutes
  b 30 minutes
  c Hour
  d 3 hours

21 A person has mitt restraints. Which will you report to the nurse at once?
  a The hands are clean, warm, and dry.
  b The person has numbness in the hands.
  c You removed the restraints for 10 minutes.
  d You felt a pulse in both arms.

22 When applying restraints, you should
  a Know when to apply and release them
  b Use force if the person is agitated
  c Allow plenty of slack in the straps
  d Apply a restraint you have not used before

23 A person has a vest restraint. To check for snugness, slide
  a A fist between the vest and the person
  b 1 finger between the vest and the person
  c An open hand between the vest and the person
  d 2 fingers between the vest and the person

24 The correct way to apply any restraint is to follow the
  a Nurse's directions
  b Doctor's orders
  c Care plan
  d Manufacturer's instructions

Answers to Chapter 15 questions are on p. 870.

FOCUS ON PRACTICE

Problem Solving

Mrs. Lopez has confusion and weakness in her legs. She uses a wheelchair and often tries to get up without help. What are some alternatives to restraints that may be tried? If a restraint is needed, how will you provide for her basic needs?

Preventing Infection

OBJECTIVES

- Define the key terms and key abbreviations in this chapter.
- Identify what microbes need to live and grow.
- List the signs and symptoms of infection.
- Explain the chain of infection.
- Describe healthcare-associated infections and the persons at risk.
- Describe the principles of medical asepsis.
- Explain how to care for equipment and supplies.

- Describe disinfection and sterilization methods.
- Describe Standard Precautions and Transmission-Based Precautions.
- Explain the Bloodborne Pathogen Standard.
- Explain the principles of surgical asepsis.
- Perform the procedures described in this chapter.
- Explain how to promote PRIDE in the person, the family, and yourself.

KEY TERMS

antibiotic A drug that kills certain microbes that cause infection

antisepsis The processes, procedures, and chemical treatments that kill microbes or prevent them from causing an infection; *anti* means *against* and *sepsis* means *infection*

asepsis The absence *(a)* of disease-producing microbes *(sepsis means infection)*

biohazardous waste Items contaminated with blood, body fluids, secretions, or excretions; *bio* means *life* and *hazardous* means *dangerous* or *harmful*

carrier A human or animal that is a reservoir for microbes but does not develop the infection

clean technique See "medical asepsis"

communicable disease A disease caused by pathogens that spread easily; contagious disease

contagious disease See "communicable disease"

contamination The process of becoming unclean

cross-contamination Passing microbes from 1 person to another by contaminated hands, equipment, or supplies

disinfectant A liquid chemical that can kill many or all pathogens except spores

disinfection The process of killing pathogens

healthcare-associated infection (HAI) An infection that develops in a person cared for in any setting where health care is given; the infection is related to receiving health care

immunity Protection against a certain disease

infection A disease state resulting from the invasion and growth of microbes in the body

infection control Practices and procedures that prevent the spread of infection

medical asepsis Practices used to reduce the number of microbes and prevent their spread from 1 person or place to another person or place; clean technique

microbe See "microorganism"

microorganism A small *(micro)* living thing *(organism)* seen only with a microscope; microbe

non-pathogen A microbe that does not usually cause an infection

normal flora Microbes that live and grow in a certain area

pathogen A microbe that is harmful and can cause an infection

reservoir The environment in which a microbe lives and grows; host

spore A bacterium protected by a hard shell

sterile The absence of *all* microbes

sterile field A work area free of *all* pathogens and non-pathogens (including spores)

sterile technique See "surgical asepsis"

sterilization The process of destroying *all* microbes

surgical asepsis The practices used to remove *all* microbes; sterile technique

vaccination Giving a vaccine to produce immunity against an infectious disease

vaccine A preparation containing dead or weakened microbes

vector A carrier (animal, insect) that transmits disease

vehicle Any substance that transmits microbes

KEY ABBREVIATIONS

AIDS	Acquired immunodeficiency syndrome		**MDRO**	Multidrug-resistant organism
CDC	Centers for Disease Control and Prevention		**MRSA**	Methicillin-resistant *Staphylococcus aureus*
cm	Centimeter		**OPIM**	Other potentially infectious materials
EPA	Environmental Protection Agency		**OSHA**	Occupational Safety and Health Administration
GI	Gastro-intestinal		**PPE**	Personal protective equipment
HAI	Healthcare-associated infection		**TB**	Tuberculosis
HBV	Hepatitis B virus		**VRE**	Vancomycin-resistant *Enterococci*
HIV	Human immunodeficiency virus			

An *infection is a disease state resulting from the invasion and growth of microbes in the body.* Infection is a major safety and health hazard. Minor infections are short-term. Some infections are serious and can cause death. Infants, older persons, and disabled persons are at risk. The health team follows certain *practices and procedures to prevent the spread of infection (infection control).* The goal is to protect patients, residents, visitors, and staff from infection.

This chapter includes measures of antisepsis. *Antisepsis is the processes, procedures, and chemical treatments that kill microbes or prevent them from causing an infection.* (Anti *means* against. Sepsis *means* infection.)

MICROORGANISMS

A *microorganism (microbe) is a small* (micro) *living thing* (organism). *It is seen only with a microscope.* Microbes, commonly called *germs*, are everywhere—mouth, nose, respiratory tract, stomach, and intestines. They are on the skin and in the air, soil, water, and food. They are on animals, clothing, and furniture.

Microbes that are harmful and can cause infections are called **pathogens.** **Non-pathogens** *are microbes that do not usually cause an infection.*

Types of Microbes

There are 5 types of microbes.
- *Bacteria*—are 1-celled organisms that multiply rapidly. They can cause an infection in any body system.
- *Fungi*—are plant-like organisms that live on other plants or animals. Mushrooms, yeasts, and mold are common fungi. Fungi can infect the mouth, vagina, skin, feet, and other body areas.
- *Protozoa*—are 1-celled animals. They can infect the blood, brain, intestines, and other body areas.
- *Rickettsiae*—are found in fleas, lice, ticks, and other insects. They are spread to humans by insect bites. Rocky Mountain spotted fever is an example. The person has fever, chills, headache, and rash.
- *Viruses*—grow in living cells. They cause many diseases. The common cold, herpes, acquired immunodeficiency syndrome (AIDS), and hepatitis are examples.

Requirements of Microbes

Microbes need a reservoir to live and grow. The *reservoir (host) is the environment in which a microbe lives and grows.* People, plants, animals, the soil, food, and water are common reservoirs. Microbes need *water* and *nourishment* from the reservoir. Most need *oxygen* to live. A *warm* and *dark* environment is needed. Most grow best at body temperature. They are destroyed by heat and light.

Normal Flora

Normal flora are microbes that live and grow in a certain area. Certain microbes are in the respiratory tract, in the intestines, and on the skin. They are non-pathogens when in or on a natural reservoir. When a non-pathogen is transmitted from its natural site to another site or host, it becomes a pathogen. For example, *Escherichia coli (E. coli)* is normally in the colon. If it enters the urinary system, it can cause an infection.

Multidrug-Resistant Organisms

Multidrug-resistant organisms (MDROs) are microbes that can resist the effects of antibiotics. *Antibiotics are drugs that kill certain microbes that cause infections.* Some microbes can change their structures, making them harder to kill. They can survive in the presence of antibiotics. Therefore the infections they cause are hard to treat.

MDROs are caused by prescribing antibiotics when not needed (over-prescribing). Not taking antibiotics for the length of time prescribed is another cause. Two common MDROs are:
- *Methicillin-resistant Staphylococcus aureus (MRSA). Staphylococcus aureus* ("staph") is found in the nose and on the skin. MRSA is resistant to antibiotics often used for "staph" infections. MRSA can cause serious wound and bloodstream infections and pneumonia.
- *Vancomycin-resistant Enterococci (VRE). Enterococcus* is found in the intestines and in feces. It can be transmitted to others by contaminated hands, toilet seats, care equipment, and other items that the hands touch. When not in the intestines, enterococci can cause urinary tract, wound, pelvic, and other infections. Vancomycin is an antibiotic used to treat such infections. Enterococci resistant to vancomycin are called vancomycin-resistant *Enterococci* (VRE).

INFECTION

A *local infection* is in a body part. A *systemic infection* involves the whole body. *(Systemic* means *entire.)* The person has some or all of the signs and symptoms listed in Box 16-1.

See *Focus on Children and Older Persons: Infection.*
See *Focus on Surveys: Infection.*

BOX 16-1   Infection—Signs and Symptoms

- Fever (elevated body temperature)
- Chills
- Pulse rate: increased
- Respiratory rate: increased
- Pain or tenderness
- Fatigue and loss of energy
- Appetite: loss of *(anorexia)*
- Nausea
- Vomiting
- Diarrhea
- Rash
- Sores on mucous membranes
- Redness and swelling of a body part
- Discharge or drainage from the infected area
- Heat or warmth in a body part
- Limited use of a body part
- Headache
- Muscle aches
- Joint pain
- Confusion

FOCUS ON CHILDREN AND OLDER PERSONS

Infection

Older Persons

The immune system protects the body from disease and infection (Chapter 10). Changes occur in this system with aging. Therefore older persons are at risk for infection.

An older person may not show the signs and symptoms listed in Box 16-1. The person may have only a slight fever or no fever at all. Redness and swelling may be very slight. The person may not complain of pain. Confusion and delirium may occur (Chapter 49).

An infection can become life-threatening before the older person has obvious signs and symptoms. Report minor changes in the person's behavior or condition at once.

Healing takes longer in older persons. Therefore an infection can prolong the rehabilitation process. Independence and quality of life are affected.

FOCUS ON SURVEYS

Infection

Infection control practices are a major focus of surveys. You may be asked:
- What do you do when you observe signs and symptoms of an infection?
- Who do you tell when you observe signs and symptoms of an infection?

The Chain of Infection

The chain of infection (Fig. 16-1) is a process involving the following.
- Source—A pathogen.
- Reservoir—The pathogen needs a place where it can grow and multiply. A **carrier** *is a human or animal that is a reservoir for microbes but does not develop the infection.* Carriers can pass pathogens to others. A **vector** *is a carrier (animal, insect) that transmits disease.* Common vectors are:
  - Dogs—carry rabies
  - Mosquitoes—carry malaria
  - Ticks—carry Rocky Mountain spotted fever
  - Mites—cause scabies (Chapter 22)
- Portal of exit—The pathogen needs a way to leave the reservoir. Exits are the respiratory, gastro-intestinal (GI), urinary, and reproductive tracts; breaks in the skin; and blood.
- Method of transmission—The pathogen is *transmitted* to another host (Fig. 16-2, p. 220). A **vehicle** *is any substance that transmits microbes.*
- Portal of entry—The pathogen enters the body. Portals of entry and exit are the same—the respiratory, GI, urinary, and reproductive tracts; breaks in the skin; and blood.
- Susceptible host—The transmitted microbe needs a host where it can grow and multiply. Susceptible hosts are persons at risk for infection.

Susceptible Hosts. Susceptible hosts include persons who:
- Are very young or who are older.
- Are ill.
- Were exposed to the pathogen.
- Do not follow practices to prevent infection.

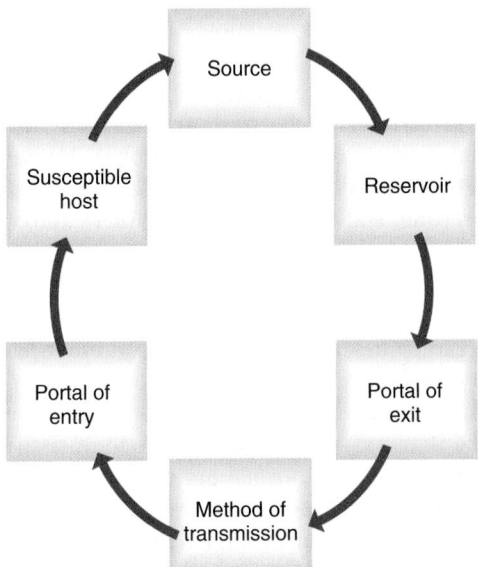

FIGURE 16-1 The chain of infection. (Redrawn from Potter PA, Perry AG, Stockert PA, Hall AM: *Fundamentals of nursing: concepts, process, and practice,* ed 8, St Louis, 2013, Mosby.)

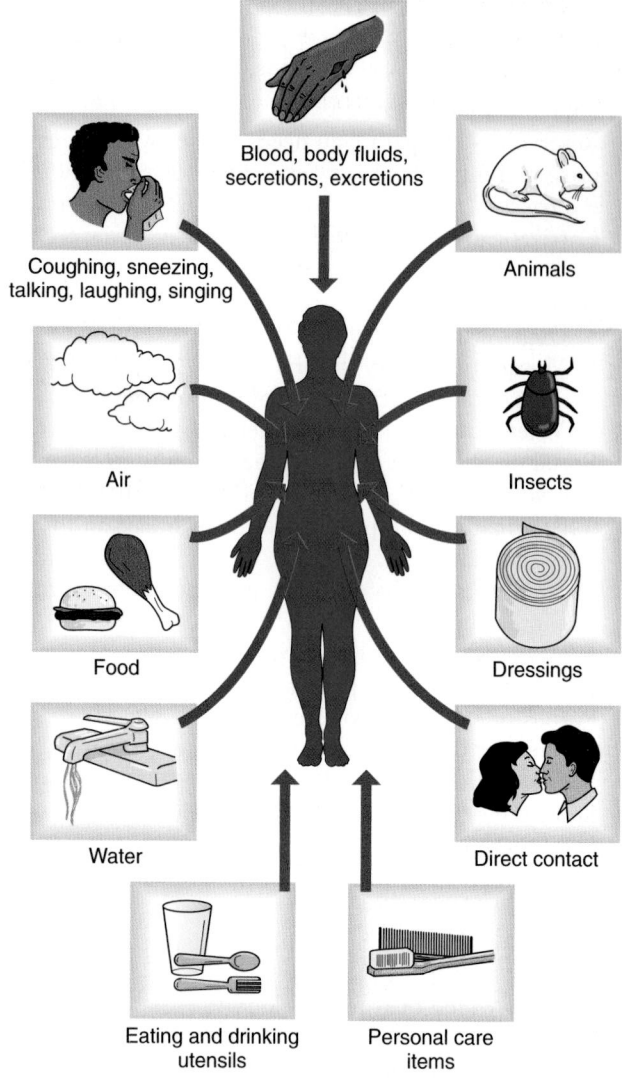

Blood, body fluids, secretions, excretions

Coughing, sneezing, talking, laughing, singing

Animals

Air

Insects

Food

Dressings

Water

Direct contact

Eating and drinking utensils

Personal care items

FIGURE 16-2 Methods of transmitting microbes.

Healthcare-Associated Infections

A *healthcare-associated infection (HAI) is an infection that develops in a person cared for in any setting where health care is given* (Box 16-2). *The infection is related to receiving health care.* Hospitals, nursing centers, clinics, and home care settings are examples. HAIs also are called nosocomial infections. (*Nosocomial* comes from the Greek word for *hospital*.)

HAIs are caused by normal flora. Or they are caused by microbes transmitted to the person from other sources. For example, *E. coli* is normally in the colon. Feces contain *E. coli*. Poor wiping after bowel movements can cause *E. coli* to enter the urinary system. With poor hand-washing, *E. coli* spreads to any body part or anything the hands touch. It also can be transmitted to other people.

Microbes can enter the body through care equipment and supplies. Such items must be free of microbes. Staff can transfer microbes from 1 person to another and from themselves to others. Common sites for HAIs are:

- The urinary system
- The respiratory system
- Wounds
- The bloodstream

Patients and residents are weak from disease or injury. Some have wounds or open skin areas. Infants and older persons have a hard time fighting infections. The health team must prevent infection by:

- Medical asepsis. This includes hand hygiene.
- Surgical asepsis, p. 244.
- Standard Precautions, p. 228.
- Transmission-Based Precautions, p. 231.
- The Bloodborne Pathogen Standard, p. 240.

See *Focus on Long-Term Care and Home Care: Healthcare-Associated Infections.*

The ability to resist infection relates to age, nutrition, stress, fatigue, and health. Drugs, disease, and injury also are factors. Severe infection can be deadly for:

- *Burn patients.* When burns destroy the skin, the wound is a portal of entry for microbes. Microbes are from the person's normal flora (p. 218), the health care setting, and the health team. MRSA and VRE are great concerns. Burns affect the immune system (Chapter 10) and the ability to fight infection.
- *Transplant patients.* A *transplant* involves transferring an organ or tissue from 1 person to another person or from 1 body part to another body part. Kidney, liver, heart, lung, bone, and skin transplants are examples. To the immune system, the new organ or tissue is a foreign object. The normal immune response is to attack (reject) the new organ or tissue. Drugs given to prevent rejection suppress (prevent) the immune system from producing antibodies. Antibodies are needed to fight infection.
- *Chemotherapy patients.* Some chemotherapy drugs affect the ability to produce white blood cells (WBCs). WBCs are needed to fight infection.

BOX 16-2	Healthcare-Associated Infections—Examples

- *Clostridium difficile*—Chapter 26
- Gastro-intestinal infections
- Hepatitis A, B, and C—Chapter 46
- Human immunodeficiency virus—Chapter 43
- Influenza—Chapter 45
- Methicillin-resistant *Staphylococcus aureus*—p. 218
- Vancomycin-resistant *Enterococci*—p. 218
- Tuberculosis—Chapter 45

Modified from Centers for Disease Control and Prevention: Healthcare-associated infections (HAIs): diseases and organisms in healthcare settings, Atlanta, updated March 26, 2014.

MEDICAL ASEPSIS

Asepsis is the absence (a) *of disease-producing microbes* (sepsis means infection). Microbes are everywhere. Measures are needed to achieve asepsis. *Medical asepsis (clean technique) is the practices used to:*

* *Reduce the number of microbes.*
* *Prevent microbes from spreading from 1 person or place to another person or place.*

Microbes cannot be present during surgery or when instruments are inserted into the body. Open wounds (cuts, burns, incisions) require the absence of microbes. They are portals of entry for microbes. *Surgical asepsis (sterile technique) is the practices used to remove all microbes. Sterile means the absence of all microbes*—pathogens and non-pathogens. *Sterilization is the process of destroying all microbes* (pathogens and non-pathogens).

Contamination is the process of becoming unclean. In medical asepsis, an item or area is *clean* when it is free of pathogens. The item or area is *contaminated* when pathogens are present. A sterile item or area is *contaminated* when pathogens or non-pathogens are present. *Cross-contamination is passing microbes from 1 person to another by contaminated hands, equipment, or supplies* (Fig. 16-3). Medical asepsis and surgical asepsis (p. 244) prevent cross-contamination.

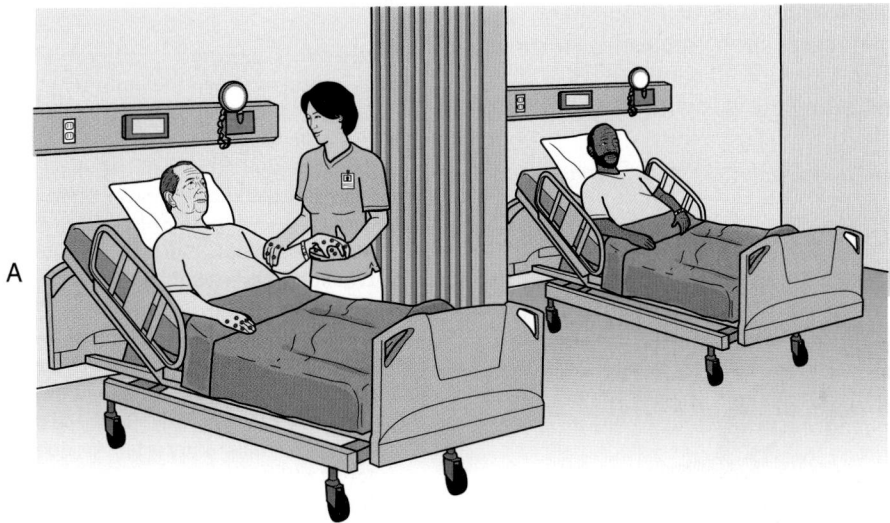

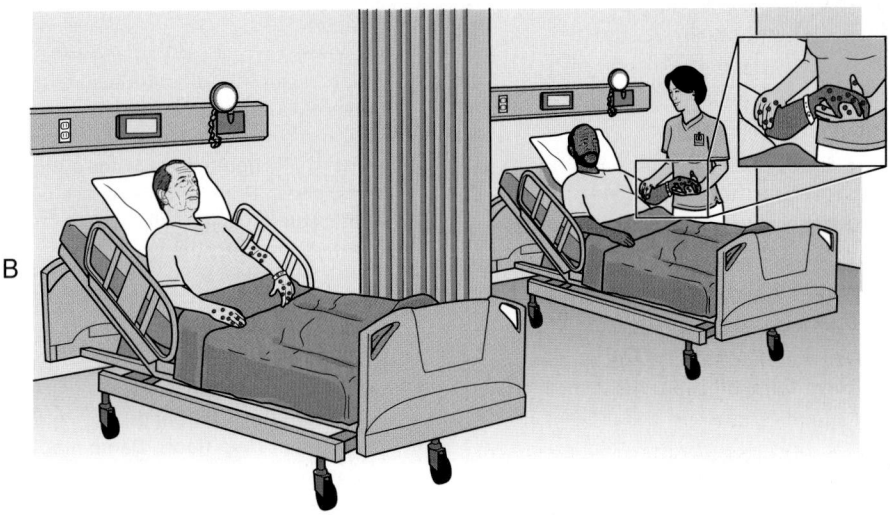

FIGURE 16-3 **Cross-contamination. A,** Microbes on the person's skin are transmitted to the nursing assistant's hands. **B,** Contaminated hands transmit microbes from 1 person to another.

Common Aseptic Practices

Aseptic practices break the chain of infection. To prevent the spread of microbes, wash your hands:
- After elimination.
- After changing tampons or sanitary pads.
- After contact with your own or another person's blood, body fluids, secretions, or excretions. This includes saliva, vomitus, urine, feces, vaginal discharge, mucus, semen, wound drainage, pus, and respiratory secretions.
- After coughing, sneezing, or blowing your nose.
- Before and after handling, preparing, or eating food.
- After smoking.

Also do the following.
- Provide all persons with their own linens and personal care items.
- Cover your nose and mouth when coughing, sneezing, or blowing your nose. If tissues are not available, cough or sneeze into your upper arm (Fig. 16-4). Do not cough or sneeze into your hands.
- Bathe, wash hair, and brush your teeth regularly.
- Wash fruit and raw vegetables before eating or serving them.
- Wash cooking and eating utensils with soap and water after use.

See *Focus on Children and Older Persons: Common Aseptic Practices.*

See *Focus on Long-Term Care and Home Care: Common Aseptic Practices.*

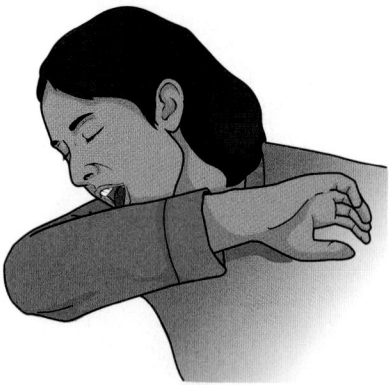

FIGURE 16-4 Sneezing into the upper arm.

FOCUS ON CHILDREN AND OLDER PERSONS

Common Aseptic Practices

Older Persons
Persons with dementia do not understand aseptic practices. The staff must protect them from infection. Assist them with hand-washing:
- After elimination
- After coughing, sneezing, or blowing the nose
- Before or after they eat or handle food
- Any time their hands are soiled

Check and clean their hands and fingernails often. They may not or cannot tell you when soiling occurs.

Hand Hygiene

Hand hygiene is the easiest and most important way to prevent the spread of microbes and infection. You use your hands for almost everything. They are easily contaminated. They can spread microbes to other persons or items (see Fig. 16-3). *Practice hand hygiene before and after giving care.* See Box 16-3 for the rules of hand hygiene.

See *Focus on Surveys: Hand Hygiene.*
See *Promoting Safety and Comfort: Hand Hygiene.*
See procedure: *Hand-Washing,* p. 225.
See procedure: *Using an Alcohol-Based Hand Rub,* p. 225.

Text continued on p. 226.

FOCUS ON LONG-TERM CARE AND HOME CARE

Common Aseptic Practices

Home Care
You must prevent the spread of microbes in home settings. Also, protect the person from microbes brought into the home. The measures on this page and others (p. 226) are needed. Also protect the person from foodborne illnesses (Chapter 27).

Microbes easily grow and spread in bathrooms. The entire family must help keep the bathroom clean. Aseptic measures are needed when the bathroom is used.
- Flush the toilet after each use.
- Rinse the sink after washing, shaving, or oral hygiene.
- Wipe out the tub or shower after each use.
- Remove and dispose of hair from the sink, tub, or shower.
- Hang towels out to dry. Or place them in a hamper.
- Wipe up spills—water, personal care products, beverages, and so on.

Wear utility gloves to clean bathrooms. Use a disinfectant or water and detergent to clean all surfaces.
- Toilet surfaces—bowl, seat, and all outside areas
- The floor
- The sides, walls, and curtain or door of the shower or tub
- Towel racks
- Toilet tissue holder, toothbrush holder, and soap holders
- The mirror (use a glass cleaner)
- The sink
- Window sills

To clean bathrooms, you also need to:
- Mop uncarpeted floors. Vacuum carpeted floors.
- Empty wastebaskets.
- Put out clean towels and washcloths.
- Open bathroom windows for a short time and use air fresheners. These actions reduce odors and give the bathroom a fresh smell.
- Wash bath mats, the wastebasket, and the laundry hamper weekly.
- Replace toilet and facial tissue as needed.

The care plan and assignment sheet tell you when to clean other areas of the home. For general housekeeping:
- Wipe up spills right away.
- Dust furniture and blinds.
- Vacuum or mop floors. Damp-mop uncarpeted floors at least weekly.
- Use a dust mop to sweep. Use a dustpan to collect dust, crumbs, and other things swept up. Sweep daily or more often if needed.
- Wash clothes and linens.

BOX 16-3   Rules of Hand Hygiene

- Wash your hands (with soap and water) at these times.
  - When they are visibly dirty or soiled with blood, body fluids, secretions, or excretions
  - Before eating and after using a restroom
  - If exposure to the anthrax spore is suspected or proven
  - If an alcohol-based hand rub is not available
- Use an alcohol-based hand rub to practice hand hygiene if your hands are not visibly soiled.
  - Before direct contact with a person.
  - After contact with the person's intact skin. After taking a pulse or blood pressure or after moving a person are examples.
  - After contact with body fluids or excretions, mucous membranes, non-intact skin, and wound dressings if hands are not visibly soiled.
  - When moving from a contaminated body site to a clean body site.
  - After contact with items in the person's care setting.
  - After removing gloves.
- Follow these rules for washing your hands with soap and water. See procedure: *Hand-Washing*, p. 225.
  - Wash your hands under warm running water. Do not use hot water.
  - Stand away from the sink. Do not let your hands, body, or uniform touch the sink. The sink is contaminated. See Figure 16-5, p. 224.
  - Do not touch the inside of the sink at any time.
  - Keep your hands and forearms lower than your elbows. Your hands are dirtier than your elbows and forearms. If you hold your hands and forearms up, dirty water runs from your hands to your elbows. Those areas become contaminated.
  - Rub your palms together (Fig. 16-6, p. 224) and interlace your fingers (Fig. 16-7, p. 224) to work up a good lather. The rubbing action helps remove microbes and dirt.
- Pay attention to areas often missed during hand-washing—thumbs, knuckles, sides of the hands, little fingers, and under the nails.
- Clean fingernails by rubbing the fingertips against your palms (Fig. 16-8, p. 224).
- Use a nail file or orangewood stick to clean under fingernails (Fig. 16-9, p. 224). Microbes grow easily under the fingernails.
- Wash your hands for at least 15 to 20 seconds. Wash your hands longer if they are dirty or soiled with blood, body fluids, secretions, or excretions. Use your judgment and follow agency policy.
- Use clean, dry paper towels to dry your hands.
- Dry your hands starting at the fingertips. Work up to your forearms (Fig. 16-10, p. 224). You will dry the cleanest area first.
- Use a clean, dry paper towel for each faucet to turn the water off (Fig. 16-11, p. 225). Faucets are contaminated. The paper towels prevent you from contaminating your clean hands.
- Follow these rules when decontaminating your hands with an alcohol-based hand rub. See procedure: *Using an Alcohol-Based Hand Rub*, p. 225.
  - Apply the product to the palm of 1 hand. Follow the manufacturer's instructions for the amount to use.
  - Rub your hands together.
  - Cover all surfaces of your hands and fingers.
  - Continue rubbing your hands together until your hands are dry.
- Apply hand lotion or cream after hand hygiene. This prevents the skin from chapping and drying. Skin breaks can occur in chapped and dry skin. Skin breaks are portals of entry for microbes.

Modified from Centers for Disease Control and Prevention: Guidelines for hand hygiene in health-care settings, Morbidity and Mortality Weekly, Report 51 (RR-16), October 2002.

FOCUS ON SURVEYS
Hand Hygiene

Hand hygiene is a focus of surveys. A surveyor may:
- Observe you washing your hands or using an alcohol-based hand rub according to agency policy.
- Observe if you practice hand hygiene:
  - After each direct patient or resident contact
  - Before and after all procedures
  - After removing gloves
  - When entering or leaving the room of a person on Transmission-Based Precautions (p. 231)
- Ask you questions about:
  - When you should wash your hands
  - When you can use an alcohol-based hand rub

PROMOTING SAFETY AND COMFORT
Hand Hygiene

Safety
You use your hands for almost every task. They can pick up microbes from a person, place, or thing. Your hands transfer them to other people, places, or things. That is why hand hygiene is so very important. Always practice hand hygiene before and after giving care.

Comfort
You will practice hand hygiene very often during your shift. Hand lotions and hand creams help prevent chapping and dry skin.

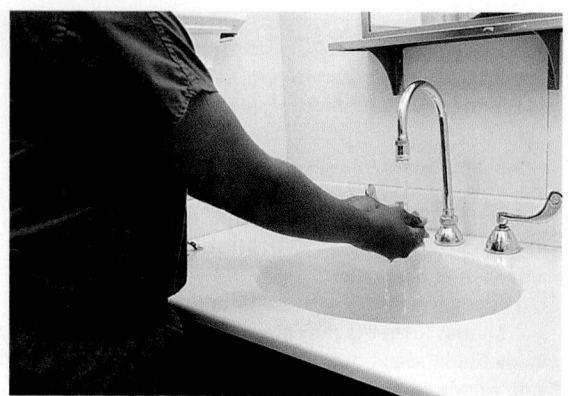

FIGURE 16-5 The uniform does not touch the sink. Soap and water are within reach. Hands are lower than the elbows. Hands do not touch the inside of the sink.

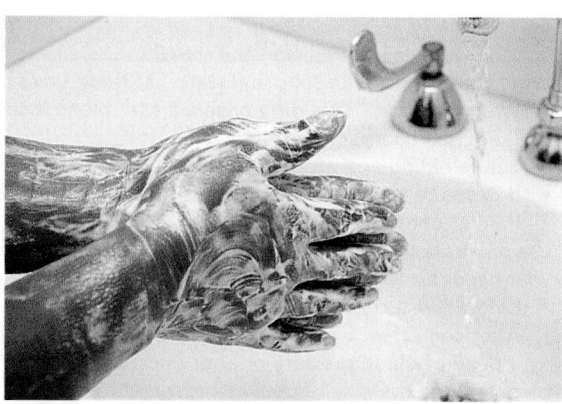

FIGURE 16-6 The palms are rubbed together to work up a good lather.

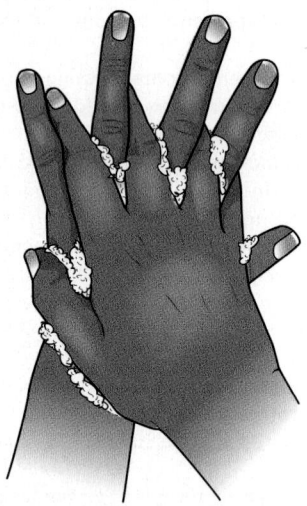

FIGURE 16-7 The fingers are interlaced to clean between the fingers.

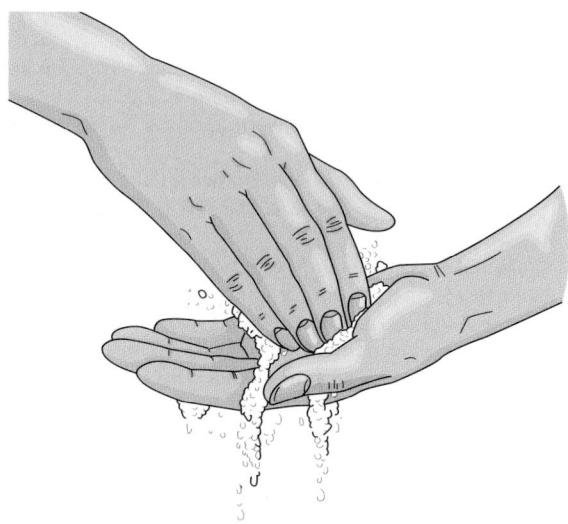

FIGURE 16-8 The fingertips are rubbed against the palms to clean under the fingernails.

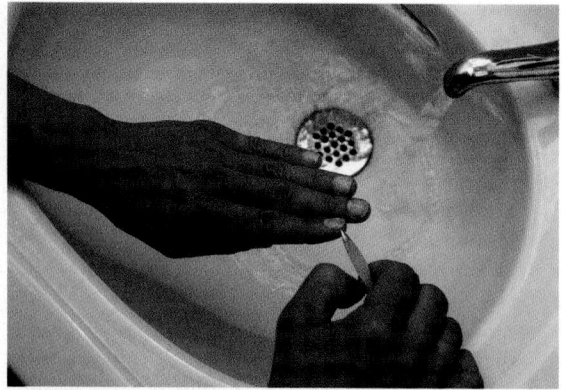

FIGURE 16-9 A nail file is used to clean under the fingernails.

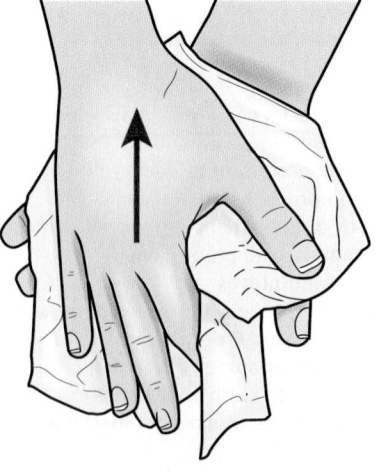

FIGURE 16-10 Hands are dried starting at the fingertips and working up to the forearms.

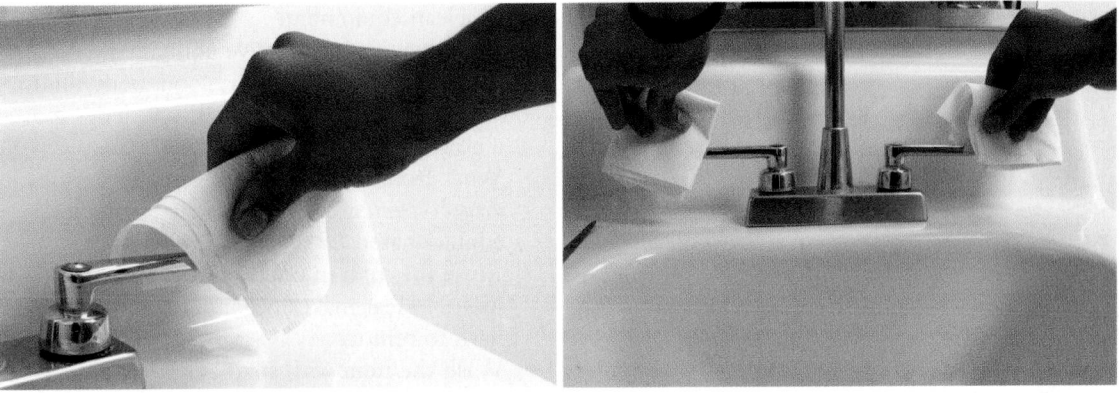

FIGURE 16-11 A paper towel is used to turn off each faucet.

Hand-Washing

PROCEDURE

1 See *Promoting Safety and Comfort: Hand Hygiene,* p. 223.
2 Make sure you have soap, paper towels, an orangewood stick or nail file, and a wastebasket. Collect missing items.
3 Push your watch up your arm 4 to 5 inches. Push long uniform sleeves up too.
4 Stand away from the sink so your clothes do not touch the sink. Stand so the soap and faucet are easy to reach (see Fig. 16-5). Do not touch the inside of the sink at any time.
5 Turn on and adjust the water until it feels warm.
6 Wet your wrists and hands. Keep your hands lower than your elbows. Be sure to wet the area 3 to 4 inches above your wrists.
7 Apply about 1 teaspoon of soap to your hands.
8 Rub your palms together and interlace your fingers to work up a good lather (see Fig. 16-6). Lather your wrists, hands, and fingers. Keep your hands lower than your elbows. This step should last at least 15 to 20 seconds.

9 Wash each hand and wrist thoroughly. Clean the back of your fingers and between your fingers (see Fig. 16-7).
10 Clean under the fingernails. Rub your fingertips against your palms (see Fig. 16-8).
11 Clean under the fingernails with a nail file or orangewood stick (see Fig. 16-9). Do this for the first hand-washing of the day and when your hands are highly soiled.
12 Rinse your wrists, hands, and fingers well. Water flows from above the wrists to your fingertips.
13 Repeat steps 7 through 12, if needed.
14 Dry your wrists and hands with clean, dry paper towels. Pat dry starting at your fingertips (see Fig. 16-10).
15 Discard the paper towels into the wastebasket.
16 Turn off faucets with clean, dry paper towels. This prevents you from contaminating your hands (see Fig. 16-11). Use a clean paper towel for each faucet. Or use knee or foot controls to turn off the faucet.
17 Discard the paper towels into the wastebasket.

Using an Alcohol-Based Hand Rub

PROCEDURE

1 See *Promoting Safety and Comfort: Hand Hygiene,* p. 223.
2 Apply a palmful of an alcohol-based hand rub into a cupped hand (Fig. 16-12, *A*, p. 226).
3 Rub your palms together (Fig. 16-12, *B*, p. 226).
4 Rub the palm of 1 hand over the back of the other (Fig. 16-12, *C*, p. 226). Do the same for the other hand.
5 Rub your palms together with your fingers interlaced (Fig. 16-12, *D*, p. 226).

6 Interlock your fingers as in Figure 16-12, *E*, p. 226. Rub your fingers back and forth.
7 Rub the thumb of 1 hand in the palm of the other (Fig. 16-12, *F*, p. 226). Do the same for the other thumb.
8 Rub the fingers of 1 hand into the palm of the other hand (Fig. 16-12, *G*, p. 226). Use a circular motion. Do the same for the fingers of the other hand.
9 Continue rubbing your hands until they are dry.

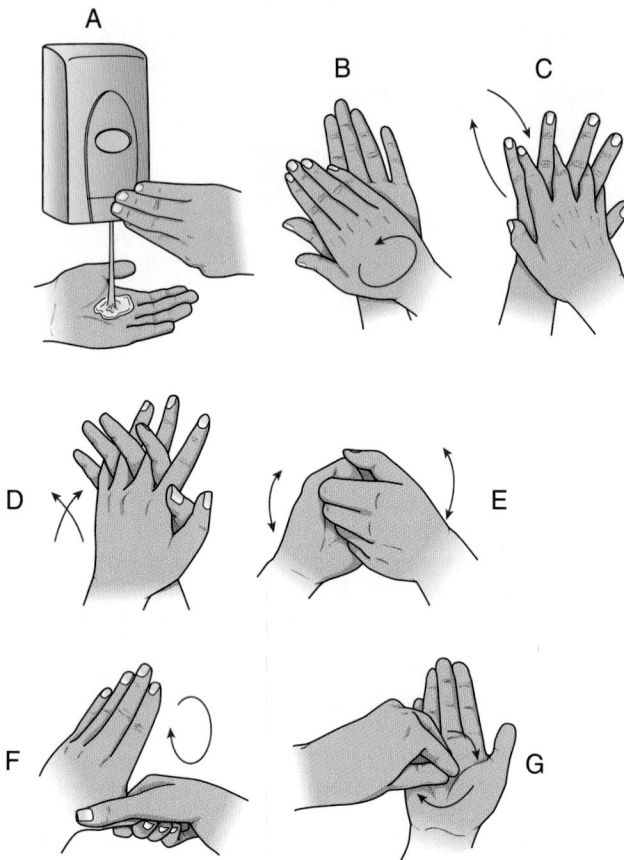

FIGURE 16-12 Using an alcohol-based hand rub. **A,** A palmful of an alcohol-based hand rub is applied into a cupped hand. **B,** The palms are rubbed together. **C,** The palm of 1 hand is rubbed over the back of the other. **D,** The palms are rubbed together with the fingers interlaced. **E,** The fingers are interlocked and rubbed back and forth. **F,** The thumb of 1 hand is rubbed in the palm of the other. **G,** The fingers of 1 hand are rubbed into the palm of the other hand with circular motions.

Supplies and Equipment

Disposable supplies and equipment help prevent the spread of infection. Discard single-use items after use. A person uses multi-use items many times. They include bedpans, urinals, wash basins, and water mugs. Label such items with the person's room and bed number. Do not "borrow" them for another person.

Non-disposable items are cleaned and then disinfected. Then they are sterilized by the supply department.

Cleaning. Cleaning reduces the number of microbes present. It also removes organic matter. *Organic matter* comes from living plants and animals and is able to decay. Blood, body fluids, secretions, and excretions are organic matter. So is food.

To clean equipment:

- Wear personal protective equipment (PPE) to clean items contaminated with blood, body fluids, secretions, or excretions. PPE includes gloves, a mask, a gown, and goggles or a face shield.
- Work from *clean* to *dirty* areas. If you work from a *dirty* to *clean* area, the *clean* area becomes contaminated *(dirty)*.
- Rinse the item in cold water to remove organic matter. Heat makes organic matter thick, sticky, and hard to remove.
- Wash the item with soap and hot water.
- Scrub thoroughly. Use a brush if necessary.
- Rinse the item in warm water. Dry the item.
- Disinfect the item. Or send it to the supply department to be sterilized.
- Disinfect equipment used and the sink.
- Discard PPE.
- Practice hand hygiene.

Agencies have *clean* and *dirty* utility rooms. Equipment is cleaned in the *dirty* utility room. Then it is disinfected or sterilized in the *clean* utility room.

Disinfection. *Disinfection is the process of killing pathogens.* Spores are not destroyed. *Spores are bacteria protected by a hard shell.* Spores are killed by very high temperatures.

Disinfectants are used to clean objects and surfaces. A *disinfectant is a liquid chemical that can kill many or all pathogens except spores.* Disinfectants are used to clean counters, tubs, showers, and re-usable items. Such items include:

- Blood pressure cuffs
- Commodes and metal bedpans
- Wheelchairs and stretchers
- Furniture

See *Focus on Long-Term Care and Home Care: Disinfection.*
See *Promoting Safety and Comfort: Disinfection.*

Sterilization. Sterilizing destroys all non-pathogens, pathogens, and spores. Very high temperatures are used. Heat destroys microbes.

Boiling water, radiation, liquid or gas chemicals, dry heat, and *steam under pressure* are sterilization methods. An autoclave (Fig. 16-13) is a pressure steam sterilizer. Glass, surgical items, and metal objects are autoclaved. High temperatures destroy plastic and rubber items. They are not autoclaved. Steam under pressure sterilizes objects in 30 to 45 minutes.

See *Focus on Long-Term Care and Home Care: Sterilization.*

Other Aseptic Measures

Hand hygiene, cleaning, disinfection, and sterilization are important aseptic measures. So are the measures listed in Box 16-4. They are useful in home and health care settings and in everyday life.

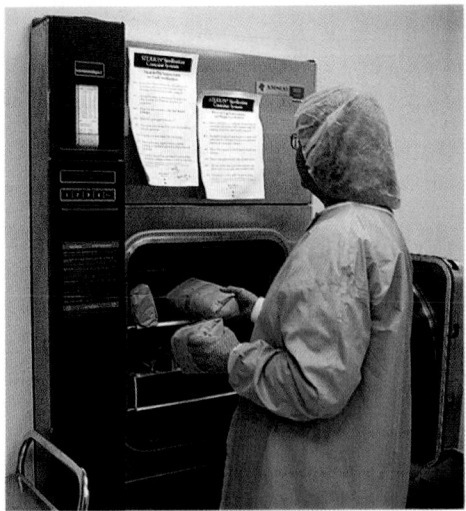

FIGURE 16-13 An autoclave.

PROMOTING SAFETY AND COMFORT
Disinfection

Safety

Disinfectants can burn and irritate the skin. Wear utility gloves or rubber household gloves to prevent skin irritation. These gloves are waterproof. Do not wear disposable gloves.

Some disinfectants have special measures for use and storage. Check the safety data sheet (SDS) before handling a disinfectant. See Chapter 13.

FOCUS ON **LONG-TERM CARE AND HOME CARE**
Sterilization

Home Care

You can use boiling water to sterilize items in the home.
1. Use a pot big enough to hold the items.
2. Wash the items with soap and hot water.
3. Fill the pot with cold water. Completely cover all items with water.
4. Bring the water to a full boil.
5. Boil the items for 10 minutes. Add 1 minute for each 1000 feet of elevation. For example, if the home is 2000 feet above sea level, boil items for 2 more minutes for a total of 12 minutes.
6. Turn off the heat.
7. Use tongs to remove the hot items to a clean towel. Remove items 1 at a time.
8. Let the items air-dry.
9. Put the items away as the family prefers or as the nurse instructs.

Many people use dishwashers for baby bottles. However, many dishwashers do not get hot enough to sterilize items.

FOCUS ON **LONG-TERM CARE AND HOME CARE**
Disinfection

Home Care

Detergent and hot water are used to clean cooking, eating, and drinking utensils and linens. Household disinfectants are used for surfaces—floors, toilets, tubs, and showers. Use the products the family prefers or as the nurse instructs.

White vinegar and water is a good, cheap disinfectant. You can use it to clean bedpans, urinals, commodes, toilets, mirrors, bathroom tiles, and so on. To make a vinegar solution:
- Mix 1 cup of white vinegar with 3 cups of water.
- Label the container as a "vinegar solution: 1 cup white vinegar, 3 cups water."
- Write the date, time, and your name on the label.

BOX 16-4   Aseptic Measures

Controlling Reservoirs (Hosts—You or the Person)
- Provide for the person's hygiene needs (Chapter 22).
- Wash contaminated areas with soap and water. Feces and urine can contain microbes. So can blood, body fluids, secretions, and excretions.
- Use leak-proof plastic bags for soiled tissues, linens, and other items.
- Keep tables, counters, wheelchair trays, and other surfaces clean and dry.
- Label bottles with the person's name and the date the bottle was opened.
- Keep bottles and fluid containers tightly capped or covered.
- Keep drainage containers below the drainage site (Chapters 25 and 36).
- Empty drainage containers and dispose of drainage following agency policy. Usually drainage containers are emptied every shift. Follow the nurse's directions if you need to empty them more often.

Controlling Portals of Exit
- Cover your nose and mouth to cough or sneeze.
- Provide the person with tissues to use when coughing or sneezing.
- Wear PPE as needed (p. 232).

Controlling Transmission
- Provide all persons with their own personal care equipment. This includes wash basins, bedpans, urinals, commodes, and eating and drinking utensils.
- Do not take equipment from 1 person's room to use for another person. Even if un-used, do not take the item from 1 room to another.
- Hold equipment and linens away from your uniform (Fig. 16-14, p. 228).
- Practice hand hygiene. See Box 16-3.

Continued

BOX 16-4   Aseptic Measures—cont'd

Controlling Transmission—cont'd
- Assist the person with hand-washing.
  - Before and after eating
  - After elimination
  - After changing tampons, sanitary napkins, or other personal hygiene products
  - After contact with blood, body fluids, secretions, or excretions
- Prevent dust movement. Do not shake linens or equipment. Use a damp cloth for dusting.
- Clean from *clean* to *dirty* areas. This prevents soiling a clean area.
- Clean away from your body. Do not dust, brush, or wipe toward yourself. Otherwise you transmit microbes to your skin, hair, and clothing.
- Flush urine and feces down the toilet. Avoid splatters and splashes.
- Pour contaminated liquids directly into sinks or toilets. Avoid splashing onto other areas.
- Do not sit on the person's bed or chair. You will pick up microbes. You will transfer them to the next surface that you sit on.
- Do not use items on the floor. The floor is contaminated.
- Follow agency disinfection procedures to clean:
  - Tubs, showers, and shower chairs after each use
  - Bedpans, urinals, and commodes after each use
- Report pests—ants, spiders, mice, and so on.

Controlling Portals of Entry
- Provide good skin care (Chapter 22). This promotes intact skin.
- Provide good oral hygiene (Chapter 22). This promotes intact mucous membranes.
- Protect the skin from injury.
  - Do not let the person lie on tubes or other items.
  - Make sure linens are dry and wrinkle-free (Chapter 21).
  - Turn and re-position the person as directed by the nurse and care plan (Chapters 17 and 18).
- Assist with or clean the genital area after elimination. (See "Perineal Care" in Chapter 22.) Wipe and clean from the urethra (cleanest area) to the rectum (dirtiest area). This helps prevent urinary tract infections.
- Make sure drainage tubes are properly connected. This prevents microbes from entering the drainage system.

Protecting the Susceptible Host
- Follow the care plan to meet nutrition and fluid needs (Chapter 27). This helps prevent infection.
- Assist with deep-breathing and coughing exercises as directed (Chapter 39). This helps prevent respiratory infections.

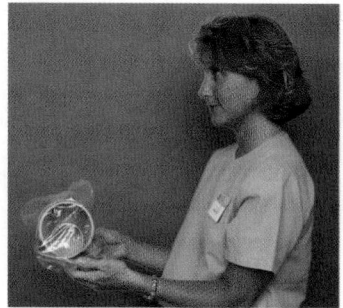

FIGURE 16-14 Hold equipment away from your uniform.

ISOLATION PRECAUTIONS

Blood, body fluids, secretions, and excretions can transmit pathogens. Sometimes barriers are needed to keep pathogens in a certain area—usually the person's room. This requires isolation precautions.

The *Guidelines for Isolation Precautions: Preventing Transmission of Infectious Agents in Healthcare Settings 2007* is followed. This is a guideline of the Centers for Disease Control and Prevention (CDC). Isolation precautions prevent the spread of **communicable diseases (contagious diseases)**. *They are diseases caused by pathogens that spread easily.*

Isolation precautions are based on *clean* and *dirty*. *Clean* areas or objects have no pathogens. They are not contaminated or *dirty*. *Dirty* areas or objects are contaminated with pathogens. If a *clean* area or object has contact with something dirty, the clean area or object is now *dirty*. *Clean* and *dirty* also depend on how the pathogen is spread.

The CDC guideline has 2 tiers of precautions.
- Standard Precautions
- Transmission-Based Precautions

Standard Precautions

Standard Precautions (Box 16-5):
- Reduce the risk of spreading pathogens.
- Reduce the risk of spreading known and unknown infections. *Standard Precautions are used for all persons whenever care is given.* They prevent the spread of infection from:
  - Blood.
  - All body fluids, secretions, and excretions (except sweat) even if blood is not visible. Sweat is not known to spread infection.
  - Non-intact skin (skin with open breaks).
  - Mucous membranes.

BOX 16-5	Standard Precautions

Hand Hygiene

- Follow the rules for hand hygiene. See Box 16-3.
- Touch surfaces close to the person only when necessary. This prevents contamination of clean hands from room or care setting surfaces. It also prevents the transmission of pathogens from contaminated hands to other surfaces.
- Do not wear fake nails or nail extenders for contact with persons at risk for infection or other adverse outcomes. (NOTE: Some agencies do not allow fake nails or nail extenders.)

Personal Protective Equipment (PPE) (p. 232)

- Wear PPE when contact with blood or body fluids is likely.
- Do not contaminate your clothing or skin when removing PPE.
- Remove and discard PPE before leaving the person's room or care setting.

Gloves (p. 233)

- Wear gloves when contact with the following is likely.
  - Blood
  - Potentially infectious materials (body fluids, secretions, and excretions are examples)
  - Mucous membranes
  - Non-intact skin
  - Skin that may be contaminated (for example, a person is incontinent of feces or urine)
- Wear gloves that fit and are needed for the task.
  - Wear disposable gloves to provide direct care.
  - Wear disposable gloves or utility gloves to clean equipment or care settings.
- Remove gloves after contact with:
  - The person
  - The person's care setting
  - Equipment used in the person's care or other care equipment
- Remove gloves after contact with a person and before going to another person.
- Do not wash gloves for re-use with different persons.
- Change gloves during care if your hands will move from a contaminated body site to a clean body site.

Gowns (p. 232)

- Wear a gown to protect your skin and clothing when contact with blood, body fluids, secretions, or excretions is likely.
- Wear a gown for direct contact with a person if he or she has uncontained secretions or excretions.
- Remove the gown and perform hand hygiene before leaving the person's room or care setting.
- Do not re-use gowns, even for repeat contact with the same person.

Mouth, Nose, and Eye Protection (p. 232)

- Wear PPE—masks, goggles, face shields—for procedures and tasks that are likely to cause splashes and sprays of blood, body fluids, secretions, and excretions.
- Wear the correct PPE—masks, goggles, face shields—for the procedure or task.
- Wear gloves, a gown, and 1 of the following for procedures or tasks likely to cause sprays of respiratory secretions.
  - A face shield that fully covers the front and sides of the face
  - A mask with attached shield
  - A mask and goggles

Respiratory Hygiene/Cough Etiquette

- Instruct persons with respiratory symptoms to:
  - Cover the nose and mouth to cough or sneeze.
  - Use tissues to contain respiratory secretions.
  - Dispose of tissues in the nearest waste container.
  - Perform hand hygiene after contact with respiratory secretions.
- Provide visitors with masks according to agency policy.

Care Equipment

- Wear the correct PPE to handle:
  - Care equipment that is visibly soiled with blood, body fluids, secretions, or excretions
  - Care equipment that may have been in contact with blood, body fluids, secretions, or excretions
- Remove organic material before disinfection and sterilization procedures. Follow agency policy for using cleaning agents.

Care of the Environment

- Follow agency procedures to clean and maintain surfaces. Care setting surfaces and care equipment are examples. Surfaces near the person may need more frequent cleaning and maintenance—door knobs, bed rails, over-bed tables, walker and cane handles, toilet surfaces and areas, and so on.
- Follow agency procedures to clean and disinfect multi-use electronic equipment. This includes:
  - Items used by patients and residents
  - Items used to give care
  - Mobile devices that are moved in and out of patient or resident rooms
- Follow these rules for children's toys. This includes toys in waiting areas.
  - Select toys that are easy to clean and disinfect.
  - Do not allow the use of stuffed, furry toys if they will be shared.
  - Clean and disinfect large stationary toys (for example, climbing equipment) at least weekly and when visibly soiled.
  - Rinse toys with water after disinfection if they are likely to be mouthed by children. Or wash them in a dishwasher.
  - Clean and disinfect a toy at once when it needs cleaning. Or store the toy in a labeled container away from toys that are clean and ready for use.

Textiles and Laundry

- Handle used textiles and fabrics (linens) with minimum agitation. This prevents contamination of air, surfaces, and other persons.

Worker Safety

- Protect yourself and others from exposure to bloodborne pathogens. This includes handling needles and other sharps. See "Bloodborne Pathogen Standard," p. 240.
- Use a mouthpiece, resuscitation bag, or other ventilation device for resuscitation to prevent contact with the person's mouth and oral secretions. See Chapter 54.

Patient or Resident Placement

- A private room is preferred if the person is at risk for transmitting the infection to others.
- Follow the nurse's directions if a private room is not available.

Modified from Siegel JD, Rhinehart E, Jackson M, Chiarello L, and the Healthcare Infection Control Practices Advisory Committee: Guideline for isolation precautions: preventing transmission of infectious agents in healthcare settings 2007, *Atlanta, 2007, Centers for Disease Control and Prevention.*

BOX 16-6	Transmission-Based Precautions

Contact Precautions
- Used for persons with known or suspected infections or conditions that increase the risk of contact transmission.
- Patient or resident placement:
  - A single room is preferred.
  - Do the following if a room is shared with another person not infected with the same agent.
    - Keep the privacy curtain between the beds closed.
    - Change PPE and practice hand hygiene between contact with persons in the same room. Do so regardless of whether 1 or both persons are on contact precautions.
- Gloves:
  - Don gloves upon entering the person's room or care setting.
  - Wear gloves to touch the person's intact skin.
  - Wear gloves to touch surfaces or items near the person.
- Gown:
  - Wear a gown when clothing may have direct contact with the person.
  - Wear a gown when contact is likely with surfaces or equipment near the person.
  - Don the gown upon entering the person's room.
  - Remove the gown and practice hand hygiene before leaving the person's room.
  - Make sure your clothing and skin do not touch potentially contaminated surfaces after removing the gown.
- Patient or resident transport:
  - Limit transport and movement of the person outside of the room to medically-necessary purposes.
  - Cover the infected area of the person's body.
  - Remove and discard contaminated PPE and practice hand hygiene before transporting the person.
  - Don clean PPE to handle the person at the transport destination.
- Care equipment:
  - Follow Standard Precautions.
  - Use disposable equipment when possible. If possible, leave non-disposable equipment in the person's room.
  - Clean and disinfect non-disposable and multiple-use equipment before use on another person.

Droplet Precautions
- Used for persons known or suspected to be infected with pathogens transmitted by respiratory droplets. Such droplets come from coughing, sneezing, or talking.
- Patient or resident placement:
  - A single room is preferred.
  - Do the following if a room is shared with another person who is not infected with the same agent.
    - Keep the privacy curtain between the beds closed.
    - Change PPE and practice hand hygiene between contact with persons in the same room. Do so regardless of whether 1 or both persons are on droplet precautions.
- PPE:
  - Don a mask upon entering the person's room.
- Patient or resident transport:
  - Limit transport and movement of the person outside of the room to medically-necessary purposes.
  - Have the person wear a mask.
  - Instruct the person to follow Respiratory Hygiene/Cough Etiquette (see Box 16-5).
  - No mask is required for staff transporting the person.

Airborne Precautions
- Used for persons known or suspected to be infected with pathogens transmitted person-to-person by the airborne route. Tuberculosis (TB), measles, chicken pox, smallpox, and severe acute respiratory syndrome (SARS) are examples.
- The person is placed in an airborne infection isolation room (AIIR). If not available, the person is transferred to an agency with an AIIR. AIIR practices include:
  - All persons entering the room wear a tuberculosis (TB) respirator.
  - The room door is kept closed except when someone enters or leaves the room.
  - Treatments and procedures are done in the room.
  - The person wears a mask during transport.
- Staff susceptible to the infection are restricted from entering the room. This is if immune staff members are available.
- PPE:
  - A mask or respirator is applied before entering the person's room.
  - An approved respirator is worn on entering the room or home of a person with TB.
  - Respiratory protection is recommended for all staff when caring for persons with smallpox.
- Patient or resident transport:
  - Limit transport and movement of the person outside of the room to medically-necessary purposes.
  - Have the person wear a surgical mask.
  - Instruct the person to follow Respiratory Hygiene/Cough Etiquette (see Box 16-5).
  - Cover skin lesions infected with the microbe.
  - No mask or respirator is required for staff transporting the person.

Modified from Siegel JD, Rhinehart E, Jackson M, Chiarello L, and the Healthcare Infection Control Practices Advisory Committee: Guideline for isolation precautions: preventing transmission of infectious agents in healthcare settings 2007, Atlanta, 2007, Centers for Disease Control and Prevention.

Transmission-Based Precautions

Some infections require Transmission-Based Precautions (Box 16-6). They are commonly called "isolation precautions." Transmission-Based Precautions require wearing PPE—gloves, gown, mask, and goggles or face shield. You must understand how certain infections are spread (see Fig. 16-2, p. 220). This helps you understand the different types of Transmission-Based Precautions.

Removing linens, trash, and equipment from the room may require double-bagging (p. 238). Follow agency procedures when collecting specimens and transporting persons.

Agency policies may differ from those in this text. The rules in Box 16-7 are a guide for giving safe care when using Transmission-Based Precautions.

See *Focus on Communication: Transmission-Based Precautions.*

See *Focus on Surveys: Transmission-Based Precautions.*

See *Delegation Guidelines: Transmission-Based Precautions.*

See *Promoting Safety and Comfort: Transmission-Based Precautions.*

FOCUS ON **COMMUNICATION**
Transmission-Based Precautions

The health team and visitors must know what PPE is needed. Signs are a common method to communicate the type of precaution and the needed PPE. Signs are posted at the person's doorway. In long-term care settings, signs may just instruct visitors to see the nurse before entering.

Visitors may ask why PPE is needed. Some visitors ignore signs or requests to wear PPE. You must communicate with the person and visitors about PPE. You can politely say:
- "Your visitors will need to wear a gown and gloves while in your room."
- "Please wear this mask. It is our policy to protect you, your family member, and others."

Tell the nurse if the person or visitors have more questions. Also tell the nurse if someone refuses to wear PPE.

Others on the health team may not wear needed PPE. Remind the person about needing PPE. Offer to get the person PPE. For example, you can say:
- "A mask is needed to care for Mrs. Stayton. I will get you one."
- "Here are gloves and a gown. They need to be worn in Mr. Parker's room."

Be polite. Tell the nurse if the person refuses.

BOX 16-7	Rules for Isolation Precautions

- Collect all needed items before entering the room.
- Do not contaminate equipment and supplies. Floors are contaminated. So is any object on the floor or that falls to the floor.
- Clean floors with mops wetted with a disinfectant solution. Floor dust is contaminated.
- Prevent drafts. Drafts can carry some microbes in the air.
- Use paper towels to handle contaminated items.
- Remove items from the room in leak-proof plastic bags.
- Double-bag items if the outside of the bag is or can be contaminated (p. 238).
- Follow agency policy to remove and transport disposable and re-usable items.
- Return re-usable dishes, drinking vessels, eating utensils, and trays to the food service (dietary) department. Discard disposable dishes, drinking vessels, eating utensils, and trays in the waste container in the person's room.
- Do not touch your hair, nose, mouth, eyes, or other body parts.
- Do not touch any clean area or object if your hands are contaminated.
- Wash your hands if they are visibly dirty or contaminated with blood, body fluids, secretions, or excretions.
- Place clean items on paper towels.
- Do not shake linens.
- Use paper towels to turn faucets on and off.
- Use a paper towel to open the door to the person's room. Discard it after use.
- Tell the nurse if you have any cuts, open skin areas, a sore throat, vomiting, or diarrhea.

FOCUS ON **SURVEYS**
Transmission-Based Precautions

When a person requires Transmission-Based Precautions, surveyors will observe if staff:
- Wash their hands correctly and at the correct times.
- Change gloves after providing personal care.
- Don, wear, and dispose of PPE correctly.

DELEGATION GUIDELINES
Transmission-Based Precautions

If a person needs Transmission-Based Precautions, review the type with the nurse. Also check with the nurse and care plan about:
- What PPE to use (p. 232)
- What special safety measures are needed

PROMOTING SAFETY AND COMFORT
Transmission-Based Precautions

Safety
Preventing the spread of infection is important. Transmission-Based Precautions protect everyone—patients, residents, visitors, staff, and you. If you are careless, everyone's safety is at risk.

Personal Protective Equipment

The PPE needed depends on tasks, procedures, care measures, and the type of Transmission-Based Precautions used. Sometimes only gloves are needed. The nurse tells you when a gown, goggles or a face shield, and a mask are needed.

See *Teamwork and Time Management: Personal Protective Equipment.*

Gowns. Gowns prevent the spread of microbes. They protect your clothes and body from contact with blood, body fluids, secretions, and excretions. They also protect against splashes and sprays.

A gown must completely cover you from your neck to your knees. The long sleeves have tight cuffs. The gown opens at the back. It is tied at the neck and waist. The gown front and sleeves are considered *contaminated.*

Gowns are used once. A wet gown is contaminated. Remove it and put on a dry one. Discard disposable gowns after use.

Masks and Respiratory Protection. You wear disposable masks:

• For protection from contact with infectious materials from the person. Respiratory secretions and sprays of blood or body fluids are examples.
• When assisting with sterile procedures. This protects the person from infectious agents carried in your mouth or nose.

A wet or moist mask is *contaminated.* Breathing can cause masks to become wet or moist. Apply a new mask when contamination occurs.

A mask fits snugly over your nose and mouth. Practice hand hygiene before putting on a mask. To remove a mask, touch only the ties or the elastic bands. The front of the mask is contaminated.

Tuberculosis respirators (Fig. 16-15) are worn when caring for persons with TB. See Chapter 45 for more information about persons with TB.

Goggles and Face Shields. Goggles and face shields protect your eyes, mouth, and nose from splashing or spraying of blood, body fluids, secretions, and excretions. Splashes and sprays can occur when you give care, clean items, or dispose of fluids.

The front (outside) of goggles or a face shield is *contaminated.* The headband, ties, or ear-pieces used to secure the device are *clean.* Use them to remove the device after hand hygiene. They are safe to touch with bare hands. Lift the ties or ear-pieces from the back when removing the device.

Discard disposable goggles or face shields after use. Re-usable eyewear is cleaned before re-use. It is washed with soap and water. Then a disinfectant is used.

See *Promoting Safety and Comfort: Goggles and Face Shields.*

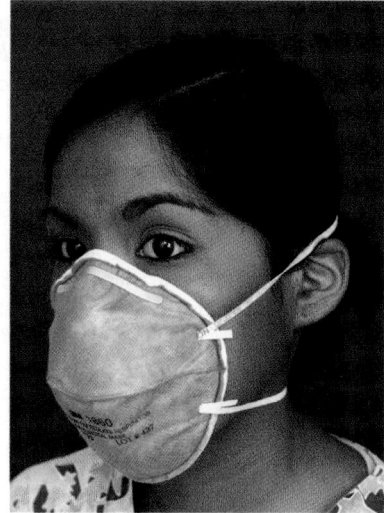

FIGURE 16-15 Tuberculosis respirator.

TEAMWORK AND TIME MANAGEMENT

Personal Protective Equipment

Donning (putting on) and removing PPE take time and effort. Once you don PPE, you must remove it before leaving the room. Therefore you need to plan your time and work so you do not need to leave the room.

• Meet the needs of other patients or residents first.
• Ask a co-worker to answer call lights for you. Ask politely and thank your co-worker for helping you.
• Gather needed care items to bring to the room.
• Make sure the person's needs are met before leaving the room.
• Complete a safety check of the room.
• Tell the person when you will return to the room.

Offer to help co-workers who care for persons needing Transmission-Based Precautions. Bring items to the room as needed. Also answer call lights. Be sure to tell them about the care given and your observations.

PROMOTING SAFETY AND COMFORT

Goggles and Face Shields

Safety

Eyeglasses and contact lenses do not provide eye protection. If you wear eyeglasses, the face shield must fit over your glasses with minimal gaps.

Goggles do not provide splash or spray protection to other parts of your face.

Gloves. A natural barrier, the skin prevents microbes from entering the body. Small skin breaks on the hands and fingers are common. Some are very small and hard to see. Disposable gloves act as a barrier. They protect:

- You from pathogens in the person's blood, body fluids, secretions, and excretions
- The person from microbes on your hands

Wear gloves when contact with blood, body fluids, secretions, excretions, mucous membranes, or non-intact skin is likely. Contact may be direct. Or contact may be with items or surfaces contaminated with blood, body fluids, secretions, or excretions.

Wearing gloves is the most common measure for Standard Precautions and Transmission-Based Precautions. When using gloves:

- Consider the outside of gloves as *contaminated.*
- Apply to dry hands. Gloves are easier to put on dry hands.
- Do not tear gloves when putting them on. Carelessness, long fingernails, and rings can tear gloves. Blood, body fluids, secretions, and excretions can enter the glove through the tear. This contaminates your hand.
- Remove and discard torn, cut, or punctured gloves at once. Practice hand hygiene. Then put on a new pair.
- Apply a new pair for every person.
- Wear gloves once. Discard them after use.
- Put on new gloves just before touching mucous membranes or non-intact skin.
- Put on new gloves when gloves become contaminated with blood, body fluids, secretions, or excretions. A task may require more than 1 pair of gloves.
- Change gloves when moving from a contaminated body site to a clean body site.
- Change gloves when touching portable computer keyboards or other mobile equipment that is transported from room to room.
- Put on gloves last when they are worn with other PPE.
- Make sure gloves cover your wrists. If you wear a gown, gloves cover the cuffs (Fig. 16-16).
- Remove gloves so the inside part is on the outside. The inside is *clean.*
- Practice hand hygiene after removing gloves.
 See *Promoting Safety and Comfort: Gloves.*

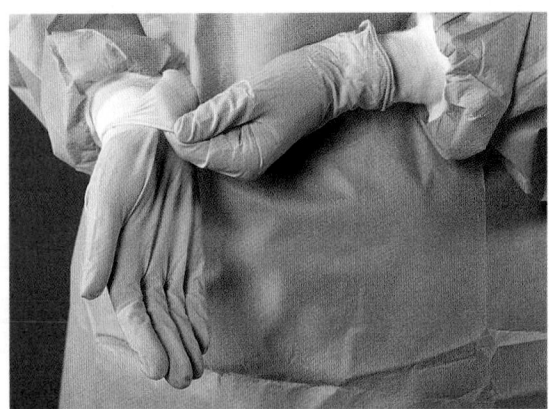
FIGURE 16-16 The gloves cover the gown cuffs.

PROMOTING SAFETY AND COMFORT
Gloves

Safety
No special method is needed to put on non-sterile gloves. To remove gloves, see procedure: *Donning and Removing Personal Protective Equipment,* p. 237.

Some gloves are made of latex (a rubber product). Latex allergies can cause skin rashes. Difficulty breathing and shock are more serious problems. Report skin rashes and breathing problems to the nurse at once.

You may have a latex allergy. Some patients and residents are allergic to latex. This is noted on the care plan and your assignment sheet. Latex-free gloves are worn for latex allergies.

Comfort
Gloves are needed when contact with blood, body fluids, secretions, excretions, mucous membranes, or non-intact skin is likely. Gloves are not needed when such contact is not likely. Back massages and brushing and combing hair are examples. To reduce exposure to latex, wear gloves only when needed.

Donning and Removing PPE. The type of PPE worn depends on the type of precautions needed. According to the CDC's isolation guidelines, gloves are always worn when gowns are worn. Sometimes other PPE is needed when gowns are worn.

See *Promoting Safety and Comfort: Donning and Removing PPE,* p. 234.

See procedure: *Donning and Removing Personal Protective Equipment,* p. 237.

Text continued on p. 238.

PROMOTING SAFETY AND COMFORT
Donning and Removing PPE

Safety

According to the CDC, PPE is donned and removed in the following order.

- Donning PPE (Fig. 16-17, A):
  1. Gown
  2. Mask or respirator
  3. Eyewear (goggles or face shield)
  4. Gloves
- Removing PPE (removed at the doorway before leaving the person's room):
  - Method 1 (Fig. 16-17, B)
    1. Gloves
    2. Eyewear (goggles or face shield)
    3. Gown
    4. Mask or respirator (respirator is removed after leaving the person's room and closing the door)
- Method 2 (Fig. 16-17, C, p. 236)
  1. Gown and gloves
  2. Eyewear (goggles or face shield)
  3. Mask or respirator (respirator is removed after leaving the person's room and closing the door)

Practice hand hygiene after removing PPE. Practice hand hygiene between steps if your hands become contaminated. Then practice hand hygiene again after removing all PPE.

(NOTE: Some state competency tests require hand hygiene after removing each PPE item. And some states use a different order for donning and removing PPE. Follow the procedures used in your state and agency.)

Some infections such as Ebola (Chapter 45) are very severe and deadly. Such infections require additional PPE—full face shield, helmet, or headpiece; coveralls with socks or special gowns; double gloving; boot or shoe covers; and aprons. Special training is needed to care for such patients and for donning and removing the PPE.

SEQUENCE FOR PUTTING ON PERSONAL PROTECTIVE EQUIPMENT (PPE)

The type of PPE used will vary based on the level of precautions required, such as standard and contact, droplet or airborne infection isolation precautions. The procedure for putting on and removing PPE should be tailored to the specific type of PPE.

1. GOWN

- Fully cover torso from neck to knees, arms to end of wrists, and wrap around the back
- Fasten in back of neck and waist

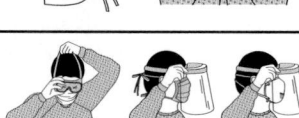

2. MASK OR RESPIRATOR

- Secure ties or elastic bands at middle of head and neck
- Fit flexible band to nose bridge
- Fit snug to face and below chin
- Fit-check respirator

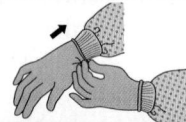

A

3. GOGGLES OR FACE SHIELD

- Place over face and eyes and adjust to fit

4. GLOVES

- Extend to cover wrist of isolation gown

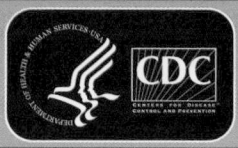

USE SAFE WORK PRACTICES TO PROTECT YOURSELF AND LIMIT THE SPREAD OF CONTAMINATION

- Keep hands away from face
- Limit surfaces touched
- Change gloves when torn or heavily contaminated
- Perform hand hygiene

CDC

CS250672-E

FIGURE 16-17 A, Donning PPE. (From Centers for Disease Control, Department of Health and Human Services.)

HOW TO SAFELY REMOVE PERSONAL PROTECTIVE EQUIPMENT (PPE) EXAMPLE 1

There are a variety of ways to safely remove PPE without contaminating your clothing, skin, or mucous membranes with potentially infectious materials. Here is one example. **Remove all PPE before exiting the patient room** except a respirator, if worn. Remove the respirator **after** leaving the patient room and closing the door. Remove PPE in the following sequence:

1. GLOVES

- Outside of gloves are contaminated!
- If your hands get contaminated during glove removal, immediately wash your hands or use an alcohol-based hand sanitizer
- Using a gloved hand, grasp the palm area of the other gloved hand and peel off first glove
- Hold removed glove in gloved hand
- Slide fingers of ungloved hand under remaining glove at wrist and peel off second glove over first glove
- Discard gloves in a waste container

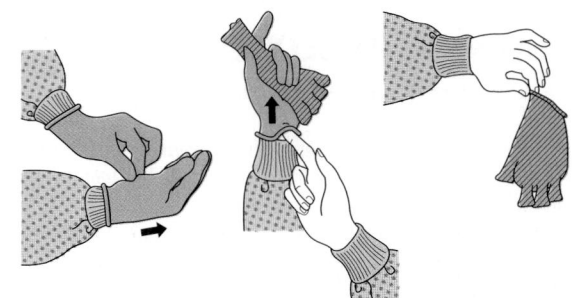

2. GOGGLES OR FACE SHIELD

- Outside of goggles or face shield are contaminated!
- If your hands get contaminated during goggle or face shield removal, immediately wash your hands or use an alcohol-based hand sanitizer
- Remove goggles or face shield from the back by lifting head band or ear pieces
- If the item is reusable, place in designated receptacle for reprocessing. Otherwise, discard in a waste container

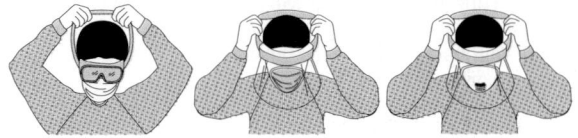

3. GOWN

- Gown front and sleeves are contaminated!
- If your hands get contaminated during gown removal, immediately wash your hands or use an alcohol-based hand sanitizer
- Unfasten gown ties, taking care that sleeves don't contact your body when reaching for ties
- Pull gown away from neck and shoulders, touching inside of gown only
- Turn gown inside out
- Fold or roll into a bundle and discard in a waste container

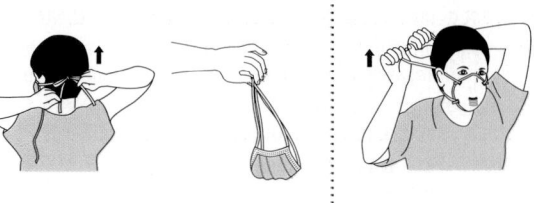

B

4. MASK OR RESPIRATOR

- Front of mask/respirator is contaminated — DO NOT TOUCH!
- If your hands get contaminated during mask/respirator removal, immediately wash your hands or use an alcohol-based hand sanitizer
- Grasp bottom ties or elastics of the mask/respirator, then the ones at the top, and remove without touching the front
- Discard in a waste container

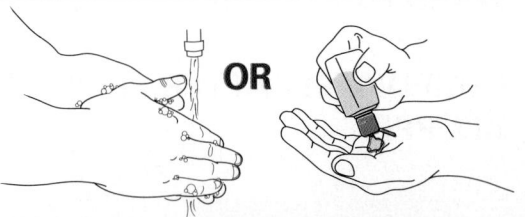

5. WASH HANDS OR USE AN ALCOHOL-BASED HAND SANITIZER IMMEDIATELY AFTER REMOVING ALL PPE

OR

PERFORM HAND HYGIENE BETWEEN STEPS IF HANDS BECOME CONTAMINATED AND IMMEDIATELY AFTER REMOVING ALL PPE

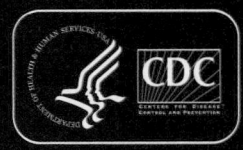

CS250672-E

FIGURE 16-17, cont'd B, Method 1: Removing PPE.

Continued

HOW TO SAFELY REMOVE PERSONAL PROTECTIVE EQUIPMENT (PPE) EXAMPLE 2

Here is another way to safely remove PPE without contaminating your clothing, skin, or mucous membranes with potentially infectious materials. **Remove all PPE before exiting the patient room** except a respirator, if worn. Remove the respirator **after** leaving the patient room and closing the door. Remove PPE in the following sequence:

1. GOWN AND GLOVES

- Gown front and sleeves and the outside of gloves are contaminated!
- If your hands get contaminated during gown or glove removal, immediately wash your hands or use an alcohol-based hand sanitizer
- Grasp the gown in the front and pull away from your body so that the ties break, touching outside of gown only with gloved hands
- While removing the gown, fold or roll the gown inside-out into a bundle
- As you are removing the gown, peel off your gloves at the same time, only touching the inside of the gloves and gown with your bare hands. Place the gown and gloves into a waste container

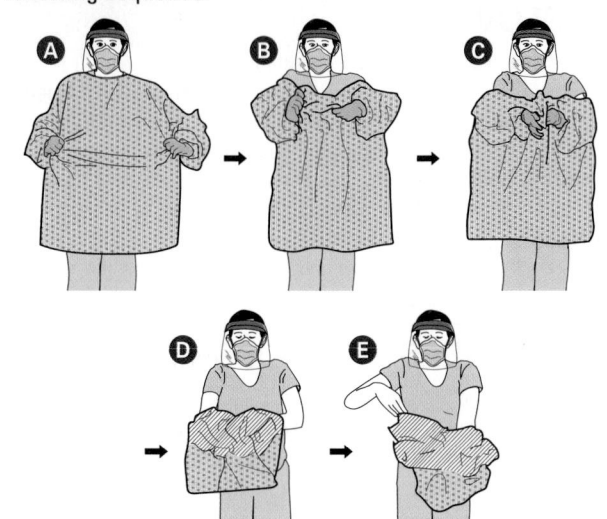

2. GOGGLES OR FACE SHIELD

- Outside of goggles or face shield are contaminated!
- If your hands get contaminated during goggle or face shield removal, immediately wash your hands or use an alcohol-based hand sanitizer
- Remove goggles or face shield from the back by lifting head band and without touching the front of the goggles or face shield
- If the item is reusable, place in designated receptacle for reprocessing. Otherwise, discard in a waste container

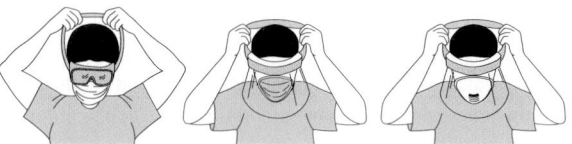

3. MASK OR RESPIRATOR

- Front of mask/respirator is contaminated — DO NOT TOUCH!
- If your hands get contaminated during mask/respirator removal, immediately wash your hands or use an alcohol-based hand sanitizer
- Grasp bottom ties or elastics of the mask/respirator, then the ones at the top, and remove without touching the front
- Discard in a waste container

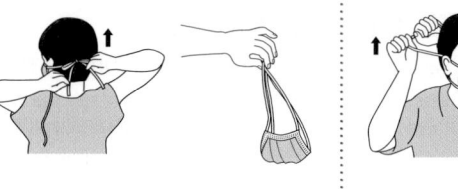

4. WASH HANDS OR USE AN ALCOHOL-BASED HAND SANITIZER IMMEDIATELY AFTER REMOVING ALL PPE

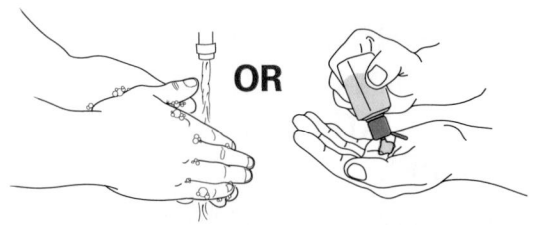

OR

PERFORM HAND HYGIENE BETWEEN STEPS IF HANDS BECOME CONTAMINATED AND IMMEDIATELY AFTER REMOVING ALL PPE

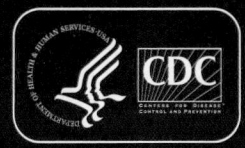

CS250672-E

FIGURE 16-17, cont'd C, Method 2: Removing PPE.

C

Donning and Removing Personal Protective Equipment
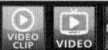

PROCEDURE

1 Follow *Delegation Guidelines: Transmission-Based Precautions*, p. 231. See *Promoting Safety and Comfort*:
  a *Transmission-Based Precautions*, p. 231.
  b *Goggles and Face Shields*, p. 232.
  c *Gloves*, p. 233.
  d *Donning and Removing PPE*, p. 234.
2 Remove your watch and all jewelry.
3 Roll up uniform sleeves.
4 Practice hand hygiene.
5 Put on a gown (see Fig. 16-17, *A*).
  a Hold a clean gown out in front of you.
  b Unfold the gown. Face the back of the gown. Do not shake it.
  c Put your hands and arms through the sleeves.
  d Make sure the gown covers you from your neck to your knees. It must cover your arms to the end of your wrists.
  e Tie the strings at the back of the neck.
  f Overlap the back of the gown. Make sure it covers your uniform. The gown should be snug, not loose.
  g Tie the waist strings. Tie them at the back or the side. Do not tie them in front.
6 Put on a mask or respirator (see Fig. 16-17, *A*).
  a Pick up a mask by its upper ties. Do not touch the part that will cover your face.
  b Place the mask over your nose and mouth (Fig. 16-18, *A*, p. 238).
  c Place the upper strings above your ears. Tie them at the back in the middle of your head (Fig. 16-18, *B*, p. 238).
  d Tie the lower strings at the back of your neck (Fig. 16-18, *C*, p. 238). The lower part of the mask is under your chin.
  e Pinch the metal band around your nose. The top of the mask must be snug over your nose. If you wear eyeglasses, the mask must be snug under the bottom of the eyeglasses.
  f Make sure the mask is snug over your face and under your chin.
7 Put on goggles or a face shield (if needed and if not part of the mask) (see Fig. 16-17, *A*).
  a Place the device over your face and eyes. Touch only the ties or the elastic bands.
  b Adjust the device to fit.
8 Put on gloves. Make sure the gloves cover the wrists of the gown.
9 Provide care.
10 Remove and discard the PPE. Practice hand hygiene between each step if your hands become contaminated.
  a *Method 1: Gloves, goggles or face shield, gown, mask or respirator* (see Fig. 16-17, *B*)
    1) Remove and discard the gloves.
      a) Make sure that glove touches only glove.
      b) Grasp a glove at the palm (Fig. 16-19, *A*, p. 238). Grasp it on the outside.
      c) Pull the glove down over your hand so it is inside out (Fig. 16-19, *B*, p. 238).
      d) Hold the removed glove with your other gloved hand.
      e) Reach inside the other glove. Use the first 2 fingers of the ungloved hand (Fig. 16-19, *C*, p. 238).
      f) Pull the glove down (inside out) over your hand and the other glove (Fig. 16-19, *D*, p. 238).
      g) Discard the gloves.

  2) Remove and discard the goggles or face shield if worn.
    a) Lift the headband from the back. Do not touch the front of the device.
    b) Discard the device. If re-usable, follow agency policy.
  3) Remove and discard the gown. Do not touch the outside of the gown.
    a) Untie the neck and then the waist strings.
    b) Pull the gown down and away from your neck and shoulders. Only touch the inside of the gown.
    c) Turn the gown inside out as it is removed. Hold it at the inside shoulder seams and bring your hands together.
    d) Fold or roll up the gown away from you. Keep it inside out. Do not let the gown touch the floor.
    e) Discard the gown.
  4) Remove and discard the mask if worn. (NOTE: Remove a respirator after leaving the room and closing the door.)
    a) Untie the lower strings of the mask.
    b) Untie the top strings.
    c) Hold the top strings. Remove the mask.
    d) Discard the mask.
  b *Method 2: Gown and gloves, goggles or face shield, mask or respirator* (see Fig. 16-17, *C*).
    1) Remove and discard the gown and gloves.
      a) Grasp the gown in front with your gloved hands. Pull away from your body so the ties break. Only touch the outside of the gown.
      b) Fold or roll the gown inside-out into a bundle while removing the gown. Keep it inside out. Do not let the gown touch the floor.
      c) Peel off your gloves as you remove the gown. Only touch the inside of the gloves and gown with your bare hands.
      d) Discard the gown and gloves.
    2) Remove and discard the goggles or face shield.
      a) Lift the headband from the back. Do not touch the front of the device.
      b) Discard the device. If re-usable, follow agency policy.
    3) Remove and discard the mask if worn. (NOTE: Remove a respirator after leaving the room and closing the door.)
      a) Untie the lower strings of the mask.
      b) Untie the top strings.
      c) Hold the top strings. Remove the mask.
      d) Discard the mask.
11 Practice hand hygiene after removing all PPE.

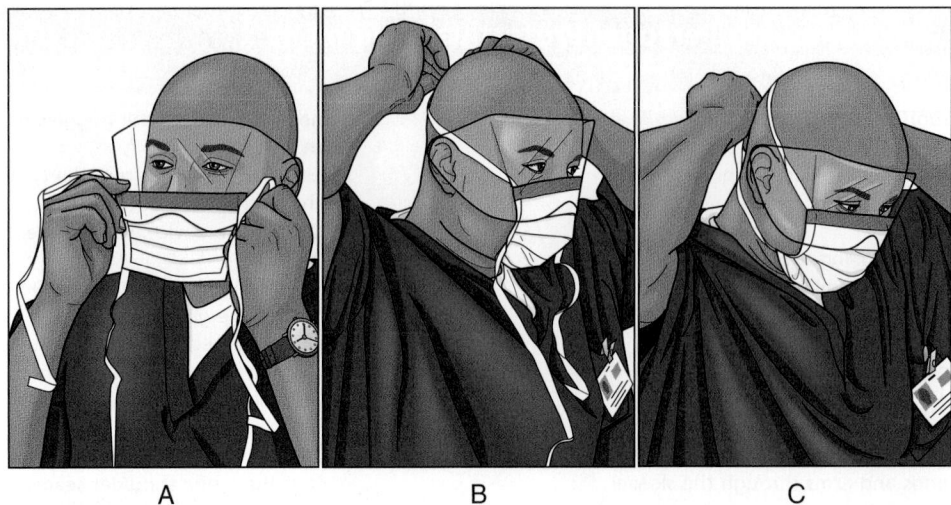

FIGURE 16-18 Donning a mask. (NOTE: The mask has a face shield.) **A,** The mask covers the nose and mouth. **B,** Upper strings are tied at the back of the head. **C,** Lower strings are tied at the back of the neck.

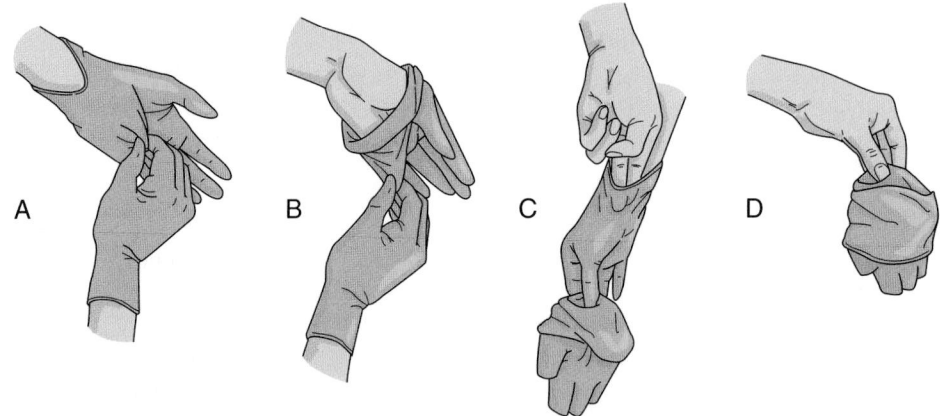

FIGURE 16-19 Removing gloves. **A,** Grasp the glove at the palm. **B,** Pull the glove down over the hand. The glove is inside out. **C,** Insert the fingers of the ungloved hand inside the other glove. **D,** Pull the glove down and over the other hand and glove. The glove is inside out.

Bagging Items. Contaminated items are bagged for removal from the person's room. Leak-proof plastic bags are used. They have the *BIOHAZARD* symbol (Fig. 16-20). *Biohazardous waste is items contaminated with blood, body fluids, secretions, or excretions.* (Bio *means* life. Hazardous *means* dangerous *or* harmful.)

Bag and transport linens following agency policy. Laundry bags with contaminated linen need a *BIOHAZARD* symbol. Melt-away bags dissolve in hot water. Once soiled linen is bagged, no one needs to handle it. Do not over-fill the bag. Tie the bag securely. Then place it in a laundry hamper lined with a biohazard plastic bag.

Trash is placed in a container labeled with the *BIOHAZARD* symbol. Follow agency policy for bagging and transporting trash, equipment, and supplies.

Usually 1 bag is needed. Double-bagging involves 2 bags. Double-bagging is needed if the outside of the bag is wet, soiled, or may be contaminated.

See procedure: *Double-Bagging.*

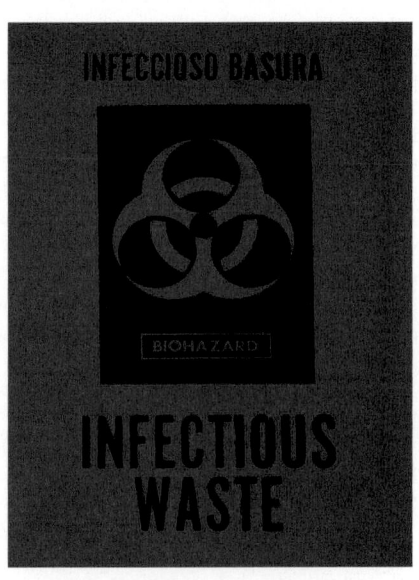

FIGURE 16-20 *BIOHAZARD* symbol.

Double-Bagging

PROCEDURE

1 Ask a co-worker to help you. He or she stands outside the doorway. You are in the room.
2 Place soiled linen, re-usable items, disposable supplies, and trash in the right containers. Containers are lined with leak-proof biohazard bags. These are the *dirty (contaminated)* bags.
3 Seal the *dirty* bag securely.
4 Ask your co-worker to make a wide cuff on a *clean* bag. It is held wide open. The cuff protects the hands from contamination (Fig. 16-21, *A*).

5 Place the *dirty* bag into the *clean* bag (Fig. 16-21, *B*). Do not touch the outside of the *clean* bag.
6 Ask your co-worker to seal the *clean* bag. Have the bag labeled with the *BIOHAZARD* symbol.
7 Repeat steps 3, 4, 5, and 6 for other *dirty* bags.
8 Ask your co-worker to take or send the bags to the appropriate department for disposal, disinfection, or sterilization.

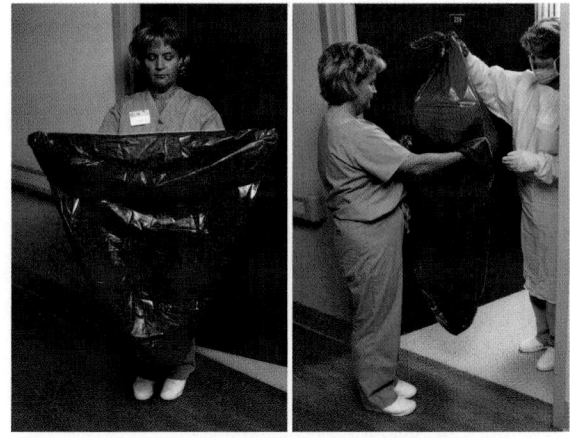

A   B

FIGURE 16-21 Double-bagging. **A,** A cuff is made on a clean bag. **B,** One nursing assistant is in the room by the doorway. The other is outside the doorway. The *dirty* bag is placed inside the *clean* bag.

Collecting Specimens. Blood, body fluids, secretions, and excretions often require laboratory testing (Chapter 34). Specimens are transported to the laboratory in biohazard specimen bags. To collect a specimen:

- Label the specimen container and biohazard specimen bag. Apply warning labels according to agency policy. Leave the biohazard bag outside the room.
- Wear gloves. Don other PPE as required.
- Put the specimen container and lid in the person's bathroom. Put them on a paper towel.
- Collect the specimen. Do not contaminate the outside of the container. Also avoid contamination when transferring the specimen from the collecting vessel to the specimen container.
- Put the lid on securely.
- Remove and discard PPE. Practice hand hygiene.
- Use a paper towel to pick up and take the container outside the room.
- Put the container in the biohazard bag. Avoid touching the outside of the bag with the specimen container.
- Discard the paper towels.
- Follow agency policy for storing the specimen.
- Practice hand hygiene.

Transporting Persons. Persons on Transmission-Based Precautions usually do not leave their rooms. Sometimes they go to other areas for treatments or tests.

Transport procedures vary among agencies. Some require transport by bed. This prevents contaminating wheelchairs and stretchers. Others use wheelchairs and stretchers.

A safe transport protects others from the infection. Follow agency procedures and these guidelines.

- Have the person wear a clean gown or pajamas and an isolation gown.
- Have the person wear a mask as required by the Transmission-Based Precautions used.
- Cover any draining wounds.
- Give the person tissues and a leak-proof bag. Used tissues are placed in the bag.
- Wear PPE as required.
- Place an extra layer of sheets and absorbent pads on the stretcher or wheelchair. This protects against draining body fluids.
- Do not let others on the elevator. This reduces exposure to infection.
- Alert staff in the receiving area about the Transmission-Based Precautions. They wear gloves and PPE as needed.
- Disinfect the stretcher or wheelchair after use.

Meeting Basic Needs

The person has love, belonging, and self-esteem needs. Often they are unmet during Transmission-Based Precautions. Visitors and staff avoid the person. Putting on PPE takes extra effort before entering the room. Some are not sure what they can touch. They may fear getting the disease.

The person may feel lonely, unwanted, and rejected. The person knows the disease can be spread to others. He or she may feel dirty and undesirable. Without intending to, visitors and staff can make the person feel ashamed and guilty for having a contagious disease.

The nurse helps the person, visitors, and staff understand the need for Transmission-Based Precautions and how they affect the person.

You can help meet love, belonging, and self-esteem needs. To help the person:
- Remember that the pathogen is undesirable, not the person.
- Treat the person with respect, kindness, and dignity.
- Provide newspapers, magazines, books, a current TV guide, and other reading matter.
- Provide hobby materials if possible.
- Place a clock in the room.
- Suggest that the person call family and friends.
- Plan your work so you can stay to visit with the person.
- Say "hello" from the doorway often.

Items brought into the person's room become contaminated. Disinfect or discard the items according to agency policy.

See *Focus on Communication: Meeting Basic Needs.*

See *Focus on Children and Older Persons: Meeting Basic Needs.*

BLOODBORNE PATHOGEN STANDARD

The human immunodeficiency virus (HIV) and the hepatitis B virus (HBV) are major health concerns (Chapters 43 and 46). The Bloodborne Pathogen Standard is intended to protect the health team from exposure to these viruses. It is a regulation of the Occupational Safety and Health Administration (OSHA). See Box 16-8 for terms used in the standard.

Found in the blood, HIV and HBV are bloodborne pathogens. They exit the body through blood. They are spread to others by blood and other potentially infectious materials (OPIM) (see Box 16-8).

Exposure Control Plan

The agency's exposure control plan identifies staff at risk for exposure to blood or OPIM. All caregivers and laundry, supply, and housekeeping staffs are at risk. The plan lists actions for an exposure incident.

Staff receive free training upon employment and yearly. Training is also done for new or changed tasks involving exposure to bloodborne pathogens. Training includes:
- An explanation of the standard, the exposure control plan, and where to get a copy of each
- The causes, signs, and symptoms of bloodborne diseases
- How bloodborne pathogens are spread
- The tasks that might cause exposure
- The use and limits of safe work practices, engineering controls, and PPE
- Information about the hepatitis B vaccination
- Who to contact and what to do in an emergency
- Information on reporting an exposure incident, post-exposure evaluation, and follow-up
- Information on warning labels and color-coding

BOX 16-8	Bloodborne Pathogen Standard Terms

Blood. Human blood, human blood components, and products made from human blood.

Bloodborne pathogens. Pathogens present in human blood that can cause disease in humans. They include but are not limited to HBV and HIV.

Contaminated. The presence or reasonably anticipated presence of blood or OPIM on an item or surface.

Contaminated laundry. Laundry soiled with blood or OPIM or that may contain sharps.

Contaminated sharps. Any contaminated object that can penetrate the skin—needles, scalpels, broken glass, broken capillary tubes, exposed ends of dental wires, and so on.

Decontamination. The use of physical or chemical means to remove, inactivate, or destroy bloodborne pathogens on a surface or item. The infectious particles can no longer be transmitted. The surface or item is safe for handling, use, or disposal.

Engineering controls. Controls that isolate or remove the bloodborne pathogen hazard from the workplace (sharps disposal containers, self-sheathing needles).

Exposure incident. Eye, mouth, other mucous membrane, non-intact skin, or parenteral contact with blood or OPIM that results from an employee's duties.

Hand-washing facilities. The adequate supply of running water, soap, single-use towels, or hot-air drying machines.

HBV. Hepatitis B virus.

HIV. Human immunodeficiency virus.

Occupational exposure. Reasonably anticipated skin, eye, mucous membrane, or parenteral contact with blood or OPIM that may result from an employee's duties.

Other potentially infectious materials (OPIM):
- Human body fluids—semen, vaginal secretions, cerebrospinal fluid, synovial fluid, pleural fluid, pericardial fluid, peritoneal fluid, amniotic fluid, saliva in dental procedures, body fluid that is visibly contaminated with blood, and all body fluids when it is difficult or impossible to differentiate between them
- Any tissue or organ (other than intact skin) from a human (living or dead)
- HIV-containing cell or tissue cultures, organ cultures, and HIV- or HBV-containing culture medium or other solutions; blood, organs, or other tissues from experimental animals infected with HIV or HBV

Parenteral. Piercing mucous membranes or the skin through needle-sticks, human bites, cuts, abrasions, and so on.

Personal protective equipment (PPE). The clothing or equipment worn by staff for protection against a hazard.

Regulated waste:
- Liquid or semi-liquid blood or OPIM
- Contaminated items that would release blood or OPIM in a liquid or semi-liquid state if compressed
- Items caked with dried blood or OPIM that can release these materials during handling
- Contaminated sharps
- Pathological and microbiological wastes containing blood or OPIM

Source individual. Any person (living or dead) whose blood or OPIM may be a source of occupational exposure to staff. Examples include but are not limited to:
- Hospital and clinic patients
- Clients in agencies for the intellectually and developmentally disabled
- Trauma victims
- Clients of drug and alcohol treatment agencies
- Hospice and nursing center residents
- Human remains
- Persons who donate or sell blood or blood components

Sterilize. The use of a physical or chemical procedure to destroy all microbes, including spores.

Work practice controls. Controls that reduce the likelihood of exposure by changing the way the task is performed.

Preventive Measures

Preventive measures reduce the risk of exposure. Such measures follow.

Hepatitis B Vaccination.

Hepatitis B is a liver disease caused by HBV. HBV is spread by the blood and sexual contact.

The hepatitis B vaccine produces immunity against hepatitis B. *Immunity means that a person has protection against a certain disease.* He or she will not get the disease.

A *vaccination* *involves giving a vaccine to produce immunity against an infectious disease.* A *vaccine* is a preparation containing dead or weakened microbes. The hepatitis B vaccination involves 3 injections (shots). Injection 2 is given 1 month after the first. Injection 3 is given at least 4 months after the first one. The vaccination can be given before or after HBV exposure.

You can receive the hepatitis B vaccination within 10 working days of being hired. The agency pays for it. You can refuse the vaccination. If so, you must sign a statement refusing the vaccine. You can have the vaccination at a later date if you want.

Work Practice Controls. *Work practice controls* reduce employee exposure in the workplace. All tasks involving blood or OPIM are done in ways to limit splatters, splashes, and sprays. Producing droplets also is avoided.

OSHA requires these work practice controls.

- Do not eat, drink, smoke, apply cosmetics or lip balm, or handle contact lenses in areas of exposure.
- Do not store food or drinks where blood or OPIM are kept.
- Practice hand hygiene after removing gloves.
- Wash hands as soon as possible after skin contact with blood or OPIM.
- Never re-cap, bend, or remove needles by hand. Use a mechanical means (forceps) or a 1-handed method.
- Never shear or break needles.
- Discard needles and sharp instruments (such as razors) in containers that are closable, puncture-resistant, and leak-proof. *Containers are color-coded in red and have the BIOHAZARD symbol.* Containers must be upright and not allowed to over-fill.

Personal Protective Equipment (PPE). This includes gloves, goggles, face shields, masks, laboratory coats, gowns, shoe covers, and surgical caps. Blood or OPIM must not pass through them. They protect your clothes, undergarments, skin, eyes, mouth, and hair.

PPE is free to staff in the correct sizes. OSHA requires these measures for PPE.

- Remove PPE before leaving the work area.
- Remove PPE when it becomes contaminated.
- Place used PPE in marked areas or containers when being stored, washed, decontaminated, or discarded.
- Wear gloves for contact with blood or OPIM.
- Wear gloves to handle or touch contaminated items or surfaces.
- Replace worn, punctured, or contaminated gloves.
- Never wash or decontaminate disposable gloves for re-use.
- Discard utility gloves that show signs of cracking, peeling, tearing, or puncturing. Utility gloves are decontaminated for re-use if the process will not ruin them.

Equipment. Contaminated equipment is cleaned and decontaminated. Decontaminate equipment and work surfaces with a proper disinfectant.

- Upon completing tasks
- At once for obvious contamination
- At the end of your work shift when surfaces became contaminated since the last cleaning

Use a brush and dustpan or tongs to clean up broken glass. Never pick up broken glass with your hands, not even with gloves. Discard broken glass into a puncture-resistant container.

Waste. Special measures are used to discard regulated waste.

- Liquid or semi-liquid blood or OPIM
- Items contaminated with blood or OPIM
- Items caked with blood or OPIM
- Contaminated sharps

Closable, puncture-resistant, leak-proof containers are used. Containers are color-coded in red. They have the *BIOHAZARD* symbol.

See *Focus on Long-Term Care and Home Care: Waste.*

Housekeeping. A cleaning schedule is required to keep the agency clean and sanitary. It includes decontamination methods and required tasks and procedures.

Laundry. OSHA requires these measures for contaminated laundry.

- Handle it as little as possible.
- Wear gloves or other needed PPE.
- Bag contaminated laundry where it is used.
- Mark laundry bags or containers with the *BIOHAZARD* symbol for laundry sent off-site.
- Place wet, contaminated laundry in leak-proof containers before transport. The containers are color-coded in red or have the *BIOHAZARD* symbol.

See *Focus on Surveys: Laundry.*

FOCUS ON SURVEYS

Laundry

Surveyors will observe how staff handle, store, process, and transport linen. For example, do staff:

- Handle linens in a way that prevents exposure of urine or feces?
- Handle linens in a way that prevents the spread of infection?
- Handle linens according to agency policies and procedures?
- Store and transport linens properly?

FOCUS ON LONG-TERM CARE AND HOME CARE

Waste

Home Care

Dressings, gloves, and other care items are used in home care. So are syringes, needles, and sharps (such as razors). The patient or family may use syringes or needles. You use safety razors for shaving (Chapter 23) and lancets for blood glucose testing (Chapter 34). Proper disposal:

- Protects neighbors, children, pets, janitors, housekeepers, sanitation workers, and sewage treatment workers from injury and infection. HIV, AIDS, and hepatitis B and C are risks.
- Prevents needle sharing and re-using sharps.
- Protects the environment.
  According to the Environmental Protection Agency (EPA):
- Do not throw loose needles, syringes, or sharps into the trash or into a recycling bin.
- Do not flush needles, syringes, or sharps down the toilet.
- Do not put needles, syringes, or sharps in recycling containers for bottles, plastics, and paper.
  Properly store used needles, syringes, and sharps.
- Put them in a commercial or household sharps container right after use. A household container can be a hard plastic, puncture-resistant container with a screw-on lid. Detergent bottles with screw-on lids are examples. Secure the lid in place with heavy tape for added protection. See Figure 16-22.
- Label the container with "Do Not Recycle" or "SHARPS" label.
- Put sharps in the container point-first.
- Do not use soda cans or bottles, milk cartons, glass bottles, coffee cans, aluminum cans, or other containers that are not puncture-resistant.
- Keep storage containers where children cannot reach them.

Many states have disposal options. The nurse and care plan tell you what to use at the person's address. The EPA describes these disposal options.

- *Drop-off collection sites.* Filled sharps containers are taken to a collection site. Hospitals, doctors' offices, clinics, pharmacies, health departments, and police and fire stations are examples. So are medical waste facilities.
- *Household hazardous waste collection sites.* Sharps containers are placed in sharps collection bins at a collection site.
- *Residential special waste pick-up services.* Used sharps are placed in a special recycling-type container. The container is placed outside the home for collection by special waste handlers. Programs have regular pick-up times or require a call for pick-up.
- *Mail-back programs.* Used sharps are placed in special containers and mailed to a collection site. U.S. Postal Service procedures are followed. The program works well for rural areas.
- *Syringe-exchange programs.* Used needles and syringes are exchanged for new ones. The agency operating the program disposes of used ones.
- *Home needle destruction devices.* Such devices clip, melt, or burn the needle. The syringe and destroyed needle are placed in the trash.
  Dressings, gloves, soiled bed protectors, and other care items also need proper disposal.
- Place them in plastic bags.
- Close the bags securely.
- Label each bag with a "Do Not Recycle" label.
- Place the bags in a trash can with a lid.
- Make sure animals cannot get into the trash can. Trash scents can attract animals.

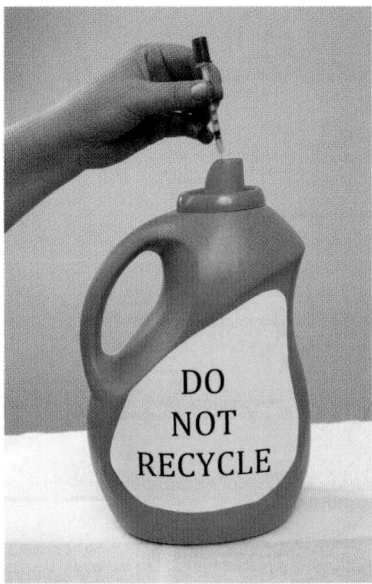

FIGURE 16-22 Household disposable sharps container labeled with "Do Not Recycle." The needle with syringe is inserted "point first."

Exposure Incidents

An *exposure incident* is any eye, mouth, other mucous membrane, non-intact skin, or parenteral contact with blood or OPIM. *Parenteral* means *piercing the mucous membranes or the skin.* Piercing occurs by needle-sticks, human bites, cuts, and abrasions.

Report exposure incidents at once. Medical evaluation, follow-up, and testing are free. Your blood is tested for HIV and HBV. If you refuse testing, the blood sample is kept for at least 90 days. Testing is done later if you desire.

Confidentiality is important. You are told about the evaluation results and any medical conditions that may need treatment. You receive a written opinion within 15 days after the evaluation is complete.

The *source individual* is the person whose blood or body fluids are the source of an exposure incident. His or her blood is tested for HIV or HBV. The agency informs you about laws affecting the source's identity and test results.

SURGICAL ASEPSIS

Surgical asepsis (sterile technique) is the practices used to remove all microbes. Sterile means the absence of all microbes. Surgical asepsis is required any time the skin or sterile tissues are entered.

Surgery and labor and delivery areas require surgical asepsis. So do many tests and nursing procedures. If a break occurs in sterile technique, microbes can enter the body. Infection is a risk.

Assisting With Sterile Procedures

You can assist with sterile procedures. You may be allowed to perform certain sterile procedures. A sterile dressing change is an example.

See *Delegation Guidelines: Assisting With Sterile Procedures.*

See *Promoting Safety and Comfort: Assisting With Sterile Procedures.*

Principles of Surgical Asepsis

All items in contact with the person are kept sterile. If an item is contaminated, infection is a risk. A sterile field is needed. A *sterile field is a work area free of all pathogens and non-pathogens (including spores).* Box 16-9 lists the principles and practices of surgical asepsis. Follow them to maintain a sterile field.

Sterile Gloving

Before donning sterile gloves, the sterile field is set up. After sterile gloves are on, you can handle sterile items within the sterile field. Do not touch anything outside the sterile field.

Sterile gloves are disposable. They come in many sizes to fit snugly. The insides are powdered for ease in donning gloves. The right and left gloves are marked on the package.

See *Promoting Safety and Comfort: Sterile Gloving.*

See procedure: *Sterile Gloving*, p. 246.

DELEGATION GUIDELINES
Assisting With Sterile Procedures

Before a sterile procedure, you need this information from the nurse.
- The name of the procedure and reason for it
- What gloves to wear—sterile or non-sterile
- What you are expected to do
- When to report observations
- What you can and cannot touch
- What patient or resident concerns to report at once

PROMOTING SAFETY AND COMFORT
Assisting With Sterile Procedures

Safety
Do not perform a sterile procedure unless:
- Your state allows you to perform the procedure.
- The procedure is in your job description.
- You received the necessary education and training.
- You review the procedure with the nurse.
- A nurse is available for questions and guidance.

BOX 16-9   Surgical Asepsis—Principles and Practices

- A sterile item can touch only another sterile item.
  - If a sterile item touches a clean item, the sterile item is contaminated.
  - If a clean item touches a sterile item, the sterile item is contaminated.
  - A sterile package is contaminated if open, torn, punctured, wet, or moist.
  - A sterile package is contaminated when the expiration date has passed.
  - Place only sterile items on a sterile field.
  - Use sterile gloves or sterile forceps to handle other sterile items (Fig. 16-23).
  - Consider any item to be contaminated if not sure of its sterility.
  - Do not use contaminated items. They are discarded or re-sterilized.
- A sterile field or sterile items are always kept within your vision and above your waist.
  - If you cannot see an item, the item is contaminated.
  - If the item is below your waist, the item is contaminated.
  - Keep sterile-gloved hands above your waist and in your sight.
  - Do not leave a sterile field unattended.
  - Do not turn your back on a sterile field.
- Airborne microbes can contaminate sterile items or a sterile field.
  - Prevent drafts. Close the door and avoid extra movements. Ask other staff in the room to avoid extra movements.
  - Avoid coughing, sneezing, talking, or laughing over a sterile field. Turn your head away from the sterile field if you must talk.
  - Wear a mask if you need to talk during the procedure.
  - Do not perform or assist with sterile procedures if you have a respiratory infection.
  - Do not reach over a sterile field.
- Fluid flows downward, in the direction of gravity.
  - Hold wet items down (see Fig. 16-23). If held up, fluid flows down into a contaminated area.
- The sterile field is kept dry, unless the area below it is sterile.
  - The sterile field is contaminated if it gets wet and the area below it is not sterile.
  - Avoid spilling and splashing when pouring sterile fluids into sterile containers.
- The edges of a sterile field are contaminated.
  - A 1-inch (2.5 centimeter [cm]) margin around the sterile field is considered contaminated (Fig. 16-24).
  - Place all sterile items inside the 1-inch (2.5 cm) margin of the sterile field.
  - Items outside the 1-inch (2.5 cm) margin are contaminated.
- Honesty is essential to sterile technique.
  - You know when you contaminate an item or sterile field. Be honest with yourself even if other staff are not present.
  - Remove the contaminated item and correct the matter. If necessary, start over with sterile supplies.
  - Report the contamination to the nurse.

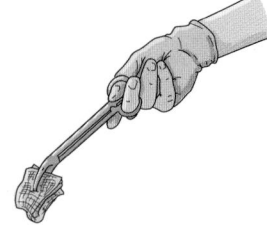

FIGURE 16-23 Sterile forceps are used to handle sterile items.

FIGURE 16-24 A 1-inch (2.5 cm) margin around the sterile field is considered contaminated. The shading and slash marks show that the 1-inch (2.5 cm) margin is contaminated.

PROMOTING SAFETY AND COMFORT

Sterile Gloving

Safety
Always keep sterile gloved hands above your waist and within your vision. Touch only items within the sterile field. If you contaminate the gloves, remove them. Tell the nurse what happened. Practice hand hygiene and put on a new pair. Replace gloves that are torn, cut, or punctured.

Comfort
If you, the nurse, or the person contaminates your gloves, they must be removed. This means leaving the bedside to get another pair. Care is delayed. The person's comfort is affected if the care is painful or involves an uncomfortable position. When collecting supplies, get an extra pair of gloves. The gloves are in the room if the first pair is contaminated. Care can continue with little delay.

Sterile Gloving

PROCEDURE

1 Follow *Delegation Guidelines: Assisting With Sterile Procedures*, p. 244. See *Promoting Safety and Comfort*:
  a *Assisting With Sterile Procedures*, p. 244
  b *Sterile Gloving*, p. 245
2 Practice hand hygiene.
3 Inspect the package of sterile gloves for sterility.
  a Check the expiration date.
  b See if the package is dry.
  c Check for tears, holes, punctures, and watermarks.
4 Arrange a work surface.
  a Make sure you have enough room.
  b Arrange the work surface at waist level and within your vision.
  c Clean and dry the work surface.
  d Do not reach over or turn your back on the work surface.
5 Open the package. Grasp the flaps. Gently peel them back.
6 Remove the inner package. Place it on your work surface.
7 Read the manufacturer's instructions on the inner package. It may be labeled *left, right, up,* and *down.*
8 Arrange the inner package for left, right, up and down. The left glove is on your left. The right glove is on your right. The cuffs are near you; the fingers point away from you.
9 Grasp the folded edges of the inner package. Use the thumb and index finger of each hand.
10 Fold back the inner package to expose the gloves (Fig. 16-25, *A*). Do not touch or otherwise contaminate the inside package or the gloves. The inside of the inner package is a sterile field.
11 Note that each glove has a cuff about 2 to 3 inches wide. The cuffs and insides of the gloves are *not sterile.*

12 Put on the right glove if you are right-handed. Put on the left glove if you are left-handed.
  a Pick up the glove with your other hand. Use your thumb and index and middle fingers (Fig. 16-25, *B*).
  b Touch only the cuff and inside of the glove.
  c Turn the hand to be gloved palm side up.
  d Lift the cuff up. Slide your fingers and hand into the glove (Fig. 16-25, *C*).
  e Pull the glove up over your hand. If some fingers get stuck, leave them that way until the other glove is on. *Do not use your ungloved hand to straighten the glove. Do not let the outside of the glove touch any non-sterile surface.*
  f Leave the cuff turned down.
13 Put on the other glove. Use your gloved hand.
  a Reach under the cuff of the second glove. Use the 4 fingers of your gloved hand (Fig. 16-25, *D*). Keep your gloved thumb close to your gloved palm.
  b Put on the second glove (Fig. 16-25, *E*). Your gloved hand cannot touch the cuff or any surface. Hold the thumb of your first gloved hand away from the second gloved palm.
14 Adjust each glove with the other hand. The gloves should be smooth and comfortable (Fig. 16-25, *F*).
15 Slide your fingers under the cuffs to pull them up (Fig. 16-25, *G*).
16 Touch only sterile items.
17 Remove and discard the gloves. See Figure 16-19.
18 Practice hand hygiene.

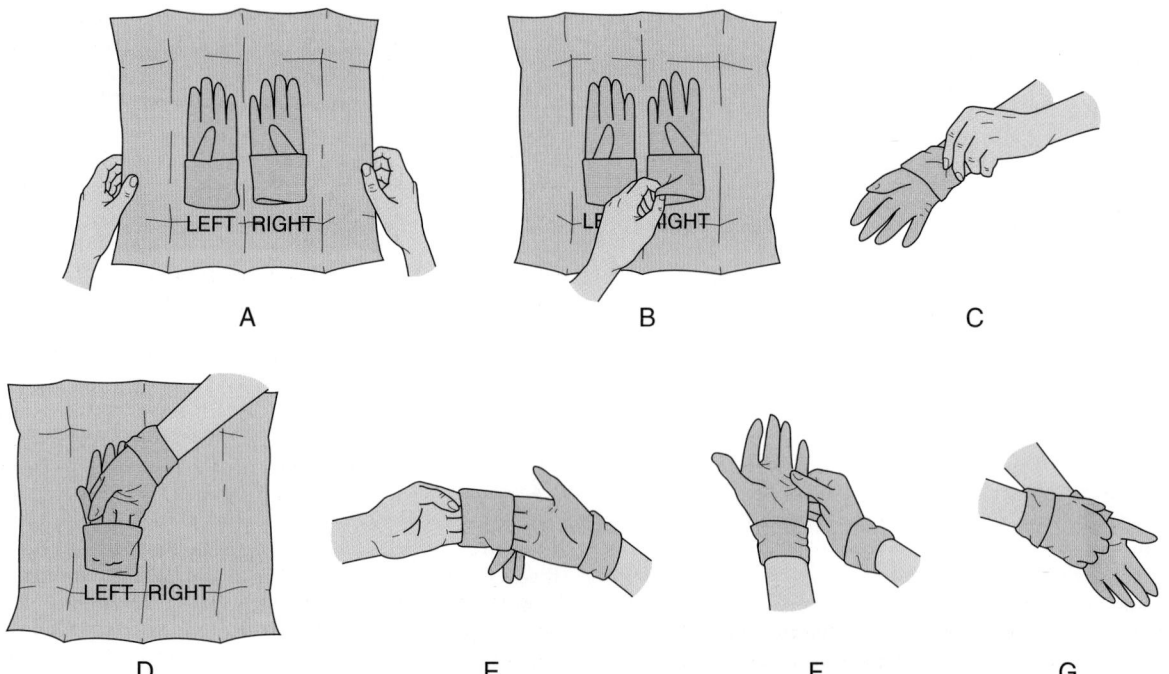

FIGURE 16-25 Sterile gloving. **A,** Open the inner wrapper to expose the gloves. **B,** Pick up the glove at the cuff with your thumb and index and middle fingers. **C,** Slide your fingers and hand into the glove. **D,** Reach under the cuff of the other glove with your fingers. **E,** Pull on the second glove. **F,** Adjust each glove for comfort. **G,** Slide your fingers under the cuff to pull them up.

FOCUS ON **PRIDE**

The Person, Family, and Yourself

Personal and Professional Responsibility

You have an important role in preventing the spread of infection. Your actions affect the person's risk for infection. You are responsible for following the guidelines in this chapter. Practice good hand hygiene before and after giving care. Follow Standard Precautions and Transmission-Based Precautions.

When assisting with or performing a procedure, remove items that become contaminated. If necessary, stop and get new supplies. Do not use a contaminated item. You may be alone. Be honest with yourself. Be responsible. Do the right thing, even if other staff are not present. Take pride in providing care that prevents the spread of infection.

Rights and Respect

Caring for persons who need Transmission-Based Precautions can be a challenge. Extra time and effort are needed to apply and remove PPE and clean equipment used in the room. You must plan carefully when gathering supplies before entering the room. If an item is forgotten, you must wait for help or remove and re-apply PPE. You may feel frustrated.

The person must not feel as if he or she is a burden. The person deserves the same kindness and respect you give others. You must:

- Watch your verbal and nonverbal communication (Chapter 9).
- Avoid complaining.
- Practice good teamwork and time management.
- Tell the nurse if you are feeling overwhelmed.

Independence and Social Interaction

Patients and residents are often unable to perform hygiene measures they would normally do alone. Hand hygiene is an example. Ask patients and residents if they would like to wash their hands often. Assist them to wash their hands before and after eating, after voiding or having a bowel movement, after coughing or sneezing, and any time the hands are dirty. Hand hygiene is not only important for you. It also is important for patients and residents. When independence is limited, protect the person and others by promoting hand hygiene.

Delegation and Teamwork

Before making delegation decisions, the nurse must assess and plan (Chapter 8). The nurse considers the person's needs and risks. Some persons are more at risk for infection than others. Burn, transplant, and chemotherapy patients are examples. The nurse must make delegation decisions carefully. If delegated care of persons at increased risk for infection, you must:

- Practice medical asepsis at all times.
- Practice surgical asepsis when assisting with sterile procedures.
- Practice hand hygiene.
- Follow Standard Precautions and the Bloodborne Pathogen Standard at all times.
- Follow any Transmission-Based Precautions ordered for the person.
- Wear PPE as directed by the nurse.
- Follow the person's care plan.
- Report any signs or symptoms of infection at once.
- Provide good oral hygiene and skin care (Chapter 22).
- Tell the nurse if you have any sign or symptom of an infection.

Communication is an important part of delegation. Do not be offended or annoyed if the nurse reminds you to perform these actions. Measures to prevent infection are very important to these persons. The nurse must make sure the person's health and safety are protected.

Ethics and Laws

The following is a real case showing how failure to follow infection control procedures led to patient harm.

A patient, Mr. Helman, had hip surgery (August 1) following a car accident in which he suffered many injuries. His roommate, Mr. Hagerup, had a back injury that caused paralysis from the waist down. The men shared a room for about 2 weeks.

Eight days after Mr. Helman's hip surgery (August 9), Mr. Hagerup complained of a boil under his right arm. (Author note: A boil is a local skin infection. The infection causes a painful red bump. When opened, purulent drainage comes from the boil. Purulent drainage is thick and green, yellow, or brown in color.) The boil was treated with hot compresses. On August 10, there was purulent drainage from the boil. On the same day, a drainage specimen was sent to the laboratory. On August 13, the laboratory report showed the boil drainage contained a type of staphylococcus. Mr. Hagerup was moved at once to an isolation room.

Between August 10 and August 13, the nursing team cared for Mr. Helman and Mr. Hagerup. They "moved from one patient to the other, changed sheets, gave sponge baths, changed dressings, administered back rubs...[and] carried out the necessary hospital routine for the care of the two men. They did not observe sterile techniques...[to be used] when infection is suspected; they did not wash their hands or leave the room between administering to the patients."

On August 13, Mr. Helman's surgical wound opened and drained a large amount of purulent drainage. Laboratory tests showed the drainage contained the same microbe found in Mr. Hagerup's wound. Mr. Helman's wound infection destroyed bone, tissue, and ligaments. He had another surgery on October 28. His hip was fused in a "nearly immovable position." (To fuse means to unite 2 or more bones together.) He was discharged from the hospital on March 14. He needed home care and doctor's care.

In a lawsuit against the hospital, the jury returned a verdict in favor of Mr. Helman. The hospital appealed the verdict. The court hearing the appeal upheld the verdict in favor of Mr. Helman.

(G. E. Helman et al. v Sacred Heart Hospital, Washington, 1963.)

The health team must prevent the spread of microbes and infection. Even one careless act can spread microbes. This affects the person's health and safety. Be very careful about your work. Take pride in providing care that protects the person from infection.

FOCUS ON **PRIDE**: *Application*

Your attitude about preventing infection affects your actions. Consider your everyday actions. Do they show that you value the health and wellness of yourself and others? Give some examples. Identify areas where you need to improve. How might your attitude affect how you prevent infection at work?

REVIEW QUESTIONS

Circle T if the statement is TRUE or F if it is FALSE.

1 T F   Microbes are pathogens in their natural sites.

2 T F   A pathogen can cause an infection.

3 T F   An infection results when microbes invade and grow in the body.

4 T F   An item is sterile if non-pathogens are present.

5 T F   You hold your hands and forearms up during hand-washing.

6 T F   A towel falls to the floor. The towel is contaminated.

7 T F   Un-used items in the person's room are used for another person.

8 T F   A person received the hepatitis B vaccine. The person will develop the disease.

9 T F   The 1-inch edge around a sterile field is considered contaminated.

10 T F   The inside and cuffs of sterile gloves are considered contaminated.

11 T F   You can flush household sharps down the toilet.

12 T F   You can throw household sharps in the trash.

Circle the BEST answer.

13 Which area is *best* for a pathogen to live and grow?
   a A cold and wet area
   b A warm and dark area
   c A hot and bright area
   d A dry area without oxygen

14 Which is a sign of infection?
   a A bruise
   b Redness in a body part
   c Warm, dry, and intact skin
   d A bleeding wound

15 To control a portal of exit
   a Cover the mouth and nose when coughing
   b Position drainage containers above the drainage site
   c Clean the genital area from the rectum to the urethra
   d Leave an open wound uncovered

16 Preventing healthcare-associated infections involves
   a Sterilizing all care items
   b Over-prescribing antibiotics
   c Hand hygiene before and after giving care
   d Using Transmission-Based Precautions for all persons

17 You have blood on your hand. What should you do?
   a Wash your hands with soap and water.
   b Use an alcohol-based hand rub.
   c Rinse your hands.
   d Tell the nurse.

18 You move from a contaminated body site to a clean body site. Your hands are not visibly soiled. What should you do?
   a Disinfect your gloves.
   b Practice hand hygiene.
   c Rinse your hands.
   d Continue care without hand hygiene.

19 To use an alcohol-based hand rub correctly
   a Wash your hands before applying the hand rub
   b Rinse your hands after applying the hand rub
   c Rub the product only on the palms of your hands
   d Rub your hands together until they are dry

20 When cleaning equipment
   a Rinse the item in hot water before cleaning
   b Wash the item with soap and cold water
   c Use a brush if necessary
   d Work from dirty to clean areas

21 Isolation precautions
   a Treat communicable diseases
   b Destroy pathogens
   c Keep pathogens within a certain area
   d Destroy all microbes

REVIEW QUESTIONS—cont'd

22 Which statement about Standard Precautions is *true?*
   a They are used for all persons.
   b The 3 types are contact, droplet, and airborne.
   c They are used only in hospitals.
   d They require a doctor's order.

23 You wear utility gloves for contact with
   a Blood
   b Body fluids
   c Secretions and excretions
   d Cleaning solutions

24 A mask
   a Can be re-used
   b Is clean on the inside
   c Is contaminated when moist
   d Should fit loosely for breathing

25 To use PPE correctly
   a Never change gloves in the person's room
   b Tie a gown's waist strings in front
   c Don gloves first when applying PPE
   d Apply new PPE for each person

26 Which task requires gloves?
   a Applying wrist restraints
   b Giving a back massage
   c Providing denture care
   d Moving the person up in bed

27 Goggles or a face shield is worn
   a When using Standard Precautions
   b When splashing body fluids is likely
   c If you have an eye infection
   d When assisting with sterile procedures

28 The Bloodborne Pathogen Standard involves microbes spread through
   a Blood and OPIM
   b Only blood
   c Droplets
   d Close contact

29 According to the Bloodborne Pathogen Standard, you should
   a Practice hand hygiene after removing gloves
   b Discard a used razor in a wastebasket
   c Tell the nurse about exposure to blood before washing your hands
   d Refuse the hepatitis B vaccine

30 You were exposed to a bloodborne pathogen. Which is *true?*
   a You do not have to report the exposure.
   b You pay for required tests.
   c You can refuse HIV and HBV testing.
   d The source individual can refuse testing.

31 These statements are about surgical asepsis. Which is *true?*
   a If a sterile item touches a clean item, the sterile item is clean.
   b Wet sterile items are held up.
   c A torn sterile package is still sterile.
   d If you cannot see an item, it is considered contaminated.

32 You have on sterile gloves. You can touch
   a Anything on your work surface
   b Anything on the sterile field
   c Anything below your waist
   d Any part of your uniform

Answers to Chapter 16 questions are on p. 870.

FOCUS ON **PRACTICE**

Problem Solving

A nurse enters the room of a person who requires contact precautions. The nurse is not wearing PPE. What do you do? What PPE is needed? What precautions are needed upon entering and leaving the room and while in the room?

Body Mechanics

OBJECTIVES

- Define the key terms and key abbreviations in this chapter.
- Explain the purpose and rules of body mechanics.
- Identify the risk factors for work-related injuries.
- Identify the activities at high risk for work-related injuries, including back injuries.

- Explain how to prevent work-related injuries.
- Identify the causes, signs, and symptoms of back injuries.
- Position persons in the basic bed positions and in a chair.
- Explain how to promote PRIDE in the person, the family, and yourself.

KEY TERMS

base of support The area on which an object rests
body alignment The way the head, trunk, arms, and legs are aligned with one another; posture
body mechanics Using the body in an efficient and careful way
dorsal recumbent position The back-lying or supine position
ergonomics The science of designing the job to fit the worker; *ergo* means *work, nomos* means *law*
Fowler's position A semi-sitting position; the head of the bed is raised between 45 and 60 degrees
lateral position The person lies on 1 side or the other; side-lying position
posture See "body alignment"

prone position Lying on the abdomen with the head turned to 1 side
semi-prone side position See "Sims' position"
side-lying position See "lateral position"
Sims' position A left side-lying position in which the upper leg (right leg) is sharply flexed so it is not on the lower leg (left leg) and the lower arm (left arm) is behind the person; semi-prone side position
supine position The back-lying or dorsal recumbent position
work-related musculo-skeletal disorders Injuries and disorders of the muscles, tendons, ligaments, joints, and cartilage; they are caused or made worse by the work setting

KEY ABBREVIATIONS

MSD   Musculo-skeletal disorder

OSHA   Occupational Safety and Health Administration

Body mechanics means using the body in an efficient and careful way. It involves good posture, balance, and using your strongest and largest muscles for work. Fatigue, muscle strain, and injury can result from the improper use and positioning of the body during activity or rest. Focus on the person's and your own body mechanics. Good body mechanics reduce the risk of injury.

See *Body Structure and Function Review: The Musculo-Skeletal System.*

PRINCIPLES OF BODY MECHANICS

Body alignment (posture) is the way the head, trunk, arms, and legs are aligned with one another. Good alignment lets the body move and function with strength and efficiency. Standing, sitting, and lying down require good alignment.

Base of support is the area on which an object rests. A good base of support is needed for balance (Fig. 17-3, p. 252). When standing, your feet are your base of support. Stand with your feet apart for a wider base of support and more balance.

Your strongest and largest muscles are in your shoulders, upper arms, hips, and thighs. Use these muscles to handle and move persons and heavy objects. Otherwise, you place strain and exertion on the smaller and weaker muscles. This causes fatigue and injury. *Back injuries are a major risk.* For good body mechanics:

- Bend your knees and squat to lift a heavy object (Fig. 17-4, p. 252). Do not bend from your waist. Bending from your waist places strain on small back muscles.
- Hold items close to your body and base of support (see Fig. 17-4). This involves upper arm and shoulder muscles. Holding objects away from your body places strain on small muscles in your lower arms.

BODY STRUCTURE AND FUNCTION REVIEW

The Musculo-Skeletal System

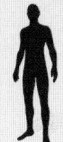

The *musculo-skeletal system:*
- Provides the framework for the body.
- Lets the body move.
- Protects internal organs.
- Gives the body shape.

Bones

Bones are hard, rigid structures. They are made up of living cells. The human body has 206 bones.
- *Long bones* bear the body's weight. Leg bones are long bones.
- *Short bones* allow skill and ease in movement. Bones in the wrists, fingers, ankles, and toes are short bones.
- *Flat bones* protect the organs. They include the ribs, skull, pelvic bones, and shoulder blades.
- *Irregular bones* are the vertebrae in the spinal column. They allow various degrees of movement and flexibility.

Joints

A *joint* is the point at which 2 or more bones meet. Joints allow movement. There are 3 major types of joints (Fig. 17-1).
- A *ball-and-socket joint* allows movement in all directions. It is made of the rounded end of 1 bone and the hollow end of another bone. The rounded end of 1 fits into the hollow end of the other. The joints of the hips and shoulders are ball-and-socket joints.
- A *hinge joint* allows movement in 1 direction. The elbow is a hinge joint.
- A *pivot joint* allows turning from side to side. A pivot joint connects the skull to the spine.

  Some joints are immovable. They connect the bones of the skull.

Muscles

The human body has more than 500 *muscles* (Fig. 17-2, p. 252).
- *Voluntary muscles* can be consciously controlled. Muscles attached to bones *(skeletal muscles)* are voluntary. Arm muscles do not work unless you move your arm; likewise for leg muscles. Skeletal muscles are *striated.* That is, they look striped or streaked.
- *Involuntary muscles* work automatically. You cannot control them. They control the action of the stomach, intestines, blood vessels, and other body organs. Involuntary muscles also are called *smooth muscles.* They look smooth, not streaked or striped.
- *Cardiac muscle* is in the heart. It is an involuntary muscle. However, it appears striated like skeletal muscle.

  Muscles have 3 functions.
- Movement of body parts
- Maintenance of posture or muscle tone
- Production of body heat

  Some muscles constantly contract to maintain the body's posture. When muscles contract, they burn food for energy. Heat is produced. The more muscle activity, the greater the amount of heat produced.

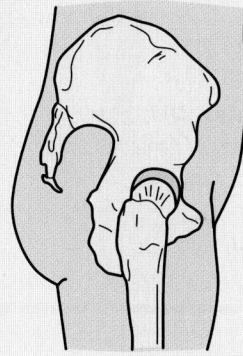

Ball-and-socket

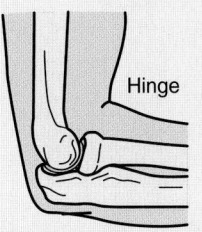

Hinge

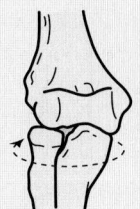

Pivot

FIGURE 17-1 Types of joints.

Continued

BODY STRUCTURE AND FUNCTION REVIEW—cont'd

The Musculo-Skeletal System

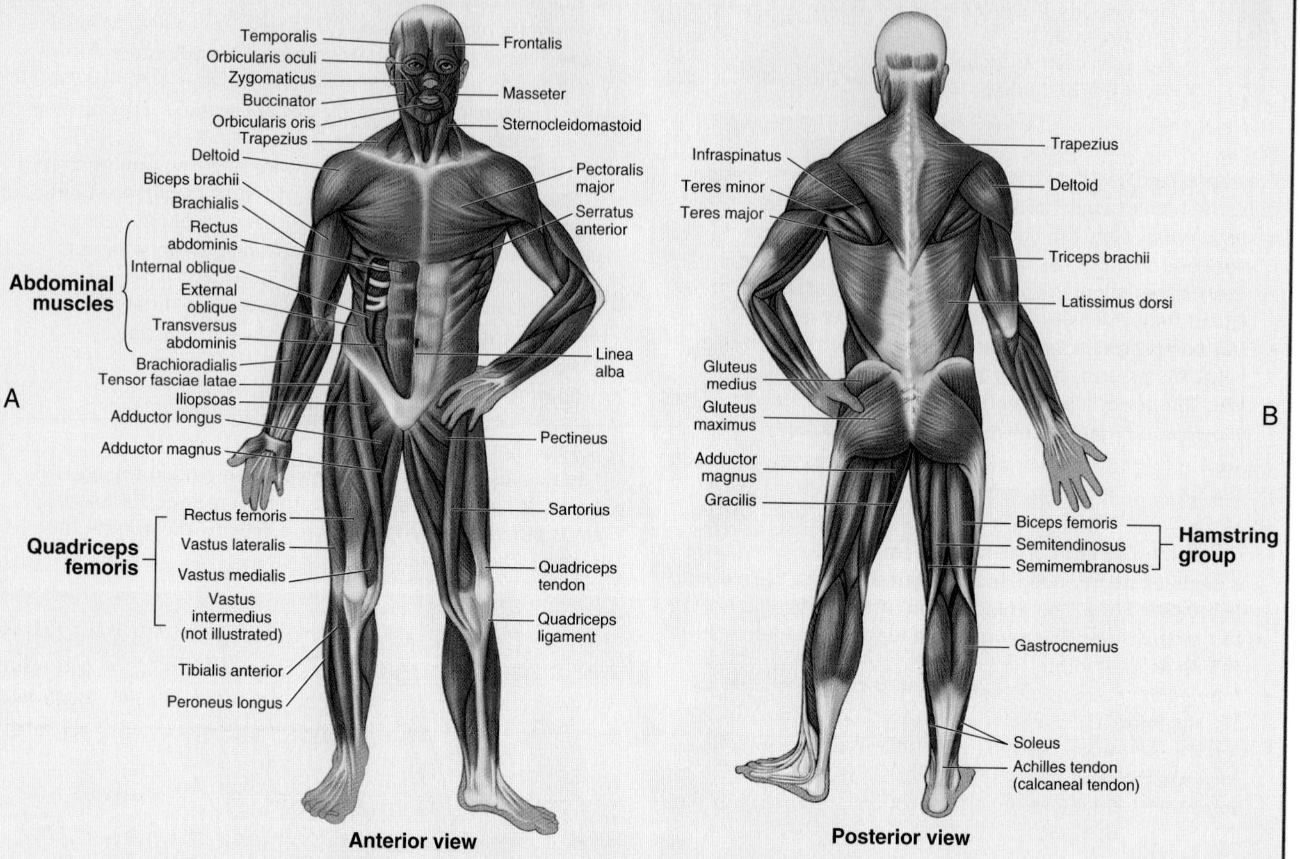

Temporalis
Orbicularis oculi
Zygomaticus
Buccinator
Orbicularis oris
Trapezius
Deltoid
Biceps brachii
Brachialis
Rectus abdominis
Internal oblique
Abdominal muscles
External oblique
Transversus abdominis
Brachioradialis
Tensor fasciae latae
Iliopsoas
Adductor longus
Adductor magnus

Frontalis
Masseter
Sternocleidomastoid
Pectoralis major
Serratus anterior
Linea alba
Pectineus
Sartorius

Quadriceps femoris
Rectus femoris
Vastus lateralis
Vastus medialis
Vastus intermedius (not illustrated)
Tibialis anterior
Peroneus longus

Quadriceps tendon
Quadriceps ligament

A

Anterior view

Infraspinatus
Teres minor
Teres major
Trapezius
Deltoid
Triceps brachii
Latissimus dorsi
Gluteus medius
Gluteus maximus
Adductor magnus
Gracilis
Biceps femoris
Semitendinosus
Semimembranosus
Hamstring group
Gastrocnemius
Soleus
Achilles tendon (calcaneal tendon)

B

Posterior view

FIGURE 17-2 A, Anterior view of the muscles of the body. **B,** Posterior view of the muscles of the body. (From Herlihy B, Maebius NK: *The human body in health and illness,* ed 4, St Louis, 2011, Elsevier.)

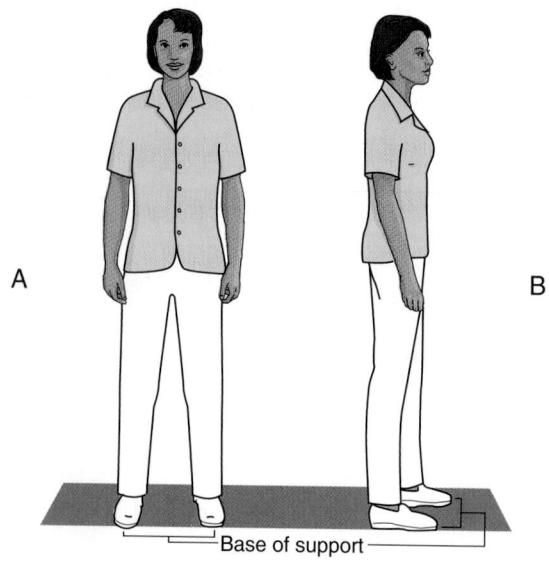

FIGURE 17-3 A, Anterior (front) view of an adult in good body alignment. The feet are apart for a wide base of support. **B,** Lateral (side) view of an adult with good posture and alignment.

A

B

Base of support

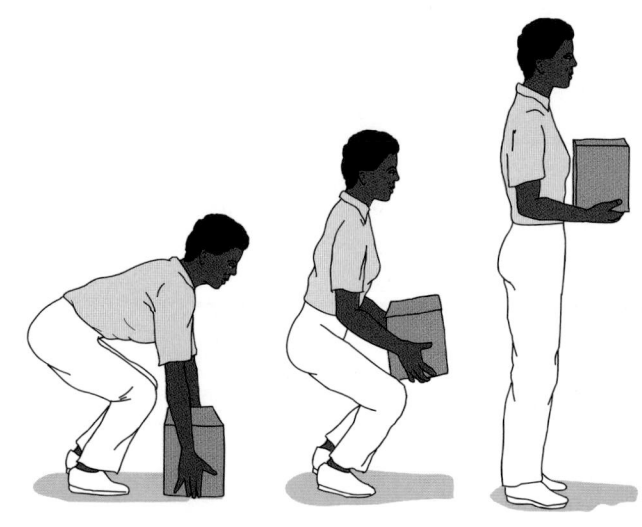

FIGURE 17-4 Picking up a box using good body mechanics.

BOX 17-1　Rules for Body Mechanics

- Keep your body in good alignment with a wide base of support. Your feet are at least 12 inches apart or shoulder-wide apart.
- Use an upright working posture. Bend your legs. Do not bend your back.
- Use the stronger and larger muscles in your shoulders, upper arms, thighs, and hips.
- Keep objects close to your body when you lift, move, or carry them (see Fig. 17-4).
- Avoid unnecessary bending and reaching. Raise the bed so it is close to your waist. Adjust the over-bed table to your waist level.
- Face your work area. This prevents unnecessary twisting.
- Push, slide, or pull heavy objects when you can rather than lifting them. Pushing is easier than pulling.
- Widen your base of support to push or pull. Move your front leg forward when pushing. Move your leg back when pulling (Fig. 17-5).
- Use both hands and arms to lift, move, or carry objects.
- Turn your whole body when changing the direction of the turn. Do not twist your body.
- Work with smooth and even movements. Avoid sudden or jerky motions.
- Do not lean over a person to give care.
- *Get help from a co-worker to move heavy objects. Do not lift or move them by yourself.*
- Bend your hips and knees to lift heavy objects from the floor (see Fig. 17-4). Straighten your back as the object reaches thigh level. Your leg and thigh muscles work to raise the item off the floor and to waist level.
- Do not lift objects higher than chest level. Do not lift above your shoulders. Use a step stool or ladder to reach an object higher than chest level.

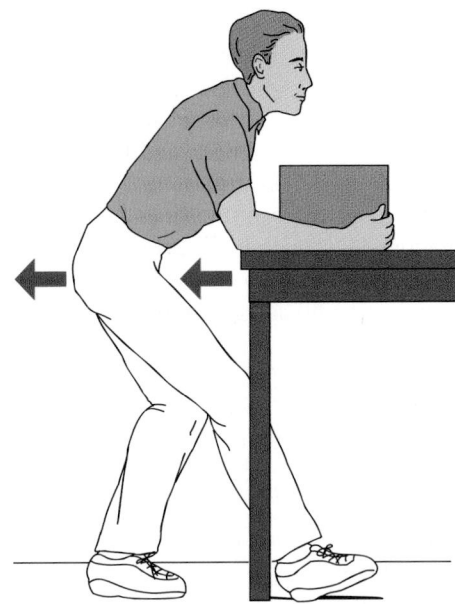

FIGURE 17-5 Move your rear leg back when pulling.

Rules for Body Mechanics

All activities require good body mechanics. You must safely and efficiently handle and move persons and heavy objects. Follow the rules in Box 17-1.

WORK-RELATED INJURIES

Work-related musculo-skeletal disorders (MSDs) are injuries and disorders of the muscles, tendons, ligaments, joints, and cartilage. They are caused or made worse by the work setting. They can involve the nervous system. The arms and back are often affected. So are the hands, fingers, neck, wrists, legs, and shoulders. MSDs are painful and disabling. They can develop slowly over weeks, months, and years. Or they can occur from 1 event. Pain, numbness, tingling, stiff joints, difficulty moving, and muscle loss can occur. Sometimes there is paralysis.

Early signs and symptoms include pain, limited joint movement, or soft tissue swelling. Time off work is often needed.

MSD Risk Factors

The Occupational Safety and Health Administration (OSHA) has identified MSD risk factors for the nursing team. An MSD is more likely if risk factors are combined. For example, a task involves both force and repeating actions.

- *Force*—the amount of physical effort needed to perform a task. Lifting or transferring heavy persons, preventing falls, and unexpected or sudden motions are examples.
- *Repeating action*—doing the same motion or series of motions continually or frequently. Re-positioning persons and transfers to and from beds, chairs, and commodes without adequate rest breaks are examples. So is frequently cranking manual beds.
- *Awkward postures*—assuming positions that place stress on the body. Examples are reaching above shoulder height, kneeling, squatting, leaning over a bed, bending, or twisting the torso while lifting.
- *Heavy lifting*—manually lifting people who cannot move themselves.

According to the U.S. Department of Labor, nursing assistants are at great risk.

The following tasks are known to be high risk for MSDs affecting the muscles, tendons, ligaments, joints, and cartilage.

- Transfers—to and from beds, chairs, wheelchairs, Geri-chairs, toilets, stretchers, and bathtubs
- Trying to stop a person from falling
- Picking up a person from the floor to the bed
- Lifting alone
- Lifting persons who are confused or uncooperative
- Lifting persons who cannot support their own weight
- Lifting heavy persons
- Weighing a person
- Moving a person up in bed
- Re-positioning a person in a bed or in a chair
- Changing an incontinence product
- Making beds
- Dressing and undressing a person
- Feeding a person in bed
- Giving a bed bath
- Applying anti-embolism stockings
- Prolonged holding of a body part for care measures— arm, leg, abdomen, skin fold

Back Injuries. Back injuries are major threats. Back injuries can occur from repeated activities or from 1 event. Signs and symptoms include:

- Pain when trying to assume a normal posture
- Decreased mobility
- Pain when standing or rising from a seated position These and other factors can lead to back disorders.
- Reaching while lifting
- Poor posture when sitting or standing
- Staying in 1 position too long
- Poor body mechanics when lifting, pushing, pulling, or carrying objects
- Poor physical condition—not having the strength or endurance to perform tasks without strain
- Repeated lifting of awkward items, equipment, or persons
- Shifting weight when a person loses balance or strength while moving
- Twisting or bending while lifting
- Maintaining a bent posture such as leaning over a bed
- Reaching over raised bed rails
- Working in a confined, crowded, or cluttered area (rooms, bathrooms, hallways)
- Fatigue
- Poor footing, such as on slippery floors
- Lifting with forceful movement

Follow the rules and safety measures in this chapter to prevent back injuries. Be extra careful when performing tasks associated with back injuries.

See *Promoting Safety and Comfort: Back Injuries.*

PROMOTING SAFETY AND COMFORT

Back Injuries

Safety

According to OSHA, these activities are associated with back injuries in nursing centers.

- Moving a person who depends totally on others for care.
- Moving a person who is combative.
- Transferring a person who is on the floor to the bed or chair.
- Re-positioning a person in bed or in a chair.
- Transferring a person from bed to chair or from chair to bed.
- Transferring a person from 1 chair to another. This includes transfers to and from the wheelchair and toilet.
- Bending to bathe, dress, or feed a person.
- Bending to make a bed or change linens.
- Weighing a person.
- Changing an incontinence product.
- Trying to stop a person from falling.
  Use good body mechanics to protect yourself from injury.

Do not work alone. Avoid lifting whenever possible.

Preventing MSDs

OSHA requires a safe work setting. The setting must be free of hazards that cause or are likely to cause death or serious physical harm to staff. The employer must make reasonable attempts to prevent or reduce the hazard. OSHA inspection teams enforce this law.

Always report a work-related injury as soon as possible. Early attention can help prevent the problem from becoming worse. Also injuries are often less serious and less costly to treat with early attention. In later stages, the problem can become more serious and harder and more costly to treat.

To prevent work-related MSDs, follow the rules in Box 17-1 and Box 17-2.

Ergonomics. *Ergonomics is the science of designing a job to fit the worker.* (Ergo *means* work. Nomos *means* law.) It involves changing the task, work station, equipment, and tools to help reduce stress on the worker's body. The goal is to eliminate a serious work-related MSD. MSDs are caused or made worse by the work setting.

BOX 17-2   Preventing Work-Related Injuries

General Guidelines

- Wear shoes with good traction. Avoid shoes with worn-down sides. Good traction helps prevent slips or falls.
- Use assist equipment and devices (Chapters 18 and 19) whenever possible instead of lifting and moving the person manually. Follow the care plan.
- Get help from other staff. The nurse and care plan tell you how many staff members are needed for a task.
- Plan and prepare for the task. For example, know what equipment is needed, where to place chairs or wheelchairs, and what side of the bed to work on.
- Schedule harder tasks early in your shift.
- Balance lighter and harder tasks. Plan your work to complete a lighter task after a harder one.
- Lock (brake) bed wheels and wheelchair or stretcher wheels.
- Tell the person how he or she can help. Give clear, simple instructions. Give the person time to respond.
- Do not hold or grab the person under the underarms.
- Do not let the person hold or grasp you around your neck.

Manual Lifting

- Minimize or eliminate manual lifting when possible.
- Stand with good posture. Keep your back straight.
- Bend your legs, not your back.
- Use the large muscles in your legs to do the work.
- Face the person.
- Do not twist or turn. Pick up your feet and pivot your whole body in the direction of the move.
- Keep what you are moving close to you.
- Move the person toward you, not away from you.
- Use a wide, balanced base of support. Stand with 1 foot slightly ahead of the other.
- Use smooth, even movements. Avoid jerking movements.
- Lift on the "count of 3" when lifting with others. Everyone lifts at the same time.

Lifting or Moving the Person in Bed

- Adjust the height of the bed to a safe and comfortable level.
- Lower the bed rail.
- Work on the side where the person will be closest to you.
- Place equipment or other items close to you at waist level.
- Use friction-reducing devices—drawsheets, turning pads, large re-usable waterproof under-pads, slide sheets (Chapters 18 and 19).

Transfer/Gait Belts

- Keep the person as close to you as possible.
- Avoid bending, reaching, or twisting to:
  - Apply or remove a transfer/gait belt.
  - Lower the person to the chair, bed, toilet, or floor.
  - Help the person walk.
- Use a gentle rocking motion to assist the person to stand. The rocking motion gives strength and force as you help the person to stand.
- See Chapter 14.

Stand and Pivot Transfers (Chapter 19)

- Use assist devices as directed. Follow the care plan.
- Use a transfer belt with handles.
- Plan the transfer so the person's strong side moves first.
- Lower the bed so the person can place his or her feet on the floor.
- Get the person close to the edge of the bed or the chair. Ask the person to lean forward as he or she stands.
- Block the person's weak leg with your legs or knees. If the position is awkward:
  - Use a transfer belt with handles.
  - Straddle your legs around the person's weak leg.
- Keep your feet at least shoulder-width apart.
- Bend your legs. Do not bend your back.
- Use a gentle rocking motion to help the person stand. The rocking motion gives strength and force as you help the person to stand.
- Pivot with your feet to turn.

Lateral Transfers (Chapter 19)

- Position surfaces close to each other.
- Adjust surfaces to about waist height. Do 1 of the following as directed by the nurse and care plan.
  - Adjust the surfaces to the same level.
  - Adjust the receiving surface so it is slightly lower (about $\frac{1}{2}$ inch) than the surface the person is on. This allows the use of gravity. For example, for a bed to stretcher transfer, the stretcher surface is lower than the bed.
- Lower bed rails and stretcher side rails.
- Use friction-reducing devices.
- Get a good hand-hold. Roll up drawsheets, turning pads, large re-usable waterproof under-pads, and slide sheets. Or use assist devices with handles.
- Kneel on the bed or stretcher. This prevents extended reaches and bending your back.
- Have staff on both sides of the bed or other surface. Move the person on the "count of 3." Use a smooth, push-pull motion. Do not reach across the person.

Transporting the Person and Equipment

- Push, do not pull.
- Keep the load close to your body.
- Use an upright posture.
- Push with your whole body, not just your arms.
- Move down the center of the hallway. This helps avoid collisions.
- Watch out for door handles and high thresholds on floors. These can cause abrupt stops.

Transferring the Person From the Floor

- See Chapter 14.

Modified from Cal/OSHA: A back injury prevention guide for health care providers, Sacramento, Calif, 1997, Author; and referenced in Occupational Safety and Health Administration: Guidelines for nursing homes: ergonomics for the prevention of musculoskeletal disorders, Washington, DC, Revised March 2009, Author.

POSITIONING THE PERSON

The person must be properly positioned at all times. Regular position changes and good alignment promote comfort and well-being. Breathing is easier. Circulation is promoted. Pressure ulcers and contractures are prevented. A *contracture* is the lack of joint mobility caused by the abnormal shortening of a muscle (Chapter 30).

For comfort, you move and turn when in bed or a chair. Many patients and residents do too. Some need reminding to adjust their positions. Others need help. Still others depend entirely on the nursing team for position changes.

Whether in bed or chair, the person is re-positioned at least every 2 hours. Some people are re-positioned more often. Follow the nurse's instructions and the care plan. To safely position a person:

- Use good body mechanics.
- Ask a co-worker to help you if needed.
- Explain the procedure to the person.
- Be gentle when moving the person.
- Provide for privacy.
- Use pillows as directed by the nurse for support and alignment.
- Provide for comfort after positioning. (See the inside of the front cover.)
- Place the call light and other needed items within reach after positioning.
- Complete a safety check before leaving the room. (See the inside of the front cover.)
  See *Focus on Communication: Positioning the Person.*
  See *Delegation Guidelines: Positioning the Person.*
  See *Promoting Safety and Comfort: Positioning the Person.*

Fowler's Positions

Fowler's position is a semi-sitting position. The head of the bed is raised between 45 and 60 degrees (Fig. 17-6). The knees may be slightly elevated. Variations on Fowler's position include:

- *Semi-Fowler's position*—the head of the bed is raised 30 degrees (Chapter 20). Some agencies define semi-Fowler's position as when the head of the bed is raised 30 degrees and the knee portion is raised 15 degrees.
- *High-Fowler's position*—the head of the bed is raised 60 to 90 degrees (Chapter 20).
  For good alignment:
- The spine is straight.
- The head is supported with a small pillow.
- The arms are supported with pillows.

The nurse may have you place small pillows under the lower back, thighs, and ankles. Persons with heart and respiratory disorders usually breathe easier in Fowler's position.

See *Focus on Math: Fowler's Positions.*

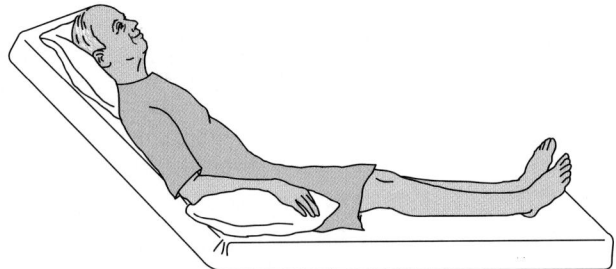

FIGURE 17-6 Fowler's position.

FOCUS ON MATH

Fowler's Positions

When 2 lines meet, an angle is formed. Angles measure how much 1 line has to turn to be in the same position as the other line. Angles are measured in degrees (°). Degrees range from 0 to 360. With bed positions, you need a basic understanding of angle measurements between 0° and 90°.

To estimate the angle:
1. Use the bed frame and the head of the bed as the 2 lines.
2. Estimate the angle from the bed frame to the head of the bed. See Figure 17-7.

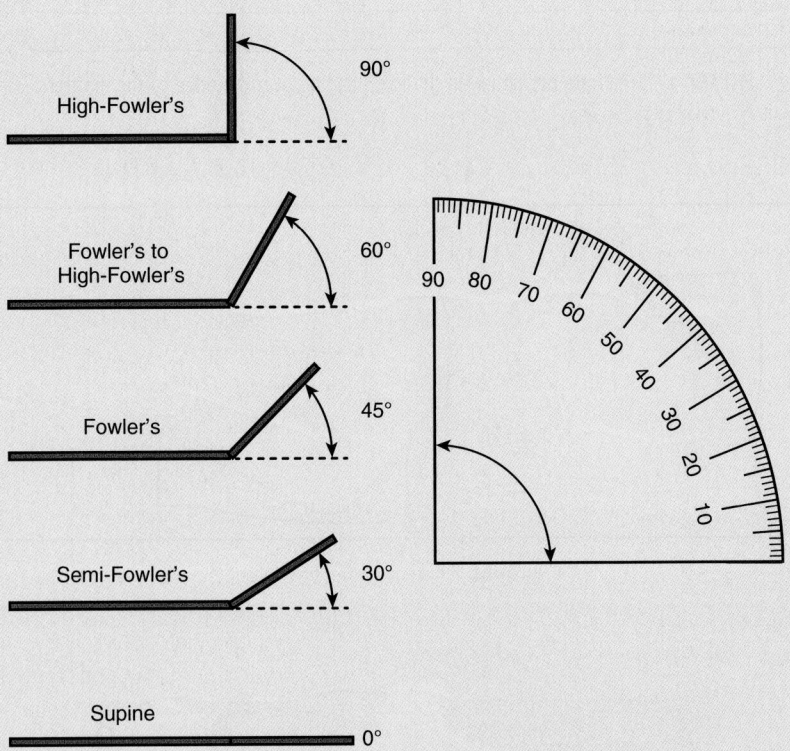

FIGURE 17-7 Measuring bed angles. The angle is measured from the bed frame to the back of the head of the bed. As the head of the bed rises, the angle increases.

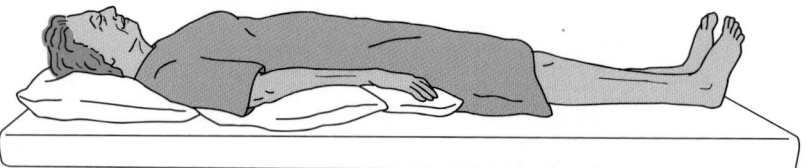

FIGURE 17-8 Supine position.

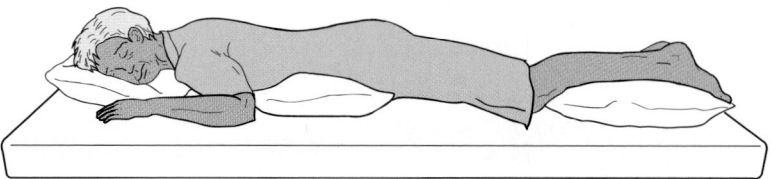

FIGURE 17-9 Prone position.

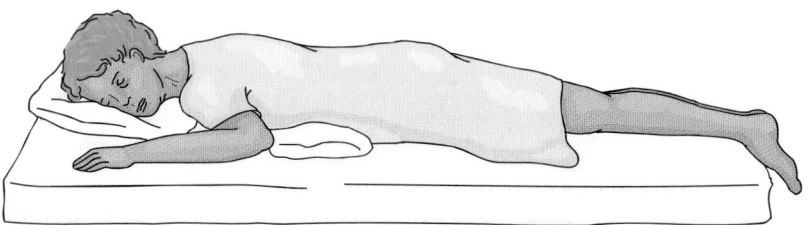

FIGURE 17-10 Prone position with the feet hanging over the edge of the mattress.

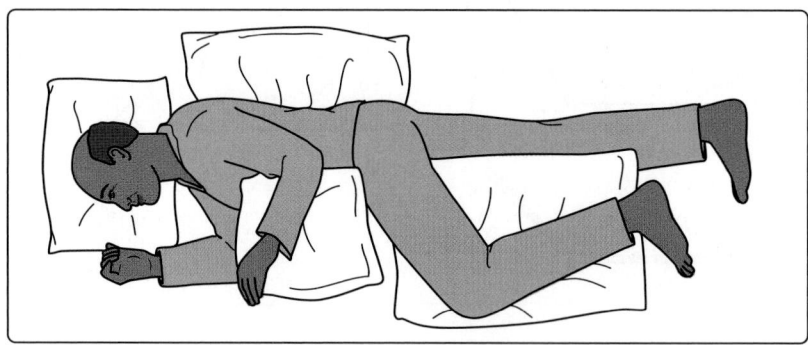

FIGURE 17-11 Lateral position.

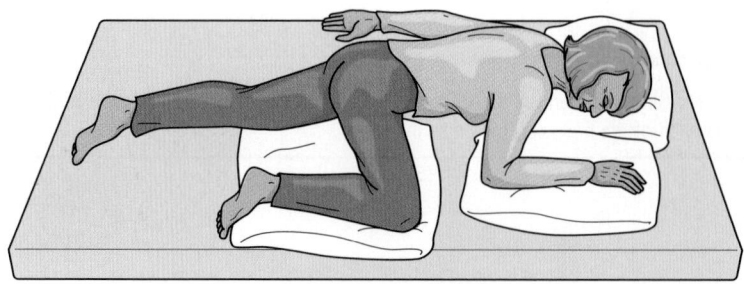

FIGURE 17-12 Sims' position.

Supine Position

The *supine position (dorsal recumbent position) is the back-lying position* (Fig. 17-8).

For good alignment:
- The bed is flat.
- The head and shoulders are supported on a pillow.
- Arms and hands are at the sides. You can support the arms with regular pillows. Or you can support the hands on small pillows with the palms down.

The nurse may have you place a folded or rolled towel under the lower back and a small pillow under the thighs. A pillow under the lower legs lifts the heels off of the bed. This prevents them from rubbing on the sheets.

Prone Position

In the *prone position, the person lies on the abdomen with the head turned to 1 side.* For good alignment:
- The bed is flat.
- Small pillows are placed under the head, abdomen, and lower legs (Fig. 17-9).
- Arms are flexed at the elbows with the hands near the head.

You also can position a person with the feet hanging over the end of the mattress (Fig. 17-10). A pillow is not needed under the feet.

Lateral Position

In the *lateral position (side-lying position), the person lies on 1 side or the other* (Fig. 17-11).
- The bed is flat.
- A pillow is under the head and neck.
- The upper leg is in front of the lower leg. (The nurse may ask you to position the upper leg behind the lower leg, not on top of it.)
- The ankle, upper leg, and thigh are supported with pillows.
- A small pillow is positioned against the person's back. The person rolls back against the pillow so that his or her back is at a 45-degree angle with the mattress.
- A small pillow is under the upper hand and arm.

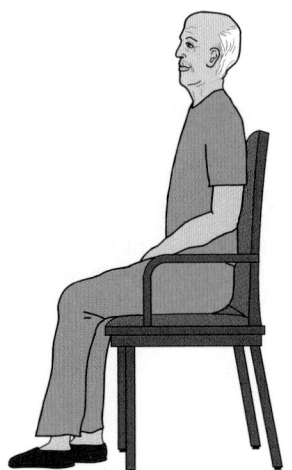

FIGURE 17-13 Chair position.

Sims' Position

The *Sims' position (semi-prone side position) is a left side-lying position. The upper leg (right leg) is sharply flexed so it is not on the lower leg (left leg). The lower arm (left arm) is behind the person* (Fig. 17-12). For good alignment:
- The bed is flat.
- A pillow is under the person's head and shoulder.
- The upper leg (right leg) is supported with a pillow.
- A pillow is under the upper arm (right arm) and hand (right hand).

Chair Position

Persons who sit in chairs must hold their upper bodies and heads erect. If not, poor alignment results. For good alignment:
- The person's back and buttocks are against the back of the chair.
- Feet are flat on the floor or wheelchair footplates. Never leave feet unsupported.
- Back of the knees and calves are slightly away from the edge of the seat (Fig. 17-13).

The nurse may have you put a small pillow between the person's lower back and the chair. This supports the lower back. *Remember, a pillow is not used behind the back if restraints are used* (Chapter 15).

Paralyzed arms are supported on pillows. Some persons have positioners (Fig. 17-14). Ask the nurse about their proper use. The nurse may have you position the wrists at a slight upward angle.

Some people require postural supports if they cannot keep their upper bodies erect (Fig. 17-15, p. 260). Postural supports help keep them in good alignment. The health team selects the best product for the person's needs. The person's safety, dignity, and function are considered.

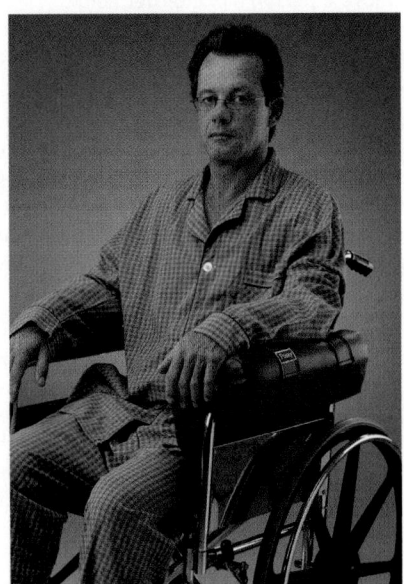

FIGURE 17-14 Elevated armrest. (Image courtesy Posey Co., Arcadia, Calif.)

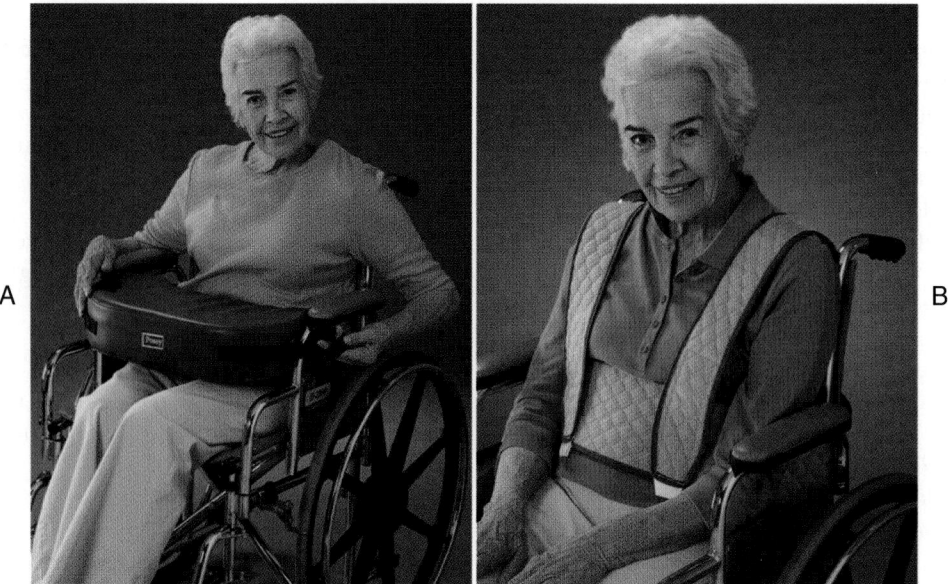

FIGURE 17-15 Postural supports. **A,** Posey Hugger. **B,** Torso support. (Images courtesy Posey Co., Arcadia, Calif.)

FOCUS ON PRIDE

The Person, Family, and Yourself

Personal and Professional Responsibility

You make decisions daily about protecting yourself. For example:

- Do you bend at the waist or the hips and knees to pick up an object?
- Do you reach or use a step stool to get high objects?
- Do you exercise to maintain strength and endurance?
- Do you raise the bed to waist level when giving bedside care?
- Do you move a person alone or get help?

Your decisions affect the safety of yourself and others. Use good judgment at home and in the workplace. Take responsibility for protecting yourself from harm.

Rights and Respect

OSHA requires that employers provide a safe work setting. You have the right to ask potential or current employers about safety plans to reduce your risk of injury. Ask about training or orientation programs related to body mechanics, safe handling of persons, and workplace hazards. Know and follow agency procedures for reporting problems.

Independence and Social Interaction

Remaining independent to the extent possible promotes dignity, self-esteem, and pride. Let the person choose bed or chair positions as allowed by the nurse and the care plan. Let the person help as much as safely possible. Talk with the person while moving him or her. Ask what he or she prefers. Doing so promotes comfort, independence, and social interaction.

Delegation and Teamwork

Many tasks strain your body. Injuries can occur. Some tasks increase your risk for injury. See "MSD Risk Factors," p. 253. Know which tasks often cause harm. Use caution when doing them. Get help when needed.

Thinking that injuries happen only to others is dangerous. Anyone can be injured. Your safety is important. Take pride in working carefully.

Ethics and Laws

Proper body mechanics help prevent injuries that could affect health and ability to function. Failure to move and position the person correctly places the person at risk. For example:

- A person is left slumped in a chair for 3 hours. The person develops a pressure ulcer.
- A person is not re-positioned as instructed in the care plan. The person's contracture worsens.
- A person is moved without enough help. The move is rough. The person is injured.

You must provide care in a manner that maintains or improves each person's quality of life, health, and safety. It is the right thing to do.

FOCUS ON PRIDE: Application

To care for others, you must take care of yourself. What changes will you make in your daily life to protect yourself from injury? How do you plan to protect yourself in the workplace?

REVIEW QUESTIONS

Circle the BEST answer.

1 Good body mechanics involve
   a Having an upright posture
   b Having a narrow base of support
   c Using the muscles in the back and lower arms
   d Lifting a heavy object alone

2 Good alignment means
   a The area on which an object rests
   b Having the head, trunk, arms, and legs aligned with one another
   c Using muscles, tendons, ligaments, and joints correctly
   d The back-lying or supine position

3 Which action shows poor body mechanics?
   a Holding an object close to your body
   b Facing the direction you are working to prevent twisting
   c Leaning over a raised bed rail to give care
   d Using both hands and arms to lift an object

4 You need to move a large chair in a resident's room. You should
   a Push or slide the chair
   b Lift and carry the chair
   c Ask the nurse to move the chair for you
   d Pull the chair using quick, jerking motions

5 The purpose of ergonomics is to
   a Reduce stress on the worker's body
   b Safely position the person
   c Promote quality of life
   d Use good body mechanics

6 Risk of MSDs decreases with
   a Repeating actions
   b Awkward postures
   c Bending your hips and knees to lift
   d Greater force

7 Which statement about back injuries is *true*?
   a Back injuries cannot be prevented.
   b Pain when assuming normal posture is a symptom.
   c Nursing center staff are at low risk.
   d Bending to change bed linens is not a cause of back injuries.

8 Which statement about positioning is *true*?
   a Re-positioning prevents pressure ulcers and contractures.
   b Circulation is not affected by positioning.
   c Position changes are avoided if moving causes pain.
   d Persons in chairs are re-positioned less often than those in bed.

9 You position a resident in the lateral position. Where do you place the call light?
   a At the head or foot of the bed
   b On either side of the bed
   c On the side of the bed facing the person's back side
   d On the side of the bed facing the person's front side

10 Patients and residents are re-positioned at least every
   a 15 minutes
   b 30 minutes
   c 2 hours
   d 3 hours

11 The back-lying position is called
   a Fowler's position
   b The supine position
   c The lateral position
   d Sims' position

12 For Fowler's position
   a The bed is flat
   b The head of the bed is raised 45 to 60 degrees
   c The person's head is turned to 1 side
   d The person's feet hang over the edge of the mattress

13 A pillow is placed against the person's back in
   a A chair while restraints are used
   b The prone position
   c The lateral position
   d Sims' position

14 When in a chair, the person's feet
   a Must be flat on the floor
   b Are positioned on footplates
   c Dangle
   d Are positioned on pillows

Answers to Chapter 17 questions are on p. 870.

FOCUS ON **PRACTICE**

Problem Solving

You are a new nursing assistant. To complete tasks quickly, you do not adjust the bed height to a comfortable working level. You move persons alone instead of getting help. You reach over raised bed rails instead of lowering them. Explain why these actions put you at increased risk for injury.

Two months later you have low back pain and numbness in a leg. Your walking is affected. How does this impact your work and daily life? How could you have avoided this problem?

OBJECTIVES

- Define the key terms and key abbreviation in this chapter.
- Identify comfort and safety measures for moving the person.
- Explain how to prevent work-related injuries when moving persons.
- Describe 5 functional status levels for bed mobility.

- Identify the delegation information needed before moving the person.
- Perform the procedures described in this chapter.
- Explain how to promote PRIDE in the person, the family, and yourself.

KEY TERMS

bed mobility How a person moves to and from a lying position, turns from side to side, and re-positions in a bed or other furniture
friction The rubbing of 1 surface against another
functional status The person's ability to perform the activities of daily living (ADL) required to meet basic needs and required for health and well-being

logrolling Turning the person as a unit, in alignment, with 1 motion
shearing When skin sticks to a surface while muscles slide in the direction the body is moving
weight-bearing To put weight on one's legs

KEY ABBREVIATION

ID   Identification

You will move persons often. You assist with bed mobility. The Centers for Medicare & Medicaid Services (CMS) defines *bed mobility* as *how a person moves to and from a lying position, turns from side to side, and re-positions in a bed or other furniture.* You also position persons in chairs and wheelchairs. You must work carefully to protect yourself and the person from injury.

See *Focus on Communication: Safely Moving the Person.*

See *Promoting Safety and Comfort: Safely Moving the Person.*

FOCUS ON **COMMUNICATION**

Safely Moving the Person

Moving can be painful after an injury or surgery. Many older persons have painful joints. Provide for comfort and avoid causing pain. You can say:
- "Please tell me when you feel pain or discomfort."
- "Do you need a pillow adjusted?"
- "Are you comfortable?"
- "How can I make you more comfortable?"

Before any move, explain the procedure. Tell the person what you and your co-workers will do. Also explain what the person needs to do. Do so as you begin the procedure. Also remind the person just before the move.

The procedures in this chapter explain how to move the person on the "count of 3." Staff move the person at the same time. The person is moved smoothly. One co-worker leads by counting. Decide who will count before the move. Be sure the person and staff know who is leading and what to do. You can say:

We will help you move up in bed. I will count "1, 2, 3." When I say "3," push against the bed with your feet and pull up with the trapeze. We will help move your body to the head of the bed when I say "3."

Safety

Many older persons have fragile bones and joints. To prevent injuries:

- Follow the rules of body mechanics (Chapter 17).
- Always have help to move the person.
- Move the person carefully.
- Keep the person in good alignment.
- Position the person in good alignment after the procedure.
- Make sure the face, nose, and mouth are not obstructed by a pillow or other device.

Comfort

To promote mental comfort when moving the person:

- Explain what you are going to do and how the person can help.
- Screen and cover the person to protect the right to privacy.
  To promote physical comfort:
- Keep the person in good alignment.
- Do not let the person's head hit the head-board when he or she is moved up in bed. If the person can be without a pillow, place it upright against the head-board.
- Use pillows to position the person as directed by the nurse and the care plan. If a pillow is allowed under the person's head, position it under the head and shoulders.
- Use other positioning devices as directed by the nurse and the care plan.

PREVENTING WORK-RELATED INJURIES

Moving procedures involve lifting, awkward postures, and repeated motions. These place you at increased risk for injury. You must prevent work-related injuries during moving procedures. See Chapter 17.

Good body mechanics alone will not prevent injury. The Occupational Safety and Health Administration (OSHA) recommends:

- Minimizing manual lifting in all cases.
- Eliminating manual lifting when possible.

Each person is different. Careful planning is needed to move the person safely. You must know:

- *The person's functional status.* **Functional status** *is the person's ability to perform the activities of daily living (ADL) required to meet basic needs and required for health and well-being.* Some persons move without help. Others depend on the staff. Know the person's functional status before you move a person. See Box 18-1. Tell the nurse about changes in the person's abilities.
- *The number of staff needed.* This depends on the person's height, weight, cognitive function, and functional status. Some persons need no help. Or they just need reminders or help with devices or equipment. Others need help from 1, 2, 3, or more staff.
- *What procedure to use.* The nurse and care plan tell you what procedure to use.
- *The equipment needed.* Assist equipment and devices are presented throughout this chapter. The nurse and care plan tell you what to use. Always follow the manufacturer's instructions. Ask for training to use the equipment and devices safely.

See *Focus on Children and Older Persons: Preventing Work-Related Injuries.*

See *Teamwork and Time Management: Preventing Work-Related Injuries*, p. 264.

See *Delegation Guidelines: Preventing Work-Related Injuries*, p. 264.

See *Promoting Safety and Comfort: Preventing Work-Related Injuries*, p. 264.

BOX 18-1   Functional Status—Bed Mobility

Level 0: Independent. The person can turn and re-position in bed, lie down, and sit up without help. The person may use a bed rail to turn. Staff may raise and lower the bed rail.

Level 1: Supervision. Staff look after, encourage, remind, or cue the person. (To *cue* means to *remind the person what to do.*) The person moves without help.

Level 2: Limited Assistance. The person is highly involved. Staff guide but do not lift the person's arms or legs. The person moves alone. Staff may encourage or cue the person to change positions.

Level 3: Extensive Assistance. The person needs help to turn, re-position, sit up, and move in bed. Two or more staff provide weight-bearing help. *(Weight-bearing means to put weight on one's legs.)* To move up in bed, a friction-reducing device is used. To assist, the person bends the knees and pushes with the legs when cued. Or a mechanical lift is used (Chapter 19).

Level 4: Total Dependence. The person is unable to sit up, lie down, turn, or re-position without help. Two or more staff turn, re-position, and move the person. A mechanical lift (Chapter 19) or friction-reducing device is used.

Modified from Centers for Medicare & Medicaid Services: RAI version 3.0 manual, October 2014.

FOCUS ON **CHILDREN AND OLDER PERSONS**
Preventing Work-Related Injuries

Older Persons

Persons with dementia may not understand what you are doing. They may resist your efforts. The person may shout, grab you, or try to hit you. Always have a co-worker help you. Do not force the person. The person's care plan has measures for safe care. For example:

- Proceed slowly.
- Use a calm, pleasant voice.
- Divert the person's attention. For example, let the person hold a washcloth or other soft object. This helps distract the person and keeps the hands busy.

Tell the nurse at once if you have problems moving the person.

TEAMWORK AND TIME MANAGEMENT
Preventing Work-Related Injuries

Patients and residents are moved, turned, and re-positioned often. These procedures are best done by at least 2 staff members.

Friendships are common among co-workers. And some working relationships are better than others. Do not ask for help just from friends or those with whom you work well. Include all co-workers. Do not help just your friends or those with whom you work well. Assist anyone who asks. This includes new staff and those from other units.

PROMOTING SAFETY AND COMFORT
Preventing Work-Related Injuries
Safety

Decide how to move the person before starting the procedure. Ask needed staff to help before you begin. Also plan how to protect drainage tubes or containers connected to the person.

Beds are raised to move persons in bed. This reduces bending and reaching. You must:
* Use the bed correctly.
* Protect the person from falling when the bed is raised.
* Follow the rules of body mechanics (Chapter 17).

DELEGATION GUIDELINES
Preventing Work-Related Injuries

Many tasks involve moving persons. Before doing so, you need this information from the nurse and the care plan.
* The person's height and weight.
* The person's functional status (see Box 18-1).
* The person's physical abilities. Does the person have strength in his or her arms and legs?
* If the person has a weak side. If yes, which side?
* If the person has problems that increase the risk of injury. Dizziness, confusion, hearing or vision problems, recent surgery, and fragile skin are examples.
* Any doctor's orders for moving the person.
* The person's ability to follow directions.
* If behavior problems are likely. Combative, agitated, uncooperative, and unpredictable behaviors are examples.
* The amount of assistance needed.
* The number of staff needed to complete the task safely.
* What procedure to use.
* What equipment to use.

PROTECTING THE SKIN

Protect the person's skin during moving procedures. Friction and shearing injure the skin. Both cause infection and pressure ulcers (Chapter 37).
* *Friction is the rubbing of 1 surface against another.* When moved in bed, the person's skin rubs against the sheet.
* *Shearing is when the skin sticks to a surface while muscles slide in the direction the body is moving* (Fig. 18-1). It occurs when the person slides down in bed or is moved in bed.

To reduce friction and shearing when moving the person in bed:
* Roll the person.
* Use friction-reducing devices. Such devices include a lift sheet (turning sheet). Drawsheets (Chapter 21) serve as lift sheets (turning sheets). Turning pads (Fig. 18-2), large re-usable waterproof under-pads (Chapter 21), and slide sheets (p. 269) are other friction-reducing devices.

See *Focus on Children and Older Persons: Protecting the Skin.*

See *Focus on Surveys: Protecting the Skin.*

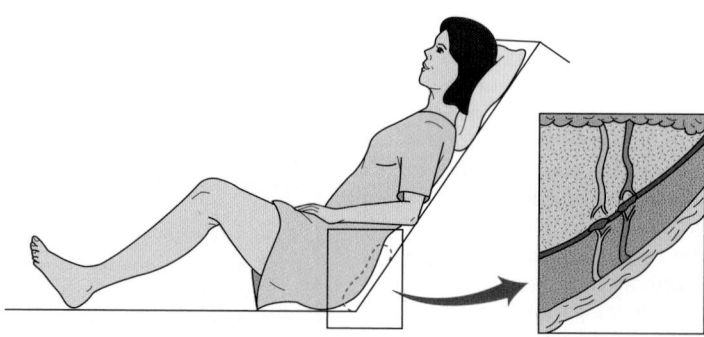

FIGURE 18-1 Shearing. When the head of the bed is raised to a sitting position, skin on the buttocks stays in place. However, internal structures move forward as the person slides down in bed. This pinches the skin between the mattress and the hip bones.

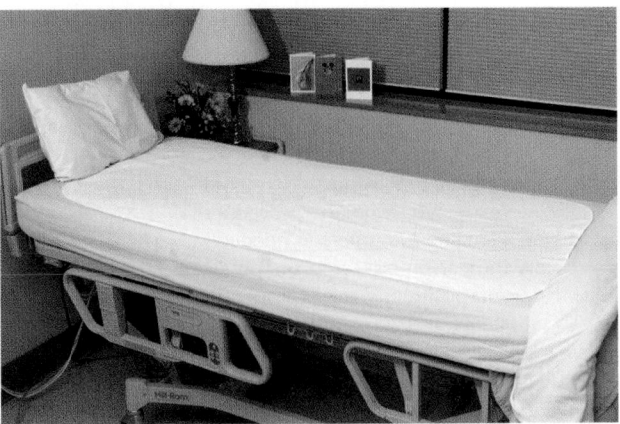

FIGURE 18-2 Turning pad.

BOX 18-2	Guidelines for Moving Persons in Bed

- Follow the rules for preventing work-related injuries in Chapter 17.
- Know how much help and what equipment or friction-reducing devices you need. Follow the nurse's directions and the care plan. The nurse uses the person's weight as a guide to plan a safe move.
  - *For persons fully able to assist*—staff assistance is not needed. Staff stand by for safety and provide cues as needed.
  - *For persons partially able to assist:*
    - *If the person weighs less than 200 pounds*—2 to 3 staff members and a friction-reducing device are used.
    - *If the person weighs more than 200 pounds*—at least 3 staff members and a friction-reducing device are used.
  - *For persons unable to assist*—a mechanical lift and at least 2 staff members are needed. See "Using a Mechanical Lift" in Chapter 19.

Modified from Occupational Safety and Health Administration: Guidelines for nursing homes: Ergonomics for the prevention of musculoskeletal disorders, Washington, DC, Revised March 2009, Author.

FOCUS ON **CHILDREN AND OLDER PERSONS**

Protecting the Skin

Older Persons

Older persons are at great risk for shearing. Their fragile skin is easily torn. Protect the skin from injury.

Ask a co-worker to help you move older persons. Use a friction-reducing device. Move older persons carefully and gently.

Persons with dementia may try to resist your efforts. Do not force the person. Work slowly. Use a calm voice. Divert the person's attention if necessary.

FOCUS ON **SURVEYS**

Protecting the Skin

Shearing and friction can easily damage the skin. Surveyors will observe the measures taken by staff to prevent or reduce shearing and friction when moving and re-positioning persons.

FOCUS ON **COMMUNICATION**

Moving Persons in Bed

The nurse observes the person and asks questions to assess the person's abilities. Your input is important. Tell the nurse what you have seen, not what you think the person may be able to do. For example:

Nurse: "How have you seen Mr. Boyd move in bed?"
You: "He can lie down and sit up alone."
Nurse: "Do you give verbal cues or move him in any way?"
You: "I remind him to use the trapeze. Once I remind him, he can do it alone. I also help him turn to his side."
Nurse: "How do you help him turn to his side?"
You: "He uses the bed rail to turn. I tell him what to do and help move his legs."

MOVING PERSONS IN BED

Some persons can move and turn in bed. Others need help from at least 1 person. Those who are weak, unconscious, paralyzed, or in casts need help. Sometimes 2 or 3 people or a mechanical lift (Chapter 19) is needed. Follow the guidelines in Box 18-2 when lifting or moving persons in bed.

See *Focus on Communication: Moving Persons in Bed.*
See *Delegation Guidelines: Moving Persons in Bed*, p. 266.

DELEGATION GUIDELINES

Moving Persons in Bed

Before moving a person, you need this information from the nurse and the care plan.
- What procedure to use
- The number of staff needed to safely move the person
- Position limits and restrictions
- How far you can lower the head of the bed
- Any limits in the person's ability to move or be re-positioned
- What pillows you can remove before moving the person
- What equipment is needed—trapeze, lift sheet, slide sheet, mechanical lift

- How to position the person
- If the person uses bed rails
- What observations to report and record:
  - Who helped you with the procedure
  - How much help the person needed
  - How the person tolerated the procedure
  - How you positioned the person
  - Complaints of pain or discomfort
- When to report observations
- What patient or resident concerns to report at once

Raising the Person's Head and Shoulders

Sometimes you raise the person's head and shoulders to give care. Simply turning or removing a pillow requires this procedure. You can raise the person's head and shoulders easily and safely by locking arms with the person. *Do not pull on the person's arm or shoulder.* Have help with older persons and with those who are heavy or hard to move. This protects the person and you from injury.

See procedure: *Raising the Person's Head and Shoulders.*

Raising the Person's Head and Shoulders

QUALITY OF LIFE

- Knock before entering the person's room.
- Address the person by name.
- Introduce yourself by name and title.

- Explain the procedure before starting and during the procedure.
- Protect the person's rights during the procedure.
- Handle the person gently during the procedure.

PRE-PROCEDURE

1 Follow *Delegation Guidelines:*
   a *Preventing Work-Related Injuries,* p. 264
   b *Moving Persons in Bed*
   See *Promoting Safety and Comfort:*
   a *Safely Moving the Person,* p. 263
   b *Preventing Work-Related Injuries,* p. 264
2 Ask a co-worker to assist if needed.

3 Practice hand hygiene.
4 Identify the person. Check the ID (identification) bracelet against the assignment sheet. Use 2 identifiers (Chapter 13). Also call the person by name.
5 Provide for privacy.
6 Lock (brake) the bed wheels.
7 Raise the bed for body mechanics. Bed rails are up if used.

PROCEDURE

8 Have your co-worker stand on the other side of the bed. Lower the bed rails if up.
9 Ask the person to put the near arm under your near arm and behind your shoulder. His or her hand rests on top of your shoulder. If you are standing on the right side, the person's right hand rests on your right shoulder (Fig. 18-3, *A*). The person does the same with your co-worker. The person's left hand rests on your co-worker's left shoulder (Fig. 18-4, *A*).
10 Put your arm nearest to the person under his or her arm. Your hand is on the person's shoulder. Your co-worker does the same.

11 Put your free arm under the person's neck and shoulders (Fig. 18-3, *B*). Your co-worker does the same (Fig. 18-4, *B*). Support the neck.
12 Help the person rise to a sitting or semi-sitting position on the "count of 3" (Figs. 18-3, *C* and 18-4, *C*).
13 Use the arm and hand that supported the person's neck and shoulders to give care (Fig. 18-3, *D*). Your co-worker supports the person (Fig. 18-4, *D*).
14 Help the person lie down. Provide support with your locked arm. Support the person's neck and shoulders with your other arm. Your co-worker does the same.

POST-PROCEDURE

15 Provide for comfort. (See the inside of the front cover.)
16 Place the call light and other needed items within reach.
17 Lower the bed to a safe and comfortable level appropriate for the person. Follow the care plan.
18 Raise or lower bed rails. Follow the care plan.

19 Unscreen the person.
20 Complete a safety check of the room. (See the inside of the front cover.)
21 Practice hand hygiene.
22 Report and record your observations.

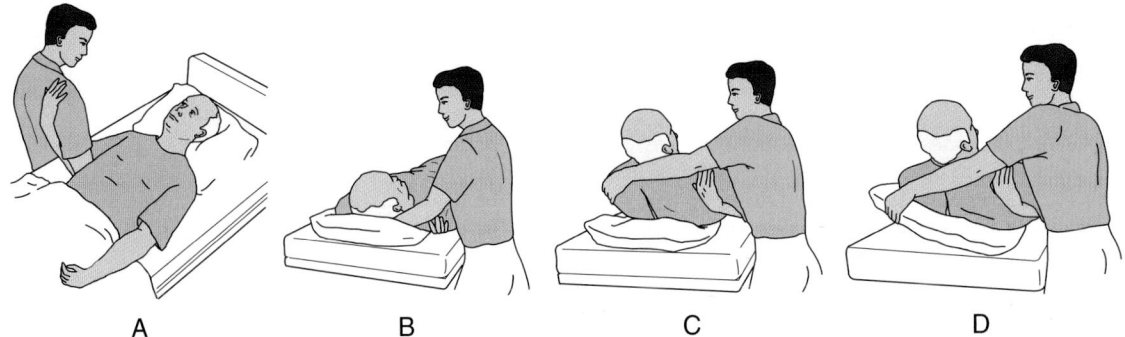

A   B   C   D

FIGURE 18-3 Raising the person's head and shoulders by locking arms with the person. **A,** The person's near arm is under the nursing assistant's near arm and behind the shoulder. **B,** The nursing assistant's far arm is under the person's neck and shoulders. The near arm is under the person's near arm. **C,** The person is raised to a semi-sitting position by locking arms. **D,** The nursing assistant lifts the pillow while the person is in a semi-sitting position.

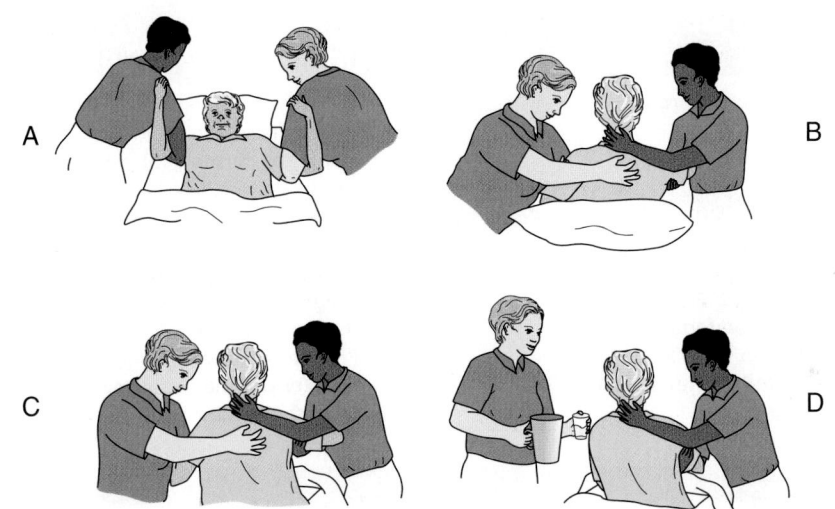

A   B

C   D

FIGURE 18-4 Raising the person's head and shoulders with a co-worker. **A,** Two nursing assistants lock arms with the person. **B,** The nursing assistants each have an arm under the person's head and neck. **C,** The nursing assistants raise the person to a semi-sitting position. **D,** One nursing assistant supports the person in the semi-sitting position. The other gives care.

Moving the Person Up in Bed

When the head of the bed is raised, it is easy to slide down toward the middle and foot of the bed (Fig. 18-5). You move the person up in bed for good alignment and comfort.

You can sometimes move light-weight adults up in bed alone if they assist using a trapeze. However, it is best done with help and an assist device (p. 269). For heavy, weak, and older persons, 2 or more staff members are needed. Always protect the person and yourself from injury.

See *Promoting Safety and Comfort: Moving the Person Up in Bed*, p. 268.

See procedure: *Moving the Person Up in Bed*, p. 268.

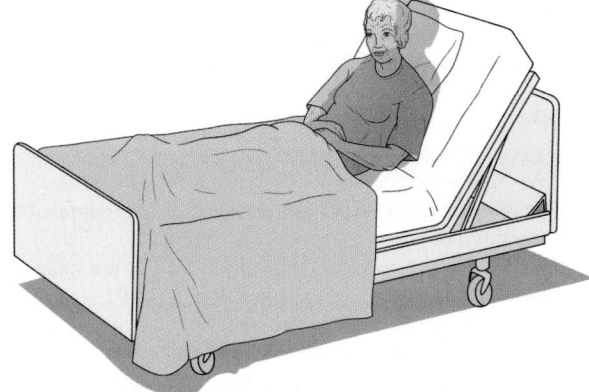

FIGURE 18-5 A person in poor alignment after sliding down in bed.

PROMOTING SAFETY AND COMFORT

Moving the Person Up in Bed

Safety

This procedure is best done with at least 2 staff members. Work from the side of the bed. *Do not pull the person from the head of the bed.* Use assist devices as directed by the nurse and the care plan. Ask any questions before you begin the procedure.

Perform the procedure alone only if:

- The person is small in size.
- The person can follow directions.
- The person can assist with much of the moving.
- The person uses a trapeze.
- The person can push against the mattress with his or her feet.
- The nurse says it is safe to do so.
- You are comfortable doing so.

Moving the Person Up in Bed

QUALITY OF LIFE

- Knock before entering the person's room.
- Address the person by name.
- Introduce yourself by name and title.

- Explain the procedure before starting and during the procedure.
- Protect the person's rights during the procedure.
- Handle the person gently during the procedure.

PRE-PROCEDURE

1 Follow *Delegation Guidelines:*
   a *Preventing Work-Related Injuries,* p. 264
   b *Moving Persons in Bed,* p. 266
   See *Promoting Safety and Comfort:*
   a *Safely Moving the Person,* p. 263
   b *Preventing Work-Related Injuries,* p. 264
   c *Moving the Person Up in Bed*
2 Ask a co-worker to help you.

3 Practice hand hygiene.
4 Identify the person. Check the ID bracelet against the assignment sheet. Use 2 identifiers (Chapter 13). Also call the person by name.
5 Provide for privacy.
6 Lock (brake) the bed wheels.
7 Raise the bed for body mechanics. Bed rails are up if used.

PROCEDURE

8 Lower the head of the bed to a level appropriate for the person. It is as flat as possible.
9 Stand on 1 side of the bed. Your co-worker stands on the other side.
10 Lower the bed rails if up.
11 Remove pillows as directed by the nurse. Place a pillow against the head-board if the person can be without it.
12 Stand with a wide base of support. Point the foot near the head of the bed toward the head of the bed. Face the head of the bed.
13 Bend your hips and knees. Keep your back straight.
14 Place 1 arm under the person's shoulder and 1 arm under the thighs. Your co-worker does the same. Grasp each other's forearms (Fig. 18-6).

15 Ask the person to grasp the trapeze.
16 Have the person flex both knees.
17 Explain that:
   a You will count "1, 2, 3."
   b The move will be on "3."
   c On "3," the person pushes against the bed with the feet if able. And the person pulls up with the trapeze.
18 Move the person to the head of the bed on the "count of 3." Shift your weight from your rear leg to your front leg (see Fig. 18-6). Your co-worker does the same.
19 Repeat steps 12 through 18 if necessary.

POST-PROCEDURE

20 Put the pillow under the person's head and shoulders. Straighten linens.
21 Position the person in good alignment. Raise the head of the bed to a level appropriate for the person.
22 Provide for comfort. (See the inside of the front cover.)
23 Place the call light and other needed items within reach.
24 Lower the bed to a safe and comfortable level appropriate for the person. Follow the care plan.

25 Raise or lower bed rails. Follow the care plan.
26 Unscreen the person.
27 Complete a safety check of the room. (See the inside of the front cover.)
28 Practice hand hygiene.
29 Report and record your observations.

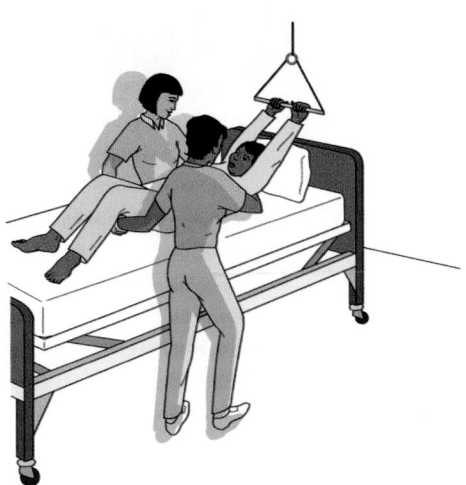

FIGURE 18-6 A person is moved up in bed by 2 nursing assistants. Each has 1 arm under the person's shoulders and the other under the thighs. They have locked arms under the person. The person grasps the trapeze and flexes the knees. The nursing assistants shift their weight from the rear leg to the front leg as the person is moved up in bed.

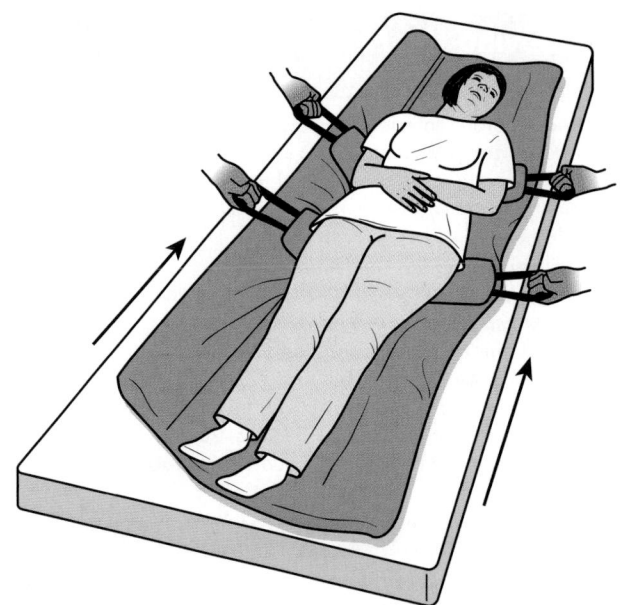

FIGURE 18-7 Slide sheet.

Moving the Person Up in Bed With an Assist Device

You use assist devices to move some persons up in bed. Such assist devices include a drawsheet (lift sheet, turning sheet), flat sheet folded in half, turning pad, slide sheet (Fig. 18-7), and large re-usable waterproof under-pad. With these devices, the person is moved more evenly. And shearing and friction are reduced.

To position the device, you must turn the person. See procedure: *Turning and Re-Positioning the Person* (p. 273). You and at least 1 co-worker:

1. Turn the person to 1 side.
2. Place the device on the bed. Open the device and fan-fold it toward the person. The device is positioned from the head to above the knees or lower.
3. Tell the person that he or she will roll over a "bump." Assure the person that he or she will not fall.
4. Turn the person to the other side. The person rolls over the device.
5. Pull the device tightly. Smooth any wrinkles.
6. Roll the person onto his or her back. The person is lying on the device.

Assist devices are used to move most patients and residents in bed. At least 2 staff members are needed. The next procedure is used:

- Following the guidelines for moving persons in bed (see Box 18-2)
- For persons recovering from spinal cord surgery or spinal cord injuries
- For older persons

See *Promoting Safety and Comfort: Moving the Person Up in Bed With an Assist Device.*

See procedure: *Moving the Person Up in Bed With an Assist Device,* p. 270.

PROMOTING SAFETY AND COMFORT

Moving the Person Up in Bed With an Assist Device

Safety

Not all waterproof under-pads are used as assist devices. Disposable, single-use under-pads are not strong enough to hold the person's weight during the move. Re-usable under-pads are stronger. Ask the nurse if the person's under-pad is safe as an assist device. For safety, the under-pad must:

- Be strong enough to support the person's weight.
- Extend from under the person's head to above the knees or lower.
- Be wide enough for you and other staff to get a firm grip.

After using a slide sheet, remove it. If left in place, the person is in danger of sliding down in bed or off the bed.

For persons with bariatric needs, the care plan may include:

- Performing the task with a friction-reducing device or bariatric lift and:
  - At least 2 staff members if the person can assist with the move.
  - At least 3 staff members if the person cannot assist with the move.
- Positioning the bed in Trendelenburg's position (Chapter 20). In this position, the head of the bed is lowered and the foot of the bed is raised. This allows the use of gravity to pull the person up in bed. The position is used only if tolerated by the person and allowed by the doctor.
- Leaving the friction-reducing device under the person. The device is covered with a drawsheet. Leaving the device under the person reduces the risk of injuries to the person and staff. The person is not turned from side to side to place and remove the friction-reducing device.

Moving the Person Up in Bed With an Assist Device

QUALITY OF LIFE

- Knock before entering the person's room.
- Address the person by name.
- Introduce yourself by name and title.

- Explain the procedure before starting and during the procedure.
- Protect the person's rights during the procedure.
- Handle the person gently during the procedure.

PRE-PROCEDURE

1 Follow *Delegation Guidelines:*
   a *Preventing Work-Related Injuries*, p. 264
   b *Moving Persons in Bed*, p. 266
   See *Promoting Safety and Comfort:*
   a *Safely Moving the Person*, p. 263
   b *Preventing Work-Related Injuries*, p. 264
   c *Moving the Person Up in Bed*, p. 268
   d *Moving the Person Up in Bed With an Assist Device*,
      p. 269

2 Ask a co-worker to help you.
3 Obtain the needed assist device.
4 Practice hand hygiene.
5 Identify the person. Check the ID bracelet against the
   assignment sheet. Use 2 identifiers (Chapter 13). Also call
   the person by name.
6 Provide for privacy.
7 Lock (brake) the bed wheels.
8 Raise the bed for body mechanics. Bed rails are up if used.

PROCEDURE

9 Lower the head of the bed to a level appropriate for the
   person. It is as flat as possible.
10 Stand on 1 side of the bed. Your co-worker stands on the
   other side.
11 Lower the bed rails if up.
12 Remove pillows as directed by the nurse. Place a pillow
   against the head-board if the person can be without it.
13 Position the assist device.
14 Stand with a wide base of support. Point the foot near the
   head of the bed toward the head of the bed. Face the
   head of the bed.

15 Roll the sides of the assist device up close to the person.
   (NOTE: Omit this step if the device has handles.)
16 Grasp the rolled-up assist device firmly near the person's
   shoulders and hips (Fig. 18-8). Or grasp it by the handles.
   Support the head.
17 Bend your hips and knees.
18 Move the person up in bed on the "count of 3." Shift your
   weight from your rear leg to your front leg.
19 Repeat steps 14 through 18 if necessary.
20 Unroll the assist device. (NOTE: Omit this step if the device
   has handles.) Remove the slide sheet if used.

POST-PROCEDURE

21 Put the pillow under the person's head and shoulders.
   Straighten linens.
22 Position the person in good alignment. Raise the head of
   the bed to a level appropriate for the person.
23 Provide for comfort. (See the inside of the front cover.)
24 Place the call light and other needed items within reach.
25 Lower the bed to a safe and comfortable level appropriate
   for the person. Follow the care plan.

26 Raise or lower bed rails. Follow the care plan.
27 Unscreen the person.
28 Complete a safety check of the room. (See the inside of
   the front cover.)
29 Practice hand hygiene.
30 Report and record your observations.

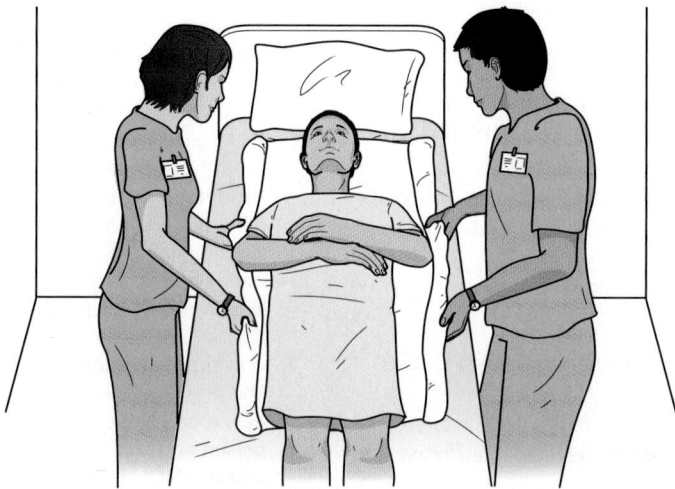

FIGURE 18-8 A drawsheet is used to move the person up in bed. It extends from the person's head to
above the knees. Rolled close to the person, the drawsheet is held near the shoulders and hips.

Moving the Person to the Side of the Bed

Re-positioning and care procedures require moving the person to the side of the bed. Move the person to the side of the bed before turning. Otherwise, after turning, the person lies on the side of the bed—not in the middle.

Sometimes you have to reach over the person. During a bed bath is an example. You reach less if the person is near you.

In 1 method, the person is moved in segments (Fig. 18-9). Sometimes you can do this alone if the person is small in size. With at least 1 co-worker, use a mechanical lift (Chapter 19) or an assist device.

- Following the guidelines for moving persons in bed (see Box 18-2)
- For older persons
- For persons with arthritis
- For persons recovering from spinal cord injuries or surgeries

Assist devices for this procedure include a drawsheet (lift sheet, turning sheet), flat sheet folded in half, turning pad, slide sheet, and large re-usable waterproof under-pad. An assist device helps prevent pain and skin damage and injury to the bones, joints, and spinal cord. The procedure that follows includes using a drawsheet.

See *Promoting Safety and Comfort: Moving the Person to the Side of the Bed.*

See procedure: *Moving the Person to the Side of the Bed,* p. 272.

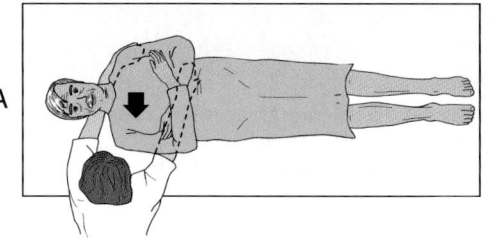
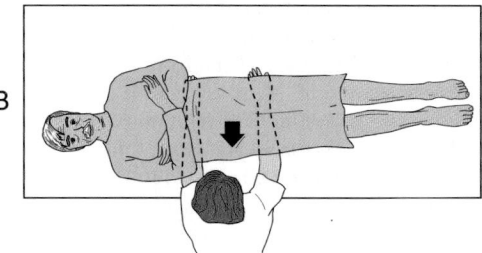
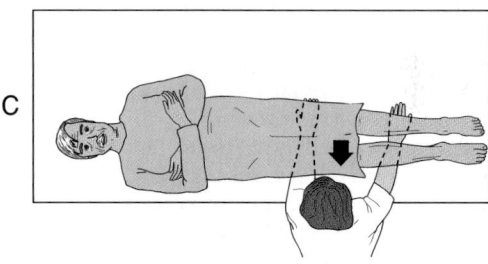

FIGURE 18-9 Moving the person to the side of the bed in segments. **A,** The upper part of the body is moved. **B,** The lower part of the body is moved. **C,** The legs and feet are moved.

Moving the Person to the Side of the Bed

QUALITY OF LIFE

- Knock before entering the person's room.
- Address the person by name.
- Introduce yourself by name and title.

- Explain the procedure before starting and during the procedure.
- Protect the person's rights during the procedure.
- Handle the person gently during the procedure.

PRE-PROCEDURE

1 Follow *Delegation Guidelines:*
   a *Preventing Work-Related Injuries,* p. 264
   b *Moving Persons in Bed,* p. 266
   See *Promoting Safety and Comfort:*
   a *Safely Moving the Person,* p. 263
   b *Preventing Work-Related Injuries,* p. 264
   c *Moving the Person to the Side of the Bed,* p. 271
2 Ask 1 or 2 co-workers to help you if using an assist device.

3 Obtain a drawsheet.
4 Practice hand hygiene.
5 Identify the person. Check the ID bracelet against the assignment sheet. Use 2 identifiers (Chapter 13). Also call the person by name.
6 Provide for privacy.
7 Lock (brake) the bed wheels.
8 Raise the bed for body mechanics. Bed rails are up if used.

PROCEDURE

9 Lower the head of the bed to a level appropriate for the person. It is as flat as possible.
10 Stand on the side of the bed to which you will move the person.
11 Lower the bed rail near you if bed rails are used. (Both bed rails are lowered for step 16.)
12 Remove pillows as directed by the nurse.
13 Cross the person's arms over the chest.
14 Stand with your feet about 12 inches apart. One foot is in front of the other. Flex your knees.
15 *Method 1—Moving the person in segments:*
   a Place your arm under the person's neck and shoulders. Grasp the far shoulder.
   b Place your other arm under the mid-back.
   c Move the upper part of the person's body toward you. Rock backward and shift your weight to your rear leg (see Fig. 18-9, *A*).
   d Place 1 arm under the person's waist and 1 under the thighs.
   e Rock backward to move the lower part of the person toward you (Fig. 18-9, *B*).
   f Repeat the procedure for the legs and feet (see Fig. 18-9, *C*). Your arms should be under the person's thighs and calves.

16 *Method 2—Moving the person with a drawsheet:*
   a Position the drawsheet.
   b Roll up the drawsheet close to the person (see Fig. 18-8).
   c Grasp the rolled-up drawsheet near the person's shoulders and hips. Your co-worker does the same. Support the person's head.
   d Rock backward on the "count of 3" moving the person toward you. Your co-worker rocks backward slightly and then forward toward you while keeping the arms straight.
   e Unroll the drawsheet. Remove any wrinkles.

POST-PROCEDURE

17 Put the pillow under the person's head and shoulders. Straighten linens.
18 Position the person in good alignment.
19 Provide for comfort. (See the inside of the front cover.)
20 Place the call light and other needed items within reach.
21 Lower the bed to a safe and comfortable level appropriate for the person. Follow the care plan.

22 Raise or lower bed rails. Follow the care plan.
23 Unscreen the person.
24 Complete a safety check of the room. (See the inside of the front cover.)
25 Practice hand hygiene.
26 Report and record your observations.

TURNING PERSONS

Turning persons onto their sides helps prevent complications from bedrest (Chapter 30). Certain procedures and care measures require the side-lying position. You also turn the person to position and to remove friction-reducing devices.

You turn the person toward you or away from you. The direction depends on the person's condition and the situation.

Many older persons have arthritis in their spines, hips, and knees. Less painful, logrolling (p. 275) is preferred for turning these persons.

See *Delegation Guidelines: Turning Persons.*
See *Promoting Safety and Comfort: Turning Persons.*
See procedure: *Turning and Re-Positioning the Person.*

DELEGATION GUIDELINES

Turning Persons

Before turning and re-positioning a person, you need this information from the nurse and the care plan.
- The person's functional status (see Box 18-1)
- How much help the person needs
- The number of staff needed for safety
- The person's comfort level and what body parts are painful
- Which procedure to use
- What assist devices to use
- What supportive devices to use for positioning (Chapter 30)
- Where to place pillows
- What observations to report and record:
  - Who helped you with the procedure
  - How much help the person needed
  - How the person tolerated the procedure
  - How you positioned the person
  - Complaints of pain or discomfort
- When to report observations
- What patient or resident concerns to report at once

PROMOTING SAFETY AND COMFORT

Turning Persons

Safety
Use good body mechanics to turn a person in bed. See Chapter 17.

The person must be in good alignment. This helps prevent musculo-skeletal injuries, skin breakdown, and pressure ulcers.

Do not turn a person away from you with the far bed rail down. Raise the bed rail on the side near you. Then go to the other side of the bed. Lower the bed rail if up. Turn the person toward you.

Comfort
After turning, position the person in good alignment. Use pillows as directed to support the person in the side-lying position (Chapter 17). Make sure the person's face, nose, and mouth are not obstructed by a pillow or other device.

Turning and Re-Positioning the Person

QUALITY OF LIFE

- Knock before entering the person's room.
- Address the person by name.
- Introduce yourself by name and title.
- Explain the procedure before starting and during the procedure.
- Protect the person's rights during the procedure.
- Handle the person gently during the procedure.

PRE-PROCEDURE

1 Follow *Delegation Guidelines:*
   a *Preventing Work-Related Injuries*, p. 264
   b *Moving Persons in Bed*, p. 266
   c *Turning Persons*
   See *Promoting Safety and Comfort:*
   a *Safely Moving the Person*, p. 263
   b *Preventing Work-Related Injuries*, p. 264
   c *Moving the Person to the Side of the Bed*, p. 271
   d *Turning Persons*

2 Practice hand hygiene.
3 Identify the person. Check the ID bracelet against the assignment sheet. Use 2 identifiers (Chapter 13). Also call the person by name.
4 Provide for privacy.
5 Lock (brake) the bed wheels.
6 Raise the bed for body mechanics. Bed rails are up if used.

Continued

Turning and Re-Positioning the Person—cont'd

PROCEDURE

7   Lower the head of the bed to a level appropriate for the person. It is as flat as possible.
8   Stand on the side of the bed opposite to where you will turn the person.
9   Lower the bed rail.
10 Move the person to the side near you. (See procedure: *Moving the Person to the Side of the Bed,* p. 272.)
11 Cross the person's arms over the chest. Cross the leg near you over the far leg.
12 *Turning the person away from you:*
    a   Stand with a wide base of support. Flex the knees.
    b   Place 1 hand on the person's shoulder. Place the other on the hip near you.
    c   Roll the person gently away from you toward the raised bed rail (Fig. 18-10, *A*).
    d   Shift your weight from your rear leg to your front leg.

13 *Turning the person toward you:*
    a   Raise the bed rail.
    b   Go to the other side of the bed. Lower the bed rail.
    c   Stand with a wide base of support. Flex your knees.
    d   Place 1 hand on the person's shoulder. Place the other on the far hip.
    e   Pull the person toward you gently (Fig. 18-10, *B*).
14 Position the person. Follow the nurse's directions and the care plan. The following are common.
    a   Place a pillow under the head and neck.
    b   Adjust the shoulder. The person should not be on an arm.
    c   Place a small pillow under the upper hand and arm.
    d   Position a pillow against the back.
    e   Flex the upper knee. Position the upper leg in front of the lower leg.
    f   Support the upper leg and thigh on pillows. Make sure the ankle is supported.

POST-PROCEDURE

15 Provide for comfort. (See the inside of the front cover.)
16 Place the call light and other needed items within reach.
17 Lower the bed to a safe and comfortable level appropriate for the person. Follow the care plan.
18 Raise or lower bed rails. Follow the care plan.

19 Unscreen the person.
20 Complete a safety check of the room. (See the inside of the front cover.)
21 Practice hand hygiene.
22 Report and record your observations.

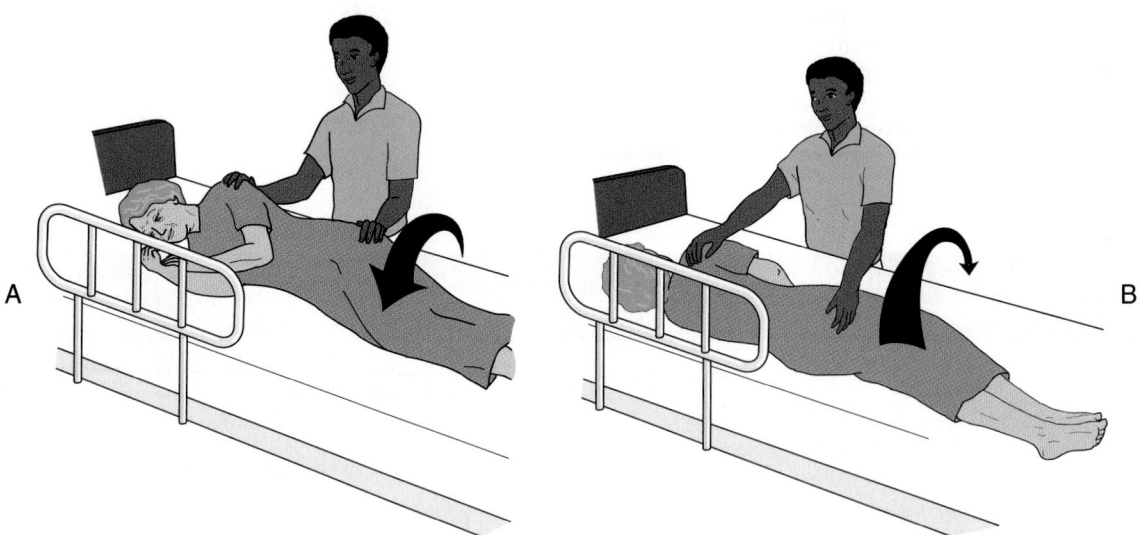

FIGURE 18-10 **Turning the person. A,** Turning the person away from you. **B,** Turning the person toward you. *(NOTE: Non-standard bed rails are used to show positioning and hand placement.)*

Logrolling

Logrolling is turning the person as a unit, in alignment, with 1 motion. The head, neck, and spine are kept straight. The procedure is used to turn:

- Older persons with arthritic spines or knees.
- Persons recovering from hip fractures.
- Persons with spinal cord injuries. The head, neck, and spine are kept straight at all times after a spinal cord injury.
- Persons recovering from spinal cord surgery. The head, neck, and spine are kept straight at all times after spinal surgery.

See *Promoting Safety and Comfort: Logrolling.*
See procedure: *Logrolling the Person.*

PROMOTING SAFETY AND COMFORT

Logrolling

Safety

For logrolling, 2 or 3 staff members are needed. If the person is tall or heavy, 3 are needed. Sometimes you use an assist device—drawsheet, turning pad, large re-usable waterproof under-pad, slide sheet.

After spinal cord injury or surgery, the head, neck, and spine are kept straight. The nurse holds the neck during moving or re-positioning. The nurse tells you what to do step-by-step. Assist the nurse as directed.

Comfort

After spinal cord injury or surgery, usually a pillow is not allowed under the head and neck. Follow the nurse's directions and the care plan to position the person and use pillows.

Logrolling the Person

VIDEO NATCEP

QUALITY OF LIFE

- Knock before entering the person's room.
- Address the person by name.
- Introduce yourself by name and title.

- Explain the procedure before starting and during the procedure.
- Protect the person's rights during the procedure.
- Handle the person gently during the procedure.

PRE-PROCEDURE

1 Follow *Delegation Guidelines:*
   a *Preventing Work-Related Injuries,* p. 264
   b *Moving Persons in Bed,* p. 266
   c *Turning Persons,* p. 273
   See *Promoting Safety and Comfort:*
   a *Safely Moving the Person,* p. 263
   b *Preventing Work-Related Injuries,* p. 264
   c *Turning Persons,* p. 273
   d *Logrolling*

2 Ask a co-worker to help you.
3 Obtain the needed assist device.
4 Practice hand hygiene.
5 Identify the person. Check the ID bracelet against the assignment sheet. Use 2 identifiers (Chapter 13). Also call the person by name.
6 Provide for privacy.
7 Lock (brake) the bed wheels.
8 Raise the bed for body mechanics. Bed rails are up if used.

PROCEDURE

9 Make sure the bed is flat.
10 Stand on the side opposite to which you will turn the person. Your co-worker stands on the other side.
11 Lower the bed rails if used.
12 Position the assist device.
13 Move the person as a unit to the side of the bed near you. Use the assist device. (If the person has a spinal cord injury or had spinal cord surgery, assist the nurse as directed.)
14 Place the person's arms across the chest. Place a pillow between the knees.
15 Raise the bed rail if used.
16 Go to the other side.
17 Stand near the shoulders and chest. Your co-worker stands near the hips and thighs.
18 Stand with a wide base of support. One foot is in front of the other.

19 Ask the person to hold his or her body rigid.
20 Roll the person toward you (Fig. 18-11, *A*, p. 276). Or use the assist device (Fig. 18-11, *B*, p. 276). Turn the person as a unit.
21 Remove the slide sheet (if used).
22 Position the person in good alignment. Use pillows as directed by the nurse and care plan. The following are common (unless the spinal cord is involved).
   a Place a pillow under the head and neck if allowed.
   b Adjust the shoulder. The person should not be on an arm.
   c Place a small pillow under the upper hand and arm.
   d Position a pillow against the back.
   e Flex the upper knee. Position the upper leg in front of the lower leg.
   f Support the upper leg and thigh on pillows. Make sure the ankle is supported.

POST-PROCEDURE

23 Provide for comfort. (See the inside of the front cover.)
24 Place the call light and other needed items within reach.
25 Lower the bed to a safe and comfortable level appropriate for the person. Follow the care plan.
26 Raise or lower bed rails. Follow the care plan.

27 Unscreen the person.
28 Complete a safety check of the room. (See the inside of the front cover.)
29 Practice hand hygiene.
30 Report and record your observations.

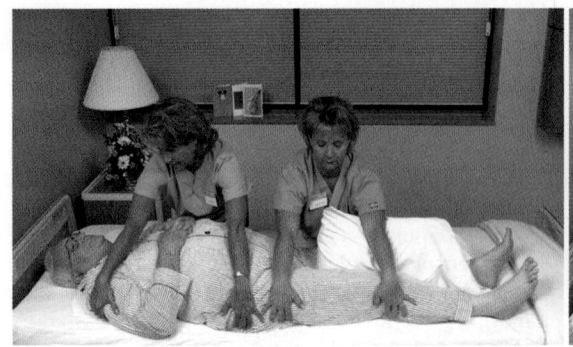
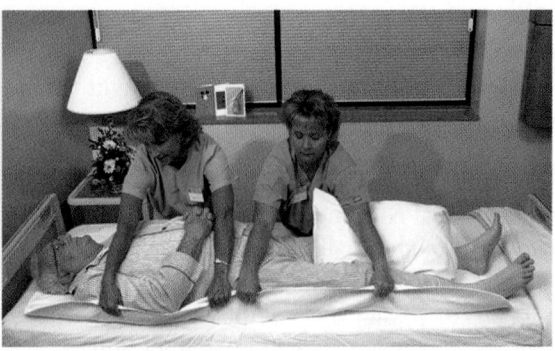

FIGURE 18-11 Logrolling. **A,** A pillow is between the person's legs. The arms are crossed on the chest. The person is on the far side of the bed. The person is turned as a unit. **B,** The assist device is used to logroll the person.

SITTING ON THE SIDE OF THE BED (DANGLING)

Patients and residents sit on the side of the bed *(dangle)* for many reasons. They may become dizzy or faint when getting out of bed too fast. They may need to sit on the side of the bed for 1 to 5 minutes before walking or transferring. Or activity may increase in stages—bedrest, to dangling, to sitting in a chair, and then to walking. This is common after surgery.

While dangling the legs, the person coughs and deep breathes. He or she moves the legs back and forth in circles. This stimulates circulation.

Two staff members may be needed. Persons with balance and coordination problems need support. If dizziness or fainting occurs, lay the person down. Tell the nurse at once.

See *Focus on Children and Older Persons: Dangling.*
See *Delegation Guidelines: Dangling.*
See *Promoting Safety and Comfort: Dangling.*
See procedure: *Sitting on the Side of the Bed (Dangling),* p. 278.

FOCUS ON CHILDREN AND OLDER PERSONS

Dangling

Older Persons
Older persons may have circulatory changes. They may become dizzy or faint when getting up too fast. Let them sit on the side of the bed for a few minutes before standing.

DELEGATION GUIDELINES

Dangling

The nurse may ask you to help a person sit on the side of the bed. The procedure is part of other tasks—assisting the person to stand, transferring from bed to chair, partial bath, and others. Before the dangling procedure, you need this information from the nurse and the care plan.

- Areas of weakness. For example, if the arms are weak, the person cannot hold on to the side of the mattress for support. If the left side is weak, turn the person onto the stronger right side. The person uses the right arm to help move from the lying to sitting position.
- The person's functional status (see Box 18-1).
- The amount of help the person needs.
- If you need a co-worker to help you.
- If the bed is raised or in a low position safe and comfortable for the person.
- How long the person needs to sit on the side of the bed.
- What exercises are to be done while dangling.
  - Range-of-motion exercises (Chapter 30)
  - Deep-breathing and coughing exercises (Chapter 39)
- If the person will walk or transfer to a chair after dangling. If yes, the bed is in a low position safe and comfortable for the person.
- What observations to report and record (Fig. 18-12):
  - Pulse and respiratory rates (Chapter 29)
  - Pale or bluish skin color *(cyanosis)*
  - Complaints of dizziness, light-headedness, or difficulty breathing
  - Who helped you with the procedure
  - How well the activity was tolerated
  - How long the person dangled
  - The amount of help needed
  - Other observations and complaints
- When to report observations.
- What patient or resident concerns to report at once.

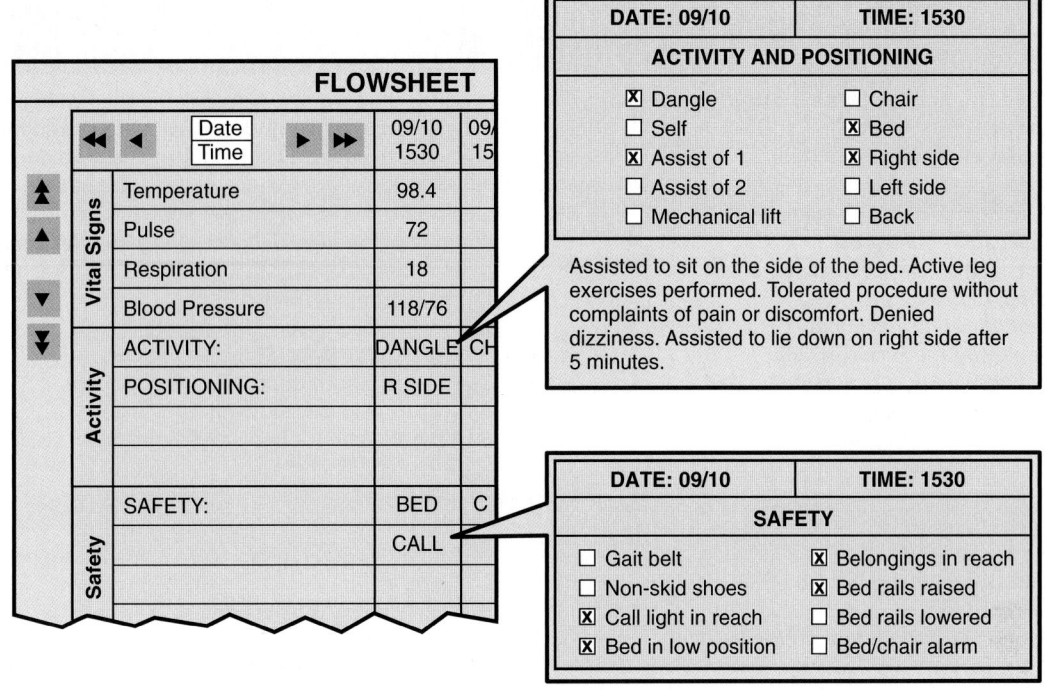

FIGURE 18-12 Charting sample—sitting on the side of the bed (dangling).

PROMOTING SAFETY AND COMFORT

Dangling

Safety

The procedure is not used for persons with:

- Level 3: Extensive Assistance
- Level 4: Total Dependence

  Sitting and balance problems can occur after illness, injury, surgery, and bedrest. Some disabilities affect sitting and balance. Support the person who is sitting on the side of the bed. Have a co-worker help you. This protects the person from falling and other injuries.

  As the person sits on the side of the bed, you check the person. Lay the person down and tell the nurse at once if the person:

- Is dizzy or light-headed.
- Has an abnormal pulse or respirations.
- Has difficulty breathing.
- Has pale or bluish skin.

Comfort

Provide for warmth during the dangling procedure. Help the person put on a robe. Or cover the person's shoulders and back with a bath blanket.

  The person may want to perform hygiene measures while sitting on the side of the bed. Oral hygiene and washing the face and hands are examples. These measures are refreshing and stimulate circulation. Follow the nurse's directions and the care plan.

Sitting on the Side of the Bed (Dangling)

QUALITY OF LIFE

- Knock before entering the person's room.
- Address the person by name.
- Introduce yourself by name and title.

- Explain the procedure before starting and during the procedure.
- Protect the person's rights during the procedure.
- Handle the person gently during the procedure.

PRE-PROCEDURE

1 Follow *Delegation Guidelines:*
  a *Preventing Work-Related Injuries,* p. 264
  b *Dangling,* p. 276
  See *Promoting Safety and Comfort:*
  a *Safely Moving the Person,* p. 263
  b *Preventing Work-Related Injuries,* p. 264
  c *Dangling,* p. 277
2 Ask a co-worker to help you.
3 Practice hand hygiene.

4 Identify the person. Check the ID bracelet against the assignment sheet. Use 2 identifiers (Chapter 13). Also call the person by name.
5 Provide for privacy.
6 Decide which side of the bed to use.
7 Move furniture to provide moving space.
8 Lock (brake) the bed wheels.
9 Raise the bed for body mechanics. Bed rails are up if used.

PROCEDURE

10 Lower the bed rail if up.
11 Position the person in a side-lying position facing you. The person lies on the strong side.
12 Raise the head of the bed to a sitting position.
13 Stand by the person's hips. Face the foot of the bed.
14 Stand with your feet apart. The foot near the head of the bed is in front of the other foot.
15 Slide 1 arm under the person's neck and shoulders. Grasp the far shoulder. Place your other hand over the thighs near the knees (Fig. 18-13, *A*).
16 Pivot toward the foot of the bed while moving the person's legs and feet over the side of the bed. As the legs go over the edge of the mattress, the trunk is upright (Fig. 18-13, *B*).
17 Ask the person to hold on to the edge of the mattress. This supports the person in the sitting position. If possible, raise a half-length bed rail (on the person's strong side) for the person to grasp. Have your co-worker support the person at all times.

18 Do not leave the person alone. Provide support at all times.
19 Check the person's condition.
  a Ask how the person feels. Ask if the person feels dizzy or light-headed.
  b Check the pulse and respirations.
  c Check for difficulty breathing.
  d Note if the skin is pale or bluish in color *(cyanosis).*
20 Reverse the procedure to return the person to bed. (Or prepare the person to walk or for a transfer to a chair or wheelchair. Lower the bed to a safe and comfortable level. The person's feet are flat on the floor. Support the person at all times.)
21 Lower the head of the bed after the person returns to bed. Help him or her move to the center of the bed.
22 Position the person in good alignment.

POST-PROCEDURE

23 Provide for comfort. (See the inside of the front cover.)
24 Place the call light and other needed items within reach.
25 Lower the bed to a safe and comfortable level appropriate for the person. Follow the care plan.
26 Raise or lower bed rails. Follow the care plan.
27 Return furniture to its proper place.

28 Unscreen the person.
29 Complete a safety check of the room. (See the inside of the front cover.)
30 Practice hand hygiene.
31 Report and record your observations.

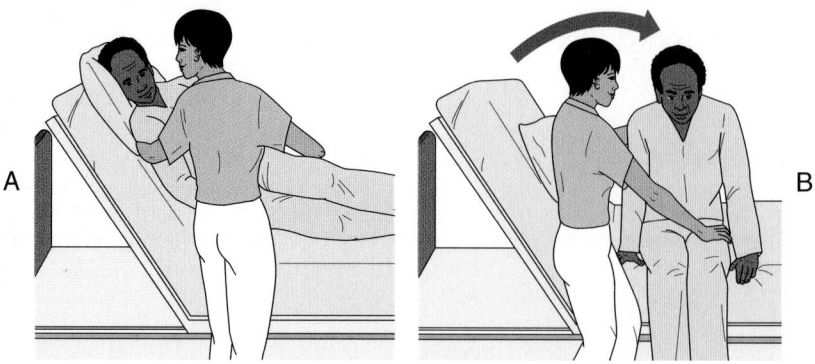

FIGURE 18-13 Helping the person sit on the side of the bed. **A,** The person's shoulders and thighs are supported. **B,** The person sits upright as the legs and feet are pulled over the edge of the bed.

RE-POSITIONING IN A CHAIR OR WHEELCHAIR

The person can slide down in a chair or wheelchair (Chapter 19). For good alignment and safety, the person's back and buttocks must be against the back of the chair.

Some persons can help with re-positioning. If the person cannot help, use a mechanical lift (Chapter 19). Follow the nurse's directions and the care plan for the best way to re-position a person in a chair or wheelchair. *Do not pull the person from behind the chair or wheelchair.*

If the person's chair reclines:
1. Ask a co-worker to help you.
2. Lock (brake) the wheels.
3. Recline the chair.
4. Position a friction-reducing device (drawsheet or slide sheet) under the person.
5. Use the device to move the person up. See procedure: *Moving the Person Up in Bed With an Assist Device*, p. 270.

Use this method if the person is alert and cooperative. The person must be able to follow directions. And the person must have the strength to help.
1. Lock (brake) the wheelchair wheels. Remove or swing front rigging out of the way. See Chapter 19 for wheelchair safety.
2. Position the person's feet flat on the floor.
3. Apply a transfer belt (Chapter 14).
4. Position the person's arms on the armrests.
5. Stand in front of the person. Block his or her knees and feet with your knees and feet.
6. Grasp the transfer belt on each side while the person leans forward.
7. Ask the person to push with his or her feet and arms on the "count of 3."
8. Move the person back into the chair on the "count of 3" as the person pushes with his or her feet and arms (Fig. 18-14).

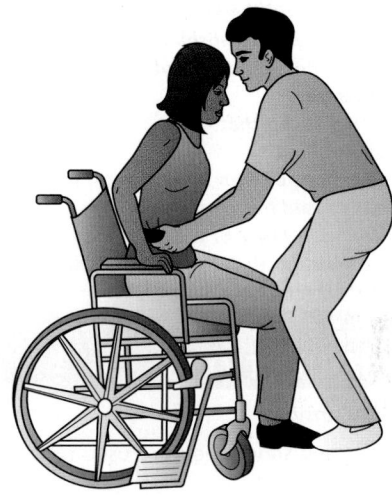

FIGURE 18-14 Re-positioning the person in a wheelchair. A transfer belt is used to move the person to the back of the chair.

Continued

FOCUS ON **P R I D E**—cont'd

The Person, Family, and Yourself

E thics and Laws

The following is a real example of a lawsuit filed against a hospital. The person accused the nurse of injuring her.

The patient had a history of shoulder injuries and surgeries. A nurse positioned the patient in a sitting position. The patient testified that she had immediate pain and heard a popping sound in her arm. The patient sued the hospital for a shoulder injury. In her lawsuit, the patient claimed that:
- *A large sign warned the staff not to touch her arms. The sign was posted by her husband.*
- *The nurse was negligent for not reading the sign and the patient's chart.*
   The hospital claimed that:
- *There was no sign.*
- *The nurse did not pull on the patient's arm.*
- *The patient caused her own injury.*
   The jury found in favor of the hospital.
   (T. Rosen v Verdugo Hills Hospital, California, 1999.)

In this case, the hospital did not have to pay damages (Chapter 5). But the lawsuit cost time, money, effort, and stress for all involved.

Always be careful. Follow delegation guidelines, the care plan, and the nurse's instructions. Also listen to the person. Ask the nurse if you are unsure how to safely move a person. Do not put yourself in a position where you may be at fault.

FOCUS ON **PRIDE**: *Application*

Most moving procedures require a team effort. How well do you work with others? What can you improve?

REVIEW QUESTIONS

Circle the BEST answer.

1 Drawsheets and slide sheets are used to
   a Remove shearing
   b Reduce friction
   c Promote independence
   d Improve posture

2 To protect the person's skin when moving in bed
   a Roll the person
   b Slide the person
   c Move the mattress
   d Use a transfer belt

3 A person is unable to turn and re-position without help. The person's functional status is
   a Independent
   b Limited Assistance
   c Total Dependence
   d Supervision

4 When moving persons in bed
   a The nurse tells you how to position the person
   b You decide which procedure to use
   c Bed rails are used at all times
   d 3 workers are needed for safety

5 To raise the person's head and shoulders
   a Pull on the person's shoulders
   b Ask for help if the person is older
   c Have the person pull on your shoulders
   d Use a slide sheet

6 As an assist device, a drawsheet is placed so that it
   a Covers the person's body
   b Extends from the mid-back to mid-thigh level
   c Is under the head to the above the knees
   d Covers the entire mattress

7 Mr. Lee needs to be moved up in bed. He is partially able to assist. You should
   a Stand by for safety but not assist
   b Move him up in bed by yourself
   c Tell him not to assist to avoid injury
   d Ask for help and get a friction-reducing device

8 Before turning a person onto his or her side, you
   a Move the person to the middle of the bed
   b Move the person to the side of the bed
   c Raise the head of the bed
   d Position pillows for comfort

9 A patient with a spinal cord injury is turned with
   a The logrolling procedure
   b A transfer belt
   c A mechanical lift
   d A pillow under the head and neck

10 To assist with dangling, you need to know
   a If a transfer belt is needed
   b Where to position pillows
   c If a mechanical lift is needed
   d Which side is stronger

11 To protect the person's rights during dangling
   a Leave the room as the person dangles
   b Perform the procedure alone
   c Ask the person what procedure to use
   d Close the privacy curtain

12 A person is able to help move. To re-position the person in a wheelchair
   a Pull the person from behind
   b Unlock the wheelchair wheels
   c Position the person's feet flat on the floor
   d Position the person's arms across the chest

Answers to Chapter 18 questions are on p. 871.

FOCUS ON PRACTICE

Problem Solving

Mr. Lazar has right-sided weakness. You need to help him sit up at the side of the bed (dangle). Which side of the bed should he sit on—right, left, or either? Why? As he dangles, his face turns pale and he says he is dizzy. What will you do?

Safely Transferring the Person

OBJECTIVES

- Define the key terms and key abbreviations in this chapter.
- Explain how to prevent work-related injuries during transfers.
- Identify the delegation information needed before transferring the person.
- Describe 5 functional status levels for transfers.

- Identify comfort and safety measures for transferring the person.
- Explain wheelchair and stretcher safety.
- Perform the procedures described in this chapter.
- Explain how to promote PRIDE in the person, the family, and yourself.

KEY TERMS

lateral transfer When a person moves between 2 horizontal surfaces

pivot To turn one's body from a set standing position

transfer How a person moves to and from surfaces—bed, chair, wheelchair, toilet, or standing position

KEY ABBREVIATIONS

ADL   Activities of daily living

ID   Identification

Patients and residents are moved to and from beds, chairs, wheelchairs, shower chairs, commodes, toilets, and stretchers. A *transfer is how a person moves to and from surfaces—bed, chair, wheelchair, toilet, or standing position.* The amount of help needed and the method used vary with the person's abilities. You will assist with transfers often.

The safety measures for preventing work-related injuries and for moving persons apply to transfers (Chapters 17 and 18). So do the rules for body mechanics (Chapter 17). Protect yourself and the person from injury. Use your body and transfer devices and equipment correctly.

See *Focus on Communication: Safely Transferring the Person.*

See *Teamwork and Time Management: Safely Transferring the Person,* p. 282.

See *Delegation Guidelines: Safely Transferring the Person,* p. 282.

See *Promoting Safety and Comfort: Safely Transferring the Person,* p. 282.

FOCUS ON COMMUNICATION

Safely Transferring the Person

Transfers can be painful for older persons and after an injury or surgery. Ask about the person's comfort. You can say:
- "Please tell me if you feel pain or discomfort."
- "Tell me to stop if you feel pain."

Before any transfer, explain the procedure. Tell the person what you and your co-workers will do. Also explain what the person needs to do. Give step-by-step instructions during the procedure.

The procedures in this chapter explain how to transfer the person on the "count of 3." You and the person or you and your co-workers move at the same time. For example:

I will help you transfer to the chair. I will count "1, 2, 3." When I say "3," push on the mattress with your hands and stand. I will steady you with the transfer belt as you stand. You will turn so your legs touch the seat's edge. Grab the chair's armrests. I will help you sit.

TEAMWORK AND TIME MANAGEMENT
Safely Transferring the Person

Some agencies have "lift teams." These teams perform most transfer procedures. They use assist equipment and do not manually lift patients and residents unless necessary.

The nurse advises the lift team of scheduled procedures. The team is called by beeper, pager, wireless phone, or other device for unscheduled transfers.

Do not assume that the lift team will transfer your assigned patients and residents. Follow agency policy for checking or adding to the lift team's schedule. Do not neglect or omit a procedure because the agency has a lift team. If the person is on the schedule, always check to make sure that the procedure was done. Unscheduled or unexpected events can cause delays. Thank the team for the work they do. Their work protects patients, residents, and you from injury.

DELEGATION GUIDELINES
Safely Transferring the Person

Many tasks involve transferring persons. Before doing so, you need this information from the nurse and the care plan.
- What procedure to use.
- The person's height and weight.
- The person's functional status (Box 19-1). *Functional status* is the person's ability to perform the activities of daily living (ADL) required to meet basic needs and required for health and well-being.
- The person's physical abilities. Can the person sit up, stand up, or walk without help? Does the person have strength in his or her arms and legs?

- If the person has a weak side. If yes, which side?
- If the person has problems that increase the risk of injury. Dizziness, confusion, hearing or vision problems, recent surgery, and fragile skin are examples.
- The person's ability to follow directions.
- If behavior problems are likely. Combative, agitated, uncooperative, and unpredictable behaviors are examples.
- The amount of assistance needed.
- The number of staff needed to complete the task safely.
- Any doctor's orders for transferring the person.
- What equipment to use.

PROMOTING SAFETY AND COMFORT
Safely Transferring the Person

Safety
Many older persons have fragile bones and joints. To prevent injuries:
- Follow the rules of body mechanics and the safety measures for preventing work-related injuries (Chapter 17).
- Always have help to transfer the person.
- Use transfer equipment and devices as directed by the nurse and the care plan.
- Transfer the person carefully.
- Keep the person in good alignment.

Decide how to transfer the person before starting the procedure. Ask needed staff to help before you begin. Arrange the room to allow enough space for a safe transfer. Correctly place the chair, wheelchair, or other device. Also plan how to protect drainage tubes or containers connected to the person.

Raise or lower the bed to a safe and comfortable level for the transfer. If the person will stand, the feet must be flat on the floor. For lateral transfers the bed is at a safe working height for staff.

Comfort
To promote mental comfort when transferring the person:
- Explain what you are going to do and how the person can help.
- Screen and cover the person to protect the right to privacy.
- Reassure the person that mechanical lifts (p. 295) are safe. To promote physical comfort:
- Keep the person in good alignment.
- Do not pull on any part of a person's body.
- Raise the head of the bed as soon as possible. Lying flat for long periods can cause discomfort and trouble breathing.
- Use pillows and other positioning devices as directed by the nurse and the care plan.

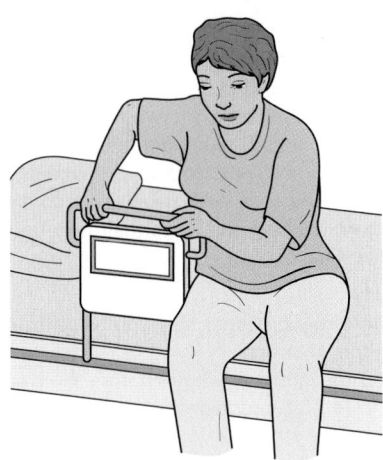

FIGURE 19-1 Stand-assist bed attachment.

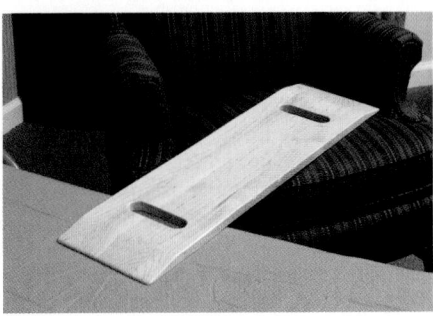

FIGURE 19-2 Sliding board for transfers to and from surfaces.

WHEELCHAIR AND STRETCHER SAFETY

Wheelchairs are useful for people who cannot walk or who have severe problems walking (Fig. 19-3). Wheelchairs are moved by:

- The person using the hand rims or his or her feet.
- The person using hand, chin, mouth, or other controls on a motorized wheelchair.
- Another person using the hand grips/push handles.

Stretchers are used to transport persons to other areas. They are used for persons who:

- Cannot sit up
- Must stay in a lying position
- Are seriously ill

The stretcher is covered with a folded flat sheet, fitted stretcher sheet, or bath blanket. A pillow and extra blankets are on hand. If the nurse allows, raise the head of the stretcher to a Fowler's or semi-Fowler's position (Chapter 17). This increases the person's comfort.

Follow the safety measures in Box 19-2 (p. 284) when using wheelchairs and stretchers. The person can fall from the wheelchair or stretcher. Or the person can fall during transfers to and from the wheelchair or stretcher.

Text continued on p. 286.

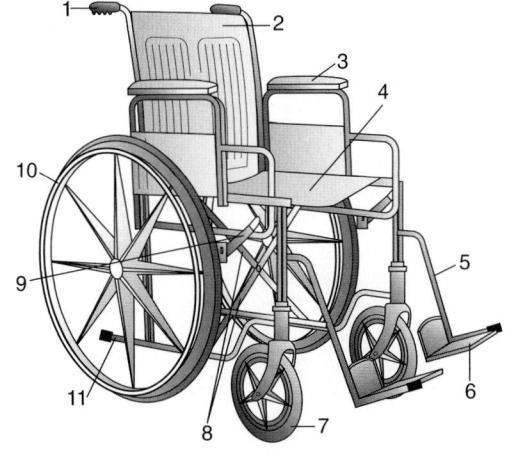

1 Hand grip/push handle
2 Back upholstery
3 Armrest
4 Seat upholstery
5 Front rigging
6 Footplate
7 Caster
8 Crossbrace
9 Wheel lock/brake
10 Wheel and hand rim
11 Tipping lever

FIGURE 19-3 Parts of a wheelchair.

BOX 19-2	Wheelchair and Stretcher Safety

Wheelchair Safety

Maintenance
- Check the wheel locks (brakes). Make sure you can lock and unlock them.
- Check for flat or loose tires. A wheel lock will not work on a flat or loose tire.
- Make sure wheel spokes are intact. Damaged, broken, or loose spokes can interfere with moving the wheelchair or locking the wheels.
- Make sure the casters point forward. This keeps the wheelchair balanced and stable.
- Clean the wheelchair according to agency policy.
- Follow the safety measures to prevent equipment accidents (Chapter 13).

Transfers
- Lock (brake) both wheels before you transfer a person to or from the wheelchair.
- Remove the armrests (if removable) when the person transfers to the bed, toilet, commode, tub, or car.
- Swing front rigging out of the way for transfers to and from the wheelchair. Some front riggings detach for transfers.
- Position the person's feet on the footplates. Make sure feet are on the footplates before moving the chair. The person's feet must not touch or drag on the floor when the chair is moving.
- Do not let the person stand on the footplates.
- Do not let the footplates fall back onto the person's legs.
- Provide needed wheelchair accessories—safety belt, pouch, tray, lap-board, cushion.

Transport
- Use good body mechanics (Chapter 17).
- Push the chair forward when transporting the person. Do not pull the chair backward unless going through a doorway or down a steep ramp or incline.
- Follow the care plan and agency policy for the number of staff needed to transport the person. This depends on:
  - The person's weight
  - If the person is cooperative
  - If the wheelchair is motorized

Wheelchair Safety—cont'd

Transport—cont'd
- Move wheelchairs up and down ramps and curbs safely (Figs. 19-4 and 19-5).
  - Going up a ramp: push the wheelchair front-first.
  - Going down a ramp: face the back of the wheelchair. Roll it backward looking behind you as you move the wheelchair.
  - Going up a curb:
    - Position the wheelchair so the front casters are at the curb.
    - Tilt the wheelchair back so the front casters are above the curb.
    - Push the wheelchair forward until you can set the wheelchair down over the curb.
    - Push the rear wheels up over the curb.
  - Going down a curb:
    - Turn the wheelchair so the rear wheels are at the curb.
    - Lower the rear wheels down the curb.
    - Lower the front casters down the curb.
- Follow the care plan for keeping the wheels locked when not moving the wheelchair. Locking the wheels prevents the chair from moving if the person wants to move to or from the chair. (Locking the wheelchair may be viewed as a restraint. See Chapter 15.)

Stretcher Safety
- Ask 2 or more co-workers to help you transfer the person to or from the stretcher.
- Lock (brake) the stretcher wheels before the transfer.
- Fasten the safety straps when the person is properly positioned on the stretcher.
- Follow the care plan and agency policy for the number of staff needed to transport the person. As many as 4 staff members may be needed. This depends on:
  - The person's weight
  - If the person is cooperative
- Raise the side rails. Keep them up during the transport.
- Do not leave the person alone.
- Make sure the person's arms, hands, legs, and feet do not dangle through the side rail bars.
- Stand at the head of the stretcher. Your co-worker stands at the foot of the stretcher.
- Move the stretcher feet first (Fig. 19-6, p. 286). This is so the staff member at the head of the stretcher can watch the person's breathing and color during the transport.
- Use good body mechanics during the transfer and transport (Chapter 17).
- Follow the safety measures to prevent equipment accidents (Chapter 13).

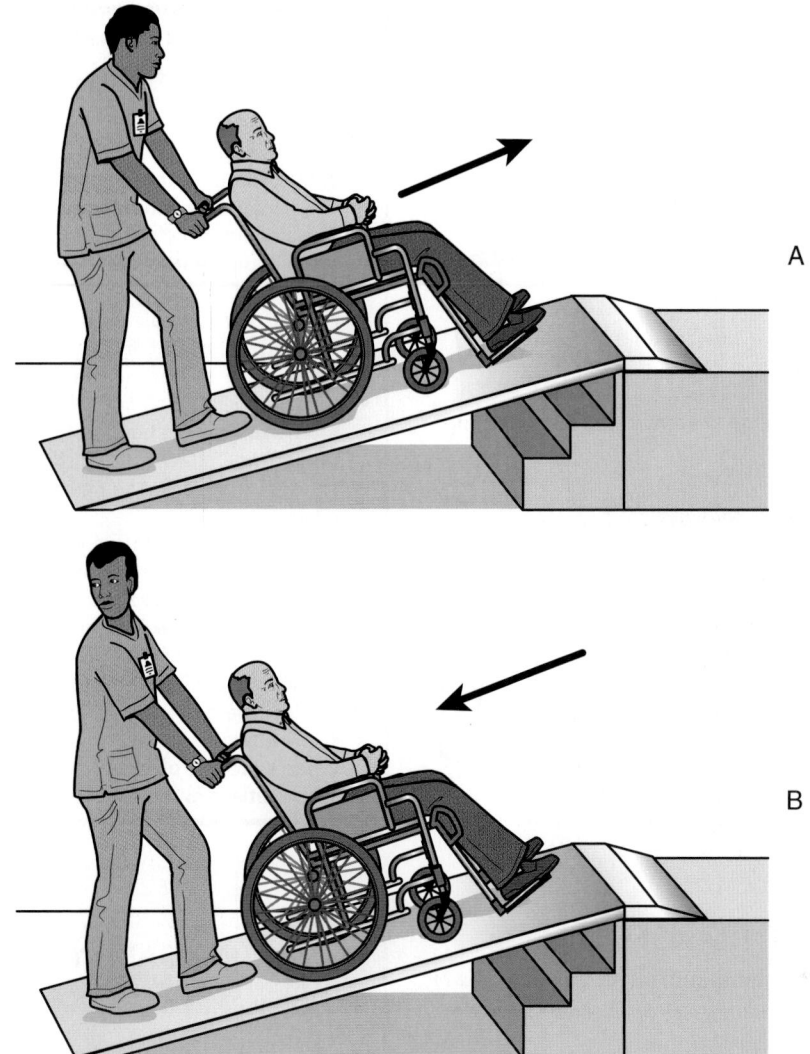

FIGURE 19-4 A, Moving a wheelchair up a ramp. **B,** Moving a wheelchair down a ramp.

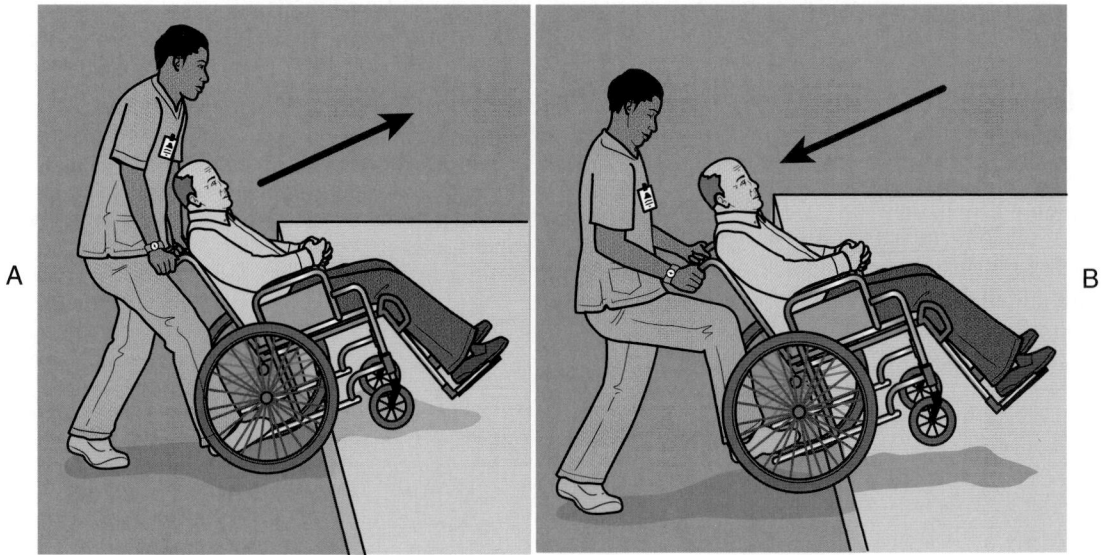

FIGURE 19-5 A, Moving a wheelchair up a curb. **B,** Moving a wheelchair down a curb.

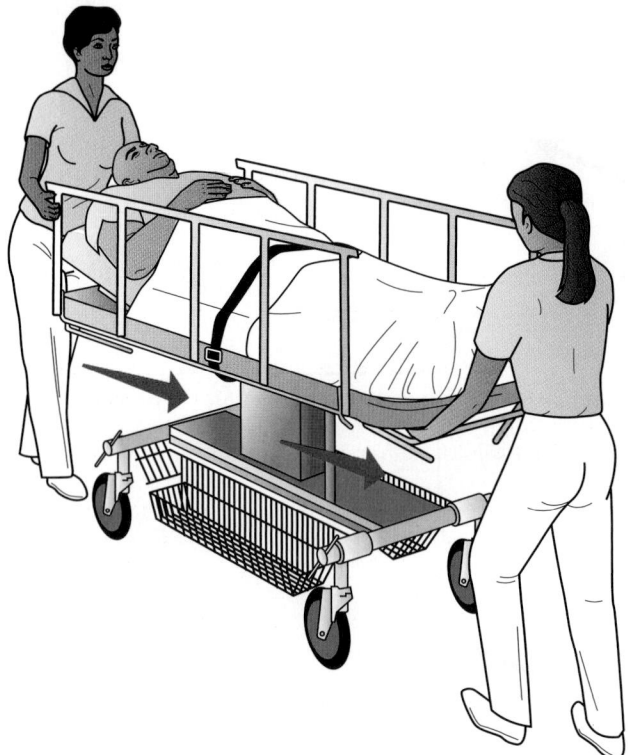

FIGURE 19-6 The stretcher is moved feet first.

STAND AND PIVOT TRANSFERS

Some persons are able to stand and pivot. *Pivot means to turn one's body from a set standing position.* A stand and pivot transfer is used if:

- The person's legs are strong enough to bear some or all of his or her weight.
- The person is cooperative and can follow directions.
- The person can assist with the transfer.
  See *Delegation Guidelines: Stand and Pivot Transfers.*
  See *Promoting Safety and Comfort: Stand and Pivot Transfers.*

Transfer Belts

Transfer belts (gait belts) are discussed in Chapter 14. They are used to:

- Support patients and residents during transfers.
- Re-position persons in chairs and wheelchairs (Chapter 18).
- Assist with ambulation (Chapter 30).
  Wider belts have padded handles. They are easier to grip and allow better control should the person fall.

DELEGATION GUIDELINES
Stand and Pivot Transfers

Before a transfer, you need this information from the nurse and the care plan.

- What procedure to use.
- The person's functional status (see Box 19-1).
- The amount of help the person needs.
- What equipment to use—transfer belt, wheelchair, stand-assist device, positioning devices, wheelchair cushion, bed or chair alarm, and so on.
- The person's height and weight.
- The number of staff needed.
- Areas of weakness. For example, if the arms are weak, the person cannot hold on to the mattress for support. If the left side is weak, he or she gets out of bed on the stronger right side. The person uses the right arm to help move.
- What observations to report and record:
  - Pulse rate before and after the transfer (Chapter 29)
  - Complaints of dizziness, pain, discomfort, difficulty breathing, weakness, or fatigue
  - The amount of help needed to transfer the person
  - Who helped you with the procedure
  - How the person helped with the procedure
  - How you positioned the person
- When to report observations.
- What patient or resident concerns to report at once.

PROMOTING SAFETY AND COMFORT
Stand and Pivot Transfers

Safety

The person wears non-skid footwear for stand and pivot transfers. Such footwear protects the person from falls. Slipping and sliding are prevented. Tie shoelaces securely. Otherwise the person can trip and fall.

Long gowns and robes can cause falls. Avoid robes with long ties. The person can trip and fall.

Lock (brake) bed and wheelchair wheels and wheels on other devices. This prevents the bed and the device from moving during the transfer. Otherwise, the person can fall. You also are at risk for injury.

Comfort

After the transfer, position the person in good alignment. Place the call light and other needed items within reach.

■ Bed to Chair or Wheelchair Transfers

Safety is important for chair, wheelchair, commode, and shower chair transfers. Help the person out of bed on his or her strong side. If the left side is weak and the right side is strong, get the person out of bed on the right side. In transferring, the strong side moves first. It pulls the weaker side along. Transfers from the weak side are awkward and unsafe.

See *Focus on Surveys: Bed to Chair or Wheelchair Transfers.*

See *Promoting Safety and Comfort: Bed to Chair or Wheelchair Transfers.*

See procedure: *Transferring the Person to a Chair or Wheelchair.*

Text continued on p. 290.

FOCUS ON **SURVEYS**

Bed to Chair or Wheelchair Transfers

Agencies must ensure that nursing assistants can safely perform the skills needed for safe care. Surveyors will observe how nursing assistants function. One skill in their focus is transferring a person from the bed to a wheelchair.

PROMOTING SAFETY AND COMFORT

Bed to Chair or Wheelchair Transfers

Safety

The chair, wheelchair, or other device must support the person's weight. The number of staff needed depends on the person's abilities, condition, and size. Sometimes you need a mechanical lift (p. 295).

The person must not put his or her arms around your neck. Otherwise the person can pull you forward or cause you to lose your balance. Neck, back, and other injuries are possible.

If not using a mechanical lift, a transfer belt is used for chair or wheelchair transfers. It is safer for the person and you. Putting your arms around the person and grasping the shoulder blades is another method. It can cause the person discomfort. And it can be stressful for you. Use this method only if instructed to do so by the nurse and the care plan.

Bed and wheelchair wheels are locked for a safe transfer. After the transfer, unlock the wheelchair wheels to position the chair as the person prefers. After positioning the chair, lock the wheels or keep them unlocked according to the care plan. Locked wheels may be viewed as restraints if the person cannot unlock them to move the wheelchair (Chapter 15). However, falls and other injuries are risks if the person tries to stand when the wheels are unlocked.

Comfort

Most wheelchairs and bedside chairs have vinyl seats and backs. Vinyl holds body heat. The person becomes warm and perspires more. If the nurse allows, cover the back and seat with a folded bath blanket. This increases the person's comfort.

Some people have wheelchair cushions or positioning devices. Ask the nurse how to use and place the devices. Also follow the manufacturer's instructions.

Transferring the Person to a Chair or Wheelchair

QUALITY OF LIFE

- Knock before entering the person's room.
- Address the person by name.
- Introduce yourself by name and title.

- Explain the procedure before starting and during the procedure.
- Protect the person's rights during the procedure.
- Handle the person gently during the procedure.

PRE-PROCEDURE

1 Follow *Delegation Guidelines:*
  a *Safely Transferring the Person,* p. 282
  b *Stand and Pivot Transfers*
  See *Promoting Safety and Comfort:*
  a *Transfer/Gait Belts,* Chapter 14
  b *Safely Transferring the Person,* p. 282
  c *Stand and Pivot Transfers*
  d *Bed to Chair or Wheelchair Transfers*
2 Collect the following.
  • Wheelchair or arm chair
  • Bath blanket
  • Lap blanket (if used)

  • Robe and non-skid footwear
  • Paper or sheet
  • Transfer belt (if needed)
  • Seat cushion (if needed)
3 Practice hand hygiene.
4 Identify the person. Check the identification (ID) bracelet against the assignment sheet. Use 2 identifiers (Chapter 13). Also call the person by name.
5 Provide for privacy.
6 Decide which side of the bed to use. Move furniture for a safe transfer.

Continued

Transferring the Person to a Chair or Wheelchair—cont'd

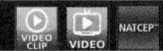

PROCEDURE

7 Raise the wheelchair footplates. Remove or swing front rigging out of the way if possible. Position the chair or wheelchair near the bed on the person's strong side.
 a If at the head of the bed, it faces the foot of the bed.
 b If at the foot of the bed, it faces the head of the bed.
 c The armrest almost touches the bed.
8 Place a folded bath blanket or cushion on the seat (if needed).
9 Lock (brake) the wheelchair wheels.
10 Fan-fold top linens to the foot of the bed.
11 Place the paper or sheet under the person's feet. (This protects linens from footwear.) Put footwear on the person.
12 Lower the bed to a safe and comfortable level for the person. Follow the care plan. Lock (brake) the bed wheels.
13 Help the person sit on the side of the bed (Chapter 18). His or her feet must be flat on the floor.
14 Help the person put on a robe.
15 Apply the transfer belt if needed (Chapter 14). It is applied at the waist over clothing.
16 *Method 1: Using a transfer belt:*
 a Stand in front of the person.
 b Have the person hold on to the mattress.
 c Make sure the person's feet are flat on the floor.
 d Have the person lean forward.
 e Grasp the transfer belt at each side. Grasp the handles or grasp the belt from underneath. See Chapter 14.
 f Prevent the person from sliding or falling. Do 1 of the following.
  1) Brace your knees against the person's knees (Fig. 19-7). Block his or her feet with your feet.
  2) Use the knee and foot of 1 leg to block the person's weak leg or foot. Place your other foot slightly behind you for balance.
  3) Straddle your legs around the person's weak leg.
 g Explain the following.
  1) You will count "1, 2, 3."
  2) The move will be on "3."
  3) On "3," the person pushes down on the mattress and stands.
 h Ask the person to push down on the mattress and to stand on the "count of 3." Assist the person to a standing position as you straighten your knees (Fig. 19-8).

17 *Method 2: No transfer belt:* (NOTE: Use this method only if directed by the nurse and the care plan.)
 a Follow steps 16, a–c.
 b Place your hands under the person's arms. Your hands are around the person's shoulder blades (Fig. 19-9).
 c Have the person lean forward.
 d Prevent the person from sliding or falling. Do 1 of the following.
  1) Brace your knees against the person's knees. Block his or her feet with your feet.
  2) Use the knee and foot of 1 leg to block the person's weak leg or foot. Place your other foot slightly behind you for balance.
  3) Straddle your legs around the person's weak leg.
 e Explain the "count of 3." See step 16, g.
 f Ask the person to push down on the mattress and to stand on the "count of 3." Assist the person to a standing position as you straighten your knees.
18 Support the person in the standing position. Hold the transfer belt or keep your hands around the person's shoulder blades. Continue to prevent the person from sliding or falling.
19 Help the person pivot (turn) so he or she can grasp the far arm of the chair or wheelchair. The legs will touch the edge of the seat (Fig. 19-10).
20 Continue to help the person pivot (turn) until the other armrest is grasped.
21 Lower him or her into the chair or wheelchair as you bend your hips and knees. To assist, the person leans forward and bends the elbows and knees (Fig. 19-11).
22 Make sure the hips are to the back of the seat. Position the person in good alignment.
23 Attach the wheelchair front rigging. Position the person's feet on the footplates.
24 Cover the person's lap and legs with a lap blanket (if used). Keep the blanket off the floor and the wheels.
25 Remove the transfer belt if used.
26 Position the chair as the person prefers. Lock (brake) the wheelchair wheels according to the care plan.

POST-PROCEDURE

27 Provide for comfort. (See the inside of the front cover.)
28 Place the call light and other needed items within reach.
29 Unscreen the person.
30 Complete a safety check of the room. (See the inside of the front cover.)
31 Practice hand hygiene.
32 Report and record your observations.
33 See procedure: *Transferring the Person From a Chair or Wheelchair to Bed* (p. 290) to return the person to bed.

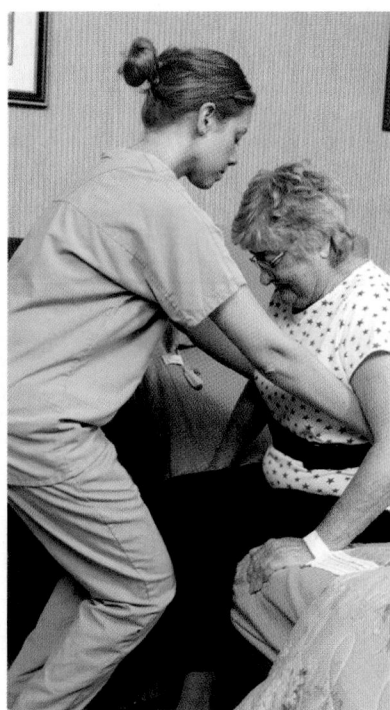

FIGURE 19-7 The person's knees are blocked by the nursing assistant's knees.

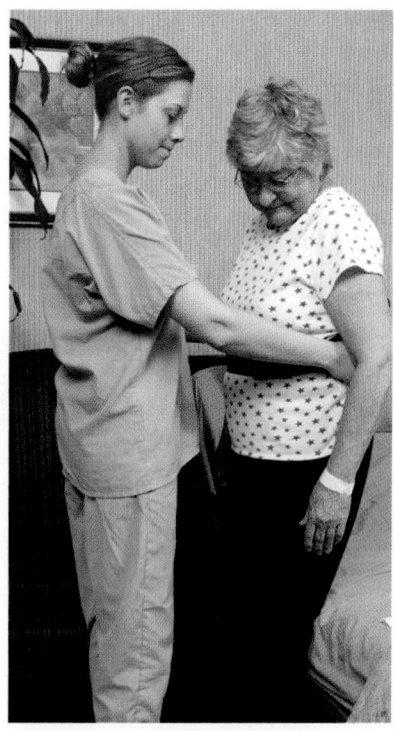

FIGURE 19-8 The person is assisted to a standing position and supported by holding the transfer belt.

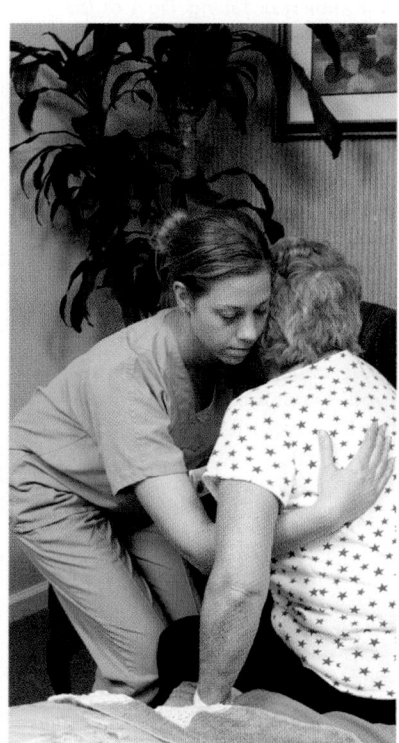

FIGURE 19-9 The person is being prepared to stand. The hands are placed under the person's arms and around the shoulder blades.

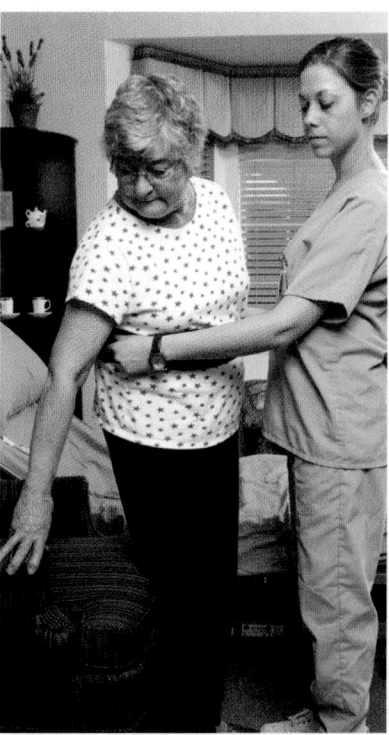

FIGURE 19-10 The person is supported as he or she grasps the far arm of the chair. The legs are against the chair.

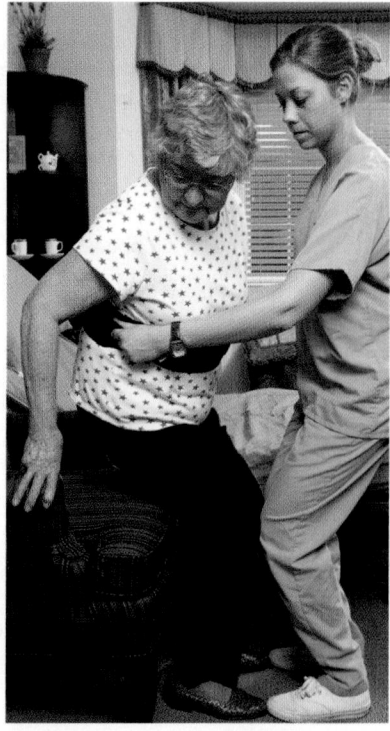

FIGURE 19-11 The person holds the armrests, leans forward, and bends the elbows and knees while being lowered into the chair.

Chair or Wheelchair to Bed Transfers

Chair or wheelchair to bed transfers have the same rules as bed to chair transfers. If the person is weak on 1 side, transfer the person so that the strong side moves first. Or position the chair or wheelchair so the person's strong side is near the bed. The strong side moves first.

For example, Mrs. Lee's right side is weak. Her left side is strong. For a bed to chair transfer, the chair was on the left side of the bed. Her left side (strong side) moved first.

Now you will transfer Mrs. Lee back to bed. With the chair on the left side of the bed, her weak right side is near the bed. Moving the weak side first is not safe. Move the chair to the other side of the bed or turn the chair around. Mrs. Lee's stronger left side will be near the bed. The stronger side moves first for a safe transfer.

See procedure: *Transferring the Person From a Chair or Wheelchair to Bed.*

Transferring the Person From a Chair or Wheelchair to Bed   NATCEP

QUALITY OF LIFE

- Knock before entering the person's room.
- Address the person by name.
- Introduce yourself by name and title.

- Explain the procedure before starting and during the procedure.
- Protect the person's rights during the procedure.
- Handle the person gently during the procedure.

PRE-PROCEDURE

1 Follow *Delegation Guidelines:*
   a *Safely Transferring the Person,* p. 282
   b *Stand and Pivot Transfers,* p. 286
   See *Promoting Safety and Comfort:*
   a *Transfer/Gait Belts* (Chapter 14)
   b *Safely Transferring the Person,* p. 282
   c *Stand and Pivot Transfers,* p. 286
   d *Bed to Chair or Wheelchair Transfers,* p. 287

2 Collect a transfer belt if needed.
3 Practice hand hygiene.
4 Identify the person. Check the ID bracelet against the assignment sheet. Use 2 identifiers (Chapter 13). Also call the person by name.
5 Provide for privacy.

PROCEDURE

6 Move furniture for moving space.
7 Raise the head of the bed to a sitting position. Lower the bed to a safe and comfortable level for the person. Follow the care plan. When the person transfers to the bed, his or her feet must be flat on the floor when sitting on the side of the bed.
8 Move the call light so it is on the strong side when the person is in bed.
9 Position the chair or wheelchair so the person's strong side is next to the bed (Fig. 19-12). Have a co-worker help you if necessary.
10 Lock (brake) the wheelchair and bed wheels.
11 Remove and fold the lap blanket.
12 Remove the person's feet from the footplates. Raise the footplates. Remove or swing front rigging out of the way. Put non-skid footwear on the person if needed.
13 Apply the transfer belt if needed.
14 Make sure the person's feet are flat on the floor.
15 Stand in front of the person.
16 Have the person hold on to the armrests. (If the nurse directs you to do so, place your arms under the person's arms. Your hands are around the shoulder blades.)
17 Have the person lean forward.
18 Grasp the transfer belt on each side if using it. Grasp underneath the belt.

19 Prevent the person from sliding or falling. Do 1 of the following.
   a Brace your knees against the person's knees. Block his or her feet with your feet.
   b Use the knee and foot of 1 leg to block the person's weak leg or foot. Place your other foot slightly behind you for balance.
   c Straddle your legs around the person's weak leg.
20 Explain the "count of 3." (See procedure: *Transferring the Person to a Chair or Wheelchair,* p. 287.)
21 Ask the person to push down on the armrests on the "count of 3." Assist the person into a standing position as you straighten your knees.
22 Support the person in the standing position. Hold the transfer belt or keep your hands around the person's shoulder blades. Continue to prevent the person from sliding or falling.
23 Help the person pivot (turn) so he or she can reach the edge of the mattress. The legs will touch the mattress.
24 Continue to help the person pivot (turn) until he or she can reach the mattress with both hands.
25 Lower him or her onto the bed as you bend your hips and knees. To assist, the person leans forward and bends the elbows and knees.
26 Remove the transfer belt.
27 Remove the robe and footwear.
28 Help the person lie down.

POST-PROCEDURE

29 Provide for comfort. (See the inside of the front cover.)
30 Place the call light and other needed items within reach.
31 Raise or lower bed rails. Follow the care plan.
32 Arrange furniture text meet the person's needs.
33 Unscreen the person.

34 Complete a safety check of the room. (See the inside of the front cover.)
35 Practice hand hygiene.
36 Report and record your observations.

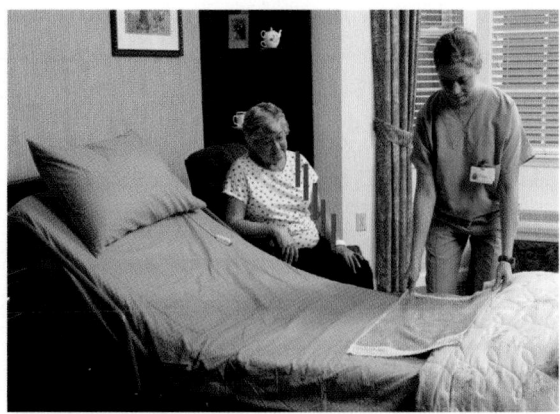

FIGURE 19-12 The chair is positioned so the person's strong side is near the bed. (*Note: The "weak" side is indicated by slash marks.*)

PROMOTING SAFETY AND COMFORT
Transferring the Person To and From the Toilet

Safety

Make sure the person has a raised toilet seat. The toilet seat and wheelchair are at the same level.

A standard toilet has a weight limit of 350 pounds. For persons with bariatric needs:
- Do not have the person use a wall-mounted toilet. A steel, floor-mounted toilet is best.
- Obtain a bariatric commode (Chapter 24) if the person's room does not have a floor-mounted toilet.

Check the grab bars by the toilet. If loose, tell the nurse. Do not transfer the person to the toilet if grab bars are not secure.

Follow Standard Precautions and the Bloodborne Pathogen Standard. Wear gloves if the person is incontinent of urine or feces.

Transferring the Person To and From the Toilet

Using the bathroom for elimination promotes dignity, self-esteem, and independence. It also is more private than using a bedpan, urinal, or bedside commode. However, getting to the toilet is hard for persons who use wheelchairs. Bathrooms are often small. There is little room for you or a wheelchair. Therefore transfers with wheelchairs and toilets are often hard. Falls and work-related injuries are risks.

Sometimes mechanical lifts are used for toilet transfers. A sliding board (see Fig. 19-2) may be used if:
- The wheelchair armrests can be removed.
- The person has upper body strength.
- The person has good sitting balance.
- There is enough room to position the wheelchair next to the toilet.

The procedure on this page can be used if the person can stand and pivot from the wheelchair to the toilet.

See *Promoting Safety and Comfort: Transferring the Person To and From the Toilet.*

See procedure: *Transferring the Person To and From the Toilet.*

Transferring the Person To and From the Toilet

QUALITY OF LIFE

- Knock before entering the person's room.
- Address the person by name.
- Introduce yourself by name and title.

- Explain the procedure before starting and during the procedure.
- Protect the person's rights during the procedure.
- Handle the person gently during the procedure.

PRE-PROCEDURE

1 Follow *Delegation Guidelines:*
   a *Safely Transferring the Person,* p. 282
   b *Stand and Pivot Transfers,* p. 286
   See *Promoting Safety and Comfort:*
   a *Transfer/Gait Belts* (Chapter 14)
   b *Safely Transferring the Person,* p. 282
   c *Stand and Pivot Transfers,* p. 286
   d *Bed to Chair or Wheelchair Transfers,* p. 287
   e *Transferring the Person To and From the Toilet*

2 Practice hand hygiene.

Continued

Transferring the Person To and From the Toilet—cont'd

PROCEDURE

3 Put non-skid footwear on the person.
4 Position the wheelchair next to the toilet if there is enough room (Fig. 19-13, *A*). If not, position the chair at a right angle (90-degree angle) to the toilet (Fig. 19-13, *B*). It is best if the person's strong side is near the toilet.
5 Lock (brake) the wheelchair wheels.
6 Raise the footplates. Remove or swing front rigging out of the way.
7 Apply the transfer belt.
8 Help the person unfasten clothing.
9 Use the transfer belt to help the person stand and to pivot (turn) to the toilet. (See procedure: *Transferring the Person to a Chair or Wheelchair*, p. 287.) The person uses the grab bars to pivot (turn) to the toilet.
10 Support the person with the transfer belt while he or she lowers clothing. Or have the person hold on to the grab bars for support. Lower the person's clothing.
11 Use the transfer belt to lower the person onto the toilet seat. Check for proper positioning on the toilet.
12 Remove the transfer belt.
13 Tell the person you will stay nearby. Remind the person to use the call light or call for you when help is needed. Stay with the person if required by the care plan.

14 Close the bathroom door for privacy.
15 Stay near the bathroom. Complete other tasks in the person's room. Check on the person every 5 minutes.
16 Knock on the bathroom door when the person calls for you.
17 Help with wiping, perineal care (Chapter 22), flushing, and hand-washing as needed. Wear gloves and practice hand hygiene after removing the gloves.
18 Apply the transfer belt.
19 Use the transfer belt to help the person stand.
20 Help the person raise and secure clothing.
21 Use the transfer belt to transfer the person to the wheelchair. (See procedure: *Transferring the Person to a Chair or Wheelchair*, p. 287.)
22 Make sure the person's buttocks are to the back of the seat. Position the person in good alignment.
23 Position the person's feet on the footplates.
24 Remove the transfer belt.
25 Cover the person's lap and legs with a lap blanket. Keep the blanket off the floor and wheels.
26 Position the chair as the person prefers. Lock (brake) the wheelchair wheels according to the care plan.

POST-PROCEDURE

27 Provide for comfort. (See the inside of the front cover.)
28 Place the call light and other needed items within reach.
29 Unscreen the person.

30 Complete a safety check of the room. (See the inside of the front cover.)
31 Practice hand hygiene.
32 Report and record your observations.

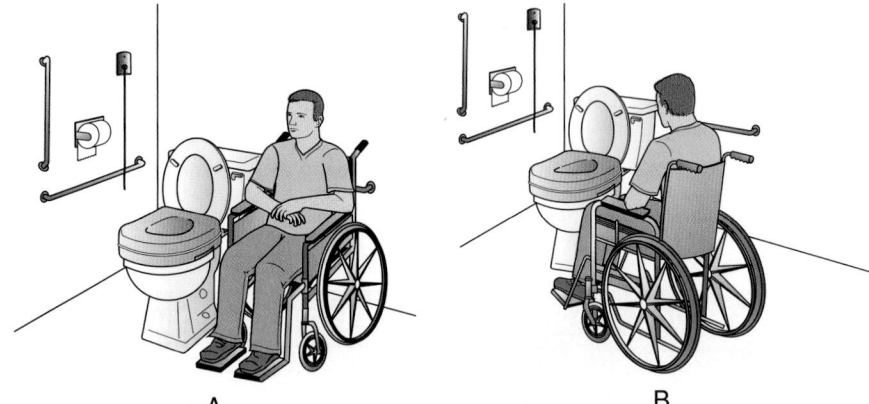

FIGURE 19-13 Wheelchair positions for a transfer to the toilet. **A,** The wheelchair is next to the toilet. **B,** The wheelchair is placed at a right angle (90-degree angle) to the toilet.

A   B

LATERAL TRANSFERS

A *lateral transfer moves a person between 2 horizontal surfaces.* The person slides from 1 surface to the other. A transfer from a bed to a stretcher is an example. A transfer from bed to a shower trolley (Chapter 22) is another example.

Protecting the Skin

Friction and shearing injure the skin (Chapter 18). Infection and pressure ulcers can result (Chapter 37).

Friction-reducing devices protect the skin from friction and shearing during lateral transfers. They also protect staff from injury. Devices include:
• Lift sheet, turning sheet, or drawsheet (Chapters 18 and 21)
• Turning pad (Chapter 18)
• Large re-usable waterproof under-pad (Chapter 21)
• Slide sheet (Fig. 19-14)
• Lateral transfer device with a slide board (Fig. 19-15)

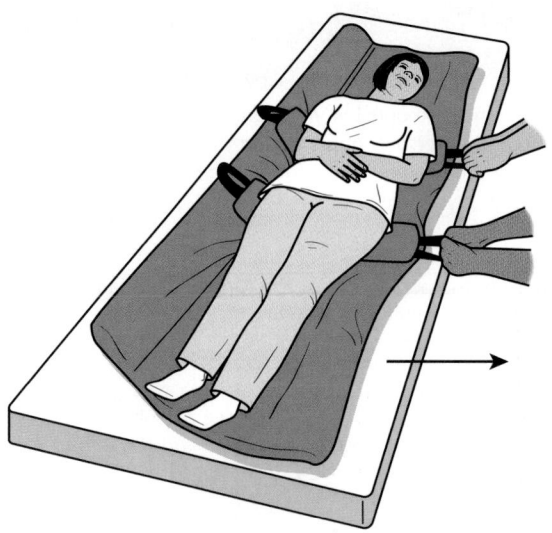

FIGURE **19-14** Slide sheet.

FIGURE **19-15** Lateral transfer device with slide board.

DELEGATION GUIDELINES

Moving the Person to a Stretcher

Before a transfer to a stretcher, you need this information from the nurse and the care plan.
- The amount of help the person needs
- What friction-reducing device to use—drawsheet (lift sheet, turning sheet), turning pad, large re-usable waterproof under-pad, slide sheet, lateral transfer device with a slide board or other device
- The person's height and weight
- The number of staff needed to complete the task safely
- What observations to report and record:
  - Complaints of light-headedness, pain, discomfort, difficulty breathing, weakness, or fatigue
  - The amount of help needed to transfer the person
  - Who helped you with the procedure
  - How you positioned the person
- When to report observations
- What patient or resident concerns to report at once

PROMOTING SAFETY AND COMFORT

Moving the Person to a Stretcher

Safety

Protect yourself and the person from injury.
- Make sure you know how to use the device. Follow the manufacturer's instructions.
- Position the stretcher and bed surfaces as close as possible to each other.
- Avoid extended reaches and bending your back. You may need to kneel on the bed or stretcher.
- Follow the rules for stretcher safety (see Box 19-2).
- Make sure the bed and stretcher wheels are locked (braked).
- Practice good body mechanics and follow the guidelines for preventing work-related injuries (Chapter 17).
- Keep the person in good alignment.
- Make sure you have enough help.
- Hold the person securely. You must not drop the person.

▪ Moving the Person to a Stretcher

A friction-reducing device is used for transfers to and from stretchers. At least 2 or 3 staff are needed for a safe transfer.
- *If the person weighs less than 200 pounds*—a friction-reducing device or lateral transfer device with a slide board is used.
- *If the person weighs more than 200 pounds*—a mechanical ceiling lift, a mechanical lateral transfer device, or other devices as directed. At least 3 staff members are needed.

For persons with bariatric needs, the nurse and care plan may direct staff to:
- Use a bariatric stretcher. Check for an "EC" (expanded capacity) sticker and the weight limit.
- Raise or lower the stretcher so that it is ½ inch lower than the bed.
- Use a friction-reducing device or a mechanical lateral transfer device.
- Transfer the person from his or her strong side.
- Apply an abdominal binder if the person's abdomen is in the way. See Chapter 36.

See *Delegation Guidelines: Moving the Person to a Stretcher.*

See *Promoting Safety and Comfort: Moving the Person to a Stretcher.*

See procedure: *Moving the Person to a Stretcher,* p. 294.

Moving the Person to a Stretcher

QUALITY OF LIFE

- Knock before entering the person's room.
- Address the person by name.
- Introduce yourself by name and title.

- Explain the procedure before starting and during the procedure.
- Protect the person's rights during the procedure.
- Handle the person gently during the procedure.

PRE-PROCEDURE

1 Follow *Delegation Guidelines:*
  a *Safely Transferring the Person,* p. 282
  b *Moving the Person to a Stretcher,* p. 293
  See *Promoting Safety and Comfort:*
  a *Safely Transferring the Person,* p. 282
  b *Moving the Person to a Stretcher,* p. 293
2 Ask 1 or 2 staff members to help you.
3 Collect the following.
  - Stretcher covered with a sheet or bath blanket
  - Bath blanket
  - Pillow(s) if needed
  - Slide sheet, lateral transfer device with slide board, drawsheet, or other assist device

4 Practice hand hygiene.
5 Identify the person. Check the ID bracelet against the assignment sheet. Use 2 identifiers (Chapter 13). Also call the person by name.
6 Provide for privacy.
7 Raise the bed and stretcher for body mechanics.

PROCEDURE

8 Position yourself and co-workers.
  a 1 or 2 workers stand on the side of the bed where the stretcher will be.
  b 1 worker stands on the other side of the bed.
9 Lower the head of the bed. It is as flat as possible.
10 Lower the bed rails if used.
11 Cover the person with a bath blanket. Fan-fold top linens to the foot of the bed.
12 Position the assist device. Or loosen the drawsheet on each side.
13 Use the assist device to move the person to the side of the bed. This is the side where the stretcher will be.
14 Protect the person from falling. Hold the far arm and leg.

15 Have your co-workers position the stretcher next to the bed. They stand behind the stretcher (Fig. 19-16, *A*).
16 Lock (brake) the bed and stretcher wheels.
17 Grasp the assist device (Fig. 19-16, *B*).
18 Transfer the person to the stretcher on the "count of 3." Center the person on the stretcher.
19 Place a pillow or pillows under the person's head and shoulders if allowed. Raise the head of the stretcher if allowed.
20 Cover the person. Provide for comfort.
21 Fasten the safety straps. Raise the side rails.
22 Unlock (release the brakes) the stretcher wheels. Transport the person.

POST-PROCEDURE

23 Practice hand hygiene.
24 Report and record:
  - The time of the transport
  - Where the person was transported to
  - Who went with him or her
  - How the transfer was tolerated

25 Reverse the procedure to return the person to bed.

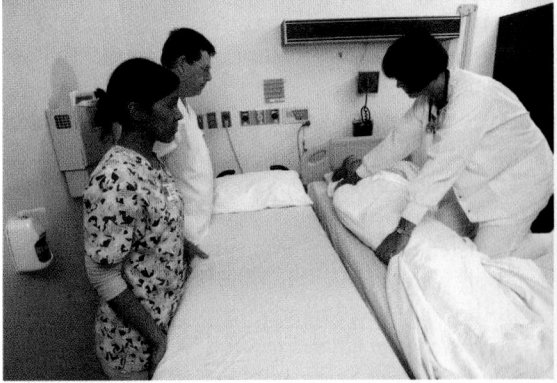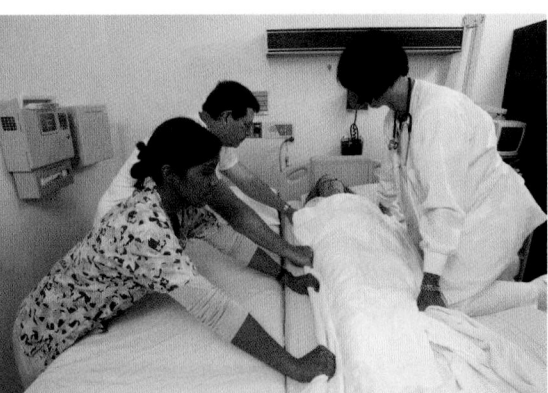

A B

FIGURE 19-16 Transferring the person to a stretcher. **A,** The stretcher is against the bed and is held in place. **B,** A drawsheet is used to transfer the person from the bed to a stretcher.

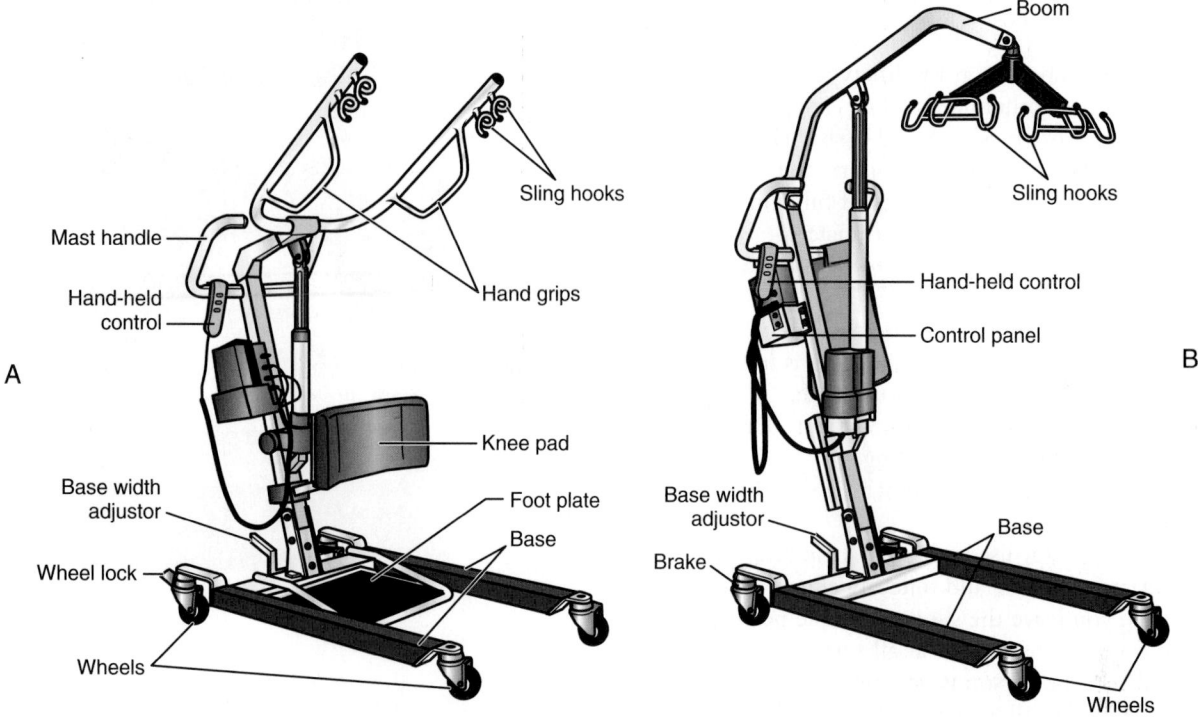

FIGURE 19-17 Mechanical lifts. **A,** Parts of a stand-assist lift. **B,** Parts of a full-sling mechanical lift.

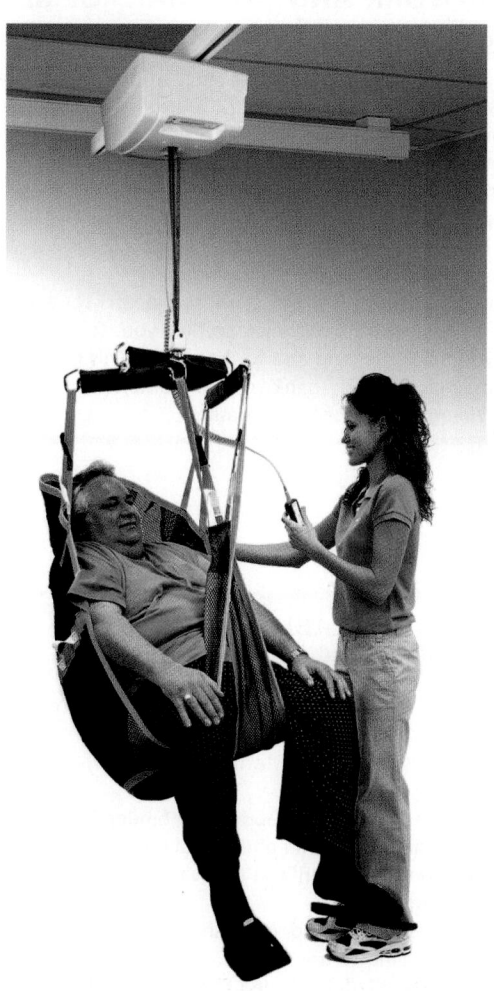

MECHANICAL LIFTS

Mechanical lifts are used for person who cannot assist with transfers. They also are used to transfer persons who are too heavy for the staff to move. Lifts are used to transfer persons to and from beds, chairs, wheelchairs, stretchers, tubs, shower chairs, toilets, commodes, whirlpools, or vehicles.

There are manual, battery-operated, and electric lifts. Two types are common (Fig. 19-17).

- Stand-assist lifts—used for persons who require some help with transfers and can:
  - Bear some weight.
  - Follow directions.
  - Sit up at the side of the bed with or without assistance.
  - Bend the hips, knees, and ankles.
- Full-sling mechanical lifts—used for persons who:
  - Cannot assist with transfers.
  - Are partially able or unable to bear weight.
  - Are heavy.
  - Have physical limits preventing other types of transfers.

Some lifts are mounted on the ceiling. Your agency may have floor or ceiling-mounted bariatric lifts (Fig. 19-18).

FIGURE 19-18 Bariatric ceiling lift. (Courtesy MedCare Products, Burnsville, Minn.)

Slings

The sling used depends on the lift type and the person's size, condition, and other needs. Slings are padded, unpadded, or made of mesh. Stand-assist slings support the upper body. Full-slings support the entire body (Fig. 19-19). There are many types of full-slings.

- *Standard full-sling*—for normal transfers.
- *Extended length sling*—for persons with extra large thighs.
- *Bathing sling*—to transfer the person directly from the bed or chair into a bathtub. The sling is left in place and attached to the lift during the bath.
- *Toileting sling*—the sling bottom is open. Each person has his or her own toileting sling.
- *Amputee sling*—for the person who has had both legs amputated.
- *Bariatric sling*—for use with a bariatric lift. There are also bariatric bathing and toileting slings. The nurse may have you leave the sling under the person when seated for short periods or at all times. If the sling is left in place, the person is not turned from side-to-side to place and remove the sling for each transfer. This reduces the risk of injury to the person and staff.

The nurse and care plan tell you what sling to use. Follow agency policy and the manufacturer's instructions for handling and washing contaminated slings. A sling is contaminated if it:

- Has any visible sign of blood, body fluids, secretions, or excretions.
- Is used on a person's bare skin.
- Is used to bathe a person.

Using a Mechanical Lift

Before using a lift:

- You must be trained in its use.
- It must work.
- The sling, straps, hooks, and chains must be in good repair.
- The person's weight must not exceed the lift's capacity.
- You need enough help. At least 2 staff members are needed for most lifts. Follow agency policy and the person's care plan.

There are different types of mechanical lifts. Always follow the manufacturer's instructions. The procedures that follow are used as a guide.

See *Teamwork and Time Management: Using a Mechanical Lift.*

See *Delegation Guidelines: Using a Mechanical Lift.*

See *Promoting Safety and Comfort: Using a Mechanical Lift.*

See procedure: *Transferring the Person Using a Stand-Assist Mechanical Lift.*

See procedure: *Transferring the Person Using a Full-Sling Mechanical Lift*, p. 299.

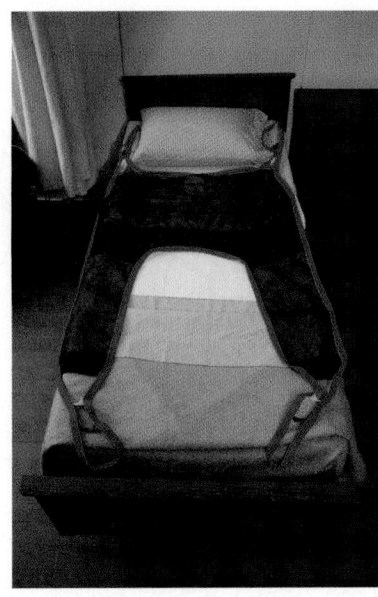

FIGURE 19-19 A full-sling supports the entire body.

TEAMWORK AND TIME MANAGEMENT

Using a Mechanical Lift

After using a mechanical lift, return it to the storage area. It needs to be there for other staff. Do not leave a device in a person's room or other area. Co-workers should not have to assume that an assist device is in use or take time looking for one.

Many mechanical lifts are battery operated. The battery must be charged for the device to work properly. Follow agency policy to charge or replace batteries.

You may need help from 1 or 2 co-workers for a safe transfer. Politely ask co-workers to help you. Tell them what time you need the help and for how long. This helps them plan their own work. Thank your co-workers for helping you. Willingly help them when asked.

DELEGATION GUIDELINES

Using a Mechanical Lift

Before using a mechanical lift, you need this information from the nurse and the care plan.

- The person's functional status (see Box 19-1).
- What lift to use.
- If you need to apply an abdominal binder. For the person with bariatric needs, an abdominal binder may be used if the person's abdomen is in the way. See Chapter 36.
- What sling to use.
- If a padded, unpadded, or mesh sling is needed.
- What size sling to use.
- The number of staff needed to perform the task safely.

PROMOTING SAFETY AND COMFORT

Using a Mechanical Lift

Safety

Always follow the manufacturer's instructions. Knowing how to use 1 lift does not mean that you know how to use others.

If you have questions, ask the nurse. If you have not used a certain lift before, ask for training. Ask the nurse to help you until you are comfortable using the lift.

The lift's base widens or opens. The base closes to fit under the bed and move through narrow areas. The lift is most stable when the base is in the open position. Lock the base in the wide or open position when lifting, lowering, and moving whenever possible. If you must narrow the base, do so only briefly. Return the base to the wide or open position as soon as possible.

For many lifts, the wheels are unlocked during lifting and lowering. This allows the lift to stabilize as the person is moved. For some stand-assist lifts, the wheels are locked when lifting and lowering. Follow the manufacturer's instructions for when to lock the lift's wheels.

Safety—cont'd

Mechanical lifts must be in good working order. Tell the nurse when a lift needs repair or is not working properly. For persons with bariatric needs:

* Make sure the receiving surface (bed, chair, wheelchair, stretcher, and so on) has expanded capacity for the person's weight.
* Use a chair or wheelchair with arms that you can remove or lower.

If the person can bear some weight, you may be able to use a stand-assist lift alone. Follow the care plan.

Two staff members are needed to safely use a full-sling mechanical lift. Federal guidelines require that at least 1 staff member be 18 years of age or older.

Comfort

The person is lifted up and off the bed or chair. Falling is a common fear. To promote mental comfort, always explain the procedure before you begin. Also show the person how the lift works.

Transferring the Person Using a Stand-Assist Mechanical Lift   NATCEP

QUALITY OF LIFE

* Knock before entering the person's room.
* Address the person by name.
* Introduce yourself by name and title.

* Explain the procedure before starting and during the procedure.
* Protect the person's rights during the procedure.
* Handle the person gently during the procedure.

PRE-PROCEDURE

1 Follow *Delegation Guidelines:*
  a *Safely Transferring the Person*, p. 282
  b *Using a Mechanical Lift*
  See *Promoting Safety and Comfort:*
  a *Safely Transferring the Person*, p. 282
  b *Using a Mechanical Lift*
2 Ask a co-worker to help you (if needed).
3 Collect the following.
  • Stand-assist mechanical lift and sling
  • Arm chair or wheelchair
  • Footwear
  • Bath blanket or cushion
  • Lap blanket (if used)

4 Practice hand hygiene.
5 Identify the person. Check the ID bracelet against the assignment sheet. Use 2 identifiers (Chapter 13). Also call the person by name.
6 Provide for privacy.

PROCEDURE

7 Place the chair (wheelchair) at the head of the bed. It is even with the head-board and about 1 foot away from the bed. Lock (brake) the wheelchair wheels. Place a folded bath blanket or cushion in the seat if needed.
8 Assist the person to a seated position on the side of the bed. See procedure: *Sitting on the Side of the Bed (Dangling)* in Chapter 18. The person is seated on the side of the bed with the feet flat on the floor. Bed wheels are locked.

9 Put footwear on the person.
10 Apply the sling.
  a Position the sling at the lower back.
  b Bring the straps around to the front of the chest. The straps are positioned under the arms.
  c Secure the waist belt around the person's waist. Adjust the belt so it is snug but not tight.
11 Position the lift in front of the person.
12 Widen the lift's base.

Continued

Transferring the Person Using a Stand-Assist Mechanical Lift—cont'd

PROCEDURE—cont'd

13 Lock (brake) the lift's wheels.
14 Direct the person to place his or her feet on the foot plate and the knees against the knee pad. Assist as needed. If the lift has a knee strap, secure the strap around the legs. Adjust the strap so it is snug but not tight.
15 Attach the sling to the sling hooks.
16 Direct the person to grasp the lift's hand grips.
17 Unlock (release the brakes) the lift's wheels.
18 Raise the person slightly off the bed. Check that the sling is secure, the feet are on the footplate, and the knees are against the knee pad (Fig. 19-20, *A*). If not, lower the person. Correct the problem before proceeding.
19 Raise the lift until the person is clear of the bed (Fig. 19-20, *B*). Or raise the person to a standing position (Fig. 19-20, *C*). Follow the care plan.
20 Adjust the base's width to move from the bed to the chair (wheelchair) if needed. Keep the base in the wide or open position as much as possible.

21 Move the lift to the chair (wheelchair). The person's back is toward the seat.
22 Lower the person into the chair (wheelchair). Guide the person into the seat. See Figure 19-20, *D* and *E*.
23 Lock (brake) the lift's wheels.
24 Unhook the sling from the sling hooks.
25 Unbuckle the waist belt. Remove the sling.
26 Unlock (release the brakes) the lift's wheels.
27 Direct the person to lift the feet off of the footplate. Assist as needed. Move the lift. Position the person's feet flat on the floor or on the wheelchair footplates.
28 Cover the person's lap and legs with a lap blanket (if used). Keep it off the floor.

POST-PROCEDURE

29 Provide for comfort. (See the inside of the front cover.)
30 Place the call light and other needed items within reach.
31 Unscreen the person.
32 Complete a safety check of the room. (See the inside of the front cover.)

33 Practice hand hygiene.
34 Report and record your observations.
35 Reverse the procedure to return the person to bed.

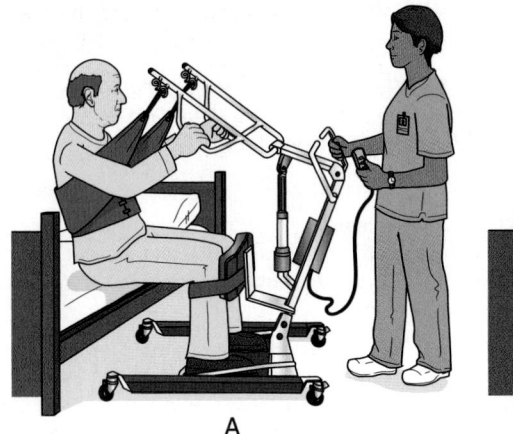
A

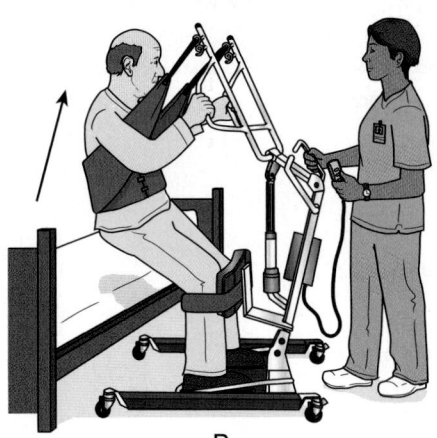
B

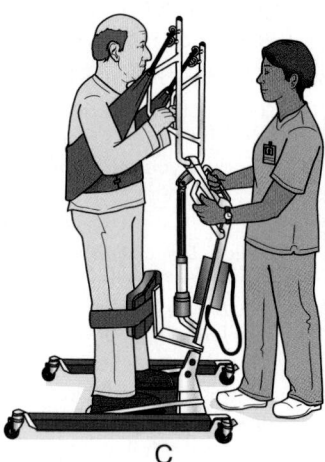
C

FIGURE 19-20 Using a stand-assist lift. **A,** The sling is around the person's lower back. The straps are under the arms. The waist belt is secure. Feet are on the footplate. The person holds the hand grips. **B,** The lift is raised. **C,** The person is in a standing position. **D,** The person is lowered into the chair. **E,** The person is seated. The back is against the back of the chair.

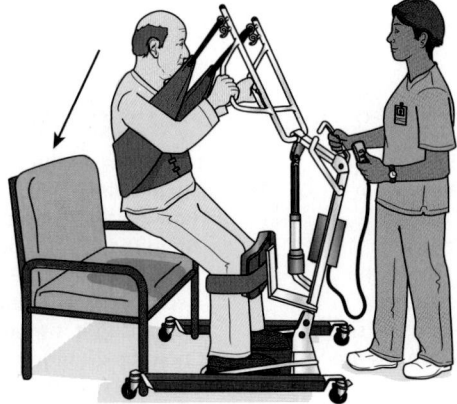
D

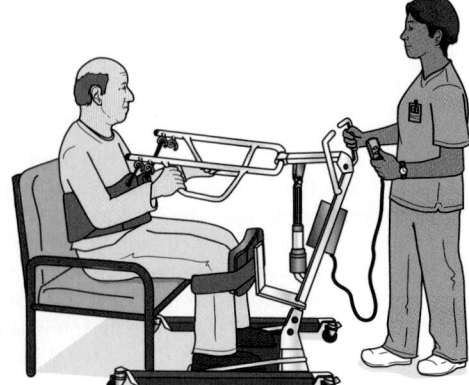
E

Transferring the Person Using a Full-Sling Mechanical Lift

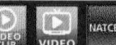

QUALITY OF LIFE

- Knock before entering the person's room.
- Address the person by name.
- Introduce yourself by name and title.

- Explain the procedure before starting and during the procedure.
- Protect the person's rights during the procedure.
- Handle the person gently during the procedure.

PRE-PROCEDURE

1 Follow *Delegation Guidelines:*
  a *Safely Transferring the Person*, p. 282
  b *Using a Mechanical Lift*, p. 296
  See *Promoting Safety and Comfort:*
  a Safely Transferring the Person, p. 282
  b Using a Mechanical Lift, p. 297
2 Ask a co-worker to help you.
3 Collect the following.
  - Full-sling mechanical lift and sling
  - Arm chair or wheelchair
  - Footwear
  - Bath blanket or cushion
  - Lap blanket (if used)

4 Practice hand hygiene.
5 Identify the person. Check the ID bracelet against the assignment sheet. Use 2 identifiers (Chapter 13). Also call the person by name.
6 Provide for privacy.
7 Raise the bed for body mechanics. Bed rails are up if used.

PROCEDURE

8 Lower the head of the bed to a level appropriate for the person. It is as flat as possible.
9 Stand on 1 side of the bed. Your co-worker stands on the other side.
10 Lower the bed rails if up. Lock (brake) the bed wheels.
11 Center the sling under the person (Fig. 19-21, *A*, p. 300). To position the sling, turn the person from side to side (Chapter 18). Follow the manufacturer's instructions to position the sling.
12 Position the person in the semi-Fowler's position.
13 Place the chair (wheelchair) at the head of the bed. It is even with the head-board and about 1 foot away from the bed. Place a folded bath blanket or cushion in the seat if needed. Lock (brake) the wheelchair wheels.
14 Lower the bed so it is level with the chair.
15 Raise the lift to position it over the person.
16 Position the lift over the person (Fig. 19-21, *B*, p. 300).
17 Widen the lift's base. Lock (brake) the lift wheels.
18 Attach the sling to the sling hooks (Fig. 19-21, *C*, p. 300).
19 Raise the head of the bed to a comfortable level for the person.
20 Cross the person's arms over the chest.
21 Unlock (release the brakes) the lift wheels.
22 Raise the person slightly from the bed. Check that the sling is secure. If not, lower the person. Correct the problem before proceeding.

23 Raise the lift until the person and sling are free of the bed (Fig. 19-21, *D*, p. 300).
24 Have your co-worker support the person's legs as you move the lift and the person away from the bed (Fig. 19-21, *E*, p. 300).
25 Adjust the base's width to move from the bed to the chair (wheelchair) if needed. Keep the base in the wide or open position as much as possible.
26 Position the lift so the person's back is toward the chair (wheelchair).
27 Adjust the position of the chair (wheelchair) as needed so you can lower the person into it. Lock (brake) the wheelchair wheels.
28 Lower the person into the chair (wheelchair). Guide the person into the seat (Fig. 19-21, *F*, p. 300).
29 Lock (brake) the lift wheels.
30 Unhook the sling. Remove the sling from under the person unless otherwise indicated.
31 Put footwear on the person. Position the person's feet flat on the floor or on the wheelchair footplates.
32 Cover the person's lap and legs with a lap blanket (if used). Keep it off the floor and wheels.
33 Position the chair (wheelchair) as the person prefers. Lock (brake) the wheelchair wheels according to the care plan.

POST-PROCEDURE

34 Provide for comfort. (See the inside of the front cover.)
35 Place the call light and other needed items within reach.
36 Unscreen the person.
37 Complete a safety check of the room. (See the inside of the front cover.)

38 Practice hand hygiene.
39 Report and record your observations.
40 Reverse the procedure to return the person to bed.

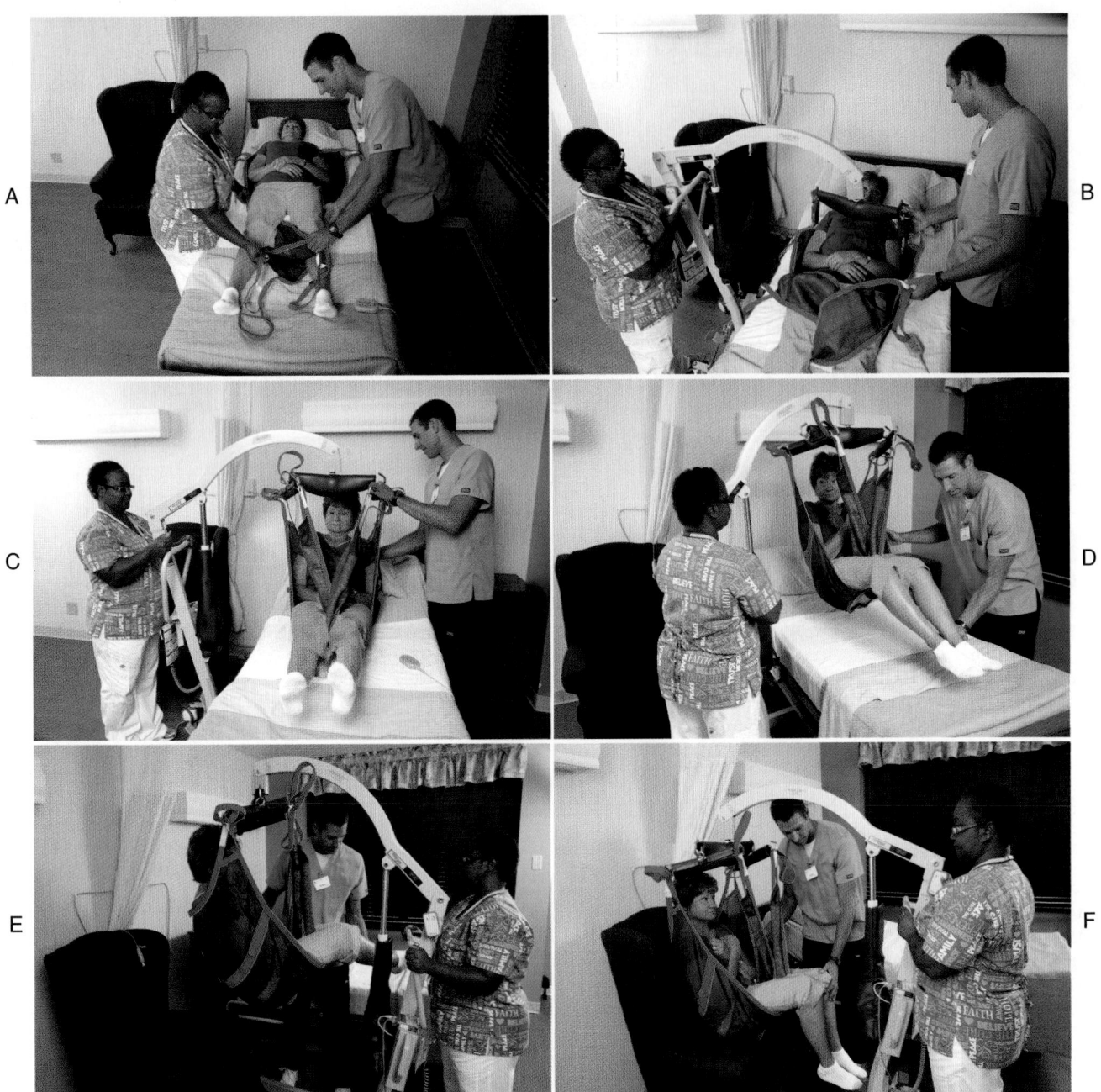

FIGURE 19-21 Using a full-sling mechanical lift. **A,** The sling is positioned under the person. **B,** The lift is over the person. **C,** The sling is attached to the lift. **D,** The lift is raised until the sling and person are off of the bed. **E,** The person's legs are supported as the person and lift are moved away from the bed. **F,** The person is guided into a chair.

FOCUS ON **PRIDE**

The Person, Family, and Yourself

Personal and Professional Responsibility

Before any procedure, take time to plan and prepare. Gather needed items. Organize the room and move or prepare equipment for a safe transfer. Remember to:
- Lock (brake) the wheels on the bed, wheelchair, stretcher, and so on.
- Remove front rigging on a wheelchair or swing it out of the way.
- Position the chair, wheelchair, stretcher, and so on for a safe transfer.
- Adjust the bed to a safe and comfortable height.
- Make sure a mechanical lift is charged.
- Move furniture or clutter out of the way.

Planning and preparing are very important for transfer procedures. Share the plan with co-workers and the person.

Rights and Respect

When transferring a person, remember to respect privacy. Close privacy curtains, doors, and window coverings. Properly cover the person. For example, a person wears a gown that opens in the back. Apply a robe or another gown to cover the person's backside. Use a covering that is safe for transfers.

Independence and Social Interaction

How you speak to the person makes a difference. When giving directions:
- Speak slowly and clearly.
- Talk loudly enough for the person to hear you.
- Give directions calmly and kindly. Never yell at or insult the person.
- Face the person and use eye contact when possible.
- Give 1 direction at a time.
- Repeat directions as needed. Be patient.
- Ask if the person has questions before proceeding.

Your speech and tone must convey dignity. Show you value the person through respectful interactions.

Delegation and Teamwork

You may need help transferring a person. Your co-workers are busy. You have a choice. Do you ask for help? Or do you try to move the person alone?

Never be afraid to ask for help. You are not bothering a co-worker by asking for help. Ask politely and say thank you. Also, willingly help others when asked. If you cannot stop what you are doing, tell your co-worker when you can help. Then help the person when you said that you would. Work as a team to ensure the person's safety and protect yourself and others from injury.

Ethics and Laws

You must transfer persons safely. Otherwise injuries can result. To avoid injury:
- Move a person with enough help.
- Position the chair or wheelchair close to the bed.
- Use the proper equipment such as a transfer belt or mechanical lift.
- Do not pull on the person's clothing or arm, underarm, or other body part.
- Do not use broken or damaged equipment.
- Do not exceed equipment weight limits.

You learned the right way to move and transfer persons. The right way is not always easy. Choose to give care correctly. Take pride in providing care in a way that prevents harm and promotes comfort and safety.

FOCUS ON **PRIDE**: *Application*

At first, explaining procedures may make you nervous. This improves with practice. Practice explaining a transfer from the bed to a chair using:
- A stand and pivot transfer
- A stand-assist mechanical lift
- A full-sling mechanical lift

REVIEW QUESTIONS

Circle the BEST answer.

1 To promote comfort during a transfer
   a Keep the head of the bed flat
   b Explain the procedure
   c Let the person choose the procedure
   d Open the privacy curtain

2 For a safe transfer to a chair
   a Tell the person to grasp you around your neck
   b Hold the person under the underarms
   c Manually lift the person
   d Move furniture and equipment as needed

3 A person can bear some weight but needs weight-bearing help to transfer. The person's functional status for transfers is
   a Independent
   b Limited Assistance
   c Extensive Assistance
   d Total Dependence

4 For chair and wheelchair transfers, the person must
   a Wear non-skid footwear
   b Have the bed rails up
   c Use a mechanical lift
   d Have a drawsheet or other assist device

5 A person uses a wheelchair. Which measure is unsafe?
   a The wheels are locked (braked) for transfers.
   b The chair is pulled backward to transport the person.
   c The feet are positioned on the footplates.
   d The casters point forward.

6 A stand and pivot transfer is unsafe for a person who
   a Is hard-of-hearing but can follow directions
   b Can bear some weight with the legs
   c Is confused and combative
   d Uses a transfer belt

7 When transferring the person to bed, a chair, or the wheelchair
   a The strong side moves first
   b The weak side moves first
   c Pillows are used for support
   d The transfer belt is removed

8 When going down a ramp with a wheelchair
   a Push the wheelchair front-first
   b Roll it backward
   c Tilt the wheelchair onto the back wheels
   d Lightly apply the brake

9 When transferring a person from a wheelchair to a toilet
   a Position the wheelchair facing the toilet
   b Remove the transfer belt when lowering clothing
   c Tell the person to hold on to the towel bar for support
   d Lock (brake) the wheelchair wheels

10 To use a stretcher safely
   a Unlock the wheels (release the brakes) for transfers to and from the stretcher
   b Fasten the safety straps
   c Lower the side rails during a transport
   d Move the stretcher head first

11 When using a mechanical lift
   a Position the lift on the person's strong side
   b Collect a sling, battery, and transfer belt
   c Compare the person's weight to the lift's weight limit
   d Allow the person to control the lift

12 To safely transfer a person with a full-sling mechanical lift, at least
   a 1 worker is needed
   b 2 workers are needed
   c 3 workers are needed
   d 4 workers are needed

13 You are using a stand-assist mechanical lift. Which is unsafe?
   a The person is holding the lift's hand grips.
   b The person's feet are on the footplate.
   c The lift's base is narrow when lifting.
   d The person's knees are against the knee pad.

14 After a transfer, which should you do *first*?
   a Place the call light within reach.
   b Return the mechanical lift to the storage area.
   c Record the procedure.
   d Report to the nurse.

Answers to Chapter 19 questions are on p. 871.

FOCUS ON PRACTICE

Problem Solving

A resident needs to go to the bathroom right away. She uses a full-sling mechanical lift to transfer safely. You do not see another staff member nearby to help. What will you do?

The Person's Unit

OBJECTIVES

- Define the key terms and key abbreviations in this chapter.
- Explain how to maintain the person's unit.
- Describe how to control temperature and drafts, odors, noise, and lighting for the person's comfort.
- Describe the basic bed positions.
- Identify the 7 hospital bed system entrapment zones.
- Identify the persons at risk for bed entrapment.
- Explain how to use the furniture and equipment in the person's unit.

- Describe how a bathroom is equipped for the person's use.
- Describe how to promote safety, privacy, and comfort in the person's unit.
- Describe OBRA and CMS requirements for resident rooms.
- Explain how to promote PRIDE in the person, the family, and yourself.

KEY TERMS

entrapment Getting caught, trapped, or entangled in spaces created by the bed rails, the mattress, the bed frame, the head-board, or the foot-board

Fowler's position A semi-sitting position; the head of the bed is raised between 45 and 60 degrees

full visual privacy Having the means to be completely free from public view while in bed

high-Fowler's position A semi-sitting position; the head of the bed is raised 60 to 90 degrees

hospital bed system The bed frame and its parts; the parts include the mattress, bed rails, head- and foot-boards, and bed attachments

person's unit The personal space, furniture, and equipment provided for the person by the agency

reverse Trendelenburg's position The head of the bed is raised and the foot of the bed is lowered

semi-Fowler's position The head of the bed is raised 30 degrees; or the head of the bed is raised 30 degrees and the knee portion is raised 15 degrees

Trendelenburg's position The head of the bed is lowered and the foot of the bed is raised

KEY ABBREVIATIONS

CMS	Centers for Medicare & Medicaid Services	**IV**	Intravenous
CNA	Certified nursing assistant	**OBRA**	Omnibus Budget Reconciliation Act of 1987
F	Fahrenheit		

The **person's unit** is the personal space, furniture, and equipment provided for the person by the agency (Fig. 20-1). The person's unit is designed to provide comfort, safety, and privacy.

A private room has 1 patient or resident unit. Semi-private rooms have 2 units. Some rooms have 3 or 4 units.

You need to keep the person's unit clean, neat, safe, and comfortable. See Box 20-1, p. 304.

See *Focus on Long-Term Care and Home Care: The Person's Unit*, p. 304.

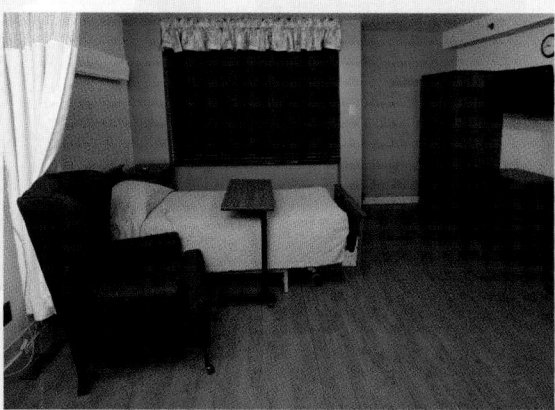

FIGURE 20-1 Furniture and equipment in a resident's unit.

BOX 20-1	Maintaining the Person's Unit

- Keep the call light within the person's reach at all times.
- Meet the needs of persons who cannot use the call system (p. 313).
- Make sure the person can reach the over-bed table (p. 312) and the bedside stand (p. 312).
- Arrange personal items as the person prefers. They are within easy reach.
- Place the phone, TV, bed, and light controls within the person's reach.
- Provide enough tissues and toilet paper.
- Adjust lighting, temperature, and ventilation for the person's comfort.
- Handle equipment carefully to prevent noise.
- Explain the causes of strange noises.
- Use room deodorizers according to agency policy.
- Empty wastebaskets at least once a day. In some agencies, they are emptied every shift. Always empty them when full.
- Respect the person's belongings. An item may not seem important to you. Yet even a scrap of paper can have great meaning to the person.
- Do not throw away any items belonging to the person.
- Do not move furniture or the person's belongings. Persons with poor vision rely on memory or feel to find items.
- Straighten bed linens and towels as often as needed.
- Complete a safety check before leaving the room. (See the inside of the front cover.)

FOCUS ON LONG-TERM CARE AND HOME CARE

The Person's Unit

Long-Term Care

The *Omnibus Budget Reconciliation Act of 1987 (OBRA)* and the Centers for Medicare & Medicaid Services (CMS) have requirements for resident rooms. See Box 20-2. Resident units must be as personal and home-like as possible. Residents are allowed to bring and use some furniture and personal items from home. This promotes dignity and self-esteem.

As space allows, the person chooses where to place personal items. However, a resident cannot take or use another person's space. Doing so violates the other person's rights.

BOX 20-2	OBRA and CMS Requirements for Resident Rooms

- Rooms are designed for 1 to 4 persons.
- Rooms have a direct access to an exit hallway.
- Rooms are designed or equipped for full visual privacy— ceiling-suspended privacy curtain that extends around the bed, movable screens, window coverings, doors.
- Rooms have at least 1 window to the outside.
- Each person has closet space with racks and shelves.
- Toilet facilities are in the room or nearby (including bathing facilities).
- Rooms, bathrooms, and bathing areas have a functioning call system.
- The person has a bed of proper height and size.
- The person has a clean, comfortable mattress.
- Bed and bath linens (towels and washcloths) are clean and in good condition.
- Bed linens are correct for the weather and climate.
- The room has furniture for clothing, personal items, and a chair for visitors.
- Rooms are clean and orderly.
- Room temperature levels are between 71°F and 81°F.
- Ventilation, humidity, and odor levels are acceptable.
- Non-smoking areas are identified.
- Sound levels are comfortable.
- Lighting is adequate and comfortable with little glare.
- Rooms have clean, orderly drawers and shelves for personal items.
- The room is free of pests and rodents.
- Hand rails are in good repair.
- Rooms are clean and dry.
- The person's setting is free of clutter.
- Personal supplies and items are correctly labeled and stored.
- Items are within reach for use in bed or bathroom.
- There is space for wheelchair or walker use.
- The person has a raised toilet seat (if needed).

COMFORT

Age, illness, and activity affect comfort. So do temperature, ventilation, noise, odors, and lighting. These factors are controlled to meet the person's needs.

See *Focus on Communication: Comfort.*

FOCUS ON COMMUNICATION

Comfort

What is comfortable for 1 person may not be comfortable for another. Ask about the person's comfort. You can say:
- "How is the temperature? Is it too hot or too cold?"
- "Is the noise level okay?"
- "Please let me know if you notice any bad odors."
- "How is the lighting? Is it too bright or too dark?"
- "Are you comfortable?"

Temperature and Ventilation

Most healthy people are comfortable with room temperatures between 68°F (Fahrenheit) and 74°F. This range may be too hot or too cold for others. Persons who are older or ill may need higher temperatures for comfort.

Less active persons usually do not like cool areas. Nor do those needing help to move about. They need warm clothing and room temperatures. You may find the rooms rather warm.

Stale room air and lingering odors affect comfort and rest. Ventilation systems provide fresh air and move room air. Drafts occur as air moves. Infants, older persons, and those who are ill are sensitive to drafts. To protect them from drafts:

- Have them wear the correct clothing.
- Have them wear enough clothing.
- Offer lap robes to those in chairs and wheelchairs. Lap robes cover the legs.
- Provide enough blankets for warmth.
- Cover them with bath blankets when giving care.
- Move them from drafty areas.

See *Focus on Children and Older Persons: Temperature and Ventilation.*

Odors

Odors occur in health care settings and in home care. Food aromas and flower scents are pleasant. Bowel movements and urine have embarrassing odors. So do draining wounds and vomitus. Body, breath, and smoke odors may offend others.

Some people are very sensitive to odors. They may become nauseated. Good nursing care, ventilation, and housekeeping practices help prevent odors. To reduce odors:

- Empty, clean, and disinfect bedpans, urinals, commodes, and kidney basins promptly.
- Make sure toilets are flushed.
- Check incontinent persons often (Chapters 24 and 26).
- Clean persons who are wet or soiled from urine, feces, vomitus, or wound drainage.
- Change wet or soiled linens and clothing promptly.
- Keep laundry containers closed.
- Follow agency policy for wet or soiled linens and clothing.
- Dispose of incontinence and ostomy products promptly (Chapters 24 and 26).
- Provide good hygiene to prevent body and breath odors (Chapter 22).
- Use room deodorizers as needed and allowed by agency policy. Do not use sprays around persons with breathing problems. Ask the nurse if you are unsure.

Smoke odors present special problems. If you smoke, follow the agency's policy. Practice hand-washing after smoking. Practice hand-washing after handling smoking materials and before giving care. Give careful attention to your uniform, hair, and breath because of smoke odors.

FOCUS ON CHILDREN AND OLDER PERSONS

Temperature and Ventilation

Older Persons

Poor circulation and loss of the skin's fatty tissue layer occur with aging. Therefore older persons are sensitive to cold (Chapter 12). They must wear enough clothing. Many wear sweaters or jackets in warm weather. Respect the person's wishes and choices.

Noise

According to the CMS, a "comfortable" sound level:

- Does not interfere with a person's hearing.
- Promotes privacy when privacy is desired.
- Allows the person to take part in social activities.

Common health care sounds may disturb some persons. Examples include:

- The clanging and clattering of equipment, dishes, and meal trays
- Loud voices, TVs, radios, music players, and so on
- Ringing phones
- Intercom systems and call lights
- Equipment or wheels needing repair or oil
- Cleaning and housekeeping equipment

Loud talking and laughter in hallways and at the nurses' station are common. Patients and residents may think that the staff are talking and laughing about them.

People want to know the cause and meaning of new sounds. This relates to safety and security needs. Some sounds seem dangerous, frightening, or irritating. Patients and residents may become upset, anxious, and uncomfortable. What is noise to 1 person may not be noise to another. For example, some people enjoy loud music. It disturbs others.

Health care agencies are designed to reduce noise. Window coverings, carpets, and acoustical tiles absorb noise. Plastic items make less noise than metal equipment (bedpans, urinals, wash basins). To decrease noise levels:

- Control your voice.
- Handle equipment carefully.
- Keep equipment in good working order.
- Answer phones, call lights, and intercoms promptly.

See *Focus on Communication: Noise*, p. 306.
See *Focus on Children and Older Persons: Noise*, p. 306.
See *Focus on Surveys: Noise*, p. 306.

Lighting

According to the CMS, comfortable lighting:
- Lessens glares.
- Lets the person control the intensity, location, and direction of light.
- Lets visually impaired persons maintain or increase independent functioning.

Good lighting is needed for safety and comfort. Glares, shadows, and dull lighting can cause falls, headaches, and eyestrain. A bright room is cheerful. Dim light is better for relaxing and rest.

Adjust lighting to meet the person's changing needs. The over-bed light provides soft, medium, or bright lighting. Ceiling lights provide soft to very bright light. Also adjust window coverings as needed.

Persons with poor vision need bright light. This is very important at meal time and when moving about in the room and agency. Bright lighting also helps the staff perform procedures.

Always keep light controls within the person's reach. This protects the right to personal choice.

See *Focus on Children and Older Persons: Lighting.*

ROOM FURNITURE AND EQUIPMENT

Rooms are furnished and equipped to meet basic needs—comfort, sleep, elimination, nutrition, hygiene, and activity. There is equipment to communicate with staff, family, and friends. The right to privacy is considered.

The Bed

Beds have electrical or manual controls. Beds are raised horizontally to give care and to reduce bending and reaching. A low horizontal position lets the person get out of bed with ease (Fig. 20-2). The head and foot of the bed are flat or raised varying degrees.

Electric beds are common. Controls are on a side panel, bed rail, or the foot-board (Fig. 20-3, *A*). Some controls are hand-held devices (Fig. 20-3, *B*). Patients and residents are taught to use the controls safely. They are warned not to raise the bed to the high position or to adjust the bed to harmful positions. They are told of position limits or restrictions.

Manual beds have cranks at the foot of the bed (Fig. 20-4). The cranks are pulled up for use. Keep them down at all other times. Cranks in the "up" position are safety hazards. Anyone walking past may bump into them.

See *Focus on Long-Term Care and Home Care: The Bed.*
See *Promoting Safety and Comfort: The Bed.*

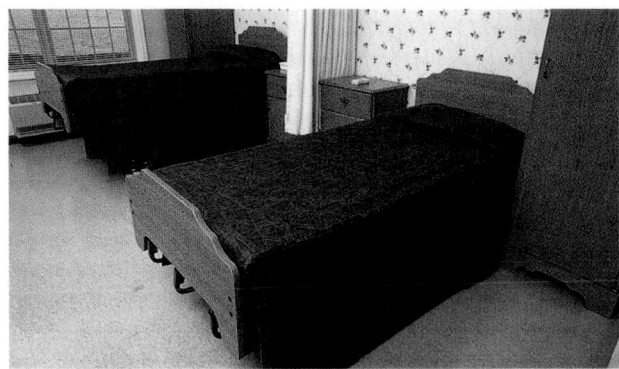

FIGURE 20-2 The far bed is in the highest horizontal position. The near bed is in a low horizontal position.

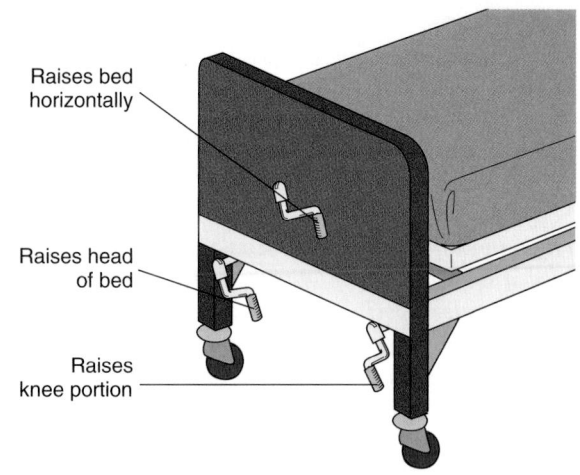

Raises bed horizontally

Raises head of bed

Raises knee portion

FIGURE 20-4 Manually operated bed.

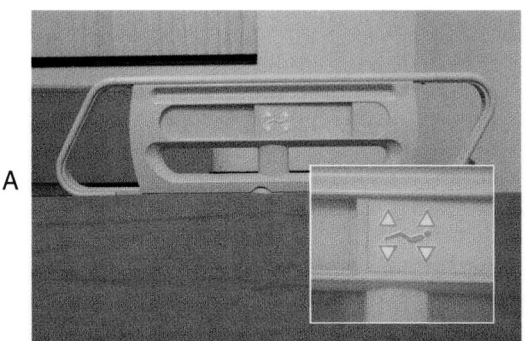

A

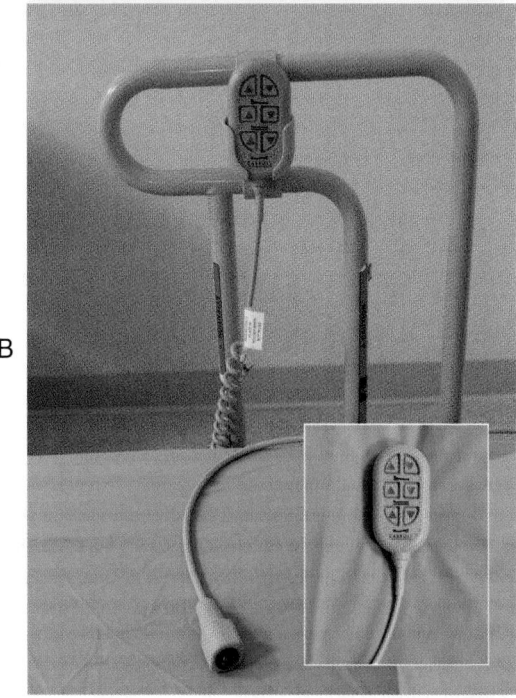

B

FIGURE 20-3 Controls for an electric bed. **A,** Controls in the bed rail. **B,** A hand-held bed control (see inset) can be attached to the bed rail.

FOCUS ON **LONG-TERM CARE AND HOME CARE**

The Bed

Home Care
Some home care patients have hospital beds. Others use their regular beds. You cannot raise regular beds to give care. You will bend more when giving care. To avoid injury, use good body mechanics.

PROMOTING SAFETY AND COMFORT

The Bed

Safety
The staff can lock most electric beds into any position. The person cannot adjust the bed to unsafe positions. Beds may be locked for persons:
- Restricted to certain positions
- With confusion or dementia

Beds have bed rails and wheels (Chapter 14). Bed wheels are locked (braked) at all times except when moving the bed. They must be locked to:
- Give bedside care.
- Transfer the person to and from the bed. The person can be injured if the bed moves. So can you.

On some beds, controls inside the bed rail adjust the head and foot of the bed (see Fig. 20-3, *A*). They are for patient or resident use. Horizontal and other controls are on the outer part of the rail. This prevents the person from raising or lowering the bed while in bed. Use the outer controls to move the bed horizontally.

Use bed rails as the nurse and care plan direct. Otherwise the person could suffer injury or harm.

Comfort
Some persons spend a lot of time in bed. Adjust the bed to meet the person's needs. Tell the nurse if the person complains about the bed or mattress.

Bed Positions. There are 6 basic bed positions.

- *Flat* is a common sleeping position. The position is used after spinal cord injury or surgery and for cervical traction.
- *Fowler's position is a semi-sitting position. The head of the bed is raised between 45 and 60 degrees* (Fig. 20-5). See Chapter 17.
- *High-Fowler's position is a semi-sitting position. The head of the bed is raised 60 to 90 degrees* (Fig. 20-6).
- *Semi-Fowler's position means the head of the bed is raised 30 degrees* (Fig. 20-7). Some agencies define semi-Fowler's position as when *the head of the bed is raised 30 degrees and the knee portion is raised 15 degrees.* This position is comfortable and prevents sliding down in bed. However, raising the knee portion can interfere with circulation in the legs. For safe care, know the definition used by your agency. Also check with the nurse before using this position.
- *Trendelenburg's position means the head of the bed is lowered and the foot of the bed is raised* (Fig. 20-8). A doctor orders the position. Blocks are placed under the legs at the foot of the bed. Or the bed frame is tilted.

- *Reverse Trendelenburg's position means the head of the bed is raised and the foot of the bed is lowered* (Fig. 20-9). A doctor orders this position. Blocks are placed under the legs at the head of the bed. Or the bed frame is tilted.

See *Focus on Long-Term Care and Home Care: Bed Positions.*

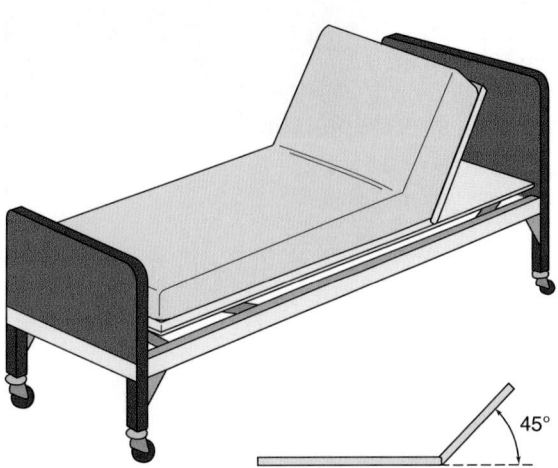

FIGURE 20-5 Fowler's position.

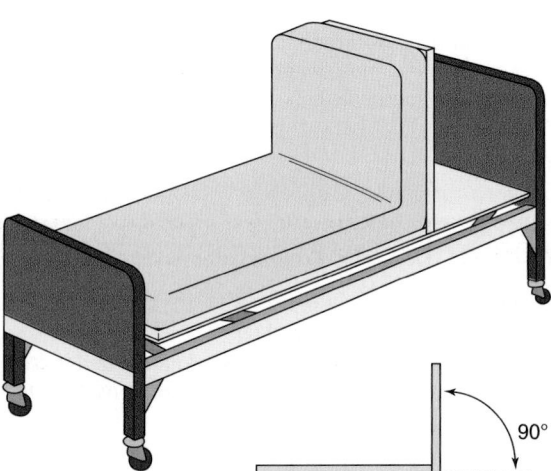

FIGURE 20-6 High-Fowler's position.

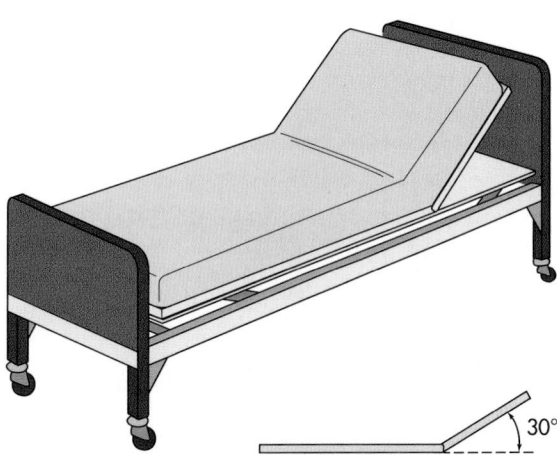

FIGURE 20-7 Semi-Fowler's position.

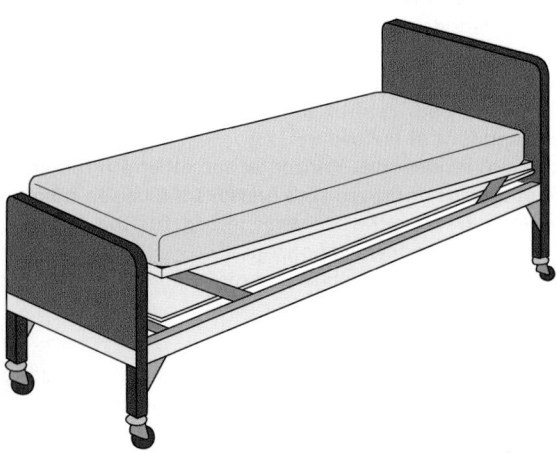

FIGURE 20-8 Trendelenburg's position.

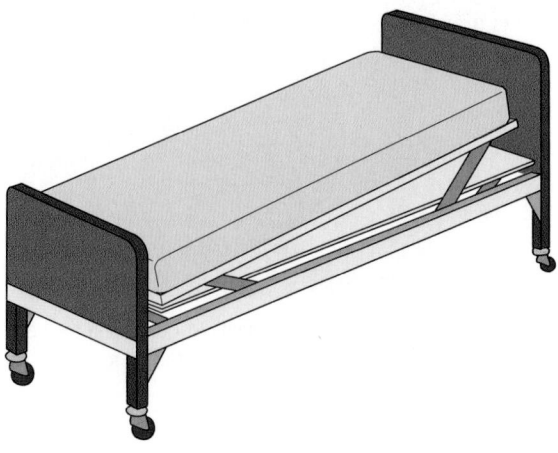

FIGURE 20-9 Reverse Trendelenburg's position.

FOCUS ON LONG-TERM CARE AND HOME CARE

Bed Positions

Home Care
Backrests are used with regular beds for Fowler's and semi-Fowler's positions (Fig. 20-10). Large, sturdy sofa pillows can be used. Check the head-board to make sure it is sturdy. It needs to provide support when the person leans against the backrest.

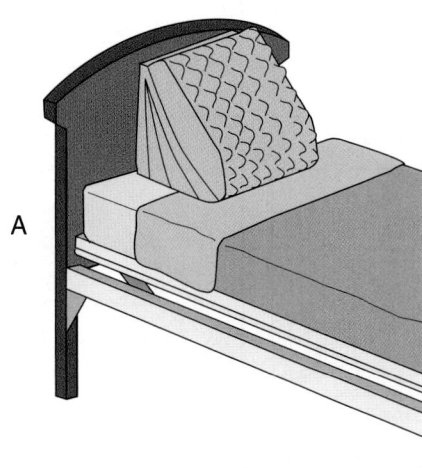

A

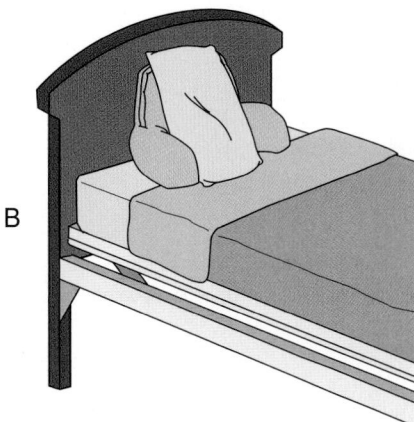

B

FIGURE 20-10 Backrests for regular beds. **A,** Wedge pillow. **B,** Study pillow (dorm pillow) with armrests. A pillow provides added support.

Bed Safety. Bed safety involves the *hospital bed system—the bed frame and its parts. The parts include the mattress, bed rails, head- and foot-boards, and bed attachments.*

Hospital bed systems have 7 entrapment zones (Fig. 20-11, p. 310). *Entrapment means getting caught, trapped, or entangled in spaces created by the bed rails, the mattress, the bed frame, the head-board, or the foot-board.* Head, neck, or chest entrapment can cause serious injuries and death. Arm and leg entrapment also can occur. Persons at greatest risk:
- Are older.
- Are frail.
- Are confused or disoriented.
- Are restless.
- Have uncontrolled body movements.
- Have poor muscle control.
- Are small in size.
- Are restrained (Chapter 15).

Always check the person for entrapment. If a person is caught, trapped, or entangled in the bed or any of its parts, try to release the person. Also call for the nurse at once.

See *Focus on Children and Older Persons: Bed Safety.*

FOCUS ON CHILDREN AND OLDER PERSONS

Bed Safety

Children
Entrapment can occur in cribs. To prevent entrapment, the mattress and crib must be the same size. When the mattress is smaller than the crib, gaps occur between:
- The crib rail and mattress
- The crib rail and head-board
- The crib rail and foot-board
  Tell the nurse if you have concerns about a baby's crib.

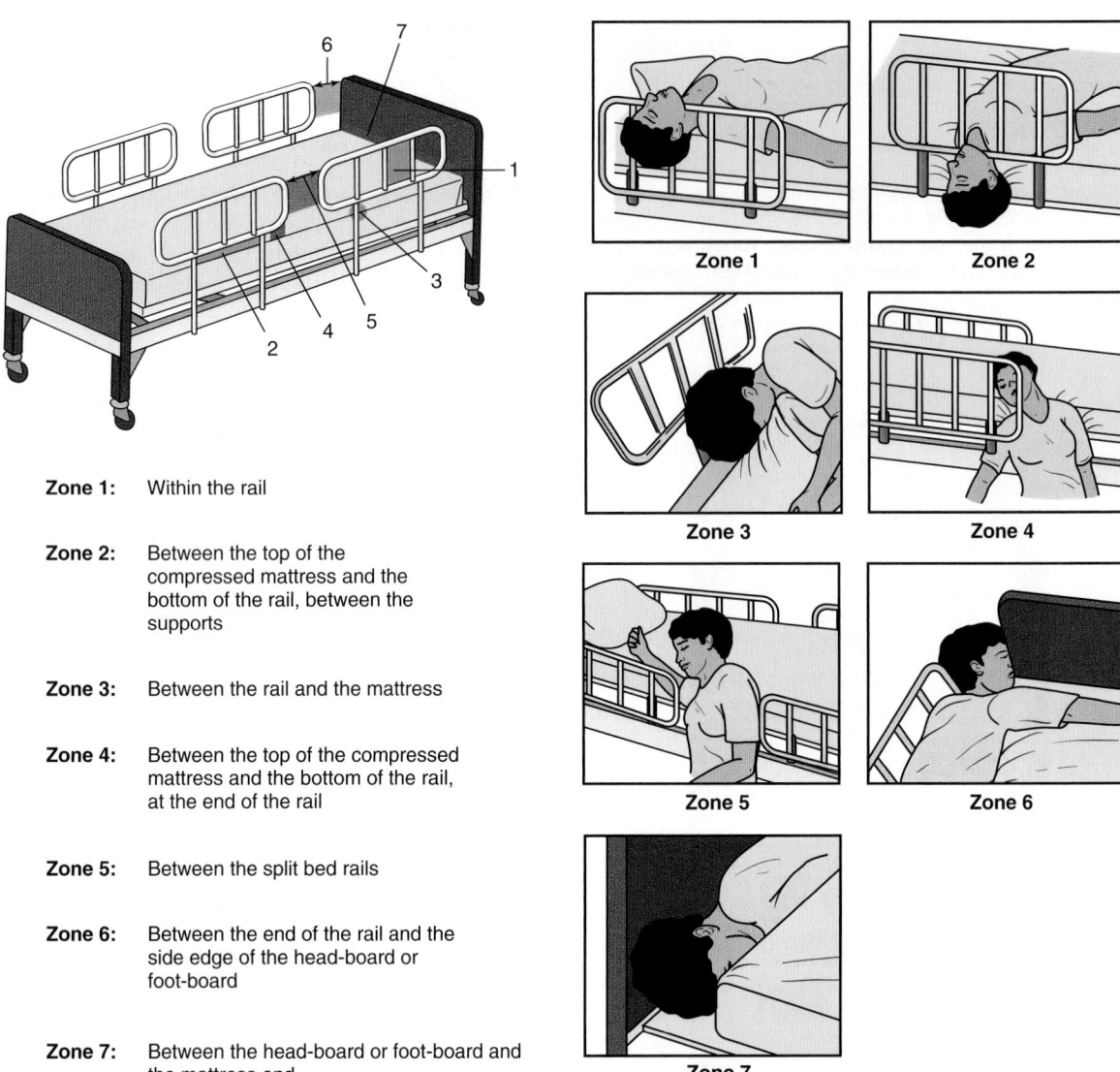

Zone 1:   Within the rail

Zone 2:   Between the top of the compressed mattress and the bottom of the rail, between the supports

Zone 3:   Between the rail and the mattress

Zone 4:   Between the top of the compressed mattress and the bottom of the rail, at the end of the rail

Zone 5:   Between the split bed rails

Zone 6:   Between the end of the rail and the side edge of the head-board or foot-board

Zone 7:   Between the head-board or foot-board and the mattress end

FIGURE 20-11 Hospital bed system entrapment zones. (Redrawn from Food and Drug Administration: *Hospital bed system dimensional and assessment guidance to reduce entrapment,* March 10, 2006, updated June 19, 2015.)

Bariatric Beds. Bariatric beds may have these and other features.

- A wide frame with a weight capacity from 500 to 1000 pounds (Fig. 20-12, *A*). Some frames can be adjusted for the person's height. For example, the bed length is shortened so the person's feet touch the foot-board. This prevents the person from sliding down in bed. Or the frame is lengthened for a taller person.
- A chair position. The bed converts into a chair without moving the person (Fig. 20-12, *B*). The foot-board becomes a footrest.
- Front and side egress positions. *Egress* means to *go out* or *leave*. By adjusting the foot-board out of the way, the person can move from a lying to sitting to standing position (Fig. 20-12, *C*). Or the person can get out of bed on the side (Fig. 20-12, *D*).

- Power transport to move the bed. The bed is used to transport the person. The person is not transferred to a stretcher.
- A pressure-relief surface to prevent pressure ulcers. The surface can be used to turn the person for care measures.
- A trapeze for the person to re-position himself or herself.
- A built-in scale.

Bariatric beds vary depending on the model. Follow the manufacturer's instructions to use the bed safely.

See *Focus on Communication: Bariatric Beds.*

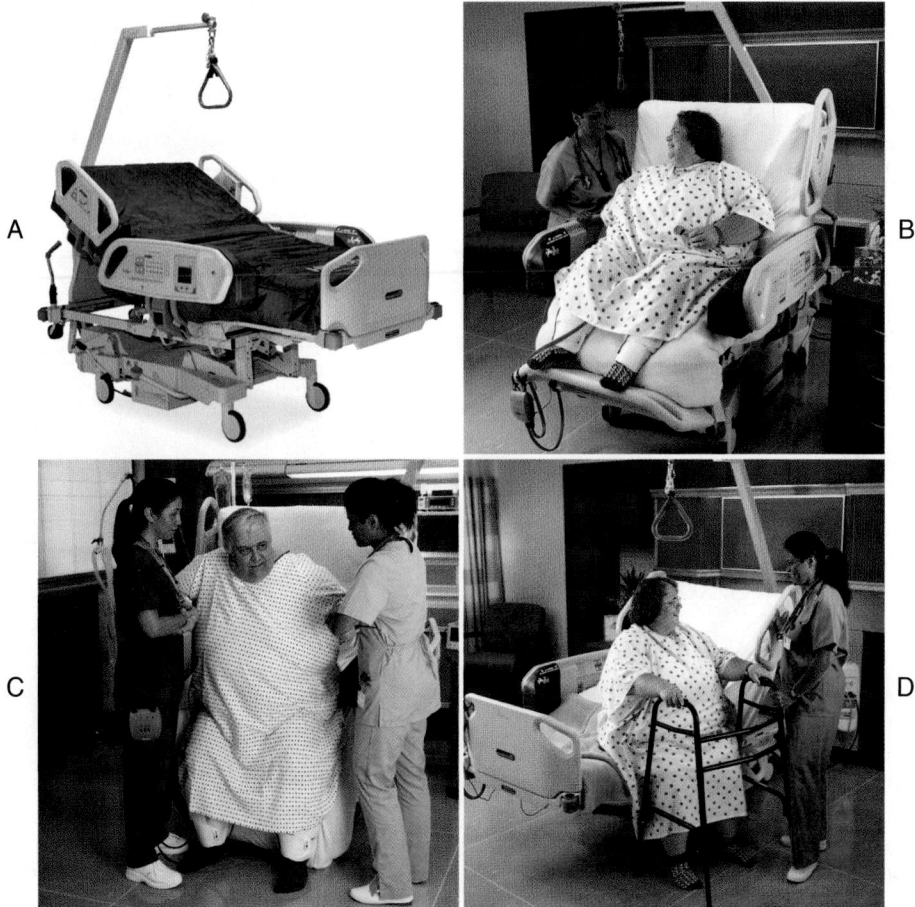

FIGURE 20-12 A, Bariatric bed with a trapeze. **B,** Bariatric bed converted to a chair. **C,** The bariatric bed allows the person to get out of bed from the chair position. **D,** The person gets out of the bariatric bed from the side. (Courtesy © Hill-Rom Services, Inc. Reprinted with permission. All rights reserved.)

FOCUS ON **COMMUNICATION**

Bariatric Beds

Many persons who are obese have been disrespected for much of their lives. They have been insulted and judged by others. This can cause low self-esteem and emotional problems. Such persons may be sensitive to comments about their weight or size.

Always think before you speak. Consider if the comment may offend the person. For example, do not say: "The nurse is trying to get a bed big enough for you." Instead, you can say: "The nurse is getting a bed that will be more comfortable for you."

Be aware of your verbal and nonverbal communication. Your words and actions must always show dignity and respect.

The Over-Bed Table

The over-bed table (see Fig. 20-1) is moved over the bed by sliding the base under the bed. The table is raised or lowered for the person in bed or in a chair. Use the handle, crank, or lever to adjust table height. Some over-bed tables have a storage area for beauty, hair care, shaving, or other personal items.

The person uses the over-bed table for meals, writing, reading, and other activities. The nursing team uses the over-bed table as a work area. Place only clean and sterile items on the table. Never place bedpans, urinals, or soiled linen on the over-bed table. Clean the table after use as a work surface. Also clean it before serving meal trays.

The Bedside Stand

By the bed, the bedside stand is used for personal items and personal care equipment. It has a top drawer and a lower cabinet with shelves or drawers (Fig. 20-13). The top drawer is used for money, eyeglasses, books, and other items.

The top shelf or middle drawer stores the wash basin. The wash basin holds personal care items—soap and soap dish, powder, lotion, deodorant, towels, washcloth, bath blanket, and sleepwear. An emesis basin or kidney basin (shaped like a kidney) holds oral hygiene items. The kidney basin is stored in the top drawer, middle drawer, or on the top shelf. The bedpan and its cover, the urinal, and toilet paper are stored on the lower shelf or in the bottom drawer.

The stand top is often used for tissues and other personal care items. A clock, photos, phone, flowers, cards, and gifts are examples. Some stands have a side or back rod for towels and washcloths.

Place only clean and sterile items on the bedside stand. Never place bedpans, urinals, or soiled linen on the top of the stand. Clean the bedside stand after use as a work surface.

Chairs

The person's unit has at least 1 chair (see Fig. 20-1). It must be comfortable, sturdy, and not move or tip during transfers. The person should be able to get in and out of the chair with ease. It should not be too low or too soft. Nursing center residents may bring chairs from home. Some agencies provide bariatric chairs. Bariatric chairs are wider and have expanded capacity.

Privacy Curtains

The person's unit has a privacy curtain extending around the bed. The curtain is pulled around the bed to provide privacy for the person (Chapter 2). Rooms with more than 1 bed have a privacy curtain between the units. *Always pull the curtain completely around the bed before giving care.*

Privacy curtains prevent others from seeing the person. They do not block sounds or voices. Others in the room can hear sounds or talking behind the curtain.

See *Focus on Long-Term Care and Home Care: Privacy Curtains.*

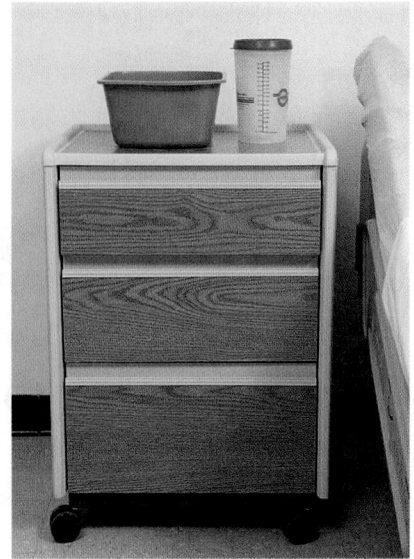

FIGURE 20-13 The bedside stand.

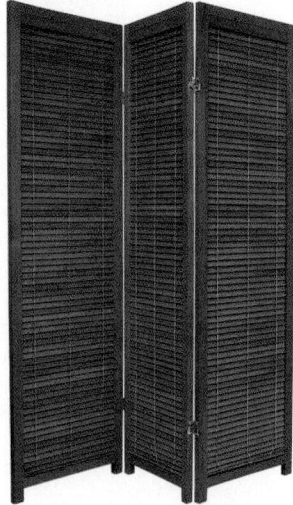

FIGURE 20-14 A portable screen provides privacy in the home. (Courtesy Oriental Furniture, Cambridge, Mass.)

Personal Care Items

Personal care items are used for hygiene and elimination. A bedpan and urinal are provided. The agency also provides a wash basin, kidney basin, water mug, and soap and soap dish (Fig. 20-15). Some provide powder, lotion, toothbrush, toothpaste, mouthwash, tissues, and a comb.

Some persons have their own oral hygiene equipment, hair care supplies, and deodorant. Some also prefer their own soap, lotion, and powder. Respect the person's choices in personal care products.

The Call System

When in their rooms, using the toilet, or in a bathing area, patients and residents must be able to contact staff at the nurses' station. The call system lets the person signal for help. The call light is at the end of a long cord (Fig. 20-16). It attaches to the bed or chair. (See p. 315 for call lights in bathrooms and shower and tub rooms.) *Always keep the call light within the person's reach—in the room, bathroom, and shower or tub room.*

To get help, the person presses a button at the end of a call light. The call light connects to a light above the room door (Fig. 20-17). The call light also connects to a computer, light panel, or intercom system at the nurses' station. These tell the staff that the person needs help. The staff member shuts off the light at the bedside when responding to the call for help.

An intercom system lets the staff talk with the person from the nurses' station. The person tells what is needed. Hard-of-hearing persons may have problems using an intercom. Remember confidentiality. When using an intercom, persons nearby can over-hear what is said.

Some call lights are turned on by tapping with a hand or fist (Fig. 20-18, p. 314). They are useful for persons with limited hand movement.

Some people cannot use call lights. Examples are persons who are confused or in a coma. The care plan lists special communication measures. Check these persons often. Make sure their needs are met.

See *Focus on Communication: The Call System*, p. 314.

See *Focus on Long-Term Care and Home Care: The Call System*, p. 314.

See *Teamwork and Time Management: The Call System*, p. 314.

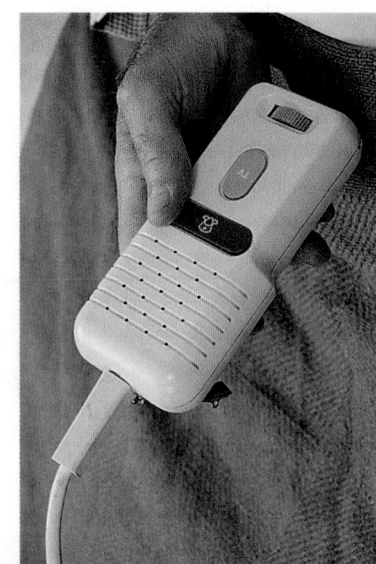
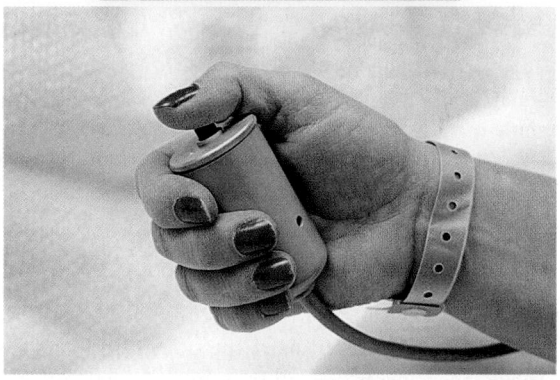

FIGURE 20-16 The call light. The call light button is pressed when help is needed. (NOTE: There are different types of call lights.)

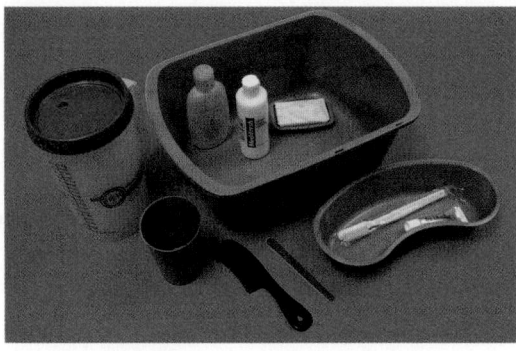

FIGURE 20-15 Personal care items.

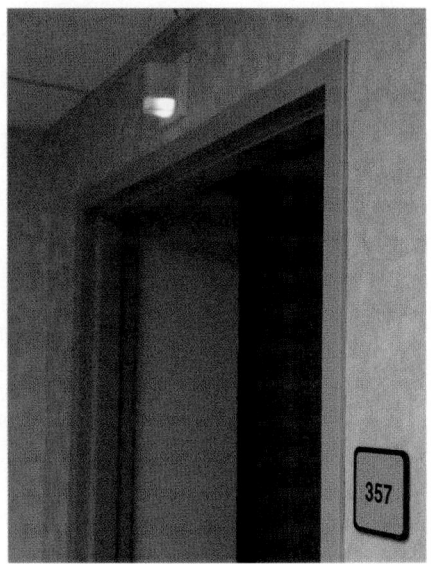

FIGURE 20-17 Light above the room door.

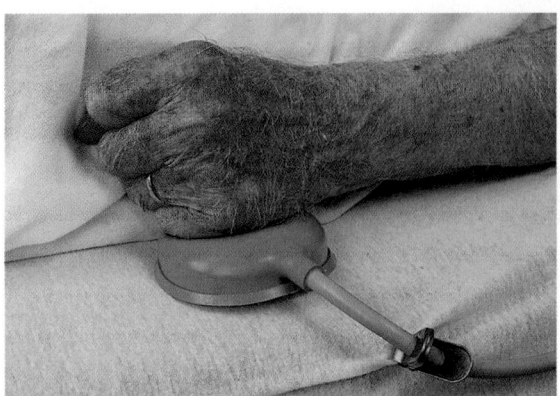

FIGURE 20-18 Call light for a person with limited hand movement.

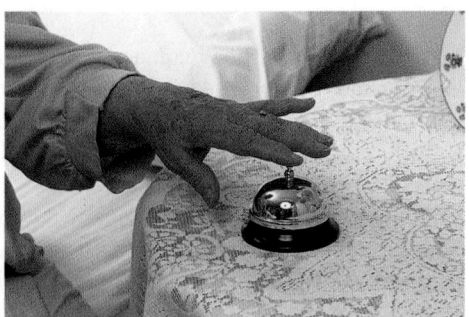

A

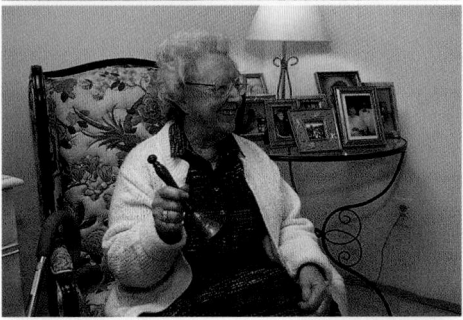

B

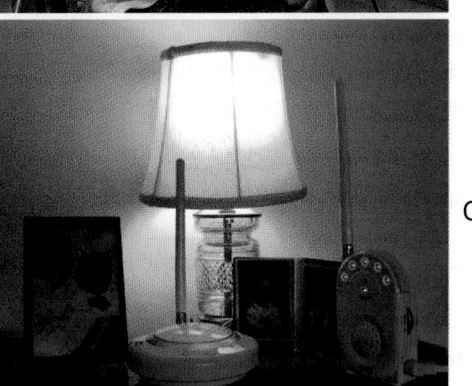

C

FIGURE 20-19 A, Tap bell. **B,** Dinner bell. **C,** Baby monitor.

FOCUS ON COMMUNICATION

The Call System

You will answer call lights for co-workers. You may not know their patients and residents and they may not know you. To promote quality of life and safe care, you can say:

- "My name is Kate Hines. I'm a nursing assistant. How can I help you?"
- "Mrs. Janz, I need to check your care plan before bringing you more salt. I'll be right back. Is there anything else I can do before I leave?"
- "Mr. Duncan, I am happy to take your meal tray. I'll tell your nursing assistant what you ate."
- "Mrs. Palmer, do you use the bathroom or the bedpan?"

Sometimes patients and residents signal for help often. Do not delay in meeting their needs. Never take call lights away from them. This is not safe. Avoid statements that make a person feel as if he or she is a burden. For example, do not say:

- "I just helped you to the bathroom. Can't you wait?"
- "I was just in your room. What do you want now?"

Do not discourage the person from asking for help. The person may try to do something alone. This could cause injury. Tell the nurse. Your co-workers can help you meet the person's needs.

FOCUS ON LONG-TERM CARE AND HOME CARE

The Call System

Home Care

Some home care patients stay in bed or in a certain part of the home. They need a way to call for help. Tap bells, dinner bells, baby monitors, and other devices are useful (Fig. 20-19). Or you can give the person a small can with a few coins inside. Children's toys with bells, horns, and whistles may be useful.

TEAMWORK AND TIME MANAGEMENT

The Call System

Patients and residents use their call lights when they need help. A person may put on a call light when you are with another person. The same may happen to other staff. If staff answer call lights for each other, lights are answered promptly. Patients and residents receive quality care. Everyone is responsible for answering call lights even if not assigned to the person.

Call System Safety. The phrase "call light" is used in this book when referring to the call system. You must:

- Keep the call light within the person's reach. Even if the person cannot use the call light, keep it within reach for use by visitors and staff. They may need to call for help.
- Place the call light on the person's strong side.
- Remind the person to signal when help is needed.
- Answer call lights promptly. For example, the person may have an urgent need to use the bathroom. Promptly helping the person to the bathroom prevents embarrassing problems. You also help prevent infection, skin breakdown, pressure ulcers, and falls.
- Answer bathroom and shower or tub room call lights at once.

The Bathroom

A toilet, sink, call system, and mirror are standard equipment in bathrooms (Fig. 20-20). Some bathrooms have showers.

Grab bars are by the toilet for safety. The person uses them for support to get on and off the toilet. Some bathrooms have higher toilets or raised toilet seats. They make wheelchair transfers easier and are helpful for persons with joint problems.

Towel racks, toilet paper, soap, paper towel dispenser, and a wastebasket are in the bathroom. They are within reach of the person.

The call light is a button or pull cord next to the toilet. The bathroom call light flashes red above the room door and at the nurses' station. To alert the staff of bathroom use, the sound at the nurses' station is different from the call light in rooms. Someone must respond at once when a person needs help in the bathroom.

Closet and Drawer Space

Closet and drawer space are provided. OBRA and the CMS require that nursing centers provide each person with closet space with shelves and a clothes rack (Fig. 20-21). The person must have free access to the closet and its contents.

Sometimes people hoard items—drugs, napkins, straws, food, sugar, salt, pepper, and so on. Hoarding can cause safety or health risks. The staff can inspect a person's closet or drawers if hoarding is suspected. The person is informed of the inspection. He or she is present when it takes place.

See *Promoting Safety and Comfort: Closet and Drawer Space.*

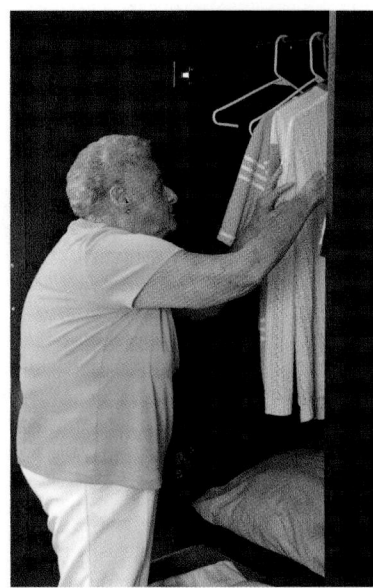

FIGURE 20-21 The resident can reach items in her closet.

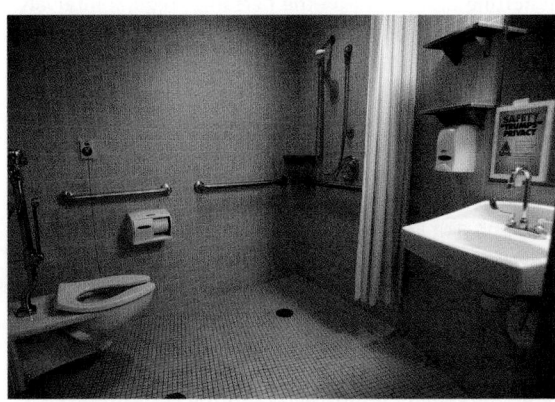

FIGURE 20-20 Bathroom in a person's room.

PROMOTING SAFETY AND COMFORT

Closet and Drawer Space

Safety

Items in closets and drawers are the person's property. You must have the person's permission to open or search closets or drawers.

The nurse may ask you to inspect a person's closet, drawers, or personal items. If so, the person must be present. Also have a co-worker with you to serve as a witness. This protects you if the person claims that something was stolen or damaged.

Other Equipment

Many agencies furnish rooms with other equipment. A TV, radio, and clock provide comfort and relaxation. Many rooms have phones, a computer, and Internet access.

Blood pressure equipment is often mounted on walls. There also are wall outlets for oxygen and suction (Fig. 20-22). Oxygen equipment and portable suction equipment are common in nursing centers and home care settings. For intravenous (IV) infusions, an IV pole (IV standard) is used to hang IV bags or feeding bags.

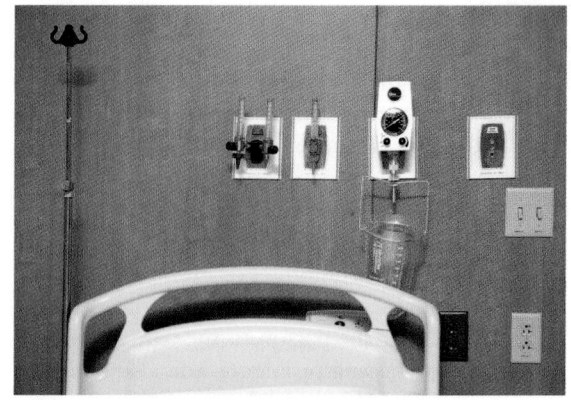

FIGURE 20-22 This room has an IV rod and oxygen and suction outlets.

FOCUS ON **PRIDE**

The Person, Family, and Yourself

Personal and Professional Responsibility

Loud talking and laughter in hallways and at the nurses' station are common. Patients, residents, and visitors over-hear this noise. They may think the staff are not working. Or they may think the staff are talking about or laughing at them. Some may be irritated or upset. Some may be anxious, uncomfortable, or angry.

Reducing noise requires cooperation from all staff. It is not your responsibility alone. But you can help. Do your part to reduce noise. Politely remind others to speak softly if needed. Take pride in providing patients and residents with a quiet and comfortable setting.

Rights and Respect

Nursing center residents have left their homes. Now the person lives in a strange place. He or she may have a roommate. Leaving one's home is a hard part of growing old with poor health.

Nursing center residents have the right to make their units as home-like as possible. Some bring personal items from home. Photos, TVs, radios, books, religious items, and plants are examples. A chair, footstool, lamp, and small table are often allowed.

Allow personal choice when arranging items. When helping the person choose the best places for items, make sure the person's choices:
- Are safe.
- Will not cause falls or other accidents.
- Do not interfere with the rights of others.

The center is the person's home. A home-like setting is important for quality of life.

Independence and Social Interaction

People want to be independent. They do not want to rely on others for simple, everyday things. Often accidents and injuries occur when the person tries to get needed items. The person has to reach too far and falls. Or he or she tries to get up without help.

The location of items in the person's unit can help prevent injuries. To promote independence and safety:
- Keep needed personal items within reach.
- Place assistive devices nearby. Walkers and canes are examples.
- Place the call light within the person's reach. Answer call lights and tend to the person's needs promptly.

Delegation and Teamwork

Some nursing units check on the person at regular intervals. For example, every hour nursing staff ask about the person's needs, positioning, comfort, and the placement of personal items. The person's needs are addressed and the person is reminded that a staff member will return in 1 hour. Nursing staff sign a form each time. The person may still use the call light for urgent needs. Non-urgent needs are met when staff return at the scheduled time. The process is explained to the person upon admission.

Some nursing units rotate assigned check times among team members. For example, a nurse checks the person on the even hours and a nursing assistant does so on the odd hours. The team works together to meet the person's needs. If your unit uses this practice:
- Be prompt. Check on the person at the correct time.
- Be honest. Do not sign the form if you did not check on the person. Also, do not sign the form early.
- Have a good attitude. Do not complain. The agency has reasons for using this practice. The agency may be trying to improve care, decrease call light use, or help nurses with time management.

FOCUS ON **P R I D E**—cont'd

The Person, Family, and Yourself

E thics and Laws

This chapter focused on how objects and surroundings in the person's unit affect comfort and well-being. You are a part of that setting. You must help the person feel safe, secure, and comfortable. The following is an example of a nursing assistant who failed to do so.

A certified nursing assistant (CNA) worked at a nursing home in Arizona. In February 2002, she was counseled to improve on her poor attendance and for having negative outbursts. In August 2002, it was noted that she gave poor care.

- *Residents were not turned and/or briefs were not changed every 2 hours according to facility policy.*
- *She continued to have negative outbursts.*

Later, reports were made that she had failed to provide care and meet a resident's needs. It was reported to the Arizona State Board of Nursing that she abused a resident by failure to provide care and not meeting his needs.

- *The resident was described as alert, paralyzed, on a ventilator for chronic respiratory failure, and totally dependent for all needs.*
- *The CNA was in his room many times during the night. She did not provide the care he requested.*
- *The CNA placed his call light out of reach. He used his head to use the call light for assistance.*

In November 2003, the CNA was terminated from employment for resident abuse. The CNA was hired by another agency in December 2003. She worked there until March 2004. On March 17 she was counseled for:

- *Telling a resident that if she did not speak English she should back go to her country*
- *Being rough, rude, and verbally abusive to residents*
- *Refusing to work on a nursing unit "because all patients stink"*
- *Being critical and judgmental with new staff*
- *Leaving a resident to "pee in their britches" rather than helping him to the bathroom*
  Her employment was terminated on March 19, 2004.

E thics and Laws—cont'd

In January 2004, the Arizona State Board of Nursing sent the CNA a questionnaire. It was returned to the Board as undeliverable. The CNA failed to notify the Board of an address change within the 30 days required by law.

The Board revoked the CNA's certificate for unprofessional conduct. She violated the following aspects of the state's Nurse Practice Act.

- *Conduct or practice that is or might be harmful or dangerous to the health of a patient or the public*
- *Failing to follow an employer's policies and procedures designed to safeguard the client*
- *Failing to respect client rights and dignity*
- *Neglecting or abusing a client physically, verbally, or financially*
- *Practice in any other manner that gives the Board reasonable cause to believe that the health of a client or the public may be harmed*
- *Failing to notify the board in writing within 30 days of any address change*
  (Arizona State Board of Nursing, 2006.)

Your words and actions are heard and seen by others. Bad conduct reduces quality of care and reflects poorly on you. You can lose your job and the ability to work as a nursing assistant. Always provide care in a way that promotes the person's comfort, safety, and quality of life.

FOCUS ON **PRIDE**: *Application*

What makes your living space comfortable and personal? How would this change if you lived in a nursing center? What would change in a hospital setting? Why is it important to provide privacy, safety, and comfort to persons in health care settings?

REVIEW QUESTIONS

Circle T if the statement is TRUE or F if it is FALSE.

1 **T F** The person's unit is considered private.

2 **T F** You should explain the cause of strange noises.

3 **T F** You can adjust the person's room temperature for your comfort.

4 **T F** Persons with dementia may have extreme reactions to strange sounds.

5 **T F** The privacy curtain prevents others from hearing conversations.

6 **T F** Soft, dim lighting is relaxing.

7 **T F** The call light must always be within the person's reach.

8 **T F** The over-bed table and bedside stand should be within the person's reach.

9 **T F** You can look through a person's closet and drawers.

10 **T F** The person must be able to reach items in the closet.

Circle the BEST answer.

11 To maintain the person's unit
   a Throw away items that do not look important
   b Remove cards from the bedside stand
   c Place personal items as you choose
   d Straighten bed linens as needed

12 Which temperature range is required by OBRA and the CMS?
   a 61°F to 68°F
   b 68°F to 74°F
   c 71°F to 81°F
   d 76°F to 82°F

13 To protect a person from drafts
   a Adjust the room temperature to 70°F
   b Provide a bath blanket during a bed bath
   c Dress the person in light-weight clothing
   d Position the person near a fan

14 To prevent odors
   a Place flowers in the room
   b Empty commodes at the end of your shift
   c Keep laundry containers open
   d Clean persons who are wet or soiled

15 To control noise
   a Answer phones after the third ring
   b Use the intercom system when possible
   c Handle equipment carefully
   d Talk with others in the hallway

16 Beds are raised horizontally to
   a Prevent bending and reaching when giving care
   b Promote the person's comfort
   c Raise the head of the bed
   d Lock the bed in position

17 The head of the bed is raised 30 degrees. This is called
   a Fowler's position
   b Semi-Fowler's position
   c Trendelenburg's position
   d Reverse Trendelenburg's position

18 Bed safety involves
   a Monitoring older and confused persons closely for entrapment
   b Removing the entrapment zones from the bed
   c Leaving the bed in the highest horizontal position
   d Restraining persons at risk for entrapment

19 Which statement about hospital bed system entrapment is *true*?
   a Bed rails present the only risk for entrapment.
   b Serious injury and death can occur.
   c A person must be small in size for entrapment to occur.
   d There are 3 entrapment zones.

20 The over-bed table is *not* used
   a For eating
   b As a working surface
   c For the urinal
   d To store shaving items

21 The bedpan is stored
   a In the closet
   b In the bedside stand
   c On the over-bed table
   d Under the bed

22 Call lights are answered
   a When you have time
   b At the end of your shift
   c Promptly
   d When you are near the person's room

Answers to Chapter 20 questions are on p. 871.

FOCUS ON PRACTICE

Problem Solving

A resident uses his call light often. Some needs are urgent. Others are not. Since your shift began, he has called for help 15 times. You just left his room and are helping another resident with her bedtime routine. His call light signals. What do you do?

The resident uses his call light more often at night, after family visits, and when he is not checked on regularly. How might this information be helpful for the nurse in care planning?

Bedmaking

Beds are made every day. Clean, dry, and wrinkle-free beds:
- Promote comfort.
- Prevent skin breakdown.
- Prevent pressure ulcers (Chapter 37).

Beds are usually made in the morning after baths. Or they are made while the person is in the shower, up in the chair, or out of the room. To keep beds neat and clean:
- Change linens when they are wet, soiled, or damp.
- Straighten linens whenever loose or wrinkled and at bedtime.
- Check for and remove food and crumbs after meals and snacks.
- Check linens for dentures, eyeglasses, hearing aids, sharp objects, and other items.
- Follow Standard Precautions and the Bloodborne Pathogen Standard. Contact with blood, body fluids, secretions, and excretions is likely.

TYPES OF BEDS

Beds are made in these ways.
- A *closed bed* is not in use. Top linens are not folded back (Fig. 21-1, p. 320). The bed is ready for a new patient or resident. In nursing centers, closed beds are made for residents who are up during the day.
- An *open bed* is in use. Top linens are fan-folded back so the person can get into bed. A closed bed becomes an open bed by fan-folding back the top linens (Fig. 21-2, p. 320).
- An *occupied bed* is made with the person in it (Fig. 21-3, p. 320).
- A *surgical bed* is made to transfer a person from a stretcher to bed (Fig. 21-4, p. 320). This includes an ambulance stretcher.

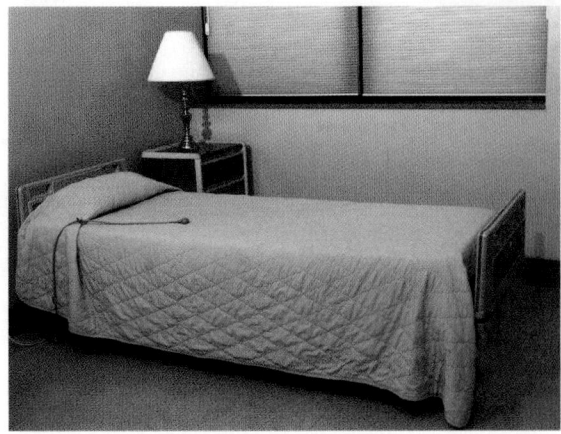

FIGURE 21-1 Closed bed.

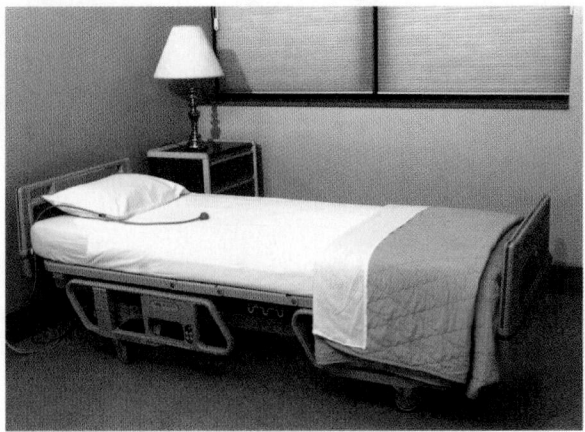

FIGURE 21-2 Open bed. Top linens are fan-folded to the foot of the bed.

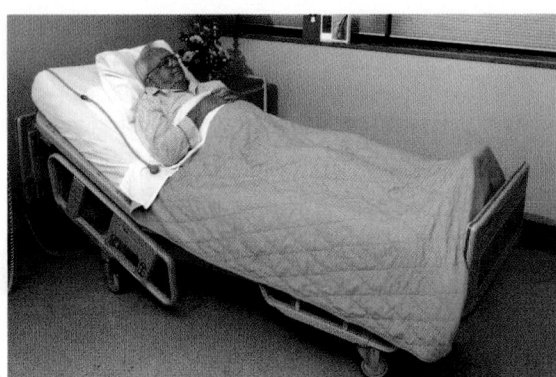

FIGURE 21-3 Occupied bed.

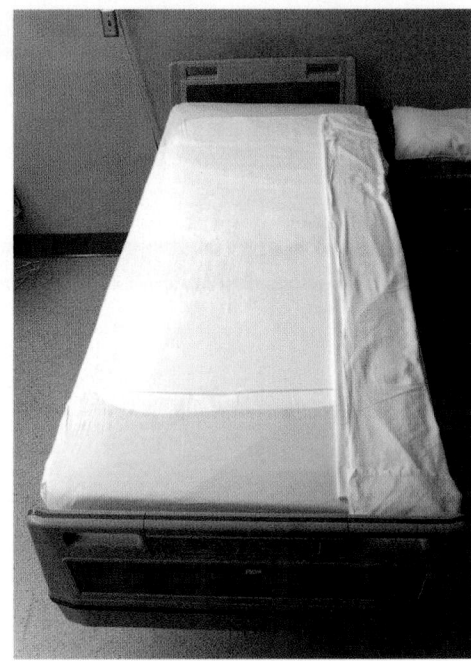

FIGURE 21-4 Surgical bed.

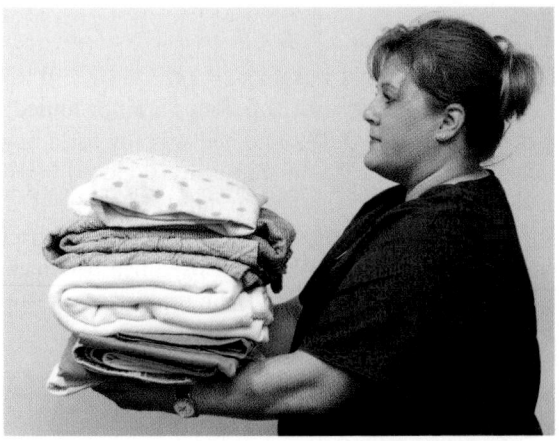

FIGURE 21-5 Hold linens away from your body and uniform.

LINENS

When handling linens and making beds, practice medical asepsis. Your uniform is considered *dirty*. Always hold linens away from your body and uniform (Fig. 21-5). Never shake linens. Shaking them spreads microbes. Place clean linens on a clean surface. Never put clean or used linens on the floor.

Collect enough linens. If the person has 2 pillows, get 2 pillowcases. The person may need extra blankets for warmth. Do not bring unneeded linens to a person's room. Once in the person's room, extra linens are considered contaminated. Do not use them for another person.

Collect linens in the order you will use them. That way you avoid fumbling with linens to find the piece you need. Linens stay neat and clean in your pile. You will use bed linens in the following order.

- Mattress pad (if needed)
- Bottom sheet (flat or fitted)
- Cotton or padded waterproof drawsheet (if needed)
- Waterproof under-pad (if needed)
- Top sheet
- Blanket
- Bedspread
- Pillowcase(s)

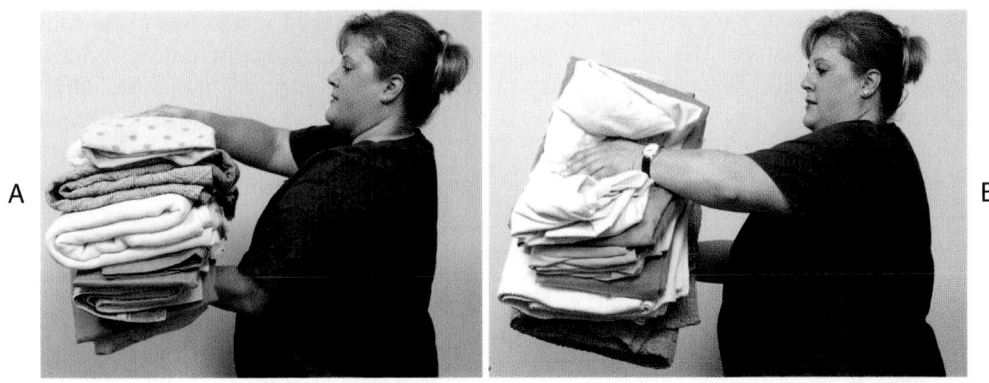

FIGURE 21-6 Collecting linens. Linens are held away from the body and uniform. **A,** The arm is placed over the top of the stack of linens. **B,** The stack of linens is turned onto the arm.

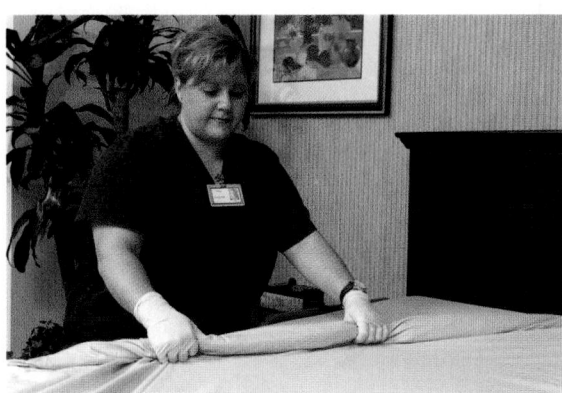

FIGURE 21-7 Roll used linens away from you.

You may also need:
- Bath towel(s)
- Hand towel
- Washcloth
- Gown or pajamas
- Bath blanket

Use 1 arm to hold the linens. Use your other hand to pick them up. The first item you will use is at the bottom of the stack. To get it on top, place your arm over the stack. Then turn the stack over onto the other arm (Fig. 21-6). The first item you will use is now on top. Place the clean linens on a clean surface.

Remove used linens 1 piece at a time. Roll each piece away from you. The side that touched the person is inside the roll and away from you (Fig. 21-7). Discard each piece into a laundry bag.

In hospitals, top and bottom sheets, the drawsheet, waterproof under-pad (if used), and pillowcases are changed daily. If still clean, the mattress pad, blanket, and bedspread are re-used for the same person. They are not re-used if soiled, wet, or wrinkled. Change wet, damp, or soiled linens right away. Wear gloves and follow Standard Precautions and the Bloodborne Pathogen Standard.

See *Focus on Long-Term Care and Home Care: Linens.*
See *Focus on Surveys: Linens.*

FOCUS ON LONG-TERM CARE AND HOME CARE

Linens

Long-Term Care
In nursing centers, linens are not changed every day. A complete linen change is usually done on the person's bath or shower day. This may be 1 or 2 times a week. Pillowcases, top and bottom sheets, and drawsheets (if used) are changed twice a week. Linens are always changed if wet, damp, soiled, or very wrinkled.

Some residents bring bedspreads, pillows, sheets, blankets, quilts, or afghans from home. Use them to make the bed. These items are the person's property. The items must be labeled with the person's name. This prevents loss or confusion with another person's property.

Some centers have colored or printed linens. If so, let the person choose what color to use. Also let him or her decide how many pillows or blankets to use. If possible, the person chooses the time when you make the bed. The resident has the right to personal choice.

Home Care
Linen changes in the home are usually done 1 or 2 times a week. Follow the person's routine. Change linens more often if the person asks you to do so. Always change linens that are wet, damp, soiled, or very wrinkled. Contact the nurse if the person refuses to have linens changed.

FOCUS ON SURVEYS

Linens

Linens may contain blood, body fluids, secretions, or excretions. They may contain microbes. You must help prevent and control the spread of infection. Surveyors will observe:
- How you transport linens.
- If you practice hand hygiene after handling soiled or used linens.
- If you double-bag linens when the outside of the laundry bag is visibly contaminated or wet.
- If you bag contaminated linens where they are used. The person's room and the shower room are examples.

Drawsheets

A *drawsheet is a small sheet placed over the middle of the bottom sheet.* The drawsheet may have tuck tails for tucking the sheet under the mattress.

* A *cotton drawsheet is made of cotton. It helps keep the mattress and bottom linens clean* (Fig. 21-8, *A*).
* A *padded waterproof drawsheet is a drawsheet made of an absorbent top and waterproof bottom* (Fig. 21-8, *B*). *It protects the mattress and bottom linens from dampness and soiling.* The waterproof side is placed down, away from the person. The absorbent top is placed up, toward the person. Other waterproof drawsheets are disposable. They are discarded when wet, soiled, or wrinkled.

Many agencies use incontinence products (Chapter 24) to keep the person and linens dry. Waterproof under-pads or disposable bed protectors also are common (Fig. 21-8, *C and D*).

Plastic-covered mattresses cause some persons to perspire heavily, causing discomfort. A drawsheet reduces heat retention and absorbs moisture. Drawsheets are often used as assist devices to move and transfer persons in bed (Chapters 18 and 19). If used as an assist device, do not tuck the drawsheet in at the sides.

See *Focus on Long-Term Care and Home Care: Drawsheets.*

MAKING BEDS

Safety and medical asepsis are important for bedmaking. Follow the rules in Box 21-1.

See *Focus on Long-Term Care and Home Care: Making Beds.*

See *Delegation Guidelines: Making Beds.*

See *Promoting Safety and Comfort: Making Beds*, p. 324.

See *Teamwork and Time Management: Making Beds*, p. 324.

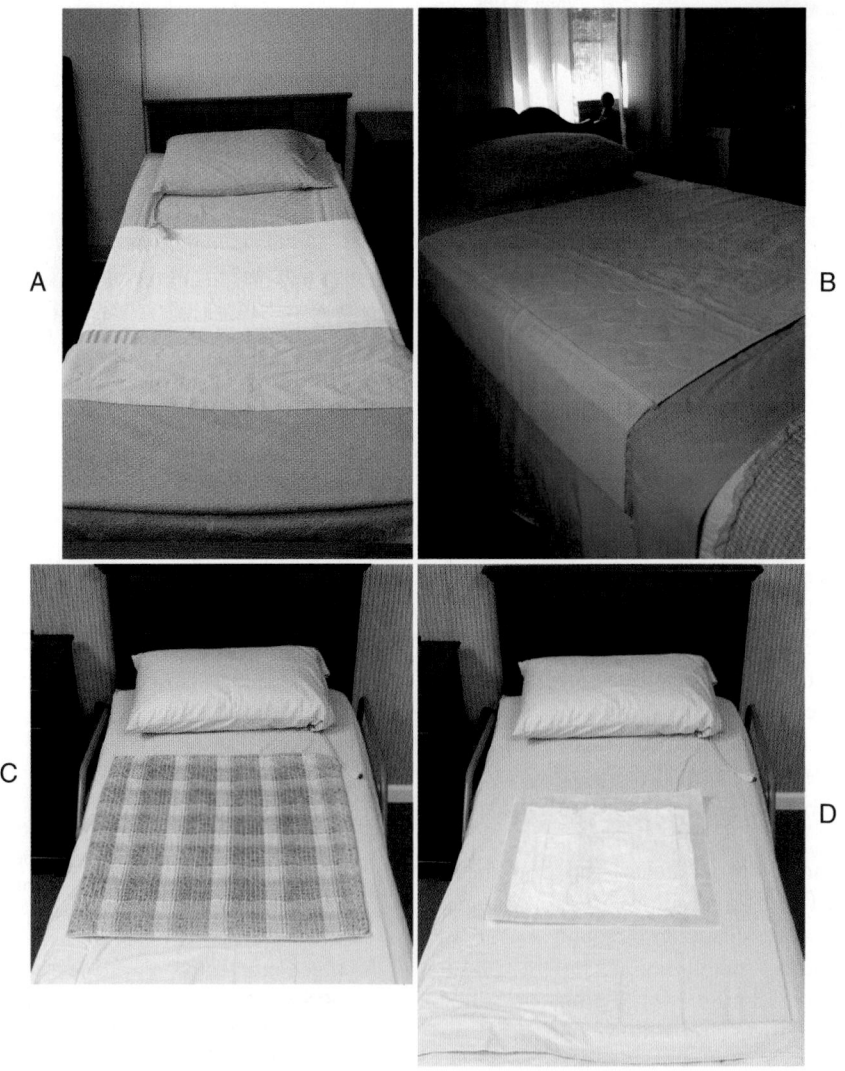

FIGURE 21-8 A, Cotton drawsheet. **B**, Padded waterproof drawsheet. **C**, Waterproof under-pad. **D**, Disposable bed protector.

FOCUS ON **LONG-TERM CARE AND HOME CARE**

Drawsheets

Home Care

A flat sheet folded in half can serve as a cotton drawsheet. A twin-sized sheet is easier to use for this purpose. The nurse tells you what to use.

Medical supply stores sell waterproof drawsheets and waterproof under-pads. The nurse discusses the need for these items with the person and family.

Some people use plastic mattress protectors. They protect mattresses but do not protect bottom linens (cotton drawsheet, bottom sheet, and mattress pad). Some people place plastic under the drawsheet. The nurse tells you what is safe for the person.

Do not use plastic trash bags or dry-cleaning bags. They are not strong enough to protect the linens and mattress. They slide easily and move out of place. Suffocation is a risk if the bag covers the person's nose and mouth.

FOCUS ON **LONG-TERM CARE AND HOME CARE**

Making Beds

Home Care

Some home care patients have hospital beds. Others do not. They have twin-, regular-, queen-, and king-sized beds. Water beds, sofa sleepers, cots, and recliners are common. Make the bed as the person wishes. Follow the rules in Box 21-1. If the person's wishes are not safe, tell the nurse.

Your assignment may include doing laundry. Wash linens when soiling is fresh to help prevent staining. Urine, feces, vomit, and blood can stain linens. Follow these guidelines.

- Wear gloves. Linens may contain blood, body fluids, secretions, or excretions.
- Rinse the item in cold water to remove the substance.
- Treat the stain. The person may use a stain-removing agent. Read and follow the manufacturer's instructions. Or follow the nurse's directions.
- Wash and dry linens as the person prefers.

BOX 21-1   Rules for Bedmaking

- Use good body mechanics at all times (Chapter 17).
- Follow the rules in Chapters 18 and 19 to safely move and transfer the person.
- Follow the rules of medical asepsis.
- Follow Standard Precautions and the Bloodborne Pathogen Standard.
- Practice hand hygiene before handling clean linens.
- Bring enough linens to the person's room. Do not bring extra linens.
- Bring only the linens that you will need. You cannot use extra linens for another person.
- Place clean linens on a clean surface. Use the bedside chair, over-bed table, or bedside stand. Place a barrier (towel, paper towel) between the clean surface and the linens if required by agency policy.
- Do not use extra linens in the person's room for another patient or resident. Extra linens are considered contaminated. Put them with the used laundry.
- Do not use torn or frayed linens.
- Never shake linens. Shaking spreads microbes.
- Hold linens away from your body and uniform. Do not let used or clean linens touch your uniform.
- Never put used linens on the floor or on clean linens. Follow agency policy for used linens.
- Bag used linens in the room where they are used. Do not carry used linens un-bagged outside of the person's room.
- Keep bottom linens tucked in and wrinkle-free.
- Straighten and tighten loose sheets, blankets, and bedspreads as needed.
- Make as much of 1 side of the bed as possible before going to the other side. This saves time and energy.
- Change wet, damp, or soiled linens right away.

DELEGATION GUIDELINES

Making Beds

Before making a bed, you need this information from the nurse and the care plan.

- What type of bed to make—closed, open, occupied, or surgical.
- If you need to use a cotton drawsheet or a padded waterproof drawsheet, waterproof under-pad, or incontinence product.
- If the person uses bed rails.
- The person's treatment, therapy, and activity schedule. For example, Mr. Smith needs a treatment in bed. Change linens after the treatment. Change Mrs. Chapman's bed while she is in physical therapy.
- Position restrictions or limits in the person's movement or activity.
- How to position the person and the positioning devices needed.
- If the bed needs to be locked into a certain position (Chapter 20).
- When to report observations.
- What patient or resident concerns to report at once.

PROMOTING SAFETY AND COMFORT
Making Beds

Safety

You need to raise the bed for body mechanics. The bed also must be as flat as possible. If the bed is locked, unlock it. Then adjust the bed. Return the bed to the correct position when you are done. Then lock the bed.

Wear gloves to remove linens from the person's bed. Also follow other aspects of Standard Precautions and the Bloodborne Pathogen Standard. Linens may contain blood, body fluids, secretions, or excretions.

After making a bed, lower the bed to the correct level for the person. Follow the care plan. For an occupied bed, raise or lower bed rails according to the care plan.

Comfort

For an occupied bed, cover the person with a bath blanket before removing the top sheet. Do not leave the person uncovered. The bath blanket provides warmth and privacy.

Adjust the person's pillow as needed during the procedure. After the procedure, position the person as directed by the nurse and the care plan. Always make sure linens are straight and wrinkle-free.

TEAMWORK AND TIME MANAGEMENT
Making Beds

Making beds with a co-worker is faster, easier, and safer for patients, residents, you, and your co-worker. Make 1 side of the bed while your co-worker makes the other. Always thank your co-worker for helping you. Also help your co-worker make beds when asked to do so.

The Closed Bed

Closed beds are made for:
- Nursing center residents and home care patients who are up for most or all of the day. Top linens are folded back at bedtime. Clean linens are used as needed.
- New patients and residents. The bed is made after the bed system (Chapter 20) is cleaned and disinfected. Clean linens are needed for the entire bed.
See procedure: *Making a Closed Bed.*

Text continued on p. 328.

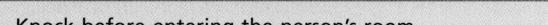

Making a Closed Bed

QUALITY OF LIFE

- Knock before entering the person's room.
- Address the person by name.
- Introduce yourself by name and title.

- Explain the procedure before starting and during the procedure.
- Protect the person's rights during the procedure.
- Handle the person gently during the procedure.

PRE-PROCEDURE

1 Follow *Delegation Guidelines: Making Beds,* p. 323. See *Promoting Safety and Comfort: Making Beds.*
2 Practice hand hygiene.
3 Collect clean linens.
- Mattress pad (if needed)
- Bottom sheet (flat sheet or fitted sheet)
- Cotton drawsheet or padded waterproof drawsheet (if needed)
- Waterproof under-pad (if needed)
- Top sheet
- Blanket
- Bedspread
- A pillowcase for each pillow

- Bath towel
- Hand towel
- Washcloth
- Gown or pajamas
- Bath blanket
- Gloves
- Laundry bag
- Paper towels (as a barrier for clean linens)

4 Place linens on a clean surface. Use the paper towels as a barrier between the clean surface and clean linens if required by agency policy.
5 Raise the bed for body mechanics. Bed rails are down.

PROCEDURE

6 Put on the gloves.
7 Remove linens. Roll each piece away from you. Place each piece in a laundry bag. (NOTE: Discard the incontinence product, disposable bed protector, and disposable drawsheet in the trash. Do not put them in the laundry bag.)
8 Clean the bed frame and mattress (if this is your job).
9 Remove and discard the gloves. Practice hand hygiene.
10 Move the mattress to the head of the bed.
11 Put the mattress pad on the mattress. It is even with the top of the mattress.

12 Place the bottom sheet on the mattress pad (Fig. 21-9). Unfold it length-wise. Place the center crease in the middle of the bed. If using a flat sheet:
a Position the lower edge even with the bottom of the mattress.
b Place the large hem at the top and the small hem at the bottom.
c Face hem-stitching downward, away from the person.

Making a Closed Bed—cont'd

PROCEDURE—cont'd

13 Open the sheet. Fan-fold it to the other side of the bed (Fig. 21-10, p. 326).
14 Tuck the corners of a fitted sheet over the mattress at the top and then foot of the bed. For a flat sheet, tuck the top of the sheet under the mattress. The sheet is tight and smooth.
15 Make a mitered corner at the top if using a flat sheet (Fig. 21-11, p. 326).
16 Place the cotton drawsheet or padded waterproof drawsheet on the bed. It is in the middle of the mattress.
    a Open the drawsheet. Fan-fold it to the other side of the bed.
    b Tuck the drawsheet under the mattress.
17 Go to the other side of the bed.
18 Miter the top corner of the flat bottom sheet.
19 Pull the bottom sheet tight so there are no wrinkles. Tuck in the sheet.
20 Pull the drawsheet tight so there are no wrinkles. (Fig. 21-12, p. 326).
21 *If using a waterproof under-pad*, place the waterproof under-pad on the bed. It is in the middle of the mattress. See Figure 21-8, *C*.
22 Go to the other side of the bed.
23 Put the top sheet on the bed.
    a Unfold it length-wise. Place the center crease in the middle.
    b Place the large hem even with the top of the mattress.
    c Open the sheet. Fan-fold it to the other side.
    d Face hem-stitching outward, away from the person.
    e Do not tuck the bottom in yet.
    f Never tuck top linens in on the sides.

24 Place the blanket on the bed.
    a Unfold it so the center crease is in the middle.
    b Put the upper hem about 6 to 8 inches from the top of the mattress.
    c Open the blanket. Fan-fold it to the other side.
    d If steps 30 and 31 are not done, turn the top sheet down over the blanket. Hem-stitching is down, away from the person.
25 Place the bedspread on the bed.
    a Unfold it so the center crease is in the middle.
    b Place the upper hem even with the top of the mattress.
    c Open and fan-fold the bedspread to the other side.
    d Make sure the bedspread facing the door is even. It covers all top linens.
26 Tuck in top linens together at the foot of the bed so they are smooth and tight. Make a mitered corner. Leave the side of the top linens untucked.
27 Go to the other side.
28 Straighten all top linens. Work from the head of the bed to the foot.
29 Tuck in top linens together at the foot of the bed. Make a mitered corner. Leave the side of the top linens untucked.
30 Turn the top hem of the bedspread under the blanket to form a cuff (Fig. 21-13, p. 326).
31 Turn the top sheet down over the bedspread. Hem-stitching is down. (Steps 30 and 31 are not done in some agencies. The bedspread covers the pillow. If so, tuck the bedspread under the pillow.)
32 Put the pillowcase on the pillow as in Figure 21-14, p. 327 or Figure 21-15, p. 327. Fold extra material under the pillow at the seam end of the pillowcase.
33 Place the pillow on the bed. The open end of the pillowcase is away from the door. The seam is toward the head of the bed.

POST-PROCEDURE

34 Provide for comfort. (See the inside of the front cover.) NOTE: Omit this step if the bed is prepared for a new patient or resident.
35 Attach the call light to the bed. Or place it within the person's reach.
36 Lower the bed to a safe and comfortable level for the person. Follow the care plan. Lock (brake) the bed wheels.

37 Put the towels, washcloth, gown or pajamas, and bath blanket in the bedside stand.
38 Complete a safety check of the room. (See the inside of the front cover.)
39 Follow agency policy for used linens.
40 Practice hand hygiene.

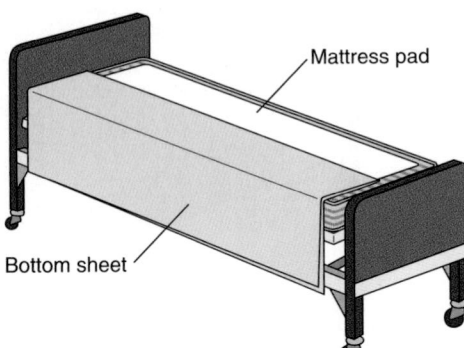

FIGURE 21-9 A flat bottom sheet is on the bed with the center crease in the middle. The lower edge of the sheet is even with the bottom of the mattress.

Mattress pad

Bottom sheet

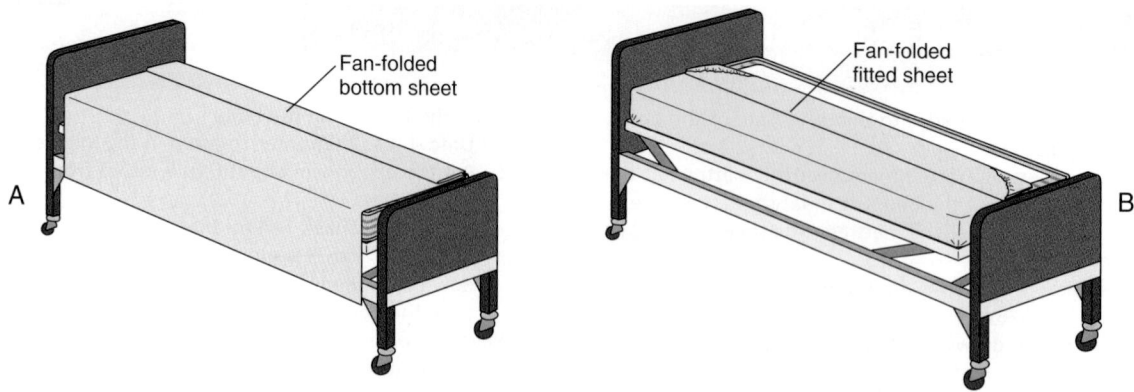

FIGURE 21-10 A, The flat bottom sheet is fan-folded to the other side of the bed. **B,** A fitted sheet is on the bed with the center crease in the middle.

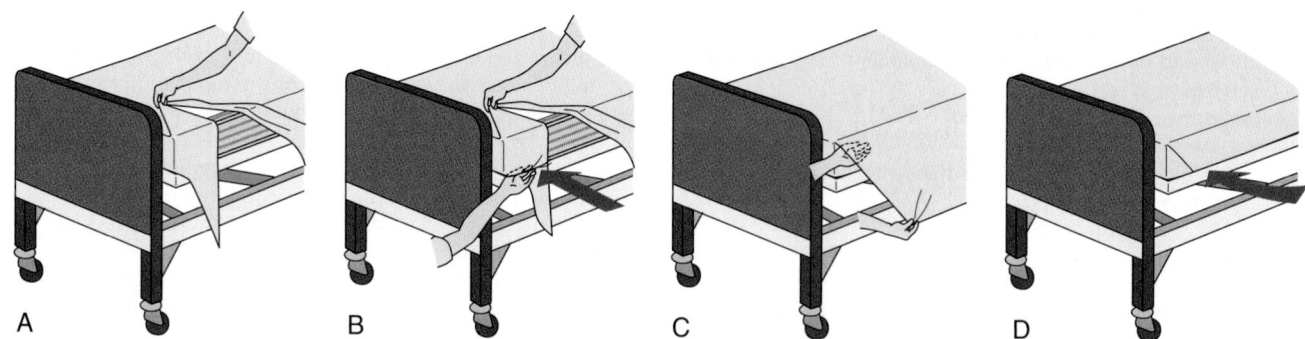

FIGURE 21-11 Making a mitered corner. A, The flat bottom sheet is tucked under the mattress at the head of the bed. The side of the sheet is raised onto the mattress. **B,** The remaining portion of the sheet is tucked under the mattress. **C,** The raised portion of the sheet is brought off the mattress. **D,** The entire side of the sheet is tucked under the mattress.

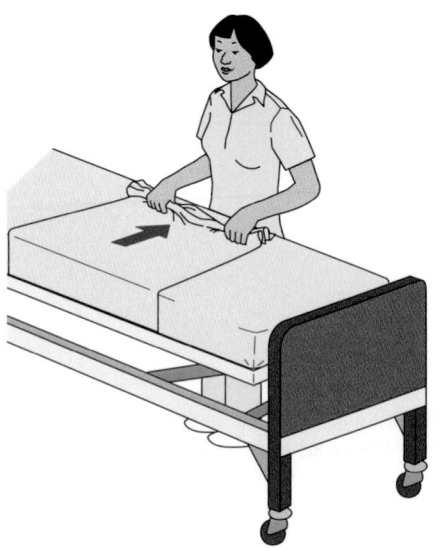

FIGURE 21-12 The drawsheet is pulled tight to remove wrinkles.

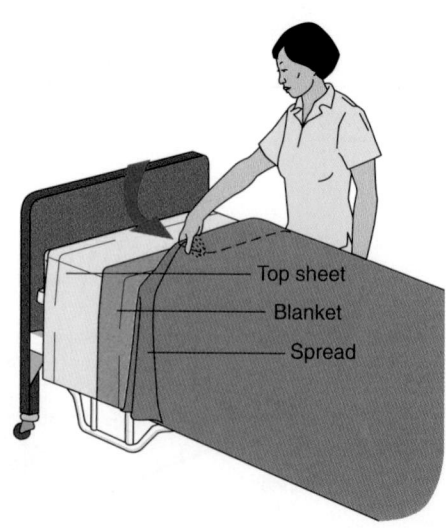

FIGURE 21-13 The top hem of the bedspread is turned under the top hem of the blanket to make a cuff.

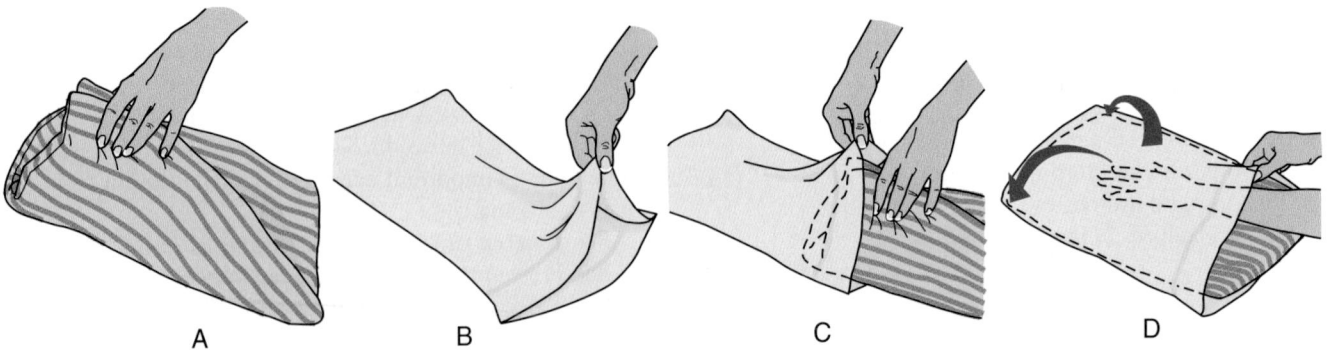

FIGURE 21-14 Putting a pillowcase on a pillow. A, Grasp the corners of the pillow at the seam end and form a "V" with the pillow. **B,** Open the pillowcase with your free hand. **C,** Guide the "V" end of the pillow into the pillowcase. **D,** Let the "V" end of the pillow fall into the corners of the pillowcase.

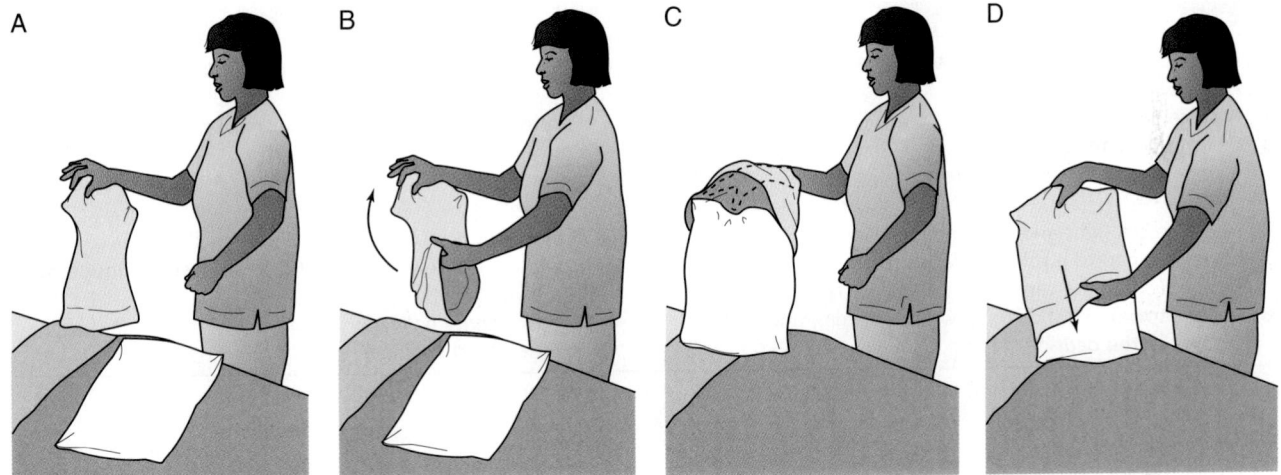

FIGURE 21-15 Putting a pillowcase on a pillow. A, Grasp the closed end of the pillowcase. **B,** Using your other hand, gather up the pillowcase. **C,** The pillowcase should cover your hand holding the closed end. Grasp the pillow with the hand covered by the pillowcase. **D,** Pull the pillowcase down over the pillow with your other hand.

The Open Bed

A closed bed becomes an open bed by fan-folding back the top linen. The person can get into bed with ease. Make this bed for:

- Newly admitted persons arriving by wheelchair
- Persons who are getting ready for bed
- Persons who are out of bed for a short time
  See procedure: *Making an Open Bed.*

The Occupied Bed

You make an occupied bed when the person stays in bed. Keep the person in good alignment. Follow restrictions or limits in the person's movement or position.

Explain each procedure step to the person before it is done. This is important even if the person cannot respond or is in a coma.

See *Focus on Communication: The Occupied Bed.*
See *Promoting Safety and Comfort: The Occupied Bed.*
See procedure: *Making an Occupied Bed.*

Making an Open Bed

QUALITY OF LIFE

- Knock before entering the person's room.
- Address the person by name.
- Introduce yourself by name and title.

- Explain the procedure before starting and during the procedure.
- Protect the person's rights during the procedure.
- Handle the person gently during the procedure.

PROCEDURE

1 Follow *Delegation Guidelines: Making Beds*, p. 323. See *Promoting Safety and Comfort: Making Beds*, p. 324.
2 Practice hand hygiene.
3 Collect linens for a closed bed (p. 324).

4 Make a closed bed. (See procedure: *Making a Closed Bed*, p. 324.)
5 Fan-fold top linens to the foot of the bed (see Fig. 21-2).

POST-PROCEDURE

6 Place the call light and other needed items within reach.
7 Lower the bed to a safe and comfortable level for the person. Follow the care plan.
8 Put the towels, washcloth, gown or pajamas, and bath blanket in the bedside stand.

9 Provide for comfort. (See the inside of the front cover.)
10 Complete a safety check of the room. (See the inside of the front cover.)
11 Follow agency policy for used linens.
12 Practice hand hygiene.

Making an Occupied Bed

QUALITY OF LIFE

- Knock before entering the person's room.
- Address the person by name.
- Introduce yourself by name and title.

- Explain the procedure before starting and during the procedure.
- Protect the person's rights during the procedure.
- Handle the person gently during the procedure.

PRE-PROCEDURE

1 Follow *Delegation Guidelines: Making Beds*, p. 323. See *Promoting Safety and Comfort:*
   a *Making Beds*, p. 324
   b *The Occupied Bed*
2 Practice hand hygiene.
3 Collect the following.
   - Gloves
   - Laundry bag
   - Clean linens (see procedure: *Making a Closed Bed*, p. 324)
   - Paper towels (as a barrier for clean linens)

4 Place linens on a clean surface. Use the paper towels as a barrier between the clean surface and clean linens if required by agency policy.
5 Identify the person. Check the ID (identification) bracelet against the assignment sheet. Use 2 identifiers (Chapter 13). Also call the person by name.
6 Provide for privacy.
7 Remove the call light.
8 Raise the bed for body mechanics. Bed rails are up if used. Bed wheels are locked (braked).
9 Lower the head of the bed. It is as flat as possible.

PROCEDURE

10 Practice hand hygiene. Put on gloves.
11 Loosen top linens at the foot of the bed.
12 Lower the bed rail near you if up.
13 Fold and remove the bedspread (Fig. 21-16, p. 330). Fold and remove the blanket the same way. Place each over the chair.
14 Cover the person with a bath blanket. Use the one in the bedside stand.
   a Unfold the bath blanket over the top sheet.
   b Ask the person to hold the bath blanket. If he or she cannot, tuck the top part under the person's shoulders.
   c Grasp the top sheet under the bath blanket at the shoulders. Bring the sheet down toward the foot of the bed. Remove the sheet from under the blanket (Fig. 21-17, p. 331).
15 Position the person on his or her side facing away from you. Adjust the pillow for comfort.
16 Loosen bottom linens from the head to the foot of the bed.
17 Fan-fold bottom linens 1 at a time toward the person. Start with the drawsheet (Fig. 21-18, p. 331). If re-using the mattress pad, do not fan-fold it.
18 Remove and discard the gloves. Practice hand hygiene. Put on clean gloves.
19 Place a clean mattress pad on the bed. Unfold it length-wise. The center crease is in the middle. Fan-fold the top part toward the person. If re-using the mattress pad, straighten and smooth any wrinkles.
20 Place the bottom sheet on the mattress pad. Hem-stitching is away from the person. Unfold the sheet so the crease is in the middle. If using a flat sheet, the small hem is even with the bottom of the mattress. Fan-fold the top part toward the person.
21 Tuck the corners of a fitted sheet over the mattress. If using a flat sheet, make a mitered corner at the head of the bed. Tuck the sheet under the mattress from the head to the foot.

22 *If using a drawsheet* (Fig. 21-19, p. 331):
   a Place the cotton drawsheet or padded waterproof drawsheet on the bed. It is in the middle of the mattress.
   b Open the drawsheet.
   c Fan-fold it toward the person.
   d Tuck in excess fabric.
23 *If using a waterproof under-pad:*
   a Place the waterproof under-pad on the bed. It is in the middle of the mattress.
   b Fan-fold it toward the person.
24 Explain to the person that he or she will roll over a "bump." Assure the person that he or she will not fall.
25 Help the person turn to the other side. Adjust the pillow for comfort.
26 Raise the bed rail. Go to the other side and lower the bed rail.
27 Loosen bottom linens. Remove 1 piece at a time. Place each piece in the laundry bag. (NOTE: Discard the disposable bed protector, incontinence product, and disposable drawsheet in the trash. Do not put them in the laundry bag.)
28 Remove and discard the gloves. Practice hand hygiene.
29 Straighten and smooth the mattress pad.
30 Pull the clean bottom sheet toward you. Tuck the corners of a fitted sheet over the mattress. If using a flat sheet, make a mitered corner at the top. Tuck the sheet under the mattress from the head to the foot of the bed.
31 Pull the drawsheet tightly toward you. Tuck in the drawsheet.
32 Position the person supine in the center of the bed. Adjust the pillow for comfort.
33 Put the top sheet on the bed. Unfold it length-wise. The crease is in the middle. The large hem is even with the top of the mattress. Hem-stitching is on the outside.
34 Ask the person to hold the top sheet so you can remove the bath blanket. Or tuck the top sheet under the person's shoulders. Remove the bath blanket. Place it in the laundry bag.

Continued

Making an Occupied Bed—cont'd

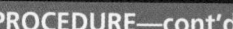

PROCEDURE—cont'd

35 Place the blanket on the bed. Unfold it so the crease is in the middle and it covers the person. The upper hem is 6 to 8 inches from the top of the mattress.

36 Place the bedspread on the bed. Unfold it so the center crease is in the middle and it covers the person. The top hem is even with the mattress top.

37 Turn the top hem of the bedspread under the blanket to make a cuff.

38 Bring the top sheet down over the bedspread to form a cuff.

39 Go to the foot of the bed.

40 Make a toe pleat. Make a 2-inch pleat across the foot of the bed. The pleat is about 6 to 8 inches from the foot of the bed.

41 Lift the mattress corner with 1 arm. Tuck all top linens under the bottom of the mattress. Make a mitered corner. Leave the side of the top linens untucked.

42 Raise the bed rail. Go to the other side and lower the bed rail.

43 Straighten and smooth top linens.

44 Tuck all top linens under the bottom of the mattress. Make a mitered corner. Leave the side of the top linens untucked.

45 Change the pillowcase(s).

POST-PROCEDURE

46 Provide for comfort. (See the inside of the front cover.)

47 Place the call light and other needed items within reach.

48 Lower the bed to a safe and comfortable level for the person. Follow the care plan. The bed wheels are locked (braked).

49 Raise or lower bed rails. Follow the care plan.

50 Put the clean towels, washcloth, gown or pajamas, and bath blanket in the bedside stand.

51 Unscreen the person.

52 Complete a safety check of the room. (See the inside of the front cover.)

53 Follow agency policy for used linens.

54 Practice hand hygiene.

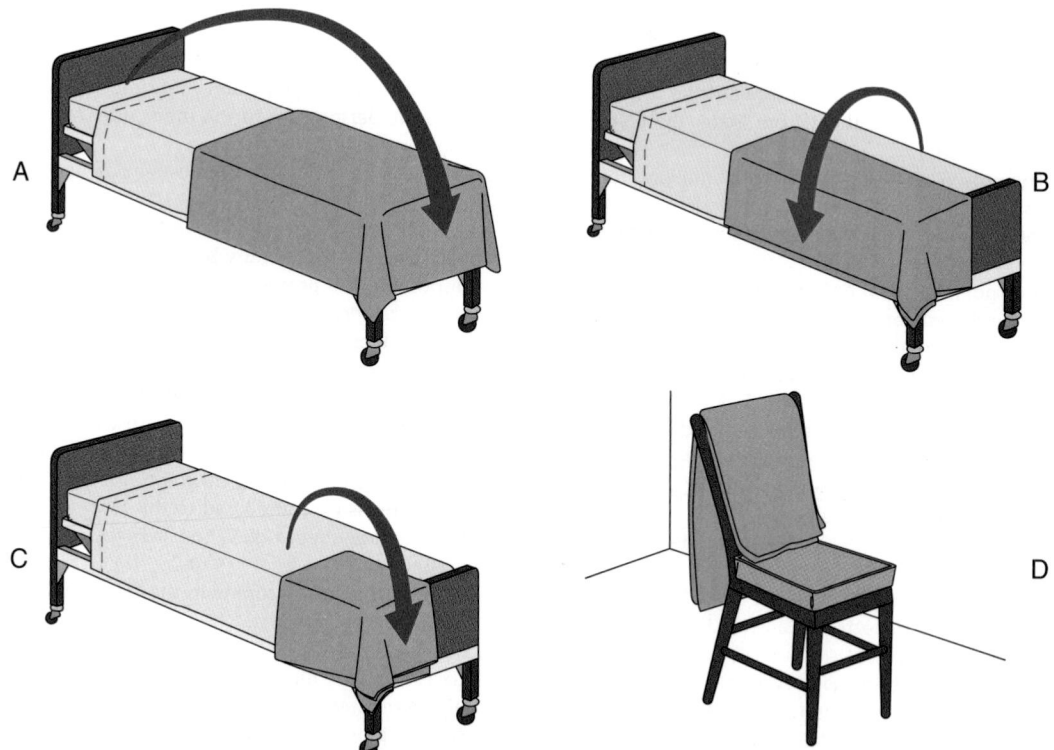

FIGURE 21-16 Folding linens for re-use. **A,** Fold the top edge of the bedspread down to the bottom edge. **B,** Fold the bedspread from the far side of the bed to the near side. **C,** Fold the top edge of the bedspread down to the bottom edge again. **D,** Place the folded bedspread over the back of the chair.

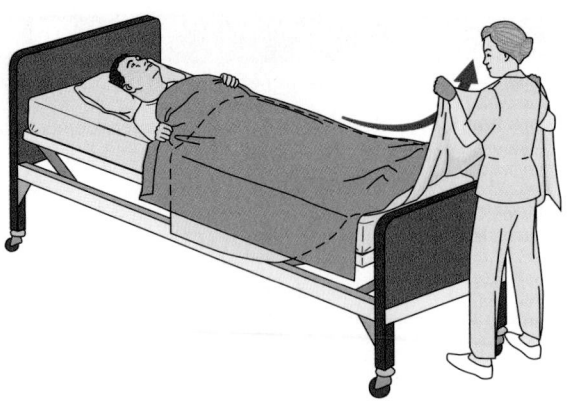

FIGURE 21-17 The person holds on to the bath blanket. The top sheet is removed from under the bath blanket. (NOTE: Bed rails are used according to the care plan.)

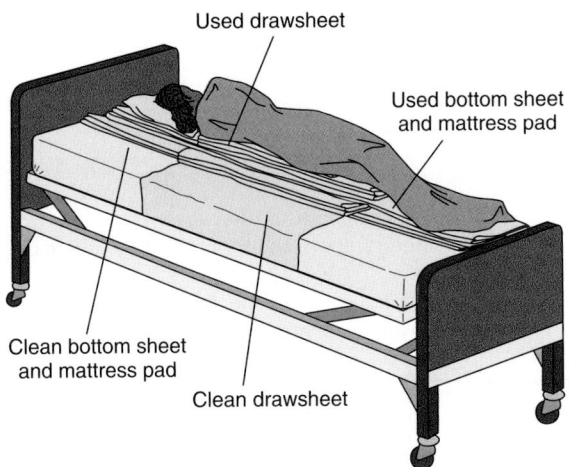

FIGURE 21-19 A clean bottom sheet and drawsheet are on the bed with both fan-folded and tucked under the person. (NOTE: Bed rails are used according to the care plan.)

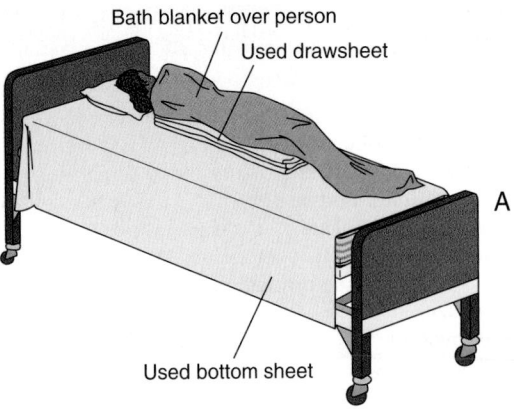

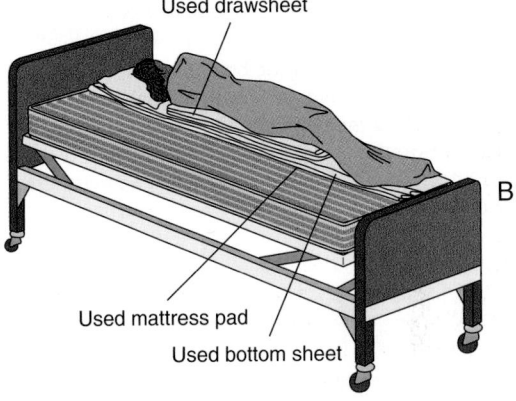

FIGURE 21-18 A, The drawsheet is fan-folded and tucked under the person. **B,** All bottom linens are tucked under the person. (NOTE: Bed rails are used according to the care plan.)

The Surgical Bed

The surgical bed also is called a *recovery bed* or *post-operative bed.* Top linens are folded to transfer the person from a stretcher to the bed. These beds are made for persons:

- Returning to their rooms from surgery. A complete linen change is needed.
- Who arrive at the agency by ambulance. A complete linen change is needed if the person:
  - Is a new patient or resident.
  - Is returning to the agency from the hospital.
- Who go by stretcher to treatment or therapy areas. A complete linen change is not needed.
- Using portable tubs (Chapter 22). Because of bathing, a complete linen change is needed.

See *Promoting Safety and Comfort: The Surgical Bed.*

See procedure: *Making a Surgical Bed,* p. 332.

PROMOTING SAFETY AND COMFORT

The Surgical Bed

Safety

Follow the rules for stretcher safety and the procedure: *Moving the Person to a Stretcher* in Chapter 19. After the transfer, lower the bed to a safe and comfortable level for the person. Lock (brake) the bed wheels. Raise or lower bed rails according to the care plan.

Making a Surgical Bed

PRE-PROCEDURE

1 Follow *Delegation Guidelines: Making Beds*, p. 323. See *Promoting Safety and Comfort*:
   a *Making Beds*, p. 324
   b *The Surgical Bed*, p. 331
2 Practice hand hygiene.
3 Collect the following.
   • Clean linens (see procedure: *Making a Closed Bed*, p. 324)
   • Gloves
   • Laundry bag
   • Equipment requested by the nurse
   • Paper towels (as a barrier for clean linens)

4 Place linens on a clean surface. Use the paper towels as a barrier between the clean surface and clean linens if required by agency policy.
5 Remove the call light.
6 Raise the bed for body mechanics.

PROCEDURE

7 Remove all linens from the bed. Place them in the laundry bag. Wear gloves. Practice hand hygiene after removing and discarding them.
8 Make a closed bed (see procedure: *Making a Closed Bed*, p. 324). Do not tuck top linens under the mattress.
9 Fold all top linens at the foot of the bed back onto the bed. The fold is even with the edge of the mattress (Fig. 21-20, *A*).

10 Know on which side of the bed the stretcher will be placed. Fan-fold linens length-wise to the other side of the bed (Fig. 21-20, *B*).
11 Put a pillowcase on each pillow.
12 Place the pillow(s) on a clean surface.

POST-PROCEDURE

13 Leave the bed in its highest position.
14 Leave both bed rails down.
15 Put the clean towels, washcloth, gown or pajamas, and bath blanket in the bedside stand.
16 Move furniture away from the bed. Allow room for the stretcher and the staff.

17 Do not attach the call light to the bed.
18 Complete a safety check of the room. (See the inside of the front cover.)
19 Follow agency policy for used linens.
20 Practice hand hygiene.

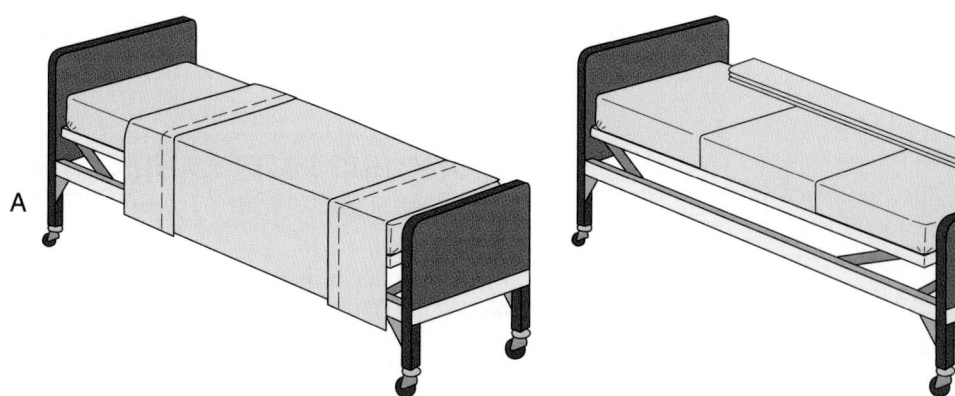

FIGURE 21-20 Surgical bed. A, The bottom of the top linens is folded back onto the bed. The fold is even with the bottom edge of the mattress. **B,** Top linens are fan-folded length-wise to the side of the bed. (NOTE: Bed rails are used according to the care plan.)

FOCUS ON PRIDE

The Person, Family, and Yourself

Personal and Professional Responsibility

The bed is the largest item in the person's room. The person, family, and visitors notice if the bed is unmade, messy, or dirty. They question the quality of care.

You are responsible for providing a neat and orderly setting. The bed must be clean and well made. If the person stays in bed, straighten and tighten linens as needed. These actions promote comfort and quality of life.

Rights and Respect

Nursing center residents have the right to make their settings as home-like as possible. Residents often bring bedspreads, blankets, quilts, and so on from home. The items have meaning and value. For example, Mr. Baker wants the afghan on his bed at night. His wife made it years ago. Mr. Baker moved into the nursing home after his wife died. The sight and smell of the afghan remind him of his wife and home.

Protect personal items from loss and damage. Handle the person's belongings with care and respect.

Independence and Social Interaction

Allow personal choice when possible. What is best for you may not be best for the person. For example, you planned to make Mrs. Beck's bed and straighten her room after breakfast. However, her family comes to visit then. Mrs. Beck wants her bed made during breakfast.

Ask about the person's preferences. Consider them when planning your day and managing your time. The more choices are allowed, the greater the person's sense of control and independence.

Delegation and Teamwork

Agencies have different ways of handling used linens. Some have containers in each room. Others have carts in the hallways. The carts are emptied each shift or as needed. Some agencies have a room where used linens are placed. Others have chutes.

When handling used linens:

* Wear gloves.
* Follow agency policy for used linens.
* Do not over-fill the bag or container. The person emptying the bag or cart may be injured.
* Work as a team. Some units assign a person to empty linen containers. Linens must not over-flow carts. If you see a full cart, empty it. Do so without complaining. The person assigned the task may be busy. If no one is assigned the task, work together to complete it.
* Clean up after yourself. If you fill a cart, empty it. If you place an item in a cart that will cause an odor, empty it.
* Place used linens in the correct location. Do not place used linens in a room or cart where they do not belong. If chutes are used, use the correct chute. Other chutes may be for trash.

Ethics and Laws

Always treat patients and residents with dignity, care, and kindness. In the following real event, the nurse ignored these values.

On August 2, 1990, a patient had back surgery. She was on complete bedrest until August 4 when the doctor changed the order. The new order was "increase activity up as tolerated with assist." According to the facts reported in the court case, the following occurred between the patient and a nurse.

* *On August 5 the patient woke up when the nurse bumped into her bed. The nurse told the patient that she had to get up and have her bed made. Despite pleas to stay in bed, the nurse said that she [the nurse] had to make the bed.*
* *The nurse then pulled the patient by her arm. The patient pleaded to be left alone. The patient said that it hurt to have her arm pulled that way. The nurse let go of the patient's arm. The patient lay down in bed.*
* *The nurse then pulled the patient's feet off the bed. In extreme pain, the patient "started to yell, to plead with the nurse not to do what she was doing and told her that it hurt."*
* *The nurse insisted that the patient had to get up. The nurse insisted that she had to make the bed. The nurse forced the patient into a standing position. The patient, in pain, told the nurse that she was going to "throw up or faint."*
* *The nurse shoved the patient "into a straight back chair using her hands to press down hard on the [patient's] shoulders."*
* *In extreme pain, the patient pleaded with the nurse and said that she was going to faint.*
* *The nurse then forced the patient's head between her knees down to her lap. The patient felt extreme pain in the middle of her back.*
* *The nurse raised the patient's back. In extreme pain, the patient could not get up when she had to do so. The patient continued to plead to be put back to bed.*
* *The nurse again told the patient that she had to make the bed. The nurse "ripped the sheet off the bed and used it to tie [the patient] to the chair with a knot towards the back."*
* *The patient "tried to reach forward to push the nurse's call button ... [The nurse] kicked and pushed the table out at the same time, away and out of the [patient's] grasp." The patient said that she wanted to call a nurse.*
* *The nurse left the room for 10 minutes. "She came back and made the bed with a laboratory technician." After making the bed, they put the patient back in bed. The patient was crying.*

The Appellate Court of Illinois, in reviewing the case, said the "negligence here was ... grossly apparent ..." The case was sent back to the trial court for a full trial.

(R. Prairie v University of Chicago Hospitals, 1998.)

If you see a person being mistreated and abused, take action. Get help. Protect the person.

FOCUS ON PRIDE: Application

What is your attitude about bedmaking? Is this a task that you will take pride in doing? Explain why the look and feel of the bed are important to the person's comfort and safety.

REVIEW QUESTIONS

Circle **T** *if the statement is* **TRUE** *or* **F** *if it is* **FALSE**.

1 T F   In nursing centers, complete linen changes are required for closed beds and surgical beds.

2 T F   In home care, complete linen changes are done daily.

3 T F   Hem-stitching faces away from the person.

4 T F   To remove crumbs from the bed, you shake linens in the air.

5 T F   The upper hem of the bedspread is even with the top of the mattress.

6 T F   Top linens are fan-folded to the foot of the bed for an open bed.

7 T F   A cotton drawsheet is used with a padded waterproof drawsheet.

8 T F   Residents can bring bed coverings from home.

Circle the **BEST** *answer*.

9 You will transfer a person from a stretcher to the bed. Which bed should you make?
   a A closed bed
   b An open bed
   c An occupied bed
   d A surgical bed

10 When handling linens
   a Put used linens on the floor
   b Hold linens away from your body and uniform
   c Shake linens to unfold them
   d Take extra linens to another person's room

11 A resident is out of bed most of the day. Which bed should you make?
   a A closed bed
   b An open bed
   c An occupied bed
   d A surgical bed

12 A complete linen change is done when
   a The bottom linens are wet or soiled
   b The bed is made for a new person
   c The person will transfer from a stretcher to a bed
   d Linens are loose or wrinkled

13 When making an occupied bed
   a Explain that the person will roll over a "bump" of linens
   b Wear the same gloves throughout the procedure
   c Lower the far bed rail if working alone
   d Fan-fold top linens to the foot of the bed

14 A surgical bed is kept
   a In Fowler's position
   b In the lowest position
   c In the highest position
   d In the supine position

Answers to Chapter 21 questions are on p. 871.

FOCUS ON **PRACTICE**

Problem Solving

You need to give a person a bath in bed (Chapter 22) and change linens. The person must remain in bed. Which type of bed will you make? Will you change linens or give the bath first? While changing linens, identify when you need to apply and remove gloves and practice hand hygiene.

Personal Hygiene

OBJECTIVES

- Define the key terms and key abbreviations in this chapter.
- Explain why personal hygiene is important.
- Describe the care given before and after breakfast, after lunch, and in the evening.
- Explain the purposes of oral hygiene.
- Describe the safety measures for giving mouth care to unconscious persons.
- Explain how to care for dentures.

- Describe the rules for bathing.
- Identify safety measures for tub baths and showers.
- Explain the purposes of perineal care.
- Identify the observations to report and record when assisting with hygiene.
- Perform the procedures described in this chapter.
- Explain how to promote PRIDE in the person, the family, and yourself.

KEY TERMS

AM care See "early morning care"
aspiration Breathing fluid, food, vomitus, or an object into the lungs
circumcised The fold of skin (foreskin) covering the glans of the penis was surgically removed
denture An artificial tooth or a set of artificial teeth
diaphoresis Profuse (excessive) sweating
early morning care Routine care given before breakfast; AM care
evening care Care given in the evening at bedtime; PM care

morning care Care given after breakfast; hygiene measures are more thorough at this time
oral hygiene Mouth care
pericare See "perineal care"
perineal care Cleaning the genital and anal areas; pericare
plaque A thin film that sticks to the teeth; it contains saliva, microbes, and other substances
PM care See "evening care"
tartar Hardened plaque
uncircumcised The male has foreskin covering the head of the penis

KEY ABBREVIATIONS

ADA American Dental Association
C Centigrade

F Fahrenheit
ID Identification

Hygiene promotes comfort, safety, and health. The skin is the body's first line of defense against disease. Intact skin prevents microbes from entering the body and causing an infection. Likewise, mucous membranes of the mouth, genital area, and anus must be clean and intact. Besides cleansing, good hygiene prevents body and breath odors. Good hygiene also is relaxing and increases circulation.

Culture and personal choice affect hygiene. (See *Caring About Culture: Personal Hygiene*, p. 336.) Some people take showers. Others take tub baths. Some bathe at bedtime. Others bathe in the morning. Some people bathe 1 or 2 times a day—before work and after work or exercise. Some people do not have water for bathing. Others cannot afford soap, deodorant, shampoo, toothpaste, or other hygiene products.

Many factors affect hygiene needs—perspiration (sweating), elimination, vomiting, drainage from wounds or body openings, bedrest, and activity. Illness and aging can affect self-care abilities. Some people need help with hygiene. The nurse uses the nursing process to meet the person's hygiene needs. Follow the nurse's directions and the care plan.

See *Body Structure and Function Review: Teeth, Gums, and Skin*, p. 336.
See *Focus on Communication: Personal Hygiene*, p. 336.
See *Focus on Children and Older Persons: Personal Hygiene*, p. 337.
See *Promoting Safety and Comfort: Personal Hygiene*, p. 337.

🌸 CARING ABOUT CULTURE

Personal Hygiene

Personal hygiene is very important to *East Indian Hindus*. Their religion requires at least 1 bath a day. Some believe bathing after a meal is harmful. Another belief is that a cold bath prevents a blood disease. Some believe that eye injuries can occur if bath water is too hot. Hot water can be added to cold water. However, cold water is not added to hot water. After bathing, the body is carefully dried with a towel.

From Giger JN: Transcultural nursing: assessment and intervention, *ed 6, St Louis, 2013, Mosby.*

FOCUS ON COMMUNICATION

Personal Hygiene

During hygiene procedures, make sure that the person is warm enough. You can ask:

- "Is the water warm enough?" "Is it too hot?" "Is it too cold?"
- "Are you warm enough?"
- "Do you need another bath blanket?"
- "Is the water starting to cool?"
- "Is the room warm enough?"

BODY STRUCTURE AND FUNCTION REVIEW

Teeth, Gums, and Skin

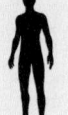

The Teeth and Gums

The *teeth* cut, chop, and grind food into small bits for digestion and swallowing. A tooth has 3 main parts: the *crown, neck,* and *root* (Fig. 22-1). The crown is the outer part. It is covered by enamel. The neck is surrounded by *gums (gingivae).* The root fits into the bone of the lower or upper jaw.

The Skin

The *skin* is the largest system. It is the body's natural covering. There are 2 skin layers (Fig. 22-2).

- The *epidermis* is the outer layer. It has living cells and dead cells. Dead cells constantly flake off and are replaced by living cells. Living cells die and flake off. Living cells of the epidermis contain *pigment* that gives skin its color. The epidermis has no blood vessels and few nerve endings.
- The *dermis* is the inner layer. It is made up of connective tissue. Blood vessels, nerves, sweat glands, oil glands, and hair roots are found in the dermis.

Sweat glands (sudoriferous glands) help regulate body temperature. Sweat is secreted through pores in the skin. The body is cooled as sweat evaporates. *Oil glands (sebaceous glands)* secrete an oily substance into the space near the hair shaft. Oil travels to the skin surface. This helps keep the hair and skin soft and shiny.

The skin has many functions.

- Provides the body's protective covering.
- Prevents microbes and other substances from entering the body.
- Prevents excess amounts of water from leaving the body.
- Protects organs from injury.
- Contains sensory structures. Nerve endings in the skin sense both pleasant and unpleasant stimulation. They sense cold, pain, touch, and pressure to protect the body from injury.
- Helps regulate body temperature. Blood vessels *dilate* (widen) when the temperature outside the body is high. More blood is brought to the body surface for cooling during evaporation. When blood vessels *constrict* (narrow), the body retains heat. This is because less blood reaches the skin.
- Stores fat and water.

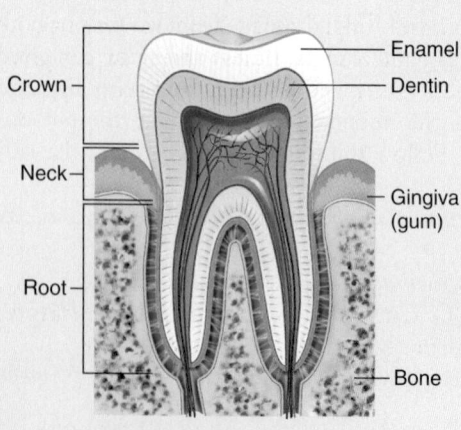

FIGURE 22-1 Parts of the tooth.

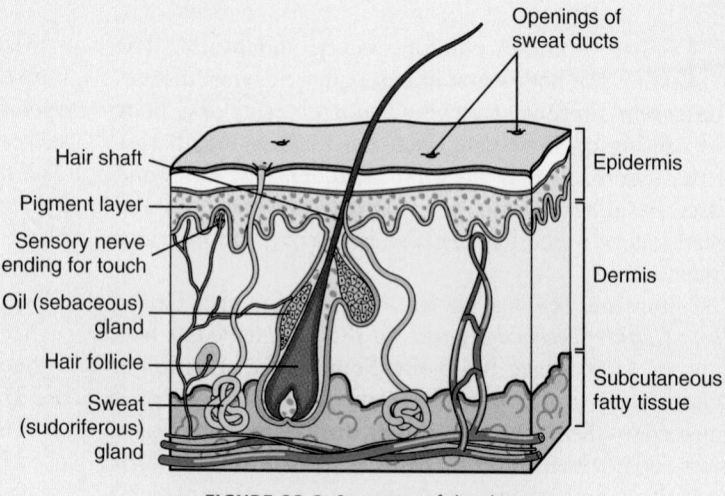

FIGURE 22-2 Structures of the skin.

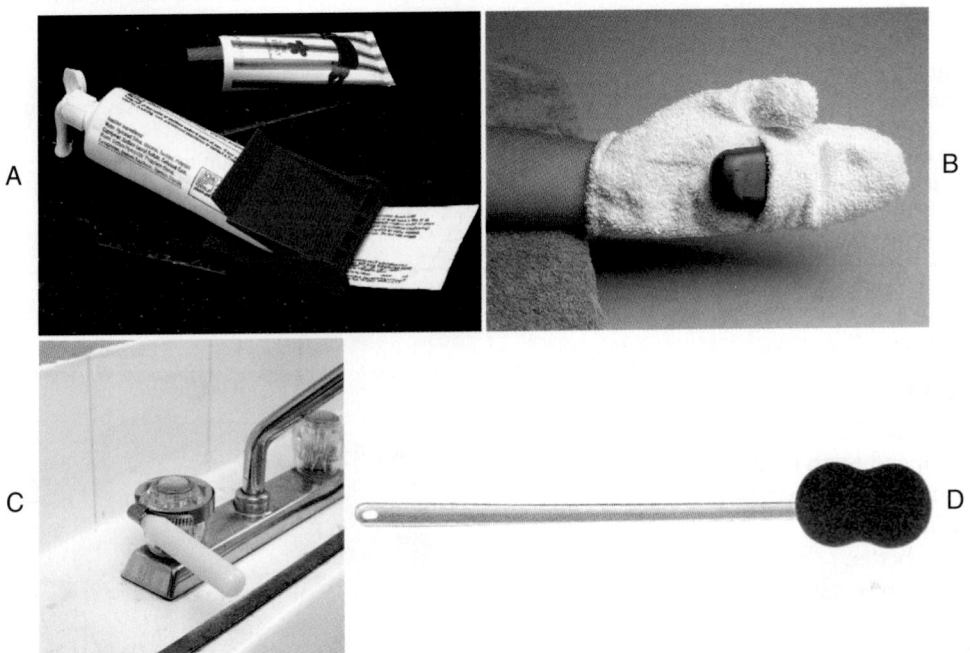

FIGURE 22-3 Adaptive (assistive) devices for hygiene. **A,** Tube squeezer for toothpaste. **B,** The wash mitt holds a bar of soap. **C,** A tap turner makes round knobs easy to turn. **D,** A long-handled sponge is used for hard-to-reach body parts. (Courtesy ElderStore, Alpharetta, Ga.)

DAILY CARE

Most people have hygiene routines and habits. For example, teeth are brushed and the face and hands washed after sleep. These and other hygiene measures are often done before and after meals and at bedtime.

Infants and young children need help with hygiene. So do some weak and disabled persons. Routine care is given during the day and evening (Box 22-1, p. 338).

- *Early morning care (AM care)—routine care given before breakfast.*
- *Morning care—care given after breakfast. Hygiene measures are more thorough at this time.*
- *Evening care (PM care)—care given in the evening at bedtime.*

You also assist with hygiene as needed. Always protect the person's right to privacy and to personal choice.

BOX 22-1 Daily Care

Before Breakfast (Early Morning Care or AM Care)
- Prepare persons for breakfast or morning tests.
- Assist with elimination.
- Clean incontinent persons.
- Change wet or soiled linens and garments.
- Assist with face- and hand-washing and oral hygiene.
- Assist with dressing and hair care.
- Assist with eyeglasses or contact lenses, hearing aids, and other needed devices.
- Position patients and residents for breakfast—dining room, bedside chair, or in bed.
- Make beds and straighten units.

After Breakfast (Morning Care)
- Assist with elimination.
- Clean incontinent persons.
- Change wet or soiled linens and garments.
- Assist with face- and hand-washing, oral hygiene, bathing, and perineal care.
- Provide back massages and other comfort measures (Chapter 31).
- Assist with hair care, shaving, dressing, and undressing.
- Assist with range-of-motion exercises and ambulation.
- Clean eyeglasses.
- Make beds and straighten rooms.

Afternoon Care
- Prepare persons for naps, visitors, or activity programs.
- Assist with elimination.
- Clean incontinent persons.
- Change wet or soiled linens and garments.
- Assist with face- and hand-washing, oral hygiene, and hair care.
- Assist with range-of-motion exercises and ambulation.
- Straighten beds and units.

Evening Care (PM Care)
- Prepare persons for sleep.
- Assist with elimination.
- Clean incontinent persons.
- Change wet or soiled linens and garments.
- Assist with face- and hand-washing and oral hygiene.
- Provide back massages and other comfort measures (Chapter 31).
- Help persons change into sleepwear.
- Store eyeglasses or contact lenses, hearing aids, and other devices.
- Straighten beds and units.

ORAL HYGIENE

Oral hygiene (mouth care):
- Keeps the mouth and teeth clean.
- Prevents mouth odors and infections.
- Increases comfort.
- Makes food taste better.
- Reduces the risk for *cavities (dental caries)* and *periodontal disease*.

Periodontal disease *(gum disease, pyorrhea)* is an inflammation of tissues around the teeth. Plaque and tartar build up from poor oral hygiene. **Plaque** *is a thin film that sticks to the teeth. It contains saliva, microbes, and other substances.* Plaque causes tooth decay *(cavities). Hardened plaque is called* **tartar**. Tartar builds up at the gum line near the neck of the tooth. Tartar buildup causes periodontal disease. The gums are red and swollen and bleed easily. Bone is destroyed and teeth loosen. Tooth loss is common.

Illness, disease, and some drugs often cause:
- A bad taste in the mouth.
- A whitish coating in the mouth and on the tongue.
- Redness and swelling in the mouth and on the tongue.
- Dry mouth. Dry mouth also is common from oxygen, smoking, decreased fluid intake, and anxiety.

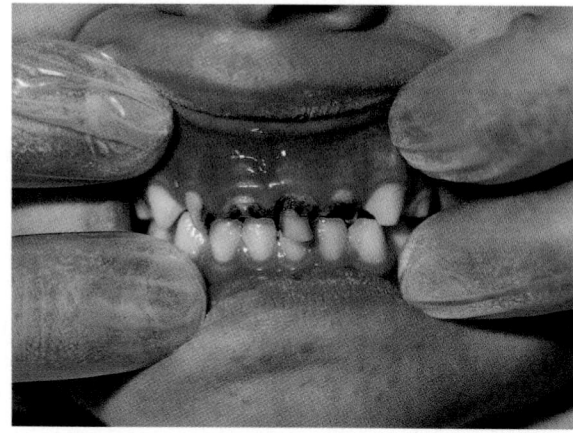

FIGURE 22-4 Baby bottle tooth decay. (From Eisen D, Lynch DP: *The mouth: diagnosis and treatment,* St Louis, 1998, Mosby.)

The nurse assesses the person's need for mouth care. So may the speech-language pathologist and the dietitian.

See *Focus on Children and Older Persons: Oral Hygiene.*
See *Delegation Guidelines: Oral Hygiene.*
See *Promoting Safety and Comfort: Oral Hygiene.*

Oral Hygiene

Children

Infants and young children need mouth care to remove food and bacteria. This helps prevent baby bottle tooth decay *(early childhood caries)*. Common in the upper front teeth, it can occur in all teeth (Fig. 22-4). Prolonged teeth exposure to liquids containing sugar is the usual cause. Such liquids include breast-milk, milk, formula, fruit juice, and other sweetened drinks. Bacteria in the mouth use sugars in such drinks for nourishment.

To prevent baby bottle tooth decay, the American Dental Association (ADA) recommends the following.
- Wipe the gums with a clean, damp gauze pad or washcloth after each feeding.
- Brush the teeth when they begin to erupt. Use a child's soft toothbrush and toothpaste. Brush gently.
  - When teeth erupt until age 3—use a smear of fluoride toothpaste. The smear is the size of a grain of rice.
  - Ages 3 to 6 years—use a pea-sized amount of fluoride toothpaste.
- Supervise brushing until the child can spit out toothpaste. This is usually until age 6 or 7.
- Fill baby bottles only with formula, milk, or breast-milk. Do not fill bottles with sugar water, juice, or soft drinks.
- Do not put the baby to bed with a bottle. Bottles should be finished before bedtime or nap-time.
- Provide a clean pacifier.
  - Do not dip a pacifier in sugar, honey, or anything sweet.
  - Do not put a pacifier in your mouth to clean it. Bacteria in your mouth can be passed to the baby.
- Encourage drinking from a cup by the first birthday.
- Discuss scheduling the first dental visit with the dentist. The first visit should be within 6 months of the first tooth erupting or by the first birthday.

Oral Hygiene

To assist with oral hygiene, you need this information from the nurse and the care plan.
- The type of oral hygiene to give. See procedures:
  - *Assisting the Person to Brush and Floss the Teeth,* p. 340
  - *Brushing and Flossing the Person's Teeth,* p. 341
  - *Providing Mouth Care for the Unconscious Person,* p. 343
  - *Providing Denture Care,* p. 345
- If flossing is needed.
- What cleaning agent and equipment to use (p. 340).
- If you apply lubricant to the lips. If yes, what lubricant to use.
- How often to give oral hygiene.
- How much help the person needs.
- What observations to report and record:
  - Dry, cracked, swollen, or blistered lips
  - Mouth or breath odor
  - Redness, swelling, irritation, sores, or white patches in the mouth or on the tongue
  - Bleeding, swelling, or redness of the gums
  - Loose teeth
  - Rough, sharp, or chipped areas on dentures
- When to report observations.
- What patient or resident concerns to report at once.

Oral Hygiene

Safety

Follow Standard Precautions and the Bloodborne Pathogen Standard. You may have contact with the person's mucous membranes. Gums may bleed during mouth care. Also, the mouth has many microbes. Pathogens spread through sexual contact may be in the mouths of some persons.

Comfort

Assist with oral hygiene after sleep, after meals, and at bedtime. Many people practice oral hygiene before meals. Some persons need mouth care every 2 hours or more often.

Flossing

Children

Flossing is started when 2 baby teeth touch. You need to floss for babies, toddlers, and pre-schoolers. You may need to remind and supervise older children when flossing.

Older Persons

Flossing was not a common oral hygiene measure many years ago. Therefore some older persons do not floss their teeth. Follow the care plan.

Flossing

Dental floss is a soft thread used to clean between the teeth. Flossing helps prevent periodontal disease and cavities by:
- Removing plaque from areas brushing cannot reach
- Removing food from between the teeth

The ADA recommends flossing at least once a day. Usually done after brushing, it can be done at other times. Some people floss after meals. If done once a day, bedtime is the best time to floss or when the person has time to floss thoroughly. You need to floss for persons who cannot do so themselves.

See *Focus on Children and Older Persons: Flossing.*

Equipment

A toothbrush, toothpaste, dental floss, and mouthwash are needed. A toothbrush with soft bristles is best.

Sponge swabs are used for persons with sore, tender mouths. They also are used for unconscious persons. Use sponge swabs with care. Check the foam pad to make sure it is tight on the stick. The person could choke on the foam pad if it comes off the stick.

You also need a kidney basin, water cup, straw, tissues, towels, and gloves. Many persons bring oral hygiene equipment from home.

Brushing and Flossing Teeth

Many people perform oral hygiene themselves. Others need help gathering and setting up oral hygiene equipment. You perform oral hygiene for persons who:

- Are very weak.
- Cannot move or use their arms.
- Are too confused to brush their teeth.

See procedure: *Assisting the Person to Brush and Floss the Teeth.*

See procedure: *Brushing and Flossing the Person's Teeth.*

Assisting the Person to Brush and Floss the Teeth

QUALITY OF LIFE

- Knock before entering the person's room.
- Address the person by name.
- Introduce yourself by name and title.

- Explain the procedure before starting and during the procedure.
- Protect the person's rights during the procedure.
- Handle the person gently during the procedure.

PRE-PROCEDURE

1 Follow *Delegation Guidelines: Oral Hygiene,* p. 339. See *Promoting Safety and Comfort: Oral Hygiene,* p. 339.
2 Practice hand hygiene.
3 Collect the following.
   - Toothbrush with soft bristles
   - Toothpaste
   - Mouthwash (or solution noted on the care plan)
   - Dental floss (if used)
   - Water cup with cool water
   - Straw
   - Kidney basin
   - Hand towel
   - Paper towels
   - Gloves

4 Place the paper towels on the over-bed table. Arrange items on top of them.
5 Identify the person. Check the ID (identification) bracelet against the assignment sheet. Use 2 identifiers (Chapter 13). Also call the person by name.
6 Provide for privacy.
7 Lower the bed rail near you if up.

PROCEDURE

8 Position the person to allow brushing with ease.
9 Place the towel over the person's chest. This protects garments and linens from spills.
10 Adjust the over-bed table in front of the person.

11 Let the person perform oral hygiene. This includes brushing the teeth and tongue, rinsing the mouth, flossing, and using mouthwash or other solution.
12 Remove the towel when the person is done.
13 Move the over-bed table to the side of the bed.

POST-PROCEDURE

14 Provide for comfort. (See the inside of the front cover.)
15 Place the call light and other needed items within reach.
16 Raise or lower bed rails. Follow the care plan.
17 Rinse the toothbrush. Clean, rinse, and dry equipment. Return the toothbrush and equipment to their proper place. Wear gloves.
18 Wipe the over-bed table with the paper towels. Discard the paper towels.

19 Unscreen the person.
20 Complete a safety check of the room. (See the inside of the front cover.)
21 Follow agency policy for used linens.
22 Remove and discard the gloves. Practice hand hygiene.
23 Report and record your observations.

Brushing and Flossing the Person's Teeth

QUALITY OF LIFE

- Knock before entering the person's room.
- Address the person by name.
- Introduce yourself by name and title.
- Explain the procedure before starting and during the procedure.
- Protect the person's rights during the procedure.
- Handle the person gently during the procedure.

PRE-PROCEDURE

1 Follow *Delegation Guidelines: Oral Hygiene*, p. 339. See *Promoting Safety and Comfort: Oral Hygiene*, p. 339.
2 Practice hand hygiene.
3 Collect the following.
   - Toothbrush with soft bristles
   - Toothpaste
   - Mouthwash (or solution noted on the care plan)
   - Dental floss (if used)
   - Water cup with cool water
   - Straw
   - Kidney basin
   - Hand towel
   - Paper towels
   - Gloves

4 Place the paper towels on the over-bed table. Arrange items on top of them.
5 Identify the person. Check the ID bracelet against the assignment sheet. Use 2 identifiers (Chapter 13). Also call the person by name.
6 Provide for privacy.
7 Raise the bed for body mechanics. Bed rails are up if used.

PROCEDURE

8 Lower the bed rail near you if up.
9 Assist the person to a sitting position or to a side-lying position near you. (NOTE: Some state competency tests require that the person is at a 75- to 90-degree angle.)
10 Place the towel across the person's chest.
11 Adjust the over-bed table so you can reach it with ease.
12 Practice hand hygiene. Put on the gloves.
13 Hold the toothbrush over the kidney basin. Pour some water over the brush.
14 Apply toothpaste to the toothbrush.
15 Brush the teeth gently (Fig. 22-5, p. 342). Brush the inner, outer, and chewing surfaces of upper and lower teeth.
16 Brush the tongue gently. Also gently brush the roof of the mouth, inside of the cheeks, and gums.
17 Let the person rinse the mouth with water. Hold the kidney basin under the person's chin (Fig. 22-6, p. 342). Repeat this step as needed.

18 Floss the person's teeth (optional).
   a Break off an 18-inch piece of dental floss from the dispenser.
   b Hold the floss between the middle fingers of each hand (Fig. 22-7, *A*, p. 342).
   c Stretch the floss with your thumbs. Hold the floss between your thumbs and index fingers.
   d Start at the upper back tooth on the right side. Work around to the left side.
   e Rub gently against the side of the tooth. Use up-and-down motions (Fig. 22-7, *B*, p. 342). Do not jerk or snap the floss against the tooth. Work from the top of the crown to the gum line.
   f Move to a new section of floss after every second tooth.
   g Floss the lower teeth. Use gentle up-and-down motions as for the upper teeth. Start on the right side. Work around to the left side.
19 Let the person use mouthwash or other solution. Hold the kidney basin under the chin.
20 Wipe the person's mouth. Remove the towel.
21 Remove and discard the gloves. Practice hand hygiene.

POST-PROCEDURE

22 Provide for comfort. (See the inside of the front cover.)
23 Place the call light and other needed items within reach.
24 Lower the bed to a safe and comfortable level for the person. Follow the care plan.
25 Raise or lower bed rails. Follow the care plan.
26 Rinse the toothbrush. Clean, rinse, and dry equipment. Return the toothbrush and equipment to their proper place. Wear gloves.

27 Wipe off the over-bed table with the paper towels. Discard the paper towels.
28 Unscreen the person.
29 Complete a safety check of the room. (See the inside of the front cover.)
30 Follow agency policy for used linens.
31 Remove and discard the gloves. Practice hand hygiene.
32 Report and record your observations.

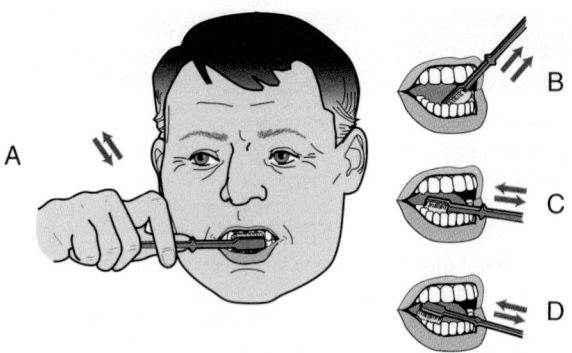

FIGURE 22-5 Brushing teeth. **A,** The brush is held at a 45-degree angle to the gums. Teeth are brushed with short strokes. **B,** The brush is at a 45-degree angle against the inside of the front teeth. Teeth are brushed from the gum to the crown of the tooth with short strokes. **C,** The brush is held horizontally against the inner surfaces of the teeth. The teeth are brushed back and forth. **D,** The brush is positioned on the chewing surfaces of the teeth. The teeth are brushed back and forth.

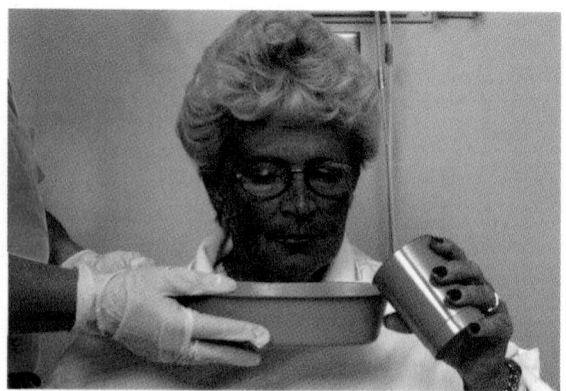

FIGURE 22-6 The kidney basin is held under the person's chin.

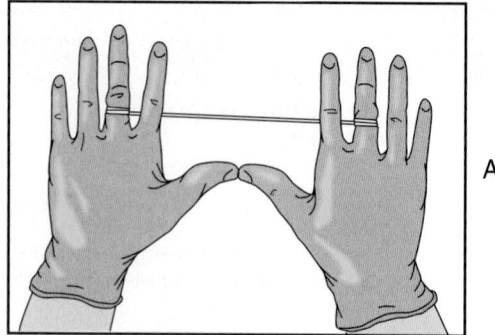

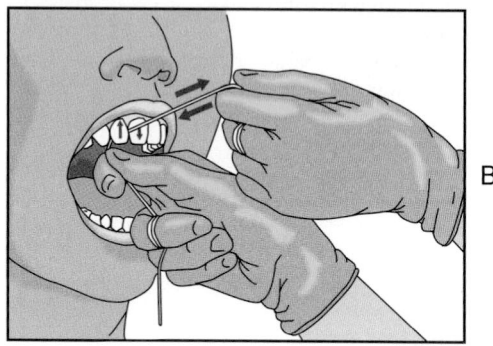

FIGURE 22-7 Flossing. **A,** Floss is wrapped around the middle fingers. **B,** Floss is moved in up-and-down motions between the teeth. Floss is moved up and down from the crown to the gum line.

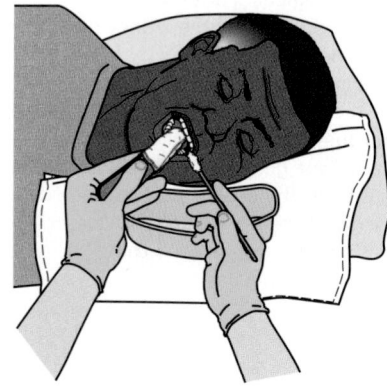

FIGURE 22-8 The unconscious person's head is turned well to the side to prevent aspiration. A padded tongue blade is used to keep the mouth open while cleaning the mouth with swabs.

Mouth Care for the Unconscious Person

Unconscious persons cannot eat or drink. Some breathe with their mouths open. Many receive oxygen. These factors cause mouth dryness. They also cause crusting on the tongue and mucous membranes. Oral hygiene keeps the mouth clean and moist. It also helps prevent infection.

The care plan tells you what cleaning agent to use. Use sponge swabs to apply the cleaning agent. Apply a lubricant (check the care plan) to the lips after cleaning. It prevents cracking of the lips.

Unconscious persons usually cannot swallow. Protect them from choking and aspiration. *Aspiration is breathing fluid, food, vomitus, or an object into the lungs.* It can cause pneumonia and death. To prevent aspiration:

- Position the person on 1 side with the head turned well to the side (Fig. 22-8). In this position, excess fluid runs out of the mouth.
- Use only a small amount of fluid to clean the mouth.
- Do not insert dentures. Dentures are not worn when the person is unconscious.

Keep the person's mouth open with a padded tongue blade (Fig. 22-9). Do not use your fingers. The person can bite down on them. The bite breaks the skin and creates a portal of entry for microbes. Infection is a risk.

Mouth care is given at least every 2 hours. Follow the nurse's directions and the care plan.

See *Focus on Communication: Mouth Care for the Unconscious Person.*

See *Promoting Safety and Comfort: Mouth Care for the Unconscious Person.*

See procedure: *Providing Mouth Care for the Unconscious Person.*

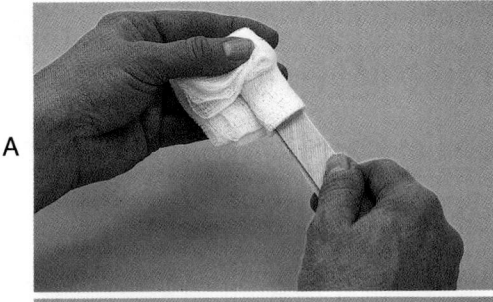

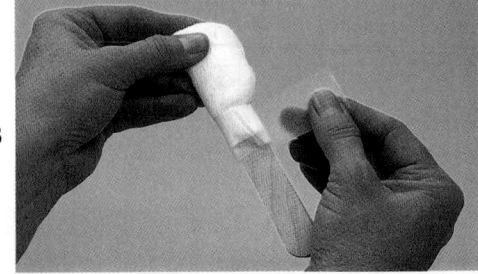

FIGURE 22-9 Making a padded tongue blade. **A,** Place 2 wooden tongue blades together. Wrap gauze around the top half. **B,** Tape the gauze in place.

FOCUS ON **COMMUNICATION**

Mouth Care for the Unconscious Person

Unconscious persons cannot speak or respond to you. However, some can hear. Always assume that unconscious persons can hear. Explain what you are doing step-by-step. Also, tell the person when you are done, when you are leaving, and when you will return.

PROMOTING SAFETY AND COMFORT

Mouth Care for the Unconscious Person

Safety
Use sponge swabs with care. Make sure the sponge pad is tight on the stick. The person could aspirate or choke on the sponge if it comes off the stick.

Comfort
Unconscious persons are re-positioned at least every 2 hours. To promote comfort, combine mouth care with skin care, re-positioning, and other comfort measures.

Providing Mouth Care for the Unconscious Person

QUALITY OF LIFE

- Knock before entering the person's room.
- Address the person by name.
- Introduce yourself by name and title.

- Explain the procedure before starting and during the procedure.
- Protect the person's rights during the procedure.
- Handle the person gently during the procedure.

PRE-PROCEDURE

1 Follow *Delegation Guidelines: Oral Hygiene*, p. 339. See *Promoting Safety and Comfort:*
  a *Oral Hygiene*, p. 339
  b *Mouth Care for the Unconscious Person*
2 Practice hand hygiene.
3 Collect the following.
  - Cleaning agent (check the care plan)
  - Sponge swabs
  - Padded tongue blade
  - Water cup with cool water
  - Hand towel

  - Kidney basin
  - Lip lubricant
  - Paper towels
  - Gloves
4 Place the paper towels on the over-bed table. Arrange items on top of them.
5 Identify the person. Check the ID bracelet against the assignment sheet. Use 2 identifiers (Chapter 13). Also call the person by name.
6 Provide for privacy.
7 Raise the bed for body mechanics. Bed rails are up if used.

PROCEDURE

8 Lower the bed rail near you.
9 Position the person in a side-lying position near you. Turn his or her head well to the side.
10 Put on the gloves.
11 Place the towel under the person's face.
12 Place the kidney basin under the chin.
13 Separate the upper and lower teeth. Use the padded tongue blade. Be gentle. Never use force. If you have problems, ask the nurse for help.

14 Clean the mouth using sponge swabs moistened with the cleaning agent (see Fig. 22-8). Squeeze out excess cleaning agent.
  a Clean the chewing and inner surfaces of the teeth.
  b Clean the gums and outer surfaces of the teeth.
  c Swab the roof of the mouth, inside of the cheek, and the lips.
  d Swab the tongue.
  e Moisten a clean swab. Swab the mouth to rinse.
  f Place used swabs in the kidney basin.
15 Remove the kidney basin and supplies.
16 Wipe the person's mouth. Remove the towel.
17 Apply lubricant to the lips.
18 Remove and discard the gloves. Practice hand hygiene.

Continued

Providing Mouth Care for the Unconscious Person—cont'd

POST-PROCEDURE

19 Provide for comfort. (See the inside of the front cover.)
20 Place the call light and other needed items within reach.
21 Lower the bed to a safe and comfortable level for the person. Follow the care plan.
22 Raise or lower bed rails. Follow the care plan.
23 Clean, rinse, dry, and return equipment to its proper place. Discard disposable items. (Wear gloves.)
24 Wipe off the over-bed table with paper towels. Discard the paper towels.
25 Unscreen the person.
26 Complete a safety check of the room. (See the inside of the front cover.)
27 Tell the person that you are leaving the room. Tell him or her when you will return.
28 Follow agency policy for used linens.
29 Remove and discard the gloves. Practice hand hygiene.
30 Report and record your observations.

Denture Care

A *denture* is an artificial tooth or a set of artificial teeth (Fig. 22-10). Often called *false teeth*, dentures replace missing teeth. Tooth loss occurs from gum disease, tooth decay, or injury. Full and partial dentures are common.

- *Full dentures.* The person has no upper or no lower natural teeth. Dentures replace the upper or lower teeth.
- *Partial dentures.* The person has some natural teeth. The partial denture replaces the missing teeth.

Mouth care is given and dentures cleaned as often as natural teeth. Dentures are slippery when wet. They easily break or chip if dropped onto a hard surface (floors, sinks, counters). Hold them firmly when removing or inserting them. During cleaning, firmly hold them over a basin of water lined with a towel. This prevents them from falling onto a hard surface.

For cleaning, a denture cleaner, denture cup, and denture brush or toothbrush are needed. Use only denture cleaning products to avoid damaging dentures.

The manufacturer's instructions tell how to use the cleaning agent and what water temperature to use. Hot water causes dentures to lose their shape (warp). If not worn after cleaning, store dentures in a container with cool or warm water or a denture soaking solution. Otherwise they can dry out and warp.

Dentures are usually removed at bedtime. Some people soak their dentures over-night in a denture cleaning solution. Rinse the dentures before they are inserted.

Some people do not wear their dentures. Others wear dentures for eating and remove them after meals. Remind patients and residents not to wrap dentures in tissues or napkins. Otherwise, they are easily discarded.

Many people clean their own dentures. Some need help collecting denture cleaning items. You clean dentures for those who cannot do so.

See *Promoting Safety and Comfort: Denture Care.*
See procedure: *Providing Denture Care.*

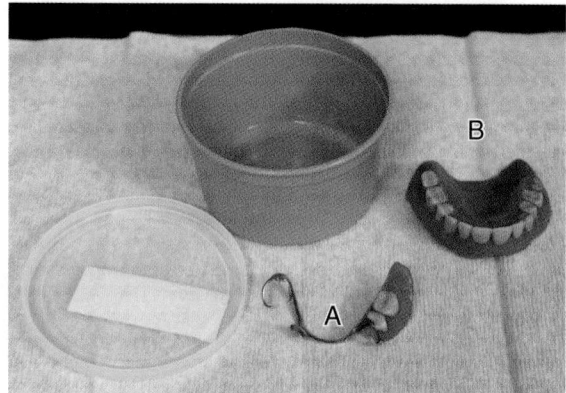

FIGURE 22-10 Dentures. A, Partial denture. **B,** Full denture.

PROMOTING SAFETY AND COMFORT

Denture Care

Safety

Dentures are the person's property. They are costly. Handle them very carefully. Label the denture cup with the person's name and room and bed number. Report lost or damaged dentures to the nurse at once. Losing or damaging dentures is negligent conduct.

Never carry dentures in your hands. Always use a denture cup or kidney basin. You could easily drop the dentures as you move to and from the bedside and sink.

Comfort

Many people do not like being seen without their dentures. Privacy is important. Allow privacy when the person cleans dentures. If you clean dentures, return them to the person as quickly as possible.

Persons with dentures may have some natural teeth. They need to brush and floss the natural teeth. See procedure: *Assisting the Person to Brush and Floss the Teeth,* p. 340. Or see procedure: *Brushing and Flossing the Person's Teeth,* p. 341.

Providing Denture Care

QUALITY OF LIFE

- Knock before entering the person's room.
- Address the person by name.
- Introduce yourself by name and title.

- Explain the procedure before starting and during the procedure.
- Protect the person's rights during the procedure.
- Handle the person gently during the procedure.

PRE-PROCEDURE

1 Follow *Delegation Guidelines: Oral Hygiene*, p. 339. See *Promoting Safety and Comfort:*
   a *Oral Hygiene*, p. 339
   b *Denture Care*
2 Practice hand hygiene.
3 Collect the following.
   - Denture brush or toothbrush (for cleaning dentures)
   - Denture cup labeled with the person's name and room and bed number
   - Denture cleaning agent
   - Soft-bristled toothbrush or sponge swabs (for oral hygiene)
   - Toothpaste
   - Water cup with cool water
   - Straw
   - Mouthwash (or other noted solution)
   - Kidney basin
   - 2 hand towels
   - Gauze squares
   - Paper towels
   - Gloves

4 Place the paper towels on the over-bed table. Arrange items on top of them.
5 Identify the person. Check the ID bracelet against the assignment sheet. Use 2 identifiers (Chapter 13). Also call the person by name.
6 Provide for privacy.

PROCEDURE

7 Line the bottom of the sink with a towel. Do not use paper towels. Fill the sink half-way with water.
8 Raise the bed for body mechanics.
9 Lower the bed rail near you if up.
10 Practice hand hygiene. Put on the gloves.
11 Place a towel over the person's chest.
12 Ask the person to remove the dentures. Carefully place them in the kidney basin.
13 Remove the dentures if the person cannot do so. Use gauze squares for a good grip on the slippery dentures.
   a Grasp the upper denture with your thumb and index finger (Fig. 22-11, p. 346). Move it up and down slightly to break the seal. Gently remove the denture. Place it in the kidney basin.
   b Grasp and remove the lower denture with your thumb and index finger. Turn it slightly and lift it out of the person's mouth. Place it in the kidney basin.
14 Follow the care plan for raising bed rails.
15 Take the kidney basin, denture cup, denture brush, and denture cleaning agent to the sink.
16 Rinse the denture cup and lid.
17 Rinse each denture under cool or warm running water. Follow agency policy for water temperature.
18 Return dentures to the kidney basin.
19 Apply the denture cleaning agent to the brush.
20 Brush the dentures as in Figure 22-12, p. 346. Brush the inner, outer, and chewing surfaces and all surfaces that touch the gums.
21 Rinse the dentures under running water. Use warm or cool water as directed by the cleaning agent manufacturer.

22 Place dentures in the denture cup. Cover the dentures with cool or warm water. Follow agency policy for water temperature.
23 Clean the kidney basin.
24 Take the denture cup and kidney basin to the over-bed table.
25 Lower the bed rail if up.
26 Position the person for oral hygiene.
27 Clean the person's gums and tongue. Brush any natural teeth. Use toothpaste and the toothbrush (or sponge swabs).
28 Have the person use mouthwash (or noted solution). Hold the kidney basin under the chin.
29 Ask the person to insert the dentures. Insert them if the person cannot.
   a Hold the upper denture firmly with your thumb and index finger. Raise the upper lip with the other hand. Insert the denture. Gently press on the denture with your index finger to make sure it is in place.
   b Hold the lower denture with your thumb and index finger. Pull the lower lip down slightly. Insert the denture. Gently press down on it to make sure it is in place.
30 Place the denture cup in the top drawer of the bedside stand if the dentures are not worn. The dentures must be in water or in a denture soaking solution.
31 Wipe the person's mouth. Remove the towel.
32 Remove and discard the gloves. Practice hand hygiene.

Continued

Providing Denture Care—cont'd

POST-PROCEDURE

33 Assist with hand-washing.
34 Provide for comfort. (See the inside of the front cover.)
35 Place the call light and other needed items within reach.
36 Lower the bed to a safe and comfortable level for the person. Follow the care plan.
37 Raise or lower bed rails. Follow the care plan.
38 Remove the towel from the sink. Drain the sink.
39 Rinse the brushes. Empty and rinse the denture cup. Clean, rinse, and dry equipment. Return the brushes and equipment to their proper place. Discard disposable items. Wear gloves for this step.

40 Wipe off the over-bed table with paper towels. Discard the paper towels.
41 Unscreen the person.
42 Complete a safety check of the room. (See the inside of the front cover.)
43 Follow agency policy for used linens.
44 Remove and discard the gloves. Practice hand hygiene.
45 Report and record your observations.

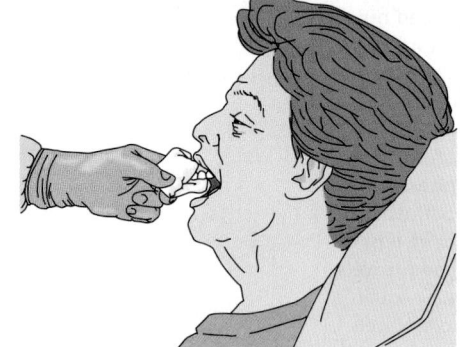

FIGURE 22-11 Remove the upper denture by grasping it with the thumb and index finger of 1 hand. Use a piece of gauze to grasp the denture.

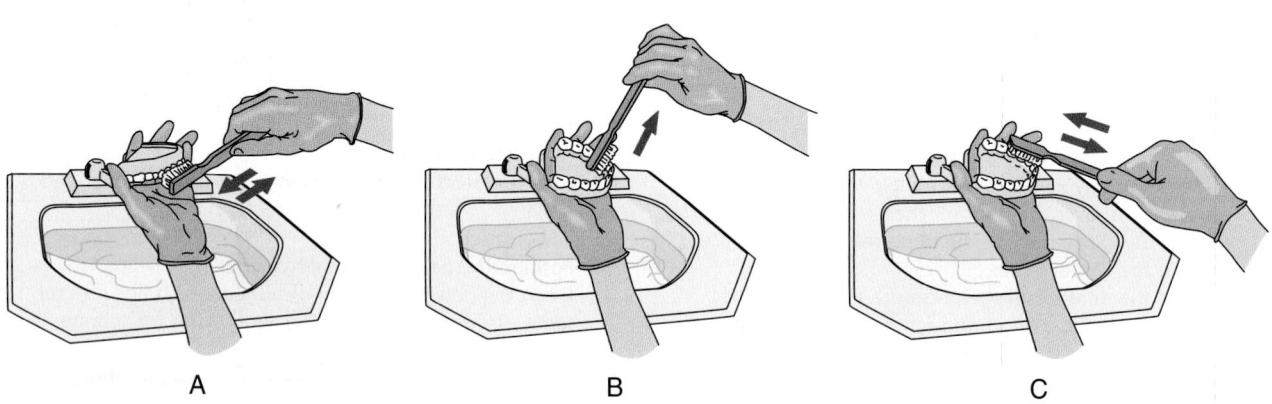

A   B   C

FIGURE 22-12 Cleaning dentures. **A,** Brush the outer surfaces of the denture with back-and-forth motions. (Note that the denture is held over the sink. The sink is lined with a towel and filled half-way with water.) **B,** Position the brush vertically to clean the inner surfaces of the denture. Use upward strokes. **C,** Brush the chewing surfaces with back-and-forth motions.

BATHING

Bathing cleans the skin. It also cleans the mucous membranes of the genital and anal areas. Microbes, dead skin, perspiration, and excess oils are removed. A bath is refreshing and relaxing. Circulation is stimulated and body parts exercised. Observations are made and you have time to talk to the person.

Complete or partial bed baths, tub baths, or showers are given. The method depends on the person's condition, self-care abilities, and personal choice. In hospitals, bathing is common after breakfast. In nursing centers, bathing usually occurs before or after breakfast or after the evening meal. The person's choice of bath time is respected when possible.

Bathing frequency is a personal matter. Some people bathe daily. Others bathe 1 or 2 times a week. Personal choice, weather, activity, and illness affect bathing. Other illnesses and dry skin may limit bathing to every 2 or 3 days.

The rules for bed baths, showers, and tub baths are listed in Box 22-2. Table 22-1 describes common skin care products.

See *Focus on Communication: Personal Hygiene*, p. 336.
See *Focus on Children and Older Persons: Bathing*, p. 348.
See *Delegation Guidelines: Bathing*, p. 348.
See *Promoting Safety and Comfort: Bathing*, p. 349.

BOX 22-2 Rules for Bathing

- Follow the care plan for bathing method and skin care products.
- Allow personal choice whenever possible.
- Follow Standard Precautions and the Bloodborne Pathogen Standard.
- Collect needed items before starting the procedure.
- Remove hearing aids before bathing. Water will damage hearing aids.
- Provide for privacy. Screen the person. Close doors and window coverings—drapes, shades, blinds, shutters, and so on.
- Assist the person with elimination. Bathing stimulates the need to urinate. Comfort and relaxation increase if the person urinates first.
- Cover the person for warmth and privacy.
- Reduce drafts. Close doors and windows.
- Protect the person from falling.
- Use good body mechanics at all times.

- Follow the rules to safely move and transfer the person (Chapters 18 and 19).
- Know what water temperature to use. See *Delegation Guidelines: Bathing*, p. 348
- Keep bar soap in the soap dish between latherings. This prevents soapy water. It also prevents slipping and falls in showers and tubs.
- Wash from the cleanest areas to the dirtiest areas.
- Encourage the person to help as much as is safely possible.
- Rinse the skin thoroughly. You must remove all soap.
- Pat dry the skin to avoid irritating or breaking the skin. Do not rub the skin.
- Dry well under the breasts, between skin folds, in the perineal area, and between the toes.
- Bathe skin when urine or feces are present. This prevents skin breakdown and odors.

TABLE 22-1 Skin Care Products

Type	Purpose	Care Considerations
Soaps	• Clean the skin • Remove dirt, dead skin, skin oil, some microbes, and perspiration	• Tend to dry and irritate the skin. Dry skin is easily injured and causes itching and discomfort. • Rinse the skin thoroughly to remove all soap. • Not needed for every bath. Plain water can clean the skin. • Plain water is often used for older persons with dry skin. • People with dry skin may use soaps with bath oils. • Not used for very dry skin.
Bath oils	• Keep the skin soft • Prevent dry skin	• Some soaps have bath oil. • Liquid bath oil can be added to bath water. • Bath oils make showers and tubs slippery. Practice safety measures to prevent falls.
Creams and lotions	• Protect the skin from the drying effect of air and evaporation	• Do not feel greasy but leave an oily film on the skin. • Lotion is applied to bony areas after bathing to prevent skin breakdown (back, elbows, knees, and heels). • Lotion is used for back massages (Chapter 31). • Most are scented.
Powders	• Absorb moisture • Prevent friction when 2 skin surfaces rub together	• May be applied under the breasts, under the arms, in the groin area, and between the toes. • Applied after drying the skin in a thin, even layer. • Excessive amounts cause caking and crusts that irritate the skin.
Deodorants	• Mask and control body odors	• Applied to the underarms. • Not applied to irritated skin. • Do not replace bathing.
Antiperspirants	• Reduce the amount of perspiration	• Applied to the underarms. • Not applied to irritated skin. • Do not replace bathing.

FOCUS ON CHILDREN AND OLDER PERSONS
Bathing

Children
The nurse collects information about the child's bathing practices. The care plan reflects the child's normal practices and needs during illness.

Many older children enjoy showers. The nurse tells you how much help and supervision the child needs. Remember, independence and privacy are important to older children.

See "Bathing an Infant" in Chapter 52.

Older Persons
Dry skin occurs with aging. Soap also dries the skin. Dry skin is easily damaged. Therefore older persons need a complete bed bath or shower only twice a week. Partial baths are taken on the other days. Some bathe daily but not with soap. Thorough rinsing is needed when using soap. Lotions and oils help keep the skin soft.

Bathing procedures can threaten persons with dementia. They do not understand what is happening or why. They may fear harm or danger. Confusion can increase. Therefore they may resist care and become agitated and combative. They may shout at you and cry out for help. You must be calm, patient, and soothing.

The nurse assesses the person's behaviors and routines. The person may be calmer and less confused or agitated during a certain time of day. Bathing is scheduled for calm times. The nurse decides the best bathing procedure for the person.

Older Persons—cont'd
The rules in Box 22-2 apply. The care plan also includes measures to help the person through the bath. For example:
- Use terms such as "cleaned up" or "washed" rather than "shower" or "bath."
- Complete pre-procedure activities. For example, ready supplies and linens. Have everything you need.
- Provide for warmth. Prevent drafts. Have extra towels and a robe nearby.
- Provide for good lighting.
- Play soft music to help the person relax.
- Provide for safety.
  - Use a hand-held shower nozzle.
  - Have the person use a shower chair or shower bench.
  - Do not use bath oil. It can make the tub or shower slippery. And it may cause a urinary tract infection.
  - Do not leave the person alone in the tub or shower.
- Draw bath water ahead of time. Test the water temperature. Add warm or cold water as needed.
- Tell the person what you are doing step-by-step. Use clear, simple statements.
- Let the person help as much as possible. For example, give the person a washcloth. Ask him or her to wash the arms. If the person does not know what to do, let the person hold the washcloth if safe to do so.
- Put a towel over the shoulders or lap (tub bath or shower). This helps the person feel less exposed.
- Do not rush the person.
- Use a calm, pleasant voice.
- Distract the person if needed.
- Calm the person.
- Handle the person gently.
- Try a partial bath if a shower or tub bath agitates the person.
- Try the bath later if the person continues to resist care.

DELEGATION GUIDELINES
Bathing

To assist with bathing, you need this information from the nurse and the care plan.
- What bath to give—complete bed bath, partial bath, tub bath, shower, towel bath, or bag bath.
- How much help the person needs.
- The person's activity or position limits.
- What water temperature to use. Bath water cools rapidly. Heat is lost to the bath basin, over-bed table, washcloth, and your hands. Therefore water temperature for complete bed baths and partial bed baths is usually between 110°F and 115°F (Fahrenheit) (43.3°C and 46.1°C [centigrade]) for adults. Older persons have fragile skin. They need lower water temperatures.
- What skin care products to use and what the person prefers.

- What observations to report and record:
  - The color of the skin, lips, nail beds, and sclera (whites of the eyes)
  - If the skin appears pale, grayish, yellow (*jaundice*—Chapter 46), or bluish *(cyanotic)*
  - The location and description of rashes
  - Skin texture—smooth, rough, scaly, flaky, dry, moist
  - *Diaphoresis—profuse (excessive) sweating*
  - Bruises or open skin areas
  - Pale, reddened, or discolored areas, particularly over bony parts
  - Drainage or bleeding from wounds or body coverings
  - Swelling of the feet and legs
  - Corns or calluses on the feet
  - Skin temperature (cold, cool, warm, hot)
  - Complaints of pain or discomfort
- When to report observations
- What patient or resident concerns to report at once

PROMOTING SAFETY AND COMFORT

Bathing

Safety

Hot water can burn the skin. Measure water temperature according to agency policy. If unsure if the water is too hot, ask the nurse to check it.

Protect the person from falls and other injuries. Practice the safety measures in Chapters 13 and 14. Also protect the person from drafts.

Use good body mechanics to protect yourself from injury (Chapter 17). The procedure that follows has you working on 1 side of the bed only. To avoid straining and reaching, you may need to wash 1 side of the body and then move to the other side to finish the bath. If room space allows, first wash the side of the body near you (eyes and face, arm, hand, chest, abdomen, leg, foot). Then move the over-bed table with equipment and supplies to the other side of the bed. Finish the bath (arm, hand, leg, foot, back, and perineal care) on that side.

Apply powder with caution. Do not use powders near persons with respiratory disorders. Inhaling powder can irritate the airway and lungs. Before using powder, check with the nurse and the care plan. To safely apply powder:

- Turn away from the person.
- Sprinkle a small amount of powder onto your hand or a cloth. Do not shake or sprinkle powder onto the person.
- Apply the powder in a thin layer.
- Make sure powder does not get on the floor. Powder is slippery and can cause falls.

Safety—cont'd

You make beds after baths. After making the bed, lower the bed to a safe and comfortable level for the person. Follow the care plan. For an occupied bed, raise or lower bed rails according to the care plan. Make sure the bed wheels are locked.

Protect the person and yourself from infection. During baths and bedmaking, contact with blood, body fluids, secretions, or excretions is likely. Follow Standard Precautions and the Bloodborne Pathogen Standard.

Comfort

Before bathing, let the person meet elimination needs (Chapters 24 and 26). Bathing stimulates the need to urinate. Comfort is greater when the bladder is empty. Also bathing is not interrupted.

Oral hygiene is common during bathing routines. Some persons do so before bathing; others do so after. Allow personal choice and follow the person's care plan.

Provide for warmth. Cover the person with a bath blanket. Make sure the water is warm enough for the person. Cool water causes chilling.

If the person prefers, remove the person's gown after washing the eyes, face, ears, and neck. Removing sleepwear at this time helps the person feel less exposed and provides more mental comfort with the bath.

If the person is able, let him or her wash the genital area. This promotes privacy and helps prevent embarrassment. See "Perineal Care," p. 358.

Persons With Bariatric Needs

Persons with bariatric needs may need help with hygiene. They may not be able to reach body parts. Skin folds are common. Good hygiene and skin care promote comfort and prevent pressure ulcers.

The rules for bathing in Box 22-2 apply. Always follow the person's care plan. The care plan includes:

- How often to bathe the person.
- The bathing method—bed bath, shower, whirlpool.
- The number of staff needed.
- The equipment needed. A bariatric shower chair is an example.
- The cleaning agent to use. Harsh soaps that dry and irritate the skin are avoided.
- When to clean under skin folds. The person may perspire heavily. Moisture can collect between skin folds, providing a place for microbes to live and grow.
- How to dry under skin folds. The nurse may have you use a hand-held hair dryer on the "cool" setting.
- What product to place under skin folds. The nurse may have you place gauze or cotton-fabric under the folds. The material reduces friction and absorbs moisture.
- What skin care products to use—powder, lotion, and so on.

See *Teamwork and Time Management: Persons With Bariatric Needs.*

TEAMWORK AND TIME MANAGEMENT

Persons With Bariatric Needs

Bathing bariatric persons requires teamwork and planning. Even if the person can assist, you will often need help from co-workers. You may need help to hold skin folds while you clean, dry, and apply skin care products. Or you need to turn or transfer the person. Ask your co-workers for help in advance. Plan a time that is best for the person, your co-workers, and you.

Also allow extra time to complete hygiene measures. Plan your work to avoid seeming rushed. The person must not feel as if he or she is a burden. If unsure how much time to allow, ask other staff who have cared for the person. They can give advice on how much time and help are needed.

The Complete Bed Bath

For a complete bed bath, you wash the person's entire body in bed. You give such baths to persons who cannot bathe themselves. Bed baths are usually needed by persons who are:

- Unconscious
- Paralyzed
- In casts or traction
- Weak from illness or surgery

A bed bath is new to some people. Some are embarrassed to have their bodies seen. Some fear exposure. Explain how you give the bath. Also explain how you cover the body for privacy.

See procedure: *Giving a Complete Bed Bath.*

Giving a Complete Bed Bath

QUALITY OF LIFE

- Knock before entering the person's room.
- Address the person by name.
- Introduce yourself by name and title.

- Explain the procedure before starting and during the procedure.
- Protect the person's rights during the procedure.
- Handle the person gently during the procedure.

PRE-PROCEDURE

1 Follow *Delegation Guidelines: Bathing,* p. 348. See *Promoting Safety and Comfort:*
  a *Personal Hygiene,* p. 337
  b *Bathing,* p. 349
2 Practice hand hygiene.
3 Identify the person. Check the ID bracelet against the assignment sheet. Use 2 identifiers (Chapter 13). Also call the person by name.
4 Collect clean linens. (See procedure: *Making a Closed Bed* in Chapter 21.) Place linens on a clean surface.
5 Collect the following.
  - Wash basin
  - Soap
  - Bath thermometer
  - Orangewood stick or nail file
  - Washcloth (and at least 4 washcloths for perineal care, p. 358)

  - 2 bath towels and 2 hand towels
  - Bath blanket
  - Clothing or sleepwear
  - Lotion
  - Powder
  - Deodorant or antiperspirant
  - Brush and comb
  - Other grooming items as requested
  - Paper towels
  - Gloves
6 Cover the over-bed table with paper towels. Arrange items on the over-bed table. Adjust the height as needed.
7 Provide for privacy.
8 Raise the bed for body mechanics. Bed rails are up if used. Lower the bed rail near you if up.

PROCEDURE

9 Practice hand hygiene. Put on gloves.
10 Remove the sleepwear. Do not expose the person. Follow agency policy for used sleepwear.
11 Cover the person with a bath blanket. Remove top linens (see procedure: *Making an Occupied Bed* in Chapter 21).
12 Lower the head of the bed. It is as flat as possible. The person has a least 1 pillow.
13 Fill the wash basin ⅔ (two-thirds) full with water. Raise the bed rail before leaving the bedside. Follow the care plan for water temperature. Water temperature is usually 110°F to 115°F (43.3°C to 46.1°C) for adults. Measure water temperature. Use the bath thermometer. Or dip your elbow or inner wrist into the basin to test the water.
14 Lower the bed rail near you if up.
15 Ask the person to check the water temperature. Adjust the water temperature if it is too hot or too cold. Raise the bed rail before leaving the bedside. Lower it when you return.
16 Place the basin on the over-bed table.
17 Place a hand towel over the person's chest.
18 Make a mitt with the washcloth (Fig. 22-13). Use a mitt for the entire bath.

19 Wash around the person's eyes with water. Do not use soap.
  a Clean the far eye. Gently wipe from the inner to the outer aspect of the eye with a corner of the mitt (Fig. 22-14, p. 352).
  b Clean around the eye near you. Use a clean part of the washcloth for each stroke.
20 Ask if the person wants you to use soap to wash the face.
21 Wash the face, ears, and neck. Rinse and pat dry with the towel on the chest.
22 Help the person move to the side of the bed near you.
23 Expose the far arm. Place a bath towel length-wise under the arm. Apply soap to the washcloth.
24 Support the arm with your palm under the person's elbow. His or her forearm rests on your forearm.
25 Wash the arm, shoulder, and underarm. Use long, firm strokes (Fig. 22-15, p. 352). Rinse and pat dry.
26 Place the basin on the towel. Put the person's hand into the water (Fig. 22-16, p. 352). Wash the hand well. Clean under the fingernails with an orangewood stick or nail file.
27 Have the person exercise the hand and fingers.

Giving a Complete Bed Bath—cont'd

PROCEDURE—cont'd

28 Remove the basin. Dry the hand well. Cover the arm with the bath blanket.
29 Repeat steps 23 to 28 for the near arm.
30 Place a bath towel over the chest cross-wise. Hold the towel in place. Pull the bath blanket from under the towel to the waist. Apply soap to the washcloth.
31 Lift the towel slightly and wash the chest (Fig. 22-17, p. 352). Do not expose the person. Rinse and pat dry, especially under the breasts.
32 Move the towel length-wise over the chest and abdomen. Do not expose the person. Pull the bath blanket down to the pubic area. Apply soap to the washcloth.
33 Lift the towel slightly and wash the abdomen (Fig. 22-18, p. 352). Rinse and pat dry.
34 Pull the bath blanket up to the shoulders. Cover both arms. Remove the towel.
35 Change soapy or cool water. Measure bath water temperature as in step 13. If bed rails are used, raise the bed rail near you before leaving the bedside. Lower it when you return.
36 Uncover the far leg. Do not expose the genital area. Place a towel length-wise under the foot and leg. Apply soap to a washcloth.
37 Bend the knee and support the leg with your arm. Wash it with long, firm strokes. Rinse and pat dry.
38 Place the basin on the towel near the foot.
39 Lift the leg slightly. Slide the basin under the foot.
40 Place the foot in the basin (Fig. 22-19, p. 352). Use an orangewood stick or nail file to clean under the toenails if necessary. If the person cannot bend the knees:
  a Wash the foot. Carefully separate the toes. Rinse and pat dry.
  b Clean under the toenails with an orangewood stick or nail file if necessary.

41 Remove the basin. Dry the leg and foot. Apply lotion to the foot if directed by the nurse and care plan. Cover the leg with the bath blanket. Remove the towel.
42 Repeat steps 36 to 41 for the near leg.
43 Change the water. Measure water temperature as in step 13. Raise the bed rail near you before leaving the bedside. Lower it when you return.
44 Turn the person onto the side away from you. The person is covered with the bath blanket.
45 Uncover the back and buttocks. Do not expose the person. Place a towel length-wise on the bed along the back. Apply soap to a washcloth.
46 Wash the back. Work from the back of the neck to the lower end of the buttocks. Use long, firm, continuous strokes (Fig. 22-20, p. 352). Rinse and dry well.
47 Turn the person onto his or her back.
48 Change water for perineal care (p. 358). See step 14 in procedure: *Giving Female Perineal Care* (p. 360) for water temperature. (Some state competency tests also require changing gloves and hand hygiene at this time.) Raise the bed rail near you before leaving the bedside. Lower it when you return.
49 Allow the person to perform perineal care if able. Provide perineal care if the person cannot do so (p. 358). At least 4 washcloths are used. (Practice hand hygiene and wear gloves for perineal care.)
50 Remove and discard the gloves. Practice hand hygiene.
51 Give a back massage (Chapter 31).
52 Apply deodorant or antiperspirant. Apply lotion and powder as requested. See *Promoting Safety and Comfort: Bathing*, p. 349.
53 Put clean garments on the person (Chapter 23).
54 Comb and brush the person's hair (Chapter 23).
55 Make the bed.

POST-PROCEDURE

56 Provide for comfort. (See the inside of the front cover.)
57 Place the call light and other needed items within reach.
58 Lower the bed to a safe and comfortable level for the person. Follow the care plan.
59 Raise or lower bed rails. Follow the care plan.
60 Put on clean gloves.
61 Empty, clean, rinse, and dry the wash basin. Return it and other supplies to their proper place.

62 Wipe off the over-bed table with paper towels. Discard the paper towels.
63 Unscreen the person.
64 Complete a safety check of the room. (See the inside of the front cover.)
65 Follow agency policy for used linens.
66 Remove and discard the gloves. Practice hand hygiene.
67 Report and record your observations.

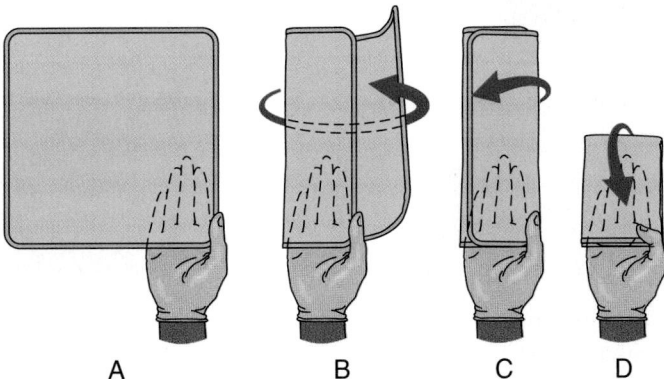

FIGURE 22-13 Making a mitted washcloth. **A,** Grasp the near side of the washcloth with your thumb. **B,** Bring the washcloth around and behind your hand. **C,** Fold the side of the washcloth over your palm as you grasp it with your thumb. **D,** Fold the top of the washcloth down and tuck it under next to your palm.

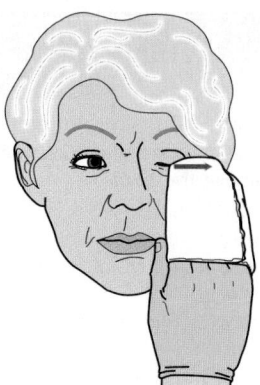

FIGURE 22-14 Wash the person's eyes with a mitted washcloth. Wipe from the inner to the outer aspect of the eye.

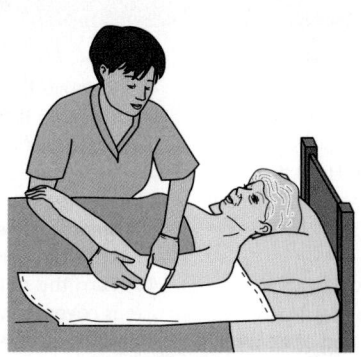

FIGURE 22-15 The person's arm is washed with firm, long strokes using a mitted washcloth.

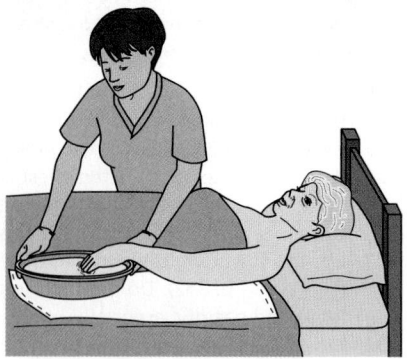

FIGURE 22-16 The person's hand is washed by placing the wash basin on the bed.

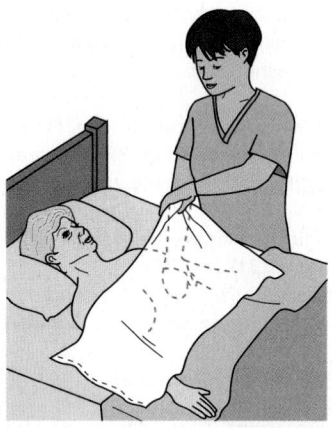

FIGURE 22-17 The person's breasts are not exposed during the bath. A bath towel is placed horizontally over the chest area. The towel is lifted slightly for reaching under to wash the breasts and chest.

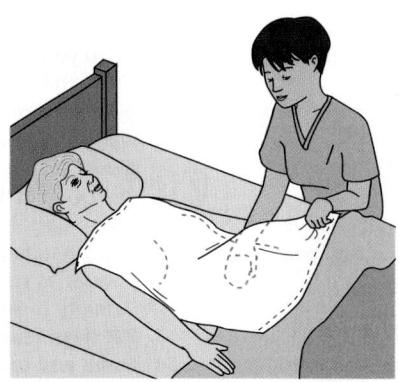

FIGURE 22-18 The bath towel is turned so that it is vertical to cover the breasts and abdomen. The towel is lifted slightly to bathe the abdomen. The bath blanket covers the pubic area.

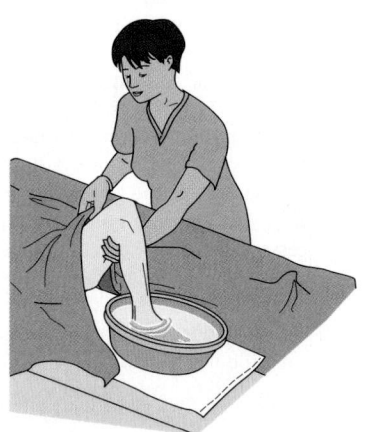

FIGURE 22-19 The foot is washed by placing it in the wash basin on the bed.

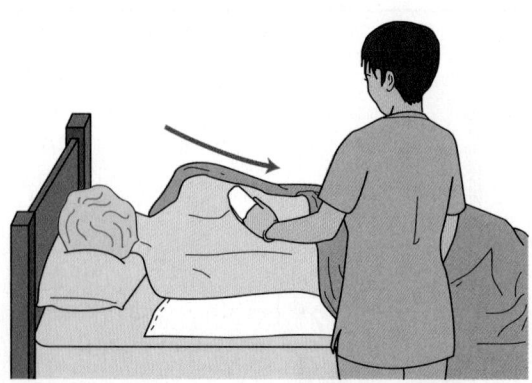

FIGURE 22-20 The back is washed with long, firm, continuous strokes. Note that the person is in a side-lying position. A towel is placed length-wise on the bed to protect the linens from water.

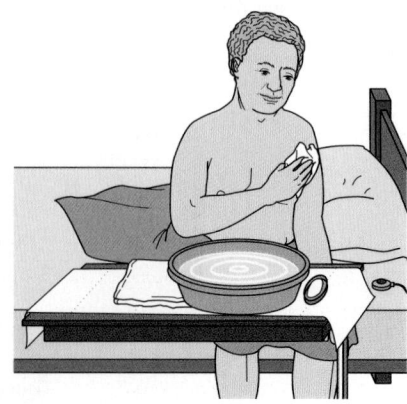

FIGURE 22-21 The person is bathing himself while sitting on the side of the bed. Needed equipment is within reach.

Towel Baths

For a towel bath, an over-sized towel covers the body from the neck to the feet. The towel is wet with a solution that does not need rinsing—water and cleaning, skin-softening, and drying agents. The drying agent lets the skin dry fast. The nurse and care plan tell you when to use a towel bath. To give a towel bath, follow agency policy.

See *Focus on Children and Older Persons: Towel Baths.*

Bag Baths

Bag baths are commercially prepared or made at the agency. A plastic bag has 8 to 10 washcloths. They are moistened with a cleansing agent that does not need rinsing. To give a bag bath:

- Warm the washcloths in a microwave oven or warmer. Follow the manufacturer's instructions for the microwave setting to use.
- Use a new washcloth for each body part.
- Let the skin air-dry. You do not need towels.
- Discard the washcloths following agency policy. Do not flush them down the toilet.

FOCUS ON **CHILDREN AND OLDER PERSONS**

Towel Baths

Older Persons

The towel bath is quick, soothing, and relaxing. Persons with dementia often respond well to towel baths.

◼ The Partial Bath

For a partial bath, the face, hands, underarms, back, buttocks, and perineal area are washed. Bathing prevents odors and discomfort in those areas. Some persons can wash in bed or at the sink. You assist as needed. Most need help washing the back. You give partial baths to persons who cannot bathe themselves.

The rules for bathing apply (see Box 22-2). So do the complete bed bath considerations.

See procedure: *Assisting With the Partial Bath.*

Assisting With the Partial Bath [VIDEO NATCEP]

QUALITY OF LIFE

- Knock before entering the person's room.
- Address the person by name.
- Introduce yourself by name and title.

- Explain the procedure before starting and during the procedure.
- Protect the person's rights during the procedure.
- Handle the person gently during the procedure.

PRE-PROCEDURE

1 Follow *Delegation Guidelines: Bathing*, p. 348. See *Promoting Safety and Comfort:*
  a *Personal Hygiene*, p. 337
  b *Bathing*, p. 349

2 Follow steps 2 through 7 in procedure: *Giving a Complete Bed Bath*, p. 350.

PROCEDURE

3 Make sure the bed is in a low position.
4 Practice hand hygiene. Put on gloves.
5 Cover the person with a bath blanket. Remove top linens.
6 Fill the wash basin ⅔ (two-thirds) full with water. Water temperature is usually 110°F to 115°F (43.3°C to 46.1°C) or as directed by the nurse. Measure water temperature with the bath thermometer. Or test bath water by dipping your elbow or inner wrist into the basin.
7 Ask the person to check the water temperature. Adjust the water temperature if it is too hot or too cold.
8 Place the basin on the over-bed table.
9 Position the person in Fowler's position. Or assist him or her to sit at the bedside.
10 Adjust the over-bed table so the person can reach the basin and supplies.
11 Help the person undress. Use the bath blanket for privacy and warmth.
12 Ask the person to wash easy-to-reach body parts (Fig. 22-21). Explain that you will wash the back and areas the person cannot reach.

13 Place the call light within reach. Ask him or her to signal when help is needed or bathing is complete.
14 Remove and discard the gloves. Practice hand hygiene. Then leave the room.
15 Return when the call light is on. Knock before entering. Practice hand hygiene.
16 Change the bath water. Measure bath water temperature as in step 6.
17 Raise the bed for body mechanics. The far bed rail is up if used.
18 Ask what was washed. Put on gloves. Wash and dry areas the person could not reach. The face, hands, underarms, back, buttocks, and perineal area are washed for the partial bath.
19 Remove and discard the gloves. Practice hand hygiene.
20 Give a back massage (Chapter 31).
21 Apply lotion, powder, and deodorant or antiperspirant as requested.
22 Help the person put on clean garments.
23 Assist with hair care and other grooming needs.
24 Make the bed.

Continued

Assisting With the Partial Bath—cont'd

POST-PROCEDURE

25 Provide for comfort. (See the inside of the front cover.)
26 Place the call light and other needed items within reach.
27 Lower the bed to a safe and comfortable level for the person. Follow the care plan.
28 Raise or lower bed rails. Follow the care plan.
29 Put on clean gloves.
30 Empty, clean, rinse, and dry the bath basin. Return the basin and supplies to their proper place.

31 Wipe off the over-bed table with the paper towels. Discard the paper towels.
32 Unscreen the person.
33 Complete a safety check of the room. (See the inside of the front cover.)
34 Follow agency policy for used linens.
35 Remove and discard the gloves. Practice hand hygiene.
36 Report and record your observations.

BOX 22-3   Tub Bath and Shower Safety

- Clean, disinfect, and dry the tub or shower before and after use.
- Dry the tub or shower room floor.
- Check hand rails, grab bars, hydraulic lifts, and other safety aids. They must be in working order.
- Place a bath mat in the tub or on the shower floor. This is not needed if there are non-skid strips or a non-skid surface.
- Cover the person for warmth and privacy. This includes during transport to and from the shower or tub room.
- Place the call light and other needed items within the person's reach.
- Show the person how to use the call light in the shower or tub room.
- Have the person use grab bars when getting in and out of the tub. Towel bars are not used for support.
- Follow the safety measures for wheelchairs when using wheeled shower chairs. See Chapter 19.
- Know what water temperature to use. See *Delegation Guidelines: Tub Baths and Showers*, p. 356.
- Turn cold water on first, then hot water. Turn hot water off first, then cold water.
- Adjust water temperature and pressure to prevent chilling or burns. Do this before the person gets into the shower.
- Direct water away from the person to adjust the water temperature and pressure.
- Fill the tub before the person gets into it. If using a tub with a side entry door, the tub is filled with the person in it. Follow the manufacturer's instructions. Closely monitor the water temperature as the tub fills.
- Measure water temperature. For showers and tub baths, use the digital display. Or you use a bath thermometer for a tub bath.
- Keep the water spray directed toward the person during the shower. This helps keep him or her warm. (NOTE: Do not direct the water spray toward the person's face. This can frighten the person.)
- Keep bar soap in the soap dish between latherings. This helps prevent slipping and falls in showers and tubs. It also prevents soapy tub water.
- Avoid using bath oils. They make tub and shower surfaces slippery.
- Do not leave weak or unsteady persons unattended.
- Stay within hearing distance if the person can be left alone. Wait outside the shower curtain or door. You must be nearby if the person calls for you or has an accident.
- Drain the tub before the person gets out of the tub. Turn off the shower before the person gets out of the shower. Cover him or her to provide privacy and prevent chilling.

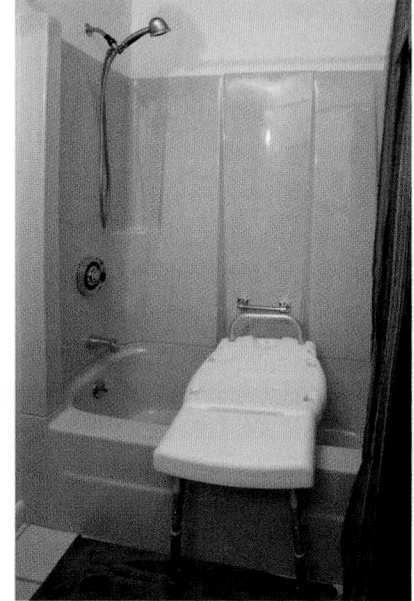

FIGURE 22-22 A shower bench.

Tub Baths and Showers

Some people like tub baths. Others like showers. Falls, burns, and chilling from water are risks. Safety is important (Box 22-3). The measures in Box 22-2 also apply. Also follow the nurse's directions and the care plan.

Some bathrooms have showers. If not, reserve the shower room for the person.

Tub Baths

Tub baths are relaxing. A tub bath can make a person feel faint, weak, or tired. These are great risks for persons who were on bedrest. A tub bath lasts no longer than 20 minutes.

To get in and out of the tub, the person may use:

- A shower bench (Fig. 22-22).
- A tub with a side entry door (Fig. 22-23).
- Bathing lift. The device transports and lifts the person into the tub (Fig. 22-24).
- Mechanical lift (Chapter 19).

Whirlpool tubs have a cleansing action. You wash the upper body. Carefully wash under the breasts and between skin folds. Also wash the perineal area. Pat dry the person with towels after the bath.

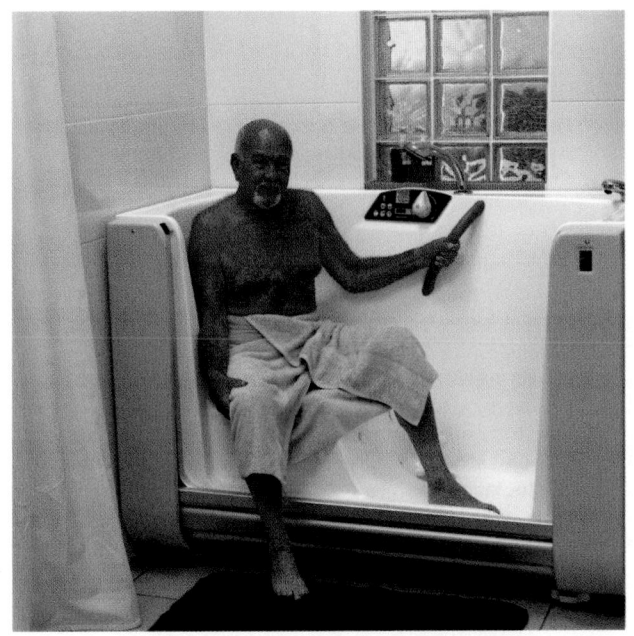

FIGURE 22-23 Tub with a side entry door. (Courtesy ARJOHUNTLEIGH, Addison, Ill., 800-307-2756.)

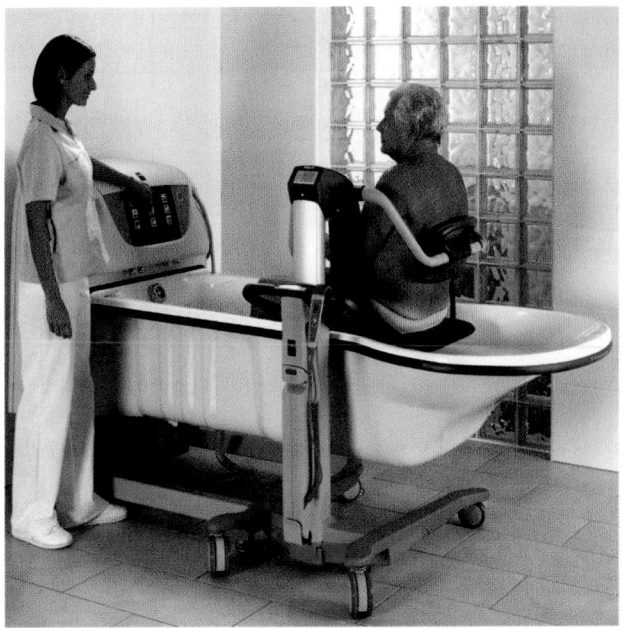

FIGURE 22-24 The lift lowers the person into the tub. (Courtesy ARJOHUNTLEIGH, Addison, Ill., 800-307-2756.)

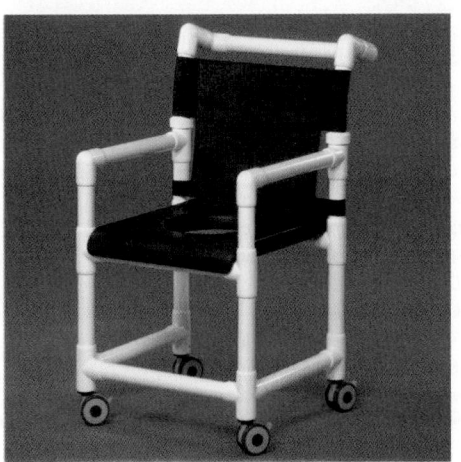

FIGURE 22-25 A shower chair. (Courtesy Innovative Products Unlimited, Niles, MI.)

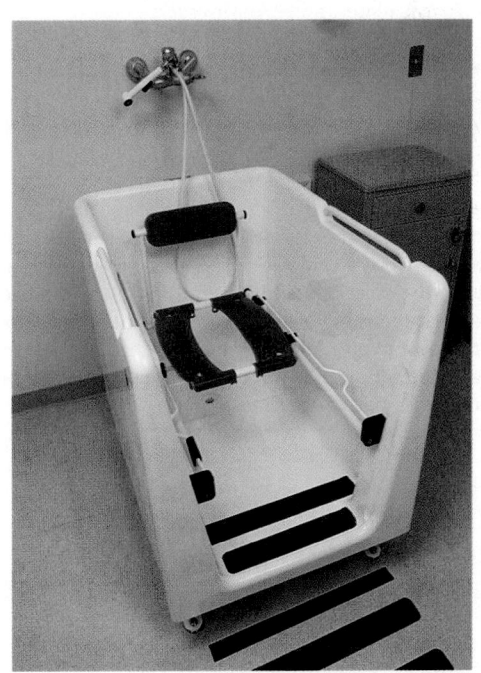

FIGURE 22-26 A shower cabinet.

Showers

Some people can stand to use a regular shower. Grab bars are used for support. Showers have non-skid surfaces. If not, a bath mat is used. Weak or unsteady persons use:

- *Shower chairs.* Water drains through an opening (Fig. 22-25). You use the chair to transport the person to and from the shower. Lock (brake) the wheels during the shower to prevent the chair from moving.
- *Shower stalls or cabinets.* The person walks into the device if able or is wheeled in a wheelchair (Fig. 22-26). Use the hand-held nozzle to give the shower.
- *Shower trolleys (portable tubs).* The person has a shower lying down (Fig. 22-27, p. 356). Lower the sides to transfer the person from the bed to the trolley. Then raise the side rails to transport the person to the tub or shower room. Use the hand-held nozzle to give the shower.

Some shower rooms have 2 or more stations. Provide for privacy. Properly screen and cover the person. Also close doors and shower curtains.

See *Focus on Long-Term Care and Home Care: Tub Baths and Showers,* p. 356.

See *Teamwork and Time Management: Tub Baths and Showers,* p. 356.

See *Delegation Guidelines: Tub Baths and Showers,* p. 356.

See *Promoting Safety and Comfort: Tub Baths and Showers,* p. 356.

See procedure: *Assisting With a Tub Bath or Shower,* p. 357.
Text continued on p. 358.

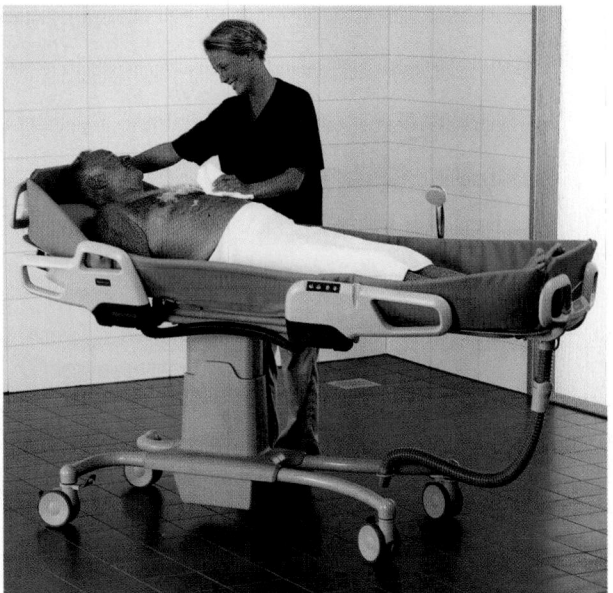

FIGURE 22-27 Shower trolley. The sides are lowered for transfers into and out of the trolley. (Courtesy ARJOHUNTLEIGH, Addison, Ill., 800-307-2756.)

TEAMWORK AND TIME MANAGEMENT
Tub Baths and Showers

You need to reserve the tub or shower room and equipment for the person. Your co-workers do the same for their patients and residents.

Consider the needs of others. For example:
- You reserve the shower room from 0945 to 1030. Do your best to follow the schedule. Have the shower room clean and ready for the next person.
- You and a co-worker schedule a shower for the same time. Plan new times with your co-worker.

All bed linens are changed on the person's bath or shower day. Ask co-workers to make the bed while you assist with the tub bath or shower. Also ask them to straighten the person's unit. The person returns to a clean bed and unit. Return the favor when your co-workers are assisting with tub baths, showers, or other care measures.

DELEGATION GUIDELINES
Tub Baths and Showers

Before assisting with a tub bath or shower, you need this information from the nurse and the care plan:
- If the person takes a tub bath or shower
- What water temperature to use (usually 105°F/40.5°C)
- What equipment is needed—bathing lift, mechanical lift, shower chair, shower cabinet, shower trolley, and so on
- How much help the person needs
- If the person can bathe himself or herself
- What observations to report and record:
  - Dizziness
  - Light-headedness
  - See *Delegation Guidelines: Bathing*, p. 348
- When to report observations
- What patient or resident concerns to report at once

FOCUS ON LONG-TERM CARE AND HOME CARE
Tub Baths and Showers

Home Care
Many homes have shower stalls or bathtub-shower units. To step into the tub or shower, have the person use the grab bars. Help the person in and out of the shower as needed.

The person can buy or rent a shower chair. The nurse helps the person and family find a safe chair for shower use.

The bathtub unit may not have a shower. A hand-held shower nozzle can be installed.

PROMOTING SAFETY AND COMFORT
Tub Baths and Showers

Safety
Some persons are very weak. At least 2 staff are needed to safely assist with tub baths and showers. If the person is heavy, 3 or more staff may be needed.

The person may use a tub with a side entry door, a shower chair, a shower trolley, or other device. Follow the manufacturer's instructions.

Protect the person from falls, chilling, and burns. Follow the safety measures in Chapters 13 and 14. Remember to measure water temperature.

Clean, disinfect, and dry the tub or shower before and after use. This prevents the spread of microbes and infection.

Comfort
Warmth and privacy promote comfort during tub baths and showers. You need to:
- Make sure the tub or shower room is warm.
- Provide for privacy. Close the room door, screen the person, and close window coverings.
- Make sure the water is warm enough for the person.
- Have the person remove his or her clothing or robe and footwear just before getting into the tub or shower. Do not have the person exposed longer than necessary.
- Leave the room if the person can be left alone. Stay within hearing distance.

Assisting With a Tub Bath or Shower

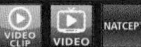

QUALITY OF LIFE

- Knock before entering the person's room.
- Address the person by name.
- Introduce yourself by name and title.

- Explain the procedure before starting and during the procedure.
- Protect the person's rights during the procedure.
- Handle the person gently during the procedure.

PRE-PROCEDURE

1 Follow *Delegation Guidelines*:
  a *Bathing*, p. 348
  b *Tub Baths and Showers*
  See *Promoting Safety and Comfort*:
  a *Personal Hygiene*, p. 337
  b *Bathing*, p. 349
  c *Tub Baths and Showers*
2 Reserve the tub or shower room.
3 Practice hand hygiene.
4 Identify the person. Check the ID bracelet against the assignment sheet. Use 2 identifiers (Chapter 13). Also call the person by name.

5 Collect the following.
  - Washcloth and 2 bath towels
  - Bath blanket
  - Soap
  - Bath thermometer (for a tub bath)
  - Clothing or sleepwear
  - Grooming items as requested
  - Robe and non-skid footwear
  - Rubber bath mat if needed
  - Disposable bath mat
  - Gloves
  - Wheelchair, shower chair, shower bench, and so on as needed

PROCEDURE

6 Place items in the tub or shower room. Use the space provided or a chair.
7 Clean, disinfect, and dry the tub or shower. Wear gloves for this step.
8 Place a rubber bath mat in the tub or on the shower floor. Do not block the drain.
9 Place the disposable bath mat on the floor in front of the tub or shower.
10 Put the OCCUPIED sign on the door.
11 Return to the person's room. Provide for privacy. Practice hand hygiene.
12 Help the person sit on the side of the bed.
13 Help the person put on a robe and non-skid footwear. Or the person can leave on clothing.
14 Assist or transport the person to the tub or shower room.
15 Have the person sit on a chair if he or she walked to the tub or shower room.
16 Provide for privacy.
17 *For a tub bath:*
  a Fill the tub half-way with warm water (usually 105°F/40.5°C). Follow the care plan for water temperature.
  b Measure water temperature. Use the bath thermometer or check the digital display.
  c Ask the person to check the water temperature. Adjust the water temperature if it is too hot or too cold.
18 *For a shower:*
  a Turn on the shower.
  b Adjust water temperature and pressure. Check the digital display.
  c Ask the person to check the water temperature. Adjust the water temperature if it is too hot or too cold.

19 Help the person undress and remove footwear.
20 Help the person into the tub or shower. Position the shower chair and lock (brake) the wheels.
21 Assist with washing as necessary. Wear gloves.
22 Ask the person to use the call light when done or when help is needed. Remind the person that a tub bath lasts no longer than 20 minutes.
23 Place a towel across the chair.
24 Leave the room if the person can bathe alone. If not, stay in the room or nearby. Remove and discard the gloves and practice hand hygiene if you will leave the room.
25 Check the person at least every 5 minutes.
26 Return when the person signals for you. Knock before entering. Practice hand hygiene.
27 Turn off the shower or drain the tub. Cover the person with the bath blanket while the tub drains.
28 Help the person out of the shower or tub and onto the chair.
29 Help the person dry off. Pat gently. Dry under the breasts, between skin folds, in the perineal area, and between the toes.
30 Assist with lotion and other grooming items as needed.
31 Help the person dress and put on footwear.
32 Help the person return to the room. Provide for privacy.
33 Assist the person to a chair or into bed.
34 Provide a back massage if the person returns to bed (Chapter 31).
35 Assist with hair care and other grooming needs.

POST-PROCEDURE

36 Provide for comfort. (See the inside of the front cover.)
37 Place the call light and other needed items within reach.
38 Raise or lower bed rails. Follow the care plan.
39 Unscreen the person.
40 Complete a safety check of the room. (See the inside of the front cover.)

41 Clean, disinfect, and dry the tub or shower. Remove soiled linens. Wear gloves.
42 Discard disposable items. Put the UNOCCUPIED sign on the door. Return supplies to their proper place.
43 Follow agency policy for used linens.
44 Remove and discard the gloves. Practice hand hygiene.
45 Report and record your observations.

PERINEAL CARE

Perineal care (pericare) involves cleaning the genital and anal areas. These areas provide a warm, moist, and dark place for microbes to grow. Cleaning prevents infection and odors and it promotes comfort.

Perineal care is done daily during the bath. It also is done when the area is soiled with urine or feces. Perineal care is very important for persons who:

- Have urinary catheters (Chapter 25).
- Have had rectal or genital surgery.
- Are menstruating (Chapter 10).
- Are incontinent of urine or feces (Chapters 24 and 26).
- Are uncircumcised (Fig. 22-28). Being *circumcised* means that the fold of skin (foreskin) covering the glans of the penis was surgically removed. Being *uncircumcised* means that the male has foreskin covering the head of the penis.

The person does perineal care if able. Otherwise, the nursing staff does so. This procedure embarrasses many people and staff, especially when it involves the other sex.

Perineal and *perineum* are not common terms. Most people understand *privates*, *private parts*, *crotch*, *genitals*, or *the area between your legs.* Use terms the person understands. The terms must be in good taste professionally.

Work from the cleanest area to the dirtiest. This is commonly called from *front to back.* Some state competency tests use *top to bottom.* The urethral area (the front or top) is the cleanest. The anal area (the back or bottom) is the dirtiest. Therefore clean from the urethra to the anal area. This prevents the spread of bacteria from the anal area to the vagina and urinary system.

The perineal area is delicate and easily injured. Use warm water, not hot. Use washcloths, towelettes, cotton balls, or swabs according to agency policy. Rinse thoroughly. Pat dry after rinsing. This reduces moisture and promotes comfort.

See *Focus on Communication: Perineal Care.*
See *Delegation Guidelines: Perineal Care.*
See *Promoting Safety and Comfort: Perineal Care.*
See procedure: *Giving Female Perineal Care.*
See procedure: *Giving Male Perineal Care*, p. 362.

Text continued on p. 363.

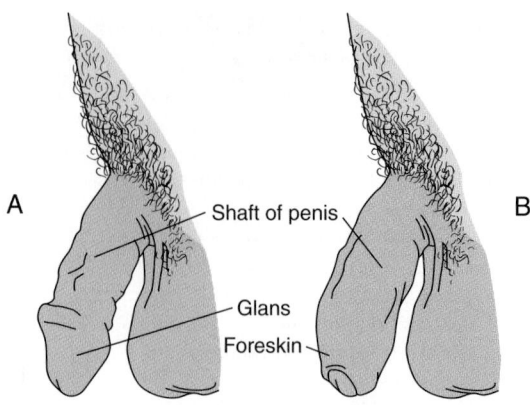

FIGURE 22-28 A, Circumcised male. **B,** Uncircumcised male.

FOCUS ON COMMUNICATION

Perineal Care

Talking to the person about perineal care may be difficult. You may be embarrassed. However, you must explain the procedure to the person. You can say:

- "Mrs. Bell, I'll give you some privacy while you finish your bath. Can you reach everything you need? Please call for me if you need help. Here is your call light."
- "Mr. Baker, I'll give you time to finish your bath. Please wash your genital and rectal areas. Signal for me when you're done or need help."
- "Mrs. Allan, next I'll clean between your legs. I'll keep you covered with the bath blanket. I'll tell you before I touch you. Please tell me if you feel any pain or discomfort."
- "Mr. Scott, I'll clean your private parts now. Please let me know if you feel any pain or discomfort."

DELEGATION GUIDELINES

Perineal Care

Before giving perineal care, you need this information from the nurse and the care plan.

- When to give perineal care.
- What terms the person understands—perineum, privates, private parts, crotch, area between the legs, and so on.
- How much help the person needs.
- What water temperature to use—usually 105°F to 109°F (40.5°C to 42.7°C). Water in a basin cools rapidly.
- What cleaning agent to use.
- Any position restrictions or limits.
- What observations to report and record:
  - Odors
  - Redness, swelling, discharge, bleeding, or irritation
  - Complaints of pain, burning, or other discomfort
  - Signs of urinary or fecal incontinence
- When to report observations.
- What patient or resident concerns to report at once.

PROMOTING SAFETY AND COMFORT
Perineal Care

Safety

Hot water can burn perineal tissues. To prevent burns, measure water temperature according to agency policy. If water seems too hot, ask the nurse to check it.

Protect yourself and the person from infection. Contact with blood, body fluids, secretions, or excretions is likely during perineal care. Follow Standard Precautions and the Bloodborne Pathogen Standard.

Persons who are incontinent need perineal care. Protect the person and dry garments and linens from wet or soiled items. Remove the wet or soiled incontinence product, garments, and linens. Then apply clean, dry ones. See Chapter 24.

Comfort

If you provide perineal care, explain how you protect privacy. Act in a professional manner at all times.

Perineal care involves touching the genital and anal areas. The person may prefer that someone of the same sex provide this care. Or the person may fear sexual assault. Always obtain the person's consent before providing perineal care. For mental comfort, the person may want a family member or another staff member present to witness the procedure. Ask if he or she wants someone present and that person's name. Also keep the call light within the person's reach. If feeling threatened, the person needs to be able to call for help.

Comfort—cont'd

If the person is able, let him or her perform perineal care. This promotes privacy and helps prevent embarrassment. You need to:

1. Provide clean water. See step 14 in procedure: *Giving Female Perineal Care.*
2. Adjust the over-bed table so the person can reach the wash basin, soap, and towels with ease.
3. Make sure the person understands what to do.
4. Place the call light and other needed items within reach. Ask the person to signal when finished.
5. Lower the bed to a safe and comfortable level for the person. Follow the care plan.
6. Remove and discard the gloves. Practice hand hygiene.
7. Leave the room.
8. Answer the call light promptly. Knock before entering the room.
9. Raise the bed for body mechanics.
10. Practice hand hygiene. Put on gloves.
11. Make sure the person has cleaned thoroughly. Assist the person with hand-washing.
12. Finish the bathing procedure.

Giving Female Perineal Care

QUALITY OF LIFE

- Knock before entering the person's room.
- Address the person by name.
- Introduce yourself by name and title.

- Explain the procedure before starting and during the procedure.
- Protect the person's rights during the procedure.
- Handle the person gently during the procedure.

PRE-PROCEDURE

1 Follow *Delegation Guidelines: Perineal Care.* See *Promoting Safety and Comfort:*
  a *Personal Hygiene,* p. 337
  b *Perineal Care*
2 Practice hand hygiene.
3 Collect the following.
- Soap or other cleansing agent as directed
- At least 4 washcloths
- Bath towel
- Bath blanket
- Bath thermometer
- Wash basin
- Waterproof under-pad
- Gloves
- Laundry bag
- Paper towels

4 Cover the over-bed table with paper towels. Arrange items on top of them.
5 Identify the person. Check the ID bracelet against the assignment sheet. Use 2 identifiers (Chapter 13). Also call the person by name.
6 Provide for privacy.
7 Raise the bed for body mechanics. Bed rails are up if used.

Continued

Giving Female Perineal Care—cont'd

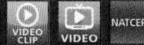

PROCEDURE

8 Lower the bed rail near you if up.
9 Practice hand hygiene. Put on gloves.
10 Cover the person with a bath blanket. Move top linens to the foot of the bed.
11 Position the person on her back.
12 Drape the person as in Figure 22-29.
13 Raise the bed rail if used.
14 Fill the wash basin. Water temperature is usually 105°F to 109°F (40.5°C to 42.7°C). Follow the care plan for water temperature. Measure water temperature according to agency policy.
15 Ask the person to check the water temperature. Adjust the water temperature if it is too hot or too cold. Raise the bed rail before leaving the bedside. Lower it when you return.
16 Place the basin on the over-bed table.
17 Lower the bed rail if up.
18 Help the person flex her knees and spread her legs. Or help her spread her legs as much as possible with the knees straight.
19 Fold the corner of the bath blanket between her legs onto her abdomen.
20 Place a waterproof under-pad under her buttocks. Remove any wet or soiled incontinence products.
21 Remove and discard the gloves. Practice hand hygiene. Put on clean gloves.
22 Wet the washcloths.
23 Squeeze out excess water from a washcloth. Make a mitted washcloth. Apply soap. (Squeeze out excess water every time you change washcloths. Do not place used washcloths back in the basin. Put used washcloths in the laundry bag.)
24 Clean the perineum. Change washcloths as needed.
   a Separate the labia.
   b Clean 1 side of the labia. Clean downward from front to back (top to bottom) with 1 stroke (Fig. 22-30, *A*). Use 1 part of a washcloth.
   c Clean the other side of the labia. Clean downward from front to back (top to bottom) with 1 stroke (Fig. 22-30, *B*). Use a clean part of a washcloth.
   d Clean the vaginal area. Clean downward from front to back (top to bottom) with 1 stroke (Fig. 22-30, *C*). Use a clean part of a washcloth.

25 Rinse the perineum using a clean washcloth. Change washcloths as needed.
   a Separate the labia.
   b Rinse 1 side of the labia. Rinse downward from front to back (top to bottom) with 1 stroke. Use 1 part of a washcloth.
   c Rinse the other side of the labia. Rinse downward from front to back (top to bottom) with 1 stroke. Use a clean part of a washcloth.
   d Rinse the vaginal area. Rinse downward from front to back (top to bottom) with 1 stroke. Use a clean part of a washcloth.
26 Pat dry the perineal area with the towel. Dry from front to back.
27 Fold the blanket back between her legs.
28 Help the person lower her legs and turn onto her side away from you.
29 Apply soap to a mitted washcloth. Use a clean washcloth.
30 Clean and rinse the rectal area.
   a Clean from the vagina to the anus with 1 stroke (Fig. 22-31). Use 1 part of the washcloth.
   b Repeat steps 29 and 30-a until the area is clean. Use a clean part of the washcloth for each stroke. Change washcloths as needed.
   c Rinse the rectal area using a clean washcloth. Rinse from the vagina to the anus. Repeat as necessary. Use a clean part of the washcloth for each stroke. Change washcloths as needed.
31 Pat dry the rectal area with the towel. Dry from the vagina to the anus.
32 Remove the waterproof under-pad.
33 Remove and discard the gloves. Practice hand hygiene. Put on clean gloves.
34 Provide clean and dry linens and incontinence products as needed.

POST-PROCEDURE

35 Cover the person. Remove the bath blanket.
36 Provide for comfort. (See the inside of the front cover.)
37 Place the call light and other needed items within reach.
38 Lower the bed to a safe and comfortable level for the person. Follow the care plan.
39 Raise or lower bed rails. Follow the care plan.
40 Empty, clean, rinse, and dry the wash basin.
41 Return the basin and supplies to their proper place.
42 Wipe off the over-bed table with the paper towels. Discard the paper towels.
43 Unscreen the person.
44 Complete a safety check of the room. (See the inside of the front cover.)
45 Follow agency policy for used linens.
46 Remove and discard the gloves. Practice hand hygiene.
47 Report and record your observations.

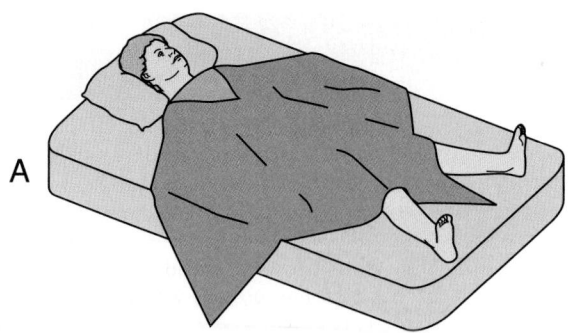
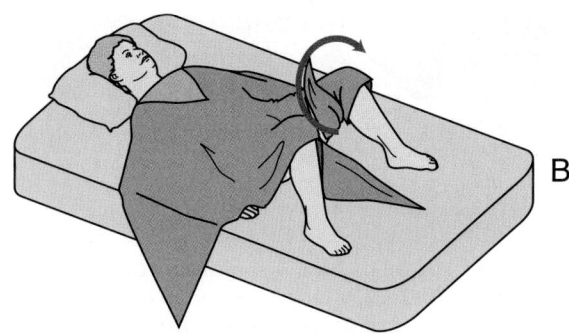

FIGURE 22-29 Draping for perineal care. A, Position the bath blanket like a diamond: 1 corner is at the neck, there is a corner at each side, and 1 corner is between the person's legs. **B,** Wrap the blanket around a leg by bringing the corner around the leg and over the top. Tuck the corner under the hip. Repeat for the other leg.

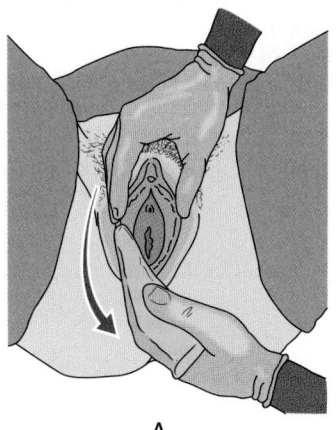
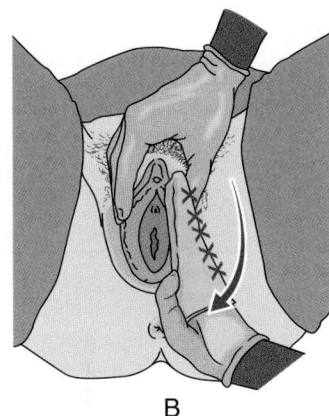
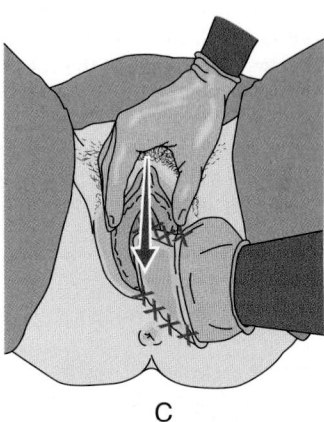

FIGURE 22-30 Cleaning the perineum. A, Separate the labia with 1 hand. Use a mitted washcloth to clean 1 side of the labia with a downward stroke. **B,** Clean the other side of the labia with a clean part of the washcloth. Use a downward stroke. **C,** Clean the vaginal area with a clean part of the washcloth. Use a downward stroke. (NOTE: Used areas of the washcloth are marked with Xs.)

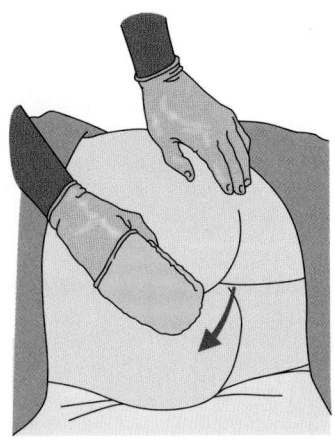

FIGURE 22-31 The rectal area is cleaned by wiping from the vagina to the anus. The side-lying position allows the anal area to be cleaned more thoroughly.

Giving Male Perineal Care

QUALITY OF LIFE

- Knock before entering the person's room.
- Address the person by name.
- Introduce yourself by name and title.

- Explain the procedure before starting and during the procedure.
- Protect the person's rights during the procedure.
- Handle the person gently during the procedure.

PROCEDURE

1 Follow steps 1 through 17 in procedure: *Giving Female Perineal Care*, p. 359. Drape the person as in Figure 22-29.
2 Fold the corner of the bath blanket between the legs onto the person's abdomen.
3 Place a waterproof under-pad under the buttocks. Remove any wet or soiled incontinence products.
4 Remove and discard the gloves. Practice hand hygiene. Put on clean gloves.
5 Retract the foreskin if the person is uncircumcised (Fig. 22-32).
6 Grasp the penis.
7 Clean the tip. Use a circular motion. Start at the meatus of the urethra and work outward (Fig. 22-33). Repeat as needed. Use a clean part of the washcloth each time.
8 Rinse the area with another washcloth. Use the same circular motion.
9 Return the foreskin to its natural position immediately after rinsing.
10 Clean the shaft of the penis. Use firm downward strokes. Rinse the area.

11 Help the person flex his knees and spread his legs. Or help him spread his legs as much as possible with his knees straight.
12 Clean the scrotum. Rinse well. Observe for redness and irritation of the skin folds.
13 Pat dry the penis and the scrotum. Use the towel.
14 Fold the bath blanket back between his legs.
15 Help him lower his legs and turn onto his side away from you.
16 Clean the rectal area. Clean from the scrotum (front or top) to the anus (back or bottom). (See procedure: *Giving Female Perineal Care*, p. 359). Rinse and dry well.
17 Remove the waterproof under-pad.
18 Remove and discard the gloves. Practice hand hygiene. Put on clean gloves.
19 Provide clean and dry linens and incontinence products.
20 Follow steps 35 through 47 in procedure: *Giving Female Perineal Care*, p. 359.

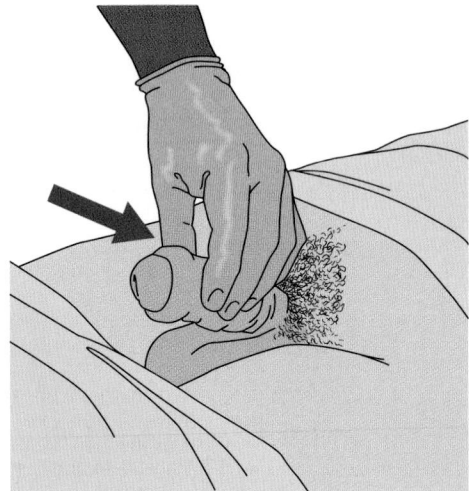

FIGURE 22-32 The foreskin of the uncircumcised male is pulled back for perineal care. It is returned to the normal position immediately after cleaning and rinsing.

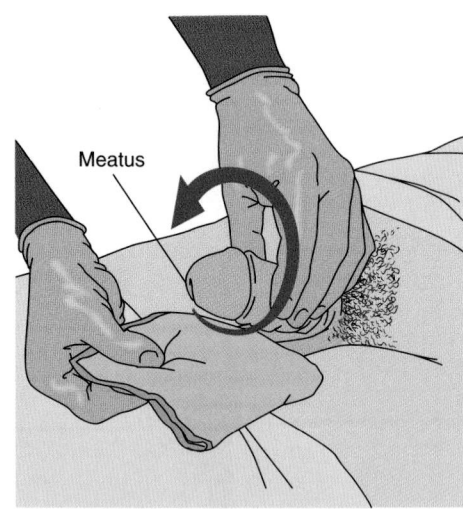

FIGURE 22-33 The penis is cleaned with circular motions starting at the meatus.

REPORTING AND RECORDING

You make many observations while assisting with hygiene. See Box 22-4 for a summary of the observations to report and record.

Also report and record the care given. If care is not recorded, it is assumed that care was not given. This can cause serious legal problems. Tell the nurse if the person refuses care or if care is not given for another reason.

BOX 22-4   Personal Hygiene Observations

Report the Following at Once
- Bleeding
- Signs of skin breakdown
- Discharge from the vagina or urinary tract
- Unusual odors
- Changes from prior observations

Oral Hygiene
- Dry, cracked, swollen, or blistered lips
- Mouth or breath odor
- Redness, swelling, irritation, sores, or white patches in the mouth or on the tongue
- Bleeding, swelling, or redness of the gums
- Loose teeth
- Rough, sharp, or chipped areas on dentures

Bathing
- The color of the skin, lips, nail beds, and sclera (whites of the eyes)
- If the skin appears pale, grayish, yellow (*jaundice*—Chapter 46), or bluish (*cyanotic*)

Bathing—cont'd
- The location and description of rashes
- Skin texture—smooth, rough, scaly, flaky, dry, moist
- *Diaphoresis*—profuse (excessive) sweating
- Bruises or open skin areas
- Pale, reddened, or discolored areas, particularly over bony parts
- Drainage or bleeding from wounds or body coverings
- Swelling of the feet and legs
- Corns or calluses on the feet
- Skin temperature (cold, cool, warm, hot)
- Complaints of pain or discomfort

Perineal Care
- Odors
- Redness, swelling, discharge, bleeding, or irritation
- Complaints of pain, burning, or other discomfort
- Signs of urinary or fecal incontinence

FOCUS ON **PRIDE**

The Person, Family, and Yourself

Personal and Professional Responsibility

Patients and residents depend on you for their hygiene needs. You are responsible for maintaining or improving the person's quality of life, health, and safety. To do so:
- Follow the guidelines and procedures in this chapter.
- Focus on the "Quality of Life" section at the beginning of each procedure.
- View the person as an individual with unique needs. Ask about the person's needs and preferences.

Take pride in providing care that benefits the person's over-all well-being.

Rights and Respect

Patients and residents have the right to choose schedules and routines. They also have the right to refuse care. Some persons refuse if it does not meet their preferences. For example:
- A resident refuses a shower because she prefers a bath.
- A patient prefers to bathe at night, not in the morning.
- A male resident prefers to be bathed by a male nursing assistant. A female is caring for him today.

Refusing care for these reasons does not mean the person refuses to be clean. The person may accept the care if preferences are met. Tell the nurse of any refusal of care. Adjust as needed to provide care and respect the person's preferences.

Independence and Social Interaction

Hygiene is a very personal matter. Allow personal choice in such matters as bath time, products used, and what to wear. Encourage the person to do as much self-care as safely possible. Doing so promotes independence and improves self-esteem.

Delegation and Teamwork

Some agencies have commercial warmers for bag baths that show which bags are warm. When you remove a pack, replace it with another pack. Then the warmer is full for other staff. If a warmer is getting low, fill it. Otherwise, staff find an empty warmer when needing a pack. They must wait for a pack to heat up. Or the warmer is almost empty and the other person has to fill it.

Avoid having the attitude that "someone else can do it." This shows poor teamwork and work ethics. Take pride in being a helpful and courteous member of the team.

Continued

FOCUS ON **P R I D E—cont'd**

The Person, Family, and Yourself

E thics and Laws

You will perform some tasks often. Bathing and other personal hygiene measures are examples. Over time, some staff become less careful with routine tasks. They may forget about dangers. Or they think that nothing bad will happen. This is very unsafe.

Accidents happen. Mistakes are made. The following examples show how harm can occur during bathing.

A patient (Mr. Genza) was paralyzed on his right side because of a stroke. He could not walk or talk. He could stand with difficulty. He died at age 51 from burns suffered during a shower.

A wrongful death suit was filed for what was claimed to be negligent care. According to the facts reported in the court case, the following occurred.

- *An attendant took the patient to the shower in a wheelchair.*
- *The attendant undressed the patient. The patient was placed on a chair and under running water in a shower.*
- *The attendant claimed that he tested the water.*
- *The shower room was supervised by an RN (registered nurse). The RN testified that an attendant was required to be present at all times while a paralyzed patient was receiving care.*
- *The attendant stated that he washed the patient's back and head. Then he went to attend to another patient 5 or 6 feet from the shower. A tub was between the attendant and Mr. Genza.*
- *When the attendant asked if he needed to get out of the shower, Mr. Genza indicated that he did not.*
- *Two minutes later, the attendant was getting another patient out of the tub. The attendant heard Mr. Genza shout and saw that the shower handle was moved from its original setting.*
- *Two days later, Mr. Genza died from burns.*
- *On the day of the accident, the hot water gauge read 171°F. It tested at 158°F to 159°F.*
- *An expert witness stated that 110°F is hot enough for shower room use.*
- *In the Court's opinion, the home was grossly negligent for:*
  - *Failing to provide the supervision needed by a helpless person*
  - *Providing water facilities that were dangerous and a threat to the lives of anyone using them*

  (Mr. Lewinsky v State of Illinois, 1967.)

E thics and Laws—cont'd

In another case, a daughter filed a complaint for the wrongful death of her mother. According to the complaint, on August 29, 1993, a nurse's aide ran water in a whirlpool bath for the nursing home resident. The nurse's aide tested the water with her bare arm and hand. She found the water satisfactory. The resident also tested the water by putting her foot into the water, which showed that the water was okay. Using a chair lift, the resident was transferred into the tub.

After the bath, the nurse's aide asked 2 co-workers to help her get the resident out of the tub. After getting her out, a co-worker noted a small spot on the resident's left hip. The resident had no burns on her body before the bath. However, redness of her extremities was noted over the next 30 minutes. Blisters began and continued to form.

The resident had second and third degree burns from her mid-back down over her buttocks, the perineal area, and lower extremities. (Author note: A first degree burn means the epidermis is damaged. A second degree burn involves the epidermis and part of the dermis. A third degree burn involves the epidermis and the entire dermis.) The resident was transferred to the hospital. She died on September 1, 1993.

The daughter sued the county, the nursing home and hospital, the nursing home administrator, hospital board members, and the nurse's aide. The trial court dismissed the case on a legal technicality. However, the Appellate Court reversed the dismissal by the trial court and returned the case to court for trial.

(D. Burton v Choctaw County Mississippi, Choctaw Hospital d/b/a Choctaw County Nursing Home, and others, 1997.)

You must always be careful. Harm can result from routine care measures. Follow the safety measures in this chapter at all times.

FOCUS ON **PRIDE**: *Application*

The care measures in this chapter are very private and personal. Needing help with hygiene can embarrass the person. At first, you may feel embarrassed. This improves with practice and experience. What concerns do you have about the procedures in this chapter? How will you stay calm and professional and ease the person's worries?

REVIEW QUESTIONS

Circle T if the statement is TRUE and F if it is FALSE.

1 T F Hygiene is needed for comfort, safety, and health.

2 T F During evening care, you prepare the person for sleep.

3 T F A toothbrush with hard bristles is good for oral hygiene.

4 T F A baby's teeth are flossed when 2 teeth touch.

5 T F Unconscious persons are supine for mouth care.

6 T F You use your fingers to keep the unconscious person's mouth open for oral hygiene.

7 T F You clean dentures over a towel on a counter.

REVIEW QUESTIONS—cont'd

8 T F Place the upper denture in the sink while cleaning the lower denture.

9 T F A person has a partial denture. Natural teeth are brushed.

10 T F Bath oils cleanse the skin.

11 T F Powders absorb moisture and prevent friction.

12 T F Deodorants reduce the amount of perspiration.

13 T F To wash the eye, wash from the inner to the outer aspect.

14 T F A tub bath lasts 30 minutes.

15 T F Washcloths are rinsed and re-used during perineal care.

16 T F Perineal care helps prevent infection.

17 T F Foreskin is returned to its normal position immediately after rinsing.

18 T F Report bleeding to the nurse at once.

Circle the BEST answer.

19 When assisting with daily care, you
  a Clean an incontinent person as often as needed
  b Give early morning care after breakfast
  c Follow your own routines and habits
  d Change soiled linens in the afternoon

20 You perform oral hygiene to
  a Prevent aspiration
  b Remove excess oils and perspiration
  c Prevent mouth odors and infection
  d Remove cavities

21 A person flosses once a day. When is the best time to floss?
  a In the morning
  b Before a meal
  c Before brushing
  d At bedtime

22 Which must you report to the nurse?
  a Clean skin
  b Moist and intact lips
  c A bruise on the arm
  d Food between the teeth

23 To apply powder
  a Turn the person toward you
  b Sprinkle a small amount onto your hand
  c Apply a thick layer of powder
  d Shake the powder onto the person

24 Soaps
  a Dry the skin
  b Replace skin oils
  c Soften the skin
  d Reduce perspiration

25 When bathing a person
  a Keep bar soap in the wash basin or tub
  b Wash from the dirtiest to the cleanest area
  c Assist with elimination after a bath
  d Rinse the skin well to remove all soap

26 Water for a complete bed bath is between
  a 100°F and 104°F
  b 105°F and 109°F
  c 110°F and 115°F
  d 120°F and 125°F

27 When drying the person
  a Dry well between skin folds
  b Rub the skin dry
  c Avoid drying between the toes
  d Allow the person to air dry

28 When assisting with a shower in a shower room
  a Direct the water spray at the person's face
  b Allow a weak person to stand if you provide support
  c Go to the person's room to make the bed during the shower
  d Clean, disinfect, and dry the shower before and after use

29 Water temperature for perineal care is between
  a 100°F and 104°F
  b 105°F and 109°F
  c 110°F and 115°F
  d 120°F and 125°F

30 These statements are about perineal care. Which is *true?*
  a Do not explain the procedure to avoid embarrassment.
  b The person does perineal care if able.
  c Clean from the back (bottom) to front (top).
  d Draping the person is not needed.

Answers to Chapter 22 questions are on p. 871.

FOCUS ON **PRACTICE**

Problem Solving

You are a student in the clinical setting. You are helping a nursing assistant position and turn a resident during perineal care. The nursing assistant does not wear gloves, does not use a clean part of the washcloth for each stroke, and wipes from the back (bottom) to the front (top). What has the nursing assistant done wrong? How you can you correct the situation?

Grooming

OBJECTIVES

- Define the key terms and key abbreviations in this chapter.
- Explain why grooming is important.
- Explain how to safely provide grooming measures—hair care, shaving, nail and foot care, and changing garments.

- Perform the procedures described in this chapter.
- Explain how to promote PRIDE in the person, the family, and yourself.

KEY TERMS

alopecia Hair loss
anticoagulant A drug that prevents or slows down (anti) blood clotting (coagulate)
dandruff Excessive amounts of dry, white flakes from the scalp
hirsutism Excessive body hair
infestation Being in or on a host
lice See "pediculosis"
mite A very small spider-like organism

pediculosis Infestation with wingless insects; lice
pediculosis capitis Infestation of the scalp (capitis) with lice
pediculosis corporis Infestation of the body (corporis) with lice
pediculosis pubis Infestation of the pubic (pubis) hair with lice
scabies A skin disorder caused by a female mite—a very small spider-like organism

KEY ABBREVIATIONS

C	Centigrade	ID	Identification
F	Fahrenheit	IV	Intravenous

Hair care, shaving, nail and foot care, and clean garments prevent infection and promote comfort. Such measures affect love, belonging, and self-esteem needs.

People differ in their grooming measures. Some want only clean hair. Others want a certain hairstyle. Some want only clean hands. Others want polished nails. Men may shave and groom their beards. Likewise, women may shave their legs and underarms. Some women use hair removal methods for facial hair.

As with hygiene, the person performs grooming measures to the extent possible. This promotes independence and quality of life. The person may use adaptive devices (Fig. 23-1).

See *Focus on Surveys: Grooming*.

See *Teamwork and Time Management: Grooming*.

FOCUS ON SURVEYS

Grooming

Grooming promotes the person's self-esteem and self-worth. Therefore surveyors will observe if patients and residents:

- Are groomed according to their wishes.
- Have hair combed and styled.
- Have beards shaved or trimmed.
- Are dressed in their own clothes.
- Are wearing the correct clothing for the time of day.
- Can reach grooming supplies.

TEAMWORK AND TIME MANAGEMENT

Grooming

Some grooming equipment is shared among patients and residents. Shampoo trays, electric shavers, nail clippers, and whirlpool foot baths are examples. Let your co-workers know when you need an item. Schedule the item following agency policy. When done, promptly clean and return the item to its proper place. Do not make your co-workers look for or clean an item.

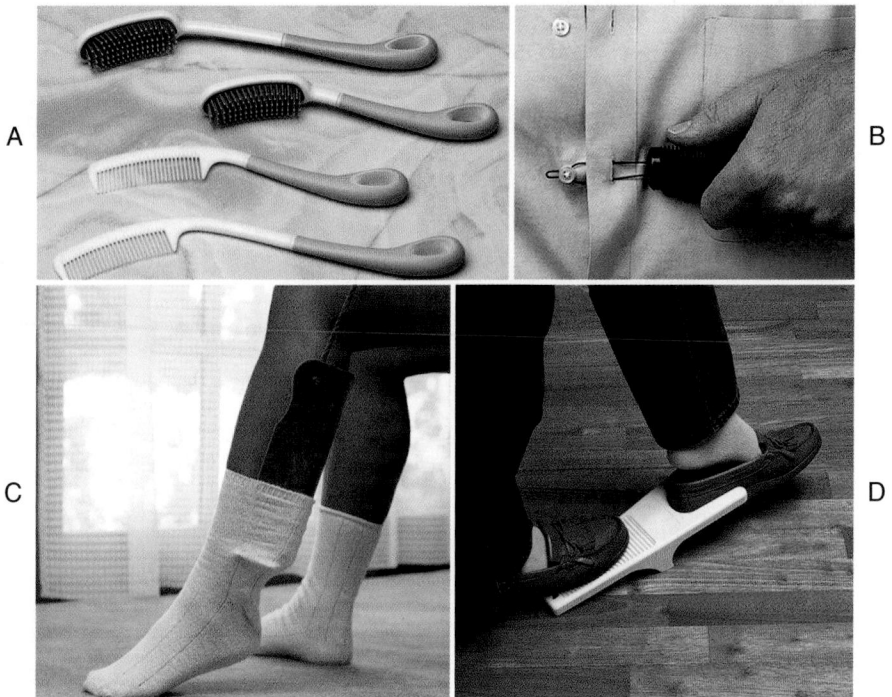

FIGURE 23-1 Grooming aids. **A,** Long-handled combs and brushes for hair care. **B,** A button hook to button and zip clothing. **C,** A sock assist to pull on socks and stockings. **D,** A shoe remover to take off shoes. (Courtesy North Coast Medical Inc., Morgan Hill, Calif.)

HAIR CARE

The look and feel of hair affect mental well-being. The nursing process reflects the person's culture, personal choice, skin and scalp conditions, health history, and self-care ability. You assist with hair care as needed.

See *Focus on Long-Term Care and Home Care: Hair Care.*

FOCUS ON **LONG-TERM CARE AND HOME CARE**
Hair Care
Long-Term Care
Beauty and barber shops are common in nursing centers (Fig. 23-2). Residents can have their hair shampooed, cut, and styled. Men can have their mustaches and beards groomed.

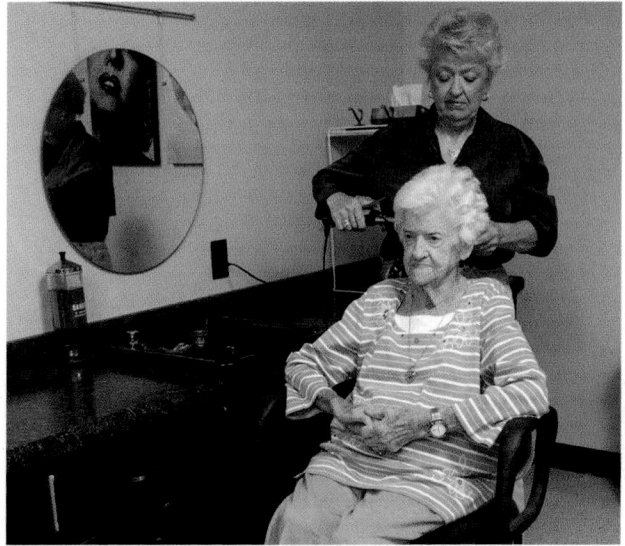

FIGURE 23-2 Beauty shop in a nursing center.

Skin and Scalp Conditions

Skin and scalp conditions include hair loss, excessive body hair, dandruff, lice, and scabies.

- *Alopecia means hair loss.* Hair loss may be complete or partial. A result of heredity, male pattern baldness occurs with aging. Hair thins in some women with aging. Cancer treatments (radiation therapy to the head and chemotherapy) may cause alopecia in all age-groups. Skin disease, stress, poor nutrition, pregnancy, some drugs, and hormone changes are other causes. Except for hair loss from aging, hair usually grows back.
- *Hirsutism is excessive body hair.* It can occur in men, women, and children. It results from heredity and abnormal amounts of male hormones.
- *Dandruff is the excessive amount of dry, white flakes from the scalp.* Itching is common. Sometimes eyebrows and ear canals are involved. Medicated shampoos correct the problem.
- *Pediculosis (lice) is the infestation with wingless insects* (Fig. 23-3). *Infestation means being in or on a host.* Lice attach their eggs *(nits)* to hair shafts. Nits are oval and yellow to white in color. They hatch in about 1 week. After hatching, they bite the scalp or skin to feed on blood. About the size of a sesame seed, adult lice are tan to gray-ish white in color. Lice easily spread to others through clothing, head coverings, furniture, beds, towels, bed linens, and sexual contact. They also are spread by sharing combs and brushes. Lice are treated with medicated shampoos, lotions, and creams specific for lice. Thorough bathing is needed. So is washing clothing and linens in hot water. Lice bites cause severe itching in the affected body area.
  - *Pediculosis capitis is the infestation of the scalp* (capitis) *with lice.* It is commonly called "head lice."
  - *Pediculosis pubis is the infestation of the pubic* (pubis) *hair with lice.* This form of lice is also called "crabs."
  - *Pediculosis corporis is the infestation of the body* (corporis) *with lice.*
- *Scabies is a skin disorder caused by a female mite* (Fig. 23-4). A *mite is a very small spider-like organism.* The female mite burrows into the skin and lays eggs. After hatching, the females produce more eggs. Infested with mites, the person has a rash and intense itching. Common sites are between the fingers, the wrists, underarm areas, thighs, and genital area. Other sites include the breasts, waist, and buttocks. Highly contagious, scabies is transmitted to others by close contact. Persons in crowded living settings are at risk. So are persons with weakened immune systems. Special creams are ordered to kill the mites. The person's room is cleaned. Clothing and linens are washed in hot water.

See *Focus on Communication: Skin and Scalp Conditions.*

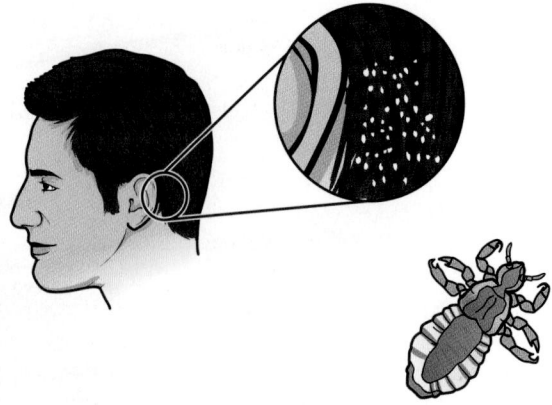

FIGURE 23-3 Head lice. (Redrawn from Medline Plus: *Head lice.* Bethesda, Md., National Institutes of Health.)

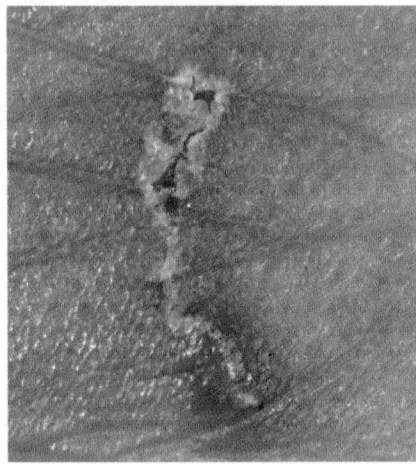

FIGURE 23-4 Scabies. (From Marks JG, Miller JJ: *Lookingbill & Marks' principles of dermatology,* ed 4, St Louis, 2006, Saunders.)

FOCUS ON **COMMUNICATION**

Skin and Scalp Conditions

Some skin or scalp conditions may alarm you. Remain professional. Do not say things that may embarrass the person.

Report an abnormal skin or scalp condition. Describe what you saw as best as you can. For example:

- "I saw some small red dots on Mr. Martin's right underarm during his bath. Would you please look at them?"
- "I saw some small white specks in Mrs. Patel's hair. Would you please look at them before I wash her hair?"

Brushing and Combing Hair

Brushing and combing hair are part of early morning care, morning care, and afternoon care. Some people also do so at bedtime. Provide hair care when needed and before visitors arrive.

Encourage patients and residents to do their own hair care. The person chooses how to brush, comb, and style hair. Assist as needed. Provide hair care for those who cannot do so.

Brushing increases blood flow to the scalp. And it brings scalp oils along the hair shaft to help keep hair soft and shiny. Daily brushing and combing prevent tangled and matted hair. To brush and comb hair, start at the scalp. Then brush or comb to the hair ends.

Braiding prevents long hair from matting and tangling. You need the person's consent to braid hair. Report matted or tangled hair to the nurse. The nurse may have you comb or brush through the matting and tangling from the hair ends to the scalp. *Never cut the person's hair.*

Special measures are needed for curly, coarse, and dry hair. For curly hair, use a wide-tooth comb. Start at the neckline. Working upward, lift and fluff hair outward. Continue to the forehead. Wet hair or apply conditioner, petroleum jelly, or other hair care product as directed. This makes combing easier. Follow the care plan for coarse and dry hair.

The person may have certain hair care practices and products. They are part of the care plan. Also, let the person guide you when giving hair care.

See *Caring about Culture: Brushing and Combing Hair.*

See *Focus on Children and Older Persons: Brushing and Combing Hair.*

See *Delegation Guidelines: Brushing and Combing Hair.*

See *Promoting Safety and Comfort: Brushing and Combing Hair.*

See procedure: *Brushing and Combing Hair*, p. 370.

DELEGATION GUIDELINES
Brushing and Combing Hair

To brush and comb hair, you need this information from the nurse and the care plan.
- How much help the person needs
- What to do for matted or tangled hair
- What to do for curly, coarse, or dry hair
- What hair care products to use
- The person's preferences and routine hair care measures
- What observations to report and record:
  - Scalp sores
  - Flaking
  - Itching
  - Rash
  - Patches of hair loss
  - Hair falling out in patches
  - Very dry or very oily hair
  - Matted or tangled hair
  - The presence of nits or lice
    - Nits (lice eggs attached to hair shafts)—oval and yellow to white in color
    - Lice—about the size of a sesame seed and gray-ish white in color
    - Itching
    - Complaints of a tickling feeling or something moving in the hair
    - Irritability
    - Sores on the head or body caused by scratching
    - Rash
- When to report observations
- What patient or resident concerns to report at once

CARING ABOUT CULTURE
Brushing and Combing Hair

Small braids (cornrows) are common in some cultural groups. The braids are left intact for shampooing. To undo these braids, the nurse obtains the person's consent.

FOCUS ON CHILDREN AND OLDER PERSONS
Brushing and Combing Hair

Children
Hairstyles are important to older children and teenagers. Do not make judgments about the hairstyle. Style hair in a way that pleases the child and parents. Do not style hair according to your standards or customs.

PROMOTING SAFETY AND COMFORT
Brushing and Combing Hair

Safety
Sharp bristles can injure the scalp. So can a comb with sharp or broken teeth. Report concerns about the person's brush or comb.

Wear gloves if the person has scalp sores. Follow Standard Precautions and the Bloodborne Pathogen Standard.

Comfort
Place a towel across the person's back and shoulders to protect garments from falling hair. If the person is in bed, give hair care before changing linens and the pillowcase. If done after a linen change, place a towel across the pillow to collect falling hair.

Brushing and Combing Hair

QUALITY OF LIFE

- Knock before entering the person's room.
- Address the person by name.
- Introduce yourself by name and title.

- Explain the procedure before starting and during the procedure.
- Protect the person's rights during the procedure.
- Handle the person gently during the procedure.

PRE-PROCEDURE

1 Follow *Delegation Guidelines: Brushing and Combing Hair,* p. 369. See *Promoting Safety and Comfort: Brushing and Combing Hair,* p. 369.
2 Practice hand hygiene.
3 Identify the person. Check the ID (identification) bracelet against the assignment sheet. Use 2 identifiers (Chapter 13). Also call the person by name.

4 Ask the person how to style hair.
5 Collect the following.
  - Comb and brush
  - Bath towel
  - Other hair care items as requested
6 Arrange items on the bedside stand.
7 Provide for privacy.

PROCEDURE

8 Lower the bed rail if up.
9 Position the person.
  a *In a chair*—Help the person to the chair. The person puts on a robe and non-skid footwear when up.
  b *In bed*—Raise the bed for body mechanics. Bed rails are up if used. Lower the bed rail near you. Assist the person to a semi-Fowler's position if allowed.
10 Place a towel across the person's back and shoulders or across the pillow.
11 Ask the person to remove eyeglasses. Put them in the eyeglass case. Put the case inside the bedside stand.

12 *Brush and comb hair that is not matted or tangled.*
  a Use the comb to part the hair.
    1) Part hair down the middle into 2 sides (Fig. 23-5, *A*).
    2) Divide 1 side into 2 smaller sections (Fig. 23-5, *B*).
  b Brush 1 of the small sections of hair. Start at the scalp and brush toward the hair ends (Fig. 23-6). Do the same for the other small section of hair.
  c Repeat steps 12, a(2) and b for the other side.
13 *Brush or comb matted or tangled hair.*
  a Take a small section of hair near the ends.
  b Comb or brush through to the hair ends.
  c Add small sections of hair as you work up to the scalp.
  d Comb or brush through each longer section to the hair ends.
14 Style the hair as the person prefers.
15 Remove the towel.
16 Let the person put on the eyeglasses.

POST-PROCEDURE

17 Provide for comfort. (See the inside of the front cover.)
18 Place the call light and other needed items within reach.
19 Lower the bed to a safe and comfortable level for the person. Follow the care plan.
20 Raise or lower bed rails. Follow the care plan.
21 Remove hair from the brush or comb. Clean and return hair care items to their proper place. Wear gloves for this step. Remove and discard the gloves. Practice hand hygiene.

22 Unscreen the person.
23 Complete a safety check of the room. (See the inside of the front cover.)
24 Follow agency policy for used linens.
25 Practice hand hygiene.

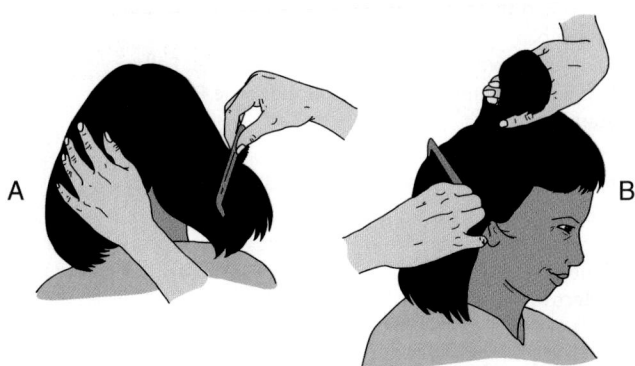

FIGURE 23-5 Part hair. A, Part hair down the middle. Divide it into 2 sides. **B,** Then part 1 side into 2 smaller sections.

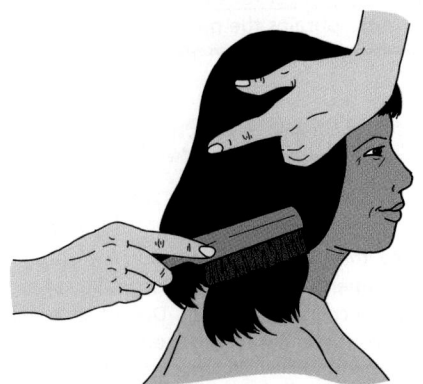

FIGURE 23-6 Brush hair by starting at the scalp. Brush down to the hair ends.

Shampooing

People vary in shampoo frequency—1, 2, or 3 times a week or daily. Factors affecting frequency include hair and scalp condition, hairstyle, and personal choice.

Some persons use certain shampoos and conditioners. Others use medicated products ordered by the doctor.

The person may need help shampooing. The nurse tells you what method to use. The shampoo method depends on the person's condition, safety factors, and personal choice.

- *Shampoo during the shower or tub bath.* You use a hand-held nozzle for persons in shower chairs or taking tub baths. Direct a spray of water at the hair.
- *Shampoo at the sink.* The person sits or lies facing away from the sink. A folded towel placed over the sink edge protects the neck. The person's head is tilted back over the sink edge (Fig. 23-7). Use a water pitcher or hand-held nozzle to wet and rinse the hair.
- *Shampoo in bed.* The person's head and shoulders are at the edge of the bed if possible. A shampoo tray is under the head to protect the linens and mattress from water. The tray drains into a basin on a chair by the bed (Fig. 23-8). Use a water pitcher to wet and rinse the hair. This method is used for persons:
  - Needing complete bed baths
  - Who cannot use a chair, wheelchair, or stretcher

Some agencies have commercial shampoo caps. The cap has a cleaning agent that does not need rinsing. Some caps also have a conditioner. To use a shampoo cap:

- Warm the package in a microwave oven or commercial warmer. Follow the manufacturer's instructions for microwave settings and warming times.
- Check the temperature. The cap should be warm. Do not use a cap that is too hot.
- Apply the cap to the person's head.
- Massage the cap gently. Follow the manufacturer's instructions for how long to massage—usually 1 to 3 minutes. Longer hair may require more time.
- Remove the cap. You do not need to rinse the hair. Dry the hair with a towel if needed.
- Comb the hair.

Dry and style hair as soon as possible after the shampoo. Women may want hair curled or rolled up before drying. Check with the nurse before doing so.

See *Focus on Children and Older Persons: Shampooing.*

See *Focus on Long-Term Care and Home Care: Shampooing,* p. 372.

See *Delegation Guidelines: Shampooing,* p. 372.

See *Promoting Safety and Comfort: Shampooing,* p. 372.

See procedure: *Shampooing the Person's Hair,* p. 373.

Text continued on p. 374.

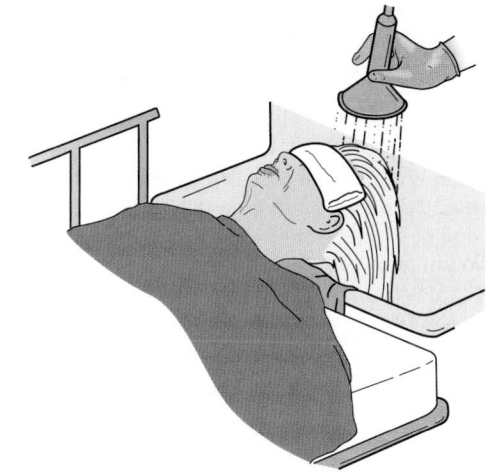

FIGURE 23-7 Shampooing while the person is on a stretcher. The stretcher is in front of the sink.

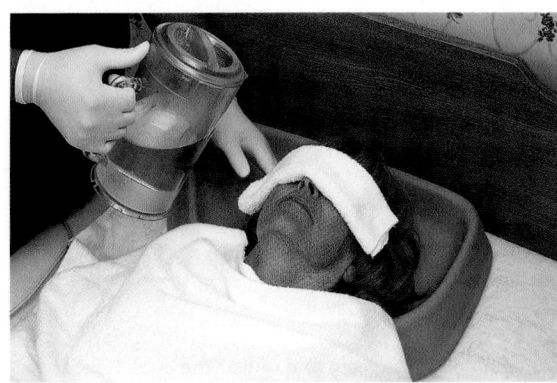

FIGURE 23-8 A shampoo tray for a person in bed. The tray is directed to the side of the bed so water drains into a collecting basin.

FOCUS ON **CHILDREN AND OLDER PERSONS**

Shampooing

Children

Oil gland secretion increases with puberty. Therefore adolescents tend to have oily hair. They may need to shampoo often.

Older Persons

Oil gland secretion decreases with aging. Therefore older persons have dry hair. They may shampoo less often than younger adults do.

FOCUS ON LONG-TERM CARE AND HOME CARE

Shampooing

Long-Term Care

Shampooing is usually done weekly on the person's bath or shower day. If a person's hair is done by a hairdresser or barber, do not shampoo the hair. The person wears a shower cap during the tub bath or shower.

Home Care

You can make a shampoo tray from a plastic shower curtain or tablecloth. Or use a sturdy plastic drop cloth for painting. Do not use plastic trash bags or dry-cleaning bags. Not sturdy, they slip and slide easily.

To make the tray, place the plastic under the person's head. Make a raised edge around the plastic to prevent water from spilling over the sides. Tape the plastic in place if necessary. Direct the ends of the plastic into a basin. Water flows into the basin.

DELEGATION GUIDELINES

Shampooing

To shampoo a person, you need this information from the nurse and the care plan.
- When to shampoo the person's hair
- What method to use
- What shampoo and conditioner to use
- What to do with medicated products after the procedure
- The person's position restrictions or limits
- What water temperature to use—usually 105°F (Fahrenheit) (40.5°C [centigrade])
- If hair is curled up or rolled before drying
- What observations to report and record:
  - Scalp sores
  - Flaking
  - Itching
  - The presence of nits or lice (p. 368)
  - Patches of hair loss
  - Hair falling out in patches
  - Very dry or very oily hair
  - Matted or tangled hair
  - How the person tolerated the procedure
- When to report observations
- What patient or resident concerns to report at once

PROMOTING SAFETY AND COMFORT

Shampooing

Safety

Keep shampoo away from and out of the eyes. Have the person hold a washcloth over the eyes. When rinsing, cup your hand at the person's forehead. This keeps soapy water from running down the forehead and into the eyes.

Remove hearing aids before shampooing. Water will damage hearing aids.

Wear gloves if the person has scalp sores. Follow Standard Precautions and the Bloodborne Pathogen Standard.

For a shampoo on a stretcher at a sink, see Chapter 19 for stretcher safety. For safe stretcher transfers, see procedure: *Moving the Person to a Stretcher* in Chapter 19. Lock (brake) the stretcher wheels and use the safety straps and side rails. The far side rail is raised during the procedure.

Some people shampoo themselves during a tub bath or shower. Place an extra towel, shampoo, and hair conditioner within the person's reach. Assist as needed.

Comfort

When shampooing during the tub bath or shower, the person tips his or her head back to keep shampoo and water out of the eyes. Support the back of the head with 1 hand. Shampoo with your other hand. Some persons cannot tip their heads back. They lean forward and hold a folded washcloth over the eyes. Support the forehead with 1 hand as you shampoo with the other. Make sure that the person can breathe easily.

Many people have limited range of motion in their necks. They are not shampooed at the sink or on a stretcher.

Shampooing the Person's Hair

QUALITY OF LIFE

- Knock before entering the person's room.
- Address the person by name.
- Introduce yourself by name and title.

- Explain the procedure before starting and during the procedure.
- Protect the person's rights during the procedure.
- Handle the person gently during the procedure.

PRE-PROCEDURE

1 Follow *Delegation Guidelines: Shampooing.* See *Promoting Safety and Comfort: Shampooing.*
2 Practice hand hygiene.
3 Collect the following.
   - 2 bath towels
   - Washcloth
   - Shampoo
   - Hair conditioner (if requested)
   - Bath thermometer
   - Pitcher or hand-held nozzle (if needed)
   - Shampoo tray (if needed)
   - Basin or pan (if needed)
   - Waterproof pad (if needed)
   - Gloves (if needed)
   - Comb and brush
   - Hair dryer
4 Arrange items nearby.
5 Identify the person. Check the ID bracelet against the assignment sheet. Use 2 identifiers (Chapter 13). Also call the person by name.
6 Provide for privacy.
7 Raise the bed for body mechanics for a shampoo in bed. Bed rails are up if used.
8 Practice hand hygiene.

PROCEDURE

9 Lower the bed rail near you if up.
10 Cover the person's chest with a bath towel.
11 Brush and comb the hair to remove snarls and tangles.
12 Position the person for the method used. For a shampoo in bed:
   a Lower the head of the bed and remove the pillow.
   b Place the waterproof pad and shampoo tray under the head and shoulders.
   c Support the head and neck with a folded towel if necessary.
13 Raise the bed rail if used.
14 Obtain water. Water temperature is usually 105°F (40.5°C). Test water temperature according to agency policy. Also ask the nurse to check the water. Adjust the water temperature as needed. Raise the bed rail before leaving the bedside.
15 Lower the bed rail near you if up.
16 Put on gloves (if needed).
17 Ask the person to hold a washcloth over the eyes. It should not cover the nose and mouth. (NOTE: A damp washcloth is easier to hold. It will not slip. However, your agency may require a dry washcloth.)
18 Use the water pitcher or nozzle to wet the hair.
19 Apply a small amount of shampoo.
20 Work up a lather with both hands. Start at the hairline. Work toward the back of the head.
21 Massage the scalp with your fingertips. Do not scratch the scalp with your fingernails.
22 Rinse the hair until the water runs clear.
23 Repeat steps 19 through 22.
24 Apply conditioner. Follow directions on the container.
25 Squeeze water from the person's hair.
26 Cover the hair with a bath towel.
27 Remove the shampoo tray, basin, and waterproof pad.
28 Dry the person's face with a towel. Use the towel on the person's chest.
29 Help the person raise the head if appropriate. For the person in bed, raise the head of the bed.
30 Rub the hair and scalp with the towel. Rub gently. Use the second towel if the first one is wet.
31 Comb the hair to remove snarls and tangles.
32 Dry and style hair.
33 Remove and discard the gloves (if used). Practice hand hygiene.

POST-PROCEDURE

34 Provide for comfort. (See the inside of the front cover.)
35 Place the call light and other needed items within reach.
36 Lower the bed to a safe and comfortable level for the person. Follow the care plan.
37 Raise or lower bed rails. Follow the care plan.
38 Unscreen the person.
39 Complete a safety check of the room. (See the inside of the front cover.)
40 Clean, rinse, dry, and return equipment to its proper place. Remember to clean the comb and brush. Wear gloves for this step. Discard disposable items. Remove and discard the gloves.
41 Follow agency policy for used linens.
42 Practice hand hygiene.
43 Report and record your observations.

■ SHAVING

Many men shave for comfort and well-being. Many women shave their legs and underarms. Some women shave facial hair. Other hair removal methods include waxing, hair removal products, plucking, and threading. See Box 23-1 for shaving rules.

Safety razors or electric shavers are used (Fig. 23-9). Some persons have their own electric shavers. If the agency's shaver is used, clean it before and after use. To brush out whiskers or hair, follow the manufacturer's instructions. Also follow agency policy for cleaning electric shavers.

Safety razors (blade razors) have razor blades. They can cause nicks and cuts. Do not use safety razors on persons with healing problems or for those taking anticoagulant drugs. An ***anticoagulant*** is a drug that prevents or slows down (anti) blood clotting (coagulate). Bleeding occurs easily and is hard to stop. A nick or cut can cause serious bleeding. Electric shavers are used.

Soften the beard before shaving. To do so, apply a moist, warm washcloth or towel for a few minutes. Then pat dry the face and apply talcum powder if using an electric shaver. For a safety razor, lather the face with soap and water or shaving cream.

See *Focus on Children and Older Persons: Shaving.*
See *Delegation Guidelines: Shaving.*
See *Promoting Safety and Comfort: Shaving.*
See procedure: *Shaving the Person's Face With a Safety Razor.*

BOX 23-1	Rules for Shaving

- Use electric shavers for persons taking anticoagulant drugs. Never use safety razors.
- Protect bed linens. Place a towel under the part being shaved. Or place a towel across the person's chest and shoulders to protect clothing.
- Soften the beard before shaving. Apply a warm, moist washcloth or towel to the face for a few minutes.
- Encourage the person to do as much as safely possible.
- Hold the skin taut as needed.
- Shave in the correct direction.
  - *Shaving the face with a safety razor*—shave in the direction of hair growth.
  - *Shaving the underarms with a safety razor*—shave in the direction of hair growth.
  - *Shaving the legs with a safety razor*—shave up from the ankles. This is against hair growth.
  - *Using an electric shaver*—shave against the direction of hair growth. If using a rotary-type shaver, move the shaver in small circles over the face. (NOTE: Some state competency tests require shaving in the direction of hair growth. Follow the manufacturer's instructions and the rules in your state and agency.)
- Do not cut, nick, or irritate the skin.
- Rinse the skin thoroughly.
- Apply direct pressure to nicks or cuts (Chapter 54).
- Report nicks, cuts, or irritation at once.

FOCUS ON CHILDREN AND OLDER PERSONS
Shaving

Older Persons
Older persons with wrinkled skin are at risk for nicks and cuts. Safety razors are not used to shave them or persons with dementia. Persons with dementia may not understand what you are doing. They may resist care and move suddenly. Serious nicks and cuts can occur. Use electric shavers for these persons.

DELEGATION GUIDELINES
Shaving

To shave a person, you need this information from the nurse and the care plan.
- What shaver to use—electric or safety
- If the person takes anticoagulant drugs
- When to shave the person
- What facial hair to shave
- If there are tender or sensitive areas on the person's face
- What observations to report and record:
  - Nicks (report at once)
  - Cuts (report at once)
  - Bleeding (report at once)
  - Irritation
- When to report observations
- What patient or resident concerns to report at once

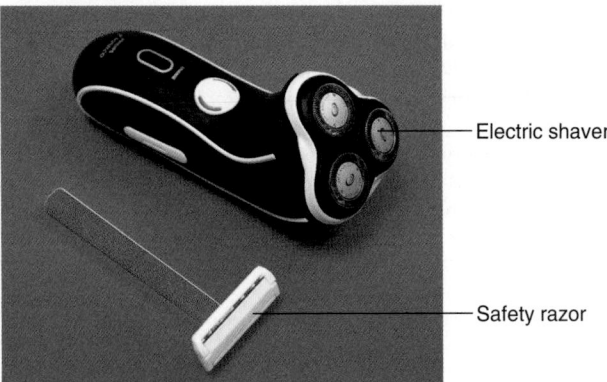

Electric shaver

Safety razor

FIGURE 23-9 Electric shaver and safety razor.

PROMOTING SAFETY AND COMFORT

Shaving

Safety

Safety razors are very sharp. Protect the person and yourself from nicks and cuts. Prevent contact with blood. For an electric shaver, follow safety measures for electrical equipment (Chapter 13).

Rinse the safety razor often during the procedure. Rinsing removes whiskers (or hair) and lather. Then wipe the razor. To protect yourself from cuts:

- Place several thicknesses of tissues or paper towels on the over-bed table. Do not hold them in your hand.
- Wipe the razor on the tissues or paper towels.

Follow Standard Precautions and the Bloodborne Pathogen Standard. Discard used razor blades and disposable shavers in the sharps container. Do not re-cap the razor.

Comfort

In some men, the neck area below the jaw is tender and sensitive. Some electric shavers become very warm or hot while in use. The heat can irritate the skin. Shave tender areas first while the shaver is cool. Then move to other areas of the face.

Some people apply lotion or after-shave to the skin after shaving. Lotion softens the skin. After-shave closes skin pores. To soften the skin and open pores, apply heat before shaving.

Shaving the Person's Face With a Safety Razor

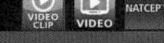

QUALITY OF LIFE

- Knock before entering the person's room.
- Address the person by name.
- Introduce yourself by name and title.
- Explain the procedure before starting and during the procedure.
- Protect the person's rights during the procedure.
- Handle the person gently during the procedure.

PRE-PROCEDURE

1 Follow *Delegation Guidelines: Shaving.* See *Promoting Safety and Comfort: Shaving.*
2 Practice hand hygiene.
3 Collect the following.
   - Wash basin
   - Bath towel
   - Hand towel
   - Washcloth
   - Safety razor
   - Mirror
   - Shaving cream, soap, or lotion
   - Shaving brush
   - After-shave or lotion
   - Tissues or paper towels
   - Gloves
4 Arrange paper towels and supplies on the over-bed table.
5 Identify the person. Check the ID bracelet against the assignment sheet. Use 2 identifiers (Chapter 13). Also call the person by name.
6 Provide for privacy.
7 Raise the bed for body mechanics. Bed rails are up if used.

PROCEDURE

8 Fill the wash basin with warm water.
9 Place the basin on the over-bed table.
10 Lower the bed rail near you if up.
11 Practice hand hygiene. Put on gloves.
12 Assist the person to semi-Fowler's position if allowed or to the supine position.
13 Adjust lighting to clearly see the person's face.
14 Place the towel over the person's chest and shoulders.
15 Adjust the over-bed table for easy reach.
16 Tighten the razor blade to the shaver if necessary.
17 Wash the person's face. Do not dry.
18 Wet the washcloth or towel. Wring it out.
19 Apply the washcloth or towel to the face for a few minutes.
20 Apply shaving cream with your hands. Or use a shaving brush to apply lather.
21 Hold the skin taut with 1 hand.
22 Shave in the direction of hair growth. Use shorter strokes around the chin and lips (Fig. 23-10, p. 376).
23 Rinse the razor often. Wipe it with tissues or paper towels.
24 Apply direct pressure to any bleeding areas (Chapter 54).
25 Wash off any remaining shaving cream or soap. Pat dry with a towel.
26 Apply after-shave or lotion if requested. (If there are nicks or cuts, do not apply after-shave or lotion.)
27 Remove and discard the towel and gloves. Practice hand hygiene.

Continued

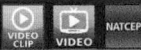

Shaving the Person's Face With a Safety Razor—cont'd

POST-PROCEDURE

28 Provide for comfort. (See the inside of the front cover.)
29 Place the call light and other needed items within reach.
30 Lower the bed to a safe and comfortable level for the person. Follow the care plan.
31 Raise or lower bed rails. Follow the care plan.
32 Clean, rinse, dry, and return equipment and supplies to their proper place. Discard the razor blade or disposable razor into the sharps container. Discard other disposable items. Wear gloves.
33 Wipe off the over-bed table with paper towels. Discard the paper towels.
34 Unscreen the person.
35 Complete a safety check of the room. (See the inside of the front cover.)
36 Follow agency policy for used linens.
37 Remove and discard the gloves. Practice hand hygiene.
38 Report nicks, cuts, irritation, or bleeding to the nurse at once. Also report and record other observations.

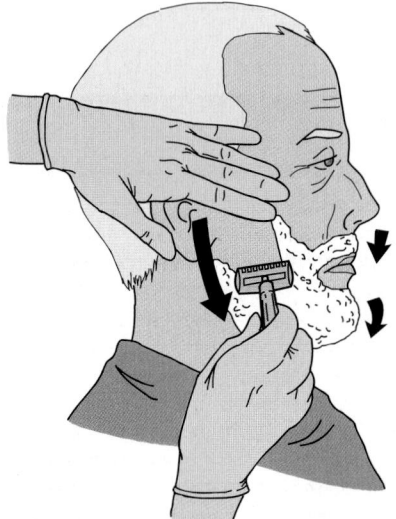

FIGURE 23-10 Shave the face in the direction of hair growth. Use long strokes on the larger areas of the face. Use short strokes around the chin and lips.

Caring for Mustaches and Beards

Mustaches and beards need daily care. Food can collect in the whiskers. So can mouth and nose drainage. Daily washing and combing are needed. Ask the person how to groom his mustache or beard. *Never trim a mustache or beard.*

Shaving Legs and Underarms

Many women shave their legs and underarms. This practice varies among cultures. Some women shave only the lower legs. Others shave to mid-thigh or the entire leg.
To shave legs and underarms:
• Follow the rules in Box 23-1.
• Collect shaving items with bath items.
• Shave after bathing. The skin is soft at this time.
• Use soap and water, shaving cream, or lotion for the lather. Follow the care plan.
• Use the kidney basin to rinse the razor. Do not use bath water.

NAIL AND FOOT CARE

Nail and foot care prevents infection, injury, and odors. Hangnails, ingrown nails (nails that grow in at the side), and nails torn away from the skin cause skin breaks. These breaks are portals of entry for microbes. Long or broken nails can scratch skin and snag clothing.

The feet are easily injured and infected. Dirty feet, socks, or stockings harbor microbes and cause odors. Shoes and socks provide a warm, moist environment for microbes to grow. Injuries occur from stubbing toes, stepping on sharp objects, or being stepped on. Poorly fitting shoes cause blisters.

Poor circulation prolongs healing. Diabetes and vascular diseases are common causes of poor circulation. Foot injuries or infections are very serious for older persons and persons with circulatory disorders. Gangrene and amputation are serious complications (Chapter 44).

Nails are easier to trim and clean right after soaking or bathing. Use nail clippers to cut fingernails. *Never use scissors.* Use extreme caution to prevent damage to nearby tissues.

Trimming and clipping toenails can easily cause injuries. *Some agencies do not let nursing assistants cut or trim toenails. Follow agency policy.*

See *Teamwork and Time Management: Nail and Foot Care.*
See *Focus on Long-Term Care and Home Care: Nail and Foot Care.*
See *Delegation Guidelines: Nail and Foot Care.*
See *Promoting Safety and Comfort: Nail and Foot Care.*
See procedure: *Giving Nail and Foot Care*, p. 378.

TEAMWORK AND TIME MANAGEMENT

Nail and Foot Care

Use your time well when giving nail and foot care. The fingernails soak for 5 to 10 minutes. The feet soak for 15 to 20 minutes. You can make the person's bed or straighten the person's unit during soak time. Or you could assist with brushing and combing hair. Check your assignment sheet for other ways to meet the person's needs.

FOCUS ON LONG-TERM CARE AND HOME CARE

Nail and Foot Care

Home Care

The feet soak during a tub bath. Or the person can sit on the side of the tub to soak the feet. Make sure the person can step into and out of the tub. Or have the person use a shower bench to get in and out of the tub (Chapter 22). Otherwise, soak the feet in a basin or a whirlpool foot bath.

If comfortable for the person, he or she can soak the fingers in the sink. Or use a bowl if you do not have a small basin.

DELEGATION GUIDELINES

Nail and Foot Care

To give nail and foot care, you need this information from the nurse and the care plan.
- What water temperature to use
- How long to soak fingernails (usually 5 to 10 minutes)
- How long to soak feet (usually 15 to 20 minutes)
- What observations to report and record:
  - Dry, reddened, irritated, or callused areas
  - Breaks in the skin
  - Corns (Chapter 36) on top of and between the toes
  - Blisters
  - Very thick nails
  - Loose nails
- When to report observations
- What patient or resident concerns to report at once

PROMOTING SAFETY AND COMFORT

Nail and Foot Care

Safety

To cut fingernails, use nail clippers. Clip the fingernails straight across (Fig. 23-11). Then file the nails.

Remember, some states and agencies do not let nursing assistants cut and trim toenails. The RN (registered nurse) or podiatrist (foot [pod] doctor) cuts toenails and provides foot care for the following persons. You do not cut or trim the toenails for persons who:
- Have diabetes
- Have poor circulation to the legs and feet
- Take drugs that affect blood clotting
- Have very thick nails or ingrown toenails

Check between the toes for cracks and sores. These areas are often overlooked. If not treated, a serious infection could occur.

The feet are easily burned. Persons with decreased sensation or circulatory problems may not feel hot temperatures.

Safety—cont'd

After soaking, apply lotion or petroleum jelly to the feet. This can cause slippery feet. Help the person put on non-skid footwear before you transfer the person or let the person walk.

Breaks in the skin and bleeding can occur. Follow Standard Precautions and the Bloodborne Pathogen Standard.

Comfort

Sometimes you just trim the fingernails. Sometimes you just give foot care. To do both, the person sits at the over-bed table (Fig. 23-12). Provide for warmth and comfort.

Promote your own comfort during nail and foot care. Sit in front of the over-bed table to clean and trim fingernails. For foot care, rest the person's lower leg and foot on your lap. Or position the feet on the floor and kneel on the floor. Lay a towel across your lap or put a bath mat on the floor to protect your uniform. Use good body mechanics. Always support the person's foot and ankle during foot care.

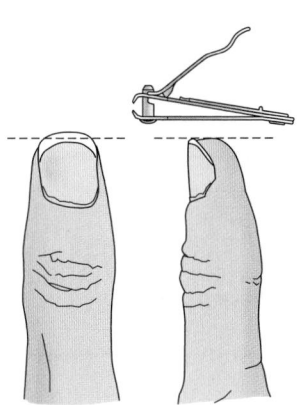

FIGURE 23-11 Clip fingernails straight across. Use nail clippers.

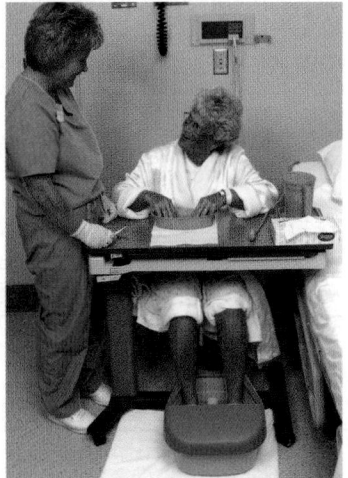

FIGURE 23-12 Nail and foot care. The feet soak in a whirlpool foot bath. The fingers soak in a kidney basin.

Giving Nail and Foot Care

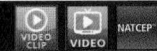

QUALITY OF LIFE

- Knock before entering the person's room.
- Address the person by name.
- Introduce yourself by name and title.

- Explain the procedure before starting and during the procedure.
- Protect the person's rights during the procedure.
- Handle the person gently during the procedure.

PRE-PROCEDURE

1 Follow *Delegation Guidelines: Nail and Foot Care*, p. 377. See *Promoting Safety and Comfort: Nail and Foot Care*, p. 377.
2 Practice hand hygiene.
3 Collect the following.
   - Wash basin or whirlpool foot bath
   - Soap
   - Bath thermometer
   - Bath towel
   - Hand towel
   - Washcloth
   - Kidney basin
   - Nail clippers
   - Orangewood stick
   - Emery board or nail file

   - Lotion for the hands
   - Lotion or petroleum jelly for the feet
   - Paper towels
   - Bath mat
   - Gloves

4 Arrange paper towels and other items on the over-bed table.
5 Identify the person. Check the ID bracelet against the assignment sheet. Use 2 identifiers (Chapter 13). Also call the person by name.
6 Provide for privacy.
7 Assist the person to the bedside chair. Remove footwear and socks or stockings. Place the call light and other needed items within reach.

PROCEDURE

8 Place the bath mat under the feet.
9 Fill the wash basin or whirlpool foot bath ⅔ (two-thirds) full with water. The nurse tells you what water temperature to use. (Measure water temperature with a bath thermometer. Or test it by dipping your elbow or inner wrist into the basin. Follow agency policy.) Also ask the person to check the water temperature. Adjust the water temperature as needed.
10 Place the basin or foot bath on the bath mat.
11 Put on gloves.
12 Help the person put his or her bare feet into the basin or foot bath. Both feet are completely covered by water.
13 Adjust the over-bed table in front of the person.
14 Fill the kidney basin ⅔ (two-thirds) full with water. See step 9 for water temperature.
15 Place the kidney basin on the over-bed table.
16 Place the person's fingers into the basin. Position the arms for comfort (see Fig. 23-12).
17 Let the fingers soak for 5 to 10 minutes. Let the feet soak for 15 to 20 minutes. Re-warm water as needed.
18 Remove the kidney basin.
19 Dry the hands and between the fingers thoroughly.
20 Clean under the fingernails with the orangewood stick. Use a towel to wipe the orangewood stick after each nail.
21 Push cuticles back with the orangewood stick or a washcloth (Fig. 23-13).

22 Clip fingernails straight across with the nail clippers (see Fig. 23-11).
23 File and shape nails with an emery board or nail file. Nails are smooth with no rough edges. Check each nail for smoothness. File as needed.
24 Apply lotion to the hands. Warm lotion before applying it.
25 Move the over-bed table to the side.
26 Remove and discard the gloves. Practice hand hygiene. Put on clean gloves. (NOTE: Some state competency tests require clean gloves for foot care.)
27 Lift a foot out of the water. Support the foot and ankle with 1 hand. With your other hand, wash the foot and between the toes with soap and a washcloth. Return the foot to the water for rinsing. Make sure you rinse between the toes.
28 Repeat step 27 for the other foot.
29 Remove the feet from the basin or foot bath. Dry thoroughly, especially between the toes. Support the foot and ankle as needed.
30 Apply lotion or petroleum jelly to the tops, soles, and heels of the feet. Do not apply between the toes. Warm lotion or petroleum jelly before applying it. Remove excess lotion or petroleum jelly with a towel. Support the foot and ankle as needed.
31 Remove and discard the gloves. Practice hand hygiene.
32 Help the person put on non-skid footwear.

POST-PROCEDURE

33 Provide for comfort. (See the inside of the front cover.)
34 Place the call light and other needed items within reach.
35 Raise or lower bed rails. Follow the care plan.
36 Clean, rinse, dry, and return equipment and supplies to their proper place. Discard disposable items. Wear gloves.
37 Unscreen the person.

38 Complete a safety check of the room. (See the inside of the front cover.)
39 Follow agency policy for used linens.
40 Remove and discard the gloves. Practice hand hygiene.
41 Report and record your observations.

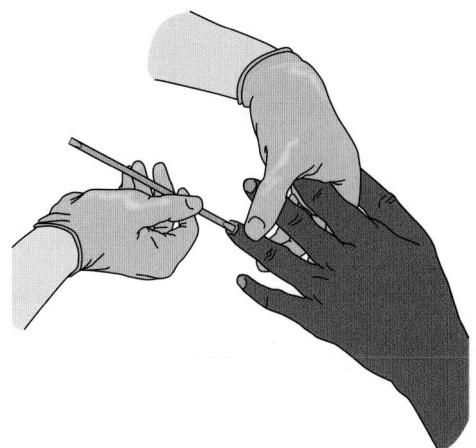

FIGURE 23-13 Push the cuticle back with an orangewood stick.

CHANGING GARMENTS

Hospital patients usually wear patient gowns or other sleepwear. Nursing center residents wear street clothes during the day and sleepwear at bedtime. Garments are changed:

- After bathing
- When wet or soiled
- On admission and discharge

◼ Dressing and Undressing

When assisting with dressing and undressing, follow the rules in Box 23-2.

See *Focus on Communication: Dressing and Undressing.*

See *Focus on Children and Older Persons: Dressing and Undressing.*

See *Focus on Long-Term Care and Home Care: Dressing and Undressing.*

See *Delegation Guidelines: Dressing and Undressing,* p. 380.

See *Promoting Safety and Comfort: Dressing and Undressing,* p. 380.

See procedure: *Undressing the Person,* p. 380.

See procedure: *Dressing the Person,* p. 382.

Text continued on p. 384.

BOX 23-2   Rules for Dressing and Undressing

- Provide for privacy. Do not expose the person.
- Encourage the person to do as much as possible.
- Let the person choose what to wear. Have the person choose the right under-garments.
- Make sure garments and footwear are the correct size.
- Remove clothing from the strong or "good" side first. This is often called the *unaffected side.*
- Put clothing on the weak side first. This is often called the *affected side.*
- Support the arm or leg to remove or put on a garment.
- Move and handle the body gently. Do not force a joint beyond its range of motion or to the point of pain. See Chapter 30.

FOCUS ON COMMUNICATION

Dressing and Undressing

Allow for personal choice and independence when assisting with dressing and undressing. You can ask:

- "What would you like to wear today?"
- "There's a concert today. Do you want to wear something special?"
- "Can I help you with those buttons?"
- "Would you like me to help you with that zipper?"

FOCUS ON CHILDREN AND OLDER PERSONS

Dressing and Undressing

Older Persons

Persons with dementia may not want to change clothes. Or they may not know how. For example, a person tries to put slacks over his or her head. Or the wrong clothes are worn for the season or weather. The Alzheimer's Disease Education and Referral Center (ADEAR) suggests the following.

- Try to assist with dressing at the same time each day. Dressing becomes part of the person's daily routine.
- Let the person dress himself or herself to the extent possible. Allow extra time. Do not rush the person.
- Let the person choose from 2 or 3 outfits. The family may buy several of the person's favorite outfit. Dressing is easier if the person insists on wearing the same thing.
- Choose comfortable clothes that are easy to get on and off. Garments with elastic waistbands and Velcro closures are examples. The person does not have to handle zippers, buttons, hooks, snaps, or other closures.
- Stack clothes in the order that they are put on. The person sees 1 item at a time. For example, underpants or under-garments are put on first. The item is on top of the stack.
- Give clear, simple, and step-by-step directions.

FOCUS ON LONG-TERM CARE AND HOME CARE

Dressing and Undressing

Long-Term Care

Some residents dress and undress themselves. Others need help. Personal choice is a resident right. Let the person choose what to wear.

Home Care

Patients often wear street clothes during the day. Or sleepwear and robes are worn. The procedures that follow apply to sleepwear, robes, and street clothes.

DELEGATION GUIDELINES

Dressing and Undressing

To assist with dressing and undressing, you need this information from the nurse and the care plan.

- How much help the person needs
- Which side is the person's strong side
- If the person needs to wear certain garments
- What observations to report and record:
  - How much help was given
  - How the person tolerated the procedure
  - Complaints by the person
  - Changes in the person's behavior
- When to report observations
- What patient or resident concerns to report at once

PROMOTING SAFETY AND COMFORT

Dressing and Undressing

Safety

When assisting with dressing and undressing, you turn the person from side to side. If the person uses bed rails, raise the far bed rail. If bed rails are not used, ask a co-worker to help turn and position the person. This protects the person from falling.

Undressing the Person

QUALITY OF LIFE

- Knock before entering the person's room.
- Address the person by name.
- Introduce yourself by name and title.

- Explain the procedure before starting and during the procedure.
- Protect the person's rights during the procedure.
- Handle the person gently during the procedure.

PRE-PROCEDURE

1 Follow *Delegation Guidelines: Dressing and Undressing.* See *Promoting Safety and Comfort: Dressing and Undressing.*
2 Ask a co-worker to help turn and position the person if needed.
3 Practice hand hygiene.
4 Collect a bath blanket and clothing as requested by the person.

5 Identify the person. Check the ID bracelet against the assignment sheet. Use 2 identifiers (Chapter 13). Also call the person by name.
6 Provide for privacy.
7 Raise the bed for body mechanics. Bed rails are up if used.
8 Lower the bed rail on the person's weak side.
9 Position him or her supine.
10 Cover the person with a bath blanket. Fan-fold linens to the foot of the bed.

PROCEDURE

11 Remove garments that open in back.
  a Raise the head and shoulders. Or turn him or her onto the side away from you.
  b Undo buttons, zippers, ties, or snaps.
  c Bring the sides of the garment to the sides of the person (Fig. 23-14). For a side-lying position, tuck the far side under the person. Fold the near side onto the chest (Fig. 23-15).
  d Position the person supine.
  e Slide the garment off the shoulder on the strong side. Remove it from the arm (Fig. 23-16).
  f Remove the garment from the weak side.
12 Remove garments that open in the front.
  a Undo buttons, zippers, ties, or snaps.
  b Slide the garment off the shoulder and arm on the strong side.
  c Assist the person to sit up or raise the head and shoulders. Bring the garment over to the weak side (Fig. 23-17).
  d Lower the head and shoulders. Remove the garment from the weak side.

  e If you cannot raise the head and shoulders:
    1) Turn the person toward you. Tuck the removed part under the person.
    2) Turn him or her onto the side away from you.
    3) Pull the side of the garment out from under the person. Make sure he or she will not lie on it when supine.
    4) Return the person to the supine position.
    5) Remove the garment from the weak side.
13 Remove pullover garments.
  a Undo any buttons, zippers, ties, or snaps.
  b Remove the garment from the strong side.
  c Raise the head and shoulders. Or turn the person onto the side away from you. Bring the garment up to the person's neck (Fig. 23-18, p. 382).
  d Bring the garment over the person's head.
  e Remove the garment from the weak side.
  f Position him or her in the supine position.

Undressing the Person—cont'd

PROCEDURE—cont'd

14 Remove pants or slacks.
  a Remove footwear and socks.
  b Position the person supine.
  c Undo buttons, zippers, ties, snaps, or buckles.
  d Remove the belt.
  e Ask the person to lift the buttocks off the bed. Slide the pants down over the hips and buttocks (Fig. 23-19, p. 382). Have the person lower the hips and buttocks.

  f If the person cannot raise the hips off the bed:
    1) Turn the person toward you.
    2) Slide the pants off the hip and buttocks on the strong side (Fig. 23-20, p. 382).
    3) Turn the person away from you.
    4) Slide the pants off the hip and buttocks on the weak side (Fig. 23-21, p. 382).
  g Slide the pants down the legs and over the feet.
15 Dress the person. See procedure: *Dressing the Person,* p. 382.

POST-PROCEDURE

16 Provide for comfort. (See the inside of the front cover.)
17 Place the call light and other needed items within reach.
18 Lower the bed to a safe and comfortable level for the person. Follow the care plan.
19 Raise or lower bed rails. Follow the care plan.
20 Unscreen the person.
21 Complete a safety check of the room. (See the inside of the front cover.)
22 Follow agency policy for soiled clothing.
23 Practice hand hygiene.
24 Report and record your observations.

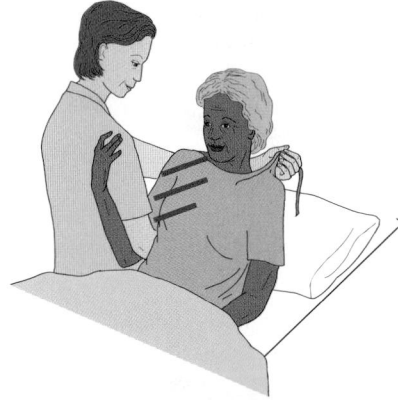

FIGURE 23-14 The sides of the garment are brought from the back to the sides of the person. (NOTE: *The "weak" side is indicated by slash marks.*)

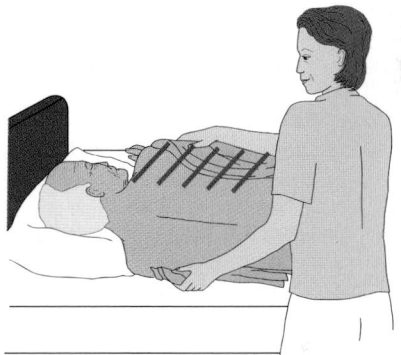

FIGURE 23-15 A garment that opens in the back is removed from the person in the side-lying position. The far side of the garment is tucked under the person. The near side is folded onto the person's chest. (NOTE: *The "weak" side is indicated by slash marks.*)

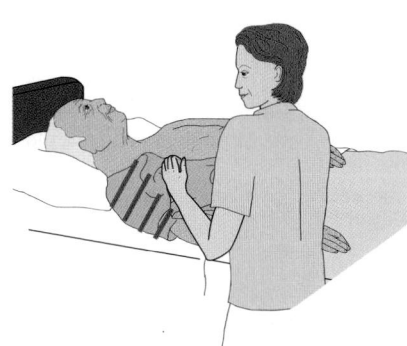

FIGURE 23-16 The garment is removed from the strong side first. (NOTE: *The "weak" side is indicated by slash marks.*)

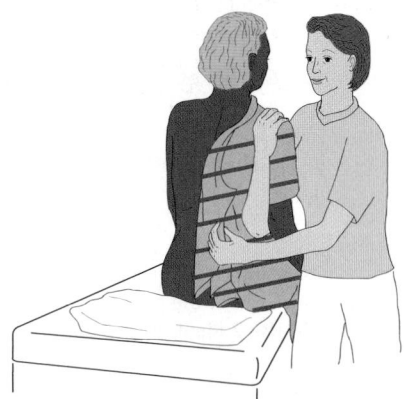

FIGURE 23-17 A front-opening garment is removed with the person's head and shoulders raised. The garment is removed from the strong side first. Then it is brought around the back to the weak side. (NOTE: *The "weak" side is indicated by slash marks.*)

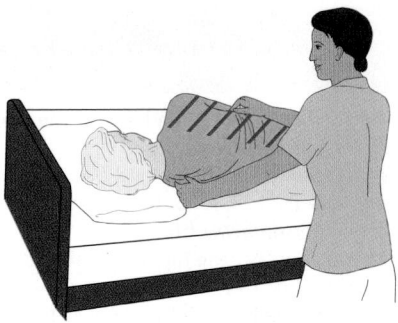

FIGURE 23-18 A pullover garment is removed from the strong side first. Then the garment is brought up to the person's neck so that it can be removed from the weak side. (NOTE: *The "weak" side is indicated by slash marks.*)

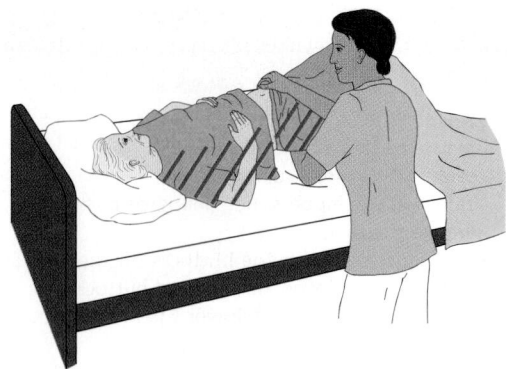

FIGURE 23-19 The person lifts the hips and buttocks to remove the pants. The pants are slid down over the hips and buttocks. (NOTE: *The "weak" side is indicated by slash marks.*)

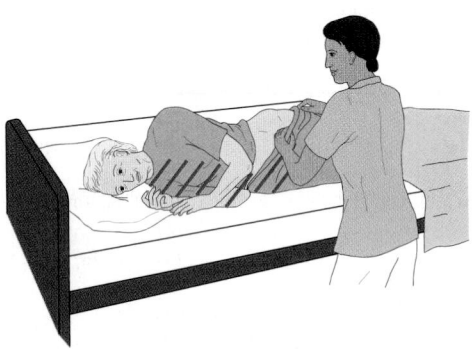

FIGURE 23-20 Pants are removed in the side-lying position. They are removed from the strong side first. They are slid over the hip and buttock. (NOTE: *The "weak" side is indicated by slash marks.*)

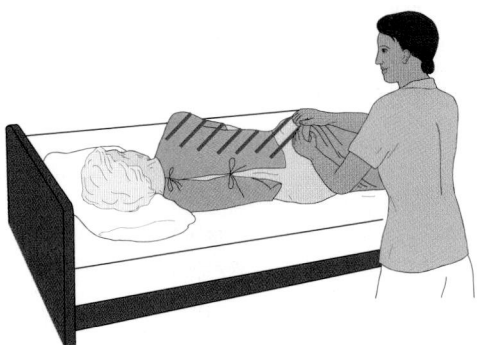

FIGURE 23-21 The person is turned onto the strong side. The pants are removed from the weak side. (NOTE: *The "weak" side is indicated by slash marks.*)

Dressing the Person

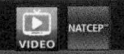

QUALITY OF LIFE

- Knock before entering the person's room.
- Address the person by name.
- Introduce yourself by name and title.

- Explain the procedure before starting and during the procedure.
- Protect the person's rights during the procedure.
- Handle the person gently during the procedure.

PRE-PROCEDURE

1. Follow *Delegation Guidelines: Dressing and Undressing,* p. 380. See *Promoting Safety and Comfort: Dressing and Undressing,* p. 380.
2. Ask a co-worker to help turn and position the person if needed.
3. Practice hand hygiene.
4. Ask the person what he or she would like to wear.
5. Get a bath blanket and clothing requested by the person.
6. Identify the person. Check the ID bracelet against the assignment sheet. Use 2 identifiers (Chapter 13). Also call the person by name.

7. Provide for privacy.
8. Raise the bed for body mechanics. Bed rails are up if used.
9. Lower the bed rail (if up) on the person's weak side.
10. Position the person supine.
11. Cover the person with a bath blanket. Fan-fold linens to the foot of the bed.
12. Undress the person. (See procedure: *Undressing the Person,* p. 380.)

Dressing the Person—cont'd

PROCEDURE

13 Put on garments that open in the back.
- a Slide the garment onto the arm and shoulder of the weak side.
- b Slide the garment onto the arm and shoulder of the strong side.
- c Raise the person's head and shoulders.
- d Bring the sides to the back.
- e If you cannot raise the person's head and shoulders:
  1) Turn the person toward you.
  2) Bring 1 side of the garment to the person's back (Fig. 23-22, *A*).
  3) Turn the person away from you.
  4) Bring the other side to the person's back (Fig. 23-22, *B*).
- f Fasten buttons, zippers, ties, snaps, or other closures.
- g Position the person supine.

14 Put on garments that open in the front.
- a Slide the garment onto the arm and shoulder on the weak side.
- b Raise the head and shoulders. Bring the side of the garment around to the back. Lower the person down. Slide the garment onto the arm and shoulder of the strong arm.
- c If the person cannot raise the head and shoulders:
  1) Turn the person away from you.
  2) Tuck the garment under him or her.
  3) Turn the person toward you.
  4) Pull the garment out from under him or her.
  5) Turn the person back to the supine position.
  6) Slide the garment over the arm and shoulder of the strong arm.
- d Fasten buttons, zippers, ties, snaps, or other closures.

15 Put on pullover garments.
- a Position the person supine.
- b Slide the arm and shoulder of the garment onto the weak side (Fig. 23-23, *A*, p. 384).

- c Raise the person's head and shoulders.
- d Bring the neck of the garment over the head.
- e Slide the arm and shoulder of the garment onto the strong side (Fig. 23-23, *B*, p. 384).
- f Bring the garment down.
- g If the person cannot assume a semi-sitting position:
  1) Bring the neck of the garment over the head.
  2) Slide the arm and shoulder of the garment onto the strong side.
  3) Turn the person onto the strong side.
  4) Pull the garment down on the person's weak side.
  5) Turn the person onto the weak side.
  6) Pull the garment down on the person's strong side.
  7) Position the person supine.

16 Put on pants or slacks:
- a Slide the pants over the feet and up the legs.
- b Ask the person to raise the hips and buttocks off the bed.
- c Bring the pants up over the buttock and hip on the weak side.
- d Pull the pants over the buttock and hip on the strong side.
- e If the person cannot raise the hips and buttocks:
  1) Turn the person onto the strong side.
  2) Pull the pants over the buttock and hip on the weak side.
  3) Turn the person onto the weak side.
  4) Pull the pants over the buttock and hip on the strong side.
  5) Position the person supine.
- f Fasten buttons, zippers, ties, snaps, a belt buckle, or other closures.

17 Put socks and non-skid footwear on the person. Make sure socks are up all the way and smooth.

18 Help the person get out of bed. If the person stays in bed, cover the person. Remove the bath blanket.

POST-PROCEDURE

19 Provide for comfort. (See the inside of the front cover.)
20 Place the call light and other needed items within reach.
21 Lower the bed to a safe and comfortable level for the person. Follow the care plan.
22 Raise or lower bed rails. Follow the care plan.
23 Unscreen the person.

24 Complete a safety check of the room. (See the inside of the front cover.)
25 Follow agency policy for soiled clothing.
26 Practice hand hygiene.
27 Report and record your observations.

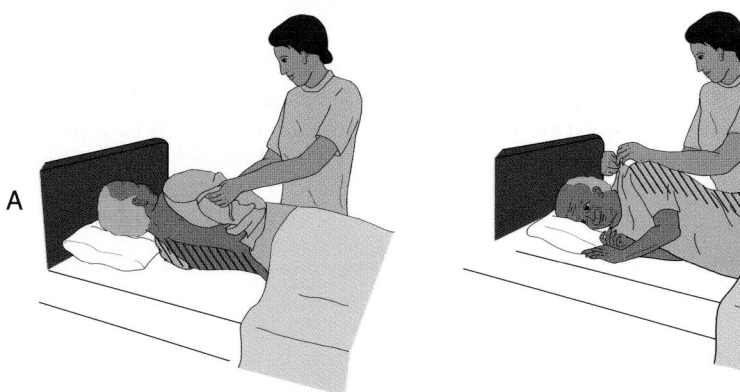

A B

FIGURE 23-22 Dressing a person. **A,** The side-lying position can be used to put on garments that open in the back. Turn the person toward you after the garment is put on the arms. The side of the garment is brought to the person's back. **B,** Then turn the person away from you. The other side of the garment is brought to the back and fastened. (NOTE: *The "weak" side is indicated by slash marks.*)

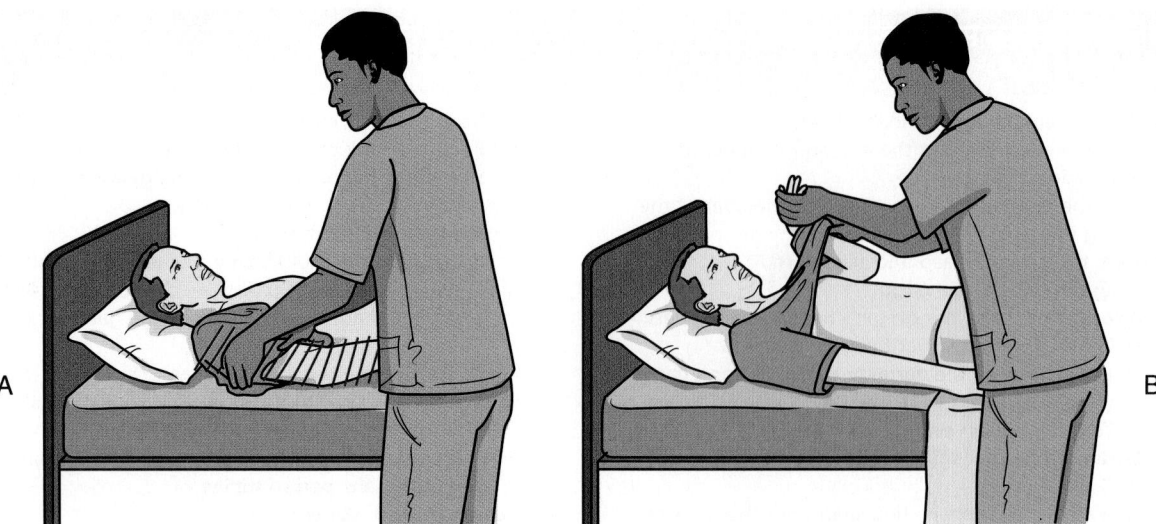

FIGURE 23-23 Applying pullover garments. **A,** The garment is applied to the weak side first. **B,** The garment is brought up over the head. The arms and shoulder of the garment are slid onto the strong side. (NOTE: *The "weak" side is indicated by slash marks.*)

Changing Patient Gowns

Many patients wear patient gowns. So do some nursing center residents. Gowns are usually worn for IV (intravenous) therapy (Chapter 28). Some agencies have IV therapy gowns that open along the sleeve and close with ties, snaps, or Velcro. Sometimes standard gowns are used.

For injury or paralysis, remove the gown from the strong arm first. Support the weak arm while removing the gown. Put the clean gown on the weak arm first and then on the strong arm.

See *Delegation Guidelines: Changing Patient Gowns.*

See *Promoting Safety and Comfort: Changing Patient Gowns.*

See procedure: *Changing a Patient Gown on a Person With an IV.*

DELEGATION GUIDELINES

Changing Patient Gowns

Before changing a gown, you need this information from the nurse and the care plan.
- Which arm has the IV
- If the person has an IV pump (see *Promoting Safety and Comfort: Changing Patient Gowns*)

PROMOTING SAFETY AND COMFORT

Changing Patient Gowns

Safety

IV pumps control the *flow rate*—how fast fluid enters a vein. If the person has an IV pump and a standard gown, do not use the procedure on the next page. The nurse handles the arm with the IV.

To change a gown, you must move the IV bag. Moving the IV bag can change the IV flow rate. Always ask the nurse to check the flow rate after you change a gown.

Do not disconnect or remove any part of the IV set-up.

Comfort

Some patient gowns tie at the upper back. The back and buttocks are exposed when the person stands. Cover the person for warmth and privacy. A robe may be used. Or a second gown can be worn backwards to cover the back and buttocks. Other gowns overlap in the back and tie at the side. These gowns provide more privacy. Because they tie at the side, uncomfortable bows and knots at the back are avoided.

Changing a Patient Gown on a Person With an IV

QUALITY OF LIFE

- Knock before entering the person's room.
- Address the person by name.
- Introduce yourself by name and title.

- Explain the procedure before starting and during the procedure.
- Protect the person's rights during the procedure.
- Handle the person gently during the procedure.

PRE-PROCEDURE

1 Follow *Delegation Guidelines: Changing Patient Gowns.* See *Promoting Safety and Comfort: Changing Patient Gowns.*
2 Practice hand hygiene.
3 Get a clean gown and bath blanket.

4 Identify the person. Check the ID bracelet against the assignment sheet. Use 2 identifiers (Chapter 13). Also call the person by name.
5 Provide for privacy.
6 Raise the bed for body mechanics. Bed rails are up if used.

PROCEDURE

7 Lower the bed rail near you (if up).
8 Cover the person with the bath blanket. Fan-fold linens to the foot of the bed.
9 Untie the gown. Free parts that the person is lying on.
10 Remove the gown from the arm with *no IV.*
11 Gather up the sleeve of the arm *with the IV.* Slide it over the IV site and tubing. Remove the arm and hand from the sleeve (Fig. 23-24, *A*).
12 Keep the sleeve gathered. Slide your arm along the tubing to the bag (Fig. 23-24, *B*).
13 Remove the bag from the pole. Slide the bag and tubing through the sleeve (Fig. 23-24, *C*). Do not pull on the tubing. Keep the bag above the person.

14 Hang the IV bag on the pole.
15 Gather the sleeve of the clean gown that will go on the arm with the IV infusion.
16 Remove the bag from the pole. Slip the sleeve over the bag at the shoulder part of the gown (Fig. 23-24, *D*). Hang the bag.
17 Slide the gathered sleeve over the tubing, hand, arm, and IV site. Then slide it onto the shoulder.
18 Put the other side of the gown on the person. Fasten the gown.
19 Cover the person. Remove the bath blanket.

POST-PROCEDURE

20 Provide for comfort. (See the inside of the front cover.)
21 Place the call light and other needed items within reach.
22 Lower the bed to a safe and comfortable level for the person. Follow the care plan.
23 Raise or lower bed rails. Follow the care plan.
24 Unscreen the person.

25 Complete a safety check of the room. (See the inside of the front cover.)
26 Follow agency policy for used linens.
27 Practice hand hygiene.
28 Ask the nurse to check the flow rate.
29 Report and record your observations.

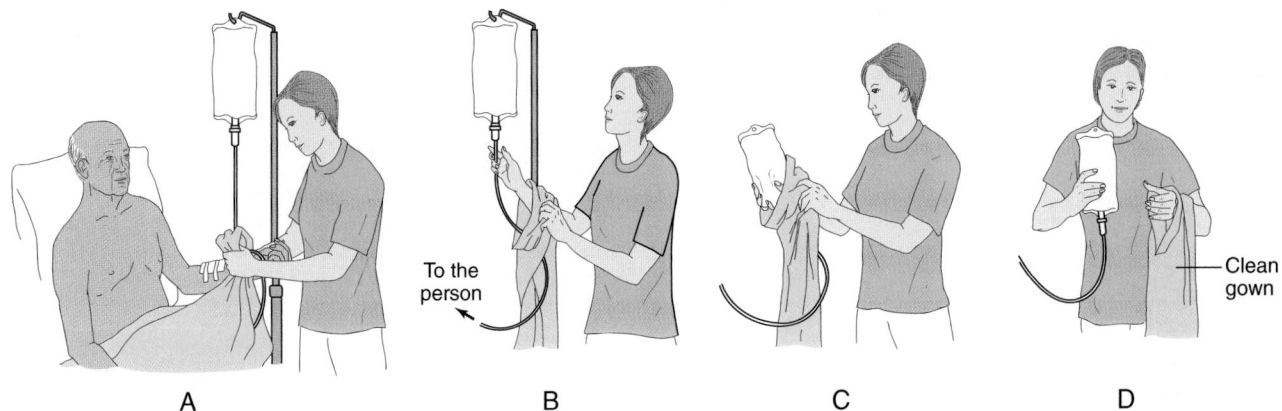

A B C D

FIGURE 23-24 Changing a gown. A, The gown is removed from the arm with no IV. The sleeve on the arm with the IV is gathered up, slipped over the IV site and tubing, and removed from the arm and hand. **B,** The gathered sleeve is slipped along the IV tubing to the bag. **C,** The IV bag is removed from the pole and passed through the sleeve. **D,** The gathered sleeve of the clean gown is slipped over the IV bag at the shoulder part of the gown.

FOCUS ON PRIDE

The Person, Family, and Yourself

P ersonal and Professional Responsibility

Grooming promotes comfort. Self-esteem and body image improve when the person likes how he or she looks. Clean hair, nails, and garments all help mental well-being. So does a clean-shaven face or a well-groomed beard or mustache.

Your attitude is reflected in the way you give care. To show that you value the person's self-esteem and comfort:

- Be pleasant. Talk with the person.
- Ask about the person's preferences. Allow personal choice.
- Avoid seeming rushed. Let the person know that you have time for him or her.
- Avoid thinking that care measures are tasks to be completed. You are caring for a *person*. Show that you care about the person's needs and feelings.
- Do a good job. Be thorough and careful.
- Clean up after yourself. Leave the person's setting neat and orderly.

Also, care for your own appearance. Patients, residents, and family members notice when others are not well groomed. If you are not groomed well, they may question the quality of care you provide. Have a professional appearance.

R ights and Respect

People have different grooming preferences. Ask what the person prefers. For example, ask what he or she would like to wear. Or ask how to style the person's hair. Follow the person's grooming routines whenever possible.

You may not like the person's hairstyle, clothing choices, or personal care products. Do not judge the person by your own standards or impose your choices on the person. Do not make the person feel badly about his or her choices. Respect the person's right to choose. Assist with grooming in a way that improves the person's self-esteem.

I ndependence and Social Interaction

Some family members want to help with grooming. For example, they want to style the person's hair. Or they want to apply lotion to the person's hands and feet.

With the person's permission, allow family members to assist with grooming measures as much as safely possible. This promotes social interaction. It also involves the family in the person's care.

D elegation and Teamwork

Grooming takes time. You, the person, the nurse, and other team members work together to plan and organize care. For example, Mr. Horn had a stroke. He needs help with grooming. He eats breakfast at 0800, has speech therapy at 0930, has physical therapy at 1030, and his wife visits during lunch. Mr. Horn prefers to comb his hair, shave, and change his clothes after breakfast but before his wife visits. He also likes to rest after physical therapy. You plan to assist Mr. Horn with grooming after breakfast and before speech therapy.

Grooming is important. Do not neglect grooming because of a busy schedule. Plan ahead to meet the person's needs at a time best for the person and the team.

E thics and Laws

Patients and residents have the right to be free from mistreatment and restraint (Chapter 2). The following is a case where a nurse did not follow these ethical principles.

A nurse told a patient that she was going to cut his hair and trim his beard. The patient repeatedly stated that he did not want a haircut or his beard trimmed. The patient protested and resisted the nurse's actions. She continued her actions while 2 other staff members restrained the patient.

The patient reported the incident to his social worker. An internal investigation was conducted.

The nurse lost her job. The United States Court of Appeals agreed that the nurse's termination was warranted because of:

- *The nature and seriousness of the offense*
- *The restraint of the patient after he repeatedly objected* (L. Taylor v Department of Veterans Affairs, 2006.)

Never force a care measure on a person. If a person resists or refuses care, stop. Do not proceed. Politely ask the person for the reason. Tell the nurse. You, the nurse, and the person can discuss a solution.

Special care measures are needed for persons with confusion or dementia who resist care. See Chapter 49. Patience, kindness, and problem solving are needed. A co-worker or family member may need to give care. Or care may need to be given at a different time. Provide care in a way that protects the person's rights and shows dignity and respect.

FOCUS ON PRIDE: Application

The family cares about the person's appearance. They notice when grooming differs from usual. The family may tell you what they expect. Why are their comments important? How can you show that you value their input?

REVIEW QUESTIONS

*Circle **T** if the statement is TRUE or **F** if it is FALSE.*

1   T   F   Scabies is contagious.

2   T   F   Mustaches are trimmed weekly.

3   T   F   Feet are soaked for 5 to 10 minutes.

4   T   F   Fingernails are clipped straight across.

5   T   F   Wear gloves when giving nail care.

6   T   F   Clothing is removed from the weak side first.

7   T   F   The person chooses what to wear.

8   T   F   A person has poor circulation in the legs and feet. You can trim the person's toenails.

9   T   F   You can cut matted hair.

Circle the BEST answer.

10   A person with alopecia has
   a   Excessive body hair
   b   Dry, white flakes from the scalp
   c   An infestation with lice
   d   Hair loss

11   Which prevents hair from matting and tangling?
   a   Bedrest
   b   Daily brushing and combing
   c   Daily shampooing
   d   Cutting hair

12   A person's hair is *not* matted or tangled. When brushing hair, start at
   a   The forehead and brush backward
   b   The hair ends
   c   The scalp
   d   The back of the neck and brush forward

13   Brushing keeps the hair
   a   Soft and shiny
   b   Clean
   c   Free of lice
   d   Long

14   A person requests a shampoo. You should
   a   Shampoo the hair during the person's shower
   b   Shampoo hair at the sink
   c   Shampoo the person in bed
   d   Follow the care plan

15   When shaving a person's face with a safety razor
   a   Discard the razor in the wastebasket when done
   b   Shave against the direction of hair growth
   c   Hold the skin taut
   d   Shave when the skin is dry

16   A person is nicked during shaving. Your *first* action is to
   a   Wash your hands
   b   Apply direct pressure
   c   Tell the nurse
   d   Apply a bandage

17   Fingernails are cut with
   a   An emery board
   b   Scissors
   c   A nail file
   d   Nail clippers

18   Fingernails are filed
   a   Before soaking
   b   After soaking
   c   Before trimming toenails
   d   After trimming toenails

19   Garments are applied
   a   To the weak side first
   b   To the strong side first
   c   To either the weak or the strong side first
   d   In the same way they are removed

20   When changing the gown on a person with an IV
   a   Keep the IV bag below the person's arm
   b   Stop the IV pump to change the gown
   c   Have the nurse check the flow rate afterward
   d   Disconnect the IV to change the gown

Answers to Chapter 23 questions are on p. 871.

FOCUS ON PRACTICE

Problem Solving

A resident with dementia has long fingernails. Some are broken and have rough edges. As you begin nail care, she resists. She swings her arms at you and yells. What do you do? Why is nail care important for this resident? How might you provide care safely?

Urinary Elimination

- Define the key terms and key abbreviations in this chapter.
- Describe normal urine.
- Describe the rules for normal urination.
- Identify the observations to report to the nurse.
- Describe urinary incontinence and the care required.
- Describe bladder training methods.
- Perform the procedures described in this chapter.
- Explain how to promote PRIDE in the person, the family, and yourself.

KEY TERMS

dysuria Painful or difficult *(dys)* urination *(uria)*; burning on urination

functional incontinence The person has bladder control but cannot use the toilet in time

hematuria Blood *(hemat)* in the urine *(uria)*

micturition See "urination"

mixed incontinence The combination of stress incontinence and urge incontinence

nocturia Frequent urination *(uria)* at night *(noc)*

oliguria Scant amount *(olig)* of urine *(uria)*; less than 500 mL in 24 hours

over-active bladder See "urge incontinence"

over-flow incontinence Small amounts of urine leak from a full bladder

polyuria Abnormally large amounts *(poly)* of urine *(uria)*

reflex incontinence Urine is lost at predictable intervals when the bladder is full

stress incontinence When urine leaks during exercise and certain movements that cause pressure on the bladder

transient incontinence Temporary or occasional incontinence that is reversed when the cause is treated

urge incontinence The loss of urine in response to a sudden, urgent need to void; the person cannot get to a toilet in time; over-active bladder

urinary frequency Voiding at frequent intervals

urinary incontinence The involuntary loss or leakage of urine

urinary retention The inability to void

urinary urgency The need to void at once

urination The process of emptying urine from the bladder; micturition or voiding

voiding See "urination"

KEY ABBREVIATIONS

BM	Bowel movement	UTI	Urinary tract infection
mL	Milliliter		

Eliminating waste is a physical need. The digestive system rids the body of solid wastes. The lungs remove carbon dioxide. Sweat contains water and other substances. Blood contains waste products from body cells burning food for energy. The urinary system removes waste products from the blood. It also maintains the body's water and electrolyte balance.

See *Body Structure and Function Review: The Urinary System.*

See *Promoting Safety and Comfort: Urinary Elimination.*

BODY STRUCTURE AND FUNCTION REVIEW

The Urinary System

The 2 *kidneys* (Fig. 24-1) lie in the upper abdomen against the back muscles on each side of the spine. Blood passes through the 2 kidneys. *Urine* is formed in the kidneys.

Urine consists of wastes and excess fluids filtered out of the blood. Urine flows through the 2 *ureters* to the urinary *bladder*. Urine is stored in the bladder. The *urethra* connects the bladder to the outside of the body. The opening at the end of the urethra is called the *meatus*. Urine passes from the body through the meatus. Urine is a clear, yellowish fluid.

See Chapter 10 for more information.

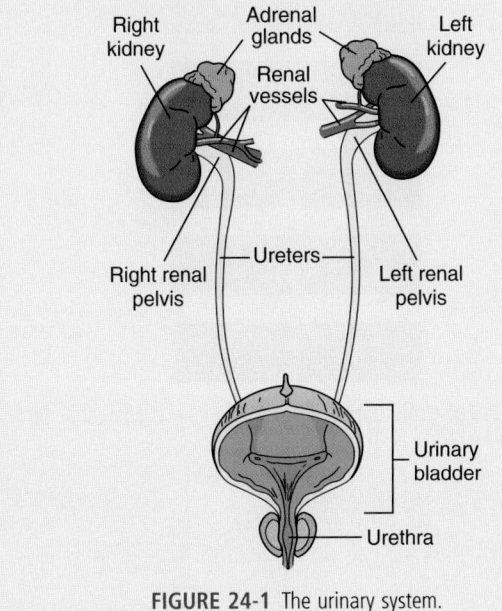

FIGURE 24-1 The urinary system.

PROMOTING SAFETY AND COMFORT

Urinary Elimination

Safety

Urinary elimination measures often involve exposing and touching private areas—the perineum and rectum. Sexual abuse has occurred in health care settings. The person may feel threatened or may actually be abused. He or she needs to call for help. Keep the call light within the person's reach at all times. And always act in a professional manner.

Urine may contain blood and microbes. Microbes can live and grow in bedpans, urinals, commodes, and urinary drainage bags (Chapter 25). Follow Standard Precautions and the Bloodborne Pathogen Standard (Chapter 16) to handle urinary devices and their contents. This includes incontinence products. Thoroughly clean and disinfect bedpans, urinals, and commodes after use. Remember to practice hand hygiene.

NORMAL URINATION

The healthy adult produces 1500 mL (milliliters) or 3 pints of urine a day. Many factors affect urine production—age, disease, the amount and kinds of fluid ingested, salt, body temperature, perspiration (sweating), and some drugs. Some substances increase urine production—coffee, tea, alcohol, and some drugs. A diet high in salt causes the body to retain water. So do some drugs. When water is retained, less urine is produced.

*Urination (**micturition** and **voiding**) means the process of emptying urine from the bladder.* The amount of fluid intake, habits, and available toilet facilities affect frequency. So do activity, work, and illness. People usually void at bedtime, after sleep, and before meals. Some people void every 2 to 3 hours. Voiding at night disturbs sleep.

Some persons need help getting to the bathroom. Others use bedpans, urinals, or commodes. Follow the rules in Box 24-1 and the person's care plan.

See *Focus on Communication: Normal Urination*, p. 390.

See *Focus on Children and Older Persons: Normal Urination*, p. 390.

See *Teamwork and Time Management: Normal Urination*, p. 390.

BOX 24-1	Rules for Normal Urination

- Practice medical asepsis.
- Follow Standard Precautions and the Bloodborne Pathogen Standard.
- Provide fluids as the nurse and care plan direct.
- Follow the person's voiding routines and habits. Check with the nurse and the care plan.
- Help the person to the bathroom upon request. Or provide the commode, bedpan, or urinal. The need to void may be urgent.
- Help the person assume a normal position for voiding if possible. Women sit or squat. Men stand.
- Warm the bedpan or urinal.
- Cover the person for warmth and privacy.
- Provide for privacy. Pull the privacy curtain around the bed, close room and bathroom doors, and close window coverings. Leave the room if the person can be alone.
- Tell the person that running water, flushing the toilet, or playing music can mask voiding sounds. Voiding with others nearby embarrasses some people.
- Stay nearby if the person is weak or unsteady.
- Place the call light and toilet tissue within reach.
- Allow enough time. Do not rush the person.
- Promote relaxation. Some people like to read.
- Run water in a sink if the person cannot start the urine stream. Or place the person's fingers in warm water.
- Provide perineal care as needed (Chapter 22).
- Assist with hand-washing after voiding. Provide a wash basin, soap, washcloth, and towel.
- Assist the person to the bathroom or offer the bedpan, urinal, or commode at regular times. Some people are embarrassed or are too weak to ask for help.

FOCUS ON **COMMUNICATION**

Normal Urination

Patients and residents may not use "voiding" or "urinating" terms. The person may not understand what you are saying. Do not ask: "Do you need to void?" or "Do you need to urinate?" Instead, you can ask these questions.
- "Do you need to use the bathroom?"
- "Do you need to use the bedpan (urinal)?"
- "Do you need to pass urine?"
- "Do you need to pass water?"
- "Do you need to pee?"

The word "pee" may offend some persons. Choose words the person understands and uses. Follow the care plan.

FOCUS ON **CHILDREN AND OLDER PERSONS**

Normal Urination

Children

Infants produce 200 to 300 mL of urine a day. The amount increases as the baby grows older. An infant can have 6 to 20 wet diapers a day. Tell the nurse at once if an infant does not have a wet diaper for several hours. This signals dehydration. It is very serious in infants.

TEAMWORK AND TIME MANAGEMENT

Normal Urination

The need to void may be urgent. Answer call lights promptly. Also, answer call lights for co-workers. Otherwise incontinence may result. The person is wet and embarrassed. Skin breakdown and infection are risks. Your co-worker has extra work—changing wet linens and garments. You like help when busy. So do your co-workers.

Observations

Normal urine is pale yellow, straw-colored, or amber (Fig. 24-2). It is clear with no particles. A faint odor is normal. Observe urine for color, clarity, odor, amount (output), particles, and blood.

Red food dyes, beets, blackberries, and rhubarb cause red-colored urine. Carrots and sweet potatoes cause bright yellow urine. Certain drugs change urine color. Asparagus causes a urine odor.

Ask the nurse to observe urine that looks or smells abnormal. Report the problems in Table 24-1. The nurse uses the information for the nursing process.

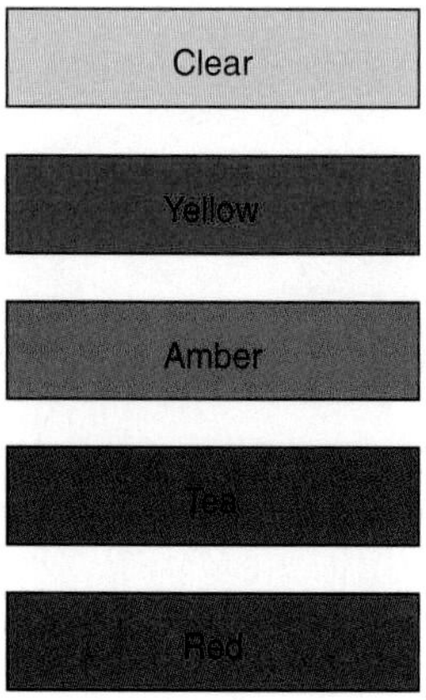

| Clear |
| Yellow |
| Amber |
| Tea |
| Red |

FIGURE 24-2 Color chart for urine. (Redrawn from Weldon, Inc., Fort Worth, Tex.)

TABLE 24-1	**Urinary Elimination Problems**	
Problem	**Definition**	**Causes**
Dysuria	*Painful or difficult (dys) urination (uria); burning on urination*	Urinary tract infection (UTI), trauma, urinary tract obstruction
Hematuria	*Blood (hemat) in the urine (uria)*	Kidney disease, UTI, trauma
Nocturia	*Frequent urination (uria) at night (noc)*	Excess fluid intake, kidney disease, prostate disease
Oliguria	*Scant amount (olig) of urine (uria); less than 500 mL in 24 hours*	Poor fluid intake, shock, burns, kidney disease, heart failure
Polyuria	*Abnormally large amounts (poly) of urine (uria)*	Drugs, excess fluid intake, diabetes, hormone imbalance
Urinary frequency	*Voiding at frequent intervals*	Excess fluid intake, UTI, pressure on the bladder, drugs
Urinary incontinence	*The involuntary loss or leakage of urine*	Trauma, disease, UTI, reproductive or urinary tract surgeries, aging, fecal impaction, constipation, not getting to the bathroom in time
Urinary retention	*The inability to void*	Prostate problems, nerve damage, UTI, drugs, surgery, kidney stones, constipation, trauma
Urinary urgency	*The need to void at once*	UTI, fear of incontinence, full bladder, stress

Bedpans

Bedpans are used by persons who cannot be out of bed. Women use bedpans for voiding and bowel movements (BMs). Men use them for BMs.

The *standard bedpan* is shown in Figure 24-3. The wide rim is placed under the buttocks. A *fracture pan* has a thin rim. It is only about $\frac{1}{2}$-inch deep at one end (see Fig. 24-3). The smaller end (flat end) is placed under the buttocks (Fig. 24-4). Fracture pans are used:

- By persons with casts
- By persons in traction
- By persons with limited back motion
- By older persons with osteoporosis (fragile bones) or arthritis (Chapter 44)
- After spinal cord injury or surgery
- After a hip fracture
- After hip replacement surgery

Like a fracture pan, the small end (flat end) of a *bariatric bedpan* is placed under the buttocks (Fig. 24-5). Some have a weight capacity of 1200 pounds.

See *Delegation Guidelines: Bedpans.*
See *Promoting Safety and Comfort: Bedpans.*
See procedure: *Giving the Bedpan,* p. 392.

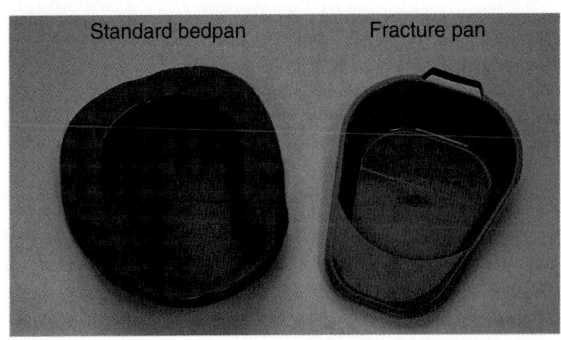

FIGURE 24-3 Standard bedpan *(left)* and the fracture pan *(right).*

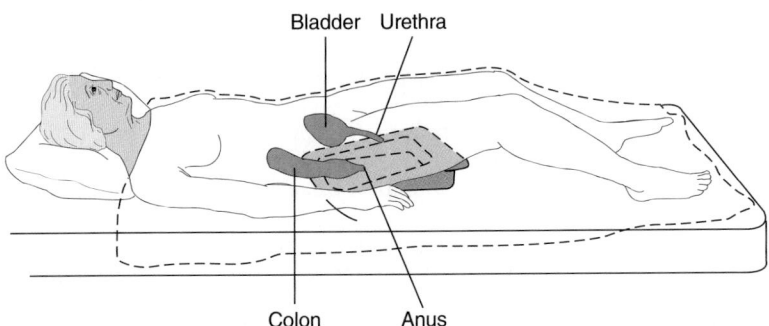

FIGURE 24-4 A person positioned on a fracture pan. The small end (flat end) is under the buttocks.

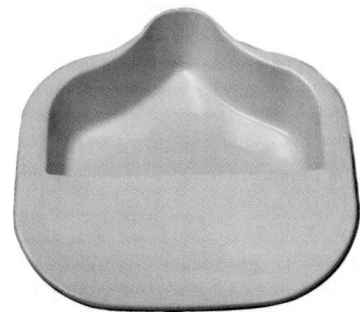

FIGURE 24-5 Bariatric bedpan. (Image courtesy AliMed, Inc., Dedham, Mass.)

DELEGATION GUIDELINES

Bedpans

To assist with a bedpan, you need this information from the nurse and the care plan.
- What bedpan to use—standard bedpan, fracture pan, bariatric bedpan
- Position or activity limits
- If you can leave the room or if you need to stay with the person
- If the nurse needs to observe the results before disposing of the contents
- What observations to report and record:
  - Urine color, clarity, and odor
  - Amount
  - Presence of particles
  - Blood in the urine
  - Cloudy urine
  - Complaints of urgency, burning, dysuria, or other problems (see Table 24-1)
  - For bowel movements, see Chapter 26
- When to report observations
- What patient or resident concerns to report at once

PROMOTING SAFETY AND COMFORT

Bedpans

Safety
Remember to raise the bed as needed for good body mechanics. Lower the bed before leaving the room. Raise or lower the bed rails according to the care plan.

Comfort
Most bedpans are plastic. Metal bedpans are often cold. Warm metal bedpans with warm water and then dry them before use.

The person must not sit on a bedpan for a long time. Bedpans are uncomfortable. They can lead to pressure ulcers from prolonged pressure (Chapter 37).

Giving the Bedpan

QUALITY OF LIFE

- Knock before entering the person's room.
- Address the person by name.
- Introduce yourself by name and title.

- Explain the procedure before starting and during the procedure.
- Protect the person's rights during the procedure.
- Handle the person gently during the procedure.

PRE-PROCEDURE

1 Follow *Delegation Guidelines: Bedpans*, p. 391. See *Promoting Safety and Comfort:*
  a *Urinary Elimination*, p. 389
  b *Bedpans*, p. 391
2 Provide for privacy.
3 Practice hand hygiene.
4 Put on gloves.

5 Collect the following.
  • Bedpan
  • Bedpan cover
  • Toilet tissue
  • Waterproof under-pad (if required by agency policy)
6 Arrange equipment on the chair or bed.

PROCEDURE

7 Lower the bed rail near you (if up).
8 Lower the head of the bed. Position the person supine. Or raise the head of the bed slightly for the person's comfort.
9 Fold the top linens and gown out of the way. Keep the lower body covered.
10 Ask the person to flex the knees and raise the buttocks. He or she does so by pushing against the mattress with the feet.
11 Slide your hand under the lower back. Help raise the buttocks. If using a waterproof under-pad, place it under the buttocks.
12 Slide the bedpan under the person (Fig. 24-6).
13 If the person cannot assist in getting on the bedpan:
  a Place the waterproof under-pad under the buttocks if using one.
  b Turn the person onto the side away from you.
  c Place the bedpan firmly against the buttocks (Fig. 24-7).
  d Hold the bedpan securely. Turn the person onto his or her back.
  e Make sure the bedpan is centered under the person.
14 Cover the person.
15 Raise the head of the bed so the person is in a sitting position (Fowler's position) for a standard bedpan. (NOTE: Some state competency tests require removing gloves and hand-washing before you raise the head of the bed.)
16 Make sure the person is correctly positioned on the bedpan (Fig. 24-8).
17 Raise the bed rail if used.
18 Place the toilet tissue and call light within reach. (NOTE: For some state competency tests you ask the person to use hand wipes to clean the hands after wiping with toilet tissue.)
19 Ask the person to signal when done or when help is needed.

20 Remove and discard the gloves. Practice hand hygiene.
21 Leave the room and close the door.
22 Return when the person signals. Or check on the person every 5 minutes. Knock before entering.
23 Practice hand hygiene. Put on gloves.
24 Raise the bed for body mechanics. Lower the bed rail (if used) and lower the head of the bed.
25 Ask the person to raise the buttocks. Remove the bedpan. Or hold the bedpan and turn him or her onto the side away from you.
26 Clean the genital area if the person cannot do so.
  a Clean from the meatus (front or top) to the anus (back or bottom) with toilet tissue. Use fresh tissue for each wipe.
  b Provide perineal care if needed.
  c Remove and discard the waterproof under-pad if using one.
27 Cover the bedpan. Take it to the bathroom. Raise the bed rail (if used) before leaving the bedside.
28 Note the color, amount (output), and character of urine or feces. See "Measuring Intake and Output" in Chapter 27.
29 Empty the bedpan contents into the toilet and flush.
30 Rinse the bedpan. Pour the rinse into the toilet and flush.
31 Clean the bedpan with a disinfectant. Pour disinfectant into the toilet and flush.
32 Remove and discard the gloves. Practice hand hygiene and put on clean gloves.
33 Return the bedpan and clean cover to the bedside stand.
34 Help the person with hand-washing. (Wear gloves for this step.)
35 Remove and discard the gloves. Practice hand hygiene.

POST-PROCEDURE

36 Provide for comfort. (See the inside of the front cover.)
37 Place the call light and other needed items within reach.
38 Lower the bed to a safe and comfortable level for the person. Follow the care plan.
39 Raise or lower bed rails. Follow the care plan.
40 Unscreen the person.

41 Complete a safety check of the room. (See the inside of the front cover.)
42 Follow agency policy for used linens.
43 Practice hand hygiene.
44 Report and record your observations.

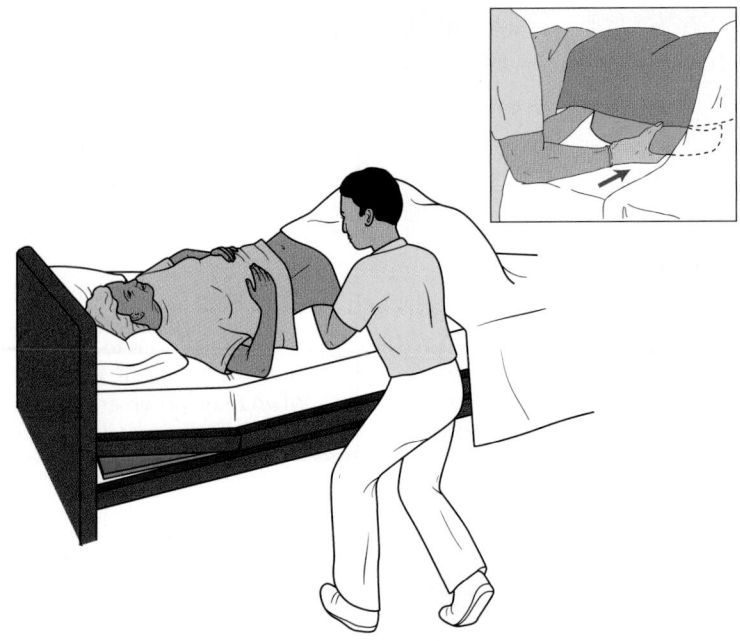

FIGURE 24-6 The person raises the buttocks off the bed with help. The bedpan is slid under the person.

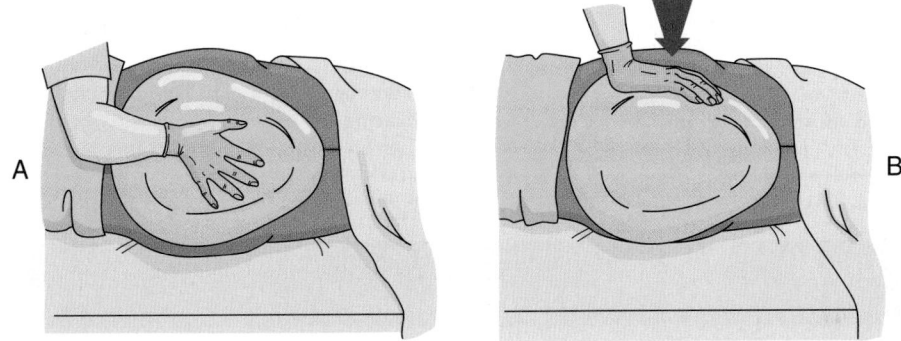

A   **B**

FIGURE 24-7 **Giving a bedpan. A,** Position the person on the side away from you. Place the bedpan firmly against the buttocks. **B,** Push downward on the bedpan and toward the person.

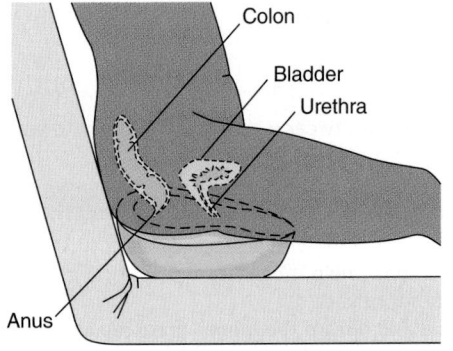

Colon

Bladder

Urethra

Anus

FIGURE 24-8 The person is positioned on the bedpan so the urethra and anus are directly over the opening.

Urinals

Men use urinals to void (Fig. 24-9, p. 394). Plastic urinals have caps and hook-type handles. The urinal hooks to the bed rail within the man's reach. He stands to use the urinal if possible. Or he sits on the side of the bed or lies in bed to use it. Some men need support when standing.

After voiding, the urinal cap is closed. This prevents urine spills. Remind men to hang urinals on bed rails and to signal after using them. Remind them not to place urinals on over-bed tables and bedside stands. Over-bed tables are used for eating and as a work surface. Bedside stands are used for personal items and supplies. These surfaces must not be contaminated with urine.

Some beds may not have bed rails. Follow agency policy for where to place urinals.

See *Focus on Communication: Urinals,* p. 394.
See *Delegation Guidelines: Urinals,* p. 394.
See *Promoting Safety and Comfort: Urinals,* p. 394.
See procedure: *Giving the Urinal,* p. 394.

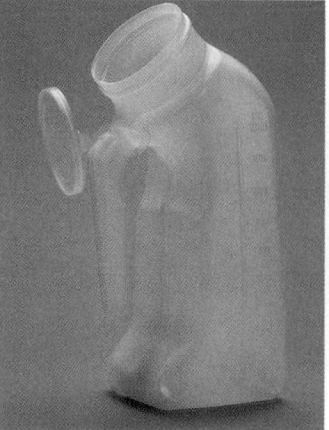

FIGURE 24-9 Male urinal.

DELEGATION GUIDELINES
Urinals

To assist with urinals, you need this information from the nurse and the care plan.
- How the urinal is used—standing, sitting, or lying in bed.
- If help is needed to place or hold the urinal.
- If the man needs support to stand. If yes, how many staff are needed.
- If you need to stay with the person.
- If the nurse will observe the urine before disposal.
- What observations to report and record (see *Delegation Guidelines: Bedpans,* p. 391).
- When to report observations.
- What patient or resident concerns to report at once.

FOCUS ON COMMUNICATION
Urinals

Some men cannot use a urinal on their own. You may need to assist. Or you may need to stay with the person. For the person's comfort, explain why you must help him. You can say:
- "Mr. Turner, I'll help you use your urinal. I need to stay with you to make sure you don't fall."
- "Mr. Gomez, I'll help you place and remove your urinal so it doesn't spill."

PROMOTING SAFETY AND COMFORT
Urinals

Safety
Empty urinals promptly to prevent odors and the spread of microbes. A filled urinal spills easily, causing hazards. Also, it is an unpleasant sight and a source of odor. Urinals are cleaned and disinfected like bedpans.

Comfort
You may have to place the urinal for some men. This means placing the penis in the urinal. This may embarrass both the person and you. Always act in a professional manner.

Giving the Urinal

QUALITY OF LIFE

- Knock before entering the person's room.
- Address the person by name.
- Introduce yourself by name and title.
- Explain the procedure before starting and during the procedure.
- Protect the person's rights during the procedure.
- Handle the person gently during the procedure.

PRE-PROCEDURE

1 Follow *Delegation Guidelines: Urinals.* See *Promoting Safety and Comfort:*
   a *Urinary Elimination,* p. 389
   b *Urinals*
2 Provide for privacy.
3 Determine if the man will stand, sit, or lie in bed.

4 Practice hand hygiene.
5 Put on gloves.
6 Collect the following.
   • Urinal
   • Non-skid footwear if the man will stand to void

PROCEDURE

7 *Using the urinal in bed:*
   a Give him the urinal if he is in bed.
   b Remind him to tilt the bottom down to prevent spills.
8 *Standing to use the urinal:*
   a Help him sit on the side of the bed.
   b Put non-skid footwear on him.
   c Help him stand. Provide support if he is unsteady.
   d Give him the urinal.
9 *Positioning the urinal (in bed or standing):*
   a Help the person stand (step 8) if he will stand.
   b Position the urinal.
   c Place the penis in the urinal if he cannot do so.
   d Cover him for privacy.

10 Place the call light within reach. Ask him to signal when done or when help is needed.
11 Provide for privacy
12 Remove and discard the gloves. Practice hand hygiene.
13 Leave the room and close the door.
14 Return when he signals for you. Or check on him every 5 minutes. Knock before entering.
15 Practice hand hygiene. Put on gloves.
16 Close the cap on the urinal. Take it to the bathroom.
17 Note the color, amount (output), and clarity of urine.
18 Empty the urinal into the toilet and flush.
19 Rinse the urinal with cold water. Pour rinse into the toilet and flush.

Giving the Urinal—cont'd

PROCEDURE—cont'd

20 Clean the urinal with a disinfectant. Pour disinfectant into the urinal and flush.
21 Return the urinal to its proper place.

22 Remove and discard the gloves. Practice hand hygiene and put on clean gloves.
23 Assist with hand-washing.
24 Remove and discard the gloves. Practice hand hygiene.

POST-PROCEDURE

25 Provide for comfort. (See the inside of the front cover.)
26 Place the call light and other needed items within reach.
27 Raise or lower bed rails. Follow the care plan.
28 Unscreen him.

29 Complete a safety check of the room. (See the inside of the front cover.)
30 Follow agency policy for used linens.
31 Practice hand hygiene.
32 Report and record your observations.

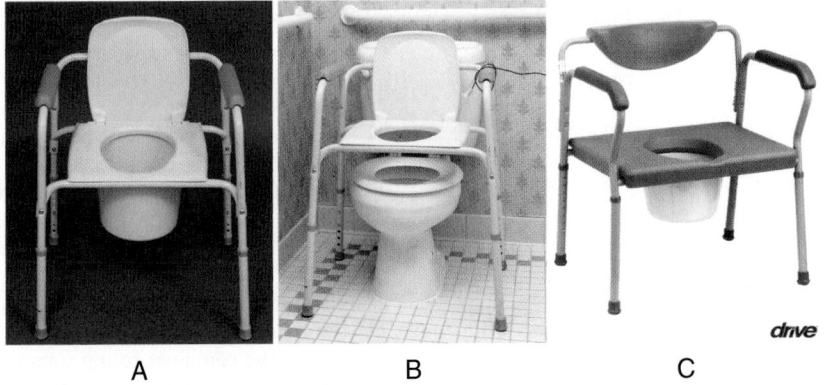

A   B   C

FIGURE 24-10 A, The commode has a toilet seat with a container. The container slides out from under the seat for emptying. **B,** The container is removed. The commode chair is placed over the toilet. **C,** Bariatric commode. (**C,** Courtesy Medical Depot, Inc., Port Washington, N.Y.)

Commodes

A commode is a chair or wheelchair with an opening for a container (Fig. 24-10). Persons unable to walk to the bathroom often use commodes. The commode allows a normal position for elimination. The commode arms and back provide support and help prevent falls.

Some commodes are wheeled into the bathrooms and placed over toilets. Remove the container if the commode is used with the toilet. Lock the wheels after the commode is positioned over the toilet.

See *Delegation Guidelines: Commodes.*
See *Promoting Safety and Comfort: Commodes.*
See procedure: *Helping the Person to the Commode*, p. 396.

DELEGATION GUIDELINES

Commodes

You need this information from the nurse and care plan when assisting with commodes.
- If the commode is used at the bedside or over the toilet
- How much help the person needs
- If you can leave the room or if you need to stay with the person
- If the nurse needs to observe urine or BMs
- What observations to report and record (see *Delegation Guidelines: Bedpans,* p. 391)
- When to report observations
- What patient or resident concerns to report at once

PROMOTING SAFETY AND COMFORT

Commodes

Safety
For commode use, transfer the person from the bed, chair, or wheelchair to the commode. Practice safe transfer procedures (Chapter 19). Use the transfer belt and lock the wheels. Remember to remove the transfer belt after the transfer. See "Transfer/Gait Belts" in Chapter 14.

Comfort
After transfer to the commode, cover the person's lap and legs with a bath blanket. This promotes warmth and privacy.

Helping the Person to the Commode

QUALITY OF LIFE

- Knock before entering the person's room.
- Address the person by name.
- Introduce yourself by name and title.

- Explain the procedure before starting and during the procedure.
- Protect the person's rights during the procedure.
- Handle the person gently during the procedure.

PRE-PROCEDURE

1 Follow *Delegation Guidelines: Commodes*, p. 395. See *Promoting Safety and Comfort:*
  a   *Urinary Elimination*, p. 389
  b   *Commodes*, p. 395
2 Provide for privacy.
3 Practice hand hygiene.
4 Put on gloves.

5 Collect the following.
- Commode
- Toilet tissue
- Bath blanket
- Transfer belt
- Robe and non-skid footwear

PROCEDURE

6 Bring the commode next to the bed.
7 Help the person sit on the side of the bed. Lower the bed rail if used.
8 Help him or her put on a robe and non-skid footwear.
9 Apply the transfer belt.
10 Assist the person to the commode. Use the transfer belt.
11 Remove the transfer belt. Cover the person with a bath blanket for warmth.
12 Place the toilet tissue and call light within reach.
13 Ask him or her to signal when done or when help is needed. (Stay with the person if necessary. Be respectful. Provide as much privacy as possible.)
14 Remove and discard the gloves. Practice hand hygiene.
15 Leave the room. Close the door.
16 Return when the person signals. Or check on the person every 5 minutes. Knock before entering.
17 Practice hand hygiene. Put on the gloves.
18 Help the person clean the genital area as needed. Remove and discard the gloves. Practice hand hygiene.
19 Apply the transfer belt. Help the person back to bed using the transfer belt. Remove the transfer belt, robe, and footwear. Raise the bed rail if used.

20 Put on clean gloves. Remove and cover the commode container. Clean the commode.
21 Take the container to the bathroom.
22 Observe urine and feces for color, amount (output), and character.
23 Empty the container contents into the toilet and flush.
24 Rinse the container. Pour the rinse into the toilet and flush.
25 Clean and disinfect the container. Pour disinfectant into the toilet and flush.
26 Return the container to the commode. Close the lid on the commode. Clean other parts of the commode if necessary.
27 Return other supplies to their proper place.
28 Remove and discard the gloves. Practice hand hygiene and put on clean gloves.
29 Assist with hand-washing.
30 Remove and discard the gloves. Practice hand hygiene.

POST-PROCEDURE

31 Provide for comfort. (See the inside of the front cover.)
32 Place the call light and other needed items within reach.
33 Raise or lower bed rails. Follow the care plan.
34 Unscreen the person.
35 Complete a safety check of the room. (See the inside of the front cover.)

36 Follow agency policy for used linens.
37 Practice hand hygiene.
38 Report and record your observations.

URINARY INCONTINENCE

Urinary incontinence is the involuntary loss or leakage of urine. Incontinence is not a normal part of aging. However, older persons are at risk for incontinence because of changes in the urinary tract, medical and surgical conditions, and drug therapy.

Types of Incontinence

Incontinence may be temporary or persistent. Risk factors and causes of incontinence are listed in Box 24-2. The common types of incontinence are:

- *Stress incontinence. Urine leaks during exercise and certain movements that cause pressure on the bladder.* Urine loss is small. Often called dribbling, it occurs with laughing, sneezing, coughing, lifting, or other activities.
- *Urge incontinence (over-active bladder). Urine is lost in response to a sudden, urgent need to void. The person cannot get to a toilet in time.* Urinary frequency, urinary urgency, and night-time voiding are common.
- *Mixed incontinence. The person has a combination of stress incontinence and urge incontinence.* Many older women have this type.
- *Over-flow incontinence. Small amounts of urine leak from a full bladder.* The person feels like the bladder is not empty. The person dribbles often or constantly and may have a weak urine stream.
- *Functional incontinence. The person has bladder control but cannot use the toilet in time.*
- *Reflex incontinence. Urine is lost at predictable intervals when the bladder is full.* The person does not feel the need to void. Nervous system disorders and injuries are common causes.
- *Transient incontinence. This refers to temporary or occasional incontinence that is reversed when the cause is treated. (Transient means for a short time.)*

Incontinence may result from a physical illness or drugs. Some causes can be reversed. Others cannot. If incontinence is a new problem, tell the nurse at once.

Managing Incontinence

The goals of managing incontinence are to:
- Prevent UTIs.
- Restore as much normal bladder function as possible.

Incontinence is embarrassing. Garments are wet and odors develop. The person is uncomfortable. Skin irritation, infection, and pressure ulcers are risks. Falling is a risk when trying to get to the bathroom quickly. Pride, dignity, and self-esteem are affected. Social isolation, loss of independence, and depression are common. Quality of life suffers.

The person's care plan may include some of the measures listed in Box 24-3, p. 398. *Good skin care and dry garments and linens are essential.* Promoting normal urinary elimination prevents incontinence in some people (see Box 24-1). Others need bladder training (p. 404). Sometimes catheters are needed (Chapter 25).

Incontinence is linked to abuse, mistreatment, and neglect. Frequent care is needed. The person may wet again right after skin care and changing wet garments and linens. Remember, incontinence is beyond the person's control. It is not something the person chooses to do. Be

patient. The person's needs are great. If you feel short-tempered, talk to the nurse at once. The person has the right to be free from abuse, mistreatment, and neglect. Kindness, empathy, understanding, and patience are needed.

See *Focus on Children and Older Persons: Managing Incontinence*, p. 398.

See *Focus on Long-Term Care and Home Care: Managing Incontinence*, p. 399.

See *Focus on Surveys: Managing Incontinence*, p. 399.

BOX 24-2 Incontinence—Risk Factors and Causes

Risk Factors
- Women—pregnancy, childbirth, menopause
- Men—prostate problems
- Age—bladder muscles lose strength with aging; the bladder holds less urine
- Over-weight—pressure on the bladder increases
- Smoking—chronic cough increases pressure on the bladder; irritates the bladder leading to over-active bladder
- Diabetes—nerve damage affects the bladder
- Kidney disease
- Immobility
- Restraint use
- Delays in voiding—unanswered call lights, no call light within reach, not knowing where to find the bathroom, trouble removing clothing, and so on
- Confusion and disorientation

Temporary Incontinence
- Alcohol—increases urine production, stimulates the bladder leading to urge incontinence.
- Bladder irritation—some drinks and foods irritate the bladder. Sodas, tea, coffee, spicy foods, citrus fruits, and tomatoes are examples.
- Caffeine—increases urine production, stimulates the bladder leading to urge incontinence.
- Constipation or fecal impaction—irritates the nerves shared by the bladder and rectum. See Chapter 26.
- Delirium—see Chapter 49.
- Drug therapies.
- Increased fluid intake—urine production increases.
- Urinary tract infection (UTI)—irritates the bladder causing an urgent need to void.

Persistent Incontinence
- Aging changes
- Alzheimer's disease and other dementias (Chapter 49)
- Bladder cancer
- Bladder stones
- Hysterectomy—removal (*ectomy*) of the uterus (*hyster*) causing damage to the pelvic muscles
- Menopause
- Nervous system disorders—multiple sclerosis, Parkinson's disease, stroke, brain tumor, spinal cord injury
- Obstruction of the urinary tract
- Pregnancy and childbirth
- Prostate problems—prostatitis (inflammation [*itis*] of the prostate [*prostat*]), enlarged prostate, prostate cancer

BOX 24-3	Urinary Incontinence—Nursing Measures

- Record the person's voidings—times and amount (output). This includes incontinent times and successful use of the toilet, commode, bedpan, or urinal.
- Answer call lights promptly. The need to void may be urgent.
- Promote normal urinary elimination (see Box 24-1).
- Promote normal bowel elimination (Chapter 26).
- Assist with elimination after sleep, before and after meals, and at bedtime.
- Follow the person's bladder training program (p. 404).
- Provide a clear pathway to the bathroom.
- Have the person wear easy-to-remove clothing. Incontinence can occur while trying to deal with buttons, zippers, other closures, and under-garments.
- Encourage the person to do pelvic muscle exercises as instructed by the nurse.
- Check the person often to make sure he or she is clean and dry.
- Help prevent UTIs.
  - Promote fluid intake as the nurse directs.
  - Have the person wear cotton underwear.
  - Keep the perineal area clean and dry.
- Decrease fluid intake at bedtime.
- Provide good skin care.
- Apply a barrier cream or moisturizer (cream, lotion, paste) to the skin or perineum as directed by the nurse. The application prevents irritation and skin damage.
- Provide dry garments and linens.
- Observe for signs of skin breakdown (Chapters 36 and 37).
- Use incontinence products as the nurse directs. Follow the manufacturer's instructions.
- Do not leave urinals in place to catch urine in men who are incontinent.
- Keep the perineal area clean and dry (Chapter 22).
  - Use soap and water or a no-rinse incontinence cleanser (perineal rinse). Follow the care plan. For soap and water, use a safe and comfortable water temperature.
  - Follow Standard Precautions and the Bloodborne Pathogen Standard.
  - Protect the person and dry garments and linens from the wet incontinence product.
  - Expose only the perineal area.
  - Dry the perineal area and buttocks.
  - Remove wet incontinence products, garments, and linens. Apply clean, dry ones.

FOCUS ON CHILDREN AND OLDER PERSONS

Managing Incontinence

Children

Urinary incontinence is common in children. Day-time wetting is more common in girls. Night-time wetting is more common in boys. After age 5, wetting at night is often called *bedwetting* or *sleep-wetting*. More common in boys, the cause is unknown. Possible factors include:

- Slower physical development
- Long sleeping periods
- Producing more urine at night
- Not recognizing a full bladder
- Anxiety
- Family history of bedwetting

Incontinence usually disappears after age 5. The bladder grows in size and holds more urine. The child learns to respond to the body's signal to void. Stress and anxiety can cause incontinence. As the child grows older, stressful and anxiety-producing events may pass.

Treatments include diet changes, moisture alarms, drugs, and bladder training.

Older Persons

Urinary incontinence is common in older persons. Complications from incontinence pose serious problems for them. These include falls, pressure ulcers, and UTIs. Long hospital or long-term care stays are often necessary.

Persons with dementia may develop incontinence. They may void in the wrong places. Trash cans, planters, heating vents, and closets are examples. Some persons remove incontinence products and throw them on the floor or in the toilet. Others resist staff efforts to keep them clean and dry.

You must provide safe care. The care plan lists needed measures. The care plan may include measures recommended by the Alzheimer's Disease Education and Referral Center (ADEAR).

- Follow the person's bathroom routine. For example, take the person to the bathroom every 2 to 3 hours during the day. Do not wait for the person to ask.
- Observe for signs that the person may need to void. Restlessness and pulling at clothes are examples. Respond quickly.
- Stay calm when the person is incontinent. Re-assure the person if he or she becomes upset.
- Tell the nurse when the person is incontinent. Report the time, what the person was doing, and other observations. A pattern to the incontinence may emerge. If so, measures are planned to prevent the problem.
- Prevent incontinence during sleep. Limit the type and amount of fluids in the evening. Follow the care plan.
- Plan ahead if the person will leave the agency. Have the person wear easy-to-remove clothing. Pack extra clothing, incontinence products, and hygiene supplies. Know where to find restrooms.

You may need a co-worker's help to keep the person clean and dry. If you have questions, ask the nurse for help.

Remember, everyone has the right to safe care. They also have the right to be treated with dignity and privacy.

Applying Incontinence Products

Incontinence products help keep the person dry. Most products are disposable—used once. They usually have 2 layers and a waterproof back. Fluid passes through the first layer. It is absorbed by the lower layer. Many products come in bariatric sizes.

Common incontinence products include:
- *Complete incontinence brief* (Fig. 24-11, *A*). The product is secured at the sides with Velcro or tape tabs.
- *Pad and under-garment* (Fig. 24-11, *B*). With styles for men and for women, the under-garment looks like regular underwear. A pad (pant liner) is inserted into the built-in pouch.
- *Pull-on underwear* (Fig. 24-11, *C*). The product looks like regular underwear. Some products are styled for men and women.
- *Belted under-garment* (Fig. 24-11, *D*). A pad is attached to a re-usable belt.

The nurse helps the person select products to meet his or her needs. To use them, follow the manufacturer's instructions and agency procedures.

See *Focus on Communication: Applying Incontinence Products*, p. 400.

See *Delegation Guidelines: Applying Incontinence Products*, p. 400.

See *Promoting Safety and Comfort: Applying Incontinence Products*, p. 400.

See procedure: *Applying Incontinence Products*, p. 401.

Text continued on p. 404.

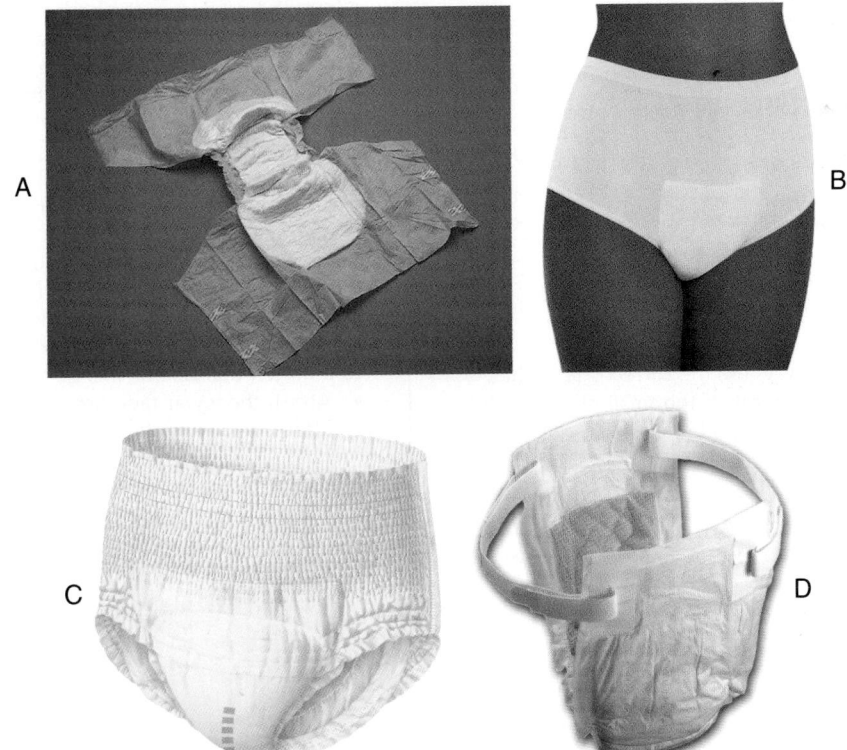

FIGURE 24-11 Disposable incontinence products. **A,** Complete incontinence brief. **B,** Pad and under-garment. **C,** Pull-on underwear. **D,** Belted under-garment. (**B,** Courtesy Hartmann USA, Inc., Rock Hill, S.C. **C,** Courtesy Hartmann Inc., Heidenheim, Germany. **D,** Courtesy Principle Business Enterprises, Dunbridge, Ohio.)

FOCUS ON COMMUNICATION

Applying Incontinence Products

Incontinence products are often called "adult diapers." The word "diaper" may offend the person or lower self-esteem. Instead, say "brief," "pad," or "underwear." Some persons prefer the brand name of the product they use. Use a term that promotes dignity and self-esteem.

DELEGATION GUIDELINES

Applying Incontinence Products

To apply an incontinence product, you need this information from the nurse and the care plan.
- What product to use.
- What size to use.
- If you need to apply a barrier cream. If yes, what cream to use.
- What observations to report and record:
  - Complaints of pain, burning, irritation, or the need to void
  - Signs and symptoms of skin breakdown:
    - Redness, irritation, blisters
    - Complaints of pain, burning, tingling, or itching
  - The amount of urine—small, moderate, large
  - Urine color
  - Blood in the urine
  - Leakage
  - A poor product fit
- When to report observations.
- What patient or resident concerns to report at once.

PROMOTING SAFETY AND COMFORT

Applying Incontinence Products

Safety

To safely apply an incontinence product, follow the manufacturer's instructions. The guidelines in Box 24-4 will help prevent:
- Leakage
- Skin irritation and blisters
- Tearing

Provide for safety if the person will stand for the procedure.
- Make sure the bed is in a low position safe and comfortable for the person.
- Lock (brake) the bed wheels.
- Have the person wear non-skid footwear.
- Provide something for the person to hold on to for balance and stability.

Comfort

For the person's comfort, always use the correct size. If the product is too large, urine can leak. If too small, the product will cause discomfort from being too tight.

BOX 24-4   Applying Incontinence Products

- Follow the manufacturer's instructions.
- Use the correct size. The nurse measures the person's hips and thighs. The largest measurement is used for the correct size.
- Note the front and back of the product.
- Center the product in the perineal area.
- Position the man's penis downward.
- Check for proper placement. The product should be in the creases between the thighs and the perineal area (groin area). It should fit the shape of the body.
- Note the amount of urine (small, moderate, large). Also note how often you change the product. An extended wear product may be needed for large amounts of urine or diarrhea (Chapter 26).
- Do not let the plastic backing touch the person's skin.
- Provide perineal care after each incontinent episode.
- Do not use the product as a turning or lift sheet.
- Attach the tabs correctly. The product will tear if you try to unfasten the tape or change the tape's position.
  - Attach the lower tape first. Stretch the tape and attach it at a slightly upward angle. Do so for both sides.
  - Attach the upper tape after the lower tape is fastened. Stretch the tape and attach it in a horizontal manner. Do so for both sides.

Applying Incontinence Products

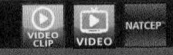

QUALITY OF LIFE

- Knock before entering the person's room.
- Address the person by name.
- Introduce yourself by name and title.

- Explain the procedure before starting and during the procedure.
- Protect the person's rights during the procedure.
- Handle the person gently during the procedure.

PRE-PROCEDURE

1 Follow *Delegation Guidelines: Applying Incontinence Products*. See *Promoting Safety and Comfort:*
   a *Urinary Elimination*, p. 389
   b *Applying Incontinence Products*
2 Practice hand hygiene.
3 Collect the following.
   - Incontinence product as directed by the nurse
   - Barrier cream or moisturizer as directed by the nurse
   - Cleanser
   - Items for perineal care (Chapter 22)
   - Waterproof under-pad
   - Paper towels
   - Trash bag
   - Gloves
   - Non-skid footwear if the person will stand

4 Cover the over-bed table with paper towels. Arrange items on top of them.
5 Identify the person. Check the ID (identification) bracelet against the assignment sheet. Use 2 identifiers (Chapter 13). Also call the person by name.
6 Mark the date, time, and your initials on the new product. Follow agency policy.
7 Provide for privacy.
8 Fill the wash basin. Water temperature is usually 105°F to 109°F (Fahrenheit) (40.5°C to 42.7°C [centigrade]). Measure water temperature according to agency policy. Ask the person to check the water temperature. Adjust water temperature as needed.
9 Raise the bed for body mechanics. Bed rails are up if used. (Omit this step if the person will stand.)

PROCEDURE

10 Lower the head of the bed. The bed is as flat as possible.
11 Lower the bed rail near you if up.
12 Practice hand hygiene. Put on the gloves.
13 Cover the person with a bath blanket. Lower top linens to the foot of the bed. Lower the pants or slacks. (Omit this step if the person will stand. See step 16.)
14 *To apply an incontinence brief with the person in bed:*
   a Place a waterproof under-pad under the buttocks. Ask the person to raise the buttocks off the bed. Or turn the person from side to side.
   b Loosen the tabs on each side of the used brief.
   c Turn the person onto the side away from you.
   d Remove the brief from front to back (top to bottom). Observe the urine as you roll the product up (Fig. 24-12, *A*, p. 402).
   e Place the used brief in the trash bag. Set the bag aside.
   f Perform perineal care (Chapter 22) wearing clean gloves. Apply the barrier cream or moisturizer.
   g Remove and discard the gloves. Practice hand hygiene. Put on clean gloves.
   h Open the new brief. Fold it in half length-wise along the center (Fig. 24-12, *B*, p. 402).
   i Insert the brief between the legs from front to back (top to bottom) (Fig. 24-12, *C*, p. 402).
   j Unfold and spread the back panel (Fig. 24-12, *D*, p. 402).
   k Center the brief in the perineal area.
   l Turn the person onto his or her back.
   m Unfold and spread the front panel. Provide a "cup" shape in the perineal area. For a man, position the penis downward.
   n Make sure the brief is positioned high in the groin folds. This allows the brief to fit the shape of the body.

   o Secure the brief (Fig. 24-12, *E*, p. 402).
      1) Pull the lower tape tab forward on the side near you. Attach it at a slightly upward angle. Do the same for the other side.
      2) Pull the upper tape tab forward on the side near you. Attach it in a horizontal manner. Do the same for the other side.
   p Smooth out all wrinkles and folds.
15 *To apply a pad and under-garment with the person in bed:*
   a Place a waterproof under-pad under the buttocks. Ask the person to raise the buttocks off the bed. Or turn the person from side to side.
   b Turn the person onto the side away from you.
   c Pull the under-garment down. The waistband is over the knee (Fig. 24-13, *A*, p. 403).
   d Remove the used pad from front to back (top to bottom). Observe the urine as you roll the product up (Fig. 24-13, *B*, p. 403).
   e Place the used pad in the trash bag. Set the bag aside.
   f Perform perineal care (Chapter 22) wearing clean gloves. Apply the barrier cream or moisturizer.
   g Remove and discard the gloves. Practice hand hygiene. Put on clean gloves.
   h Fold the new pad in half length-wise along the center (Fig. 24-13, *C*, p. 403).
   i Insert the pad between the legs from front to back (top to bottom) (Fig. 24-13, *D*, p. 403).
   j Unfold and spread the back panel (Figure 24-13, *E*, p. 403).
   k Center the pad in the perineal area.
   l Pull the garment up at the back (Fig. 24-13, *F*, p. 403).
   m Turn the person onto his or her back.
   n Unfold and spread the front panel (Fig. 24-13, *G*, p. 403). For a man, position the penis downward.
   o Pull the garment up in front (Fig. 24-13, *H*, p. 403).
   p Check and adjust the pad and under-garment for a good fit.

Continued

Applying Incontinence Products—cont'd

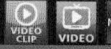

PROCEDURE—cont'd

16 *To apply pull-on underwear with the person standing:*
  a Help the person stand. Remove the pants or slacks.
  b Tear the side seams to remove the used underwear (Fig. 24-14, *A*, p. 404).
  c Remove the underwear from front to back (top to bottom) (Fig. 24-14, *B*, p. 404). Observe the urine as you roll the underwear up.
  d Place the used underwear in the trash bag. Set the bag aside.
  e Perform perineal care (Chapter 22) wearing clean gloves. Apply the barrier cream or moisturizer.
  f Remove and discard the gloves. Practice hand hygiene. Put on clean gloves.
  g Have the person sit on the side of the bed.
  h Slide the new underwear over the feet to past the knees (Fig. 24-14, *C*, p. 404).
  i Help the person stand.
  j Pull the underwear up (Fig. 24-14, *D*, p. 404).
  k Check for a good fit.

17 Ask about comfort. Ask if the product feels too loose or too tight. Check for wrinkles or creases. Make sure the product does not rub or irritate the groin. Adjust the product as needed.

18 Remove and discard the gloves. Practice hand hygiene.

19 Raise or put on pants or slacks.

POST-PROCEDURE

20 Provide for comfort. (See the inside of the front cover.)
21 Place the call light and other needed items within reach.
22 Lower the bed to a safe and comfortable level for the person. Follow the care plan.
23 Raise or lower bed rails. Follow the care plan.
24 Unscreen the person.
25 Practice hand hygiene. Put on clean gloves.
26 Estimate the amount of urine in the used product: small, moderate, large. Open the product to observe for urine color and blood.
27 Clean, rinse, dry, and return the wash basin and other equipment. Return items to their proper place.
28 Remove and discard the gloves. Practice hand hygiene.
29 Complete a safety check of the room. (See the inside of the front cover.)
30 Report and record your observations.

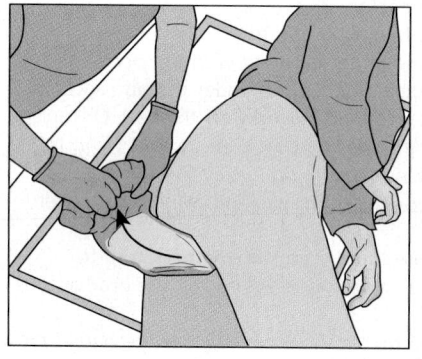

A

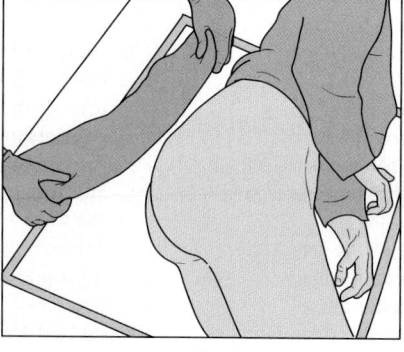

B

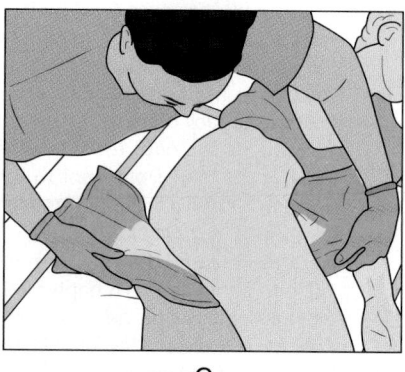

C

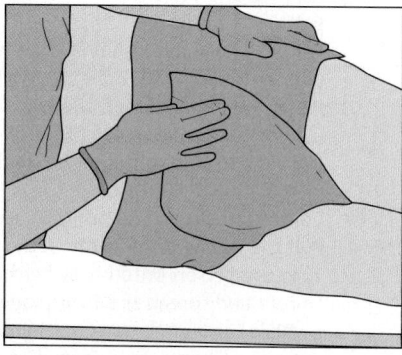

D

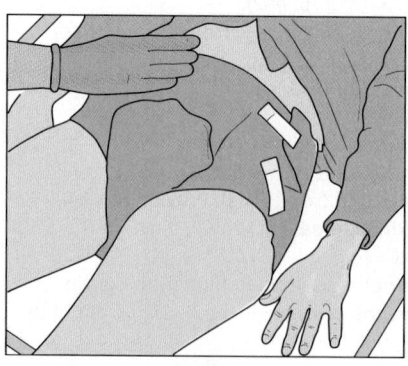

E

FIGURE 24-12 Applying an incontinence brief. **A,** The used brief is removed from front to back (top to bottom). **B,** The new brief is opened length-wise. **C,** The new brief is inserted length-wise between the legs from front to back (top to bottom). **D,** The back panel is spread open. **E,** The lower tape tab is attached at a slightly upward angle. The upper tape tab is attached in a horizontal manner.

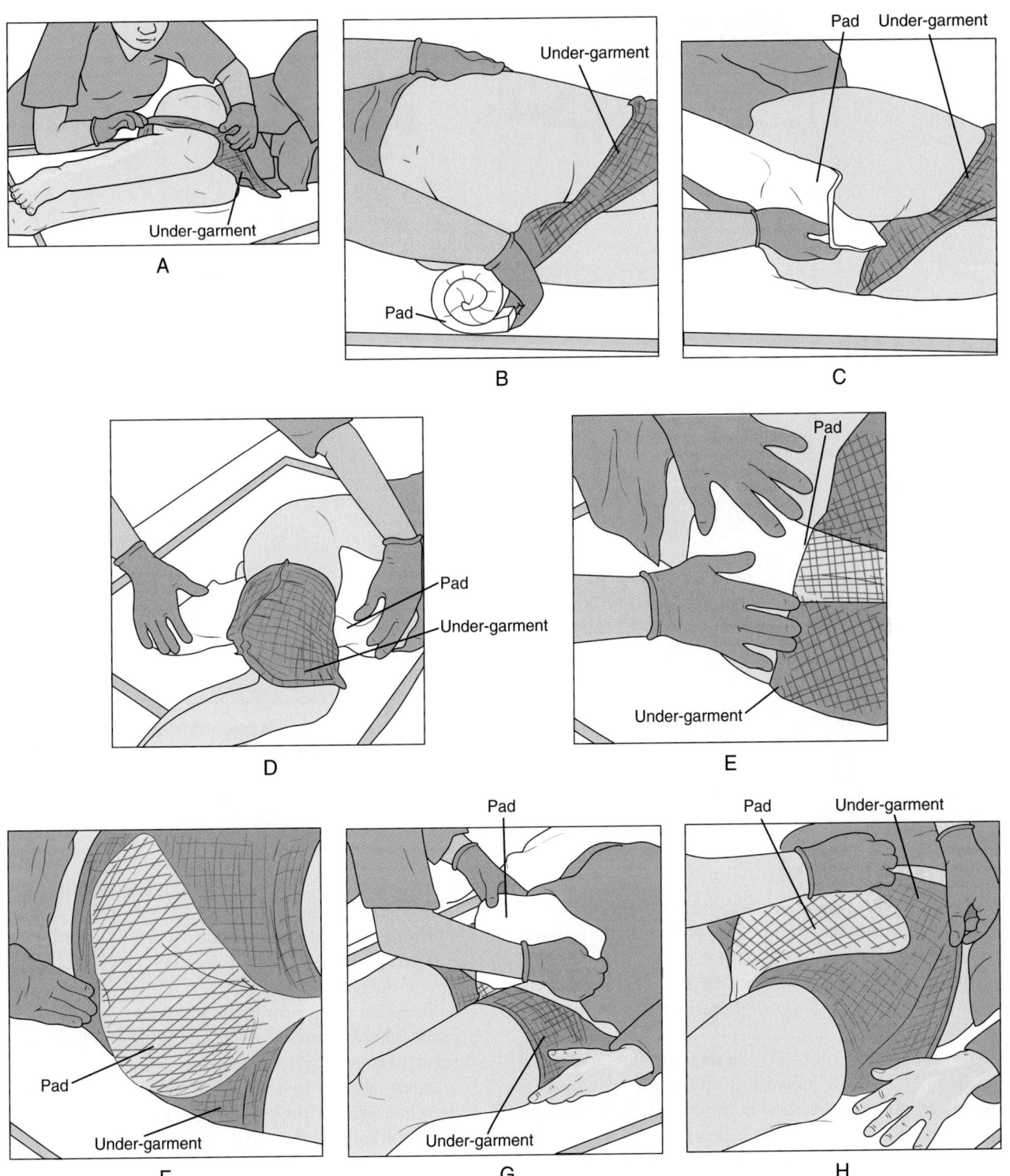

FIGURE 24-13 Applying a pad and under-garment. A, The used under-garment is pulled down. The waistband is over the knee. **B,** The pad is rolled up as it is removed from front to back (top to bottom). **C,** The new pad is folded in half length-wise along the center. **D,** The pad is inserted between the legs from the front to back (top to bottom). **E,** The back panel is unfolded and spread out. **F,** The under-garment is pulled up at the back. **G,** The front panel is unfolded and spread open. **H,** The under-garment is pulled up in front.

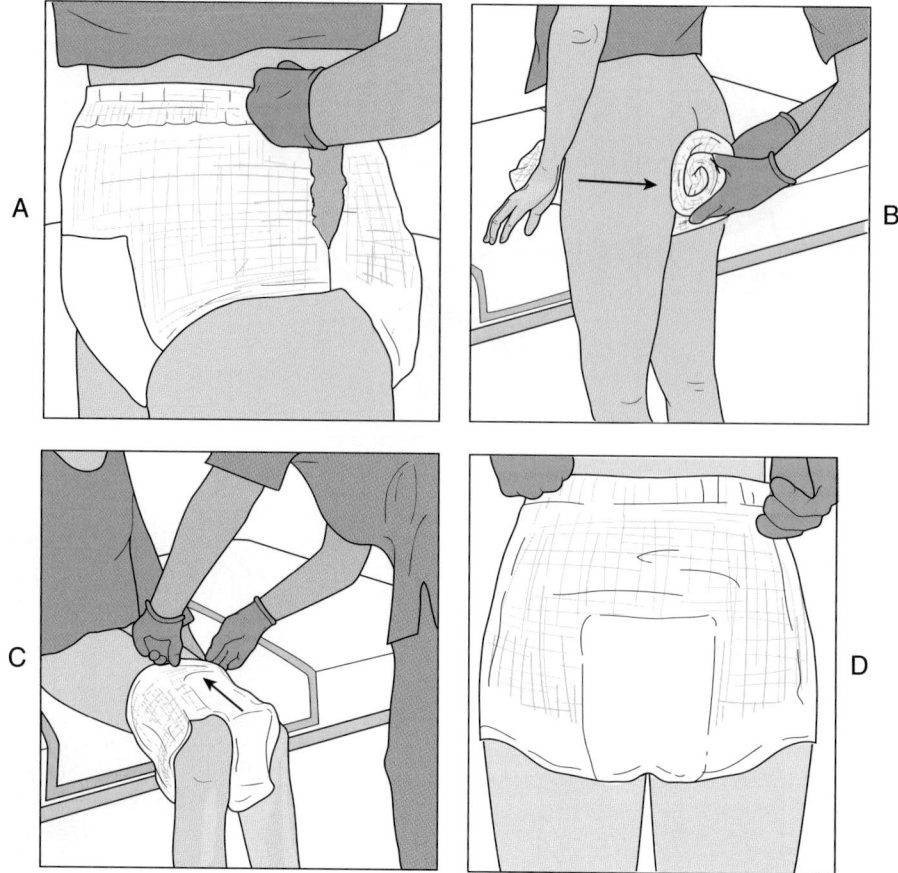

FIGURE 24-14 Applying pull-on underwear. **A,** The side seams are torn to remove the used underwear. **B,** The underwear is removed from front to back (top to bottom). **C,** The underwear is slid over the feet to past the knees. **D,** The underwear is pulled up.

BLADDER TRAINING

Bladder training may help with urinary incontinence. Some persons need bladder training after catheter removal (Chapter 25). Control of urination is the goal. Bladder control promotes comfort and quality of life. It also increases self-esteem. Successful bladder re-training may take many weeks.

The rules for normal elimination are followed (see Box 24-1). The normal position for urinating is assumed if possible. Privacy is important. The person's care plan may include 1 of the following.

- *Bladder re-training (bladder rehabilitation).* The person needs to:
  - Resist or ignore the strong desire to urinate.
  - Postpone or delay voiding.
  - Urinate following a schedule rather than the urge to void.

  The time between voidings increases as bladder re-training progresses.

- *Prompted voiding.* The person voids at scheduled times. The person is taught to:
  - Recognize when the bladder is full.
  - Recognize the need to void.
  - Ask for help.
  - Respond when prompted to void.
- *Habit training/scheduled voiding.* Voiding is scheduled at regular times to match the person's voiding habits. This is usually every 3 to 4 hours while awake. The person does not delay or resist voiding. Timed-voiding is based on the person's usual voiding patterns.
- *Catheter clamping.* The catheter is clamped to prevent urine flow from the bladder (Chapter 25). See Figure 24-15. It is usually clamped for 1 hour at first. Over time, it is clamped for 3 to 4 hours. Urine drains when the catheter is unclamped. When the catheter is removed, voiding is encouraged every 3 to 4 hours or as directed by the nurse and the care plan.

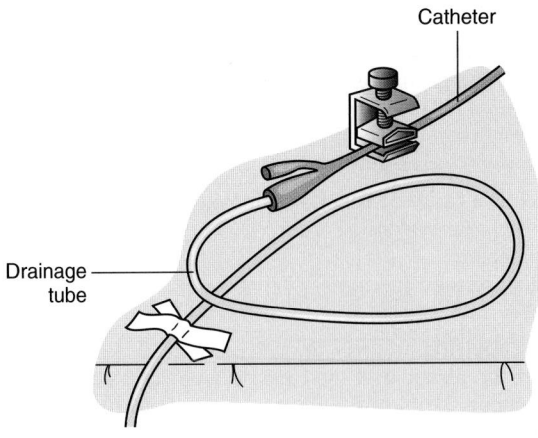

Catheter

Drainage tube

FIGURE 24-15 The clamped catheter prevents urine from draining out of the bladder. The clamp is applied directly to the catheter, not to the drainage tube.

FOCUS ON PRIDE

The Person, Family, and Yourself

Personal and Professional Responsibility

You observe and talk about urine as part of your work. Neither are odd or uncommon. They are expected.

For some, it is easy to talk about urinary elimination. Others are shy or embarrassed. Pay attention to the person's verbal and nonverbal communication (Chapter 9). Modify your communication based on the person's comfort level. Always be professional. Speak with confidence. This puts the person at ease.

Rights and Respect

People usually void in private. Illness, disease, and aging can affect this very private act. Respect the right to privacy. Allow as much privacy as safely possible. Pull privacy curtains and close doors and window coverings. If you must stay in the room, allow as much privacy as possible. Stand just outside the bathroom door in case the person needs you. Or stand on the other side of the privacy curtain if safe to do so. The nurse helps you with ways to protect the person's privacy. Follow the nurse's directions and the care plan.

Empty urinals, bedpans, and commodes promptly. Urine-filled devices in the person's room do not respect the person's right to a neat and clean setting. It also may cause embarrassment. Do your best to promote comfort, dignity, and respect when assisting with elimination needs.

Independence and Social Interaction

Some persons can place bedpans and urinals themselves. Some can get on and off the bedside commodes themselves. Others need some help but can be left alone to void. Allow persons to do as much as safely possible.

Keep devices within reach for persons who use them without help. For persons who need some help, check on them often. Do not leave a person sitting on a bedpan or commode for a long time. Discomfort, odors, and skin breakdown are likely. Also, the person may think you forgot about him or her. The person may try to get off the bedpan or commode alone and be harmed. Make sure the call light is within reach. Respond promptly when the person calls for you.

Delegation and Teamwork

Reporting and recording what you have done and observed are parts of delegation. Accurate reporting and recording are important. The nurse needs to know about urine appearance, odor, and amount (output). Changes in urination may lead to changes in the person's care. Report urinary problems and abnormal urine to the nurse. If you are unsure what to report or record, ask the nurse.

Ethics and Laws

Negligence occurs when a person does not act in a reasonable and careful manner and the person or the person's property is harmed (Chapter 5). Although the error is not intentional, the negligent person is responsible. The following is a real example of negligent care.

A patient was admitted to the hospital with a diagnosis of mild pneumonia. He was to be in the hospital for 24 to 48 hours. While in the hospital, he was left on the bedpan for 4 hours. Pressure ulcers resulted. He died of pneumonia after 41 days in the hospital.

His family sued the hospital. The jury awarded the family $800,000.

(Estate of D. Roberts v William Beaumont Hospital, Mich., 2002.)

The following practices can help you avoid this mistake.

- Be careful and focused when performing all procedures. Avoid distractions.
- Remind the person to use the call light if you do not return promptly.
- Report and record promptly. When you report, the nurse knows what you did. When you record, there is a record of the care provided.
- Use reminders. This is very important when you are busy. For example, set a timer on your watch or write yourself a note.

Take pride in developing good habits that promote safety and quality of care.

FOCUS ON PRIDE: Application

Incontinence often lowers the person's dignity. How can it be prevented? Explain how your words and actions promote dignity when incontinence cannot be prevented.

REVIEW QUESTIONS

Circle the BEST answer.

1 Which is abnormal?
  a Clear, amber urine
  b Urine with a faint odor
  c Cloudy urine with particles
  d Urine output of 1500 mL in 24 hours

2 Which prevents normal elimination?
  a Helping the person assume a normal position for voiding
  b Providing privacy
  c Helping the person to the bathroom as soon as requested
  d Staying with the person who uses a bedpan

3 Which definition is correct?
  a Dysuria means painful or difficult urination.
  b Oliguria means a large amount of urine.
  c Urinary retention means the need to void at once.
  d Urinary incontinence means the inability to void.

4 The person using a standard bedpan is in
  a Fowler's position
  b The supine position
  c The prone position
  d The side-lying position

5 When using a fracture pan
  a The person is in the Fowler's position
  b The smaller end (flat end) is under the buttocks
  c The nurse must position the pan
  d The pan can be left in place for a long time

6 After using the urinal, the man should
  a Put it on the bedside stand
  b Use the call light
  c Put it on the over-bed table
  d Empty it

7 After a person uses a commode, you should
  a Empty, clean, and disinfect the commode
  b Return the commode to the supply area
  c Get a new container
  d Get a new commode

8 Urinary incontinence
  a Is always permanent
  b Requires bladder training
  c Is a normal part of aging
  d Requires good skin care

9 Which is a cause of functional incontinence?
  a A nervous system disorder
  b Sneezing
  c Unanswered call light
  d UTI

10 When applying an incontinence product
  a Let the plastic backing touch the person's skin
  b Remove the old product from back to front
  c Apply the new product from front to back
  d Use the product to turn and position the person

11 The goal of bladder training is to
  a Control the amount voided daily
  b Promote voiding at times convenient for staff
  c Allow the person to walk to the bathroom
  d Gain control of urination

12 A person is taught to ignore the urge to void. This type of bladder training is called
  a Bladder re-training
  b Prompted voiding
  c Habit training
  d Scheduled voiding

Answers to Chapter 24 questions are on p. 871.

FOCUS ON PRACTICE

Problem Solving

You assist a patient onto the commode. The person is unsteady and is not to be left alone. The person says: "I can't go with you standing here." What do you do? How will you provide privacy and safe care?

Urinary Catheters

OBJECTIVES

- Define the key terms and key abbreviations in this chapter.
- Explain why urinary catheters are used.
- Describe 2 types of urinary catheters.
- Explain the purpose and rules for catheter care.
- Describe how to use 2 urine drainage systems.

- Explain how to remove an indwelling catheter.
- Explain how to apply a condom catheter.
- Perform the procedures described in this chapter.
- Explain how to promote PRIDE in the person, the family, and yourself.

KEY TERMS

catheter A tube used to drain or inject fluid through a body opening
catheterization The process of inserting a catheter
condom catheter A soft sheath that slides over the penis and is used to drain urine
Foley catheter See "indwelling catheter"

indwelling catheter A catheter left in the bladder so urine drains constantly into a drainage bag; retention or Foley catheter
retention catheter See "indwelling catheter"
straight catheter A catheter that drains the bladder and then is removed

KEY ABBREVIATIONS

BM	Bowel movement	**mL**	Milliliter
IV	Intravenous	**UTI**	Urinary tract infection

A *catheter is a tube used to drain or inject fluid through a body opening.* Inserted through the urethra into the bladder, a urinary catheter drains urine. *Catheterization is the process of inserting a catheter.* With proper training and supervision, some states and agencies let nursing assistants insert and remove urinary catheters.

See *Focus on Surveys: Urinary Catheters.*
See *Promoting Safety and Comfort: Urinary Catheters.*

FOCUS ON SURVEYS

Urinary Catheters

Surveys are done to determine if the person is receiving appropriate treatment and services. The surveyor may ask you questions about:

- Your understanding of the person's bladder management program
- Your training related to handling catheters, catheter tubing, drainage bags, catheter care, urinary tract infections (UTIs), catheter-related injuries, dislodgment, and skin breakdown
- What observations to report, when to report them, and to whom you should report observations

Answer questions the best you can. If you do not know an answer, tell the surveyor who you would ask or where you would find the answer.

PROMOTING SAFETY AND COMFORT

Urinary Catheters

Safety

Urinary catheter procedures often involve exposing and touching the perineum. Sexual abuse has occurred in health care settings. The person may feel threatened or actually may be abused. He or she needs to call for help. Keep the call light within the person's reach at all times. And always act in a professional manner.

Urine may contain microbes and blood. Follow Standard Precautions and the Bloodborne Pathogen Standard when performing the procedures in this chapter.

PURPOSES AND TYPES OF CATHETERS

These types of catheters are common.

- A *straight catheter* drains the bladder and then is removed.
- An *indwelling catheter (retention* or *Foley catheter) is left in the bladder. Urine drains constantly into a drainage bag.* A balloon near the tip is inflated with sterile water after the catheter is inserted. The balloon prevents the catheter from slipping out of the bladder (Fig. 25-1).

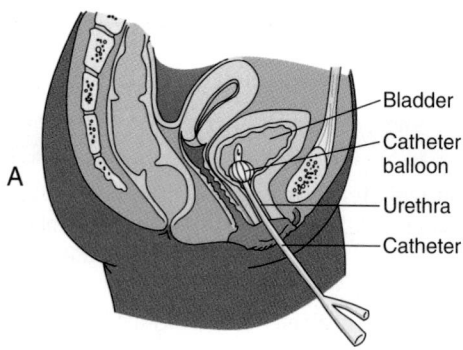

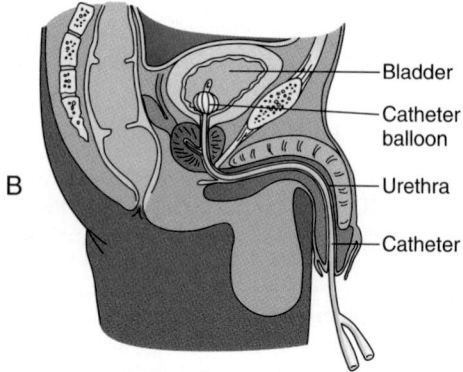

FIGURE 25-1 Indwelling catheter. **A,** Indwelling catheter is in the female bladder. The inflated balloon at the tip prevents the catheter from slipping out through the urethra. **B,** Indwelling catheter with the balloon inflated in the male bladder.

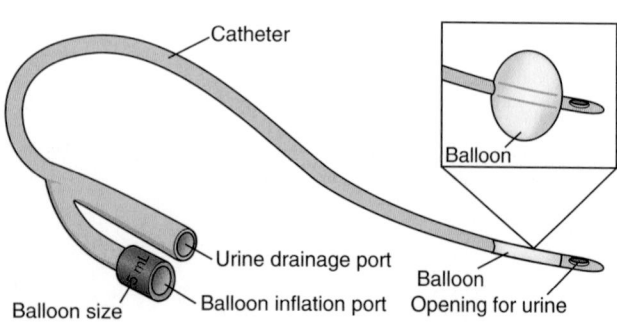

FIGURE 25-2 Parts of a Foley catheter (indwelling catheter).

See Figure 25-2 for parts of an indwelling catheter. Tubing connects the catheter to the urine drainage bag. See Figure 25-3 for the parts of the urine drainage system.

Catheters create a risk for UTIs. However, they are used:

- To keep the bladder empty before, during, and after surgery. This reduces the risk of bladder injury during surgery. Also, the amount of urine can be monitored. After surgery, a full bladder causes pressure on nearby organs. Such pressure can lead to pain or discomfort.
- To promote comfort. Some people are too weak or disabled to use the bedpan, urinal, commode, or toilet. Dying persons are examples. For them, catheters can promote comfort and prevent incontinence.
- To protect wounds and pressure ulcers from contact with urine.
- For hourly urine output measurements.
- To collect sterile urine specimens.
- To measure the amount of urine in the bladder after the person voids. This is called *residual urine.*

Catheters do not treat the cause of incontinence. They are a last resort for incontinence.

▶ CATHETER CARE

You will care for persons with indwelling catheters. The risk of UTI is high. Follow the rules in Box 25-1 to promote safety and comfort.

See *Delegation Guidelines: Catheter Care,* p. 410.
See *Promoting Safety and Comfort: Catheter Care,* p. 410.
See procedure: *Giving Catheter Care,* p. 411.

Text continued on p. 412.

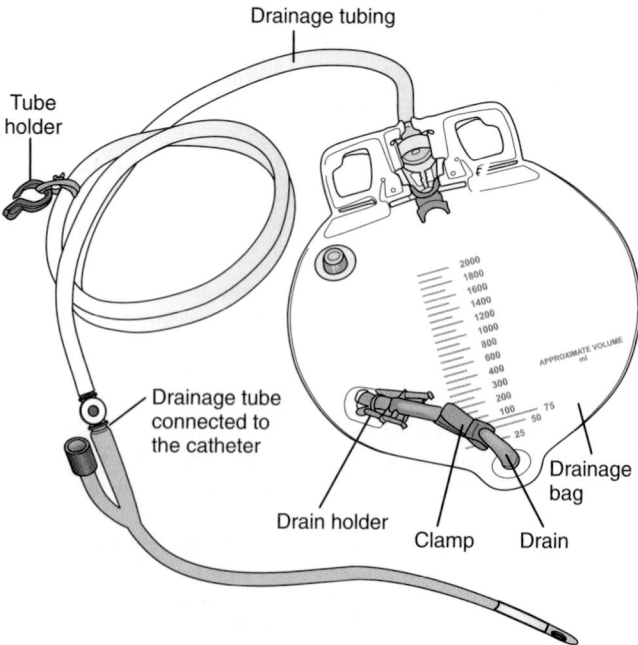

FIGURE 25-3 Parts of the urine drainage system.

BOX 25-1   Indwelling Catheter Care

Preventing Infection
- Follow the rules of medical asepsis.
- Follow Standard Precautions and the Bloodborne Pathogen Standard.
- Encourage fluid intake as directed by the nurse and the care plan.

The Drainage System
- Allow urine to flow freely through the catheter and drainage tube. Tubing should not have kinks. The person should not lie on the tubing.
- Keep the catheter connected to the drainage tube. Follow the measures on p. 412 if the catheter and drainage tube are disconnected.
- Keep the drainage tube and bag below the bladder. This prevents urine from flowing backward into the bladder. When transferring the person to or from the bed or chair, keep the drainage bag lower than the bladder. Secure the drainage bag to the bed or chair after the transfer. See Figure 25-4.
- Move the drainage bag to the other side of the bed when the person is turned and re-positioned on his or her other side.
- Hang the bag from the bed frame, back of the chair or wheelchair, or lower part of the IV (intravenous) pole.
- *Do not hang the drainage bag on a bed rail.* Otherwise the bag is higher than the bladder when the bed rail is raised.
- Hold the bag lower than the bladder when the person walks.
- Do not let the drainage bag touch or rest on the floor. This can contaminate the system.
- Position drainage tubing in a straight line or coil the drainage tubing on the bed. Secure it to the bottom linens (Fig. 25-5, p. 410). Follow the nurse's directions and agency policy. Use a clip, bed sheet clamp, tape, or other device as the nurse directs. Tubing must not loop below the drainage bag.

The Catheter
- Secure the catheter as the nurse directs. The nurse tells you where to secure the catheter.
  - Females: to the thigh (Fig. 25-5, *A*).
  - Males:
    - To the abdomen (Fig. 25-5, *B*). This site is common for long-term catheter use. The drainage bag remains below the bladder. Drainage is not affected.
    - To the thigh (Fig. 25-5, *C*)

The Catheter—cont'd
- Use a tube holder, tape, or other device to secure the catheter to the thigh or abdomen. The nurse tells you what to use. Securing the catheter prevents excess catheter movement and friction at the insertion site (meatus). Catheter movement and friction can damage the meatus.
- Check for leaks. Check the connections to the drainage tube and the drainage bag. Report any leaks to the nurse at once.
- Provide perineal care and catheter care according to the care plan—daily, twice a day, after bowel movements (BMs), or when vaginal discharge is present. (See procedure: *Giving Catheter Care,* p. 411.)

Measuring Urine (Output)
- Empty the drainage bag and measure urine:
  - At the end of the shift
  - When changing to and from a leg bag and a standard drainage bag (p. 413)
  - When the bag is becoming full
- Report an increase or decrease in urine amount.
- Use a separate measuring container for each person. This prevents the spread of microbes from 1 person to another.
- Do not let the drain on the drainage bag touch any surface.
- See procedure: *Emptying a Urine Drainage Bag,* p. 415.

Observations
- Report complaints to the nurse at once—pain, burning, the need to void, or irritation. Also report the color, clarity, and odor of urine and the presence of particles or blood.
- Observe for signs and symptoms of a UTI. Report the following at once.
  - Fever.
  - Chills.
  - Flank pain or tenderness. The flank area is in the back between the ribs and the hip (Fig. 25-6, p. 410).
  - Change in the urine—blood, foul smell, particles, cloudiness, oliguria.
  - Change in mental or functional status—confusion, decreased appetite, falls, decreased activity, tiredness, and so on.
- Urine leakage around the catheter.

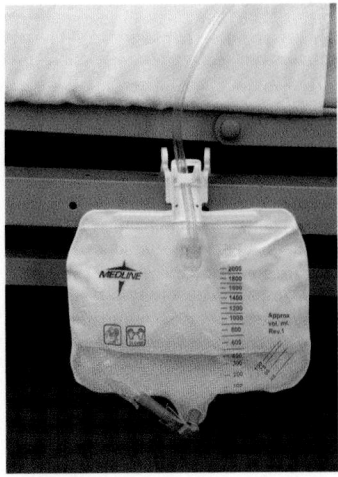

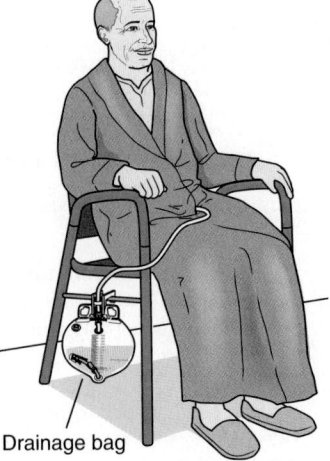

Drainage bag

A   B

FIGURE 25-4 A, Urine drainage bag secured to the bed frame. **B,** Urine drainage bag secured to a chair.

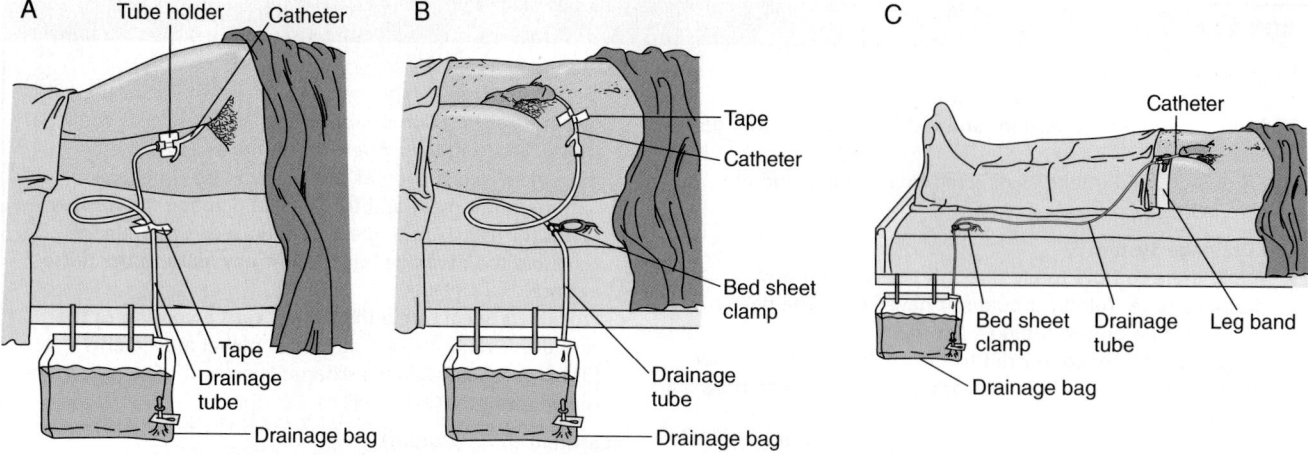

FIGURE 25-5 Securing catheters. **A,** The catheter is secured to the thigh with a tube holder. The drainage tube is coiled on the bed and secured to bottom linens with tape. **B,** The catheter is secured to the man's abdomen with tape. Drainage tubing is secured to bottom linens with a bed sheet clamp. **C,** The catheter is secured to the man's thigh with a leg band. Drainage tubing is in a straight line and secured to bottom linens with a bed sheet clamp. The drainage bag is at the foot of the bed.

DELEGATION GUIDELINES

Catheter Care

When delegated catheter care, you need this information from the nurse and the care plan.
- When to give catheter care—daily, twice a day, after BMs, or when vaginal discharge is present
- What water temperature to use for perineal care
- Where to secure the catheter—thigh or abdomen
- How to secure the catheter—tube holder, tape, or other device
- How to position the drainage tubing—straight line or coiled on the bed
- How to secure drainage tubing—clip, bed sheet clamp, tape, or other device
- What observations to report and record:
  - Complaints of pain, burning, irritation, or the need to void (report at once)
  - Crusting, abnormal drainage, or secretions
  - The color, clarity, and odor of urine
  - Particles in the urine
  - Blood in the urine
  - Cloudy urine
  - Urine leaking at the insertion site
  - Drainage system leaks
- When to report observations
- What patient or resident concerns to report at once

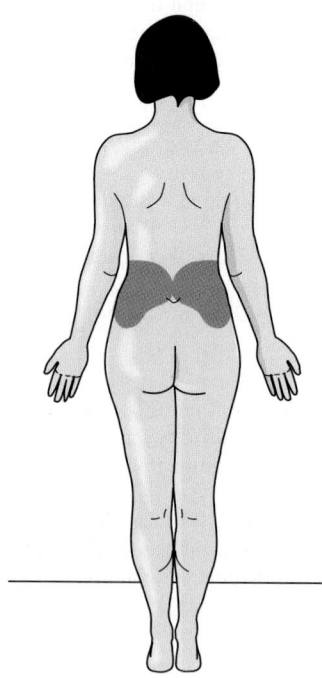

FIGURE 25-6 *Shading* shows the flank area.

PROMOTING SAFETY AND COMFORT

Catheter Care

Comfort

The catheter must not pull at the insertion site. This causes discomfort and irritation. Hold the catheter securely during catheter care. Then properly secure the catheter. Make sure the tubing is not under the person. Besides obstructing urine flow, lying on the tubing is uncomfortable. It can also cause skin breakdown. To promote comfort, see Box 25-1.

Giving Catheter Care   NATCEP

QUALITY OF LIFE

- Knock before entering the person's room.
- Address the person by name.
- Introduce yourself by name and title.

- Explain the procedure before starting and during the procedure.
- Protect the person's rights during the procedure.
- Handle the person gently during the procedure.

PRE-PROCEDURE

1 Follow *Delegation Guidelines:*
  - *Perineal Care* (Chapter 22)
  - *Catheter Care*
  See *Promoting Safety and Comfort:*
  - *Perineal Care* (Chapter 22)
  - *Urinary Catheters,* p. 407
  - *Catheter Care*
2 Practice hand hygiene.
3 Collect the following.
  - Items for perineal care (Chapter 22)
  - Gloves
  - Bath blanket

4 Cover the over-bed table with paper towels. Arrange items on top of them.
5 Identify the person. Check the ID (identification) bracelet against the assignment sheet. Use 2 identifiers (Chapter 13). Also call the person by name.
6 Provide for privacy.
7 Fill the wash basin. Water temperature is about 105°F to 109°F (40.5°C to 42.7°C). Measure water temperature according to agency policy. Ask the person to check the water temperature. Adjust water temperature as needed.
8 Raise the bed for body mechanics. Bed rails are up if used.
9 Lower the bed rail near you if up.

PROCEDURE

10 Practice hand hygiene. Put on the gloves.
11 Cover the person with a bath blanket. Fan-fold top linens to the foot of the bed.
12 Position and drape the person for perineal care (Chapter 22).
13 Fold back the bath blanket to expose the perineal area.
14 Ask the person to flex the knees and raise the buttocks off the bed. Place the waterproof under-pad under the buttocks.
15 Check the drainage tubing. Make sure it is not kinked and that urine can flow freely.
16 Separate the labia (female). In an uncircumcised male, retract the foreskin (Chapter 22). Check for crusts, abnormal drainage, or secretions.
17 Give perineal care (Chapter 22). Keep the foreskin of the uncircumcised male retracted until step 25.
18 Apply soap to a clean, wet washcloth.
19 Hold the catheter at the meatus. Do so for steps 20 through 24.
20 Wash around the catheter at the meatus. Use a circular motion (Fig. 25-7, *A*, p. 412).
21 Clean the catheter from the meatus down the catheter at least 4 inches (Fig. 25-7, *B*, p. 412). Clean downward, away from the meatus with 1 stroke. Do not tug or pull on the catheter. Repeat as needed with a clean area of the washcloth. Use a clean washcloth if needed.

22 Rinse around the catheter at the meatus with a clean washcloth.
23 Rinse the catheter from the meatus down the catheter at least 4 inches. Rinse downward, away from the meatus with 1 stroke. Do not tug or pull on the catheter. Repeat as needed with a clean area of the washcloth. Use a clean washcloth if needed.
24 Pat dry the areas washed. Dry from the meatus down the catheter at least 4 inches. Do not tug or pull on the catheter.
25 Return the foreskin (uncircumcised male) to its natural position.
26 Pat dry the perineal area. Dry from front to back (top to bottom).
27 Secure the catheter. Position the tubing in a straight line or coiled on the bed. Follow the nurse's directions. Secure the tubing to the bottom linens (see Fig. 25-5).
28 Remove the waterproof under-pad.
29 Cover the person. Remove the bath blanket.
30 Remove and discard the gloves. Practice hand hygiene.

POST-PROCEDURE

31 Provide for comfort. (See the inside of the front cover.)
32 Place the call light and other needed items within reach.
33 Lower the bed to a safe and comfortable level for the person. Follow the care plan.
34 Raise or lower bed rails. Follow the care plan.
35 Clean, rinse, dry, and return equipment to its proper place. Discard disposable items. (Wear gloves for this step.)

36 Unscreen the person.
37 Complete a safety check of the room. (See the inside of the front cover.)
38 Follow agency policy for used linens.
39 Remove and discard the gloves. Practice hand hygiene.
40 Report and record your observations.

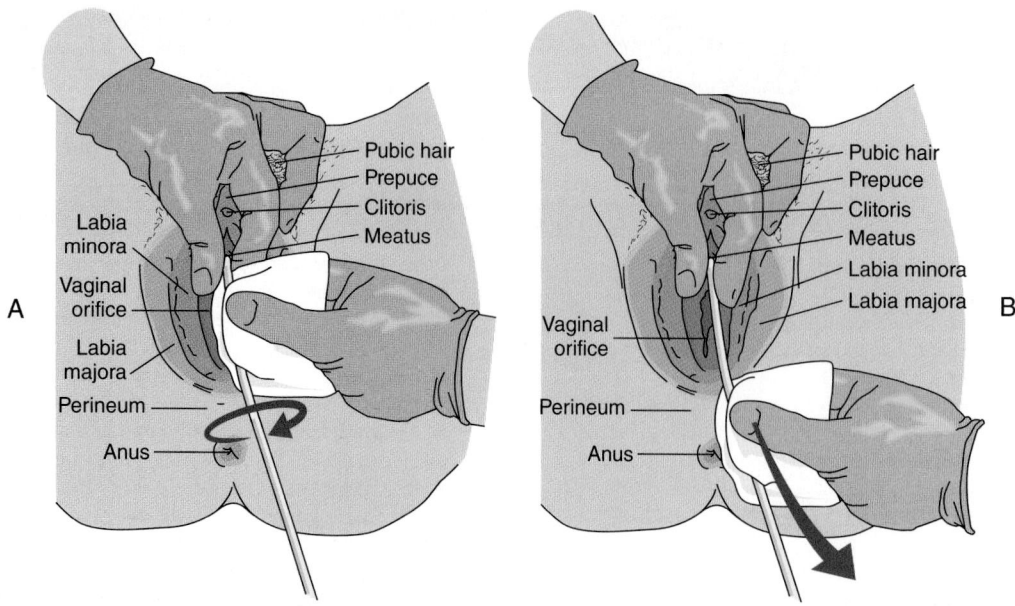

FIGURE 25-7 Cleaning the catheter. **A,** The catheter is cleaned with a circular motion at the meatus. **B,** The catheter is cleaned starting at the meatus. At least 4 inches of the catheter are cleaned.

URINE DRAINAGE SYSTEMS

A closed drainage system is used for indwelling catheters. Only urine should enter the system from the catheter to the urine drainage bag. The urinary system is sterile. Infection can occur if microbes enter the drainage system. The microbes travel up the tubing or catheter into the bladder and kidneys. A UTI can threaten health and life. See Box 25-1 to prevent infection and for proper care of the drainage system.

There are 2 types of urine drainage bags.
- *Standard drainage bags* usually hold at least 2000 mL (milliliters) of urine.
- *Leg bags* attach to the thigh or calf with elastic bands or Velcro (p. 418). Leg bags hold less than 1000 mL of urine. Some people wear leg bags when up.

Sometimes drainage systems become disconnected. If that happens, tell the nurse at once. Do not touch the ends of the catheter or tubing. Box 25-2 lists the steps for reconnecting the catheter and tubing.

Leg bags are changed to standard drainage bags when the person is in bed. The drainage bags stay lower than bladder level. You need to open the closed drainage system. You must prevent microbes from entering the system.

See *Delegation Guidelines: Urine Drainage Systems.*

See *Promoting Safety and Comfort: Urine Drainage Systems.*

See procedure: *Changing a Leg Bag to a Standard Drainage Bag.*

See procedure: *Emptying a Urine Drainage Bag,* p. 415.

Text continued on p. 416.

BOX 25-2	Re-Connecting a Catheter and Drainage Tube

1. Practice hand hygiene. Put on gloves.
2. Wipe the end of the drainage tube with an antiseptic wipe.
3. Wipe the end of the catheter with another antiseptic wipe.
4. Do not put the ends down. Do not touch the ends after you clean them.
5. Connect the drainage tubing to the catheter.
6. Discard the wipes into a biohazard bag.
7. Remove the gloves. Practice hand hygiene.

DELEGATION GUIDELINES

Urine Drainage Systems

Delegated tasks may involve urine drainage systems. If so, you need this information from the nurse and the care plan.
- When to empty the urine drainage bag
- If the person uses a leg bag
- What leg bag straps to use—elastic or Velcro
- When to switch a urine drainage bag and leg bag
- If you should clean or discard the urine drainage bag or leg bag
- What observations to report and record:
  - The amount of urine measured (see Chapter 27)
  - The color, clarity, and odor of urine
  - Particles in the urine
  - Blood in the urine
  - Cloudy urine
  - Complaints of pain, burning, irritation, or the need to urinate
  - Drainage system leaks
- When to report observations
- What patient or resident concerns to report at once

PROMOTING SAFETY AND COMFORT

Urine Drainage Systems

Safety

For the procedure: *Changing a Leg Bag to a Standard Drainage Bag,* you will open sterile packages. You must keep sterile items free from contamination. Review "Surgical Asepsis" in Chapter 16.

Leg bags fill faster than standard drainage bags. Check leg bags often. Empty the leg bag if it is becoming half full. Measure, report, and record the amount of urine.

Comfort

Urine in a drainage bag embarrasses some people. Visitors can see the urine. To promote mental comfort, have visitors sit on the side away from the drainage bag. Sometimes you can empty the bag before visitors arrive. Make sure you measure, report, and record the amount of urine.

Some agencies have drainage bag holders. The drainage bag is placed inside the holder. Urine cannot be seen.

Changing a Leg Bag to a Standard Drainage Bag

QUALITY OF LIFE

- Knock before entering the person's room.
- Address the person by name.
- Introduce yourself by name and title.

- Explain the procedure before starting and during the procedure.
- Protect the person's rights during the procedure.
- Handle the person gently during the procedure.

PRE-PROCEDURE

1 Follow *Delegation Guidelines: Urine Drainage Systems.* See *Promoting Safety and Comfort:*
   - *Urinary Catheters,* p. 407
   - *Urine Drainage Systems*
2 Practice hand hygiene.
3 Collect the following.
   - Gloves
   - Standard drainage bag and tubing
   - Antiseptic wipes
   - Waterproof under-pad
   - Sterile cap and plug

   - Catheter clamp
   - Paper towels
   - Bedpan
   - Bath blanket
4 Arrange paper towels and equipment on the over-bed table.
5 Identify the person. Check the ID bracelet against the assignment sheet. Use 2 identifiers (Chapter 13). Also call the person by name.
6 Provide for privacy.

PROCEDURE

7 Have the person sit on the side of the bed.
8 Practice hand hygiene. Put on the gloves.
9 Expose the catheter and leg bag.
10 Clamp the catheter (Fig. 25-8, p. 414). This prevents urine from draining from the catheter into the drainage tubing.
11 Let urine drain from below the clamp into the drainage tubing. This empties the lower end of the catheter.
12 Help the person lie down.
13 Raise the bed rails if used. Raise the bed for body mechanics.
14 Lower the bed rail near you if up.
15 Cover the person with a bath blanket. Fan-fold top linens to the foot of the bed. Expose the catheter and leg bag.
16 Place the waterproof under-pad under the person's leg.
17 Open the antiseptic wipes. Set them on the paper towels.
18 Open the package with the sterile cap and plug. Set the package on the paper towels. Do not let anything touch the sterile cap or plug (Fig. 25-9, p. 414).
19 Open the package with the standard drainage bag and tubing.
20 Attach the standard drainage bag to the bed frame.
21 Disconnect the catheter from the drainage tubing. Do not let anything touch the ends.

22 Insert the sterile plug into the catheter end (Fig. 25-10, p. 414). Touch only the end of the plug. Do not touch the part that goes inside the catheter. (If you contaminate the end of the catheter, wipe the end with an antiseptic wipe. Do so before inserting the sterile plug.)
23 Place the sterile cap on the end of the leg bag drainage tube (see Fig. 25-10). (If you contaminate the tubing end, wipe the end with an antiseptic wipe. Do so before you put on the sterile cap.)
24 Remove the cap from the new standard drainage bag tubing.
25 Remove the sterile plug from the catheter.
26 Insert the end of the drainage tubing into the catheter.
27 Remove the clamp from the catheter.
28 Position drainage tubing in a straight line or coiled on the bed. Follow the nurse's directions. Secure the tubing to the bottom linens.
29 Remove the leg bag. Place it in the bedpan.
30 Remove and discard the waterproof under-pad.
31 Cover the person. Remove the bath blanket.
32 Take the bedpan to the bathroom.
33 Remove and discard the gloves. Practice hand hygiene.

Continued

Changing a Leg Bag to a Standard Drainage Bag—cont'd

POST-PROCEDURE

34 Provide for comfort. (See the inside of the front cover.)
35 Place the call light and other needed items within reach.
36 Lower the bed to a safe and comfortable level for the person. Follow the care plan.
37 Raise or lower bed rails. Follow the care plan.
38 Unscreen the person.
39 Put on clean gloves. Discard disposable items.
40 Empty the drainage bag. See procedure: *Emptying a Urine Drainage Bag*.
41 Discard the drainage tubing and leg bag following agency policy. Or clean the bag following agency policy.

42 Clean and disinfect the bedpan. Place it in a clean cover.
43 Return the bedpan and other supplies to their proper place.
44 Remove and discard the gloves. Practice hand hygiene.
45 Complete a safety check of the room. (See the inside of the front cover.)
46 Follow agency policy for used linens.
47 Practice hand hygiene.
48 Report and record your observations.

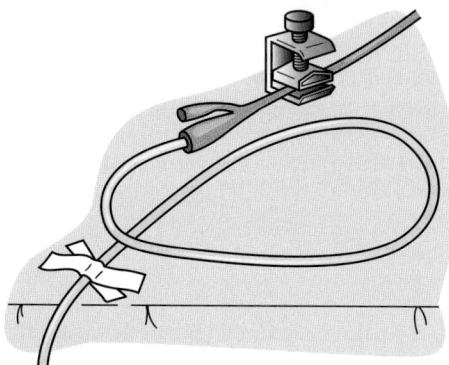

FIGURE 25-8 The clamped catheter prevents urine from draining out of the bladder. The clamp is applied directly to the catheter—not to the drainage tube.

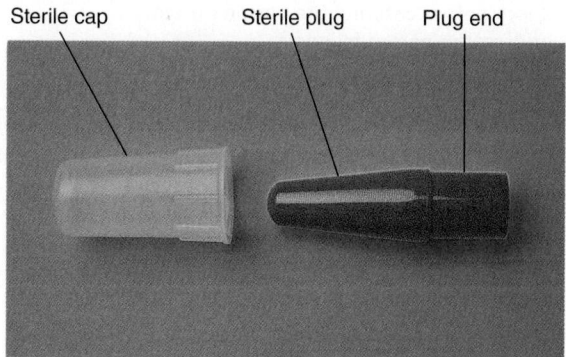

FIGURE 25-9 Sterile cap and catheter plug. The inside of the cap is sterile. Touch only the end of the plug.

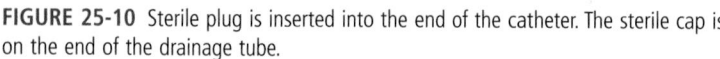
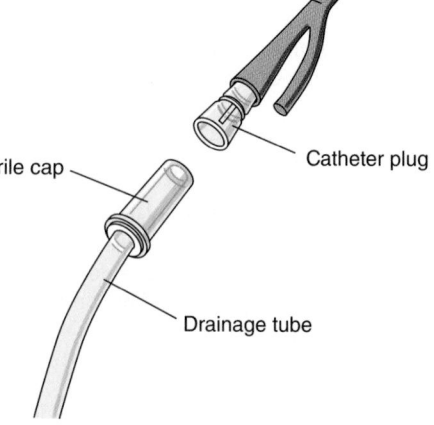

FIGURE 25-10 Sterile plug is inserted into the end of the catheter. The sterile cap is on the end of the drainage tube.

Emptying a Urine Drainage Bag

QUALITY OF LIFE

- Knock before entering the person's room.
- Address the person by name.
- Introduce yourself by name and title.

- Explain the procedure before starting and during the procedure.
- Protect the person's rights during the procedure.
- Handle the person gently during the procedure.

PRE-PROCEDURE

1 Follow *Delegation Guidelines: Urine Drainage Systems,* p. 412. See *Promoting Safety and Comfort:*
   - *Urinary Catheters,* p. 407
   - *Urine Drainage Systems,* p. 413
2 Collect the following.
   - Graduate (measuring container)
   - Gloves

   - Paper towels
   - Antiseptic wipes
3 Practice hand hygiene.
4 Identify the person. Check the ID bracelet against the assignment sheet. Use 2 identifiers (Chapter 13). Also call the person by name.
5 Provide for privacy.

PROCEDURE

6 Put on the gloves.
7 Place a paper towel on the floor. Place the graduate on top of it.
8 Position the graduate under the drainage bag.
9 Open the clamp on the drain.
10 Let all urine drain into the graduate. Do not let the drain touch the graduate (Fig. 25-11).
11 Clean the end of the drain with an antiseptic wipe.
12 Close and position the clamp (Fig. 25-12).
13 Measure urine. See procedure: *Measuring Intake and Output* in Chapter 27.

14 Remove and discard the paper towel.
15 Empty the contents of the graduate into the toilet and flush.
16 Rinse the graduate. Empty the rinse into the toilet and flush.
17 Clean and disinfect the graduate.
18 Return the graduate to its proper place.
19 Remove and discard the gloves. Practice hand hygiene.
20 Record the time and amount of urine on the intake and output (I&O) record (Chapter 27).

POST-PROCEDURE

21 Provide for comfort. (See the inside of the front cover.)
22 Place the call light and other needed items within reach.
23 Unscreen the person.

24 Complete a safety check of the room. (See the inside of the front cover.)
25 Report and record the amount of urine and other observations.

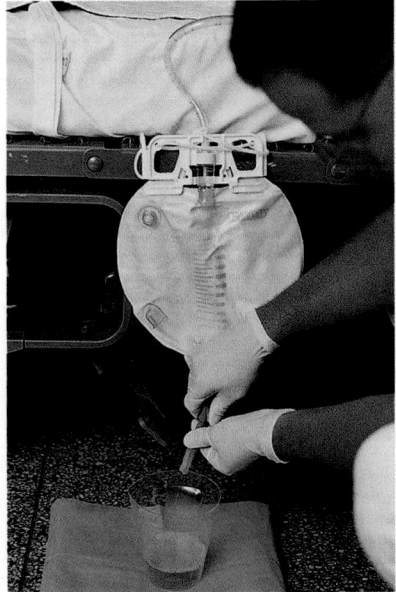

FIGURE 25-11 The clamp on the drainage bag is opened. The drain is directed into the graduate. The drain must not touch the inside of the graduate. (From Potter PA, Perry AG, Stockert PA, Hall, AM: *Fundamentals of nursing,* ed 8, St Louis, 2013, Mosby.)

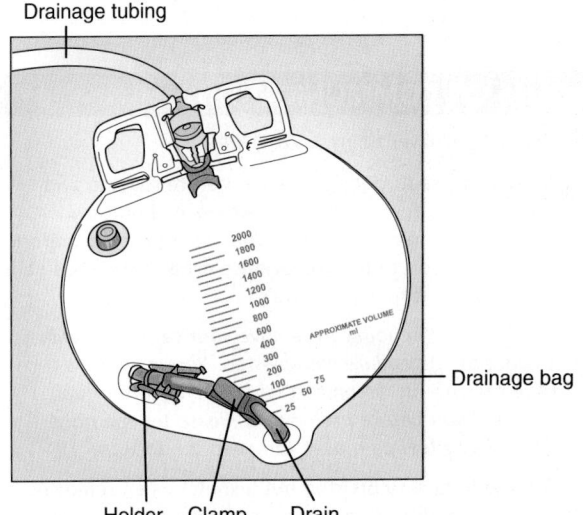

FIGURE 25-12 The clamp is closed and positioned in the holder on the drainage bag.

REMOVING INDWELLING CATHETERS

An indwelling catheter has 2 lumens (passage-ways). Sterile water is injected through 1 lumen to inflate the balloon (Fig. 25-13). The water is injected with a syringe. Urine drains from the bladder through the other lumen.

To remove the catheter, the balloon is deflated—the water is removed. You need a syringe large enough to hold all the water in the balloon. The nurse tells you what size syringe to use.

The doctor orders catheter removal. The person may need bladder training first (Chapter 24). Dysuria and urinary frequency are common after removing catheters (Chapter 24).

See *Focus on Communication: Removing Indwelling Catheters.*
See *Focus on Math: Removing Indwelling Catheters.*
See *Delegation Guidelines: Removing Indwelling Catheters.*
See *Promoting Safety and Comfort: Removing Indwelling Catheters.*
See procedure: *Removing an Indwelling Catheter.*

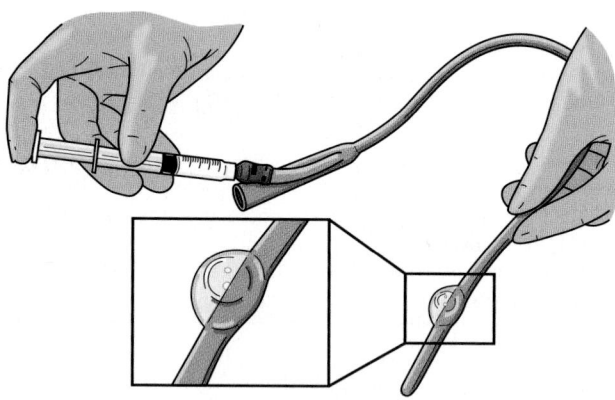

FIGURE 25-13 The balloon of an indwelling catheter is inflated with water. A syringe is used to inject the water. A syringe also is used to remove the water.

FOCUS ON COMMUNICATION

Removing Indwelling Catheters

Explain the procedure to the person before starting and during the procedure. Also, tell the person about any discomfort that may be felt and when to expect discomfort. Instruct the person to tell you at once if he or she feels pain or needs you to stop. For example:

Mrs. Turner, I'm going to remove your catheter. I will explain the procedure step-by-step. You may feel a little pressure or discomfort when I remove the tube. I will tell you before I remove it. Please tell me right away if you feel pain or if you need me to stop.

Ask the person to breathe out (exhale) when removing the catheter to distract the person and promote relaxation. Explain each step in a calm and professional manner to reduce anxiety and provide comfort. Avoid seeming bossy or hurried. Politely tell the person what you will do and what he or she needs to do.

FOCUS ON MATH

Removing Indwelling Catheters

To remove indwelling catheters, you must know how to measure liquid using a syringe. Syringes are marked in milliliters (mL). An mL is a unit used to measure liquid. Read the syringe at the top of the plunger. See Figure 25-14.

The amount of water removed should equal the amount injected. The nurse tells you the amount used for balloon inflation. Subtract the amount removed from the amount injected. If there is a difference, tell the nurse before removing the catheter. For example:

- An indwelling catheter balloon is filled with 10 mL. You remove 7 mL. The difference is 3 mL. Do not remove the catheter. Call for the nurse.

$$10 \text{ mL} - 7 \text{ mL} = 3 \text{ mL}$$

- An indwelling catheter balloon is filled with 10 mL. You remove 10 mL. The difference is 0 mL. You can safely remove the catheter.

$$10 \text{ mL} - 10 \text{ mL} = 0 \text{ mL}$$

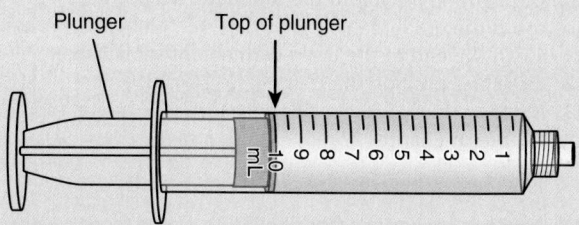

FIGURE 25-14 A syringe is read at the top of the plunger. This syringe measures 10 mL.

DELEGATION GUIDELINES

Removing Indwelling Catheters

Before removing a catheter, make sure that:
- Your state allows you to perform the procedure.
- The procedure is in your job description.
- You know how to use the supplies and equipment.
- You review the procedure with the nurse.
- A nurse is available to answer questions and to supervise you.

If the above conditions are met, you need this information from the nurse.
- When to remove the catheter
- The amount of water used for balloon inflation
- Syringe size needed
- What observations to report and record:
    - Amount of water removed from the balloon
    - The amount of urine in the drainage bag
    - Color, clarity, and odor of urine
    - Particles in the urine
    - Blood in the urine
    - How the person tolerated the procedure
    - Complaints of pain, burning, irritation, or the need to void
    - Any other observations
- When to report observations
- What patient or resident concerns to report at once

PROMOTING SAFETY AND COMFORT

Removing Indwelling Catheters

Safety

Before removing the catheter, you must know the amount of water in the balloon. The nurse tells you the amount. See Figure 25-15. You must remove all water from the balloon. If the balloon is filled with 10 mL, 10 mL must be removed. Otherwise, injury to the urethra is likely as the catheter is removed. Do not remove the catheter if water remains in the balloon. Call for the nurse at once.

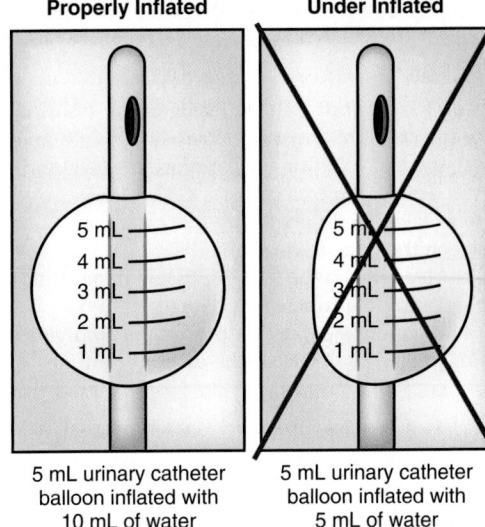

Properly Inflated | **Under Inflated**

5 mL urinary catheter balloon inflated with 10 mL of water

5 mL urinary catheter balloon inflated with 5 mL of water

FIGURE 25-15 The balloon must be inflated properly to avoid drainage and deflation problems. The balloon size marked on the catheter may not equal the amount of water in the balloon. The nurse tells you the amount of water in the balloon.

Removing an Indwelling Catheter

QUALITY OF LIFE

- Knock before entering the person's room.
- Address the person by name.
- Introduce yourself by name and title.
- Explain the procedure before starting and during the procedure.
- Protect the person's rights during the procedure.
- Handle the person gently during the procedure.

PRE-PROCEDURE

1 Follow *Delegation Guidelines: Removing Indwelling Catheters.* See *Promoting Safety and Comfort:*
 • *Urinary Catheters,* p. 407
 • *Removing Indwelling Catheters*
2 Practice hand hygiene.
3 Collect the following.
 • Disposable towel
 • Syringe in the size as directed by the nurse
 • Disposable bag
 • Gloves
 • Bath blanket
4 Identify the person. Check the ID bracelet against the assignment sheet. Use 2 identifiers (Chapter 13). Also call the person by name.
5 Provide for privacy.
6 Raise the bed for body mechanics. Bed rails are up if used.

PROCEDURE

7 Lower the bed rail near you if up.
8 Practice hand hygiene. Put on the gloves.
9 Position and drape the person as for perineal care (Chapter 22).
10 Cover the person with a bath blanket.
11 Check the size of the syringe. Know the amount of water in the balloon. Make sure the syringe is large enough to withdraw all the water from the balloon.
12 Remove the tape or tube holder securing the catheter to the person.
13 Position the towel.
 a Female—between her legs
 b Male—over his thighs
14 Remove all of the water from the balloon. (NOTE: You must know how much water is in the balloon. For example, if the balloon is filled with 10 mL of water, you must remove 10 mL of water.)
 a Slide the syringe plunger up and down several times. This loosens the plunger.
 b Pull the plunger back to the 0.5 (one-half) mL mark.
 c Attach the syringe to the catheter's balloon port gently. Use only enough force to get the syringe to stay in the port.
 d Allow the water to drain into the syringe. Wait at least 30 seconds to allow the full amount to drain. Do not pull back on the plunger. If the water is draining slowly or not at all, call for the nurse. Do not remove the catheter if there is water in the balloon. The nurse may have you
  (1) Gently re-position the syringe in the port.
  (2) Re-position the person.
  (3) Pull back on the syringe gently and slowly. Forceful pulling can collapse the catheter.
15 Pull the catheter straight out once all of the water is removed. Remove the catheter gently.
16 Discard the catheter into the bag.
17 Dry the perineal area with the towel. Discard the disposable towel in the bag.
18 Remove and discard the gloves. Practice hand hygiene.
19 Cover the person. Remove the bath blanket.

Continued

Removing an Indwelling Catheter—cont'd

POST-PROCEDURE

20 Provide for comfort. (See the inside of the front cover.)
21 Place the call light and other needed items within reach.
22 Lower the bed to a safe and comfortable level for the person. Follow the care plan.
23 Raise or lower bed rails. Follow the care plan.
24 Unscreen the person.
25 Put on clean gloves. Discard disposable items. Discard the syringe according to agency policy.
26 Empty the drainage bag. See procedure: *Emptying a Urine Drainage Bag*, p. 415. Note the amount of urine.

27 Discard the drainage tubing and bag following agency policy.
28 Remove and discard the gloves. Practice hand hygiene.
29 Complete a safety check of the room. (See the inside of the front cover.)
30 Practice hand hygiene.
31 Report and record your observations.

Condom Catheters

Condom catheters are often used for incontinent men. They also are called external catheters, Texas catheters, and urinary sheaths. A *condom catheter is a soft sheath that slides over the penis and is used to drain urine.* Tubing connects the condom catheter to the drainage bag. Many men prefer leg bags (Fig. 25-16).

Condom catheters are changed daily after perineal care. To apply a condom catheter, follow the manufacturer's instructions. Thoroughly wash the penis with soap and water. Then dry it before applying the catheter.

Some condom catheters are self-adhering. Adhesive inside the catheter adheres to the penis. Other catheters are secured in place with elastic tape. Use the elastic tape packaged with the catheter. This allows blood flow to the penis. *Only use elastic tape. Never use adhesive tape or other tape to secure catheters. They do not expand. Blood flow to the penis is cut off, injuring the penis.*

See *Delegation Guidelines: Condom Catheters.*
See *Promoting Safety and Comfort: Condom Catheters.*
See procedure: *Applying a Condom Catheter.*

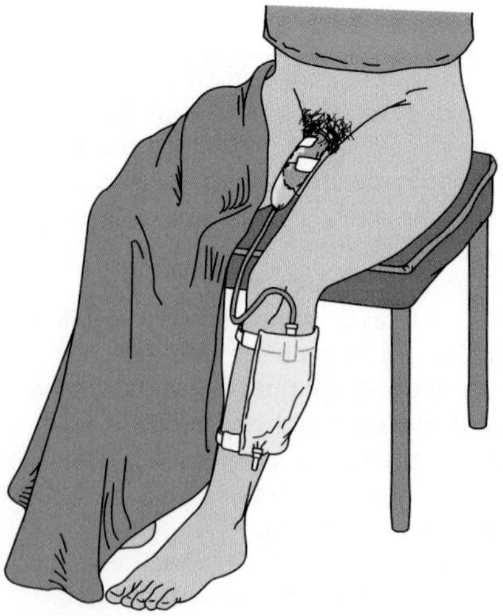

DELEGATION GUIDELINES
Condom Catheters

To remove or apply a condom catheter, you need this information from the nurse and the care plan.
- What size to use—small, medium, or large
- When to remove the catheter and apply a new one
- If a leg bag or standard drainage system is used
- What leg bag straps to use—elastic or Velcro
- What water temperature to use for perineal care
- What observations to report and record:
  - Reddened or open areas on the penis
  - Swelling of the penis
  - Color, clarity, and odor of urine
  - Particles in the urine
  - Blood in the urine
  - Cloudy urine
- When to report observations
- What patient or resident concerns to report at once

PROMOTING SAFETY AND COMFORT
Condom Catheters

Safety
Do not apply a condom catheter if the penis is red, irritated, or shows signs of skin breakdown. Report your observations to the nurse at once.

If you do not know how to use your agency's condom catheters, ask the nurse to show you the correct application. Then ask the nurse to observe you applying the catheter.

Blood must flow to the penis. If tape is needed, use the elastic tape packaged with the catheter. Apply it in a spiral.

Comfort
To apply a condom catheter, you need to touch and handle the penis. This can embarrass the man. Some men become sexually aroused. Always act in a professional manner. If necessary, allow the man privacy. Provide for safety and place the urinal within reach. Tell him when you will return and then leave the room. Or ask him to use the call light when ready for you to finish the procedure. Knock before entering the room again.

FIGURE 25-16 Condom catheter attached to a leg bag.

Applying a Condom Catheter

QUALITY OF LIFE

- Knock before entering the person's room.
- Address the person by name.
- Introduce yourself by name and title.

- Explain the procedure before starting and during the procedure.
- Protect the person's rights during the procedure.
- Handle the person gently during the procedure.

PRE-PROCEDURE

1 Follow *Delegation Guidelines:*
   - *Perineal Care* (Chapter 22)
   - *Condom Catheters*
   See *Promoting Safety and Comfort:*
   - *Perineal Care* (Chapter 22)
   - *Urinary Catheters*, p. 407
   - *Condom Catheters*
2 Practice hand hygiene.
3 Collect the following.
   - Condom catheter
   - Elastic tape
   - Standard drainage bag or leg bag
   - Cap for the drainage bag
   - Basin of warm water (see procedure: *Giving Male Perineal Care* in Chapter 22)

- Soap
- Towel and washcloths
- Bath blanket
- Gloves
- Waterproof under-pad
- Paper towels

4 Cover the over-bed table with paper towels. Arrange items on top of them.
5 Identify the person. Check the ID bracelet against the assignment sheet. Use 2 identifiers (Chapter 13). Also call the person by name.
6 Provide for privacy.
7 Raise the bed for body mechanics. Bed rails are up if used.

PROCEDURE

8 Lower the bed rail near you if up.
9 Practice hand hygiene. Put on the gloves.
10 Cover the person with a bath blanket. Lower top linens to the knees.
11 Ask the person to raise his buttocks off the bed. Or turn him onto his side away from you.
12 Slide the waterproof under-pad under his buttocks.
13 Have the person lower his buttocks. Or turn him onto his back.
14 Secure the standard drainage bag to the bed frame. Or have a leg bag ready. Close the drain.
15 Expose the genital area.
16 Remove the condom catheter.
   a Remove the tape. Roll the sheath off the penis.
   b Disconnect the drainage tubing from the condom. Cap the drainage tube.
   c Discard the tape and condom.
17 Provide perineal care (Chapter 22). Observe the penis for reddened areas, skin breakdown, and irritation.
18 Remove and discard the gloves. Practice hand hygiene. Put on clean gloves.

19 Remove the protective backing from the condom. This exposes the adhesive strip.
20 Hold the penis firmly. Roll the condom onto the penis. Leave a 1-inch space between the penis and the end of the catheter (Fig. 25-17, p. 420).
21 Secure the condom.
   a *For a self-adhering condom:* press the condom to the penis.
   b *For a condom secured with elastic tape:* apply elastic tape in a spiral. See Figure 25-17. Do not apply tape completely around the penis.
22 Make sure the penis tip does not touch the condom. Make sure the condom is not twisted.
23 Connect the condom to the drainage tubing. Coil and secure excess tubing on the bed. Or attach a leg bag.
24 Remove the waterproof under-pad and gloves. Discard them. Practice hand hygiene.
25 Cover the person. Remove the bath blanket.

POST-PROCEDURE

26 Provide for comfort. (See the inside of the front cover.)
27 Place the call light and other needed items within reach.
28 Lower the bed to a safe and comfortable level for the person. Follow the care plan.
29 Raise or lower bed rails. Follow the care plan.
30 Unscreen the person.
31 Practice hand hygiene. Put on clean gloves.
32 Measure and record the amount of urine in the bag. Clean or discard the drainage bag.

33 Clean, rinse, dry, and return the wash basin and other equipment. Return items to their proper place.
34 Remove and discard the gloves. Practice hand hygiene.
35 Complete a safety check of the room. (See the inside of the front cover.)
36 Report and record your observations.

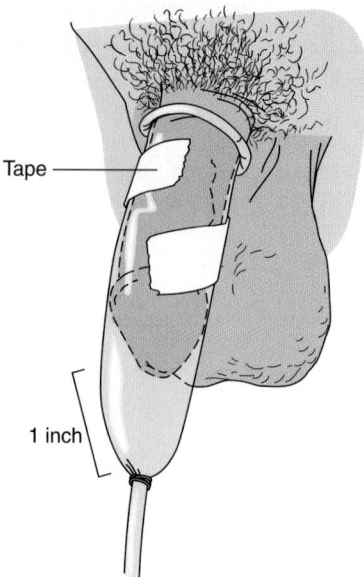

Tape

1 inch

FIGURE 25-17 A condom catheter applied to the penis. A 1-inch space is between the penis and the end of the catheter. Elastic tape is applied in a spiral to secure the condom catheter to the penis.

FOCUS ON **PRIDE**

The Person, Family, and Yourself

P ersonal and Professional Responsibility

With urinary catheters, the risk of UTIs is high. How you give care can decrease the risk of UTI. For example:

- Do you prevent urine from flowing back into the bladder when moving the drainage bag?
- Do you use a clean area of the washcloth for each stroke during catheter care?
- Do you keep the drain from touching the graduate or other surface?
- Do you use a clean, separate graduate to empty each person's drainage bag?

UTIs can be very serious. They can be life-threatening in older persons. You are responsible for giving care in a way that promotes quality of life, health, and safety. Be careful when handling and caring for catheters. Your care makes a difference.

R ights and Respect

Providing privacy promotes comfort. Show respect for the right to privacy. Simple actions make a difference. For example, knock before entering the person's room. Before any procedure, explain how you will provide privacy. This is very important for procedures that involve exposing and touching private areas.

I ndependence and Social Interaction

Urinary catheters are short-term or long-term. Some persons in home settings manage their own catheters. The nurse teaches the person to insert and remove the catheter and to provide catheter care. You:

- Give encouragement. Having a urinary catheter is stressful for the person and family. Be kind, patient, and professional.
- Reinforce the nurse's instructions.
- Tell the nurse if the person has questions or if you think the person needs more teaching.

D elegation and Teamwork

When delegated a task, consider all the person's care needs. For example, you are to turn and re-position Ms. Paul every 2 hours. She has a urinary catheter. Plan how to handle the catheter. The drainage bag needs to be moved to the other side of the bed. You must:

- Keep the catheter and drainage tube free of kinks.
- Keep the drainage bag below bladder level.
- Make sure she is not lying on the drainage tube.
- Avoid resting the bag on the floor.

Tasks become more complex as more care equipment is needed. As you study, think of how care equipment and the person's needs affect delegated tasks.

E thics and Laws

Some states and agencies allow nursing assistants to remove urinary catheters. Others do not. With more training, some allow nursing assistants to insert catheters. Follow state and agency rules to protect the person from harm. *Never* perform a task outside your role limits.

FOCUS ON **PRIDE**: *Application*

How might needing a urinary catheter affect the person mentally? How can you promote mental comfort?

REVIEW QUESTIONS

Circle the BEST answer.

1 Urinary catheters are used
   a To prevent urinary tract infections
   b To treat the cause of incontinence
   c To keep the bladder empty for surgery
   d For staff convenience with incontinent persons

2 A person has a catheter. Which is safe?
   a Keeping the drainage bag above the level of the bladder
   b Taping a leak at the connection site
   c Attaching the drainage bag to the bed rail
   d Removing a kink from the drainage tubing

3 A person has a catheter. Which is correct?
   a Report pain, burning, the need to void, or irritation at once.
   b Allow the tubing to hang below the drainage bag.
   c Empty the drainage bag once daily.
   d Use the same measuring container for all persons.

4 A person has a catheter. You are going to the turn the person from the left to the right side. What should you do with the drainage bag?
   a Move it to the right side.
   b Keep it on the left side.
   c Hang it from an IV pole.
   d Remove the catheter and the drainage bag.

5 To secure a catheter on a female
   a Tape the catheter to her lower abdomen
   b Use a safety pin to secure it to her gown
   c Secure it to her thigh with tape or a tube holder
   d Secure the catheter to the bottom linens with a bed sheet clamp

6 When giving catheter care
   a Clean from the drainage tube connection up the catheter at least 4 inches
   b Clean from the meatus down the catheter at least 4 inches
   c Pull on the catheter to make sure it is secure
   d Clamp the catheter to prevent leaking

7 Which statement about drainage systems is *true?*
   a A leg bag holds about 2000 mL.
   b A standard drainage bag holds less than a leg bag.
   c A closed drainage system means the drain cannot be opened.
   d Microbes in the drainage system can cause a UTI.

8 A drainage system becomes accidentally disconnected? You need
   a A new drainage bag and paper towels
   b A sterile cap and catheter plug
   c Gloves and an antiseptic wipe
   d A waterproof under-pad and a catheter clamp

9 When emptying a standard drainage bag
   a Do not let the drain touch the graduate
   b Gloves are not needed
   c Clamp the catheter
   d Clean the end of the catheter with an antiseptic wipe

10 You are going to remove a urinary catheter. You
   a Attach a needle to the syringe
   b Ask the nurse how much water is in the balloon
   c Tug on the catheter to see if it will come out
   d Use an antiseptic swab to clean the meatus

11 You are going to remove an indwelling catheter. The balloon is filled with 10 mL. You withdraw 6 mL. What should you do?
   a Call for the nurse.
   b Inject the water.
   c Pull the catheter out gently.
   d Cut the catheter.

12 For a condom catheter, you apply elastic tape
   a Completely around the penis
   b To the thigh
   c To the abdomen
   d In a spiral

Answers to Chapter 25 questions are on p. 871.

FOCUS ON PRACTICE

Problem Solving

Mrs. Riley has a urinary catheter. She tells you: "I feel like I have to pee, and I feel pressure down there." She points to her lower abdomen. There is no urine in her drainage bag. Is this normal? What do you do?

Bowel Elimination

- Define the key terms and key abbreviations in this chapter.
- Describe normal defecation and the observations to report.
- Identify the factors affecting bowel elimination.
- Explain how to promote comfort and safety during defecation.
- Describe the common bowel elimination problems.
- Describe bowel training.
- Explain why enemas are given.
- Describe the common enema solutions.
- Describe the rules for giving enemas.
- Describe how to care for a person with an ostomy.
- Perform the procedures described in this chapter.
- Explain how to promote PRIDE in the person, the family, and yourself.

KEY TERMS

colostomy A surgically created opening *(stomy)* between the colon *(colo)* and the body's surface

constipation The passage of a hard, dry stool

defecation The process of excreting feces from the rectum through the anus; a bowel movement

dehydration The excessive loss of water from tissues

diarrhea The frequent passage of liquid stools

enema The introduction of fluid into the rectum and lower colon

fecal impaction The prolonged retention and buildup of feces in the rectum

fecal incontinence The inability to control the passage of feces and gas through the anus

feces The semi-solid mass of waste products in the colon that is expelled through the anus; also called a *stool* or *stools*

flatulence The excessive formation of gas or air in the stomach and intestines

flatus Gas or air passed through the anus

ileostomy A surgically created opening *(stomy)* between the ileum (small intestine *[ileo]*) and the body's surface

ostomy A surgically created opening that connects an internal organ to the body's surface; see "colostomy" and "ileostomy"

peristalsis The alternating contraction and relaxation of intestinal muscles

stoma A surgically created opening seen on the body's surface; see "colostomy" and "ileostomy"

stool Excreted feces

suppository A cone-shaped, solid drug that is inserted into a body opening; it melts at body temperature

KEY ABBREVIATIONS

BM	Bowel movement	**IV**	Intravenous
CMS	Centers for Medicare & Medicaid Services	**mL**	Milliliter
GI	Gastro-intestinal	**oz**	Ounce
ID	Identification	**SSE**	Soapsuds enema

Bowel elimination is a basic physical need. Wastes are excreted from the gastro-intestinal (GI) system (Chapter 10). Many factors affect bowel elimination—privacy, habits, age, diet, exercise and activity, fluids, drugs,

disability. Problems easily occur. Normal bowel elimination is important. You assist patients and residents to meet elimination needs.

See *Body Structure and Function Review: The Gastro-Intestinal Tract.*

See *Delegation Guidelines: Bowel Elimination.*

See *Promoting Safety and Comfort: Bowel Elimination.*

BODY STRUCTURE AND FUNCTION REVIEW

The Gastro-Intestinal Tract

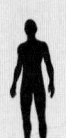

The GI tract is part of the digestive system (Chapter 10). Bowel elimination is the excretion of wastes through the GI tract. Food and fluids are normally taken in through the *mouth*. They are partially digested in the *stomach*. The partially digested food and fluids are called *chyme*.

Chyme passes from the stomach into the *small intestine* (*small bowel*). Further digestion and absorption of nutrients occur as the chyme passes through the small bowel. The chyme enters the *large intestine* (*large bowel* or *colon*) where fluid is absorbed. Chyme becomes less fluid and more solid in consistency. *Feces* (stool or stools) *refers to the semi-solid mass of waste products in the colon that is expelled through the anus.*

Feces move through the intestines by peristalsis. *Peristalsis is the alternating contraction and relaxation of intestinal muscles.* The feces move through the large intestine to the *rectum*. Feces are stored in the rectum and excreted from the body (Fig. 26-1). *Defecation* (bowel movement) *is the process of excreting feces from the rectum through the anus. Stool refers to excreted feces.*

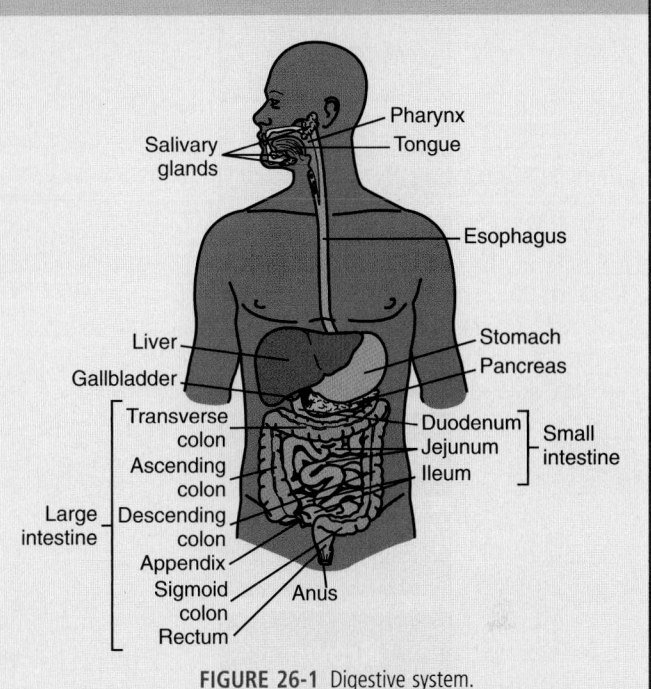

FIGURE 26-1 Digestive system.

DELEGATION GUIDELINES

Bowel Elimination

Your state and agency may not allow you to perform the procedures in this chapter. Before performing a procedure, make sure that:
- Your state allows you to perform the procedure.
- The procedure is in your job description.
- You have the necessary education and training.
- You review the procedure with a nurse.
- A nurse is available to answer questions and to supervise you.

PROMOTING SAFETY AND COMFORT

Bowel Elimination

Safety
Assisting with bowel elimination may involve exposing and touching the rectum, a private area. And you may have to give perineal care. Sexual abuse has occurred in health care settings. The person may feel threatened or may actually be abused. He or she needs to call for help. Always keep the call light within the person's reach. And always act in a professional manner.

Contact with feces is likely when assisting with bowel elimination. Feces contain microbes and may contain blood. Follow Standard Precautions and the Bloodborne Pathogen Standard (Chapter 16).

NORMAL BOWEL ELIMINATION

Some people have a bowel movement (BM) every day. Others do so every 2 to 3 days. Some people have 2 or 3 BMs a day. Many people have a BM after breakfast. Others do so in the evening.

Stools are normally brown. Bleeding in the stomach and small intestine causes black or tarry stools. Bleeding in the lower colon and rectum causes red-colored stools. So do beets, tomato juice or soup, red Jell-O, and foods with red food coloring. Green vegetables can cause green stools. Diseases and infection can cause clay-colored or white, pale, orange-colored, or green-colored stools and stools with mucus. Figure 26-2, p. 424 shows a color chart for stools.

Stools are normally soft, formed, moist, and shaped like the rectum. They have a normal odor caused by bacteria in the intestines. Certain foods and drugs also cause odors.

See *Focus on Children and Older Persons: Normal Bowel Elimination*, p. 424.

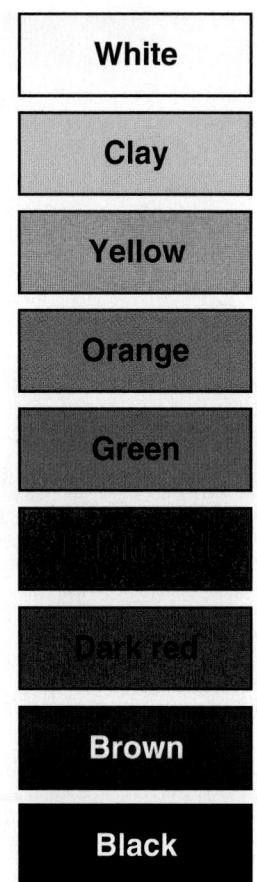

FIGURE 26-2 Color chart for stools.

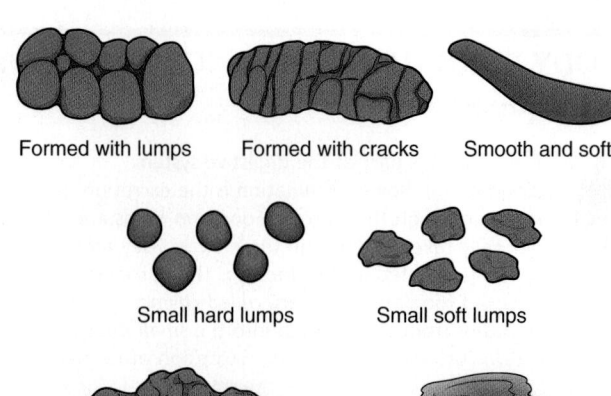

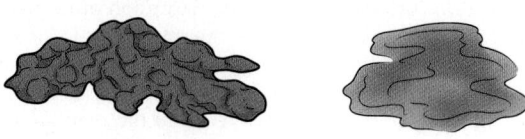

FIGURE 26-3 Stool shapes and consistencies.

FOCUS ON **CHILDREN AND OLDER PERSONS**

Normal Bowel Elimination

Children
Breast-fed infants have yellow stools that are thick liquid to very soft. Bottle-fed infants have yellowish-brown liquid stools or greenish-brown, pasty stools. Stool color and consistency change with solid foods.

Newborns usually have a BM with every feeding. Frequency changes as they grow older. Some infants have 2 or 3 BMs a day. Others have just 1.

Observations

Your observations are used for the nursing process. Ask the nurse to observe abnormal stools. Report and record the following.

- Color (see Fig. 26-2)
- Amount
- Presence of mucus
- Signs of bleeding
- Odor
- Shape and consistency (Fig. 26-3)
- The time the person had a BM
- Frequency of BMs
- Complaints of pain or discomfort
  See *Focus on Communication: Observations.*

FOCUS ON **COMMUNICATION**

Observations

Many patients and residents tend to their own bowel elimination needs. However, information is needed for the person's record and the nursing process. You may need to ask about BMs. You can say:

- "Did you have a BM today?"
- "Please tell me about your BM."
- "When did you have a BM?"
- "What was the amount?"
- "Were the stools soft or hard?"
- "Were the stools formed or loose?"
- "What was the color?"
- "Did you have any bleeding, pain, or problems having a BM?"
- "Did you pass any gas?"
- "Do you need to pass more gas?"
- "Do you need help cleaning yourself?"

For some people and children, *poop* is the common term for a BM. Follow the care plan for what word to use with the person.

Report and record what the person said or what you observed. Some agencies have forms for recording BMs (Fig. 26-4). Or you may need to record in the person's chart. For example:

Mr. Jansen stated that he had a medium-sized, soft, formed, brown BM after breakfast today. He denied bleeding, pain, straining, or other problems. Mr. Jansen performed his own perineal care.

Follow agency policy for reporting and recording BMs.

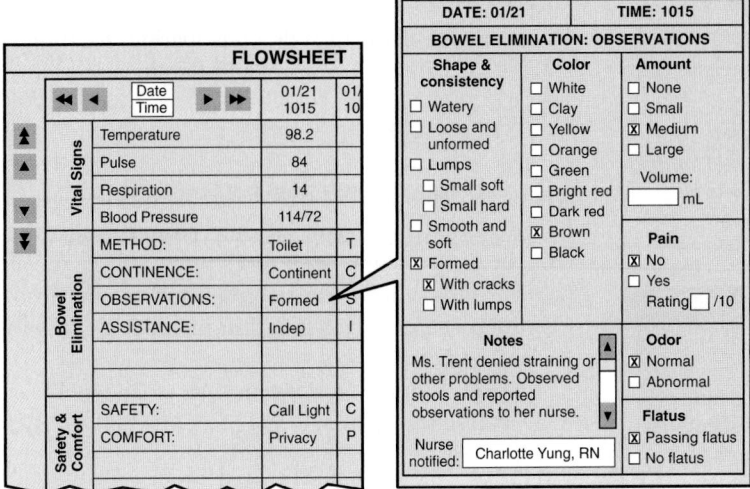

FIGURE 26-4 Bowel elimination record.

FACTORS AFFECTING BMs

These factors affect BM frequency, consistency, color, and odor. They are part of the nursing process to meet the person's elimination needs. Normal, regular elimination is the goal.

- *Privacy.* Lack of privacy can prevent a BM despite the urge. Odors and sounds are embarrassing. Some people ignore the urge when people are present.
- *Habits.* Many people have a BM after breakfast. Some drink a hot beverage, read, or take a walk. These activities are relaxing. A BM is easier when a person is relaxed, not tense.
- *Diet—high-fiber foods.* High-fiber foods leave a residue for needed bulk to prevent constipation (p. 426). Fruits, vegetables, and whole-grain cereals and breads are high in fiber. Many people do not eat enough fruits and vegetables. Some cannot chew these foods. They may not have teeth. Or dentures fit poorly. Some people think that they cannot digest fruits and vegetables. So they refuse to eat them. Sometimes bran is added to cereal, prunes, or prune juice.
- *Diet—other foods.* Milk and milk products can cause constipation in some people and diarrhea in others. Chocolate and other foods cause similar reactions. Spicy foods can irritate the intestines, causing frequent stools or diarrhea. Gas-forming foods stimulate peristalsis, aiding BMs. Such foods include onions, beans, cabbage, cauliflower, radishes, and cucumbers.
- *Fluids.* Feces contain water. Stool consistency depends on the amount of water absorbed in the colon. Fluid intake, urine output, and vomiting are factors. Feces harden and dry when large amounts of water are absorbed or from poor fluid intake. Hard, dry feces move slowly through the colon. Constipation can occur. Drinking 6 to 8 glasses of water daily promotes normal BMs. Warm fluids—coffee, tea, hot cider, warm water—increase peristalsis.

- *Activity.* Exercise and activity maintain muscle tone and stimulate peristalsis. Constipation is a risk from inactivity and bedrest. Inactivity may result from disease, surgery, injury, and aging.
- *Drugs.* Drugs can prevent constipation or control diarrhea. Other drugs have diarrhea or constipation as side effects. Pain-relief drugs often cause constipation. Antibiotics (used to fight or prevent infections) often cause diarrhea. Diarrhea occurs when the antibiotics kill normal flora in the colon. Normal flora is needed to form feces. (See "Normal Flora" in Chapter 16.)
- *Disability.* Some people cannot control BMs. They have a BM whenever feces enter the rectum. A bowel training program is needed (p. 430).
- *Aging.* Age affects bowel elimination.
See *Focus on Children and Older Persons: Factors Affecting BMs.*

FOCUS ON CHILDREN AND OLDER PERSONS

Factors Affecting BMs

Children
Infants and toddlers cannot control BMs. They have a BM whenever feces enter the rectum. Bowel training is learned between 2 and 3 years of age.

Older Persons
Aging causes GI changes. Feces pass through the intestines at a slower rate. Constipation is a risk. Some older persons lose bowel control. Older persons are at risk for GI tumors and disorders.

Older persons may not completely empty the rectum. They often have a BM about 30 to 45 minutes after the first BM.

Many older persons are very concerned if they do not have a BM every day. The nurse teaches them about normal elimination.

Safety and Comfort

The care plan has measures for meeting elimination needs. It may involve diet, fluids, and exercise. The measures in Box 26-1 promote safety and comfort.

See *Focus on Communication: Safety and Comfort.*

See *Teamwork and Time Management: Safety and Comfort.*

FOCUS ON COMMUNICATION

Safety and Comfort

Odors and sounds are common with BMs. You must control your verbal and nonverbal responses. Always be professional. Do not laugh at or make fun of a person. Your words and actions must promote comfort, dignity, and self-esteem.

TEAMWORK AND TIME MANAGEMENT

Safety and Comfort

BM needs may be urgent. Answer call lights promptly. Also help co-workers answer call lights. Listen closely for bathroom call lights. The sound and color are different from call lights in rooms. Respond at once. Do not leave patients and residents sitting on toilets, commodes, or bedpans. Do not leave them sitting or lying in stools.

COMMON PROBLEMS

Common problems include constipation, fecal impaction, diarrhea, fecal incontinence, and flatulence.

Constipation

Constipation is the passage of a hard, dry stool. The person strains to have a BM. Stools are large or marble-sized. Large stools cause pain as they pass through the anus. Constipation occurs when feces move slowly through the bowel. This allows more time for water absorption. Common causes of constipation include:

- A low-fiber diet
- Ignoring the urge to have a BM
- Decreased fluid intake
- Inactivity
- Drugs
- Aging
- Certain diseases

Diet changes, fluids, and activity prevent or relieve constipation. The doctor may order 1 or more of the following.

- Stool softeners. These drugs soften feces. A BM is easier when feces are soft.
- Laxatives. *Laxative* comes from the Latin word that means *to loosen.* A *laxative* is a drug that promotes bowel elimination. It increases the bulk of feces, softens feces, and lubricates the intestinal wall.
- Suppositories (p. 430).
- Enemas (p. 431).

BOX 26-1	Safety and Comfort During Bowel Elimination

- Follow Standard Precautions and the Bloodborne Pathogen Standard.
- Provide for privacy.
  - Ask visitors to leave the room.
  - Close doors, privacy curtains, and window coverings.
- Help the person to the toilet or commode. Or provide the bedpan upon request.
- Wheel the person into the bathroom on the commode if possible. This provides privacy. Remove the container and position the commode over the toilet. Remember to lock the commode wheels.
- Warm the bedpan.
- Position the person in a normal sitting or squatting position.

- Cover the person for warmth and privacy.
- Allow enough time for a BM.
- Place the call light and toilet tissue within reach.
- Leave the room if the person can be alone. Check on the person every 5 minutes.
- Stay nearby if the person is weak or unsteady.
- Provide perineal care.
- Dispose of stools promptly. This reduces odors and prevents the spread of microbes.
- Assist the person with hand-washing after elimination.
- Follow the care plan if the person has fecal incontinence. The care plan tells you when to assist with elimination.

Fecal Impaction

A *fecal impaction is the prolonged retention and buildup of feces in the rectum.* Feces are hard or putty-like. Fecal impaction results if constipation is not relieved. The person cannot have a BM. More water is absorbed from the already hard feces. Liquid feces pass around the hardened fecal mass in the rectum and seep from the anus.

The person tries many times to have a BM. Abdominal discomfort, abdominal distention (swelling), nausea, cramping, and rectal pain are common. Older persons may have poor appetite or confusion. Some persons have a fever. Report such signs and symptoms to the nurse.

The nurse does a digital (finger) exam to check for an impaction. A lubricated, gloved finger is inserted into the rectum to feel for a hard mass in the lower rectum (Fig. 26-5). Sometimes it is out of reach higher in the colon. The digital exam often causes the urge to have a BM. The doctor may order drugs, suppositories, or enemas to remove the impaction.

Sometimes *digital removal of an impaction* is done. A lubricated, gloved finger is hooked around a piece of feces. Then the finger and feces are removed. The stool is dropped into the bedpan. The process is repeated as needed. The procedure can be uncomfortable and embarrassing.

Checking for and removing impactions are very dangerous. The vagus nerve can be stimulated. Stimulation of the vagus nerve slows the heart rate. The heart rate can slow to unsafe levels in some persons.

See *Focus on Long-Term Care and Home Care: Fecal Impaction.*

See *Delegation Guidelines: Fecal Impaction.*

See *Promoting Safety and Comfort: Fecal Impaction.*

See procedure: *Checking For and Removing a Fecal Impaction*, p. 428.

FOCUS ON LONG-TERM CARE AND HOME CARE

Fecal Impaction

Long-Term Care
The Centers for Medicare & Medicaid Services (CMS) monitors for problem areas in nursing centers. These are known as "quality measures" or "quality indicators."

Fecal impaction is a quality indicator. A serious problem, fecal impaction must be prevented. Tell the nurse if the resident is concerned about constipation. Follow center policy for recording BMs.

DELEGATION GUIDELINES

Fecal Impaction

If checking for or removing fecal impactions is delegated to you, make sure the conditions in *Delegation Guidelines: Bowel Elimination* (p. 423) are met. If those conditions are met, you need this information from the nurse.
- What the doctor's order says
- If you should remove the impaction if you feel one
- When to take the person's pulse
- What pulse rates to report at once
- If the nurse needs to observe removed feces or the BM
- What observations to report and record:
  - Color, amount, consistency, and odor of feces
  - Signs of bleeding
  - Complaints of pain or discomfort
  - How the person tolerated the procedure
- When to report observations
- What patient or resident concerns to report at once

PROMOTING SAFETY AND COMFORT

Fecal Impaction

Safety
You must be very careful and gentle. Rectal bleeding can occur.

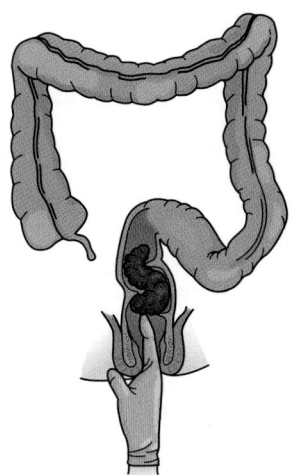

FIGURE 26-5 A gloved index finger is used to check for and remove a fecal impaction.

Checking For and Removing a Fecal Impaction

QUALITY OF LIFE

- Knock before entering the person's room.
- Address the person by name.
- Introduce yourself by name and title.

- Explain the procedure before starting and during the procedure.
- Protect the person's rights during the procedure.
- Handle the person gently during the procedure.

PRE-PROCEDURE

1 Follow *Delegation Guidelines:*
   a *Bowel Elimination,* p. 423
   b *Fecal Impaction,* p. 427
   See *Promoting Safety and Comfort:*
   a *Bowel Elimination,* p. 423
   b *Fecal Impaction,* p. 427
2 Practice hand hygiene.
3 Collect the following.
   - Bedpan and cover
   - Bath blanket
   - Toilet tissue
   - Gloves

   - Lubricant
   - Waterproof under-pad
   - Basin of warm water
   - Soap
   - Washcloth
   - Bath towel
4 Practice hand hygiene.
5 Identify the person. Check the ID (identification) bracelet against the assignment sheet. Use 2 identifiers (Chapter 13). Also call the person by name.
6 Provide for privacy.
7 Raise the bed for body mechanics. Bed rails are up if used.

PROCEDURE

8 Lower the bed rail near you if up.
9 Cover the person with a bath blanket. Fan-fold top linens to the foot of the bed.
10 Position the person in Sims' position or in a left side-lying position (Chapter 17).
11 Check the person's pulse (Chapter 29). Note the rate and rhythm.
12 Practice hand hygiene. Put on the gloves.
13 Place the waterproof under-pad under the buttocks.
14 Expose the anal area.
15 Lubricate your gloved index finger.
16 Ask the person to take a deep breath through his or her mouth.
17 Insert the gloved finger while the person is taking a deep breath.
18 Check for a fecal mass. Remove your finger and go to step 20 if:
   a You do not feel a fecal mass.
   b You feel a fecal mass but will not remove the impaction.
19 Remove the impaction.
   a Hook your index finger around a small piece of feces.
   b Remove your finger and the feces.
   c Drop the stool into the bedpan.
   d Clean your finger with toilet tissue. Place the toilet tissue in the bedpan.
   e Repeat steps 19, a-d until you no longer feel feces.
   f *Check the person's pulse at intervals. Use your clean gloved hand. Note the rate and rhythm. Stop the procedure if the pulse rate has slowed or if the rhythm is irregular.*

20 Wipe the anal area with toilet tissue.
21 Remove and discard the gloves. Practice hand hygiene. Put on clean gloves.
22 Help the person onto the bedpan. Raise the head of the bed and raise the bed rail if used. Or assist the person to the bathroom or commode. The person wears a robe and non-skid footwear when up. The bed is in a low position safe and comfortable for the person.
23 Place the call light and toilet tissue within reach. Remind the person not to flush the toilet.
24 Discard disposable items.
25 Remove and discard the gloves. Practice hand hygiene.
26 Leave the room if the person can be left alone.
27 Return when the person signals. Or check on the person every 5 minutes. Knock before entering.
28 Practice hand hygiene and put on gloves. Lower the bed rail if up.
29 Observe stools for amount, color, consistency, shape, and odor.
30 Provide perineal care as needed.
31 Remove the waterproof under-pad.
32 Empty, rinse, clean, and disinfect equipment. If the person had a BM, flush the toilet after the nurse observes it.
33 Return equipment to its proper place.
34 Remove and discard the gloves. Practice hand hygiene after removing and discarding the gloves.
35 Assist with hand-washing. Wear gloves for this step. Practice hand hygiene after removing and discarding the gloves.
36 Cover the person. Remove the bath blanket.

POST-PROCEDURE

37 Provide for comfort. (See the inside of the front cover.)
38 Place the call light and other needed items within reach.
39 Lower the bed to a safe and comfortable level for the person. Follow the care plan.
40 Raise or lower bed rails. Follow the care plan.
41 Unscreen the person.

42 Complete a safety check of the room. (See the inside of the front cover.)
43 Follow agency policy for used linens and used supplies.
44 Practice hand hygiene.
45 Report and record your observations.

Diarrhea

Diarrhea is the frequent passage of liquid stools. Feces move through the intestines rapidly. This reduces the time for fluid absorption. The need for a BM is urgent. Some people cannot get to a bathroom in time. Abdominal cramping, nausea, and vomiting may occur.

Causes of diarrhea include infections, some drugs, irritating foods, and microbes in food and water. Diet and drugs are ordered to reduce peristalsis. You need to:

- Assist with elimination needs promptly.
- Dispose of stools promptly. This prevents odors and the spread of microbes.
- Give good skin care. Liquid stools irritate the skin. So does frequent wiping with toilet tissue. Skin breakdown and pressure ulcers are risks.

Fluid lost through diarrhea must be replaced to prevent dehydration. *Dehydration is the excessive loss of water from tissues.* The person has pale or flushed skin, dry skin, and a coated tongue. Urine is dark and scant in amount *(oliguria)*. Thirst, weakness, dizziness, and confusion also occur. Falling blood pressure and increased pulse and respirations are serious signs. Death can occur. The nursing process is used to meet fluid needs. The doctor may order IV (intravenous) fluids in severe cases (Chapter 28).

Microbes can cause diarrhea. Preventing the spread of infection is important. Always follow Standard Precautions and the Bloodborne Pathogen Standard when in contact with stools.

See *Focus on Children and Older Persons: Diarrhea.*
See *Promoting Safety and Comfort: Diarrhea.*

Fecal Incontinence

Fecal incontinence is the inability to control the passage of feces and gas through the anus. Causes include:

- Intestinal diseases.
- Nervous system diseases and injuries.
- Fecal impaction or diarrhea.
- Some drugs.
- Chronic illness.
- Aging.
- Mental health problems or dementia (Chapters 48 and 49). The person may not recognize the need for or the act of having a BM.
- Unanswered call lights.
- Not getting to the bathroom in time. The person may have mobility problems or may walk slowly. The bathroom may be too far away or occupied by another person.
- Problems removing clothes.
- Not finding the bathroom in a new setting.

FOCUS ON CHILDREN AND OLDER PERSONS

Diarrhea

Children
Infants and children have large amounts of body water. Dehydration is a risk. Death can be rapid. Report any liquid or watery stool at once. Ask the nurse to observe the stool. Note the number of wet diapers. Infants wet less when dehydrated.

Older Persons
Older persons are at risk for dehydration. The amount of body water decreases with aging. Many diseases common in older persons affect body fluids. So do many drugs. Report signs of diarrhea at once. Ask the nurse to observe the stool. Death is a risk when dehydration is not recognized and treated.

PROMOTING SAFETY AND COMFORT

Diarrhea

Safety
Clostridium difficile (C. difficile) is a microbe that causes diarrhea and intestinal infections. Commonly called *C. diff,* it can cause death. Persons at risk are older, are ill, or need prolonged use of antibiotics. Older persons in hospitals and nursing centers are at high risk. Signs and symptoms include:

- Watery diarrhea
- Fever
- Loss of appetite
- Nausea
- Abdominal pain or tenderness

The microbe is found in feces. A person becomes infected by touching items or surfaces contaminated with feces and when touching his or her mouth or mucous membranes. *C. diff* can be found on bed linens, bed rails, toilets, bathroom fixtures, sinks, care supplies and equipment, walker handles, cart handles, bedside and over-bed tables, phones, TV remotes, and so on. You can spread the microbe if your contaminated hands or gloves:

- Touch a person.
- Contaminate surfaces.

Contact precautions are required (Chapter 16). You must practice good hand hygiene. Alcohol-based hand rubs are not as effective against *C. difficile* as soap and water. When caring for persons with *C. difficile,* wash your hands with soap and water. Care items and surfaces are disinfected with a bleach solution. Also follow Standard Precautions.

Fecal incontinence affects the person emotionally. Frustration, embarrassment, anger, and humiliation are common. The person may need:

- Bowel training
- Help with elimination after meals and every 2 to 3 hours
- Incontinence products to keep garments and linens clean
- Good skin care

See *Focus on Children and Older Persons: Fecal Incontinence.*

Flatulence

Gas and air are normally in the stomach and intestines. They are expelled through the mouth (burping, belching, eructating) and anus. *Gas or air passed through the anus is called **flatus**. **Flatulence** is the excessive formation of gas or air in the stomach and intestines.* Causes include:

- Swallowing air while eating and drinking. This includes chewing gum, eating fast, drinking through a straw, and drinking carbonated beverages. Tense or anxious people may swallow large amounts of air when drinking.
- Bacterial action in the intestines.
- Gas-forming foods—onions, beans, cabbage, cauliflower, radishes, and cucumbers.
- Constipation.
- Bowel and abdominal surgeries.
- Drugs that decrease peristalsis.

If flatus is not expelled, the intestines swell or enlarge (distend) from the pressure of gases. Abdominal cramping or pain, shortness of breath, and a swollen abdomen occur. *Bloating* is a common complaint. Exercise, walking, moving in bed, and the left side-lying position often expel flatus. Doctors may order enemas and drugs to relieve flatulence.

BOWEL TRAINING

Bowel training has 2 goals.

- To gain control of BMs.
- To develop a regular pattern of elimination. Fecal impaction, constipation, and fecal incontinence are prevented.

Meals, especially breakfast, stimulate the urge for a BM. The person's usual time for a BM is noted on the care plan. So is toilet, commode, or bedpan use. Offer help with elimination at the times noted. The care plan includes a high-fiber diet, increased fluids, warm fluids, activity, and privacy. The nurse tells you about a person's bowel training program.

SUPPOSITORIES

A **suppository** *is a cone-shaped, solid drug that is inserted into a body opening. It melts at body temperature.* A rectal suppository is inserted into the rectum (Fig. 26-6). A BM occurs about 30 minutes later.

The doctor may order a suppository for:

- Constipation
- Fecal impaction
- Bowel training

See *Delegation Guidelines: Suppositories.*

See *Promoting Safety and Comfort: Bowel Elimination,* p. 423.

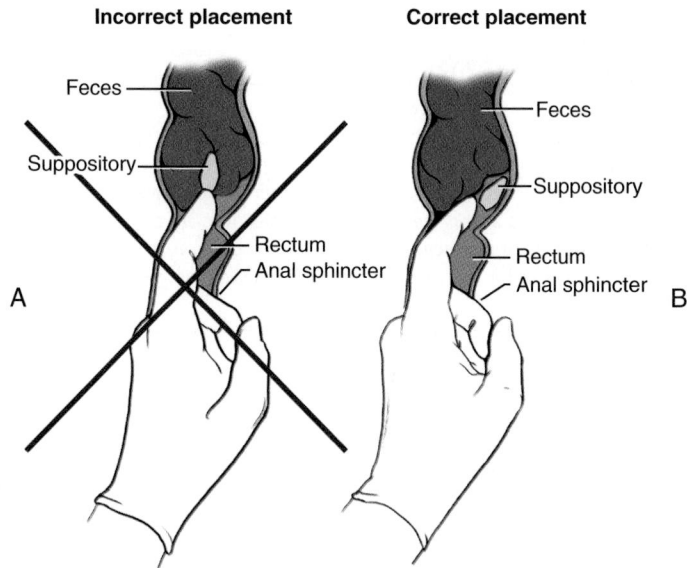

FIGURE 26-6 A, The rectal suppository is *not* inserted into feces. **B,** The suppository is inserted along the rectal wall. (Modified from deWit SC: *Fundamental concepts and skills for nursing,* ed 3, Philadelphia, 2009, Saunders.)

DELEGATION GUIDELINES

Suppositories

Because they are drugs, nurses insert suppositories. However, some states and agencies allow nursing assistants to insert suppositories. Before inserting a suppository, make sure that the conditions in *Delegation Guidelines: Bowel Elimination* (p. 423) are met. If those conditions are met, you need this information from the nurse.

- How to position the person to insert the suppository—Sims' or left side-lying position
- How to position the person after inserting the suppository and for how long—usually the Sims' or left side-lying position for 15 to 20 minutes
- What lubricant to use
- How soon to expect the urge for a BM
- What observations to report and record:
  - Bleeding or resistance when inserting the suppository
  - How long the person retained the suppository
  - Color, amount, consistency, shape, and odor of stools
  - Complaints of cramping, pain, or discomfort
  - Complaints of nausea or weakness
  - How the person tolerated the procedure
- How to record the procedure
- When to report observations
- What patient or resident concerns to report at once

ENEMAS

An *enema is the introduction of fluid into the rectum and lower colon*. Doctors order enemas to:

- Remove feces.
- Relieve constipation, fecal impaction, or flatulence.
- Clean the bowel of feces before certain surgeries and diagnostic procedures.

Safety and comfort measures for bowel elimination are practiced when giving enemas (see Box 26-1). So are the rules in Box 26-2.

The doctor orders the enema solution. The solution depends on the enema's purpose—cleansing, constipation, fecal impaction, or flatulence.

- *Tap water enema*—is obtained from a faucet.
- *Saline enema*—a solution of salt and water. For adults, 1 or 2 teaspoons of table salt is added to 500 to 1000 mL (milliliters) of tap water.
- *Soapsuds enema (SSE)*—for adults, 3 to 5 mL of castile soap is added to 500 to 1000 mL of tap water.
- *Small-volume enema*—the adult size has about 120 mL (4 ounces [oz]) of solution. The child size has about 60 mL (2 oz).
- *Oil-retention enema*—has mineral, olive, or cottonseed oil. The adult size has about 120 mL (4 oz) of solution. Children usually receive 60 mL (2 oz).

Other enema solutions may be ordered. Consult with the nurse and use the agency's procedure manual to safely prepare and give enemas. You do not give enemas that contain drugs. Nurses give them.

See *Focus on Math: Enemas.*
See *Delegation Guidelines: Enemas*, p. 432.
See *Promoting Safety and Comfort: Enemas*, p. 432.

BOX 26-2   Giving Enemas

- Have the person void first. This increases comfort during the procedure.
- Measure solution temperature with a bath thermometer. See *Delegation Guidelines: Enemas*, p. 432.
- Give the amount of solution ordered.
- Position the person as the nurse directs. The Sims' position or the left side-lying position is preferred.
- Ask the nurse and check the procedure manual for how far to insert the enema tubing. It is usually inserted 2 to 4 inches in adults.
- Lubricate the enema tip before inserting it.
- Stop tube insertion if you feel resistance, the person complains of pain, or bleeding occurs.
- Ask the nurse how high to raise the enema bag. For adults, it is usually held 12 inches above the anus.
- Give the amount of solution ordered. Give the solution slowly. Usually it takes 10 to 15 minutes to give 750 to 1000 mL.
- Hold the enema tube in place while giving the solution.
- Ask the nurse how long the person should retain the solution. The length of time depends on the amount and type of solution.
- Make sure the bathroom will be vacant when the person needs to have a BM. Make sure that another person will not use the bathroom. If the person uses the bedpan or commode, have the device ready.
- Ask the nurse to observe the enema results.

FOCUS ON MATH

Enemas

Cleansing enemas are given over 10 to 15 minutes. The nurse tells you the amount of solution to give and the amount of time to give it in. As you give the solution, monitor how fast the fluid flows. To calculate the amount to give per minute, divide the total amount (in mL) by the time (in minutes). Each minute as you give the enema, subtract this amount to gauge if the rate is too fast or too slow.

For example, you are to give a 750 mL saline enema over 15 minutes. Divide 750 mL by 15 minutes. The fluid in the bag should decrease by about 50 mL each minute.

$$750 \text{ mL} \div 15 \text{ minutes} = 50 \text{ mL/minute}$$

Note the start time. Check the amount at least each minute. At 1 minute, the solution should be at the 700 mL mark.

$$750 \text{ mL} - 50 \text{ mL} = 700 \text{ mL (at 1 minute)}$$

At 2 minutes, the solution should be about half-way between the 700 mL and 600 mL marks (650 mL).

$$700 \text{ mL} - 50 \text{ mL} = 650 \text{ mL (at 2 minutes)}$$

At 3 minutes, the solution should be at the 600 mL mark, and so on.

$$650 \text{ mL} - 50 \text{ mL} = 600 \text{ mL (at 3 minutes)}$$

If the solution is flowing too fast, clamp the tube and call for the nurse. The nurse may lower the bag to slow the flow. If the solution is flowing too slowly, call for the nurse. The nurse may adjust the tube or raise the bag to quicken the flow.

DELEGATION GUIDELINES

Enemas

If giving an enema to an adult is delegated to you, make sure the conditions in *Delegation Guidelines: Bowel Elimination* (p. 423) are met. If those conditions are met, you need this information from the nurse.

- What enema to give—cleansing, small-volume, or oil-retention
- What size enema tube to use
- What lubricant to use
- When to give the enema
- How many times to repeat the enema
- The amount of solution ordered—usually 500 to 1000 mL for a cleansing enema (for adults)
- How much castile soap to use for an SSE
- How much salt to use for a saline enema
- What the solution temperature should be—usually 98.6°F to 100°F (Fahrenheit) (37.0°C to 37.8°C [centigrade]); sometimes warmer temperatures (105°F/40.5°C) are used for adults

- What position to use—Sims' or left side-lying position
- How far to insert the enema tubing—usually 2 to 4 inches for adults
- How high to hold the solution container—usually 12 inches above the anus
- How fast to give the solution—750 to 1000 mL are usually given over 10 to 15 minutes
- How long the person should try to retain the solution
- What observations to report and record:
  - The amount of solution given
  - Bleeding or resistance when inserting the tube
  - How long the person retained the enema solution
  - Color, amount, consistency, shape, and odor of stools
  - Complaints of cramping, pain, or discomfort
  - Complaints of nausea or weakness
  - How the person tolerated the procedure
- When to report observations
- What patient or resident concerns to report at once

PROMOTING SAFETY AND COMFORT

Enemas

Safety

Enemas are usually safe procedures. Many people give themselves enemas at home. However, enemas are dangerous for older persons and those with certain heart and kidney diseases.

Comfort

Before the procedure, make sure that the bathroom is ready for the person's use. If the person will use the commode or bedpan, have the device ready. Always keep a bedpan nearby in case the enema solution and stools are expelled. You promote mental comfort when the person knows the bathroom, commode, or bedpan is ready for use.

The person should retain the solution as long as possible. Provide for a comfortable Sims' or left side-lying position. When comfortable, it is easier to tolerate the procedure.

To prevent cramping:
- Use the correct water temperature. Cool water causes cramping.
- Give the solution slowly.

FOCUS ON **CHILDREN AND OLDER PERSONS**

The Cleansing Enema

Children

Saline enemas are used for cleansing enemas in children. Check with the nurse for the amount of solution to give. These are guidelines.
- Less than 18 months—50 to 200 mL
- 18 months to 5 years—200 to 300 mL
- 5 to 12 years—300 to 500 mL

The nurse tells you to insert the enema tube usually 2 to 3 inches in children and 1 to 1½ inches in infants.

Infants cannot tell you they hurt. If cramping occurs, the child draws up the knees. The child's cry is higher-pitched than normal.

In children, cleansing enemas take effect in about 2 to 5 minutes.

▉ The Cleansing Enema

Cleansing enemas clean the bowel of feces and flatus. They relieve constipation and fecal impaction. They are given before certain surgeries and diagnostic procedures. Cleansing enemas take effect in 10 to 20 minutes.

The doctor orders a tap water, saline, or soapsuds enema. An *enemas until clear* order means that enemas are given until the return solution is clear and free of stools. Agency policy may allow repeating enemas 2 or 3 times.

The nurse tells you what enema to give and how many times to repeat the enema.

- *Tap water enema.* The colon may absorb some of the water into the bloodstream. This creates a fluid imbalance. *Only 1 tap water enema is given. Do not repeat the enema.* Repeated enemas increase the risk of excessive fluid absorption.
- *Saline enema.* The solution is similar to body fluid. However, some of the salt solution may be absorbed, causing a fluid imbalance. The body retains water from the excess salt.
- *Soapsuds enema. The SSE irritates* the bowel's mucous lining. Repeated enemas can damage the bowel. So can using more than 3 to 5 mL of castile soap or stronger soaps.

See *Focus on Children and Older Persons: The Cleansing Enema.*

See procedure: *Giving a Cleansing Enema.*

Giving a Cleansing Enema

QUALITY OF LIFE

- Knock before entering the person's room.
- Address the person by name.
- Introduce yourself by name and title.

- Explain the procedure before starting and during the procedure.
- Protect the person's rights during the procedure.
- Handle the person gently during the procedure.

PRE-PROCEDURE

1 Follow *Delegation Guidelines:*
   a *Bowel Elimination,* p. 423
   b *Enemas*
   See *Promoting Safety and Comfort:*
   a *Bowel Elimination,* p. 423
   b *Enemas*
2 Practice hand hygiene.
3 Collect the following before going to the person's room.
   - Disposable enema kit as directed by the nurse (enema bag, tube, clamp, and waterproof under-pad)
   - Bath thermometer
   - Waterproof under-pad (if not in the enema kit)
   - Water-soluble lubricant
   - 3 to 5 mL (1 teaspoon) castile soap or 1 to 2 teaspoons of salt (if needed)
   - IV (intravenous) pole
   - Gloves

4 Arrange items in the person's room and bathroom.
5 Practice hand hygiene.
6 Identify the person. Check the ID bracelet against the assignment sheet. Use 2 identifiers (Chapter 13). Also call the person by name.
7 Put on gloves.
8 Collect the following.
   - Commode or bedpan and cover
   - Toilet tissue
   - Bath blanket
   - Robe and non-skid footwear
   - Paper towels
9 Remove and discard the gloves. Practice hand hygiene. Put on clean gloves.
10 Provide for privacy.
11 Raise the bed for body mechanics. Bed rails are up if used.

PROCEDURE

12 Lower the bed rail near you if up.
13 Cover the person with a bath blanket. Fan-fold top linens to the foot of the bed.
14 Position the IV pole so the enema bag is 12 inches above the anus. Or it is at the height directed by the nurse.
15 Raise the bed rail if used.
16 Prepare the enema.
   a Close the clamp on the tube.
   b Adjust water flow until it is lukewarm.
   c Fill the enema bag for the amount ordered.
   d Measure water temperature with the bath thermometer. The nurse tells you what water temperature to use.
   e Prepare the solution as directed by the nurse.
      1) *Tap water:* add nothing.
      2) *Saline enema:* add salt as directed.
      3) *SSE:* add castile soap as directed.
   f Stir the solution with the bath thermometer. Scoop off any suds (SSE).
   g Seal the bag.
   h Hang the bag on the IV pole.

17 Lower the bed rail near you if up.
18 Position the person in Sims' position or in a left side-lying position.
19 Place a waterproof under-pad under the buttocks.
20 Expose the anal area.
21 Place the bedpan behind the person.
22 Position the enema tube in the bedpan. Remove the cap from the tubing.
23 Open the clamp. Let solution flow through the tube to remove air. Clamp the tube.
24 Lubricate the tube 2 to 4 inches from the tip.
25 Separate the buttocks to see the anus.
26 Ask the person to take a deep breath through the mouth.
27 Insert the tube gently 2 to 4 inches into the adult's rectum (Fig. 26-7). Do this when the person is exhaling. Stop if the person complains of pain, you feel resistance, or bleeding occurs.
28 Check the amount of solution in the bag.
29 Unclamp the tube. Give the solution slowly (Fig. 26-8).

Continued

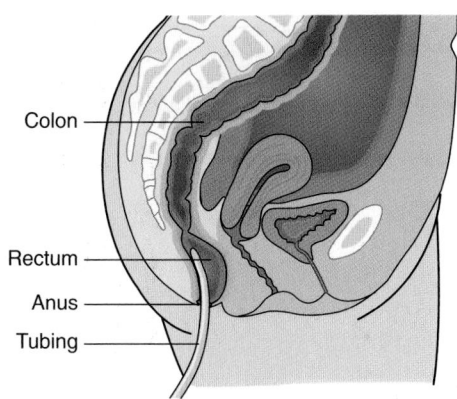

FIGURE 26-7 Enema tubing inserted into the adult rectum.

Colon
Rectum
Anus
Tubing

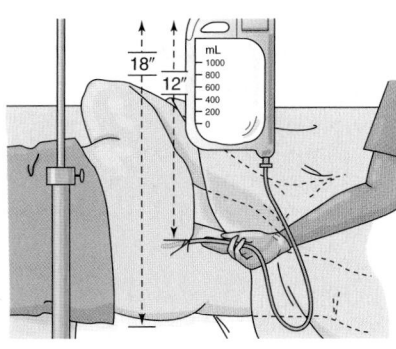

FIGURE 26-8 Giving an enema. The person is in Sims' position. The enema bag hangs from an IV pole. The bag is 12 inches above the anus and 18 inches above the mattress.

Giving a Cleansing Enema—cont'd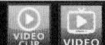

PROCEDURE—cont'd

30 Ask the person to take slow, deep breaths. This helps the person relax.
31 Clamp the tube if the person needs to have a BM, has cramping, or starts to expel the solution. Also, clamp the tube if the person is sweating or complains of nausea or weakness. Unclamp when symptoms subside.
32 Give the amount of solution ordered. Stop if the person cannot tolerate the procedure.
33 Clamp the tube before it is empty. This prevents air from entering the bowel.
34 Hold toilet tissue around the tube and against the anus. Remove the tube.
35 Discard toilet tissue into the bedpan.
36 Wrap the tubing tip with paper towels. Place it inside the enema bag.
37 Encourage retention of the enema for the time ordered.
38 Assist the person to the bathroom or commode. The person wears a robe and non-skid footwear when up. The bed is at a low level that is safe and comfortable for the person. Or help the person onto the bedpan. Raise the head of the bed. Raise or lower bed rails according to the care plan.

39 Place the call light and toilet tissue within reach. Remind the person not to flush the toilet.
40 Discard disposable items.
41 Remove and discard the gloves. Practice hand hygiene.
42 Leave the room if the person can be left alone.
43 Return when the person signals. Or check on the person every 5 minutes. Knock before entering the room or bathroom.
44 Practice hand hygiene and put on gloves. Lower the bed rail if up.
45 Observe enema results for amount, color, consistency, shape, and odor. Call the nurse to observe the results.
46 Provide perineal care as needed.
47 Remove the waterproof under-pad.
48 Empty, rinse, clean, and disinfect equipment. Flush the toilet after the nurse observes the results.
49 Return equipment to its proper place.
50 Remove and discard the gloves. Practice hand hygiene.
51 Assist with hand-washing. Wear gloves for this step. Practice hand hygiene after removing and discarding the gloves.
52 Cover the person. Remove the bath blanket.

POST-PROCEDURE

53 Provide for comfort. (See the inside of the front cover.)
54 Place the call light and other needed items within reach.
55 Lower the bed to a safe and comfortable level for the person. Follow the care plan.
56 Raise or lower bed rails. Follow the care plan.
57 Unscreen the person.

58 Complete a safety check of the room. (See the inside of the front cover.)
59 Follow agency policy for used linens and used supplies.
60 Practice hand hygiene.
61 Report and record your observations.

The Small-Volume Enema

Small-volume enemas irritate and distend the rectum. This causes a BM. They are ordered for constipation or when the bowel does not need complete cleansing.

These enemas are ready to give. This solution is usually given at room temperature. To give the enema, squeeze and roll up the plastic container from the bottom. Do not release pressure on the bottle. Otherwise, solution is drawn from the rectum back into the bottle.

Urge the person to retain the solution until he or she needs to have a BM. This usually takes 5 to 10 minutes. Staying in the Sims' or left side-lying position helps retain the enema.

See procedure: *Giving a Small-Volume Enema.*

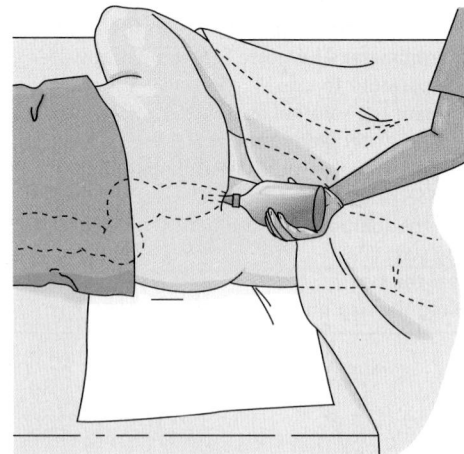

FIGURE 26-9 The small-volume enema tip is inserted 2 inches into the rectum.

Giving a Small-Volume Enema

VIDEO

QUALITY OF LIFE

- Knock before entering the person's room.
- Address the person by name.
- Introduce yourself by name and title.

- Explain the procedure before starting and during the procedure.
- Protect the person's rights during the procedure.
- Handle the person gently during the procedure.

PRE-PROCEDURE

1 Follow *Delegation Guidelines:*
   a *Bowel Elimination,* p. 423
   b *Enemas,* p. 432
   See *Promoting Safety and Comfort:*
   a *Bowel Elimination,* p. 423
   b *Enemas,* p. 432
2 Practice hand hygiene.
3 Collect the following before going to the person's room.
   - Small-volume enema
   - Waterproof under-pad
   - Gloves
4 Arrange items in the person's room.
5 Practice hand hygiene.

6 Identify the person. Check the ID bracelet against the assignment sheet. Use 2 identifiers (Chapter 13). Also call the person by name.
7 Put on gloves.
8 Collect the following.
   - Commode or bedpan
   - Toilet tissue
   - Robe and non-skid footwear
   - Bath blanket
9 Remove and discard the gloves. Practice hand hygiene. Put on clean gloves.
10 Provide for privacy.
11 Raise the bed for body mechanics. Bed rails are up if used.

PROCEDURE

12 Lower the bed rail near you if up.
13 Cover the person with a bath blanket. Fan-fold top linens to the foot of the bed.
14 Position the person in Sims' or left side-lying position.
15 Place the waterproof under-pad under the buttocks.
16 Expose the anal area.
17 Position the bedpan near the person.
18 Remove the cap from the enema tip.
19 Separate the buttocks to see the anus.
20 Ask the person to take a deep breath through the mouth.
21 Insert the enema tip 2 inches into the adult's rectum (Fig. 26-9). Do this when the person is exhaling. Insert the tip gently. Stop if the person complains of pain, you feel resistance, or bleeding occurs.
22 Squeeze and roll up the container gently. Release pressure on the bottle after you remove the tip from the rectum.
23 Put the container into the box, tip first. Discard the container and box.
24 Assist the person to the bathroom or commode when he or she has the urge to have a BM. The person wears a robe and non-skid footwear when up. The bed is at a low level that is safe and comfortable for the person. Or help the person onto the bedpan and raise the head of the bed. Raise or lower bed rails according to the care plan.

25 Place the call light and toilet tissue within reach. Remind the person not to flush the toilet.
26 Discard disposable items.
27 Remove and discard the gloves. Practice hand hygiene.
28 Leave the room if the person can be left alone.
29 Return when the person signals. Or check on the person every 5 minutes. Knock before entering the room or bathroom.
30 Practice hand hygiene. Put on gloves.
31 Lower the bed rail if up.
32 Observe enema results for amount, color, consistency, shape, and odor. Call the nurse to observe the results.
33 Provide perineal care as needed.
34 Remove the waterproof under-pad.
35 Empty, rinse, clean, and disinfect equipment. Flush the toilet after the nurse observes the results.
36 Return equipment to its proper place.
37 Remove and discard the gloves. Practice hand hygiene.
38 Assist with hand-washing. Wear gloves for this step. Practice hand hygiene after removing and discarding the gloves.
39 Cover the person. Remove the bath blanket.

POST-PROCEDURE

40 Provide for comfort. (See the inside of the front cover.)
41 Place the call light and other needed items within reach.
42 Lower the bed to a safe and comfortable level for the person. Follow the care plan.
43 Raise or lower bed rails. Follow the care plan.
44 Unscreen the person.

45 Complete a safety check of the room. (See the inside of the front cover.)
46 Follow agency policy for used linens and used supplies.
47 Practice hand hygiene.
48 Report and record your observations.

The Oil-Retention Enema

Oil-retention enemas relieve constipation and fecal impaction. The oil softens feces and lubricates the rectum so feces pass with ease. The oil is retained for 30 minutes to 1 to 3 hours. Most oil-retention enemas are ready-to-use.

See *Promoting Safety and Comfort: The Oil-Retention Enema.*

See procedure: *Giving an Oil-Retention Enema.*

PROMOTING SAFETY AND COMFORT

The Oil-Retention Enema

Safety

The oil-retention enema is retained for at least 30 minutes. Leave the room after giving the enema. Check on the person often. Then tell him or her when you will return. Remind the person to signal for you if help is needed. Report any problems to the nurse at once.

Giving an Oil-Retention Enema

QUALITY OF LIFE

- Knock before entering the person's room.
- Address the person by name.
- Introduce yourself by name and title.

- Explain the procedure before starting and during the procedure.
- Protect the person's rights during the procedure.
- Handle the person gently during the procedure.

PRE-PROCEDURE

1 Follow *Delegation Guidelines:*
  a *Bowel Elimination,* p. 423
  b *Enemas,* p. 432
  See *Promoting Safety and Comfort:*
  a *Bowel Elimination,* p. 423
  b *Enemas,* p. 432
  c *The Oil-Retention Enema*
2 Practice hand hygiene.
3 Collect the following.
  • Oil-retention enema

  • Waterproof under-pads
  • Gloves
  • Bath blanket
4 Arrange items in the person's room.
5 Practice hand hygiene.
6 Identify the person. Check the ID bracelet against the assignment sheet. Use 2 identifiers (Chapter 13). Also call the person by name.
7 Provide for privacy.
8 Raise the bed for body mechanics. Bed rails are up if used.

PROCEDURE

9 Put on gloves.
10 Follow steps 12 through 23 in procedure: *Giving a Small-Volume Enema,* p. 435.
11 Cover the person. Leave him or her in the Sims' or left side-lying position.

12 Encourage retention of the enema for the time ordered.
13 Place more waterproof under-pads on the bed if needed.
14 Remove and discard the gloves. Practice hand hygiene.

POST-PROCEDURE

15 Provide for comfort. (See the inside of the front cover.)
16 Place the call light and other needed items within reach.
17 Lower the bed to a safe and comfortable level for the person. Follow the care plan.
18 Raise or lower bed rails. Follow the care plan.
19 Unscreen the person.

20 Complete a safety check of the room. (See the inside of the front cover.)
21 Follow agency policy for used linens and used supplies.
22 Practice hand hygiene.
23 Report and record your observations.
24 Check the person often.

THE PERSON WITH AN OSTOMY

Sometimes part of the intestines is removed surgically. Cancer, bowel disease, and trauma (stab or bullet wounds) are common reasons. An ostomy is sometimes necessary. An **ostomy** *is a surgically created opening that connects an internal organ to the body's surface. The surgically created opening seen on the body's surface is called a* **stoma** (Fig. 26-10). A pouch is worn over the stoma to collect stools and flatus.

Colostomy

A **colostomy** *is a surgically created opening* (stomy) *between the colon* (colo) *and the body's surface.* Part of the colon is brought out onto the body's surface and a stoma is made. Feces and flatus pass through the stoma instead of the anus.

With a permanent colostomy, the diseased part of the colon is removed. A temporary colostomy gives the diseased or injured bowel time to heal. After healing, the bowel is surgically reconnected. The colostomy site

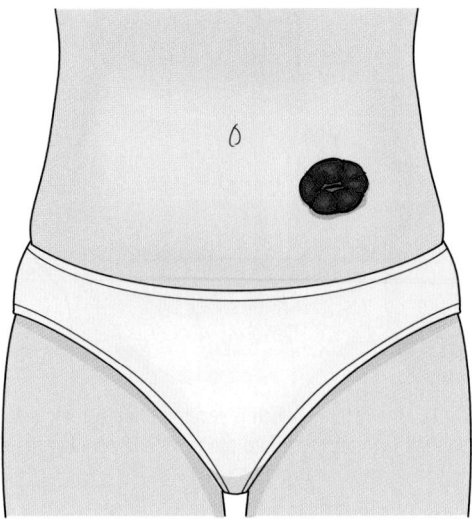

FIGURE 26-10 A stoma on the surface of the body.

depends on the site of disease or injury (Fig. 26-11). Stool consistency—liquid to formed—depends on the colostomy site. The more colon remaining to absorb water, the more solid and formed the stool. If the colostomy is near the end of the colon, stools are formed.

Stools irritate the skin. Skin care prevents skin breakdown around the stoma. The skin is washed and dried. Then a skin barrier is applied around the stoma. It prevents stools from having contact with the skin. The skin barrier is part of the pouch or a separate device.

Ileostomy

An ***ileostomy*** *is a surgically created opening* (stomy) *between the ileum* (small intestine [ileo]) *and the body's surface.* Part of the ileum is brought out onto the body's surface and a stoma is made. The entire colon is removed (Fig. 26-12, p. 438).

Liquid stools drain constantly from an ileostomy. Water is not absorbed because the colon was removed. Feces in the small intestine contain digestive juices that are very irritating to the skin. The ileostomy pouch must fit well. Stools must not touch the skin. Good skin care is required.

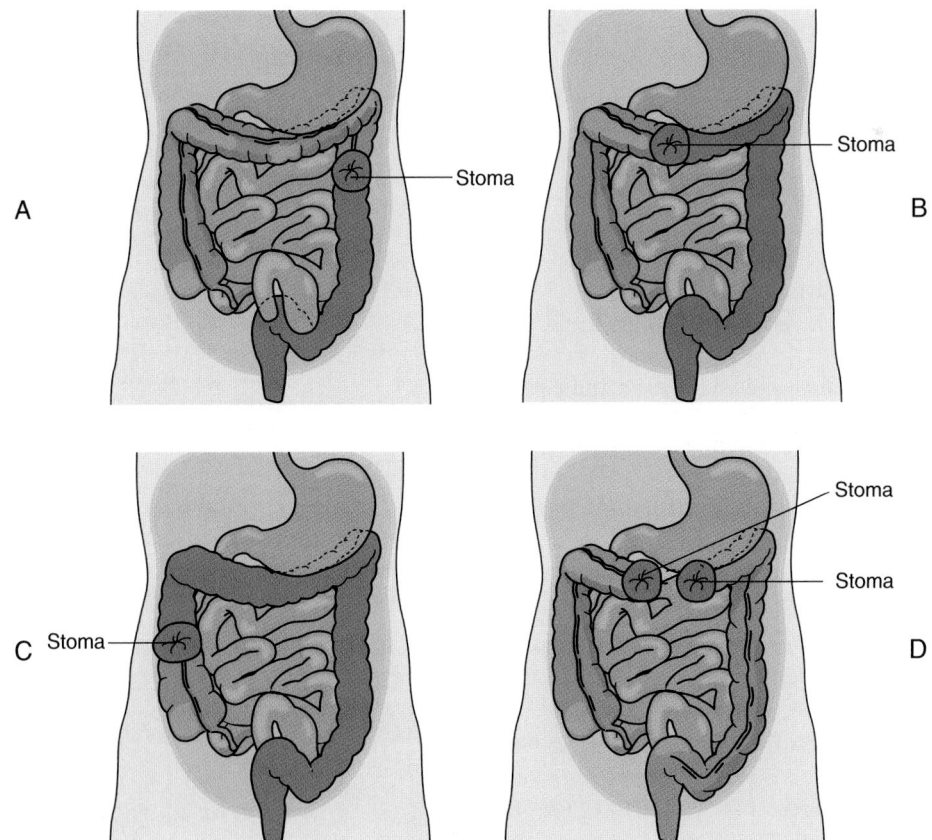

FIGURE 26-11 Colostomy sites. *Shading* shows the part of the bowel surgically removed. **A,** Sigmoid or descending colostomy. **B,** Transverse colostomy. **C,** Ascending colostomy. **D,** Double-barrel colostomy has 2 stomas. One allows for the excretion of feces. The other is for the introduction of drugs to help the bowel heal. This type is usually temporary.

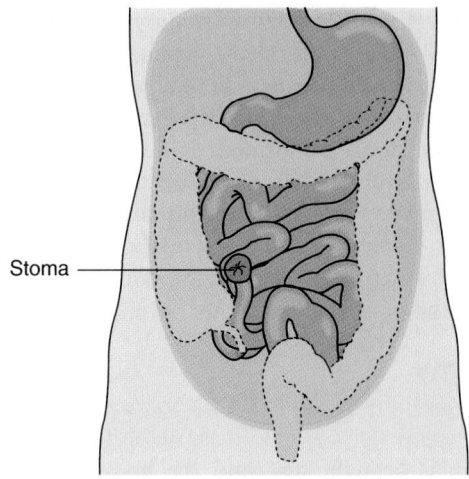

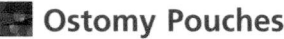

FIGURE 26-12 An ileostomy. The entire large intestine is surgically removed.

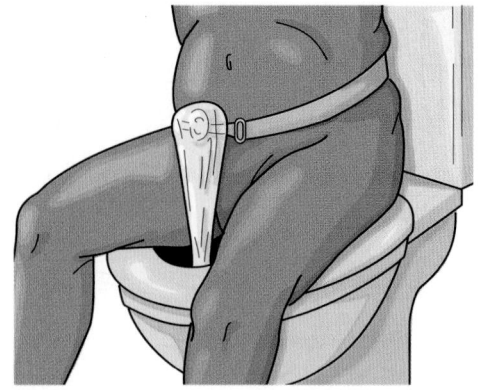

FIGURE 26-13 The ostomy pouch is secured to an ostomy belt. The pouch is emptied by directing it into the toilet and opening the end.

Ostomy Pouches

A plastic pouch with an adhesive backing is applied to the skin. Some pouches are secured to ostomy belts (Fig. 26-13).

Pouches have a drain at the bottom that closes with a clip, clamp, or wire closure. The drain is opened to empty the pouch. The pouch is emptied when stools are present. It is opened when it balloons or bulges to release flatus. The drain is wiped with toilet tissue before closing.

The pouch is changed every 2 to 7 days and when it leaks. Frequent pouch changes can damage the skin.

Odors are prevented by:
- Using odor-free pouches.
- Performing good hygiene.
- Emptying the pouch.
- Avoiding gas-forming foods.
- Putting deodorants into the pouch. The nurse tells you what to use.

The person wears normal clothes. However, tight garments can prevent feces from entering the pouch. Also, bulging from stools and flatus can be seen with tight clothes.

Peristalsis increases after eating and drinking. Therefore stomas are usually quiet after sleep. That is, expelling feces is less likely at this time. If the person showers or bathes with the pouch off, it is best done before breakfast. Showers and baths are delayed for 1 to 2 hours after applying a new pouch. This gives adhesive time to seal to the skin.

Do not flush pouches down the toilet. Follow agency policy for disposal.

See *Focus on Children and Older Persons: Ostomy Pouches.*
See *Delegation Guidelines: Ostomy Pouches.*
See *Promoting Safety and Comfort: Ostomy Pouches.*
See procedure: *Changing an Ostomy Pouch.*

FOCUS ON **CHILDREN AND OLDER PERSONS**
Ostomy Pouches

Children
Children of all ages can have ostomies, even premature infants. If changing or emptying a child's ostomy pouch is delegated to you, the nurse gives you the necessary information.

DELEGATION GUIDELINES
Ostomy Pouches

Many people manage their own ostomies. If the nurse delegates changing an ostomy pouch to you, make sure that the conditions in *Delegation Guidelines, Bowel Elimination* (p. 423) are met. If those conditions are met, you need this information from the nurse and the care plan.
- If the person has a colostomy or ileostomy
- When to change the pouch
- What equipment and supplies to use
- What soap or cleaning agent to use
- Drying time for the skin barrier (usually 1 to 2 minutes)
- What pouch deodorant to use (if needed)
- What observations to report and record:
  - Signs of skin breakdown (a normal stoma is red like a mucous membrane)
  - Color, amount, consistency, and odor of stools
  - Complaints of pain or discomfort
- When to report observations
- What patient or resident concerns to report at once

PROMOTING SAFETY AND COMFORT
Ostomy Pouches

Safety
When changing an ostomy pouch, the stoma may bleed slightly when washed. Follow Standard Precautions and the Bloodborne Pathogen Standard.

Comfort
The stoma does not have sensation. Touching the stoma does not cause pain or discomfort.

Changing an Ostomy Pouch

QUALITY OF LIFE

- Knock before entering the person's room.
- Address the person by name.
- Introduce yourself by name and title.

- Explain the procedure before starting and during the procedure.
- Protect the person's rights during the procedure.
- Handle the person gently during the procedure.

PRE-PROCEDURE

1 Follow *Delegation Guidelines:*
  a *Bowel Elimination*, p. 423
  b *Ostomy Pouches*
  See *Promoting Safety and Comfort:*
  a *Bowel Elimination*, p. 423
  b *Ostomy Pouches*
2 Practice hand hygiene.
3 Collect the following before going to the person's room.
  • Clean pouch with skin barrier
  • Pouch clamp, clip, or wire closure
  • Clean ostomy belt (if used)
  • Gauze pads or washcloths
  • Adhesive remover wipes
  • Skin paste (optional)
  • Pouch deodorant
  • Disposable bag
  • Waterproof under-pad

  • Gloves
  • Paper towels
4 Place the paper towels on the over-bed table. Arrange supplies on top of the paper towels.
5 Practice hand hygiene.
6 Identify the person. Check the ID bracelet against the assignment sheet. Use 2 identifiers (Chapter 13). Also call the person by name.
7 Put on gloves.
8 Collect the following.
  • Bedpan with cover
  • Bath blanket
  • Wash basin with warm water
9 Remove and discard the gloves. Practice hand hygiene. Put on clean gloves.
10 Provide for privacy.
11 Raise the bed for body mechanics. Bed rails are up if used.

PROCEDURE

12 Lower the bed rail near you if up.
13 Cover the person with a bath blanket. Fan-fold linens to the foot of the bed.
14 Place the waterproof under-pad under the buttocks.
15 Disconnect the pouch from the belt if one is worn. Remove the belt.
16 Remove and place the pouch and skin barrier in the bedpan. Gently push the skin down and lift up on the barrier. Use adhesive remover wipes if necessary.
17 Wipe the stoma and around it with a gauze pad. This removes excess stool and mucus. Discard the gauze pad into the disposable bag.
18 Wet the gauze pads or washcloth.
19 Wash the stoma and the skin around it with a gauze pad or washcloth. Wash gently. Do not scrub or rub the skin.
20 Pat dry with a gauze pad or the towel.
21 Observe the stoma and the skin around the stoma. Report bleeding, skin irritation, or skin breakdown.
22 Remove the backing from the new pouch.
23 Apply a thin layer of paste around the pouch opening. Let it dry following the manufacturer's instructions.

24 Pull the skin around the stoma taut. The skin must be wrinkle-free.
25 Center the pouch over the stoma. The drain is downward.
26 Press around the pouch and skin barrier so it seals to the skin. Apply gentle pressure with your fingers. Start at the bottom and work up around the sides to the top.
27 Maintain the pressure for 1 to 2 minutes. This allows the adhesive on the skin barrier to activate. Follow the manufacturer's instructions.
28 Tug downward on the pouch gently. Make sure the pouch is secure.
29 Add deodorant to the pouch (if needed).
30 Close the pouch at the bottom. Use a clamp, clip, or wire closure.
31 Attach the ostomy belt if used. The belt should not be too tight. You should be able to slide 2 fingers under the belt.
32 Remove the waterproof under-pad.
33 Discard disposable supplies into the disposable bag.
34 Remove and discard the gloves. Practice hand hygiene.
35 Cover the person. Remove the bath blanket.

POST-PROCEDURE

36 Provide for comfort. (See the inside of the front cover.)
37 Place the call light and other needed items within reach.
38 Lower the bed to a safe and comfortable level for the person. Follow the care plan.
39 Raise or lower bed rails. Follow the care plan.
40 Unscreen the person.
41 Practice hand hygiene. Put on gloves.
42 Take the bedpan and disposable bag into the bathroom.
43 Empty the pouch and bedpan into the toilet. Observe the color, amount, consistency, and odor of stools. Flush the toilet.

44 Discard the pouch into the disposable bag. Discard the disposable bag.
45 Empty, rinse, clean, and disinfect equipment. Return equipment to its proper place.
46 Remove and discard the gloves. Practice hand hygiene.
47 Complete a safety check of the room. (See the inside of the front cover.)
48 Follow agency policy for used linens.
49 Practice hand hygiene.
50 Report and record your observations.

FOCUS ON PRIDE

The Person, Family, and Yourself

P ersonal and Professional Responsibility

You are responsible for knowing the legal limits of your role. Some states and agencies allow nursing assistants to insert some types of suppositories. If your state and agency allow this, you must know your limits. You cannot insert all types.

For example, you may be allowed to insert suppositories only in persons who use them regularly for constipation. You cannot give a suppository for fever or vomiting. Know what you are and are not allowed to do. Never perform a task beyond the legal limits of your role.

R ights and Respect

Bowel elimination is typically done in private. Illness, disease, surgery, and aging can affect this private act. Some persons may feel embarrassed to have a BM in a strange setting. To promote comfort and privacy:

- Ask others to leave the room.
- Close doors, privacy curtains, and window coverings.
- Turn on water or music to mask sounds.
- Cover the person.
- Allow enough time. Place the call light nearby and instruct the person to call if help is needed.
- Knock before entering the room. Tell the person who you are. Ask if you can enter before opening the door completely.
- Use an agency-approved spray for odors.

I ndependence and Social Interaction

Persons with ostomies manage their care if able. Some have had ostomies for a long time. They may have special routines or care measures. Do not react to things that seem odd to you. When you assist, ask what they prefer. Listen to their requests. Follow their choices in ostomy care. To promote independence, allow personal choice and control as much as safely possible.

D elegation and Teamwork

The nurse may delegate a task to you that you have not done before. Giving an enema is an example. Never attempt a task that you are not comfortable doing. Make sure your state and agency allow you to perform the procedure. If those conditions are met, you can politely say: "I'm sorry, but I have never done that task before. I am not comfortable doing it on my own. Would you please show me how it is done?" Take pride in making the right choice to tell the nurse about your delegation concern.

E thics and Laws

Leaving a person sitting or lying in urine or feces is neglect. It is a form of physical abuse. State laws, the Omnibus Budget Reconciliation Act of 1987 (OBRA), and the CMS require the reporting and investigating of abuse.

If found guilty of abuse, neglect, or mistreatment, you will lose your job. The offense is noted on your registry. You cannot work in a nursing center or on a skilled care nursing unit in a hospital. Protect yourself from being accused of neglect. Check on your patients or residents often. Do not leave them sitting or lying in urine or feces.

FOCUS ON PRIDE: Application

You are asked to do an unfamiliar task. Do you seek help? Do you try to do it alone? Does asking for help bother you?

Supervision is part of the nurse's role in delegation. The nurse needs to know your comfort level with tasks. Never be ashamed to ask for supervision.

REVIEW QUESTIONS

Circle the BEST answer

1 Which is *true*?
   a A person must have a BM every day.
   b Stools are normally brown, soft, and formed.
   c Diarrhea occurs when feces move slowly through the bowel.
   d Constipation occurs when feces move quickly through the bowel.

2 Which should you ask the nurse to observe?
   a A black and tarry stool
   b The person's first BM of the day
   c Stool with an odor
   d Liquid stool from an ileostomy

3 The prolonged retention and buildup of feces in the rectum is called
   a Constipation
   b Fecal impaction
   c Diarrhea
   d Fecal incontinence

4 These measures promote normal BMs. Which is outside your role limits?
   a Provide oral fluids according to the care plan.
   b Assist with activity according to the care plan.
   c Give drugs to control diarrhea.
   d Provide privacy for bowel elimination.

5 A person has *C. difficile*. You should
   a Disinfect care items with soap and water
   b Use an alcohol-based hand rub before leaving the room
   c Wear a gown and gloves
   d Refuse to care for the person

6 Bowel training is aimed at
   a Bowel control and regular elimination
   b Ostomy control
   c Promoting toilet use
   d Preventing bleeding

7 Your state and agency allow you to insert rectal suppositories. You insert a suppository
   a Into the feces
   b Into the stoma
   c Along the rectal wall
   d With an enema tube

8 Which is used for a cleansing enema?
   a Mineral, olive, or cottonseed oil
   b A suppository
   c A 120 mL bottle of solution
   d Tap water, saline, or a soapsuds enema

9 Which is used for cleansing enemas in children?
   a Soapsuds
   b Saline
   c Oil
   d Tap water

10 When giving an enema
   a Use a cool solution
   b Place the person in the supine position
   c Have the person void after giving the enema
   d Give the solution slowly

11 In adults, the enema tube is inserted
   a 2 to 4 inches
   b 6 to 8 inches
   c 12 inches
   d Until you feel resistance

12 A small-volume enema is retained
   a For 2 minutes
   b At least 10 to 20 minutes
   c At least 30 minutes
   d Until the urge to have a BM is felt

13 Which care measure for an ostomy should you question?
   a Use deodorant in the pouch.
   b Perform good skin care around the stoma.
   c Change the pouch daily.
   d Apply a skin barrier around the stoma.

14 An ostomy pouch is usually emptied
   a Every 4 to 6 hours
   b When it is full
   c Every 2 to 7 days
   d When stools are present

Answers to Chapter 26 questions are on p. 871.

FOCUS ON PRACTICE

Problem Solving

A resident shares a bathroom with a roommate. You respond to the resident's call light. He says he needs to have a BM urgently. The bathroom is occupied. What do you do?

Nutrition and Fluids

OBJECTIVES

- Define the key terms and key abbreviations in this chapter.
- Explain the purpose and use of the MyPlate symbol.
- Describe the functions and sources of nutrients.
- Explain how to read and use food labels.
- Describe the factors that affect eating and nutrition.
- Describe OBRA requirements for serving food.
- Describe the special diets and between-meal snacks.
- Identify the signs, symptoms, and precautions for aspiration and regurgitation.
- Explain how to assist with measuring food intake.

- Describe fluid requirements and the causes of dehydration.
- Explain how to assist with special fluid orders.
- Explain the purpose of intake and output records.
- Identify what to count as fluid intake and output.
- Explain how to assist with food and fluid needs.
- Explain how to provide drinking water.
- Explain how to prevent foodborne illness.
- Perform the procedures described in this chapter.
- Explain how to promote PRIDE in the person, the family, and yourself.

KEY TERMS

anorexia The loss of appetite
aspiration Breathing fluid, food, vomitus, or an object into the lungs
calorie The fuel or energy value of food
cholesterol A soft, waxy substance found in the bloodstream and all body cells
dehydration A decrease in the amount of water in body tissues
dysphagia Difficulty (dys) swallowing (phagia)
edema The swelling of body tissues with water

graduate A measuring container for fluid
hydration Having an adequate amount of water in body tissues
intake The amount of fluid taken in; input
nutrient A substance that is ingested, digested, absorbed, and used by the body
nutrition The processes involved in the ingestion, digestion, absorption, and use of foods and fluids by the body
output The amount of fluid lost

KEY ABBREVIATIONS

F	Fahrenheit	**mL**	Milliliter
FDA	Food and Drug Administration	**NPO**	*Non per os;* nothing by mouth
GI	Gastro-intestinal	**OBRA**	Omnibus Budget Reconciliation Act of 1987
ID	Identification	**oz**	Ounce
I&O	Intake and output	**USDA**	United States Department of Agriculture
mg	Milligram		

Food and water are necessary for life. The person's diet affects physical and mental well-being and function. A poor diet and poor eating habits:
- Increase the risk for disease and infection
- Cause chronic illnesses to become worse
- Cause healing problems
- Increase the risk for accidents and injuries

Eating and drinking provide pleasure. They often are part of social times with family and friends. A friendly, social setting for meals is important. Otherwise, the person may eat poorly.

Many factors affect dietary practices. They include culture, finances, and personal choice. (See *Caring About Culture: Meal Time Practices.*) Dietary practices also include selecting, preparing, and serving food. The health team includes these factors in planning the person's nutrition needs.

See *Body Structure and Function Review: The Digestive System.*

See *Focus on Long-Term Care and Home Care: Nutrition and Fluids.*

See *Focus on Surveys: Nutrition and Fluids,* p. 444.

✿ CARING ABOUT CULTURE

Meal Time Practices

Many cultural groups have their main meal at mid-day. Persons from *Austria* and *Brazil* do so. They eat light meals in the evening. A main meal at lunch also is common in *Finland, Germany,* and *Greece.* In *Iran,* the most important meal is eaten at mid-day.

Modified from D'Avanzo CE: Pocket guide to cultural health assessment, ed 4, St Louis, 2008, Mosby.

FOCUS ON LONG-TERM CARE AND HOME CARE

Nutrition and Fluids

Long-Term Care
The Centers for Medicare & Medicaid Services (CMS) requires that the health team assess the resident's nutritional status. This will include:
- Drugs that affect taste or cause dry mouth, nausea, confusion, and so on
- Weight and height (Chapter 32)
- Appearance
- Food intake (p. 454)
- Fluid balance (p. 456)
- Factors affecting eating and nutrition (p. 449)

BODY STRUCTURE AND FUNCTION REVIEW

The Digestive System

The digestive system *(gastro-intestinal [GI] system)* breaks down food so it can be absorbed for use by the cells. This process is called *digestion.* The system also removes solid wastes from the body.

The digestive system involves the *alimentary canal (GI tract)* and the accessory organs of digestion (Fig. 27-1). The GI tract extends from the mouth to the anus.

Digestion begins in the *mouth (oral cavity).* It receives food and prepares it for digestion. Using chewing motions, the *teeth* cut, chop, and grind food into small particles for digestion and swallowing. The *tongue* aids in chewing and swallowing. *Taste buds* on the tongue contain nerve endings. Taste buds allow for sensing sweet, sour, bitter, and salty tastes. *Salivary glands* in the mouth secrete saliva. Saliva moistens food particles to ease swallowing and begin digestion. During swallowing, the tongue pushes food into the pharynx.

The *pharynx (throat)* is a muscular tube. Swallowing continues as the pharynx contracts. Contraction of the pharynx pushes food into the esophagus. The *esophagus* is a muscular tube about 10 inches long. It extends from the pharynx to the stomach. Involuntary muscle contractions called *peristalsis* move food down the esophagus through the GI tract.

The *stomach* is a muscular, pouch-like sac. Strong stomach muscles stir and churn food to break it up into even smaller particles. A mucous membrane lines the stomach. It contains glands that secrete *gastric juices.* Food is mixed and churned with the gastric juices to form a semi-liquid substance called *chyme.* Through peristalsis, the chyme is pushed from the stomach into the small intestine.

The *small intestine* is about 20 feet long with 3 parts. The first part is the *duodenum.* There, more digestive juices are added to the chyme. One is called *bile.* Bile is a greenish liquid made in the *liver.* Bile is stored in the *gallbladder.* Juices from the *pancreas* and small intestine are added to the chyme. Digestive juices chemically break down food for absorption.

Peristalsis moves the chyme through the other parts of the small intestine: *jejunum* and *ileum.* Tiny projections called *villi* line the small intestine. Villi absorb the digested food into the capillaries. Most food absorption takes place in the jejunum and the ileum.

Some chyme is not digested. Undigested chyme passes from the small intestine into the *large intestine (large bowel* or *colon).* More fluid is absorbed. The solid waste that remains is eliminated through the *anus.* See Chapters 10 and 26.

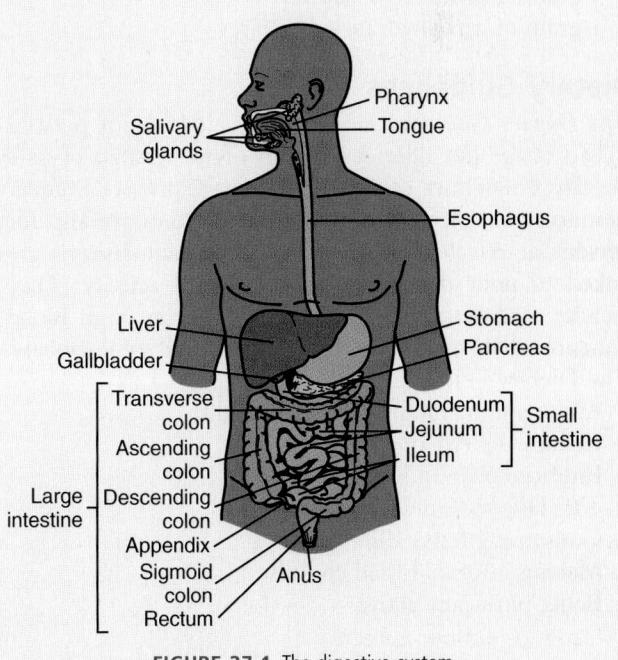

FIGURE 27-1 The digestive system.

BASIC NUTRITION

Nutrition is the processes involved in the ingestion, digestion, absorption, and use of food and fluids by the body. Good nutrition is needed for growth, healing, and body functions. A well-balanced diet and correct calorie intake are needed. A high-fat, high-calorie diet causes weight gain and obesity. A low-calorie diet promotes weight loss.

Foods and fluids contain nutrients. A *nutrient is a substance that is ingested, digested, absorbed, and used by the body.* Nutrients are grouped into fats, proteins, carbohydrates, vitamins, minerals, and water (p. 447).

Fats, proteins, and carbohydrates give the body fuel for energy. The amount of energy provided by a nutrient is measured in calories. A *calorie is the fuel or energy value of food.*

• 1 gram of fat—9 calories
• 1 gram of protein—4 calories
• 1 gram of carbohydrate—4 calories

Dietary Guidelines

The *Dietary Guidelines for Americans, 2015* is for persons 2 years of age and older. A summary of the most up-to-date Dietary Guidelines can be found on the Evolve Student Resources for this textbook. The Guidelines are also for persons at risk for chronic disease. Certain diseases are linked to poor diet and lack of physical activity. They include cardiovascular disease, hypertension (high blood pressure), diabetes, obesity, osteoporosis, and some cancers. The Dietary Guidelines help people:

• Attain and maintain a healthy weight.
• Reduce the risk of chronic disease.
• Promote over-all health.
  The Dietary Guidelines focus on:
• Consuming fewer calories
• Making informed food choices
• Being physically active

MyPlate

The MyPlate symbol (Fig. 27-2) encourages well-balanced meals with foods from 5 food groups. Issued by the United States Department of Agriculture (USDA), MyPlate helps you make wise food choices by:

• Balancing calories
  • Eating less
  • Avoiding over-sized portions
• Increasing certain foods
  • Making half of your plate fruits and vegetables
  • Making at least half of your grains whole grains
  • Drinking fat-free or low-fat (1%) milk
• Reducing certain foods
  • Choosing low-sodium foods
  • Drinking water instead of sugary drinks

The amount needed from each food group depends on age, sex, and physical activity (Table 27-1). Activity should be moderate or vigorous (Box 27-1). The USDA recommends that adults do at least 1 of the following.

• 2 hours and 30 minutes each week of moderate physical activity
• 1 hour and 15 minutes each week of vigorous physical activity

Physical activity at least 3 days a week is best. Each activity should be for at least 10 minutes at a time. Adults also should do strengthening activities at least 2 days a week. Push-ups, sit-ups, and weight-lifting are examples.

See *Focus on Children and Older Persons: MyPlate.*

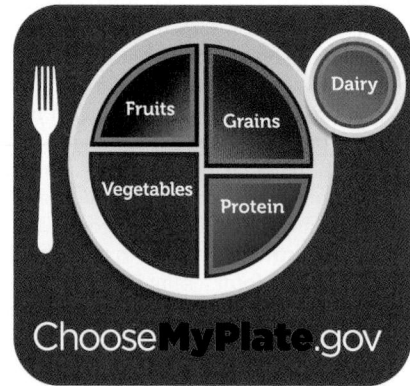

FIGURE 27-2 The MyPlate symbol. (Courtesy U.S. Department of Agriculture, Center for Nutrition and Policy Promotion, 2011.)

TABLE 27-1	MyPlate Serving Sizes	
Group	**Daily Servings**	**Serving Sizes**
Grains	• Adult women: 5 to 6 ounces (oz); at least 3 oz from whole grains • Adult men: 6 to 8 oz; at least 3 to 4 oz from whole grains	• 1 oz = 1 slice of bread • 1 oz = 1 cup breakfast cereal • 1 oz = ½ cup cooked rice, cereal, or pasta
Vegetables	• Adult women: 2 to 2½ cups • Adult men: 2½ to 3 cups	• 1 cup = 1 cup raw or cooked vegetables or vegetable juice • 1 cup = 2 cups raw leafy greens
Fruits	• Adult women: 1½ to 2 cups • Adult men: 2 cups	• 1 cup = 1 cup fruit • 1 cup = 1 cup fruit juice • 1 cup = ½ cup dried fruit
Dairy	• Adult women: 3 cups • Adult men: 3 cups	• 1 cup = 1 cup milk or yogurt • 1 cup = 1½ oz natural cheese • 1 cup = 2 oz processed cheese
Protein foods	• Adult women: 5 to 5½ oz • Adult men: 5½ to 6½ oz	• 1 oz = 1 oz lean meat, poultry, or fish • 1 oz = 1 egg • 1 oz = 1 tablespoon peanut butter • 1 oz = ¼ cup cooked dry beans • 1 oz = ½ oz nuts or seeds

Modified from U.S. Department of Agriculture: MyPlate, *June 2011.*

BOX 27-1	Physical Activities

Moderate Physical Activities
• Walking briskly (about 3½ miles per hour)
• Bicycling (less than 10 miles per hour)
• Gardening (raking, trimming bushes)
• Dancing
• Golf (walking and carrying clubs)
• Water aerobics
• Canoeing
• Tennis (doubles)

Vigorous Physical Activities
• Running and jogging (5 miles per hour)
• Walking very fast (4½ miles per hour)
• Bicycling (more than 10 miles per hour)
• Heavy yard work (chopping wood)
• Swimming (freestyle laps)
• Aerobics
• Basketball (competitive)
• Tennis (singles)

From U.S. Department of Agriculture: What is physical activity? *June 4, 2011.*

FOCUS ON CHILDREN AND OLDER PERSONS

MyPlate

Children

The USDA offers these tips to help children eat vegetables and fruits. Some measures depend on the child's age.
• Serve vegetables and fruits with meals and as snacks.
• Let children choose vegetables, fruits, and what goes in salads.
• Let children help shop for vegetables and fruits. Let them choose new ones to try.
• Let children clean, peel, or cut up vegetables and fruits.
• Do not mix vegetables. Serve them separately. For example, do not combine peas and carrots.
• Decorate plates and serving dishes with fruit slices.
• Top cereal with berries.
• Make a "smiley face" with fruit. You can use banana slices for the eyes, raisins for the nose, and an orange slice for the mouth.
• Offer dried fruits and raisins in place of candy and chewy fruit snacks.
• Make fruit kabobs. Use pineapple chunks, bananas, grapes, and berries.
• Offer 100% fruit juices instead of soda or other drinks with sugar.
 For physical activity, the USDA recommends the following for children 6 to 17 years of age.
• 60 minutes or more each day of moderate to vigorous physical activity.
• Vigorous activity at least 3 days a week.
• Muscle strengthening activities daily. Climbing and jumping are examples.

Grains Group. Foods made from wheat, rice, oats, cornmeal, barley, or other cereal grains are grain products. Bread, pasta, oatmeal, breakfast cereals, tortillas, and grits are examples.

- *Whole grains* have the entire grain kernel. Whole-wheat flour, bulgur (cracked wheat), oatmeal, whole cornmeal, and brown rice are examples.
- *Refined grains* were processed to remove the grain kernel. They have a fine texture. White flour, white bread, and white rice are examples. They have less dietary fiber than whole grains.
  Grains have these health benefits.
- Reduce the risk of heart disease.
- May prevent constipation.
- May help with weight management.
- May prevent certain birth defects.
- Contain these nutrients—dietary fiber, several B vitamins (thiamin, riboflavin, niacin, folate), and minerals (iron, magnesium, and selenium).

Vegetable Group. Vegetables can be eaten raw or cooked. They may be fresh, frozen, canned, dried, or juice.

- *Dark green vegetables*—bok choy, broccoli, collard greens, dark green leafy lettuce, kale, mesclun, mustard greens, romaine lettuce, spinach, turnips, watercress
- *Red and orange vegetables*—acorn, butternut, and hubbard squashes; carrots; pumpkin; red peppers; sweet potatoes; tomatoes; tomato juice
- *Beans and peas*—black beans, black-eyed peas, garbanzo beans (chickpeas), kidney beans, lentils, navy beans, pinto beans, soybeans, split peas, and white beans
- *Starchy vegetables*—corn, green bananas, green peas, green lima beans, plantains, potatoes, taro, water chestnuts
- *Other vegetables*—artichokes, asparagus, bean sprouts, beets, Brussels sprouts, cabbage, cauliflower, celery, cucumbers, eggplant, green beans, green peppers, iceberg (head) lettuce, mushrooms, okra, onions, parsnips, turnips, wax beans, zucchini
  Vegetables have these health benefits.
- May reduce the risk for stroke, high blood pressure, heart and cardiovascular diseases, and type 2 diabetes.
- May protect against certain cancers. Cancers of the mouth, stomach, and colon-rectum are examples.
- May reduce the risk of kidney stones.
- May reduce the risk of bone loss.
- May help lower calorie intake. Most vegetables are low in fat and calories.
- Contain no cholesterol. (**Cholesterol** *is a soft, waxy substance. It is found in the bloodstream and all body cells.* Dietary sources are from animal foods—egg yolks, meat, poultry, shellfish, milk, and milk products.)
- May prevent certain birth defects.
- Contain these nutrients—potassium, dietary fiber, folate (folic acid), vitamins A and C.

Fruit Group. Any fruit or 100% fruit juice counts as part of the fruit group. Fruits may be fresh, frozen, canned, or dried. Avoid fruits canned in syrup. Syrup contains added sugar. Choose fruits canned in 100% fruit juice or water.
Fruits have these health benefits.

- May reduce the risk for stroke, heart disease, high blood pressure, cardiovascular diseases, obesity, and type 2 diabetes.
- May protect against certain cancers. Cancers of the mouth, stomach, and colon-rectum are examples.
- May reduce the risk of kidney stones.
- May reduce the risk of bone loss.
- May help prevent constipation.
- May help lower calorie intake. Most fruits are low in fat and calories.
- Contain no cholesterol.
- Are low in sodium.
- May prevent certain birth defects.
- Contain these nutrients—potassium, dietary fiber, vitamin C, and folate (folic acid).

Dairy Group. All fluid milk products are part of the dairy group. So are many foods made from milk. Low-fat or fat-free choices are best. The milk group includes all fluid milk, yogurt, and cheese. (Cream, cream cheese, and butter are not in this group.) Health benefits include:

- Helps build and maintain bone mass throughout life. This may reduce the risk of osteoporosis.
- May reduce the risk of cardiovascular disease, type 2 diabetes, and high blood pressure.
- Contains these nutrients—calcium, potassium, and vitamin D.

Protein Foods Group. This group includes all foods made from meat, poultry, seafood, eggs, processed soy products, nuts, and seeds. Beans and peas are included in this group as well as the vegetable group.
When selecting foods from this group, remember:

- To choose lean or low-fat meat and poultry. Higher fat choices include regular ground beef (75% to 80% lean) and chicken with skin.
- Using fat for cooking increases the calories. Fried chicken and eggs fried in butter are examples.
- Salmon, trout, and herring are rich in substances that may reduce the risk of heart disease.
- Liver and other organ meats are high in cholesterol.
- Egg yolks are high in cholesterol. Egg whites are cholesterol-free.
- Processed meats have added sodium (salt). They include ham, sausage, hot dogs, and luncheon and deli meats.
  Many proteins are high in fat and cholesterol. Heart disease is a major risk. However, this group provides nutrients needed for health and body maintenance.
- Protein
- B vitamins (niacin, thiamin, riboflavin, and B_6) and vitamin E
- Iron, zinc, and magnesium

Oils. Oils are fats that are liquid at room temperature. Vegetable oils for cooking are examples. They include canola oil, corn oil, and olive oil. Oils come from plants and fish. Because they have nutrients, the USDA includes oils in food patterns. However, *oils are not a food group.*

Adult women are allowed 5 to 6 teaspoons daily. Adult men are allowed 6 to 7 teaspoons daily. Some foods are high in oil—nuts, olives, some fish, and avocados.

When making oil choices, remember:
* Oils are high in calories.
* The best oil choices come from fish, nuts, and vegetables.
* Some foods are mainly oil. Mayonnaise, certain salad dressings, and soft margarine (tub or squeeze) are examples.
* Oils from plant sources do not contain cholesterol.
* *Solid fats* are solid at room temperature. Common solid fats include butter, milk fat, beef fat (tallow, suet), chicken fat, pork fat (lard), stick margarine, and shortening.
* Oils and solid fats have about 120 calories in each tablespoon.
* Enough oil is usually consumed daily from nuts, fish, cooking oil, and salad dressings.

Nutrients

No food or food group has every essential nutrient. A well-balanced diet ensures an adequate intake of essential nutrients.
* *Protein*—is the most important nutrient. It is needed for tissue growth and repair. Sources include meat, fish, poultry, eggs, milk and milk products, cereals, beans, peas, and nuts.
* *Carbohydrates*—provide energy and fiber for bowel elimination. They are found in fruits, vegetables, breads, cereals, and sugar. Fiber is not digested. It provides the bulky part of chyme for elimination.
* *Fats*—provide energy. They provide flavor and help the body use certain vitamins. Sources include meats, lard, butter, shortening, oils, milk, cheese, egg yolks, and nuts. Unneeded dietary fat is stored as body fat (*adipose tissue*).
* *Vitamins*—are needed for certain body functions. The body stores vitamins A, D, E, and K. Vitamins C and the B complex vitamins are not stored. They must be ingested daily. The lack of a certain vitamin results in illness. See Table 27-2.
* *Minerals*—are needed for bone and tooth formation, nerve and muscle function, fluid balance, and other body processes. Foods containing calcium help prevent musculo-skeletal changes. See Table 27-3, p. 448.
* *Water*—is needed for all body processes (p. 456).

TABLE 27-2	Common Vitamins	
Vitamin	Major Functions	Sources
Vitamin A	Growth; vision; healthy hair, skin, and mucous membranes; resistance to infection	Liver, spinach, green leafy and yellow vegetables, yellow fruits, fish liver oils, egg yolks, butter, cream, whole milk
Vitamin B1 (thiamin)	Muscle tone, nerve function, digestion, appetite, normal elimination, carbohydrate use	Pork, fish, poultry, eggs, liver, breads, pastas, cereals, oatmeal, potatoes, peas, beans, soybeans, peanuts
Vitamin B2 (riboflavin)	Growth, healthy eyes, protein and carbohydrate metabolism, healthy skin and mucous membranes	Milk and milk products, liver, green leafy vegetables, eggs, breads, cereals
Vitamin B3 (niacin)	Protein, fat, and carbohydrate metabolism; nervous system function; appetite; digestive system function	Meat, pork, liver, fish, peanuts, breads and cereals, green vegetables, dairy products
Vitamin B12	Forming red blood cells, protein metabolism, nervous system function	Liver, meats, poultry, fish, eggs, milk, cheese
Folate (folic acid)	Forming red blood cells, intestinal function, protein metabolism	Liver, meats, fish, poultry, green leafy vegetables, whole grains
Vitamin C (ascorbic acid)	Forming substances that hold tissues together; healthy blood vessels, skin, gums, bones, and teeth; wound healing; preventing bleeding; resistance to infection	Citrus fruits, tomatoes, potatoes, cabbage, strawberries, green vegetables, melons
Vitamin D	Absorbing and metabolizing calcium and phosphorus, healthy bones	Fish liver oils, milk, butter, liver, exposure to sun light
Vitamin E	Normal reproduction, forming red blood cells, muscle function	Vegetable oils, milk, eggs, meats, cereals, green leafy vegetables
Vitamin K	Blood clotting	Liver, green leafy vegetables, egg yolks, cheese

TABLE 27-3	Common Minerals	
Mineral	Major Functions	Sources
Calcium	Forming teeth and bones, blood clotting, muscle contraction, heart function, nerve function	Milk and milk products, green leafy vegetables, whole grains, egg yolks, dried peas and beans, nuts
Phosphorus	Forming bones and teeth; use of proteins, fats, and carbohydrates; nerve and muscle function	Meat, fish, poultry, milk and milk products, nuts, egg yolks, dried peas and beans
Iron	Allows red blood cells to carry oxygen	Liver, meat, eggs, green leafy vegetables, breads and cereals, dried peas and beans, nuts
Iodine	Thyroid gland function, growth, metabolism	Iodized salt, seafood, shellfish
Sodium	Fluid balance, nerve and muscle function	Almost all foods
Potassium	Nerve function, muscle contraction, heart function	Fruits, vegetables, cereals, meats, dried peas and beans

Food Labels

Food labels are used to make informed food choices for a healthy diet (Fig. 27-3). Food labels contain information about:

- Serving size and the number of servings in each package.
- Calories. The number of servings eaten determines the number of calories of that food.
- Nutrients—total fat (saturated fat and trans fat), cholesterol, sodium, carbohydrate (dietary fiber, sugars, and added sugar), protein, vitamin D, calcium, iron, and potassium.

How a serving fits into the daily diet is called the *Daily Value (DV)*. The DV is a percent (%). The percent is based on 2000 calories daily. The % DV helps you decide if a food is high or low in a nutrient. According to the Food and Drug Administration (FDA), a 5% DV is low. A DV of 20% or more is high.

MEETING NUTRITIONAL NEEDS

A team approach is needed to meet a person's nutritional needs. The person, nursing team, doctor, dietitian, speech-language pathologist, and occupational therapist are involved. So is the family if necessary. The person's likes, dislikes, and life-long habits are part of the nutritional care plan.

See *Focus on Long-Term Care and Home Care: Meeting Nutritional Needs.*

Nutrition Facts
Serving size 2/3 cup (55g)
Servings Per Container About 8

Amount Per Serving
Calories 230   Calories from Fat 72

	% Daily Value*
Total Fat 8g	12%
Saturated Fat 1g	5%
Trans Fat 0g	
Cholesterol 0mg	0%
Sodium 160mg	7%
Total Carbohydrate 37g	12%
Dietary Fiber 4g	16%
Sugars 1g	
Protein 3g	
Vitamin A	10%
Vitamin C	8%
Calcium	20%
Iron	45%

*Percent Daily Values are based on a 2,000 calorie diet. Your daily value may be higher or lower depending on your calorie needs.

	Calories:	2,000	2,500
Total Fat	Less than	65g	80g
Sat Fat	Less than	20g	25g
Cholesterol	Less than	300mg	300mg
Sodium	Less than	2,400mg	2,400mg
Total Carbohydrate		300g	375g
Dietary Fiber		25g	30g

A

Nutrition Facts
8 servings per container
Serving size   2/3 cup (55g)

Amount per 2/3 cup
Calories   **230**

% DV*	
12%	**Total Fat** 8g
5%	Saturated Fat 1g
	Trans Fat 0g
0%	**Cholesterol** 0mg
7%	**Sodium** 160mg
12%	**Total Carbs** 37g
14%	Dietary Fiber 4g
	Sugars 1g
	Added Sugars 0g
	Protein 3g
10%	**Vitamin D** 2mcg
20%	**Calcium** 260mg
45%	**Iron** 8mg
5%	**Potassium** 235mg

* Footnote on Daily Values (DV) and calories reference to be inserted here.

B

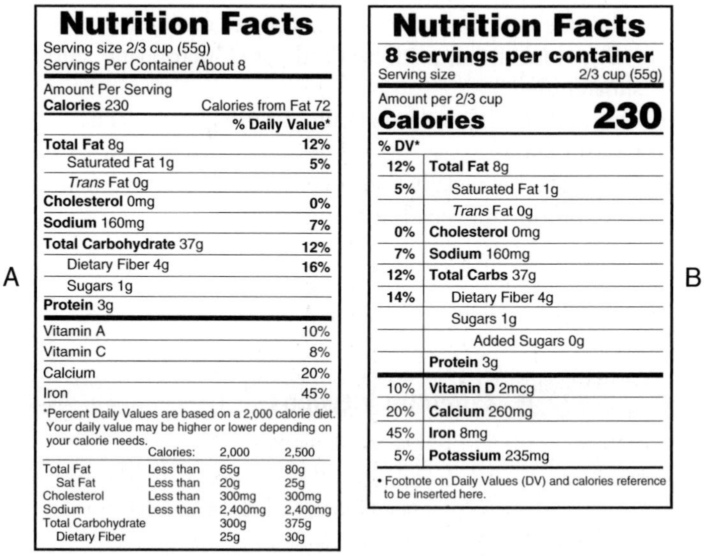

FIGURE 27-3 A, 2015 Nutrition Facts Label. **B,** FDA's proposed Nutrition Facts Label. (NOTE: FDA regulations issued in 2015 and 2016 require updated labels by January 1, 2018.) (From U.S. Food and Drug Administration, *Protecting and Promoting Your Health,* 2015.)

✿ CARING ABOUT CULTURE

Food Practices

Rice, corn, and beans are protein sources in *Mexico.* In the *Philippines,* rice is a main food. And fish, vegetables, and native fruits are preferred. A diet high in sugar and animal fat is common in *Poland.* In *China,* a meal of rice with meat, fish, and vegetables is common. High sodium content is from the use of soy sauce and dried and preserved foods.

Eating beef is common in the *United States.* In *India,* Hindus do not eat beef.

Modified from D'Avanzo CE: Pocket guide to cultural health assessment, ed 4, St Louis, 2008, Mosby.

FOCUS ON LONG-TERM CARE AND HOME CARE

Meeting Nutritional Needs

Long-Term Care

The *Omnibus Budget Reconciliation Act of 1987 (OBRA)* has requirements for food served in nursing centers.

- Each person's nutritional and dietary needs are met.
- The person's diet is well-balanced. It is nourishing and tastes good. Food is well-seasoned. It is not too salty or too sweet.
- Food is appetizing. It has an appealing aroma and is attractive.
- Hot food is served hot. Cold food is served cold. Food servers keep food at the correct temperature.
- Food is served promptly. If not, hot food cools and cold food warms.
- Food is prepared to meet each person's needs. Some people need food cut, ground, or chopped. Others have special diets ordered by the doctor.
- Other foods are offered to residents who refuse the food served. The substituted food must have a similar nutritional value to the first foods served.
- Each person receives at least 3 meals a day. A bedtime snack is offered.
- The center provides needed adaptive equipment (assistive devices) and utensils.

Home Care

You may be assigned to shop for groceries, plan meals, and cook. You need to understand the MyPlate symbol, basic nutrition, and food labels. You also need to know the person's food likes and dislikes and eating habits. For example, some people have the same breakfast every day. Some people have their large meal in the evening, others at noon.

The nurse and dietitian advise you about what to prepare. Remember to:

- Review the person's allowed diet (p. 451).
- Use a good cookbook to plan and prepare meals.
- Plan menus for a full week.
- Check recipe ingredients. Place needed items on your shopping list.
- Try to save money. Check newspapers and the Internet for sales and coupons.
- Give all receipts to the person or family member.
- Store food properly. Refrigerate dairy products and most fresh fruits and vegetables right away. Do the same for meat, fish, or poultry that you will use that day. Freeze the rest and any frozen foods. Dried, packaged, canned, and bottled foods keep well in cabinets.
- See p. 468 for preventing "Foodborne Illness."

Factors Affecting Eating and Nutrition

Many factors affect eating and nutrition.

- *Culture.* Culture influences dietary practices, food choices, and food preparation. Frying, baking, smoking, or roasting food and eating raw food are cultural practices. So is using sauces, herbs, and spices. See *Caring About Culture: Food Practices.*
- *Religion.* Selecting, preparing, and eating food often involve religious practices (Box 27-2, p. 450). A person may follow all, some, or none of the dietary practices of his or her faith. Respect the person's religious practices.
- *Finances.* People with limited incomes often buy the cheaper carbohydrate foods. Their diets often lack protein and certain vitamins and minerals.
- *Appetite.* Appetite relates to the desire for food. Aromas and thoughts of food can stimulate the appetite. *Loss of appetite* (**anorexia**) can occur. Causes include illness, drugs, anxiety, pain, and depression. Unpleasant sights, thoughts, and smells are other causes.
- *Personal choice.* Food likes and dislikes are personal. They begin in childhood with foods served in the home. Food choices depend on how food looks, how it is prepared, its smell, and ingredients. Usually food likes expand with age and social experiences.
- *Body reactions.* People usually avoid foods that cause allergic reactions. They also avoid foods that cause nausea, vomiting, diarrhea, indigestion, gas, or headaches.

- *Illness.* Appetite usually decreases during illness and recovery from injuries. However, nutritional needs increase. The body must fight infection, heal tissue, and replace lost blood cells. Nutrients lost through vomiting and diarrhea need replacement.
- *Drugs.* Drugs can cause loss of appetite, confusion, nausea, constipation, impaired taste, or changes in GI function. They can cause inflammation of the mouth, throat, esophagus, and stomach.
- *Chewing problems.* Mouth, teeth, and gum problems can affect chewing. Examples include oral pain, dry or sore mouth, gum disease (Chapter 22), and dentures that fit poorly. Broken, decayed, or missing teeth also affect chewing, especially the meat group.
- *Swallowing problems.* Stroke; pain; confusion; dry mouth; and diseases of the mouth, throat, and esophagus can affect swallowing. See "The Dysphagia Diet" on p. 454.
- *Disability.* Disease or injury can affect the hands, wrists, and arms. Adaptive equipment (assistive devices) let the person eat independently (Fig. 27-4, p. 450). The speech-language pathologist and occupational therapist teach the person how to use them. Make sure each person has needed devices.
- *Impaired cognitive function.* Impaired cognitive function may affect the person's ability to use eating utensils. And it may affect eating, chewing, and swallowing. Follow the care plan to assist the person.
- *Age.* Many GI changes occur with aging. See *Focus on Children and Older Persons: Factors Affecting Eating and Nutrition,* p. 450.

BOX 27-2	Religion and Dietary Practices

Church of Jesus Christ of Latter-Day Saints (Mormon)
- Alcohol and hot drinks (coffee and tea) are avoided. Caffeine is often avoided.
- Meats are avoided or limited.
- Grains are an important part of the diet.

Greek Orthodox
- Fasting is required during the Great Lent and before other holy days.
- Meat, fish, and dairy products are not eaten during a fast.

Hinduism
- Pork, fowl, ducks, snails, and crabs are avoided.
- No beef is eaten. The cow is a sacred animal to Hindus.
- Products from cows—milk, yogurt, and butter—are allowed.
- Days of fast include Hindu holidays, Sundays, birthdays, and marriage and death anniversaries.

Islam
- All pork and pork products are forbidden.
- Tea, coffee, and alcohol are discouraged.
- Alcohol is not allowed.
- Fasting is practiced on Mondays and Thursdays, for 6 days during the Shawwal (the tenth month of the Islamic calendar), and during the entire month of Ramadan (the ninth month of the Islamic calendar). Fasting means no food or drink from sunrise to sunset.

Judaism (Jewish Faith)
- Foods must be kosher. (*Kosher* means *fit, proper, or correct.*) Food must be prepared according to Jewish law.
- Meat of kosher animals can be eaten—cows, goats, and lambs.
- Chickens, ducks, and geese are kosher fowl.
- Kosher fish have scales and fins—tuna, sardines, carp, salmon, herring, whitefish, and so on. Lobster, shrimp, and clams are not allowed.
- Milk, milk products, and eggs from kosher animals and fowl are allowed.
- Meat and milk cannot be cooked together.
- Meat and milk products cannot be eaten at the same meal. They cannot be served on the same plate.
- Meat and milk products are not prepared or served with the same utensils and dishes. Two sets of utensils and dishes are needed. They are washed and stored separately.
- Fermented grain products are not consumed during Passover—cookies, noodles, alcohol, and so on.

Roman Catholic
- Fasting from meat is required on Ash Wednesday, Good Friday, and all Fridays during Lent.
- Not eating food is required for 1 hour before receiving Holy Communion. Water and drugs are allowed.

Seventh-Day Adventist
- Coffee, tea, and alcohol are avoided.
- Beverages with caffeine (colas) are avoided.
- Some groups have restrictions about meat, fish, and fowl.
- A vegetarian diet is encouraged.

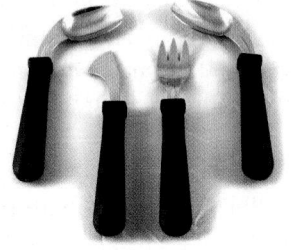 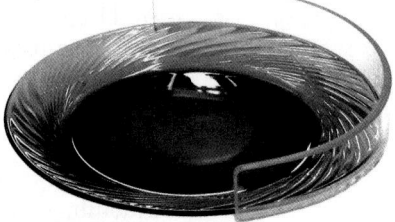 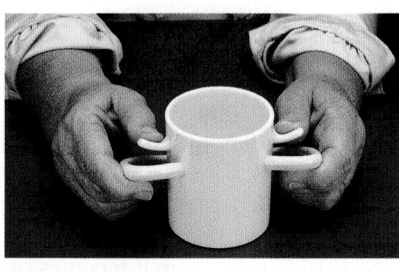

A   B   C

FIGURE 27-4 Adaptive equipment (assistive devices) for eating. **A,** Eating utensils have tapered and angled handles. The knife cuts with slicing and rocking motions. **B,** The plate guard helps keep food on the plate. **C,** The thumb grips on the cup help prevent spilling. (Images courtesy Elderstore, Alpharetta, Ga.)

FOCUS ON CHILDREN AND OLDER PERSONS

Factors Affecting Eating and Nutrition

Older Persons
With aging, changes occur in the GI system.
- Taste and smell dull.
- Appetite decreases.
- Secretion of digestive juices decreases. Hard to digest, fried and fatty foods may cause indigestion.

Some people avoid the high-fiber foods needed for bowel elimination—apricots, celery, and fruits and vegetables with skins and seeds. High-fiber foods are hard to chew and can irritate the intestines.

Foods providing soft bulk are often ordered for persons with chewing problems or constipation. Whole-grain cereals and cooked fruits and vegetables are examples.

Calorie needs are lower. Energy and activity levels are lower. Foods that contain calcium help prevent musculo-skeletal changes. Protein is needed for tissue growth and repair. Because of cost, diets may lack high-protein foods.

SPECIAL DIETS

Doctors may order special diets (Table 27-4).

- For a nutritional deficiency or a disease
- For weight control (gain or loss)
- To remove or decrease certain substances in the diet

The health team considers the need for dietary changes, personal choices, religion, culture, and eating problems. They also consider food allergies and sensitivities. The nurse and dietitian teach the person and family about the diet.

Regular diet, *general diet*, and *house diet* mean no dietary limits or restrictions. Persons with diseases of the heart, kidneys, gallbladder, liver, stomach, or intestines often need special diets. High-protein diets are needed to heal wounds and pressure ulcers. Some persons have bran added to their food. It provides fiber for bowel elimination. Allergies, excess weight, and other disorders also require special diets.

The sodium-controlled diet is often ordered (p. 452). So is a diabetes meal plan (p. 453). Persons with swallowing problems may need a dysphagia diet (p. 454).

TABLE 27-4	Special Diets	
Diet	**Use**	**Foods Allowed/Restricted**
Clear liquid—foods liquid at body temperature and that leave small amounts of residue; non-irritating and non-gas forming	After surgery; for acute illness, infection, nausea and vomiting; and to prepare for GI exams	Water, tea, and coffee (without milk or cream); carbonated drinks; gelatin; fruit juices without pulp (apple, grape, cranberry); fat-free broth; hard candy, sugar, and Popsicles
Full liquid—foods liquid at room temperature or that melt at body temperature	Advance from clear-liquid diet after surgery; for stomach irritation, fever, nausea, and vomiting; for persons unable to chew, swallow, or digest solid foods	Foods on the clear-liquid diet; custard; eggnog; strained soups; strained fruit and vegetable juices; milk and milk-shakes; cooked cereals; plain ice cream and sherbet; pudding; yogurt
Mechanical soft—semi-solid foods that are easily digested	Advance from full-liquid diet; chewing problems, GI disorders, and infections	All liquids; eggs (not fried); broiled, baked, or roasted meat, fish, or poultry that is chopped or shredded; mild cheeses (American, Swiss, cheddar, cream, cottage); strained fruit juices; refined bread (no crust) and crackers; cooked cereal; cooked or pureed vegetables; cooked or canned fruit without skin or seeds; pudding; plain cakes and soft cookies without fruit or nuts
Fiber- and residue-restricted—foods that leave a small amount of residue in the colon	Diseases of the colon and diarrhea	Coffee, tea, milk, carbonated drinks, strained fruit and vegetable juices; refined bread and crackers; creamed and refined cereal; rice; cottage and cream cheese; eggs (not fried); plain puddings and cakes; gelatin; custard; sherbet and ice cream; canned or cooked fruit without skin or seeds; potatoes (not fried); strained cooked vegetables; plain pasta; *no raw fruits or vegetables*
High-fiber—foods that increase residue and fiber in the colon to stimulate peristalsis	Constipation and GI disorders	All fruits and vegetables; whole-wheat bread; whole-grain cereals; fried foods; whole-grain rice; milk, cream, butter, and cheese; meats
Bland—foods that are non-irritating and low in roughage; foods served at moderate temperatures; no strong spices or condiments	Ulcers, gallbladder disorders, and some intestinal disorders; after abdominal surgery	Lean meats; white bread; creamed and refined cereals; cream or cottage cheese; gelatin; plain puddings, cakes, and cookies; eggs (not fried); butter and cream; canned fruits and vegetables without skin and seeds; strained fruit juices; potatoes (not fried); pastas and rice; strained or soft cooked carrots, peas, beets, spinach, squash, and asparagus tips; creamed soups from allowed vegetables; *no fried or spicy foods*
High-calorie—3000 to 4000 calories daily; includes 3 full meals and between-meal snacks	Weight gain and some thyroid problems	Dietary increases in all foods; large portions of regular diet with 3 between-meal snacks
Calorie-controlled—adequate nutrients while controlling calories to promote weight loss and reduce body fat	Weight loss	Foods low in fats and carbohydrates and lean meats; *avoid butter, cream, rice, gravies, salad oils, noodles, cakes, pastries, carbonated and alcoholic drinks, candy, potato chips, and similar foods*

Continued

TABLE 27-4	Special Diets—cont'd	
Diet	Use	Foods Allowed/Restricted
High-iron—foods high in iron	Anemia; after blood loss; for women during the reproductive years	Liver and other organ meats; lean meats; egg yolks; shellfish; dried fruits; dried beans; green leafy vegetables; lima beans; peanut butter; enriched breads and cereals
Fat-controlled (low cholesterol)—foods low in fat and prepared without adding fat	Heart, gallbladder, and liver diseases; disorders of fat digestion; diseases of the pancreas	Skim milk (fat-free) or buttermilk; cottage cheese (*no other cheeses allowed);* gelatin; sherbet; fruit; lean meat, poultry, and fish (baked, broiled, or roasted); fat-free broth; soups made with skim milk (fat-free); margarine; rice, pasta, breads, and cereals; vegetables; potatoes
High-protein—aids and promotes tissue healing	Burns, high fever, infection, and some liver diseases	Meat, milk, eggs, cheese, fish, poultry; breads and cereals; green leafy vegetables
Sodium-controlled—a certain amount of sodium is allowed	Heart disease, fluid retention, liver diseases, and some kidney diseases	Fruits and vegetables and unsalted butter are allowed; *adding salt at the table is not allowed; highly salted foods and foods high in sodium are not allowed; the use of salt during cooking may be restricted*
Gluten-free—foods without the gluten protein	Celiac disease	Beans; seeds; nuts; eggs; meats, fish, and poultry (*without breading, batter, or marinade);* fruits and vegetables; most dairy foods; gluten-free grains and starches (arrowroot, corn, cornmeal, hominy, flax, millet, rice, soy, and tapioca); gluten-free flours (rice, soy, corn, potato, bean); *no foods containing wheat, barley, triticale, or rye*
Diabetes meal plan—the same amount of carbohydrates, protein, and fat are eaten at the same time each day	Diabetes	Determined by nutritional and energy requirements

The Sodium-Controlled Diet

The average amount of sodium in the daily diet is greater than 3000 mg (milligrams). The body needs no more than 2400 mg a day. Healthy people excrete excess sodium in the urine.

The USDA recommends that sodium intake be reduced to 1500 mg daily for:

- Persons aged 51 and older
- African-Americans of any age (including children)
- Persons who have hypertension, diabetes, or chronic kidney disease (including children)

According to the USDA, persons needing to lower blood pressure should:

- Consume no more than 2400 mg of sodium daily.
- Lower sodium intake to 1500 mg daily to lower blood pressure more.
- Lower sodium intake by at least 1000 mg daily even if the goals above cannot be met.

Heart, liver, and kidney diseases and certain drugs cause the body to retain extra sodium. Sodium causes the body to retain water. With too much sodium, water is retained. Tissues swell with water. There is excess fluid in the blood vessels. The heart works harder. With heart disease, the extra workload can cause serious problems or death.

Sodium-control decreases the amount of sodium in the body. Less water is retained. Less water in the tissues and blood vessels reduces the heart's workload.

The doctor orders the amount of sodium allowed. Sodium-controlled diets involve:

- Omitting high-sodium foods (Box 27-3)
- Not adding salt to food at the table
- Limiting the amount of salt used in cooking
- Diet planning

BOX 27-3	High-Sodium Foods

Grains
- Baked goods—biscuits, muffins, cakes, cookies, pies, pastries, sweet rolls, donuts, and so on
- Breads and rolls
- Cereals—cold, instant hot
- Noodle mixes
- Pancakes
- Salted snack foods—pretzels, corn chips, popcorn, crackers, chips, and so on
- Stuffing mixes
- Waffles

Vegetables
- Canned vegetables
- Olives
- Pickles and other pickled vegetables
- Relish
- Sauerkraut
- Tomato sauce or paste
- Vegetable juices—tomato, V8, Bloody Mary mixes
- Vegetables with sauces, creams, or seasonings

Fruits
- None—fruits are not high in sodium

Dairy Group
- Buttermilk
- Cheese
- Commercial dips made with sour cream

Protein Foods
- Bacon and Canadian bacon
- Canned meats and fish—chicken, tuna, salmon, anchovies, sardines
- Caviar
- Chipped, dried, and corned beef and other meats
- Deli meats—turkey, ham, bologna, salami, pastrami, and so on

Protein Foods—cont'd
- Dried fish
- Ham
- Herring
- Hot dogs (frankfurters)
- Liverwurst
- Lox and smoked salmon
- Mackerel
- Pepperoni
- Salt pork
- Sausages
- Scrapple
- Shellfish—shrimp, crab, clams, oysters, scallops, lobster

Other
- Asian foods—Chinese, Japanese, East Indian Thai, Vietnamese
- Baking soda and baking powder
- Catsup (ketchup)
- Cocoa mixes
- Commercially prepared dinners—frozen, canned, boxed, and so on
- Mayonnaise
- Mexican foods
- Mustard
- Pasta dishes—lasagna, manicotti, ravioli
- Peanut butter
- Pizzas
- Pot pies
- Salad dressings
- Salted nuts or seeds
- Sauces—soy, teriyaki, Worcestershire, steak, barbecue, pasta, chili, cocktail
- Seasoning salts—garlic, onion, celery, meat tenderizers, monosodium glutamate (MSG), and so on
- Soups—canned, packaged, instant, dried, bouillon

Diabetes Meal Plan

Diabetes is a chronic illness in which the body cannot produce or use insulin properly (Chapter 46). The pancreas produces and secretes insulin. Insulin lets the body use sugar. Without enough insulin, sugar builds up in the bloodstream. It is not used by cells for energy. Diabetes is usually treated with insulin or other drugs, diet, and exercise.

A meal plan for healthy eating is developed. Consistency is key. It involves:

- Food preferences (likes, eating habits, meal times, culture, and life-style). Food amounts and preparation methods may be restricted.
- Calories needed. The same amount of carbohydrates, protein, and fat are eaten each day.
- Eating meals and snacks at regular times. The person eats at regular times every day to maintain a certain blood sugar level.

Serve meals and snacks on time. Always check what was eaten. Report what the person did and did not eat. A between-meal snack makes up for what was not eaten (p. 466). The nurse tells you what to provide. The amount of insulin given depends on daily food intake. Report changes in the person's eating habits.

The Dysphagia Diet

Dysphagia means *difficulty* (dys) *swallowing* (phagia). See Box 27-4 for signs and symptoms.

- A *slow swallow* means the person has difficulty getting enough food and fluids for good nutrition and fluid balance.
- An *unsafe swallow* means that food enters the airway (aspiration). *Aspiration is breathing fluid, food, vomitus, or an object into the lungs* (Chapter 28).

Food thickness is changed to meet the person's needs (see Box 27-4). The doctor, speech-language pathologist, occupational therapist, dietitian, and nurse choose the right food thickness.

Safety and comfort are important when feeding a person with dysphagia. You must:

- Know the signs and symptoms of dysphagia (see Box 27-4).
- Feed the person according to the care plan.
- Follow aspiration precautions (Box 27-5) and the care plan.
- Report changes in how the person eats.
- Observe for signs and symptoms of aspiration: choking, coughing, or difficulty breathing during or after meals, and abnormal breathing or respiratory sounds. Report these observations at once.

BOX 27-5	Aspiration Precautions

- Help the person with meals and snacks. Follow the care plan.
- Position the person upright as the nurse and care plan direct. The person maintains this position for at least 1 hour after eating.
- Support the upper back, shoulders, and neck with a pillow.
- Observe for signs and symptoms of aspiration during meals and snacks.
- Check the person's mouth after eating for pocketing. Check inside the cheeks, under the tongue, and on the roof of the mouth. Remove any food.
- Provide mouth care after eating.
- Report and record your observations.

FOOD INTAKE

Food intake is measured in different ways. Follow agency policy for the method used.

- *Percentage of food eaten.* Intake ranges from 0 to 100 percent (%). Some agencies record the percent of the whole meal tray. Others record the percent of each food item eaten. See Figure 27-5.
- *Calorie counts.* Note what the person ate and how much. For example, a chicken breast, rice, beans, a roll, pudding, and 2 pats of butter were served. The person ate all the chicken, half the rice, and the roll. One pat of butter was used. The beans and pudding were not eaten. Note these on the flow sheet. A nurse or dietitian converts these portions into calories. See *Focus on Math: Food Intake.*

BOX 27-4	Dysphagia

Signs and Symptoms

The person:

- Avoids food that needs chewing.
- Avoids food with certain textures and temperatures.
- Tires during a meal.
- Has food spill out of the mouth while eating.
- "Pockets" or "squirrels" food in the cheeks. This means that food remains or is hidden in the mouth.
- Eats slowly, especially solid foods.
- Complains that food will not go down or that the food is stuck.
- Coughs or chokes before, during, or after swallowing.
- Regurgitates food after eating (Chapter 28).
- Spits out food suddenly and almost violently.
- Has food come up through the nose.
- Has hoarseness—especially after eating.
- Makes gurgling sounds while talking or breathing after swallowing.
- Has a runny nose, sneezes, or has excessive drooling.
- Complains of frequent heartburn.
- Has a decreased appetite.

Dysphagia Diet

- *Thickened liquid*—No lumps. Pureed with milk, gravy, or broth to thickness of baby food. Thickener is added to some foods and fluids as needed. Does not mound on a plate. May be called *creamy* or a *sauce*. Stir before serving if the food settles.
- *Medium thick (nectar-like)*—The thickness of nectar or V8 juice (does not hold its shape). Stir right before serving.
- *Extra thick (honey-like)*—Thick like honey. Mounds a bit on a spoon. Can drink from a cup. Stir before serving.
- *Yogurt-like*—Thick like yogurt or pudding. Holds its shape. Served with a spoon.
- *Puree*—No lumps; mounds on a plate. May be thick like mashed potatoes.

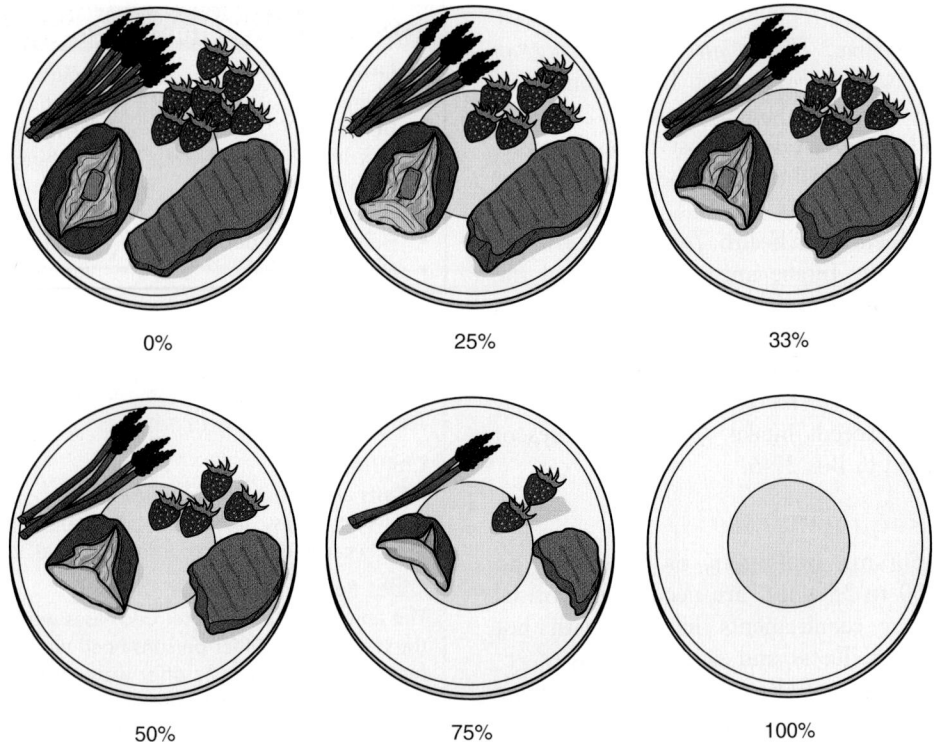

FIGURE 27-5 Percent of food eaten.

FOCUS ON **MATH**

Food Intake

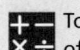 To measure food intake, you need a basic understanding of percents. Percents measure parts of a whole (Fig. 27-6). The "whole" is written as 100%.

To measure food intake, compare the food left to what was served. Depending on agency policy and the food type, *estimate* or *calculate* food intake. To estimate, record the approximate amount of food eaten. See Figure 27-5. To calculate:

1 Subtract the amount of food left from the amount served. (This is the amount the person ate.)
2 Divide the number from step 1 by the amount served (the number of pieces that make up the whole).
3 Multiply the number from step 2 by 100 to convert it into a percent. (*Percent* means *out of 100*.)

For example, a person was served 8 apple slices with 2 slices remaining on the tray.

8 slices – 2 slices = 6 slices
The person ate 6 apple slices; 8 were served.
6 slices ÷ 8 slices = 0.75 of the slices served
$0.75 \times 100 = 75\%$
75% of the apple slices were eaten.

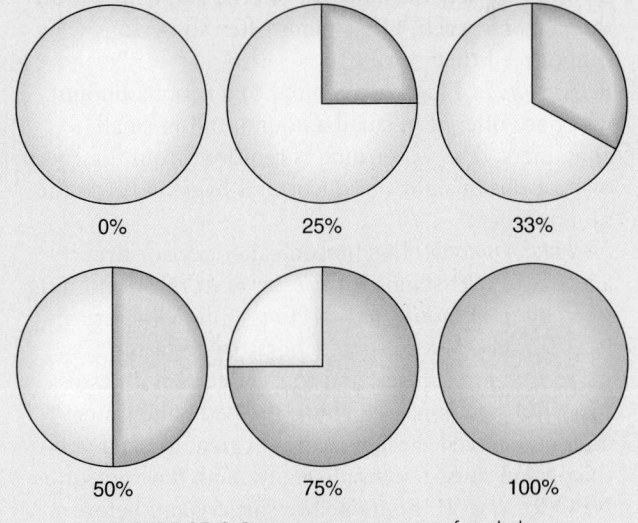

FIGURE 27-6 Percents measure parts of a whole.

FLUID BALANCE

Water is needed to live. *Hydration means having an adequate amount of water in body tissues.* Death can result from too much or too little water. Water is ingested through fluids and foods. Water is lost through urine, feces, and vomit. It is also lost through the skin (perspiration) and the lungs (expiration).

Fluid balance is needed for health. *Intake (input) is the amount of fluid taken in.* Intake must roughly equal the *amount of fluid lost (output).* When fluid intake exceeds fluid output *body tissues swell with water (edema).* Edema is common in people with heart and kidney diseases. *Dehydration is a decrease in the amount of water in body tissues.* Fluid output exceeds intake. Common causes of dehydration are listed in Box 27-6.

Normal Fluid Requirements

An adult needs 1500 mL (milliliters) of water daily to survive. About 2000 to 2500 mL are needed for normal fluid balance. Water requirements increase with hot weather, exercise, fever, illness, and excess fluid losses.

See *Focus on Children and Older Persons: Normal Fluid Requirements.*

Special Fluid Orders

The doctor may order the amount of fluid a person can have during a 24-hour period. This is done to maintain fluid balance. Intake and output (I&O) records are kept. Common fluid orders are:

- *Encourage fluids.* The person drinks an increased amount of fluid. The order states the amount to ingest. A variety of fluids are offered and kept within the person's reach. Offer fluids often to persons who cannot feed themselves.
- *Restrict fluids.* Fluids are limited to a certain amount. They are offered in small amounts and in small containers. The water mug is removed from the room or kept out of sight. Frequent oral hygiene keeps the mouth moist.
- *Nothing by mouth.* The person cannot eat or drink anything. *NPO* stands for *non per os.* It means nothing *(non)* by *(per)* mouth *(os).* NPO is ordered before and after surgery, before some laboratory tests and diagnostic procedures, and to treat certain illnesses. An NPO sign is posted above the bed. The water mug is removed. Frequent oral hygiene is needed but the person must not swallow any fluid. The person is NPO for 6 to 10 hours before surgery and before some laboratory tests and diagnostic procedures. Follow agency policy.
- *Thickened liquids.* All fluids are thickened, including water. The thickness depends on the person's ability to swallow (see Box 27-4). Thickener is added before fluids are served. Or thickened commercial fluids are used.

BOX 27-6	Dehydration—Common Causes
• Bleeding • Coma • Dementia • Diarrhea • Drug therapy • Fever • Fluid intake: poor • Fluid restriction	• Fluids: refusing • Functional impairments: difficulty drinking, reaching fluids, communicating fluid needs • Sweating: excess • Urine production: increased • Vomiting

FOCUS ON CHILDREN AND OLDER PERSONS

Normal Fluid Requirements

Children
Infants and young children have more body water than adults do. Excess fluid losses cannot be tolerated. They quickly cause death in an infant or child.

Older Persons
The amount of body water decreases with age. So does the thirst sensation. Older persons need water but they may not feel thirsty. You need to offer water often. Older persons are at risk for diseases that affect fluid balance. Examples include heart disease, kidney disease, cancer, and diabetes. Some drugs cause the body to lose fluids. Others cause the body to retain water. Dehydration and edema are risks. Some persons have special fluid orders.

Intake and Output Records

The doctor or nurse may order I&O (intake and output) measurements.

- *Intake.* All fluids taken by mouth are recorded. All oral fluids are measured and recorded—water, milk, coffee, tea, juices, soups, and soft drinks. So are foods that melt at room temperature—ice cream, sherbet, custard, pudding, gelatin, and Popsicles. The nurse measures and records intravenous (IV) fluids and tube feedings (Chapter 28).
- *Output.* Urine, vomitus, diarrhea, and wound drainage amounts are recorded.

I&O records are used to evaluate fluid balance and kidney function. They help in planning medical treatment. They also are kept when the person has special fluid orders.

Measuring Intake and Output. Intake and output are measured in milliliters (mL). See Box 27-7 for amounts to know.

BOX 27-7	I&O Converting Measures
1 cubic centimeter (cc) = 1 mL 1 teaspoon = 5 mL 1 tablespoon = 15 mL 1 oz = 30 mL	1 cup = 240 mL 1 pint = about 500 mL 1 quart = about 1000 mL 1 liter (L) = 1000 mL

You also need to know the serving sizes of bowls, dishes, cups, pitchers, mugs, glasses, and other containers. This information may be on the I&O record (Fig. 27-7). Or the serving size is on the container.

A measuring container for fluid is called a **graduate.** It is used to measure left-over fluids, urine, vomitus, and drainage from suction. Like a measuring cup, the graduate is marked in ounces (oz) and milliliters (Fig. 27-8, p. 458). Plastic urinals and kidney basins also have amounts marked. Hold the measuring device at eye level to read the amount (Fig. 27-9, p. 458).

An I&O record is kept. When intake or output is measured, the amount is recorded in the correct column (see Fig. 27-7). Amounts are totaled at the end of the shift and 24-hour day. The totals are recorded in the person's chart. They also are shared during the end-of-shift report.

The purpose of measuring I&O and how to help are explained to the person. Some persons measure and record their intake. Family members may help. The urinal, commode, bedpan, or specimen pan is used to void. Remind the person not to void in the toilet. Also remind the person not to put toilet tissue into the receptacle.

See *Focus on Math: Measuring Intake and Output*, p. 458.

See *Delegation Guidelines: Measuring Intake and Output*, p. 459.

See *Promoting Safety and Comfort: Measuring Intake and Output*, p. 459.

See procedure: *Measuring Intake and Output*, p. 459.

Text continued on p. 460.

FLUID BALANCE CHART

OSF℠
ST. JOSEPH MEDICAL CENTER
Bloomington, Illinois

DATE 6/15

Water Glass	250mL
Styrofoam Cup	180mL
Cup (coffee)	250mL
Milk Carton	240mL
Pop (1 can)	360mL
Broth-Soup	175mL
Juice Carton	120mL
Juice Glass	120mL
Jello	120mL
Ice Cream / Ice Chips	120mL / 1/2 amt. of mL's in cup
Pitcher (Yellow)	1000mL

	INTAKE			OUTPUT					
					URINE		OTHER		CONT. IRRIGATION
TIME	ORAL	Parenteral	Amt. mL Absbd.		Method Collected	Amt. (mL)	Method Collected	Amt. (mL)	In	Out
2400-0100		mL from previous shift			V	150				
0100-0200							Vom.	150		
0200-0300										
0300-0400										
0400-0500										
0500-0600	125				V	200				
0600-0700										
0700-0800										
	125	8 - hour Sub-total			8-hr T	350	8-hr T	150		
0800-0900	400	mL from previous shift			V	250				
0900-1000	100									
1000-1100										
1100-1200										
1200-1300	400				V	250				
1300-1400										
1400-1500	200									
1500-1600										
	1100	8 - hour Sub-total			8-hr T	500	8-hr T			
1600-1700		mL from previous shift			V	270				
1700-1800	350									
1800-1900	50									
1900-2000	200									
2000-2100					V	400				
2100-2200										
2200-2300										
2300-2400										
	600	8 - hour Sub-total			8-hr T	670	8-hr T			
	1825	24 - hour Sub-total			24-hr T	1520	24-hr T	150		

310' Marie Mills

Source Key:		Source Key:	
URINE		**OTHER**	
V	- Voided	G.I.T.	- Gastric Intestinal Tube
C	- Catheter	T.T.	- T. Tube
INC	- Incontinent	Vom.	- Vomitus
U.C.	- Ureteral Catheter	Liq S.	- Liquid Stool
		H.V.	- Hemovac

Form No. MF36722 (Rev. 5/97) **MFI**

FIGURE 27-7 A sample intake and output (I&O) record. (Modified from OSF St. Joseph Medical Center, Bloomington, Ill.)

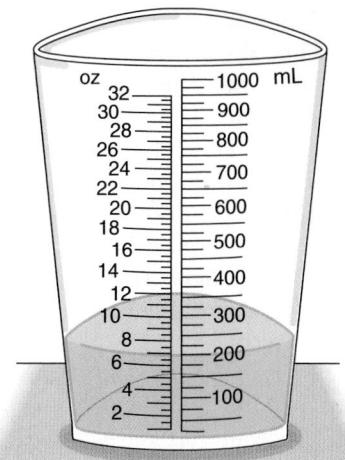

FIGURE 27-8 A graduate marked in ounces (oz) and milliliters (mL).

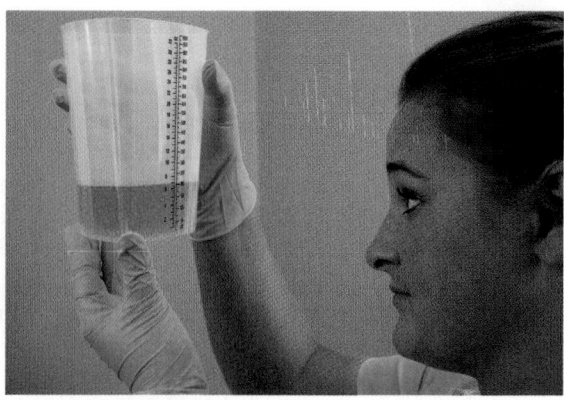

FIGURE 27-9 A graduate is held at eye level to read the amount.

FOCUS ON MATH

Measuring Intake and Output

To measure I&O, you must accurately read the container measurements. And you may have to do some math.

Measuring Intake
To measure intake, subtract the amount left in each liquid served from the full serving amount. Add the intake amounts from each liquid together.

Intake is measured in mL (milliliters). Some containers show the serving amount in oz (ounces). You need to convert (change) the serving amount from oz to mL. One oz equals 30 mL (1 oz = 30 mL). To convert, multiply the number of oz by 30. For example:

A coffee cup holds 8 oz. Multiply 8 oz by 30 (the number of mL in each oz). The full serving amount is 240 mL.

$$8 \text{ oz} \times 30 \text{ mL/oz} = 240 \text{ mL}$$
(mL/oz is read as "milliliters per ounce")

You measured 90 mL left in the cup. Now subtract 90 mL (amount left) from 240 mL (serving amount). The person drank 150 mL.

$$240 \text{ mL (full serving)} - 90 \text{ mL (amount left)} = 150 \text{ mL intake}$$

Measuring Output
Graduates, urinals, specimen pans, and other containers are marked in oz and mL. Not all lines are labeled. To calculate unlabeled measurements (Fig. 27-10):

1. Choose the labeled line above the fluid level and the labeled line below it.

$$400 \text{ mL and } 300 \text{ mL}$$

2. Subtract these 2 numbers. The result is called the *difference*.

$$400 \text{ mL} - 300 \text{ mL} = 100 \text{ mL}$$

3. Count the number of spaces between the 2 labeled lines in step 1.

4 spaces

4. Divide the difference in step 2 by the number of spaces.

$$100 \text{ mL} \div 4 \text{ spaces} = 25 \text{ mL}$$
Each line increases by 25 mL.

Totaling Intake and Output
Intake and output amounts are each totaled at the end of the shift and 24-hour day. See Figure 27-7. Add the amounts for intake and the amounts for output. For example:

- *For a total shift output amount:* A person voided 3 times during your shift—200 mL, 250 mL, and 100 mL. The total output for your shift is 550 mL.

$$200 \text{ mL} + 250 \text{ mL} + 100 \text{ mL} = 550 \text{ mL}$$

- *For a total 24-hour intake amount:* A person had 125 mL during the first shift, 1100 mL during the second shift, and 600 mL during the third shift. The total 24-hour day amount is 1825 mL.

$$125 \text{ mL} + 1100 \text{ mL} + 600 \text{ mL} = 1825 \text{ mL}$$

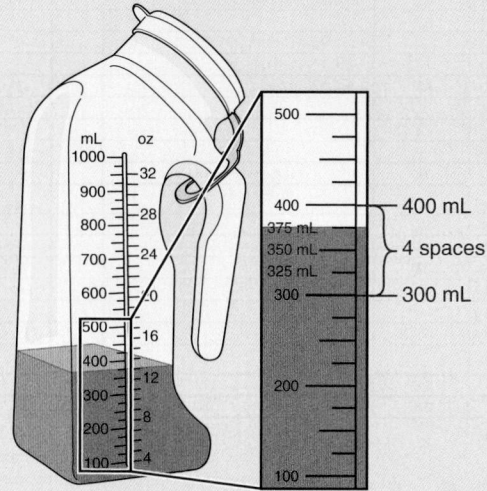

$$400 \text{ mL} - 300 \text{ mL} = 100 \text{ mL}$$
$$100 \text{ mL} \div 4 = 25 \text{ mL}$$
Each line increases by 25 mL

FIGURE 27-10 Calculating unlabeled measurements. Divide the difference between 2 labeled lines by the number of spaces between the 2 lines. For example, each line on the urinal increases by 25 mL. The measurements between 300 mL and 400 mL are 325 mL, 350 mL, and 375 mL.

DELEGATION GUIDELINES
Measuring Intake and Output

When measuring I&O, you need this information from the nurse and the care plan.
- If the person has a special fluid order (p. 456)
- When to report measurements—hourly or end-of-shift
- What the person uses for voiding—urinal, bedpan, commode, or specimen pan (Chapter 24)
- If the person has a catheter (Chapter 25)
- What patient or resident concerns to report at once

PROMOTING SAFETY AND COMFORT
Measuring Intake and Output

Safety
Urine may contain microbes and blood. Microbes can grow in urinals, commodes, bedpans, specimen pans, and drainage systems. Follow Standard Precautions and the Bloodborne Pathogen Standard to handle such equipment. Thoroughly clean the item with a disinfectant after it is used.

Comfort
Promptly measure the contents of urinals, bedpans, commodes, and specimen pans. This helps prevent or reduce odors. Odors can disturb the person.

Measuring Intake and Output

QUALITY OF LIFE
- Knock before entering the person's room.
- Address the person by name.
- Introduce yourself by name and title.
- Explain the procedure before starting and during the procedure.
- Protect the person's rights during the procedure.
- Handle the person gently during the procedure.

PRE-PROCEDURE
1. Follow *Delegation Guidelines: Measuring Intake and Output.* See *Promoting Safety and Comfort: Measuring Intake and Output.*
2. Practice hand hygiene.
3. Collect the following.
   - I&O record
   - Graduates
   - Gloves

PROCEDURE
4. Put on gloves.
5. Measure intake.
   a. Pour liquid remaining in the container into the graduate. Avoid spills and splashes on the outside of the graduate.
   b. Measure the amount at eye level (see Fig. 27-9). Keep the graduate level.
   c. Check the serving amount on the I&O record. Or check the serving size of each container.
   d. Subtract the remaining amount from the full serving amount. Note the amount. (For example, a cup holds 250 mL. The amount in the graduate is 50 mL. 250 mL − 50 mL = 200 mL.)
   e. Pour fluid in the graduate back into the container.
   f. Repeat steps 5, a-e for each liquid.
   g. Add the amounts from each liquid together.
   h. Record the time and amount on the I&O record.
6. Measure output as follows.
   a. Pour the fluid into the graduate used to measure output. Avoid spills and splashes on the outside of the graduate.
   b. Measure the amount at eye level. Keep the graduate level.
   c. Dispose of fluid in the toilet. Avoid splashes.
7. Clean and rinse the graduates. Dispose of rinse in the toilet and flush. Return the graduates to their proper place.
8. Clean, rinse, and disinfect the voiding receptacle or drainage container. Dispose of rinse in the toilet and flush. Return the item to its proper place.
9. Remove and discard the gloves. Practice hand hygiene.
10. Record the output amount on the person's I&O record.

POST-PROCEDURE
11. Provide for comfort. (See the inside of the front cover.)
12. Place the call light and other needed items within reach.
13. Complete a safety check of the room. (See the inside of the front cover.)
14. Report and record your observations.

MEETING FOOD AND FLUID NEEDS

Weakness, illness, and confusion can affect appetite and ability to eat. So can unpleasant odors, sights, and sounds. An uncomfortable position, oral hygiene needs, elimination needs, and pain also affect appetite.

See *Focus on Communication: Meeting Food and Fluid Needs.*

Preparing for Meals

Preparing patients and residents for meals promotes comfort. To promote comfort:

- Assist with elimination needs.
- Provide oral hygiene. Make sure dentures are in place.
- Make sure eyeglasses and hearing aids are in place.
- Make sure incontinent persons are clean and dry.
- Position the person in a comfortable position.
- Assist the person with hand-washing.
  See *Delegation Guidelines: Preparing for Meals.*
  See *Promoting Safety and Comfort: Preparing for Meals.*
  See procedure: *Preparing the Person for a Meal.*

Preparing the Person for a Meal

QUALITY OF LIFE

- Knock before entering the person's room.
- Address the person by name.
- Introduce yourself by name and title.

- Explain the procedure before starting and during the procedure.
- Protect the person's rights during the procedure.
- Handle the person gently during the procedure.

PRE-PROCEDURE

1 Follow *Delegation Guidelines: Preparing for Meals.* See *Promoting Safety and Comfort: Preparing for Meals.*
2 Practice hand hygiene.
3 Collect the following.
   - Equipment for oral hygiene (Chapter 22)
   - Bedpan and cover, urinal, commode, or specimen pan
   - Toilet tissue

   - Wash basin
   - Soap
   - Washcloth
   - Towel
   - Gloves
4 Provide for privacy.

PROCEDURE

5 Make sure eyeglasses and hearing aids are in place.
6 Assist with oral hygiene. Make sure dentures are in place. Wear gloves and practice hand hygiene after removing and discarding them.
7 Assist with elimination. Make sure the incontinent person is clean and dry. Wear gloves and practice hand hygiene after removing and discarding them.
8 Assist with hand-washing. Wear gloves and practice hand hygiene after removing and discarding them.
9 *If the person will eat in bed:*
   a Raise the head of the bed to a comfortable position—Fowler's (45 to 60 degrees) or high-Fowler's (60 to 90 degrees). (NOTE: Some state competency tests require that the person sit upright at least 45 degrees to eat, others require 75 to 90 degrees.)
   b Remove items from the over-bed table. Clean the table.
   c Adjust the over-bed table in front of the person.

10 *If the person will sit in a chair:*
   a Position the person in a chair or wheelchair.
   b Remove items from the over-bed table. Clean the table.
   c Adjust the over-bed table in front of the person.
11 Assist the person to the dining area. (This step is for the person who eats in a dining area.)

POST-PROCEDURE

12 Provide for comfort. (See the inside of the front cover.)
13 Place the call light and other needed items within reach.
14 Empty, clean, rinse, and disinfect equipment. Return equipment to its proper place. Wear gloves and practice hand hygiene after removing and discarding them.
15 Straighten the room. Eliminate unpleasant noise, odors, or equipment.

16 Unscreen the person.
17 Complete a safety check of the room. (See the inside of the front cover.)
18 Practice hand hygiene.

Serving Meals

Food is served in containers with covers that keep foods at the correct temperature. Hot food is kept hot. Cold food is kept cold. Uncover food just before the person eats. Uncovered food changes temperature quickly.

Serve meals after preparing patients and residents for meals. If they are ready to eat, you can serve meals promptly. Doing so keeps food at the correct temperature.

Some agencies have "room service" meal programs. A full menu (breakfast, lunch, dinner) is in the person's room. When ready to eat, the person calls the dietary department to place an order. Food is served a short while later. This program allows the person to eat when hungry. For a fee, visitors can order food to dine with the person.

Serve meals in the assigned order. In nursing centers, residents seated at tables are served at the same time.

If food is not served within 15 minutes, re-check food temperatures. Follow agency policy. If not at the correct temperature, get fresh food. Temperature guides and food thermometers are in dining rooms and in nursing unit kitchens. Some agencies allow re-heating in microwave ovens.

See *Focus on Long-Term Care and Home Care: Serving Meals.*

See *Delegation Guidelines: Serving Meals.*

See *Promoting Safety and Comfort: Serving Meals.*

See *Teamwork and Time Management: Serving Meals.*

See procedure: *Serving Meal Trays.*

FOCUS ON LONG-TERM CARE AND HOME CARE

Serving Meals

Long-Term Care

The following dining programs are common in nursing centers.

- *Social dining.* A table seats 4 to 6 residents (Fig. 27-11). Food is served as in a restaurant. Residents are oriented and can feed themselves. Some are quietly confused. Residents must be able to feed themselves and not disrupt others.
- *Family dining.* Food is served in bowls and on platters. Residents serve and feed themselves as at home.
- *Low-stimulation dining.* Meal time distractions are prevented. The health team decides on the best place for each person to sit.
- *Restaurant-style menus.* The person selects food from a menu. This program allows more food choices. The person is served as in a restaurant.
- *Open dining.* A buffet is open for several hours. Residents can eat any time while the buffet is open.

DELEGATION GUIDELINES

Serving Meals

To serve meal trays, you need this information from the nurse and the care plan.

- The person's food allergies (if any)
- What adaptive equipment (assistive devices) the person uses
- If the person needs help opening cartons, cutting food, buttering bread, and so on
- If the person's food intake (p. 454) and fluid intake (p. 456) are measured
- If calorie counts are done (p. 454)
- When to report observations
- What patient or resident concerns to report at once

PROMOTING SAFETY AND COMFORT

Serving Meals

Safety

Always check food temperature after re-heating. Food that is too hot can cause burns.

Comfort

Check the person's position when serving a meal. The position may have changed after the person was prepared to eat. Provide other comfort measures as needed. See the inside of the front cover.

TEAMWORK AND TIME MANAGEMENT

Serving Meals

Meal trays are served in the order set by the health team. You will serve trays to your patients and residents and to those assigned to other nursing assistants. Your co-workers will do the same. The goal is to serve trays quickly. This keeps food at the desired temperature.

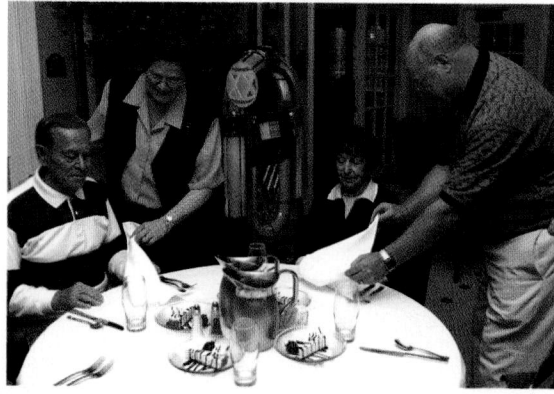

FIGURE 27-11 These residents are eating in the dining room. Volunteers help as needed.

Serving Meal Trays

QUALITY OF LIFE

- Knock before entering the person's room.
- Address the person by name.
- Introduce yourself by name and title.

- Explain the procedure before starting and during the procedure.
- Protect the person's rights during the procedure.
- Handle the person gently during the procedure.

PRE-PROCEDURE

1 Follow *Delegation Guidelines: Serving Meals.* See *Promoting Safety and Comfort: Serving Meals.*

2 Practice hand hygiene.

PROCEDURE

3 Make sure the tray is complete. Check items on the tray with the dietary card. Makes sure adaptive equipment (assistive devices) are included.

4 Identify the person. Check the ID (identification) bracelet against the dietary card. Use 2 identifiers (Chapter 13). Also call the person by name.

5 Place the tray within the person's reach. Adjust the over-bed table as needed.

6 Remove food covers. Open cartons, cut food into bite-sized pieces, butter bread, and so on as needed (Fig. 27-12). Season food as the person prefers and is allowed on the care plan.

7 Place the napkin, clothes protector, adaptive equipment (assistive devices), and eating utensils within reach.

8 Place the call light within reach.

9 Do the following when the person is done eating.
  a Measure and record fluid intake if ordered (p. 456).
  b Note the amount and type of foods eaten (p. 454).
  c Check for and remove any food in the mouth (pocketing). Wear gloves. Practice hand hygiene after removing and discarding them.
  d Remove the tray.
  e Clean spills. Change used linens and soiled clothing.
  f Help the person return to bed if needed.
  g Assist with oral hygiene and hand-washing. Wear gloves. Practice hand hygiene after removing and discarding the gloves.

POST-PROCEDURE

10 Provide for comfort. (See the inside of the front cover.)

11 Place the call light and other needed items within reach.

12 Raise or lower bed rails. Follow the care plan.

13 Complete a safety check of the room. (See the inside of the front cover.)

14 Follow agency policy for used linens.

15 Practice hand hygiene.

16 Report and record your observations.

Feeding the Person

Weakness, paralysis, casts, confusion, and other limits can make self-feeding impossible. These persons are fed.

Serve food and fluids in the order the person prefers. Offer fluids during the meal. Fluids help the person chew and swallow.

Use teaspoons to feed the person. They are less likely to cause injury than forks. The teaspoon should be only one-third (⅓) full. This portion is chewed and swallowed easily. Some people need smaller portions. Follow the care plan.

Persons who need to be fed are often angry, humiliated, and embarrassed. Some are depressed, resentful, or refuse to eat. Let them do what they can. Some can manage "finger foods" (bread, cookies, crackers). If strong enough, let them hold milk or juice cups (never hot drinks). Follow activity limits ordered by the doctor. Provide support. Encourage them to try, even if food is spilled.

Visually impaired persons are often very aware of food aromas. They may know the food served. Describe what is on the tray and what you are offering. For persons who feed themselves, describe foods and fluids and their place on the tray. Use the numbers on a clock for the location of foods (Fig. 27-13).

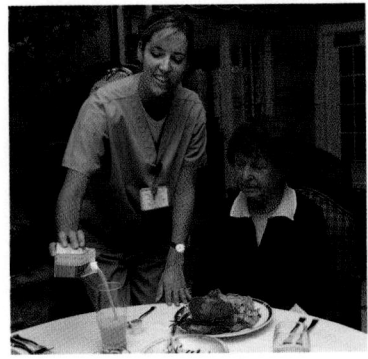

FIGURE 27-12 Cartons and containers are opened for the person.

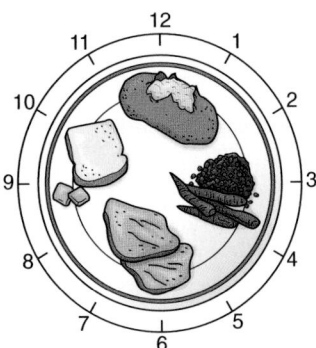

FIGURE 27-13 The numbers on a clock are used to help a visually impaired person locate food.

Many people pray before eating. Allow time and privacy for prayer. This shows respect and caring.

Meals provide social contact with others. Engage the person in pleasant conversation. However, allow time for chewing and swallowing. Also, sit facing the person. Sitting is more relaxing. It shows that you have time for the person. By facing the person, you can see how well the person is eating. You can also see swallowing problems.

See *Focus on Children and Older Persons: Feeding the Person.*

See *Focus on Surveys: Feeding the Person.*

See *Delegation Guidelines: Feeding the Person.*

See *Promoting Safety and Comfort: Feeding the Person.*

See procedure: *Feeding the Person.*

FOCUS ON CHILDREN AND OLDER PERSONS
Feeding the Person

Older Persons

Persons with dementia may become distracted during meals. Some cannot sit long enough for a meal. Others forget how to use eating utensils. Some persons resist your efforts to assist them with eating. A confused person may throw or spit food.

The Alzheimer's Disease Education and Referral Center (ADEAR) recommends the following. The measures may be part of the person's care plan.

- Provide a calm, quiet setting. Limit noise and other distractions. This helps the person focus on the meal.
- Limit the number of food choices.
- Offer several small meals throughout the day instead of larger ones.
- Use straws or cups with lids. These make drinking easier.
- Provide finger foods if the person has problems with utensils. A bowl may be easier to use than a plate.
- Provide healthy snacks. Keep snacks where the person can see them.

You must be patient. Talk to the nurse if you feel upset or impatient. The person has the right to be treated with dignity and respect.

FOCUS ON SURVEYS
Feeding the Person

Surveyors will focus on nutritional needs. They will observe if staff:

- Provide assistance with eating.
- Encourage the person to eat.
- Help the person use adaptive equipment (assistive devices).
- Feed the person if necessary.

DELEGATION GUIDELINES
Feeding the Person

Before feeding a person, you need this information from the nurse and the care plan.

- The person's food allergies (if any)
- Why the person needs help
- How much help the person needs
- How to position the person
- If the person can manage finger foods
- The person's activity limits
- The person's dietary restrictions
- What size portion to feed the person—$\frac{1}{3}$ teaspoonful or less
- Needed safety measures if the person has dysphagia
- If the person can use a straw
- What observations to report and record:
  - The amount and kind of food eaten
  - Complaints of nausea or dysphagia
  - Signs and symptoms of dysphagia
  - Signs and symptoms of aspiration
- When to report observations
- What patient or resident concerns to report at once

PROMOTING SAFETY AND COMFORT
Feeding the Person

Safety

Check food temperature. Very hot foods and fluids can burn the person.

Prevent aspiration. Check the person's mouth before offering more food or fluids. The person's mouth must be empty between bites and swallows.

Comfort

The person will eat better if not rushed. Sit to show that you have time. Standing communicates that you are in a hurry.

Wipe the person's hands, face, and mouth as needed during the meal. Use the napkin. If necessary, use a wet washcloth. Then dry the person with a towel.

Feeding the Person

QUALITY OF LIFE

- Knock before entering the person's room.
- Address the person by name.
- Introduce yourself by name and title.

- Explain the procedure before starting and during the procedure.
- Protect the person's rights during the procedure.
- Handle the person gently during the procedure.

PRE-PROCEDURE

1 Follow *Delegation Guidelines: Feeding the Person.* See *Promoting Safety and Comfort: Feeding the Person.*
2 Practice hand hygiene.

3 Position the person in a comfortable position for eating—sitting in a chair or in Fowler's (45 to 60 degrees) or high-Fowler's (60 to 90 degrees). (NOTE: Some state competency tests require that the person sit upright at least 45 degrees, others require 75 to 90 degrees.)
4 Get the tray. Place the tray on the over-bed table or dining table where the person can reach it.

PROCEDURE

5 Make sure the tray is complete. Check items on the tray with the dietary card.
6 Identify the person. Check the ID bracelet against the dietary card. Use 2 identifiers (Chapter 13). Also call the person by name.
7 Drape a napkin across the person's chest and underneath the chin. Clean the person's hands with a hand wipe.
8 Tell the person what foods and fluids are on the tray.
9 Prepare food for eating. Cut food into bite-sized pieces. Season food as the person prefers and is allowed on the care plan.
10 Place the chair where you can sit comfortably. Sit facing the person at eye level.
11 Serve foods in the order the person prefers. Identify foods as you serve them. Alternate between solid and liquid foods. Use a spoon for safety (Fig. 27-14). Allow enough time for chewing and swallowing. Do not rush the person. Also offer water, coffee, tea, or other fluids on the tray.
12 Check the person's mouth before offering more food or fluids. Make sure the person's mouth is empty between bites and swallows. Ask if the person is ready for the next bite or drink.

13 Use straws (if allowed) for liquids if the person cannot drink out of a glass or cup. Have 1 straw for each liquid. Provide short straws for weak persons. Follow the care plan for using straws.
14 Wipe the person's hands, face, and mouth as needed during the meal. Use the napkin or a hand wipe.
15 Follow the care plan if the person has dysphagia. (Some persons with dysphagia do not use straws.) Give thickened liquid with a spoon.
16 Talk with the person in a pleasant manner.
17 Encourage him or her to eat as much as possible.
18 Wipe the person's mouth with a napkin or a hand wipe. Discard the napkin or hand wipe.
19 Note how much and which foods were eaten (p. 454).
20 Measure and record fluid intake if ordered (p. 456).
21 Remove the tray.
22 Take the person back to his or her room (if in a dining area).
23 Assist with oral hygiene and hand-washing. Provide for privacy. Wear gloves. Practice hand hygiene after removing and discarding gloves.

POST-PROCEDURE

24 Provide for comfort. (See the inside of the front cover.)
25 Place the call light and other needed items within reach.
26 Raise or lower bed rails. Follow the care plan.
27 Complete a safety check of the room. (See the inside of the front cover.)

28 Return the food tray to the food cart.
29 Practice hand hygiene.
30 Report and record your observations.

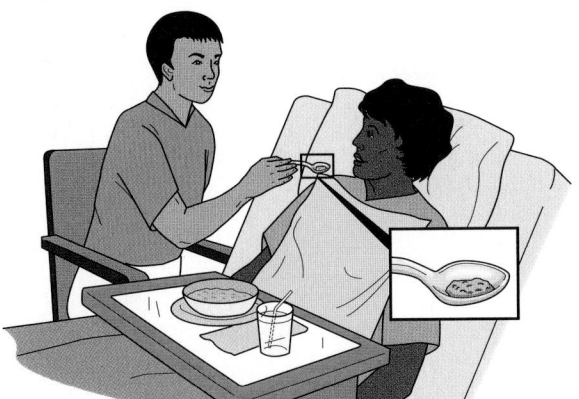

FIGURE 27-14 A spoon is used to feed the person. The spoon is one-third ($\frac{1}{3}$) full.

Between-Meal Snacks

Many special diets involve between-meal snacks. Also called *supplemental feedings*, snacks supplement (add to) the person's diet. Snacks provide extra nutrients. Common snacks are crackers, milk, juice, a milk-shake, cake, wafers, a sandwich, gelatin, and custard.

Snacks are served upon arrival on the nursing unit. Provide needed utensils, a straw, and a napkin. Follow the same considerations and procedures for serving meals and feeding the person.

Providing Drinking Water

Patients and residents need fresh drinking water each shift. They also need water when the water mug is empty (Fig. 27-15).

Some agencies do not use the procedure that follows. Each person's mug is filled as needed. The mug is taken to an ice and water dispenser. If so, fill the mug with ice first. Then add water. Follow the agency's procedure for providing fresh drinking water.

See *Focus on Communication: Providing Drinking Water.*

See *Delegation Guidelines: Providing Drinking Water.*

See *Promoting Safety and Comfort: Providing Drinking Water.*

See procedure: *Providing Drinking Water.*

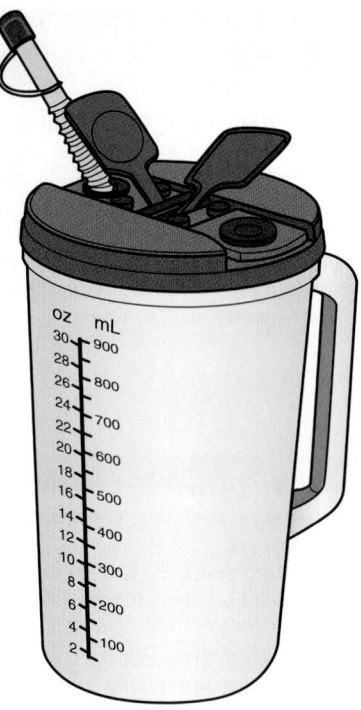

FIGURE 27-15 Water mug with straw. The mug is marked in milliliters (mL) and ounces (oz).

FOCUS ON COMMUNICATION

Providing Drinking Water

Some persons do not like ice in their water. Others like mostly ice with little water. Ask what the person prefers. You can say:
- "How much ice do you want in your water?"
- "Do you like more ice or more water?"

Also ask where to place the mug. Be sure the person can reach it.

DELEGATION GUIDELINES

Providing Drinking Water

To provide water, you need this information from the nurse and the care plan.
- The person's fluid orders
- If the person can have ice
- If the person uses a straw

PROMOTING SAFETY AND COMFORT

Providing Drinking Water

Safety

Water mugs can spread microbes. To prevent the spread of microbes:
- Make sure the mug is labeled with the person's name and room and bed number.
- Do not touch the rim or inside of the mug or lid.
- Do not let the ice scoop touch the mug, lid, or straw.
- Do not place the ice scoop in the ice container or dispenser. Place it in the scoop holder or on a towel for the scoop.
- Keep the ice chest closed when not in use.
- Make sure the mug is clean. Also check for cracks and chips. Provide a new mug as needed.

Providing Drinking Water

QUALITY OF LIFE

- Knock before entering the person's room.
- Address the person by name.
- Introduce yourself by name and title.
- Explain the procedure before starting and during the procedure.
- Protect the person's rights during the procedure.
- Handle the person gently during the procedure.

PRE-PROCEDURE

1 Follow *Delegation Guidelines: Providing Drinking Water.* See *Promoting Safety and Comfort: Providing Drinking Water.*
2 Obtain a list of persons who have special fluid orders from the nurse. Or use your assignment sheet.
3 Practice hand hygiene.
4 Collect the following.
   - Cart
   - Ice chest filled with ice
   - Cover for the ice chest
   - Scoop
   - Paper towels
   - Water mugs for patient or resident use
   - Large water pitcher filled with cold water (optional depending on agency procedure)
   - Towel for the scoop
5 Cover the cart with paper towels. Arrange equipment on top of the paper towels.

PROCEDURE

6 Take the cart to the person's room door. Do not take the cart into the room.
7 Check the person's fluid orders. Use the list from the nurse.
8 Identify the person. Check the ID bracelet against the fluid orders sheet or your assignment sheet. Use 2 identifiers (Chapter 13). Also call the person by name.
9 Take the mug from the person's over-bed table. Empty it into the bathroom sink.
10 Determine if a new mug is needed.
11 Use the scoop to fill the mug with ice (Fig. 27-16). Do not let the scoop touch the mug, lid, or straw.
12 Place the ice scoop on the towel.
13 Fill the mug with water. Get water from the room sink or bathroom sink or the large water pitcher on the cart.
14 Place the mug on the over-bed table.
15 Make sure the mug is within the person's reach.

POST-PROCEDURE

16 Provide for comfort. (See the inside of the front cover.)
17 Place the call light and other needed items within reach.
18 Complete a safety check of the room. (See the inside of the front cover.)
19 Practice hand hygiene.
20 Repeats steps 6 through 19 for each person.

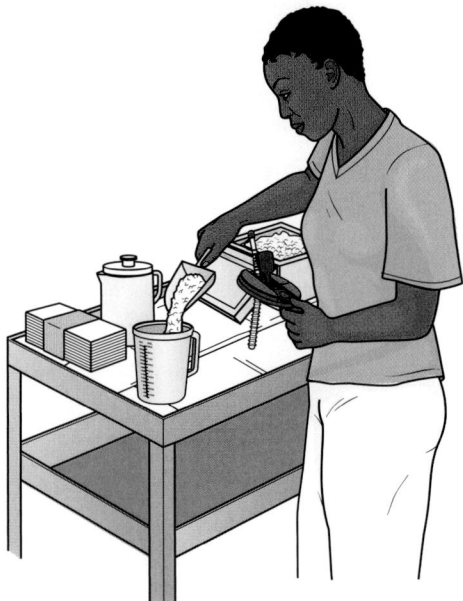

FIGURE 27-16 Providing drinking water.

FOODBORNE ILLNESS

A foodborne illness (food poisoning) is caused by pathogens in food and fluids. Report the signs and symptoms listed in Box 27-8 to the nurse at once.

Food is not sterile. Therefore pathogens are present in food. Cooked and ready-to-eat foods can become contaminated from other food. For example, meat juices can spill or splash onto other food. Food handlers with poor hygiene can contaminate the food.

Pathogens grow rapidly between 40°F and 140°F (Fahrenheit). This range is called the "danger zone" by the USDA. You must keep food out of the "danger zone." To do so, keep cold food cold and hot food hot.

To keep food safe, the USDA recommends these 4 safety tips.

- *Clean*. Wash hands, utensils, and counter tops often.
- *Separate*. Avoid cross-contamination. Do not let raw meat, poultry, or their juices touch other foods that will not be cooked.
- *Cook*. Cook food to a safe internal temperature (Fig. 27-17). Use a food thermometer to check the internal temperature. When re-heating cooked food, re-heat to 165°F.
- *Chill*. Refrigerate or freeze food within 2 hours. If the air is 90°F or above, chill food within 1 hour.

See *Focus on Long-Term Care and Home Care: Foodborne Illness*.

BOX 27-8	Foodborne Illness—Signs and Symptoms

- Abdominal cramps or pain
- Backache
- Breathing problems
- Chills
- Diarrhea (may be bloody)
- Eyelids: droopy
- Fever
- Headache
- Muscle pain
- Nausea
- Speaking problems
- Swallowing problems
- Vision: double
- Vomiting

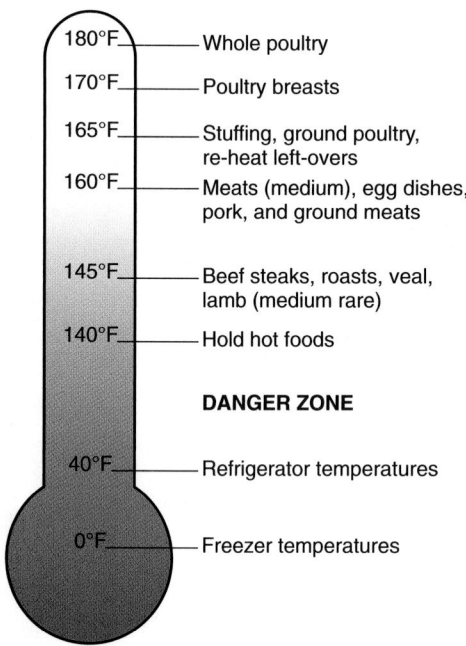

FIGURE 27-17 Food temperature guide. (Redrawn from U.S. Department of Health and Human Services and U.S. Department of Agriculture: Dietary Guidelines for Americans 2010.)

FOCUS ON LONG-TERM CARE AND HOME CARE

Foodborne Illness

Home Care

You need to protect the patient and family from foodborne illnesses. Follow the clean, separate, cook, and chill safety tips.

Clean

- Wash your hands with soap and warm water.
  - Before and after preparing food. Do so especially after handling raw seafood, meat, poultry, and eggs.
  - Before eating.
  - After elimination.
  - After changing diapers.
  - After coughing or sneezing.
  - Before and after providing care.
  - After touching animals.
  - After handling garbage.
- Wash surfaces with hot, soapy water. Use a solution of 1 tablespoon of unscented, liquid chlorine bleach in 1 gallon of water to sanitize surfaces.
  - Tables and counter tops.
  - Sinks.
  - Utensils.
  - Cutting boards.
  - The inside and outside of appliances and microwave ovens. This includes buttons and handles.
- Discard refrigerated foods.
  - Cooked left-overs after 4 days
  - Raw poultry and ground meats after 1 or 2 days
- Wipe up spills at once.
- Clean food contact surfaces often.
- Rinse all fruits and vegetables thoroughly. Products labeled as "pre-washed" or "ready-to-eat" do not need further rinsing.
  - Rinse under running water before eating, peeling, cutting, or cooking.
  - Do not use soap or detergent.
  - Scrub firm produce (melons, cucumbers, potatoes, and so on) with a clean produce brush while rinsing.
  - Dry produce with a clean towel or paper towel.
- Do not rinse raw seafood, meat, and poultry. Bacteria in the raw juices can spread to other foods, utensils, and surfaces.

Separate

- Place raw seafood, meat, and poultry in plastic bags. Separate them from other foods in the grocery cart and in bags.
- Store raw seafood, meat, and poultry in the refrigerator. Store them below ready-to-eat foods.
- Clean re-usable grocery bags.
  - Wash canvas and cloth bags in the washing machine.
  - Wash plastic bags with hot, soapy water.
- Use a clean cutting board for fresh produce.
- Use a separate cutting board for raw seafood, meat, and poultry.
- Use a clean plate to serve and eat food.
- Do not place cooked food back on a plate or cutting board that held raw food.

Cook and Chill

- Cook seafood, meat, poultry, and egg dishes to the correct internal temperature.
- Use a food thermometer to make sure that:
  - Food is safely cooked.
  - Cooked food is held at safe temperatures until eaten.
- Place the food thermometer in the thickest part of the food. It should not touch bone, fat, or gristle.
- Follow the manufacturer's instructions for using the food thermometer.
- Clean food thermometers with hot, soapy water before and after each use.
- Stir, rotate, or flip foods for even cooking in a microwave oven. Follow package instructions.
- Keep foods at a safe temperature.
  - Keep cold foods at 40°F or below.
  - Keep hot foods at 140°F or above.
  - Do not eat or serve foods when they have been in the "danger zone" (see Fig. 27-17) of 40°F to 140°F for more than 2 hours. Or 1 hour if the temperature is above 90°F. This time frame includes:
    - The amount of time food is in the grocery cart, car, and at home.
    - When frozen foods begin to thaw and become warmer than 40°F.
- Thaw foods in 1 of these ways.
  - In the refrigerator.
  - In a leak-proof bag in cold water. Change the water every 30 minutes.
  - In the microwave.
- Never thaw food on the counter.
- Keep the refrigerator at 40°F or below. Keep the freezer at 0°F or below.

Modified from U.S. Department of Agriculture and U.S. Department of Health and Human Services: Dietary guidelines for Americans, 2010, ed 7, Washington, DC, U.S. Government Printing Office, December 2010. See the Evolve Student Resources for this textbook for a summary of the most up-to-date Dietary Guidelines.

FOCUS ON PRIDE

The Person, Family, and Yourself

Personal and Professional Responsibility

Many agencies serve food in new ways. For example:

- 24-hour catering. Meals and snacks are served 24 hours a day. This is for persons who cannot or do not want to eat at the usual meal times. Food is ordered directly from the food service department. Food choices must be allowed on the person's ordered diet.
- Mobile food carts. Food service staff bring a food cart to the nursing unit. The person selects food and a tray is prepared.

With such systems, you may have new responsibilities. You may have to serve food trays more often. Or you may need to read and fill out menus. Know your role in the agency's food ordering and delivery system. Take pride in helping others meet their nutritional needs.

Rights and Respect

The right to personal choice is important to meet food and fluid needs. Cultural, social, religious, medical, and personal factors affect food choices throughout life. These do not change when in a hospital or nursing center. People often comment about food likes and dislikes. A person may say that the food is cold. Or it is bland. Or the food tastes bad.

People have the right to express what they prefer. Do not become angry or upset. The person should not feel as if he or she is complaining or being picky. Learning the person's likes and dislikes can improve nutrition. It also shows interest and concern for the person. Respect the person's right to express personal food choices.

Independence and Social Interaction

Meals provide a time for social contact with others. A friendly, social setting is important. Some nursing centers have areas where residents can dine with guests. They can enjoy holidays, birthdays, anniversaries, and other events. Food is provided by guests or the dietary department.

Families and friends may bring food from home. This helps meet love and belonging needs. The agency may not provide everything the person likes. The person usually enjoys having home-made food. Tell the nurse when the person receives food. The food must not interfere with the person's diet.

Delegation and Teamwork

Some agencies deliver trays in meal carts. Each tray is in a slot. Trays are served in the order that they appear in the cart. The entire nursing team serves trays. The team works together to serve food promptly.

Ethics and Laws

Proper food and fluid intake are needed to live. The person must be closely observed for changes in nutrition and hydration. The case below is a real example of how poor hydration resulted in harm.

Mr. Phillip Caruso was admitted to a nursing center on January 22 after needing hospital care for about 5 weeks. He had nervous and urinary system disorders. A doctor examined him on January 23. The doctor found him to be in stable condition. He showed signs of adequate hydration and responded to the doctor's commands.

The nursing center "did not keep a chart of Phillip's intake or output of fluids." According to the nurses, Mr. Caruso received:

- *3 meals a day.*
- *3 snacks [a day] with juice or milk.*
- *Drugs 4 times a day. He was given 4 oz of water with the drugs.*
- *Offers of something to drink every 2 hours during the night.*

Seven days after being admitted to the nursing center (January 29), Mr. Caruso was taken to the hospital. The emergency room doctor diagnosed severe dehydration. He was weak, confused, had tremors, and had dry skin with poor turgor. (Author note: Poor skin turgor means that the skin slowly returns to its normal position after being grasped between 2 fingers.) In the hospital, Mr. Caruso was treated with IV fluids and a catheter. He was also treated for a urinary tract infection caused by the catheter.

Mr. Caruso returned to the nursing center on February 19. He died on May 14.

His family sued and charged the nursing center with negligence, abuse, and neglect for failing to give Mr. Caruso enough water. They claimed that the dehydration led to declines in his physical and mental condition.

The jury found in favor of Mr. Caruso's family. The jury awarded the family $195,000 and attorney fees. The nursing home appealed the case. Because of a legal technicality, a judge ordered a new trial.

(I. Caruso v Pine Manor Nursing Center, Ill., 1989.)

You can do your part to promote good nutrition and fluid intake. Follow the person's care plan and dietary preferences. Carefully record intake and output as ordered. Tell the nurse if you notice a change in the person's intake.

FOCUS ON PRIDE: Application

Meal time should be as pleasant as possible. Sights, sounds, and smells have an impact. The person's preferences are important. For example, some prefer meals to be a social time. Others enjoy a quiet meal. How can you make meal time pleasant?

REVIEW QUESTIONS

*Circle **T** if the statement is **TRUE** or **F** if it is **FALSE**.*

1 T F You should wash fruits before serving them.

2 T F Raw meat can touch other foods.

3 T F Refrigerated left-over foods should be eaten within 4 days.

4 T F Poultry is washed and rinsed before cooking.

5 T F A cutting board can be used for all foods.

6 T F Raw meat is stored on the top shelf of the refrigerator.

7 T F Ground beef can be placed on a counter top to thaw.

8 T F Left-over foods should be refrigerated within 2 hours.

9 T F Hot, soapy water is used to clean kitchen surfaces.

*Circle the **BEST** answer.*

10 Nutrition is
a Fats, proteins, carbohydrates, vitamins, and minerals
b The many processes involved in the ingestion, digestion, absorption, and use of food and fluids by the body
c The MyPlate food guidance system
d The balance between calories taken in and used by the body

11 MyPlate encourages
a The same diet for everyone
b Eating less
c Increasing the amount of high-sodium foods
d Eating more refined grains

12 On a 2000 calorie diet, what is the amount of grains needed for an adult woman?
a 1 oz
b 2 to 2½ oz
c 3 oz
d 5 to 6 oz

13 On a 2000 calorie diet, which would meet an adult male's daily dairy needs?
a 1 slice of bread, 1 cup of cheese, and ½ oz of nuts
b 2 cups of milk and 1 cup of cooked rice
c 1 cup of milk, 1 cup of yogurt, and 1½ oz of cheese
d 2 tablespoons of peanut butter and 1 egg

14 Which food group contains the *most* cholesterol?
a Grains
b Vegetables
c Fruit
d Protein foods

15 These statements are about oils. Which is *true?*
a The best oil choices come from fish, nuts, and vegetable oils.
b Oils are low in calories.
c Oils from plant sources contain cholesterol.
d Oils are a food group.

16 Protein is needed for
a Tissue growth and repair
b Energy and the fiber for bowel elimination
c Body heat and to protect organs from injury
d Improving the taste of food

17 Which foods provide the *most* protein?
a Butter and cream
b Tomatoes and potatoes
c Meats and fish
d Corn and lettuce

18 The sodium-controlled diet involves
a Omitting high-sodium foods
b Adding salt to food at the table
c Using 3000 mg of salt in cooking
d A sodium-intake flow sheet

19 Diabetes meal planning involves
a Changing the thickness of foods
b Varying the amount of carbohydrates each day
c Controlling sodium
d Eating at regular times

20 Which does OBRA require?
a 2 meals a day and a bedtime snack
b Serving food promptly
c Serving food at room temperature to avoid burns
d A sodium-controlled diet

21 For normal fluid balance, an adult requires
a 500 to 1000 mL daily
b 1500 mL daily
c 2000 to 2500 mL daily
d 5000 mL daily

22 A person is NPO. You should
a Provide a variety of fluids
b Remove the water mug from the room
c Offer fluids in small amounts and in small containers
d Remove oral hygiene equipment from the room

23 A resident eats half of the food on his meal tray. His food intake for this meal is
a 25%
b 33%
c 50%
d 75%

24 Which are counted as fluid intake?
a Broths and ice cream
b Sauces and melted cheese
c Thick stews and mashed potatoes
d Butter and syrup

25 A person drank all of an 8 oz carton of milk. How many mL of fluid would you chart on the I&O record?
a 8 mL
b 60 mL
c 120 mL
d 240 mL

26 A person was served 250 mL of coffee and 120 mL of juice. You measure 50 mL of coffee and 60 mL of juice left. What do you chart for intake on the I&O record?
a 110 mL
b 260 mL
c 370 mL
d 480 mL

Continued

REVIEW QUESTIONS—cont'd

27 Persons with dysphagia
  a Use straws for all liquids
  b Have a regular diet
  c Are fed according to the care plan
  d Eat alone in their rooms

28 A person coughs and drools while eating. You should
  a Give the person a drink
  b Puree the person's food
  c Give mouth care and continue feeding
  d Tell the nurse

29 Which is a sign of a swallowing problem?
  a Edema
  b Sore throat
  c Coughing while eating
  d Increased appetite

30 When feeding a person
  a Ask in what order the person likes foods served
  b Use a fork
  c Stand facing the person
  d Talk with your co-workers

31 Before providing fresh drinking water, you need to know the person's
  a Intake
  b Fluid orders
  c Diet
  d Preferred beverages

32 You are re-heating cooked food. The food temperature should be
  a 40°F
  b 90°F
  c 140°F
  d 165°F

Answers to Chapter 27 questions are on p. 871.

FOCUS ON PRACTICE

Problem Solving

Mr. Lund has Parkinson's disease (Chapter 44). This affects movement, swallowing, and speech. When you try to feed him, he closes his mouth and shakes his head. He takes only small sips of thickened liquid. What do you do? What measures might be included in his care plan to meet nutrition and fluid needs?

Nutritional Support and IV Therapy

OBJECTIVES

- Define the key terms and key abbreviations in this chapter.
- Identify the reasons for nutritional support and IV therapy.
- Explain how tube feedings are given.
- Describe scheduled and continuous feedings.
- Explain how to prevent aspiration.
- Describe the comfort measures for the person with a feeding tube.
- Describe parenteral nutrition.
- Describe the IV therapy sites.

- Identify the equipment used in IV therapy.
- Describe how to assist with the IV flow rate.
- Identify the safety measures for IV therapy.
- Identify the observations to report when a person has nutritional support or IV therapy.
- Explain how to assist with nutritional support and IV therapy.
- Explain how to promote PRIDE in the person, the family, and yourself.

KEY TERMS

aspiration Breathing fluid, food, vomitus, or an object into the lungs

enteral nutrition Giving nutrients into the gastro-intestinal (GI) tract *(enteral)* through a feeding tube

flow rate The number of drops per minute *(gtt/min)* or milliliters per hour *(mL/hr)*

gastrostomy tube A doctor inserts a feeding tube through a surgically created opening *(stomy)* in the stomach *(gastro)*; stomach tube

gavage The process of giving a tube feeding

intravenous (IV) therapy Giving fluids through a needle or catheter inserted into a vein; IV and IV infusion

jejunostomy tube A feeding tube inserted into a surgically created opening *(stomy)* in the *jejunum* of the small intestine

naso-enteral tube A feeding tube inserted through the nose *(naso)* into the small bowel *(enteral)*

naso-gastric (NG) tube A feeding tube inserted through the nose *(naso)* into the stomach *(gastro)*

parenteral nutrition Giving nutrients through a catheter inserted into a vein; *para* means *beyond*; *enteral* relates to the *bowel*

percutaneous endoscopic gastrostomy (PEG) tube A feeding tube inserted into the stomach *(gastro)* through a small incision *(stomy)* made through *(per)* the skin *(cutaneous)*; a lighted instrument *(scope)* is used to see inside a body cavity or organ *(endo)*

regurgitation The backward flow of stomach contents into the mouth

KEY ABBREVIATIONS

GI	Gastro-intestinal	**NG**	Naso-gastric
gtt	Drops	**NPO**	Nothing by mouth
gtt/min	Drops per minute	**oz**	Ounce
IV	Intravenous	**PEG**	Percutaneous endoscopic gastrostomy
mL	Milliliter	**TPN**	Total parenteral nutrition
mL/hr	Milliliters per hour		

Many persons cannot eat or drink because of illness, surgery, or injury. They may have chewing, swallowing, or other eating problems. Aspiration is a risk. *Aspiration is breathing fluid, food, vomitus, or an object into the lungs.* Some persons refuse to eat or drink. Others cannot eat enough to meet their nutritional needs. The doctor may order nutritional support or intravenous (IV) therapy to meet food and fluid needs.

See *Delegation Guidelines: Nutritional Support and IV Therapy.*

ENTERAL NUTRITION

Some persons cannot or will not ingest, chew, or swallow food. Or food cannot pass from the mouth into the esophagus and into the stomach or small intestine. Poor nutrition results. Common causes are:

* Cancer, especially cancers of the head, neck, and esophagus
* Trauma to the face, mouth, head, or neck
* Coma
* Dysphagia
* Dementia
* Eating disorders
* Nervous system disorders (Chapter 44)
* Prolonged vomiting
* Major trauma or surgery
* Acquired immunodeficiency syndrome (AIDS) (Chapter 43)
* Illnesses and disorders affecting eating and nutrition

Enteral nutrition is giving nutrients into the gastrointestinal (GI) tract (enteral) through a feeding tube. Gavage is the process of giving a tube feeding. Tube feedings replace or supplement normal nutrition.

Types of Feeding Tubes

These feeding tubes are common.

* *Naso-gastric (NG) tube. A feeding tube is inserted through the nose* (naso) *into the stomach* (gastro) (Fig. 28-1). A doctor or an RN inserts the tube.
* *Naso-enteral tube. A feeding tube is inserted through the nose* (naso) *into the small bowel* (enteral) (Fig. 28-2). A doctor or RN inserts the tube.
* *Gastrostomy tube. A doctor inserts a feeding tube through a surgically created opening* (stomy) *in the stomach* (gastro). It is also called a stomach tube. See Figure 28-3.
* *Jejunostomy tube. A feeding tube is inserted into a surgically created opening* (stomy) *in the* jejunum *of the small intestine* (Fig. 28-4).
* *Percutaneous endoscopic gastrostomy (PEG) tube. A doctor inserts a feeding tube into the stomach* (gastro) *through a small incision* (stomy) *made through* (per) *the skin* (cutaneous). *A lighted instrument* (scope) *is used to see inside a body cavity or organ* (endo). See Figure 28-5.

NG and naso-enteral tubes are used for short-term nutritional support—usually less than 6 weeks. Gastrostomy, jejunostomy, and PEG tubes are used for long-term nutritional support—usually longer than 6 weeks.

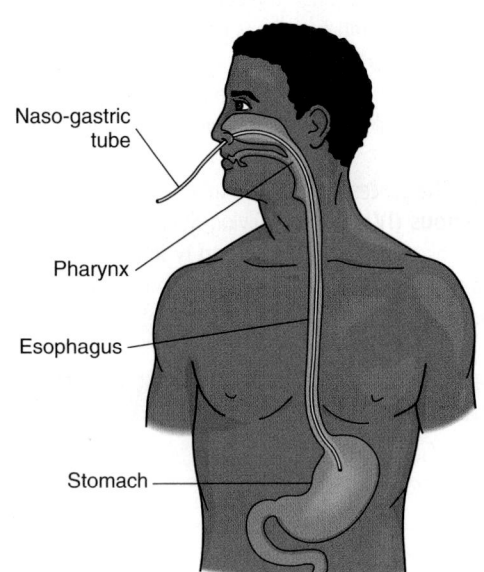

FIGURE 28-1 A naso-gastric (NG) tube is inserted through the nose and esophagus and into the stomach.

DELEGATION GUIDELINES

Nutritional Support and IV Therapy

Your state and agency may not allow you to assist with some of the care measures in this chapter or perform procedures involving nutritional support and IV therapy. Before assisting with a care measure or performing a procedure, make sure that:

* Your state allows you to perform the task.
* The task is in your job description.
* You have had the necessary education and training.
* You know how to use the agency's equipment and supplies.
* You review the task in the agency's procedure manual.
* You review the task with the nurse.
* A nurse is available to answer questions and to supervise you.
* An RN (registered nurse) has identified and labeled all tubes, catheters, and needles.

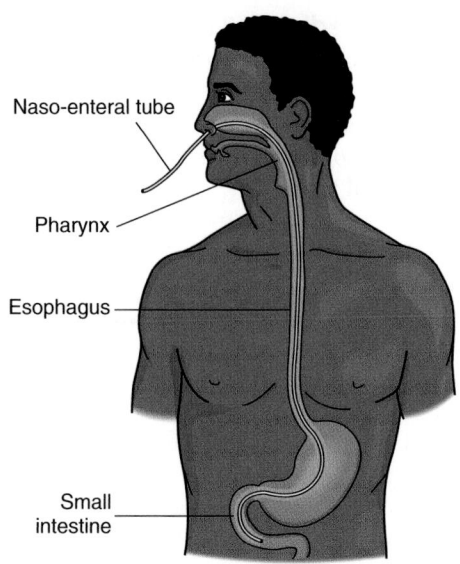

FIGURE 28-2 A naso-enteral tube is inserted through the nose and into the small intestine.

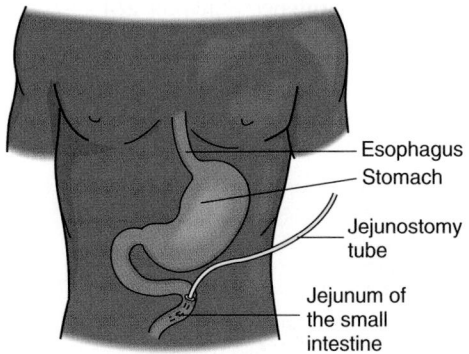

FIGURE 28-4 A jejunostomy tube.

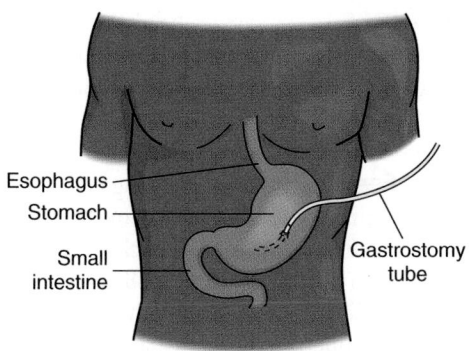

FIGURE 28-3 A gastrostomy tube.

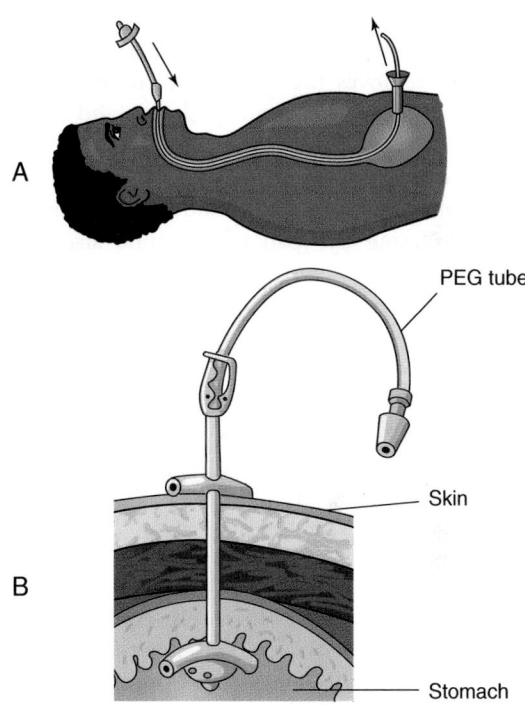

FIGURE 28-5 A, A percutaneous endoscopic gastrostomy (PEG) tube is inserted. B, PEG tube in place.

Formulas

The doctor orders the type of formula, the amount to give, and when to give tube feedings. Most formulas contain proteins, carbohydrates, fats, vitamins, and minerals. Commercial formulas are common.

Formula is given at room temperature. Cold fluids can cause cramping. Opened formula can remain at room temperature for about 8 hours. Microbes can grow in warm formula.

See *Teamwork and Time Management: Formulas.*

TEAMWORK AND TIME MANAGEMENT
Formulas

Refrigerated formula is warmed to room temperature. To warm formula, place the container in a wash basin filled with warm water. If warmed in the sink, other staff cannot use the sink. They waste time and energy going elsewhere. Or someone may remove the container to use the sink. The container does not warm in a timely manner. That affects the person, you, and the nurse.

The nurse and manufacturer's instructions tell you how long formula can hang. Check the time that the feeding started. Remind the nurse when the time limit is near. For example, a feeding that started at 0800 can hang for 8 hours. At 1530 or 1545, tell the nurse how much time is left. Also report the amount of formula left.

Feeding Times

Tube feedings are given at certain times (scheduled feedings). Or they are given over a 24-hour period (continuous feedings).

Scheduled Feedings.
Such feedings also are called intermittent feedings. (*Intermittent* means *to start, stop, and then start again.*) Feeding times are scheduled. At least 4 feedings are given each day. Usually 8 to 12 ounces (oz) (240 to 360 milliliters [mL]) are given over about 30 minutes. The frequency, amount, and time are like a normal eating pattern.

The nurse uses a syringe or a feeding bag (Fig. 28-6). The syringe attaches to the feeding tube. Connecting tubing connects the feeding bag to the tube. Formula is added to the syringe or to the feeding bag. Then it slowly flows through the feeding tube into the stomach.

The nurse removes the syringe or connecting tubing after the feeding. Then the nurse clamps and covers the end of the feeding tube with a cap or gauze. Gauze is secured in place with a rubber band. Clamping prevents air from entering the tube and fluid from leaking out of the tube. Covering the end of the tube also prevents leaking.

Continuous Feedings.
These feedings are usually given over 24 hours. A feeding pump is used (Fig. 28-7). Formula drips into the feeding tube at a certain rate per minute. The person receives a certain amount each hour.

A pump alarm sounds if something is wrong. When you hear an alarm, tell the nurse.

Observations

Diarrhea, constipation, delayed stomach emptying, and aspiration are risks. Report the following at once.

- Nausea
- Discomfort during the feeding
- Vomiting
- Distended (enlarged and swollen) abdomen
- Coughing
- Complaints of indigestion or heartburn
- Redness, swelling, drainage, odor, or pain at the ostomy site
- Fever
- Signs and symptoms of respiratory distress (Chapter 39)
- Increased pulse rate
- Complaints of flatulence (Chapter 26)
- Diarrhea (Chapter 26)

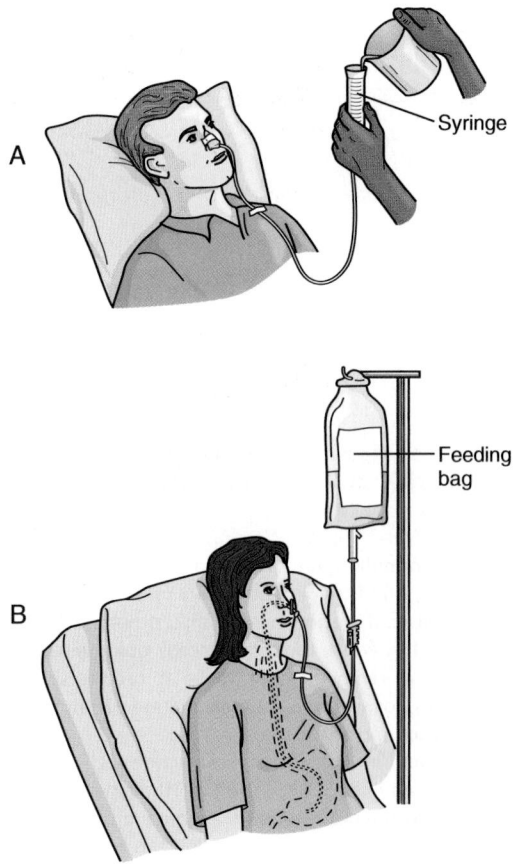

FIGURE 28-6 A, A tube feeding is given with a syringe. **B,** Formula drips from a feeding bag into the feeding tube.

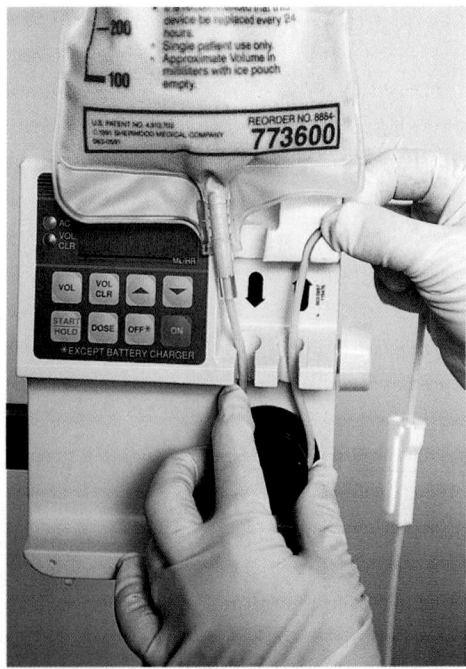

FIGURE 28-7 Feeding pump. (From Potter PA, Perry AG, Stockert PA, Hall AM: *Fundamentals of nursing,* ed 8, St Louis, 2013, Mosby.)

Preventing Aspiration

Aspiration is a major risk from tube feedings. It can cause pneumonia and death. Aspiration can occur:

- *During insertion.* NG tubes and naso-enteral tubes are passed through the nose into the esophagus and then into the stomach or small intestine. The tube can slip into the airway. An x-ray is taken after insertion to check tube placement.
- *From tube movement out of place.* Coughing, sneezing, vomiting, suctioning, and poor positioning are common causes. A tube can move from the stomach or intestines into the esophagus and then into the airway. The RN checks tube placement before every scheduled tube feeding. With continuous feedings, the RN checks tube placement every 4 hours. To do so, the RN attaches a syringe to the tube. GI secretions are withdrawn through the syringe. Then the pH of the secretions is measured (Chapter 34). *You never check feeding tube placement.*
- *From regurgitation. Regurgitation is the backward flow of stomach contents into the mouth.* Delayed stomach emptying and over-feeding are common causes.

To help prevent regurgitation and aspiration:

- Position the person in Fowler's or semi-Fowler's position before the feeding. Follow the care plan and the nurse's directions.
- Maintain Fowler's or semi-Fowler's position after the feeding. This allows formula to move through the GI tract. The position is required for 1 to 2 hours after the feeding or at all times. Follow the care plan and the nurse's directions.
- Avoid the left side-lying position. It prevents the stomach from emptying into the small intestine.

Persons with NG or gastrostomy tubes are at great risk for regurgitation. The risk is less with intestinal tubes. Formula passes directly into the small intestine and is given at a slow rate. During digestion, food slowly passes from the stomach into the small intestine. The stomach handles larger amounts of food at one time than does the small intestine.

Before a tube feeding, the nurse checks tube placement and residual stomach contents. *Residual* means *what remains*. For an NG tube or gastrostomy tube, the nurse aspirates stomach contents and measures the amount. Depending on the amount, the nurse decides if the feeding should be given or delayed. The intent is to prevent aspiration from regurgitation caused by over-feeding.

See *Focus on Children and Older Persons: Preventing Aspiration.*

FOCUS ON CHILDREN AND OLDER PERSONS

Preventing Aspiration

Older Persons

Digestion slows with aging. Stomach emptying also slows. Older persons are at risk for regurgitation and aspiration. Less formula and longer feeding times prevent over-feeding.

Comfort Measures

Persons with feeding tubes usually are not allowed to eat or drink. They are NPO—nothing by mouth (Chapter 27). Dry mouth, dry lips, and sore throat cause discomfort. Sometimes hard candy or gum is allowed. These measures are common every 2 hours while the person is awake.

- Oral hygiene
- Lubricant for the lips
- Mouth rinses

Feeding tubes can irritate and cause pressure on the nose. They can change the shape of the nostrils or cause pressure ulcers. These measures are common.

- Clean the nose and nostrils every 4 to 8 hours.
- Secure the tube to the nose (Fig. 28-8). Use tape or a tube holder. Tube holders have foam cushions that prevent pressure on the nose. Re-taping is not needed. Re-taping irritates the nose.
- Secure the tube to the person's garment at the shoulder area. This prevents the tube from pulling or dangling. Both can cause pressure on the nose. Do 1 of the following according to agency policy.
  - Loop a rubber band around the tube. Then pin the rubber band to the garment with a safety pin.
  - Tape the tube to the garment.

Assisting With Tube Feedings

You assist the nurse with tube feedings. With more training, some states and agencies allow nursing assistants to give tube feedings and remove NG tubes. *Remember, you never insert feeding tubes, check their placement, or check residual stomach contents. They are the RN's responsibility.*

See *Delegation Guidelines: Assisting With Tube Feedings,* p. 478.

See *Promoting Safety and Comfort: Assisting With Tube Feedings,* p. 478.

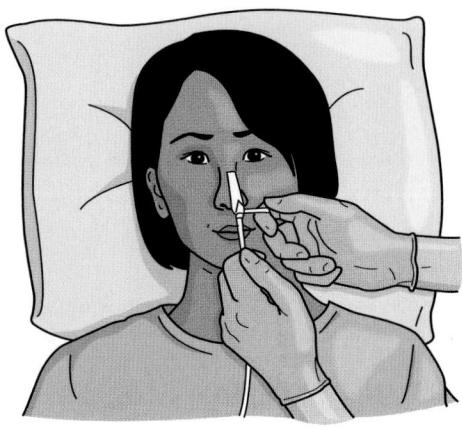

FIGURE 28-8 The feeding tube is secured to the nose.

PARENTERAL NUTRITION

Parenteral nutrition is giving nutrients through a catheter inserted into a vein (Fig. 28-9). (Para *means* beyond. Enteral *relates to the* bowel.) A nutrient solution is given directly into the bloodstream. Nutrients do not enter the GI tract. Parenteral nutrition is often called *total parenteral nutrition (TPN)* or *hyperalimentation. (Hyper means high or excessive. Alimentation means nourishment.)*

The solution contains water, proteins, carbohydrates, vitamins, and minerals. It drips through a catheter inserted into a large vein. TPN is used when the person cannot receive oral or enteral feedings. Or it is used when oral or enteral feedings are not enough to meet the person's needs.

Common reasons for TPN include:
- Disease, injury, or surgery to the GI tract
- Severe trauma, infection, or burns
- Being NPO for more than 5 to 7 days
- GI side effects from cancer treatments (Chapter 43)
- Prolonged coma
- Prolonged anorexia (loss of appetite)

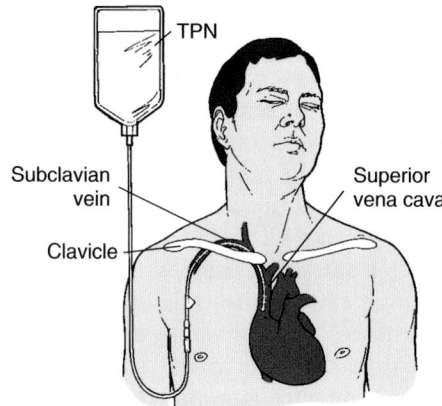

FIGURE 28-9 Parenteral nutrition. (Modified from *Mosby's dictionary of medicine, nursing, and health professions,* ed 8, St Louis, 2009, Mosby.)

Observations

TPN risks include infection, fluid imbalances, and blood sugar imbalances. Report the following to the nurse at once.

- Fever, chills, and other signs and symptoms of infection (Chapter 16)
- Signs and symptoms of sugar imbalances (see "Diabetes" in Chapter 46)
- Chest pain
- Difficulty breathing or shortness of breath
- Cough
- Nausea and vomiting
- Diarrhea
- Thirst
- Rapid heart rate or an irregular heartbeat
- Weakness or fatigue
- Sweating
- Pallor (pale skin)
- Trembling
- Confusion or behavior changes

Assisting with TPN

The nurse is responsible for all aspects of TPN. To assist, carefully observe the person. Also assist with the person's basic needs and activities of daily living. The person may be NPO. Provide frequent oral hygiene, lubricant to the lips, and mouth rinses as the nurse and care plan direct. Also follow other aspects of the person's care plan.

Many aspects of IV therapy apply to TPN.

IV THERAPY

Intravenous (IV) therapy (IV, IV infusion) is giving fluids through a needle or catheter inserted into a vein (Fig. 28-10). Fluid flows directly into the bloodstream. Doctors order IV therapy to:

- Provide fluids when they cannot be taken by mouth.
- Replace minerals and vitamins lost because of illness or injury.
- Provide sugar for energy.
- Give drugs and blood.

RNs are responsible for IV therapy. They start and maintain the infusion as ordered. RNs also give IV drugs and administer blood. State laws vary about your role and that of LPNs/LVNs in IV therapy.

IV Sites

Peripheral and central venous sites are used. *Peripheral* means *around (peri)* a *boundary (pheral)*. The boundary is the center of the body near the heart. *Peripheral IV sites* are away from the center of the body. For adults, the back of the hand and inner forearm are useful sites (Fig. 28-11).

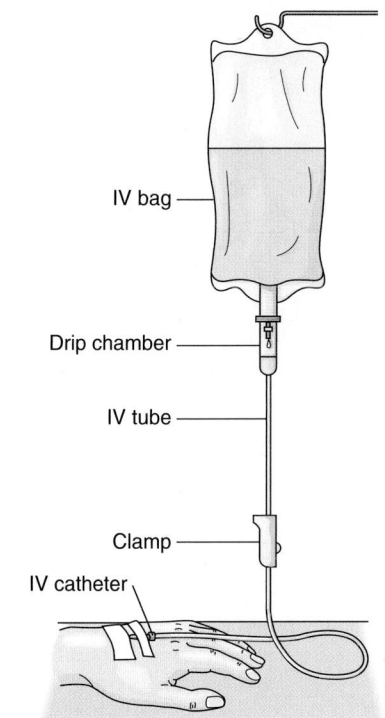

FIGURE 28-10 Equipment for IV therapy.

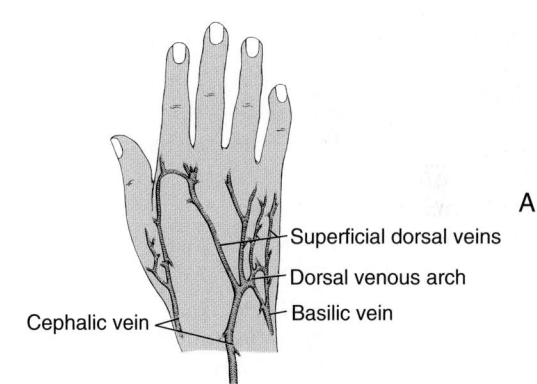
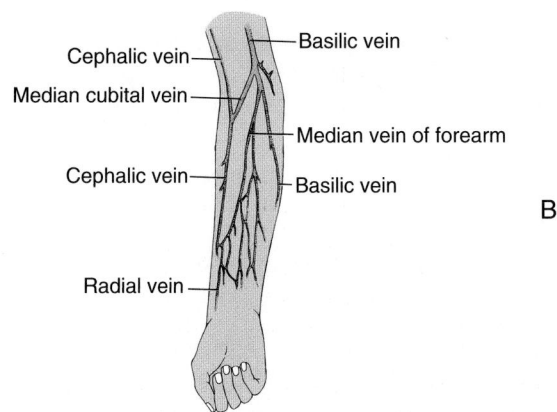

FIGURE 28-11 Peripheral IV sites. A, Back of the hand. **B,** Inner forearm. (From Potter PA, Perry AG, Stockert PA, Hall AM: *Fundamentals of nursing*, ed 8, St Louis, 2013, Mosby.)

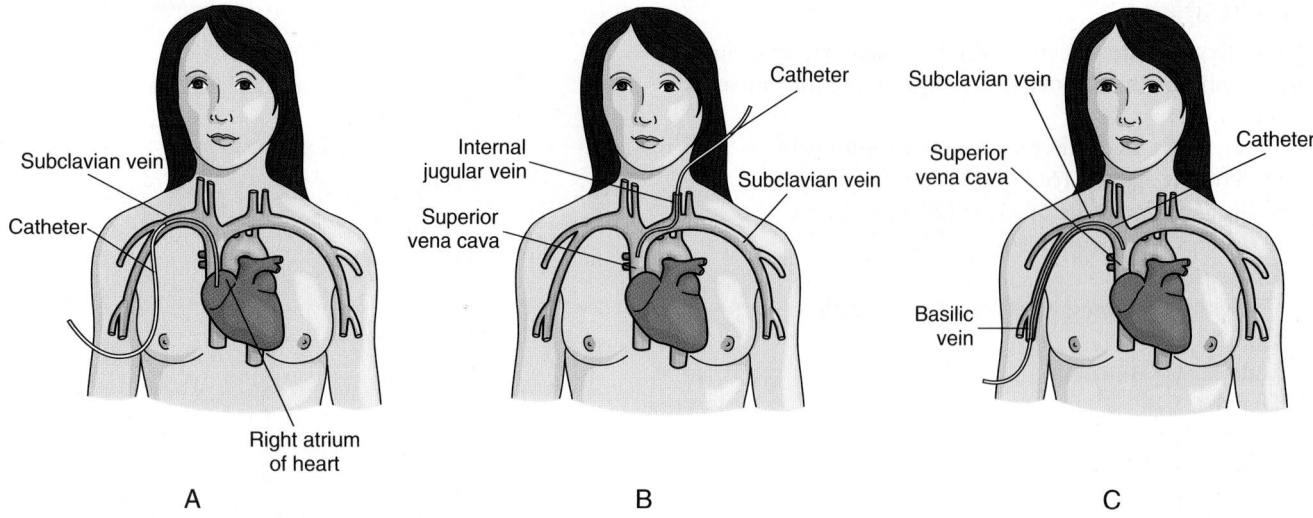

FIGURE 28-12 Central venous sites. **A,** Subclavian vein. The catheter tip is in the right atrium. **B,** Internal jugular vein. The catheter tip is in the superior vena cava. **C,** Basilic vein. This is a peripherally inserted central catheter (PICC).

The subclavian vein and the internal jugular vein are *central venous sites*. They are close to the heart. A catheter is threaded into the superior vena cava or right atrium (Fig. 28-12, *A and B*). The catheter is called a *central venous catheter* or a *central line*. The cephalic and basilic veins in the arm also are used. Catheters inserted into these sites are called *peripherally inserted central catheters (PICCs)*. The catheter is threaded into the subclavian vein or the superior vena cava (Fig. 28-12, *C*).

Central venous sites are used:
- For parenteral nutrition
- To give large amounts of fluid
- For long-term IV therapy
- To give drugs that irritate peripheral veins.
  See *Focus on Children and Older Persons: IV Sites.*
  See *Focus on Long-Term Care and Home Care: IV Sites.*

FOCUS ON CHILDREN AND OLDER PERSONS

IV Sites

Children
See Figure 28-13 for the IV sites in children. The hand, wrist, and inner arm sites are commonly used. The site selected depends on:
- The child's age. For example, scalp veins are sometimes used in infants. For a toddler, foot veins are avoided. IVs in foot veins prevent walking.
- The amount and kind of fluid ordered.
- How long the IV will be needed.

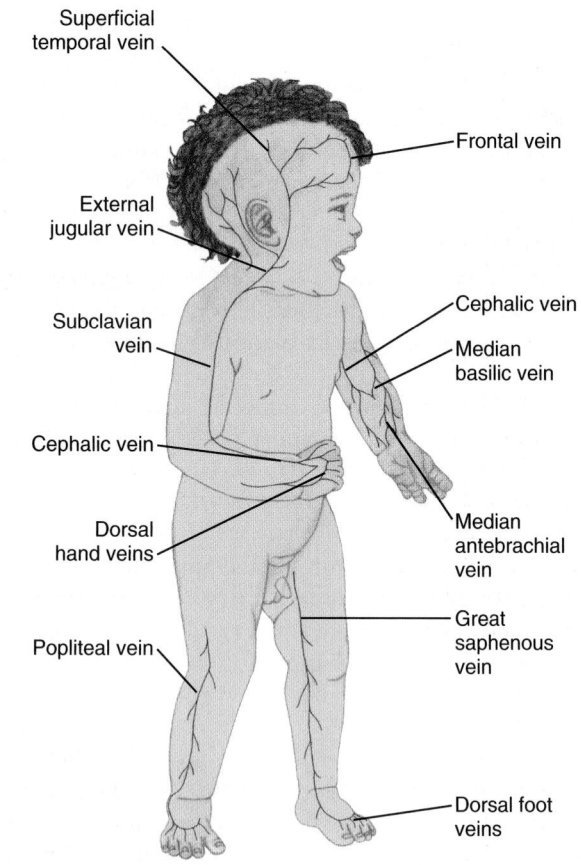

FIGURE 28-13 IV sites in children. (Modified from James SR, Ashwill JW: *Nursing care of children: principles and practice,* ed 3, St Louis, 2007, Saunders.)

IV Equipment

The basic equipment used in IV therapy is shown in Figure 28-10.

- The solution container is a plastic bag. It is called the *IV bag*.
- A *catheter* or *needle* is inserted into a vein (Fig. 28-14).
- The *IV tube* or *infusion tubing* connects the IV bag to the catheter or needle. Fluid drips from the bag into the *drip chamber*. The *clamp* is used to regulate the flow rate.
- The IV bag hangs from an IV pole (IV standard) or ceiling hook.

Flow Rate

The doctor orders the amount of fluid to give (infuse) and the amount of time to give it in. With this information, the RN figures the flow rate. The ***flow rate*** *is the number of drops per minute (gtt/min) or milliliters per hour (mL/hr)*. The abbreviation *gtt* means *drops*. The Latin word *guttae* means *drops*.

The RN sets the clamp for the flow rate. Or an electronic pump is used (Fig. 28-15). The flow rate is displayed in mL/hr. An alarm sounds if something is wrong. Tell the nurse at once if you hear an alarm. *Never change the position of the clamp or adjust any controls on IV pumps.*

You can check the flow rate if a pump is not used. The RN tells you the number of drops per minute (gtt/min). To check the flow rate, count the number of drops in 1 minute (Fig. 28-16). Tell the RN at once if:

- No fluid is dripping.
- The rate is too fast.
- The rate is too slow.
- The bag is empty or close to being empty.

The time tape shows how much fluid to give over a period of time (Fig. 28-17, p. 482). For example, the doctor orders 1000 mL of fluid over 8 hours. The RN marks the tape in 8 one-hour intervals. To check if the infusion is on time, compare the fluid line with the time line on the tape. If the fluid line is above or below the time line, the flow rate is too slow or too fast. Tell the RN at once if too much or too little fluid was given.

See *Promoting Safety and Comfort: Flow Rate*, p. 482.

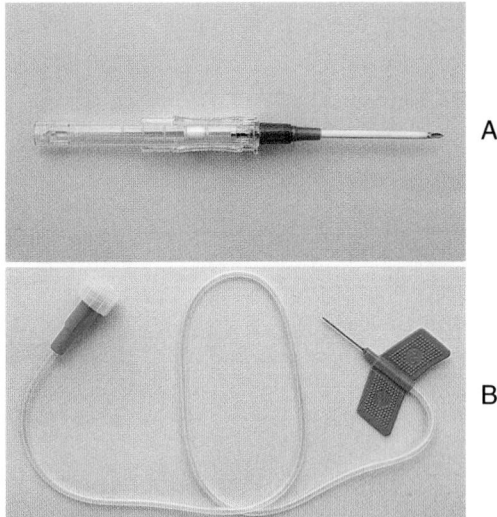

FIGURE 28-14 A, Intravenous catheter. **B,** Butterfly needle.

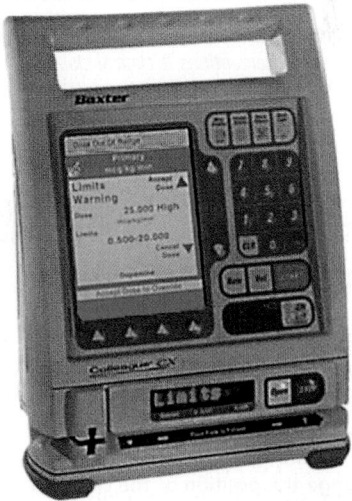

FIGURE 28-15 Electronic IV pump. (Courtesy Baxter Healthcare Corporation, Round Lake, Ill.)

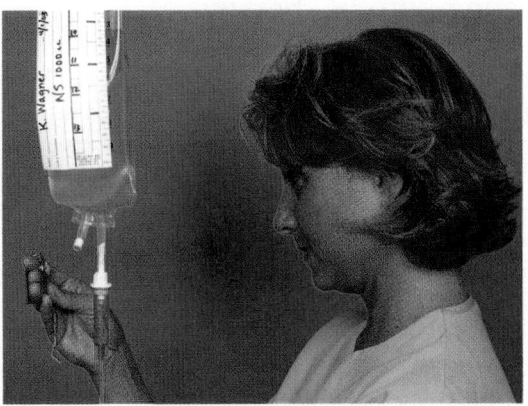

FIGURE 28-16 The flow rate is checked by counting the number of drops per minute.

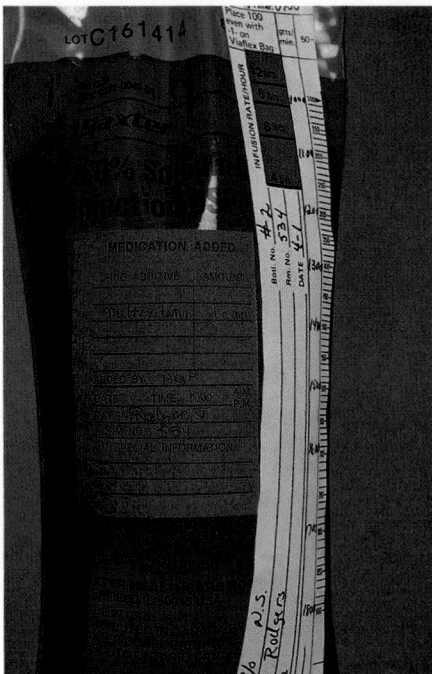

FIGURE 28-17 Time tape applied to an IV bag. (From Elkin MK, Perry AG, Potter PA: *Nursing interventions & clinical skills,* ed 4, St Louis, 2007, Mosby.)

PROMOTING SAFETY AND COMFORT

Flow Rate

Safety
The person can suffer serious harm if the flow rate is too fast or too slow. The flow rate can change from:
- Position changes
- Kinked tubes
- Lying on the tube
  Never change the position of the clamp or adjust any controls on infusion pumps. Tell the nurse at once if there is a problem with the flow rate.

BOX 28-1	IV Therapy

- Follow Standard Precautions and the Bloodborne Pathogen Standard.
- Do not move the needle or catheter. Correct position must be maintained. If the needle or catheter is moved, it may come out of the vein. Then fluid flows into tissues (infiltration). Or the flow stops.
- Follow the safety measures for restraints (Chapter 15). The nurse may splint or restrain the extremity to prevent movement (Fig. 28-18). Or the nurse may apply a protective device (Fig. 28-19). This helps prevent the needle or catheter from moving.
- Protect the IV bag, tubing, and needle or catheter when the person walks. Portable IV standards are rolled next to the person (Fig. 28-20).
- Assist the person with turning and re-positioning. Move the IV bag to the side of the bed on which the person is lying. Always allow enough slack in the tubing. The needle or catheter can move from pressure on the tube.
- Tell the nurse at once if bleeding occurs at the insertion site.
- Report signs and symptoms of IV therapy complications. Report the following at once.
  - Local—at the IV site
    - Bleeding
    - Blood backing up into the IV tube
    - Puffiness or swelling
    - Pale or reddened skin
    - Complaints of pain at or above the IV site
    - Hot or cold skin near the site
  - Systemic—involving the whole body
    - Fever
    - Itching
    - Drop in blood pressure
    - Pulse rate greater than 100 beats per minute
    - Irregular pulse
    - Cyanosis (bluish color)
    - Confusion or changes in mental function
    - Loss of consciousness
    - Difficulty breathing
    - Shortness of breath
    - Decreasing or no urine output
    - Chest pain
    - Nausea

Assisting with IV Therapy

You help meet the safety, hygiene, and activity needs of persons with IVs. Follow the safety measures in Box 28-1. Report any of the signs and symptoms listed in Box 28-1 at once.

Your state and agency may allow you to change dressings at peripheral IV sites. They also may let you discontinue (remove) a peripheral IV.

You never start or maintain IV therapy. Nor do you regulate the flow rate or change IV bags. You never give blood or IV drugs.

See *Focus on Communication: Assisting With IV Therapy.*

See *Teamwork and Time Management: Assisting With IV Therapy.*

See *Delegation Guidelines: Assisting With IV Therapy.*

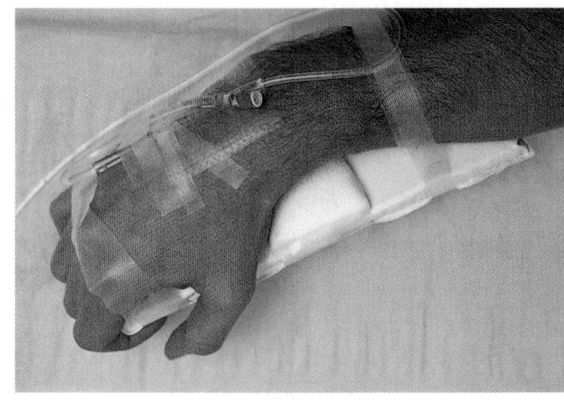

FIGURE 28-18 An armboard prevents movement at an IV site. (From Elkin MK, Perry AG, Potter PA: *Nursing interventions & clinical skills,* ed 4, St Louis, 2007, Mosby.)

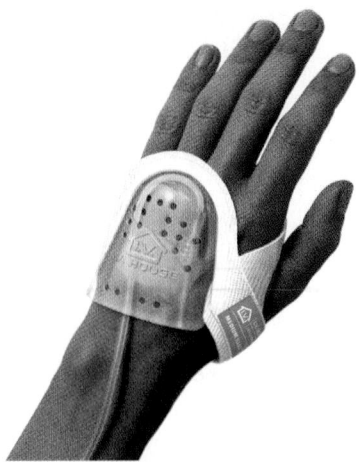

FIGURE 28-19 I.V. House Protective Device. (Courtesy I.V. House, St Louis, Mo.)

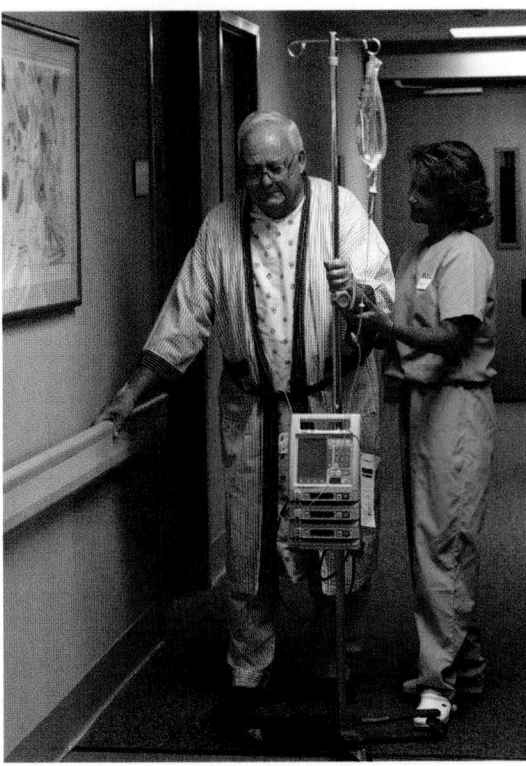

FIGURE 28-20 A person walking with an IV.

FOCUS ON COMMUNICATION

Assisting With IV Therapy

The nurse may instruct the person how to position the arm during IV therapy. You may need to remind the person:
- To position his or her arm a certain way
- About position limits

For example, Mr. Winn has an IV in his arm. If he bends his arm, the tubing is kinked. The flow of fluid stops. You can say: "Mr. Winn, please keep your arm straight. The fluid will not flow through your IV when your arm is bent."

TEAMWORK AND TIME MANAGEMENT

Assisting With IV Therapy

If assigned to a person with an IV, you must know the flow rate. When with the person, check the flow rate. Report any problems to the nurse at once.

Also check the amount of fluid in the bag. Tell the nurse at once if the bag is empty or almost empty.

Patients and residents cared for by other staff may have IVs. When near the person or walking past the person's room, make sure the IV is dripping. Also check the amount of fluid in the bag. Report any problems to a nurse at once.

DELEGATION GUIDELINES

Assisting With IV Therapy

Before changing a peripheral IV dressing or discontinuing a peripheral IV, make sure that the conditions in *Delegation Guidelines: Nutritional Support and IV Therapy* (p. 474) are met. If those conditions are met, you need this information from the nurse and the care plan.
- When to change the IV dressing
- If the person has an IV needle or catheter
- When to discontinue the IV
- If the person has 2 or more IVs, which IV to discontinue
- What supplies to use
- What observations to report and record (see Box 28-1)
- When to report observations
- What patient or resident concerns to report at once

FOCUS ON **PRIDE**

The Person, Family, and Yourself

Personal and Professional Responsibility

Being attentive is a valuable quality for nursing assistants. When you are attentive, you pay close attention. You are careful, alert, exact, and thorough. You meet the person's needs. You report problems at once.

These qualities are very important when assisting with nutritional support or IV therapy. The more complex the person's needs, the more attentive you must be.

Rights and Respect

Persons needing nutritional support or IV therapy are often very ill. Sometimes decisions are made to stop therapy and allow the person to die. The person or family makes the decision after talking to the doctor. See Chapter 55.

You may disagree with such choices. Your beliefs must not interfere with the person's right to choose and to refuse treatment. The person's or family's wishes and doctor's orders must be followed. Tell the nurse if you have a problem with the decision. The nurse may need to change your assignment.

Independence and Social Interaction

The need for a feeding tube affects the person as a whole. Physical changes are obvious. Emotional and social changes also occur. The person may miss the taste of food and social contact during meals. Feelings of sadness, loss, dependence, and loneliness can occur. You can:

* Listen.
* Provide emotional support.
* Encourage social contact.
* Tell the nurse about any concerns.

Delegation and Teamwork

Before any task, you must know how to protect feeding tubes and IVs. For example:

* A patient has an IV and needs a tub bath. The IV site must be kept clean and dry. The nurse may have you apply a plastic bag, plastic wrap, or glove. Follow agency policy and the nurse's instructions.
* A patient with a continuous tube feeding needs to be re-positioned in bed. You need to plan how to protect the feeding tube during the move.

Ethics and Laws

IV pump alarms can sound for many reasons.

* There is air in the tubing.
* The infusion is done.
* The pump's battery is low.
* Fluid flow is blocked. Kinks in the tubing and closed clamps are common reasons.

When you hear an IV pump alarm, tell the nurse. Do so even if you are not assigned to the person. If the battery is low, you may plug in the pump. If the person needs to re-position his or her arm, you may ask the person to do so. You do not adjust controls on IV pumps or clamps on IV tubing.

Know the limits of your role. If asked to do something outside those limits, politely refuse and explain why. Doing tasks outside the limits of your role can harm the person. Legal action can be taken. You can lose your ability to work as a nursing assistant.

FOCUS ON **PRIDE**: *Application*

Consider the emotional impact of 1 treatment in this chapter. Describe how the person might feel. How can you provide mental comfort?

REVIEW QUESTIONS

Circle the BEST answer.

1 Enteral nutrition
   a Requires an NG tube
   b Is given into a central venous site
   c Is given into the GI tract
   d Requires an IV

2 The process of giving a tube feeding is called
   a Gavage
   b Parenteral nutrition
   c Aspiration
   d Regurgitation

3 For a tube feeding, the person is positioned in
   a Fowler's or semi-Fowler's position
   b The left side-lying position
   c The right side-lying position
   d The supine position

4 Formula for a tube feeding is given
   a At body temperature
   b At room temperature
   c Hot
   d Cold

5 Continuous feedings are given with a
   a Syringe
   b Feeding bag
   c PEG tube
   d Feeding pump

6 The nurse checks feeding tube placement to prevent
   a Aspiration
   b Bleeding
   c Over-feeding
   d Cramping

7 Which position prevents regurgitation after a tube feeding?
   a Fowler's or semi-Fowler's position
   b The supine position
   c The left or right side-lying position
   d The prone position

8 The risk of regurgitation is greatest with
   a Naso-enteral tubes
   b Total parenteral nutrition
   c NG and gastrostomy tubes
   d A jejunostomy tube

9 A person with a feeding tube is NPO. Which measure should you question?
   a Provide oral hygiene
   b Provide mouth rinses
   c Give clear liquids
   d Apply lubricant to the lips

10 A person has an NG tube. To prevent nasal irritation
   a Clean the tube every 4 to 8 hours
   b Replace the tape on the nose every 4 hours
   c Remove the tube every 4 hours
   d Secure the tube to the person's gown

11 A nurse asks you to give a tube feeding. The procedure is not in your job description. What should you do?
   a Give the tube feeding.
   b Refuse to perform the task.
   c Tell the director of nursing.
   d Ask another nurse what you should do.

12 A person is receiving TPN. The person complains of chest pain and difficulty breathing. What should you do?
   a Put the person in Fowler's position.
   b Call for the nurse.
   c Stop the TPN.
   d Provide oral hygiene.

13 A person is receiving TPN. You know that TPN
   a Involves a nutrient solution
   b Is given through a feeding tube
   c Can cause pressure ulcers on the nose
   d Requires that the person be NPO

14 Which is a peripheral IV site?
   a Subclavian vein
   b Superior vena cava
   c Jugular vein
   d A vein on the back of the hand

15 A nurse asks you to check an IV flow rate. A pump is not used. What should you do?
   a Count the drops in 30 seconds. Multiply the number by 2.
   b Count the drops for 1 minute.
   c Check if the fluid is dripping too fast or slow.
   d Measure the amount of fluid.

16 The IV flow rate is
   a The number of gtt/hr
   b The amount of fluid given in 1 minute
   c The number of gtt/min or mL/hr
   d The amount of fluid in the IV bag

17 You note that the IV bag is almost empty. You should
   a Clamp the IV tubing
   b Tell the nurse
   c Remove the IV
   d Adjust the flow rate

18 You see bleeding from an IV site. You should
   a Tell the nurse
   b Move the needle or catheter
   c Remove the IV
   d Clamp the IV tubing

Answers to Chapter 28 questions are on p. 871.

FOCUS ON PRACTICE

Problem Solving

Mrs. Stenson is receiving a continuous tube feeding. You hear her feeding pump alarm sound. You go to check on her. The head of her bed is flat and she says: "My mouth is dry." What do you do first? What do you do next? What can you do within your role limits? What does the nurse need to do?

OBJECTIVES

- Define the key terms and key abbreviations in this chapter.
- Explain why vital signs are measured.
- List the factors affecting vital signs.
- Identify the normal ranges for each temperature site.
- Explain when to use each temperature site.
- Explain how to use thermometers.
- Identify the pulse sites.

- Describe a normal pulse and normal respirations.
- Describe the practices to follow when measuring blood pressure.
- Perform the procedures described in this chapter.
- Know the normal vital signs for the different age-groups.
- Explain how to promote PRIDE in the person, the family, and yourself.

KEY TERMS

afebrile Without (a) a fever (febrile)

apical-radial pulse Taking the apical and radial pulses at the same time

blood pressure (BP) The amount of force exerted against the walls of an artery by the blood

body temperature The amount of heat in the body that is a balance between the amount of heat produced and the amount lost by the body

bradycardia A slow (brady) heart rate (cardia); less than 60 beats per minute

diastole The period of heart muscle relaxation; the heart is at rest

diastolic pressure The pressure in the arteries when the heart is at rest

febrile With a fever

fever Elevated body temperature

hypertension When the systolic pressure is 140 mm Hg or higher (hyper) or the diastolic pressure is 90 mm Hg or higher

hypotension When the systolic pressure is below (hypo) 90 mm Hg or the diastolic pressure is below 60 mm Hg

pulse The beat of the heart felt at an artery as a wave of blood passes through the artery

pulse deficit The difference between the apical and radial pulse rates

pulse rate The number of heartbeats or pulses in 1 minute

respiration Breathing air into (inhalation) and out of (exhalation) the lungs

sphygmomanometer A cuff and measuring device used to measure blood pressure (sphygmo means pulse; manometer is a device for measuring pressure)

stethoscope An instrument used to listen to the sounds produced by the heart, lungs, and other body organs

systole The period of heart muscle contraction; the heart is pumping blood

systolic pressure The pressure in the arteries when the heart contracts

tachycardia A rapid (tachy) heart rate (cardia); more than 100 beats per minute

thermometer A device used to measure (meter) temperature (thermo)

vital signs Temperature, pulse, respirations, and blood pressure; and pain in some agencies

KEY ABBREVIATIONS

BP	Blood pressure	ID	Identification
C	Centigrade	IV	Intravenous
DUS	Doppler ultrasound stethoscope	mm	Millimeter
F	Fahrenheit	mm Hg	Millimeters of mercury
Hg	Mercury	TPR	Temperature, pulse, and respirations

Vital signs reflect the function of 3 body processes essential for life: regulation of body temperature, breathing, and heart function. The *vital signs of body function are:*

- *Temperature*
- *Pulse*
- *Respirations*
- *Blood pressure*
- *Pain (in some agencies)* (Chapter 31)

Vital signs are often called TPR (temperature, pulse, and respirations) and BP (blood pressure). Some agencies include "pain" as a vital sign (p. 511 and Chapter 31). Also see "Pulse Oximetry" in Chapter 39.

MEASURING AND REPORTING VITAL SIGNS

A person's vital signs vary within certain limits. See Box 29-1 for the factors affecting vital signs.

Vital signs are measured to detect changes in normal body function. They tell about treatment response. They often signal life-threatening events. Vital signs are part of the assessment step in the nursing process. Vital signs are measured:

- During physical exams
- When the person is admitted to a health care agency
- As often as the person's condition requires
- Before and after surgery, complex procedures, and diagnostic tests
- After some care measures, such as ambulation (walking)
- After a fall or other injury
- When drugs affect the respiratory or circulatory system
- When the person complains of pain, dizziness, light-headedness, feeling faint, shortness of breath, a rapid heart rate, or not feeling well
- As stated on the care plan (usually daily, twice a day, or weekly in nursing centers)

Vital signs show even minor changes in the person's condition. Accuracy is essential when you measure, record, and report vital signs. If unsure of your measurements, promptly ask the nurse to take them again. Unless otherwise ordered, take vital signs with the person at rest—lying or sitting. Report the following at once.

- Any vital sign that is changed from a prior measurement
- An abnormal vital sign (a vital sign above or below the normal range)

Vital signs are recorded in the person's medical record. If measured often, a flow sheet may be used. The doctor or nurse compares past and current measurements.

See *Focus on Communication: Measuring and Reporting Vital Signs.*

See *Focus on Children and Older Persons: Measuring and Reporting Vital Signs.*

BOX 29-1	Factors Affecting Vital Signs	
• Activity	• Exercise	• Pain
• Age	• Fear	• Sleep
• Anger	• Gender (male	• Smoking
• Anxiety	or female)	• Stress
• Drugs	• Illness	• Weather
• Eating	• Noise	• Weight

FOCUS ON COMMUNICATION

Measuring and Reporting Vital Signs

Some persons like to know their vital signs. If agency policy allows, share the measurements with the person. With the person's consent, you can tell family members if they ask. Remember, this information is private and confidential. Roommates and visitors must not hear what you are saying. For greater privacy, write the measurements for the person.

A measurement may be abnormal. Or you may not be able to feel a pulse or hear a blood pressure. Do not alarm the person. You can say:

- "I'm not sure that I counted your pulse correctly. I'll ask the nurse to take it."
- "I'm not sure that I heard your blood pressure correctly. I'll ask the nurse to take it again."
- "Your pulse is a little slow (or fast). I'll ask the nurse to check it."
- "Your temperature is higher than normal. I'll use another thermometer and ask the nurse to check you."

FOCUS ON CHILDREN AND OLDER PERSONS

Measuring and Reporting Vital Signs

Children

How you measure vital signs varies with the child's age. Equipment also varies. Agency policy and the nurse direct what you do.

The order for measuring vital signs is important. Measuring blood pressure and temperature can upset young children. Stress, fear, and anger affect vital signs. If the child is crying, report this along with the vital sign measurements. In young children, measure vital signs in the following order.

1. Respirations
2. Pulse
3. Blood pressure
4. Temperature

Older Persons

Measuring vital signs on persons with dementia may be difficult. The person may move about, hit at you, and grab equipment. This is not safe for the person or you. Two staff may be needed. One uses touch and a soothing voice to calm and distract the person. The other measures the vital signs.

Trying the procedure when the person is calmer may help. Or take the respirations and pulse at one time. Then take the temperature and blood pressure later.

Always approach the person calmly. Use a soothing voice. Tell the person what you will do. Do not rush. Follow the care plan. If you cannot measure vital signs, tell the nurse at once.

BODY TEMPERATURE

Body temperature is the amount of heat in the body. It is a balance between the amount of heat produced and the amount lost by the body. Heat is produced as cells use food for energy. It is lost through the skin, breathing, urine, and feces. Body temperature is fairly stable. It is lower in the morning and higher in the afternoon and evening. Body temperature is affected by the factors listed in Box 29-1, pregnancy, and the menstrual cycle.

You use thermometers to measure temperature. Temperature is measured using the Fahrenheit (F) and centigrade (C) scales. The degrees symbol (°) is used to record temperatures.

Temperature Sites

Temperature sites are the mouth, rectum, axilla (underarm), tympanic membrane (ear), and temporal artery (forehead) (Box 29-2). Each site has a normal range (Table 29-1). Always report temperatures above or below the normal range.

Fever means an elevated body temperature. These terms are used to describe the person.
- *Febrile*—*with a fever.* (The Latin word *febris* means *fever.*)
- *Afebrile*—*without a fever.* (The prefix *a* means *without.*)
  See *Focus on Communication: Temperature Sites.*
  See *Focus on Children and Older Persons: Temperature Sites.*
  See *Promoting Safety and Comfort: Temperature Sites.*

TABLE 29-1	Normal Body Temperatures	
Site	**Baseline**	**Normal Range**
Oral	98.6°F (37.0°C)	97.6°F to 99.6°F (36.5°C to 37.5°C)
Rectal	99.6°F (37.5°C)	98.6°F to 100.6°F (37.0°C to 38.1°C)
Axillary	97.6°F (36.5°C)	96.6°F to 98.6°F (35.9°C to 37.0°C)
Tympanic membrane	98.6°F (37.0°C)	98.6°F (37.0°C)
Temporal artery	99.6°F (37.5°C)	99.6°F (37.5°C)

BOX 29-2	Temperature Sites

Oral Site
Oral temperatures are *not* taken if the person:
- Is under 4 or 5 years of age.
- Is unconscious.
- Has had surgery or an injury to the face, neck, nose, or mouth.
- Is receiving oxygen.
- Breathes through the mouth.
- Has a naso-gastric tube.
- Is delirious, restless, confused, or disoriented.
- Is paralyzed on 1 side of the body.
- Has a sore mouth.
- Has a convulsive (seizure) disorder.

Rectal Site
The rectal site is used for infants and children under 3 years old. Rectal temperatures are taken when the oral site cannot be used. Rectal temperatures are *not* taken if the person:
- Has diarrhea.
- Has a rectal disorder or injury.
- Has heart disease.
- Had rectal surgery.
- Is confused or agitated.

Tympanic Membrane Site
The site has fewer microbes than the mouth or rectum. The risk of spreading infection is reduced. This site is *not* used if the person has:
- An ear disorder
- Ear drainage

Temporal Artery Site
Measures body temperature at the temporal artery in the forehead. The site is non-invasive.

Axillary Site
Less reliable than the other sites. It is used when the other sites cannot be used.

FOCUS ON COMMUNICATION

Temperature Sites

Checking a rectal temperature can be embarrassing and uncomfortable. Be professional. Explain what you will do and why you must use the rectal site. For example:

> *Mr. Presney, I need to check your temperature. I must check a rectal temperature because your oxygen changes the temperature in your mouth. This electronic thermometer has to stay in place until the thermometer beeps. This will be about 10 seconds. Please tell me if you feel pain.*

A glass thermometer (p. 490) remains in the rectum for at least 2 minutes. This can cause discomfort. To promote comfort, talk the person through the procedure. You can say: "I'm almost done. There's about 1 minute left. Are you doing okay?"

FOCUS ON CHILDREN AND OLDER PERSONS

Temperature Sites

Children
The oral site is not used for infants and children younger than 4 to 5 years. Use other routes as directed by the nurse and the care plan. See Box 29-2.

Older Persons
Older persons have lower body temperatures than younger persons. An oral temperature of 98.6°F may signal fever in an older person.

Thermometers

A *thermometer* *is a device used to measure* (meter) *temperature* (thermo). Follow the manufacturer's instructions and agency procedures to use, clean, and store thermometers.

Electronic Thermometers. Electronic thermometers show the temperature on the front of the device. Probe covers prevent the spread of infection. Battery operated, they are kept in chargers when not in use.

- *Standard electronic thermometers*—measure body temperature at the oral, rectal, and axillary sites in a few seconds. They have oral (blue) and rectal (red) probes. The oral (blue) probe is also used for axillary temperatures. A disposable cover (sheath) protects the probe. See Figure 29-1, *A*.
- *Tympanic membrane thermometers*—measure body temperature at the tympanic membrane in the ear in 1 to 3 seconds (Fig. 29-1, *B*). They are comfortable and not invasive. There are fewer microbes in the ear than in the mouth or rectum. The risk of spreading infection is reduced. These devices are not used if there is ear drainage. To use one, gently insert the covered probe into the ear.
- *Temporal artery thermometers*—measure body temperature at the temporal artery in the forehead in 3 to 4 seconds (Fig. 29-1, *C*). Non-invasive, they measure the temperature of the blood in the temporal artery. It is the same temperature of the blood coming from the heart. To use one:
  1. Use the side of the head that is exposed. Do not use the side covered by hair, a dressing, a hat, or other covering. Do not use the side that was on a pillow.
  2. Place a disposable cap or cover on the thermometer.
  3. Place the device in the center of the forehead.
  4. Press the scan button.
  5. Slide the device across the forehead and across the temporal artery (see Fig. 29-1, *C*).
  6. Release the scan button.
  7. Read the temperature display.
- *Digital thermometers*—measure body temperature at the oral, rectal, and axillary sites. Depending on the type, the temperature is measured in 6 to 60 seconds. See Figure 29-1, *D*.
- *Pacifier thermometers*—look like a baby's pacifier (Fig. 29-1, *E*). The baby sucks on the device for 90 seconds. The temperature is displayed on the front. See *Teamwork and Time Management: Electronic Thermometers.*

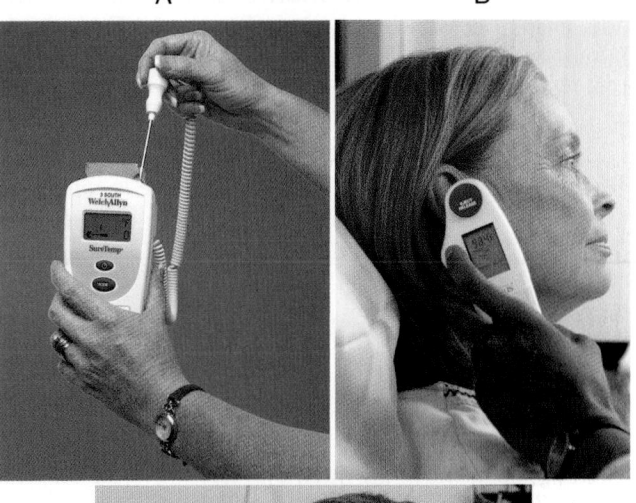
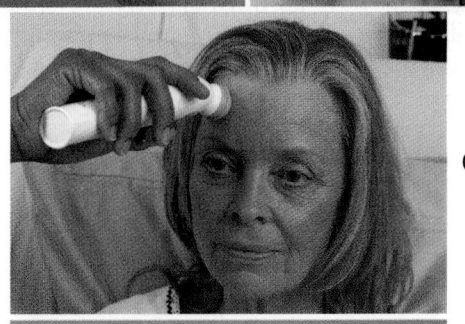
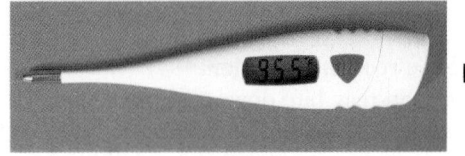
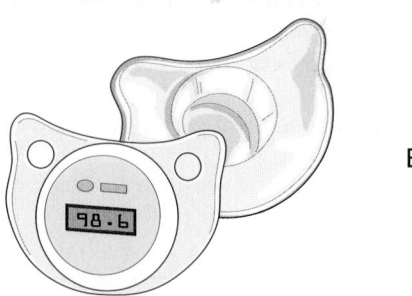

FIGURE 29-1 Electronic thermometers. **A,** Standard electronic thermometer. **B,** Tympanic membrane thermometer. **C,** Temporal artery thermometer. **D,** Digital thermometer. **E,** Pacifier thermometer.

Disposable Oral Thermometers. Small chemical dots change color when heated (Fig. 29-2). Each dot is heated to a certain temperature before it changes color. Used once, these thermometers measure temperature in 45 to 60 seconds.

Temperature-Sensitive Tape. The tape is applied to the forehead and changes color in response to body heat (Fig. 29-3). The measurement takes about 15 seconds.

Glass Thermometers. Glass thermometers have a hollow glass tube and a bulb tip (Fig. 29-4). The device is filled with a substance. When heated, the substance expands and rises in the tube. When cooled, the substance contracts and moves down the tube.

Long- or slender-tip thermometers are used for oral and axillary temperatures. So are thermometers with stubby and pear-shaped tips. Rectal thermometers have stubby tips. See Figure 29-4.

Glass thermometers are color-coded.
• Blue—oral and axillary thermometers
• Red—rectal thermometers

Glass thermometers are re-usable. However, the following are problems.
• They take a long time to register—3 to 10 minutes depending on the site (p. 494).
• They break easily. Broken rectal thermometers can injure the rectum and colon.
• The person may bite down and break an oral thermometer. Cuts in the mouth are risks. If the thermometer contains mercury, swallowed mercury can cause mercury poisoning.

See *Focus on Long-Term Care and Home Care: Glass Thermometers.*

See *Promoting Safety and Comfort: Glass Thermometers.*

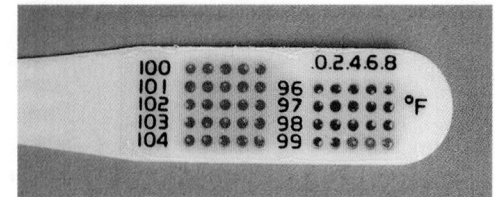

FIGURE 29-2 Disposable oral thermometer with chemical dots.

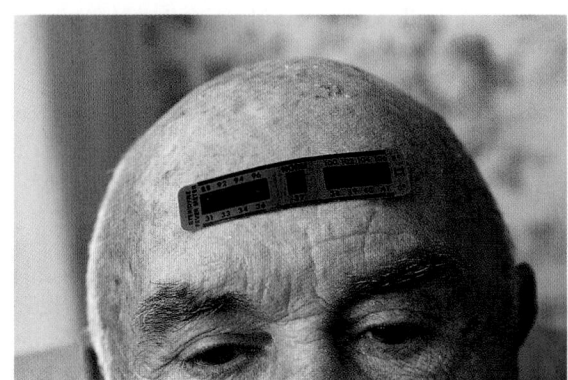

FIGURE 29-3 Temperature sensitive tape.

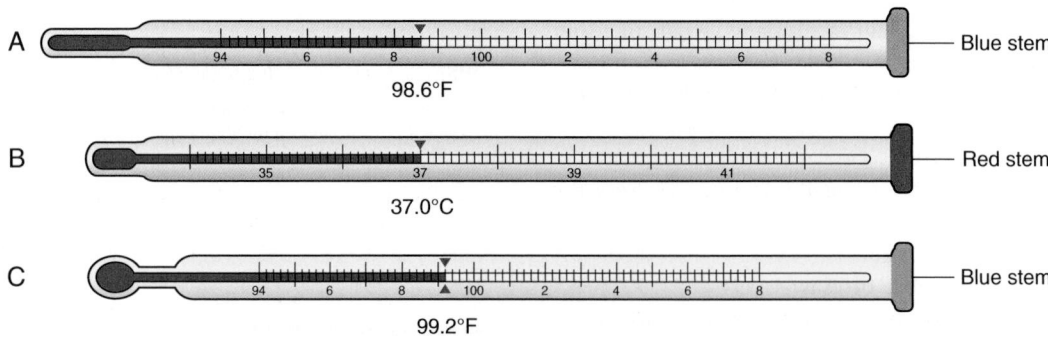

FIGURE 29-4 Glass thermometers. **A,** A Fahrenheit thermometer with a long or slender tip. The temperature measurement is 98.6°F. **B,** Centigrade thermometer with a stubby tip (rectal thermometer). The temperature measurement is 37.0°C. **C,** Fahrenheit thermometer with a pear-shaped tip. The temperature measurement is 99.2°F.

FOCUS ON LONG-TERM CARE AND HOME CARE

Glass Thermometers

Home Care

Your home care agency may supply you with a digital thermometer. However, patients in home settings may have mercury-glass thermometers. If so, tell the nurse. The nurse can suggest that the person buy a digital thermometer or a glass thermometer with a mercury-free substance.

You may care for children in home settings. Do not use a mercury-glass thermometer to measure a child's temperature.

FOCUS ON CHILDREN AND OLDER PERSONS

Taking Temperatures

Older Persons

Tympanic membrane and temporal artery thermometers are used for persons who are confused and resist care. They are fast and comfortable. Oral and rectal thermometers are unsafe because:

- A glass thermometer can easily break if the person moves, resists care, or bites down on it. Serious injury can occur.
- A standard electronic thermometer can injure the mouth and teeth if the person bites down on it. It also can cause injury if the person moves quickly and without warning.

PROMOTING SAFETY AND COMFORT

Glass Thermometers

Safety

Mercury-glass thermometers are rarely used today. Safer chemicals have replaced mercury. However, do not assume that a glass thermometer contains a mercury-free mixture. If a thermometer breaks, tell the nurse at once.

Mercury is a hazardous substance. Do not touch the substance. Do not let the person do so. The agency follows special procedures for handling all hazardous materials. See Chapter 13.

DELEGATION GUIDELINES

Taking Temperatures

Before taking temperatures, you need this information from the nurse and the care plan.

- What site to use for each person—oral, rectal, axillary, tympanic membrane, or temporal artery
- What thermometer to use for each person
- How long to leave a glass thermometer in place (p. 494)
- When to take temperatures
- Which persons are at risk for a fever
- What observations to report and record
- When to report observations
- What patient or resident concerns to report at once:
    - A temperature that is changed from a past measurement
    - A temperature above or below the normal range for the site used

Taking Temperatures

The nurse and care plan tell you:

- When to take the person's temperature
- What site to use
- What thermometer to use

See *Focus on Children and Older Persons: Taking Temperatures.*

See *Delegation Guidelines: Taking Temperatures.*

See *Promoting Safety and Comfort: Taking Temperatures.*

Taking Temperatures With Electronic Thermometers. There are many types of electronic thermometers. Follow the manufacturer's instructions. The procedure that follows is used as a guide.

See procedure: *Taking a Temperature With an Electronic Thermometer*, p. 492.

Text continued on p. 494.

PROMOTING SAFETY AND COMFORT

Taking Temperatures

Safety

Thermometers are inserted into the mouth, rectum, axilla, and ear. Each area has many microbes. The area may contain blood. Therefore each person has his or her own glass or digital thermometer. This prevents the spread of microbes and infection. Follow Standard Precautions and the Bloodborne Pathogen Standard when taking temperatures.

With rectal temperatures, your gloved hands may have contact with feces. If so, remove gloves and practice hand hygiene. Then note the temperature on your note pad or assignment sheet. Put on clean gloves to complete the procedure.

Comfort

Remove the thermometer in a timely manner. Do not leave it in place longer than needed. This affects the person's comfort. For example, an oral glass thermometer is left in place for 2 to 3 minutes. Do not leave it in place longer than that.

Taking a Temperature With an Electronic Thermometer

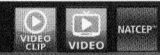

QUALITY OF LIFE

- Knock before entering the person's room.
- Address the person by name.
- Introduce yourself by name and title.

- Explain the procedure before starting and during the procedure.
- Protect the person's rights during the procedure.
- Handle the person gently during the procedure.

PRE-PROCEDURE

1 Follow *Delegation Guidelines: Taking Temperatures,* p. 491. See *Promoting Safety and Comfort: Taking Temperatures,* p. 491.
2 For an oral temperature, ask the person not to eat, drink, smoke, or chew gum for at least 15 to 20 minutes before the measurement or as required by agency policy.
3 Practice hand hygiene.
4 Collect the following.
   - Thermometer—electronic or tympanic membrane
   - Probe (blue for an oral or axillary temperature; red for a rectal temperature)

   - Probe covers
   - Toilet tissue (rectal temperature)
   - Water-soluble lubricant (rectal temperature)
   - Gloves
   - Towel (axillary temperature)
5 Plug the probe into the thermometer if using a standard electronic thermometer.
6 Practice hand hygiene.
7 Identify the person. Check the identification (ID) bracelet against the assignment sheet. Use 2 identifiers (Chapter 13). Also call the person by name.

PROCEDURE

8 Provide for privacy. Position the person for an oral, rectal, axillary, or tympanic membrane temperature. The Sims' position is used for a rectal temperature.
9 Put on gloves if contact with blood, body fluids, secretions, or excretions is likely.
10 Insert the probe into a probe cover.
11 *To take an oral temperature:*
   a Ask the person to open the mouth and raise the tongue.
   b Place the covered probe at the base of the tongue and to 1 side (Fig. 29-5).
   c Ask the person to lower the tongue and close the mouth.
12 *To take a rectal temperature:*
   a Place some lubricant on toilet tissue.
   b Lubricate the end of the covered probe.
   c Expose the anal area.
   d Raise the upper buttock (Fig. 29-6).
   e Insert the probe ½ inch into the rectum.
   f Hold the probe in place.
13 *To take an axillary temperature:*
   a Help the person remove an arm from the gown. Do not expose the person.
   b Dry the axilla with the towel.
   c Place the covered probe in the center of the axilla (Fig. 29-7).
   d Place the person's arm over the chest.
   e Hold the probe in place.

14 *To take a tympanic membrane temperature:*
   a Ask the person to turn his or her head so the ear is in front of you.
   b Pull up and back on the adult's ear to straighten the ear canal (Fig. 29-8).
   c Insert the covered probe gently.
15 Start the thermometer.
16 Hold the probe in place until you hear a tone or see a flashing or steady light.
17 Read the temperature on the display.
18 Remove the probe. Press the eject button to discard the cover.
19 Note the person's name, temperature, and temperature site on your note pad or assignment sheet.
20 Return the probe to the holder.
21 Help the person put the gown back on (axillary temperature). For a rectal temperature:
   a Wipe the anal area with toilet tissue to remove lubricant.
   b Cover the person.
   c Dispose of used toilet tissue.
   d Remove and discard the gloves. Practice hand hygiene.

POST-PROCEDURE

22 Provide for comfort. (See the inside of the front cover.)
23 Place the call light and other needed items within reach.
24 Unscreen the person.
25 Complete a safety check of the room. (See the inside of the front cover.)

26 Return the thermometer to the charging unit.
27 Practice hand hygiene.
28 Report and record the temperature. Note the temperature site when reporting and recording. Report an abnormal temperature at once.

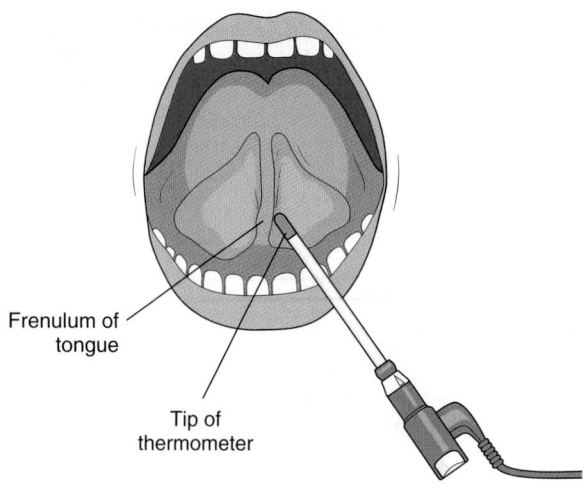

FIGURE 29-5 The thermometer is placed at the base of the tongue and to 1 side.

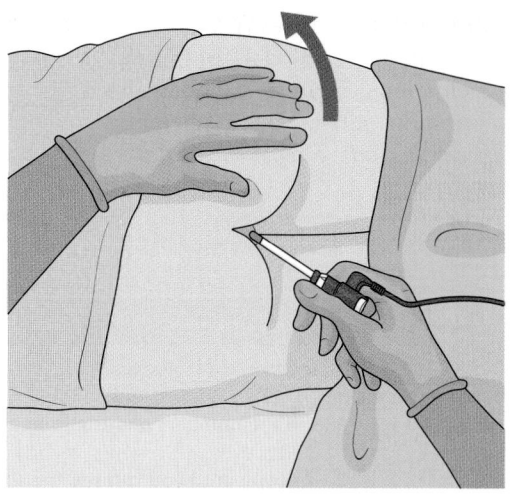

FIGURE 29-6 The rectal temperature is taken with the person in Sims' position. The buttock is raised to expose the anus.

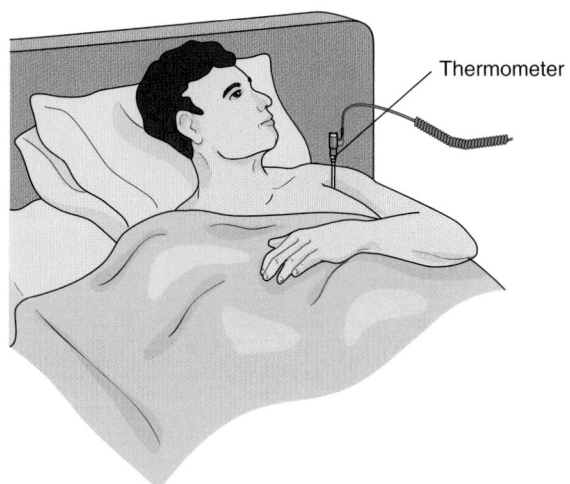

FIGURE 29-7 The thermometer is held in place in the axilla by bringing the person's arm over the chest.

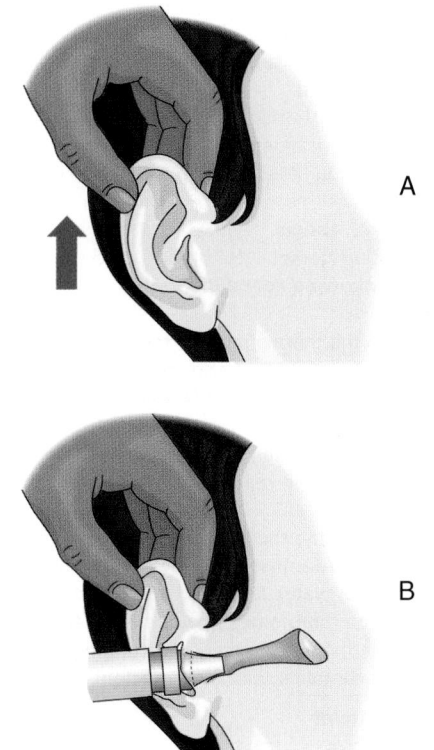

FIGURE 29-8 Using a tympanic membrane thermometer. **A,** The adult's ear is pulled up and back. **B,** The probe is inserted into the ear canal.

Taking Temperatures With Glass Thermometers.

While uncommon in hospitals and nursing centers, glass thermometers may be used in homes. See Box 29-3 for how to use and read glass thermometers.

See *Focus on Math: Taking Temperatures With Glass Thermometers.*

See procedure: *Taking a Temperature With a Glass Thermometer.*

BOX 29-3	Glass Thermometers

Reading a Glass Thermometer
- Hold it at the stem (Fig. 29-9). Bring it to eye level.
- Turn it until you can see the numbers and the long and short lines.
- Turn it back and forth slowly until you can see the silver or red line.
- Read from the tip toward the stem.
- Read the nearest degree (long line) to the left of the silver or red line.
- Read the nearest tenth of a degree (short line)—an even number on a Fahrenheit thermometer.

Using a Glass Thermometer
- Follow Standard Precautions and the Bloodborne Pathogen Standard.
- Use the person's thermometer.
- Use a rectal thermometer only for rectal temperatures.
- Rinse the thermometer under cold, running water if it was soaking in a disinfectant. Dry it from the stem to the bulb end with tissues.
- Check the thermometer for breaks, cracks, and chips. Discard it following agency policy if it is broken, cracked, or chipped.
- Shake down the thermometer to move the substance down in the tube. Hold it at the stem and stand away from walls, tables, or other hard surfaces. Flex and snap your wrist until the substance is below 94°F or 34°C. See Figure 29-10.
- Insert the thermometer into a plastic cover (Fig. 29-11). Remove the cover to read the device. Discard the cover after use.
- Clean and store the thermometer following agency policy. Wipe it with tissues first to remove mucus, feces, or sweat. Do not use hot water. It causes the substance to expand so much that the thermometer could break. After cleaning, rinse the thermometer under cold, running water. Then store it in a container with a disinfectant solution.

Taking Temperatures
- The oral site:
  - The glass thermometer remains in place 2 to 3 minutes or as required by agency policy.
- The rectal site:
  - Provide for privacy. The buttocks and anus are exposed. The procedure embarrasses many people.
  - Lubricate the bulb end of the rectal thermometer for easy insertion and to prevent injury.
  - Hold the device in place so it is not lost into the rectum or broken.
  - Leave the thermometer in the rectum for 2 minutes or as required by agency policy.
- The axillary site:
  - Make sure the axilla (underarm) is dry. Do not use the site right after bathing.
  - Leave the thermometer in place for 5 to 10 minutes or as required by agency policy.

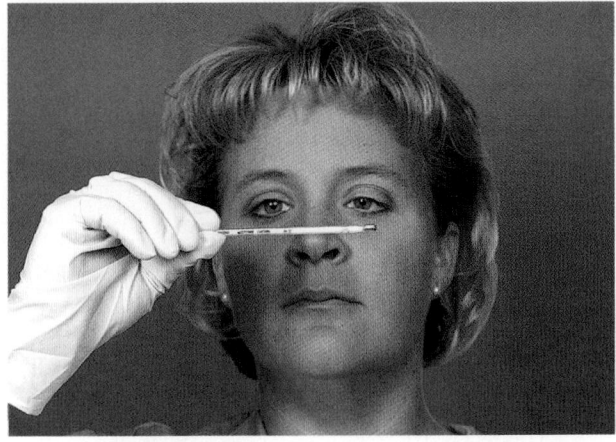

FIGURE 29-9 The thermometer is held at the stem. It is read at eye level.

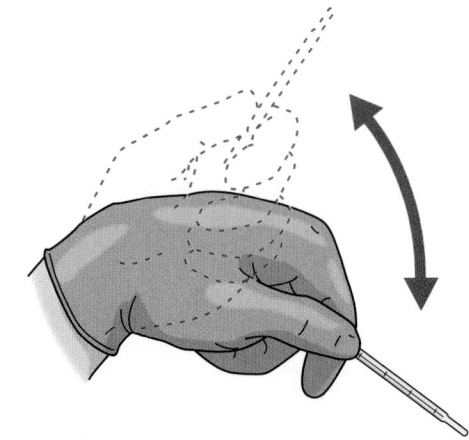

FIGURE 29-10 The wrist is snapped to shake down the thermometer.

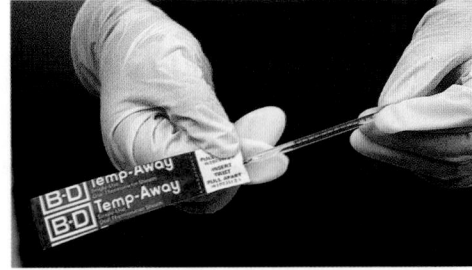

FIGURE 29-11 The thermometer is inserted into a plastic cover.

FOCUS ON MATH

Taking Temperatures With Glass Thermometers

To read a thermometer, you must understand whole numbers and decimals. Whole numbers are 0, 1, 2, 3, and so on. They are to the *left* of the decimal point. The numbers to the right of the decimal point are part of a whole number. Thermometers are read to 1 number past the decimal point (the "tenths" place). See Figure 29-12.

To read a glass thermometer (Fig. 29-13):

1 Read the nearest long line to the left of the silver or red line.
   * Fahrenheit—every other long line is an even degree (ending in 0, 2, 4, 6, or 8) from 94°F to 108°F.
   * Centigrade—every long line is 1 degree from 34°C to 42°C.
2 Read the nearest tenth of a degree (short line).
   * Fahrenheit—the short lines mean 0.2 (two-tenths) of a degree.
   * Centigrade—each short line means 0.1 (one-tenth) of a degree.

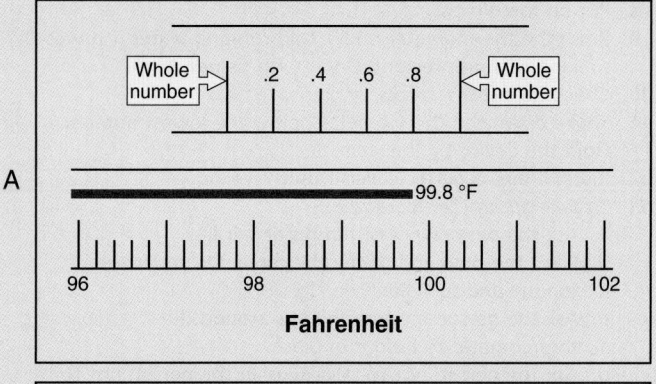

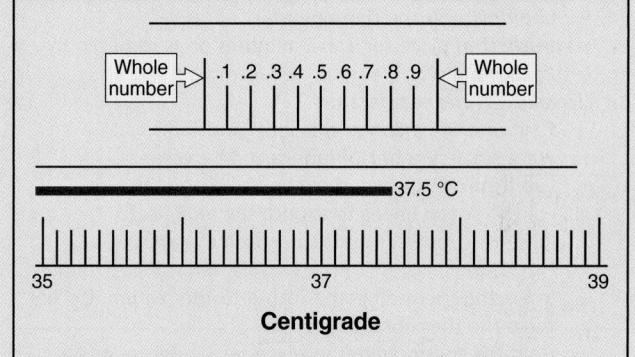

FIGURE 29-13 Reading thermometers. A, Fahrenheit thermometer. Every other long line is marked in even degrees. Each long line increases by 1 degree. Each short line increases by 0.2 (two-tenths) of a degree. **B,** Centigrade thermometer. Each long line increases by 1 degree. Each short line increases by 0.1 (one-tenth) of a degree.

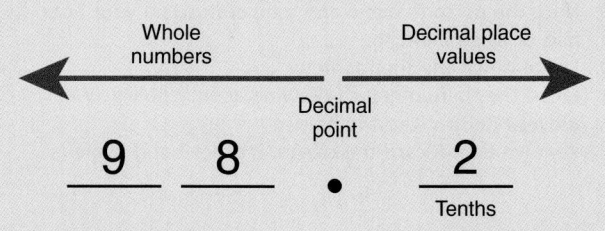

FIGURE 29-12 Values used to read thermometers.

Taking a Temperature With a Glass Thermometer

QUALITY OF LIFE

* Knock before entering the person's room.
* Address the person by name.
* Introduce yourself by name and title.

* Explain the procedure before starting and during the procedure.
* Protect the person's rights during the procedure.
* Handle the person gently during the procedure.

PRE-PROCEDURE

1 Follow *Delegation Guidelines: Taking Temperatures,* p. 491. See *Promoting Safety and Comfort:*
   a *Glass Thermometers,* p. 491
   b *Taking Temperatures,* p. 491
2 For an oral temperature, ask the person not to eat, drink, smoke, or chew gum for at least 15 to 20 minutes before the measurement or as required by agency policy.
3 Practice hand hygiene.

4 Collect the following.
   * Oral or rectal thermometer and holder
   * Tissues
   * Plastic covers if used
   * Gloves
   * Toilet tissue (rectal temperature)
   * Water-soluble lubricant (rectal temperature)
   * Towel (axillary temperature)
5 Practice hand hygiene.
6 Identify the person. Check the ID bracelet against the assignment sheet. Use 2 identifiers (Chapter 13). Also call the person by name.
7 Provide for privacy.

Continued

Taking a Temperature With a Glass Thermometer—cont'd

PROCEDURE

8   Put on the gloves.

9   Rinse the thermometer under cold running water if it was soaking in a disinfectant. Dry it with tissues.

10 Check for breaks, cracks, or chips.

11 Shake down the thermometer below the lowest number. Hold the device by the stem. See Figure 29-10.

12 Insert it into a plastic cover if used (see Fig. 29-11).

13 *To take an oral temperature:*
   a Ask the person to moisten his or her lips.
   b Place the bulb end of the thermometer under the tongue and to 1 side (see Fig. 29-5).
   c Ask the person to close the lips around the thermometer to hold it in place.
   d Ask the person not to talk. Remind the person not to bite down on the thermometer.
   e Leave it in place for 2 to 3 minutes or as required by agency policy.

14 *To take a rectal temperature:*
   a Position the person in the Sims' position.
   b Put a small amount of lubricant on a tissue.
   c Lubricate the bulb end of the thermometer.
   d Fold back top linens to expose the anal area.
   e Raise the upper buttock to expose the anus (see Fig. 29-6).
   f Insert the thermometer 1 inch into the rectum. Do not force the thermometer.
   g Hold the thermometer in place for 2 minutes or as required by agency policy. Do not let go of it while it is in the rectum.

15 *To take an axillary temperature:*
   a Help the person remove an arm from the gown. Do not expose the person.
   b Dry the axilla with the towel.
   c Place the bulb end of the thermometer in the center of the axilla.
   d Ask the person to place the arm over the chest to hold the thermometer in place (see Fig. 29-7). Hold it and the arm in place if he or she cannot help.
   e Leave the thermometer in place for 5 to 10 minutes or as required by agency policy.

16 Remove the thermometer.

17 *After taking an oral or axillary temperature:*
   a Use a tissue to remove the plastic cover.
   b Wipe the thermometer with a tissue if no cover was used. Wipe from the stem to the bulb end.
   c Discard the tissue and cover (if used).
   d Read the thermometer.
   e Help the person put the gown back on (axillary temperature).

18 *After taking a rectal temperature:*
   a Use toilet tissue to remove the plastic cover.
   b Wipe the thermometer with toilet tissue if no cover was used. Wipe from the stem to the bulb end.
   c Place used toilet tissue on several thicknesses of clean toilet tissue. Discard the cover (if used).
   d Read the thermometer.
   e Place the thermometer on clean toilet tissue.
   f Wipe the anal area with toilet tissue to remove lubricant and any feces. Set the used toilet tissue on several thicknesses of clean toilet tissue.
   g Cover the person.
   h Dispose of toilet tissue in the toilet.
   i Remove and discard the gloves. Practice hand hygiene.

19 Note the person's name and temperature on your note pad or assignment sheet.

20 Shake down the thermometer.

21 Clean the thermometer following agency policy. (Wear gloves.) Return it to the holder.

22 Remove and discard the gloves. Practice hand hygiene.

POST-PROCEDURE

23 Provide for comfort. (See the inside of the front cover.)

24 Place the call light and other needed items within reach.

25 Unscreen the person.

26 Complete a safety check of the room. (See the inside of the front cover.)

27 Practice hand hygiene.

28 Report and record the temperature. Note the temperature site when reporting and recording. Report an abnormal temperature at once.

PULSE

Arteries carry blood from the heart to all parts of the body. The *pulse* is the beat of the heart felt at an artery as a wave of blood passes through the artery. A pulse is felt when the heart beats.

See *Body Structure and Function Review: The Heart and Blood Vessels.*

Pulse Sites

The temporal, carotid, brachial, radial, femoral, popliteal, posterior tibial, and dorsalis pedis (pedal) pulses are on each side of the body (Fig. 29-16, p. 498). The arteries are close to the body surface and lie over a bone. Therefore they are easy to feel.

The radial pulse is used most often. It is easy to reach and find. The person is not exposed. The carotid pulse is taken during cardiopulmonary resuscitation (CPR) and other emergencies (Chapter 54).

The apical pulse is felt over the heart. The apex (apical) of the heart is at the tip of the heart, just below the left nipple (p. 501). This pulse is taken with a stethoscope (p. 499).

See *Focus on Children and Older Persons: Pulse Sites,* p. 498.

BODY STRUCTURE AND FUNCTION REVIEW

The Heart and Blood Vessels

The heart is a muscle. It pumps blood through the blood vessels to the tissues and cells. The heart lies in the middle to lower part of the chest cavity toward the left side (Fig. 29-14).

The heart has 4 chambers. Upper chambers receive blood and are called the *atria*. The *right atrium* receives blood from body tissues. The *left atrium* receives blood from the lungs. Lower chambers are called *ventricles*. Ventricles pump blood. The *right ventricle* pumps blood to the lungs for oxygen. The *left ventricle* pumps blood to all parts of the body.

There are 2 phases of heart action. *Diastole* is the resting phase. Heart chambers fill with blood. *Systole* is the working phase. The heart contracts. Blood is pumped through the blood vessels when the heart contracts.

Blood flows to body tissues and cells through the blood vessels. *Arteries* carry blood away from the heart. Arterial blood is rich in oxygen. The *aorta* is the largest artery. The aorta receives blood directly from the left ventricle. The aorta branches into other arteries that carry blood to all parts of the body (Fig. 29-15). *Veins* return blood to the heart.

See Chapter 10 for more detailed information.

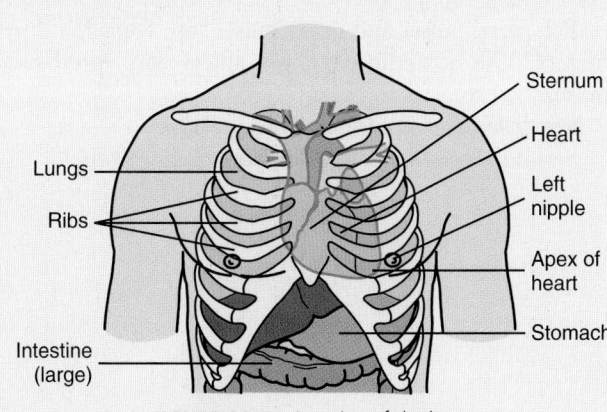

FIGURE 29-14 Location of the heart.

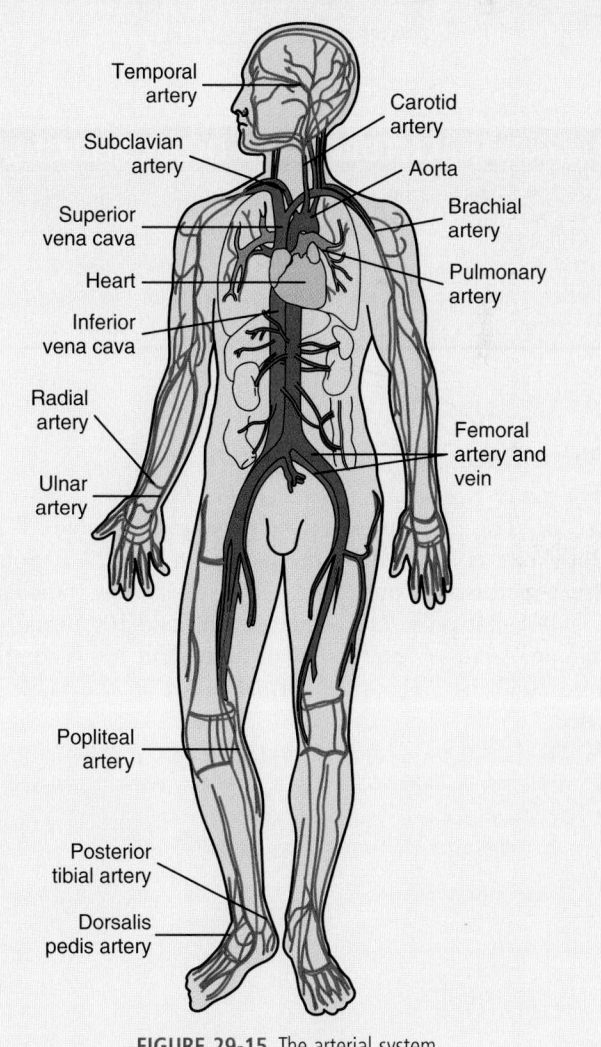

FIGURE 29-15 The arterial system.

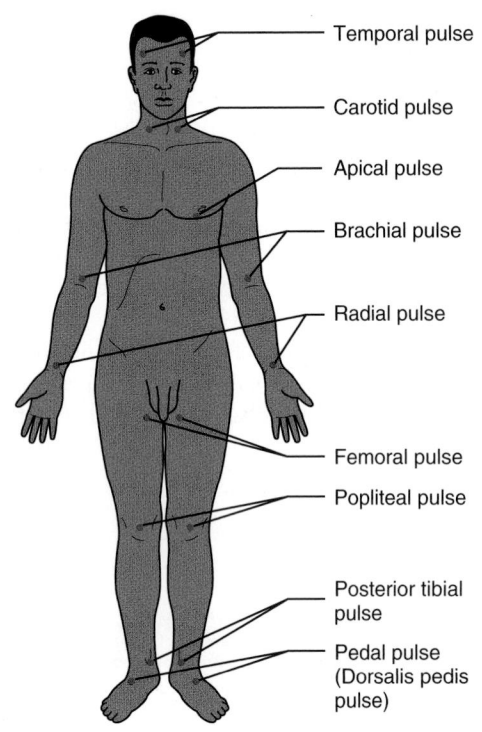

FIGURE 29-16 The pulse sites.

TABLE 29-2	Pulse Ranges by Age
Age	Pulse Rate per Minute
Birth to 1 year	80-190
2 years	80-160
6 years	75-120
10 years	70-110
12 years and older	60-100

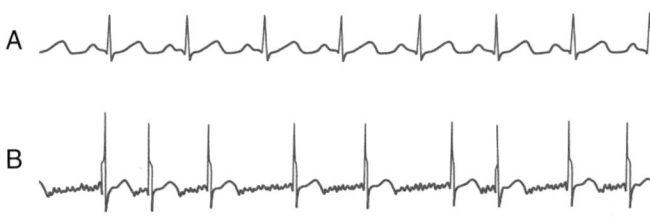

FIGURE 29-17 A, The electrocardiogram shows a regular pulse. The beats occur at regular intervals. **B,** These beats are at irregular intervals.

FOCUS ON CHILDREN AND OLDER PERSONS

Pulse Sites

Children
The apical pulse is used for infants and children under 2 years. The nurse may ask you to use the radial site for children older than 2 years.

Pulse Rate

The **pulse rate** *is the number of heartbeats or pulses in 1 minute.* The rate varies for each age-group (Table 29-2). Pulse rate is affected by the factors in Box 29-1. Some drugs increase the pulse rate. Other drugs slow the pulse.

The adult pulse rate is between 60 and 100 beats per minute. A rate of less than 60 or more than 100 is considered abnormal. Report abnormal pulses to the nurse at once.

- **Tachycardia** *is a rapid* (tachy) *heart rate* (cardia). *The heart rate is more than 100 beats per minute.*
- **Bradycardia** *is a slow* (brady) *heart rate* (cardia). *The heart rate is less than 60 beats per minute.*

Pulse Rhythm and Force

The pulse *rhythm* should be regular. There is a pattern. The same interval occurs between beats. An irregular pulse occurs when the beats are not evenly spaced or beats are skipped (Fig. 29-17).

Force relates to pulse strength. A forceful pulse is easy to feel. It is described as *strong, full,* or *bounding.* Hard-to-feel pulses are described as *weak, thready,* or *feeble.*

Electronic blood pressure equipment (p. 507) can also count pulses. The pulse rate and blood pressures are shown. Some show if the pulse is regular or irregular. However, you need to feel the pulse to determine its force.

Taking Pulses

You will take radial, apical, and apical-radial pulses. You must count, report, and record accurately.

For radial pulses and other pulses, use your first 2 or 3 fingers. Use a stethoscope for apical and apical-radial pulses.

See *Delegation Guidelines: Taking Pulses.*
See *Promoting Safety and Comfort: Taking Pulses.*

Using a Stethoscope. A *stethoscope is an instrument used to listen to the sounds produced by the heart, lungs, and other body organs* (Fig. 29-18). It is used for apical pulses and blood pressures. The device makes sounds louder for easy hearing. See Box 29-4 for how to use a stethoscope.

See *Focus on Communication: Using a Stethoscope*, p. 500.

See *Promoting Safety and Comfort: Using a Stethoscope*, p. 500.

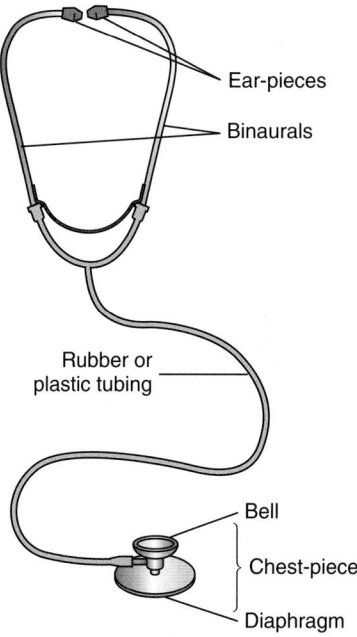

FIGURE 29-18 Parts of a stethoscope.

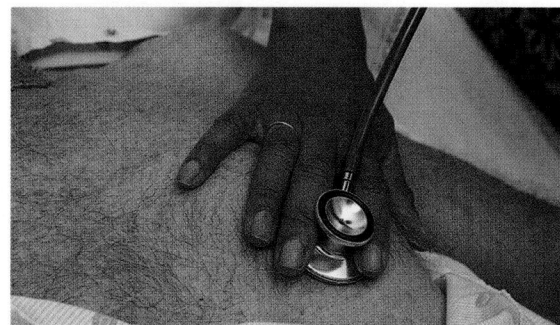

FIGURE 29-19 The stethoscope is held in place with the fingertips of the index and middle fingers.

Taking Radial Pulses. The radial pulse is used for routine vital signs. Place the first 2 or 3 fingertips of 1 hand against the radial artery. The radial artery is on the thumb side of the wrist (Fig. 29-21).

Follow agency policy for how long to count pulses. The following is common.

- Regular pulses—count the pulse for 30 seconds. Multiply by 2 for the number of pulses in 1 minute.
- Irregular pulses—count the pulse for 1 minute.

In some agencies, all pulses are taken for 1 minute. Some state competency tests require that pulses are taken for 1 minute.

See *Focus on Math: Taking Radial Pulses.*
See procedure: *Taking a Radial Pulse.*

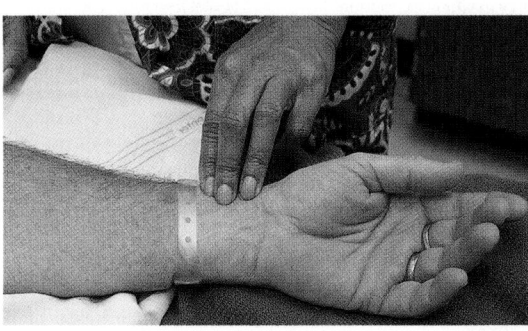

FIGURE 29-21 The 3 middle fingers are used to take the radial pulse.

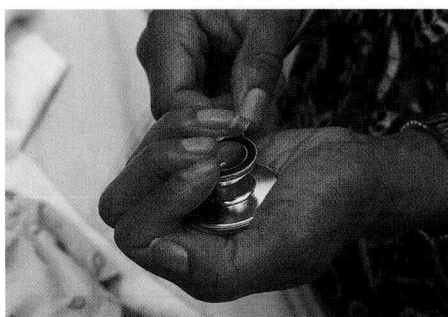

FIGURE 29-20 The diaphragm of the stethoscope is warmed in the palm of the hand.

Taking a Radial Pulse

QUALITY OF LIFE

- Knock before entering the person's room.
- Address the person by name.
- Introduce yourself by name and title.

- Explain the procedure before starting and during the procedure.
- Protect the person's rights during the procedure.
- Handle the person gently during the procedure.

PRE-PROCEDURE

1 Follow *Delegation Guidelines: Taking Pulses,* p. 499. See *Promoting Safety and Comfort: Taking Pulses,* p. 499.
2 Practice hand hygiene.

3 Identify the person. Check the ID bracelet against the assignment sheet. Use 2 identifiers (Chapter 13). Also call the person by name.
4 Provide for privacy.

PROCEDURE

5 Have the person sit or lie down.
6 Locate the radial pulse on the thumb side of the person's wrist. Use your first 2 or 3 middle fingertips (see Fig. 29-21).
7 Note if the pulse is strong or weak and regular or irregular.
8 Count the pulse for 30 seconds. Multiply the number of beats by 2 for the number of pulses in 60 seconds (1 minute). For example:
   - You count 45 beats in 30 seconds.
   - Multiply 45 beats by 2.
   - 45 beats × 2 = 90 beats per minute.

9 Count the pulse for 1 minute if:
   a Directed by the nurse and the care plan.
   b Required by agency policy.
   c The pulse was irregular.
   d Required for your state competency test.
10 Note the following on your note pad or assignment sheet.
   a The person's name
   b Pulse rate
   c Pulse strength
   d If the pulse was regular or irregular

POST-PROCEDURE

11 Provide for comfort. (See the inside of the front cover.)
12 Place the call light and other needed items within reach.
13 Unscreen the person.
14 Complete a safety check of the room. (See the inside of the front cover.)

15 Practice hand hygiene.
16 Report and record the pulse rate and your observations. Report an abnormal pulse at once.

Taking Apical and Apical-Radial Pulses. The apical pulse is on the left side of the chest slightly below the nipple (Fig. 29-22). Apical pulses are taken on persons who:

- Have heart disease.
- Have irregular heart rhythms.
- Take drugs that affect the heart.

The apical and radial pulse rates should be the same. Sometimes heart contractions are not strong enough to create pulses in the radial artery. Then the radial rate is less than the apical rate. Heart disease is a common cause.

To see if the apical and radial pulses are equal, 2 staff members are needed. One takes the radial pulse; the other takes the apical pulse (Fig. 29-23, p. 502). *Taking the apical and radial pulses at the same time is called the* **apical-radial pulse.** The **pulse deficit** *is the difference between the apical and radial pulse rates.*

A stethoscope is used to take apical and apical-radial pulses. Count the pulse for 1 minute. The heartbeat normally sounds like a *lub-dub.* Count each *lub-dub* as 1 beat. Do not count the *lub* as 1 beat and the *dub* as another.

See *Focus on Math: Taking Apical and Apical-Radial Pulses,* p. 502.

See procedure: *Taking an Apical Pulse,* p. 502.

See procedure: *Taking an Apical-Radial Pulse,* p. 503.

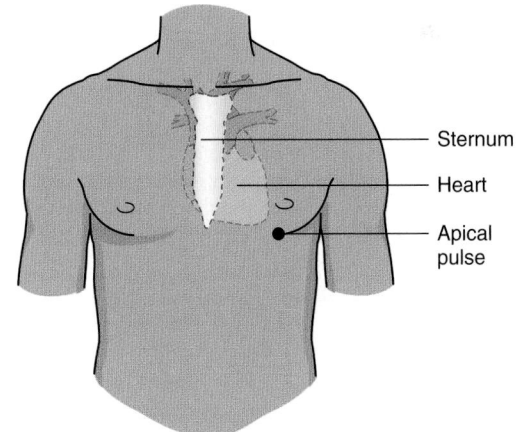

FIGURE 29-22 The apical pulse is located 2 to 3 inches to the left of the sternum (breastbone) and below the left nipple.

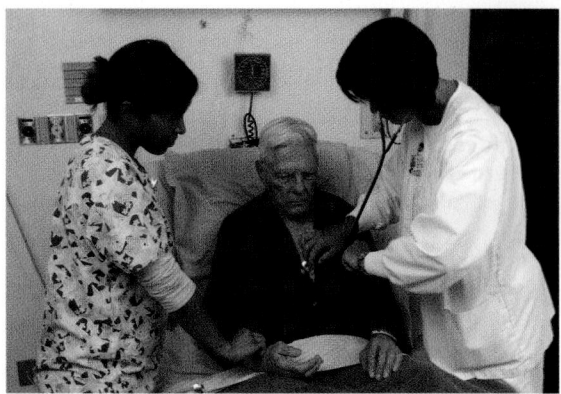

FIGURE 29-23 Taking an apical-radial pulse. One worker takes the apical pulse. The other takes the radial pulse.

FOCUS ON MATH

Taking Apical and Apical-Radial Pulses

For the *pulse deficit,* subtract the radial rate from the apical rate. (The radial rate is never greater than the apical rate.) For example:

- The apical rate is 84 beats per minute. The radial rate is 84 beats per minute.

$$84 \text{ apical beats} - 84 \text{ radial beats} = 0$$
The pulse deficit is 0.

- The apical rate is 90 beats per minute. The radial rate is 86 beats per minute.

$$90 \text{ apical beats} - 86 \text{ radial beats} = 4$$
The pulse deficit is 4.

Taking an Apical Pulse

QUALITY OF LIFE

- Knock before entering the person's room.
- Address the person by name.
- Introduce yourself by name and title.

- Explain the procedure before starting and during the procedure.
- Protect the person's rights during the procedure.
- Handle the person gently during the procedure.

PRE-PROCEDURE

1 Follow *Delegation Guidelines: Taking Pulses,* p. 499. See *Promoting Safety and Comfort: Using a Stethoscope,* p. 500.
2 Practice hand hygiene.
3 Collect a stethoscope and antiseptic wipes.

4 Practice hand hygiene.
5 Identify the person. Check the ID bracelet against the assignment sheet. Use 2 identifiers (Chapter 13). Also call the person by name.
6 Provide for privacy.

PROCEDURE

7 Clean the stethoscope ear-pieces and chest-piece with the wipes.
8 Have the person sit or lie down.
9 Expose the nipple area of the left chest. Expose a woman's breasts only to the extent necessary.
10 Warm the diaphragm in your palm.
11 Place the stethoscope ear-pieces in your ears.
12 Find the apical pulse. Place the diaphragm 2 to 3 inches to the left of the breastbone and below the left nipple (see Fig. 29-22).

13 Count the pulse for 1 minute. Note if it was regular or irregular.
14 Cover the person. Remove the stethoscope ear-pieces.
15 Note the person's name and pulse on your note pad or assignment sheet. Note if the pulse was regular or irregular.

POST-PROCEDURE

16 Provide for comfort. (See the inside of the front cover.)
17 Place the call light and other needed items within reach.
18 Unscreen the person.
19 Complete a safety check of the room. (See the inside of the front cover.)
20 Clean the stethoscope ear-pieces and chest-piece with the wipes.

21 Return the stethoscope to its proper place.
22 Practice hand hygiene.
23 Report and record your observations. Record the pulse rate with *Ap* for apical. Report an abnormal pulse at once.

Taking an Apical-Radial Pulse

QUALITY OF LIFE

- Knock before entering the person's room.
- Address the person by name.
- Introduce yourself by name and title.

- Explain the procedure before starting and during the procedure.
- Protect the person's rights during the procedure.
- Handle the person gently during the procedure.

PRE-PROCEDURE

1 Follow *Delegation Guidelines: Taking Pulses*, p. 499. See *Promoting Safety and Comfort:*
   a *Taking Pulses*, p. 499
   b *Using a Stethoscope*, p. 500
2 Ask a co-worker to help you.
3 Practice hand hygiene.

4 Collect a stethoscope and antiseptic wipes.
5 Practice hand hygiene.
6 Identify the person. Check the ID bracelet against the assignment sheet. Use 2 identifiers (Chapter 13). Also call the person by name.
7 Provide for privacy.

PROCEDURE

8 Clean the stethoscope ear-pieces and chest-piece with the wipes.
9 Have the person sit or lie down.
10 Expose the nipple area of the left chest. Expose a woman's breasts only to the extent necessary.
11 Warm the diaphragm in your palm.
12 Place the stethoscope ear-pieces in your ears.
13 Find the apical pulse. Your co-worker finds the radial pulse (see Fig. 29-23).
14 Give the signal to begin counting.
15 Count the apical pulse for 1 minute. Your co-worker counts the radial pulse for 1 minute.

16 Give the signal to stop counting. Ask your co-worker for the radial pulse rate.
17 Cover the person. Remove the stethoscope ear-pieces.
18 Note the person's name and the apical and radial pulses on your note pad or assignment sheet. Subtract the radial pulse from the apical pulse for the pulse deficit. For example:
   - You counted 72 apical beats per minute.
   - Your co-worker counted 66 radial beats per minute.
   - Subtract 66 (radial pulse) from 72 (apical pulse).
   - 72 apical beats – 66 radial beats = 6. The pulse deficit is 6.

POST-PROCEDURE

19 Provide for comfort. (See the inside of the front book cover.)
20 Place the call light and other needed items within reach.
21 Unscreen the person.
22 Complete a safety check of the room. (See the inside of the front book cover.)
23 Clean the stethoscope ear-pieces and chest-piece with the wipes.

24 Return the stethoscope to its proper place.
25 Practice hand hygiene.
26 Report and record your observations. (Report an abnormal pulse at once.) Include:
   - The apical and radial pulse rates
   - The pulse deficit
   - If the pulses were regular or irregular

Checking Pedal Pulses. The pedal (dorsalis pedis) pulse is used to check circulation in the foot. The dorsalis pedis artery is over a foot bone (Fig. 29-24). Often a nurse will mark the skin with an X where the pulse is found. This is so that all staff use the same site. When the pedal pulse cannot be felt, a *Doppler ultrasound stethoscope (DUS)* is used (Fig. 29-25, p. 504).

- Doppler—the device is named after Christian J. Doppler. He developed the ultrasound method.
- Ultrasound—*ultra* means *beyond* or *farther. Sound* relates to *sound waves*. Blood flowing in an artery creates sound waves.

Your role may include using a DUS. If so, make sure that you:
- Have received the necessary training.
- Follow the nurse's directions.
- Follow the manufacturer's instructions.

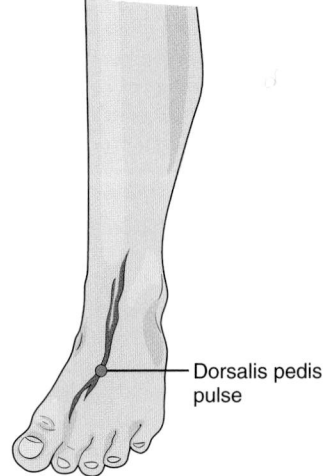

Dorsalis pedis pulse

FIGURE 29-24 The pedal pulse.

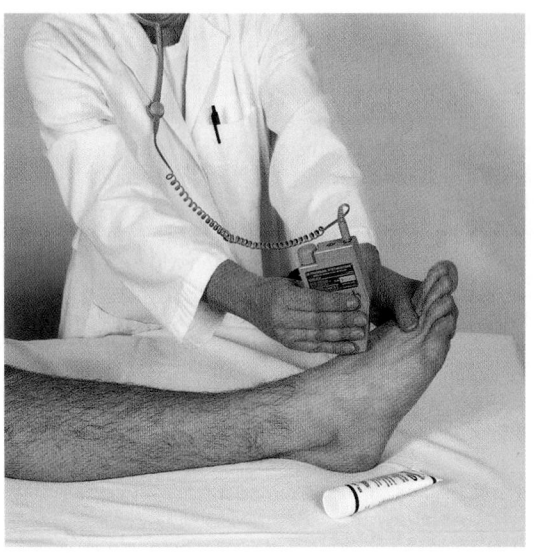

FIGURE 29-25 A Doppler ultrasound stethoscope is used to check a pedal pulse. (From Jarvis C: *Physical examination and health assessment,* ed 4, Philadelphia, 2004, Saunders.)

RESPIRATIONS

Respiration means breathing air into (inhalation) *and out of* (exhalation) *the lungs.* Oxygen enters the lungs during inhalation. Carbon dioxide leaves the lungs during exhalation. Each respiration involves 1 inhalation and 1 exhalation. The chest rises during inhalation. It falls during exhalation.

See *Body Structure and Function Review: The Respiratory System.*

Counting Respirations

The healthy adult has 12 to 20 respirations per minute. See Box 29-1 for the factors affecting vital signs. Heart and respiratory diseases often increase the respiratory rate.

Respirations are normally quiet, effortless, and regular. Both sides of the chest rise and fall equally. See Chapter 39 for abnormal respiratory patterns.

Count respirations when the person is at rest. Position the person so you can see the chest rise and fall. To some extent, a person can control the rate and depth of breathing. People tend to change their breathing patterns when they know their respirations are being counted. Therefore do not tell the person that you are counting them.

BODY STRUCTURE AND FUNCTION REVIEW

The Respiratory System

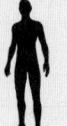

Oxygen is needed for life. Every cell needs oxygen. The respiratory system (Fig. 29-26) brings oxygen into the lungs and rids the body of carbon dioxide. *Respiration* is the process of supplying the cells with oxygen and removing carbon dioxide from them. Respiration involves *inhalation* (breathing in) and *exhalation* (breathing out). The terms *inspiration* (breathing in) and *expiration* (breathing out) are also used.

Air enters the body through the nose. The air then passes into the *pharynx* (throat), a tube-shaped passage-way for both air and food. Air passes from the pharynx into the *larynx* (voice box). Air passes from the larynx into the *trachea* (windpipe). The trachea divides at its lower end into the *right bronchus* and *left bronchus.* Each bronchus enters a lung.

On entering the lungs, the bronchi divide many times into smaller branches called *bronchioles.* Eventually the bronchioles further divide. They end in tiny 1-celled air sacs called *alveoli.* They are supplied by capillaries.

Oxygen and carbon dioxide are exchanged between the alveoli and capillaries. Blood in the capillaries picks up oxygen from the alveoli. Then the blood returns to the left side of the heart and is pumped to the rest of the body. Alveoli pick up carbon dioxide from the capillaries for exhalation.

Each lung is divided into lobes. The right lung has 3 lobes, the left lung has 2. The lungs are separated from the abdominal cavity by a muscle called the *diaphragm.* A bony framework made up of the ribs, sternum, and vertebrae protects the lungs.

See Chapter 10 for more detailed information.

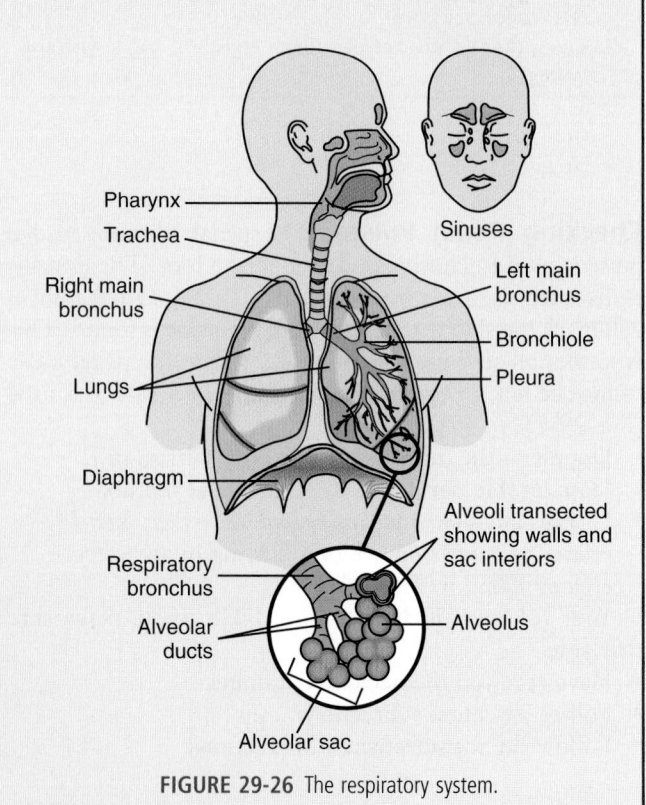

FIGURE 29-26 The respiratory system.

Count respirations right after taking a pulse. Keep your fingers or stethoscope over the pulse site. (The person assumes you are taking the pulse.) To count respirations, watch the chest rise and fall. Count them for 30 seconds. Multiply the number by 2 for the number of respirations in 1 minute. If you note an abnormal pattern, count the respirations for 1 minute.

In some agencies, respirations are counted for 1 minute. Follow agency policy. Some state competency tests require that respirations are counted for 1 minute.

See *Focus on Math: Counting Respirations.*

See *Focus on Children and Older Persons: Counting Respirations.*

See *Delegation Guidelines: Counting Respirations.*

See procedure: *Counting Respirations.*

FOCUS ON MATH

Counting Respirations

Respirations are measured in breaths per minute. When you count regular respirations for 30 seconds, multiply the number by 2. This gives the number of respirations per minute (60 seconds). For example, you count 8 breaths in 30 seconds. For the number of breaths per minute, multiply 8 by 2.

$$8 \text{ breaths} \times 2 = 16 \text{ breaths}$$
The respiratory rate is 16 breaths per minute.

FOCUS ON CHILDREN AND OLDER PERSONS

Counting Respirations

Children
Infants and children have higher respiratory rates than adults. Count an infant's respirations for 1 minute.

Age	Respirations per Minute
Newborn	35
1 year	30
2 years	25
4 years	23
6 years	21
8 years	20
10-12 years	19
14 years	18
16 years	17
18 years	16–18

Modified from Hockenberry MJ, Wilson D: Wong's essentials of pediatric nursing, ed 9, St Louis, 2013, Mosby.

DELEGATION GUIDELINES

Counting Respirations

Before counting respirations, you need this information from the nurse and the care plan.
- How long to count respirations for each person—30 seconds or 1 minute
- When to count respirations
- If the nurse has concerns about certain patients or residents
- What other vital signs to measure

- What observations to report and record:
  - The respiratory rate
  - Equality and depth of respirations
  - If the respirations were regular or irregular
  - If the person has pain or difficulty breathing
  - Any respiratory noises
  - An abnormal respiratory pattern (Chapter 39)
- When to report observations
- What patient or resident concerns to report at once

Counting Respirations

PROCEDURE

1 Follow *Delegation Guidelines: Counting Respirations.*
2 Keep your fingers or stethoscope over the pulse site.
3 Do not tell the person you are counting respirations.
4 Begin counting when the chest rises. Count each rise and fall of the chest as 1 respiration.
5 Note the following.
  a If respirations are regular
  b If both sides of the chest rise equally
  c The depth of respirations
  d If the person has any pain or difficulty breathing
  e An abnormal respiratory pattern

6 Count respirations for 30 seconds. Multiply the number by 2 for the number of respirations in 60 seconds (1 minute). For example:
  - You count 9 breaths in 30 seconds.
  - Multiply 9 breaths by 2.
  - 9 breaths × 2 = 18 breaths per minute.
7 Count respirations for 1 minute if:
  a Directed by the nurse and the care plan.
  b Required by agency policy.
  c They are abnormal or irregular.
  d Required for your state competency test.
8 Note the person's name, respiratory rate, and other observations on your note pad or assignment sheet.

Continued

Counting Respirations—cont'd

POST-PROCEDURE

9 Provide for comfort. (See the inside of the front cover.)
10 Place the call light and other needed items within reach.
11 Unscreen the person.
12 Complete a safety check of the room. (See the inside of the front cover.)

13 Practice hand hygiene.
14 Report and record the respiratory rate and your observations. Report abnormal respirations at once.

BLOOD PRESSURE

Blood pressure (BP) is the amount of force exerted against the walls of an artery by the blood. BP is controlled by:

- The force of heart contractions
- The amount of blood pumped with each heartbeat
- How easily the blood flows through the blood vessels

Systole is the period of heart muscle contraction. The heart is pumping blood. Diastole is the period of heart muscle relaxation. The heart is at rest.

You measure systolic and diastolic pressures. The **systolic pressure** *is the pressure in the arteries when the heart contracts.* It is the higher pressure. The **diastolic pressure** *is the pressure in the arteries when the heart is at rest.* It is the lower pressure.

BP is measured in millimeters (mm) of mercury (Hg). The systolic pressure is recorded over the diastolic pressure. A systolic pressure of 120 mm Hg (millimeters of mercury) and a diastolic pressure of 80 mm Hg are written as 120/80 mm Hg. This is read as "120 over 80 millimeters of mercury."

Normal and Abnormal Blood Pressures

BP can change from minute to minute. Factors affecting BP are listed in Box 29-5.

BP has normal ranges.

- *Systolic pressure*—90 mm Hg or higher but lower than 120 mm Hg
- *Diastolic pressure*—60 mm Hg or higher but lower than 80 mm Hg

Treatment is indicated for:

- **Hypertension**—*The systolic pressure is 140 mm Hg or higher* (hyper) *or the diastolic pressure is 90 mm Hg or higher.* Report any systolic measurement at or above 120 mm Hg. Also report a diastolic pressure at or above 80 mm Hg.
- **Hypotension**—*The systolic pressure is below* (hypo) *90 mm Hg or the diastolic pressure is below 60 mm Hg.* Report a systolic pressure below 90 mm Hg. Also report a diastolic pressure below 60 mm Hg. Some people normally have low blood pressures. However, hypotension can signal a life-threatening problem.

See *Focus on Communication: Normal and Abnormal Blood Pressures.*

See *Focus on Children and Older Persons: Normal and Abnormal Blood Pressures.*

BOX 29-5   Factors Affecting Blood Pressure

- *Age.* BP increases with age. It is lowest in infants and children. It is highest in adults.
- *Gender (male or female).* Women usually have lower blood pressures than men do. Blood pressures rise in women after menopause.
- *Blood volume.* This is the amount of blood in the system. Severe bleeding lowers the blood volume. Therefore BP lowers. Giving IV (intravenous) fluids rapidly increases the blood volume. The BP rises.
- *Stress.* Stress includes anxiety, fear, and emotions. BP increases as the body responds to stress.
- *Pain.* Pain generally increases BP. However, severe pain can cause shock. BP is seriously low in the state of shock (Chapter 54).
- *Exercise.* BP increases. BP is usually measured at rest.
- *Weight.* BP is higher in over-weight persons. It lowers with weight loss.

- *Race.* Black persons generally have higher blood pressures than white persons do.
- *Diet.* A high-sodium diet increases the amount of water in the body. The extra fluid volume increases BP.
- *Drugs.* Drugs can be given to raise or lower BP. Other drugs have the side effects of high or low BP.
- *Position.* BP is higher when lying down. It is lower in the standing position. Sudden changes in position can cause a sudden drop in BP (orthostatic hypotension). When standing suddenly, the person may have a sudden drop in BP. Dizziness and fainting can occur.
- *Smoking.* BP increases. Nicotine in cigarettes causes blood vessels to narrow. The heart must work harder to pump blood through narrowed vessels.
- *Alcohol.* Excessive alcohol intake can raise BP.

Normal and Abnormal Blood Pressures

Many persons want to know their blood pressures. If agency policy allows, tell the person the BP. If the BP is high or low, the person may worry. He or she may say: "That is higher (lower) than normal for me." Be calm and professional. You can say: "Yes, I noticed it was a little high (low). I will tell your nurse." Report abnormal blood pressures to the nurse.

You must report some concerns at once. For example, you take Mr. Carter's BP. It is 82/58. Mr. Carter says he is dizzy. You assist him to a lying position. You need to stay with Mr. Carter and report the concern. You press the call light and identify yourself. You say: "Please have Mr. Carter's nurse come to room 216 right away." When the nurse arrives, you say: "I checked Mr. Carter's blood pressure. It was 82/58. He said he was dizzy. Would you please check him?"

Normal and Abnormal Blood Pressures

Children

Age, sex, and height are used to determine a child's normal BP. Young children can have high blood pressure. Overweight children usually have higher blood pressures than do children with a normal weight. Children 3 years of age and older are screened for high blood pressure.

Older Persons

Older persons also are at risk for orthostatic hypotension (Chapter 30).

Blood Pressure Equipment

A *sphygmomanometer* has a cuff and a measuring device for measuring blood pressure. Sphygmo *means* pulse. *A device for measuring pressure is called a* manometer.

- The *aneroid type* has a round dial and a needle that points to the numbers (Fig. 29-27, *A*).
- The *mercury type* has a column of mercury within a calibrated tube (Fig. 29-27, *B*).
- The *electronic type* shows the systolic and diastolic pressures and the pulse rate (Fig. 29-27, *C*).
- The *wrist monitor* (Fig. 29-27, *D*) measures blood pressure at the wrist. This type is sometimes used for persons with bariatric needs. This type is very sensitive to body position.

You wrap the blood pressure cuff around the upper arm. Tubing connects the cuff to the manometer. The inflated cuff causes pressure over the brachial artery. BP is measured as the cuff deflates.

- *Aneroid and mercury types. A* tube connects the cuff to a small, hand-held bulb. See Figure 29-28, p. 508. To inflate the cuff, turn the valve on the bulb clockwise to close the valve. Squeeze the bulb. To deflate the cuff, turn the valve counter-clockwise. Using a stethoscope, listen and measure BP as the cuff deflates. Blood flowing through the arteries produces sounds.
- *Electronic type.* A stethoscope is not needed. A button is pressed to inflate the cuff. The cuff deflates automatically. The BP is displayed. Follow the manufacturer's instructions to use electronic BP equipment.

See *Focus on Children and Older Persons: Blood Pressure Equipment*, p. 508.

See *Promoting Safety and Comfort: Blood Pressure Equipment*, p. 508.

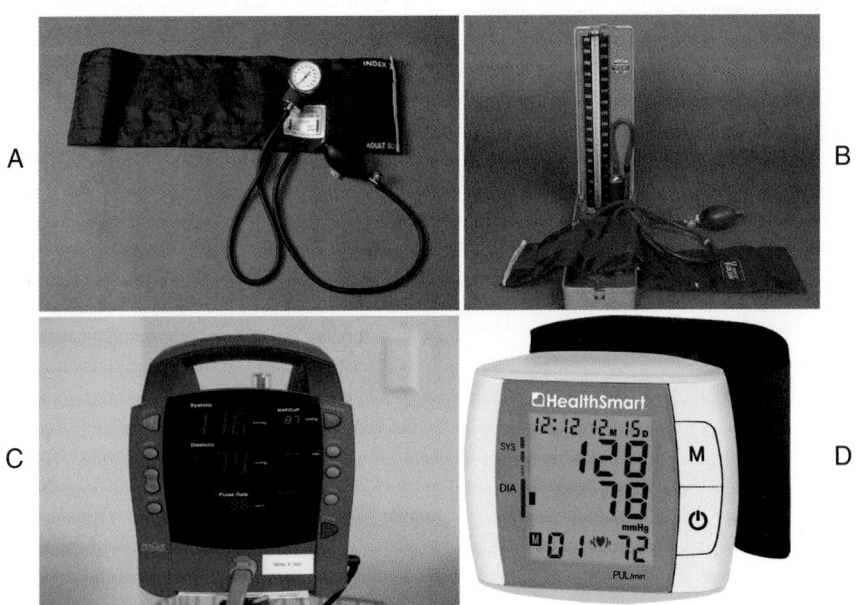

FIGURE 29-27 Blood pressure equipment. **A,** Aneroid manometer and cuff. **B,** Mercury manometer and cuff. **C,** Electronic manometer. **D,** Wrist monitor. (**D,** Courtesy Briggs Medical Service Company, Des Moines, Iowa.)

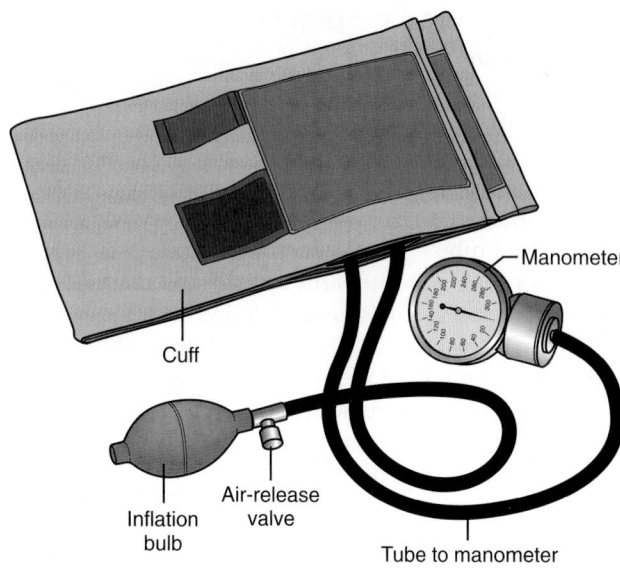

FIGURE 29-28 Parts of an aneroid sphygmomanometer.

FOCUS ON CHILDREN AND OLDER PERSONS

Blood Pressure Equipment

Children
Pediatric blood pressure cuffs are used for children. Infant and child sizes are available. The nurse tells you what size to use.

PROMOTING SAFETY AND COMFORT

Blood Pressure Equipment

Safety
Mercury is a hazardous substance. Mercury manometers are being phased out of health care. Some agencies may still use them. Handle mercury manometers carefully. If one breaks, call for the nurse at once. Do not touch the mercury. Do not let the person touch it. The agency follows special procedures for handling all hazardous substances. See Chapter 13.

Comfort
Inflate the cuff only to the extent necessary (see procedure: *Measuring Blood Pressure*). The inflated cuff causes discomfort. The higher the inflation, the greater the discomfort.

Measuring Blood Pressure

You measure blood pressure in the brachial artery. Box 29-6 lists the guidelines for measuring blood pressure.

See *Focus on Math: Measuring Blood Pressure.*
See *Delegation Guidelines: Measuring Blood Pressure.*
See procedure: *Measuring Blood Pressure.*

BOX 29-6	Measuring Blood Pressure—Guidelines

- Do not take BP on an arm:
  - With an IV infusion
  - With an arm cast
  - With a dialysis access site
  - On the side of breast surgery
  - That is injured
- Ask the nurse if you are not sure which arm to use.
- Let the person rest for 10 to 20 minutes before measuring BP.
- Measure BP with the person sitting or lying. Sometimes BP is measured in the standing position.
- Apply the cuff to the bare upper arm. Clothing can affect the measurement.
- Make sure the cuff is snug. The reading will be wrong if the cuff is loose.
- Use a larger cuff if the person is obese or has a large arm. Use a small cuff if the person has a very small arm. Ask the nurse what size to use. Also check the care plan.
- Make sure the room is quiet. Talking, TV, music, and sounds from the hallway can affect an accurate measurement.
- Place the diaphragm of the stethoscope firmly over the brachial artery. The entire diaphragm must have contact with the skin.
- Have the manometer where you can clearly see it.
- Measure the systolic and diastolic pressures.
  - Expect to hear the first sound at the point where you last felt the radial or brachial pulse (see procedure: *Measuring Blood Pressure*). The first sound is the systolic pressure.
  - The point where the sound disappears is the diastolic pressure.
- Take the BP again if you are not sure of accuracy. Wait 30 to 60 seconds to repeat the measurement. Ask the nurse to take the BP if you are unsure of the measurement.
- Tell the nurse at once if you cannot hear the blood pressure.

FOCUS ON MATH

Measuring Blood Pressure

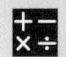 Manometers are marked with long and short lines (Fig. 29-29).

- Long lines mark 10 mm Hg values.
- Short lines mark 2 mm Hg values.

Read the manometer as the cuff deflates. The needle or mercury column is dropping.

- If the needle or mercury column is at a long line, note this value. Long line values end in 0. For example: 70, 80, 90, 100, 110, 120, and so on.
- If the needle or mercury column is between 2 long lines:
  - Note the value of the long line below the needle or mercury column.
  - Note the short line. Count up from the long line below by even numbers. Short line values end with 2, 4, 6, or 8. See Figure 29-29.

For example, the needle is at the 3rd short line between 90 and 100. Count up by even numbers from 90. Line 1 is 92. Line 2 is 94. Line 3 is 96. The value is 96.

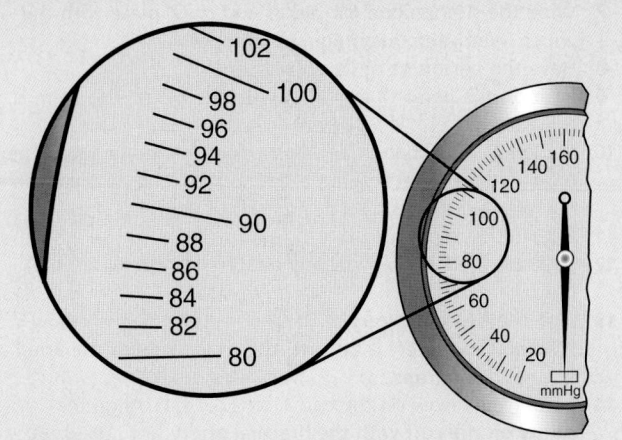

FIGURE 29-29 Reading the manometer. Long lines mark 10 mm Hg values. Short lines mark 2 mm Hg values.

DELEGATION GUIDELINES

Measuring Blood Pressure

Before measuring BP, you need this information from the nurse and the care plan.

- When to measure BP
- What arm to use
- The person's normal blood pressure range
- If the nurse has concerns about certain patients or residents

- If the person needs to be lying down, sitting, or standing
- What size cuff to use—regular, child-sized, extra-large, bariatric
- What observations to report and record
- When to report the BP measurement
- What patient or resident concerns to report at once

Measuring Blood Pressure

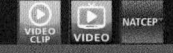

QUALITY OF LIFE

- Knock before entering the person's room.
- Address the person by name.
- Introduce yourself by name and title.

- Explain the procedure before starting and during the procedure.
- Protect the person's rights during the procedure.
- Handle the person gently during the procedure.

PRE-PROCEDURE

1. Follow *Delegation Guidelines: Measuring Blood Pressure.* See *Promoting Safety and Comfort:*
   a *Using a Stethoscope,* p. 500
   b *Blood Pressure Equipment*
2. Practice hand hygiene.
3. Collect the following.
   - Sphygmomanometer
   - Stethoscope
   - Antiseptic wipes

4. Practice hand hygiene.
5. Identify the person. Check the ID bracelet against the assignment sheet. Use 2 identifiers (Chapter 13). Also call the person by name.
6. Provide for privacy.

Continued

Measuring Blood Pressure—cont'd

PROCEDURE

7   Wipe the stethoscope ear-pieces and chest-piece with the wipes. Warm the diaphragm in your palm.

8   Have the person sit or lie down.

9   Position the person's arm level with the heart. The palm is up.

10 Stand no more than 3 feet away from the manometer. The mercury type is vertical, on a flat surface, and at eye level. The aneroid type is directly in front of you.

11 Expose the upper arm.

12 Squeeze the cuff to expel any air. Close the valve on the bulb.

13 Find the brachial artery at the inner aspect of the elbow. (The brachial artery is on the little finger side of the arm.) Use your fingertips.

14 Locate the arrow on the cuff (Fig. 29-30, *A*). Align the arrow on the cuff with the brachial artery (Fig. 29-30, *B*). Wrap the cuff around the upper arm at least 1 inch above the elbow. It is even and snug.

15 Place the stethoscope ear-pieces in your ears. Place the diaphragm over the brachial artery (Fig. 29-30, *C*). Do not place it under the cuff.

16 Find the radial pulse. This step is for Methods 1 and 2.

17 *Method 1:*
  a Inflate the cuff until you cannot feel the pulse. Note this point.
  b Inflate the cuff 30 mm Hg beyond where you last felt the pulse.

18 *Method 2:*
  a Inflate the cuff until you cannot feel the pulse. Note this point.
  b Inflate the cuff 30 mm Hg beyond where you last felt the pulse.
  c Deflate the cuff slowly. Note the point when you feel the pulse.
  d Wait 30 seconds.
  e Inflate the cuff again, 30 mm Hg beyond where you felt the pulse return.

19 *Method 3:*
  a Inflate the cuff 160 mm Hg to 180 mm Hg.
  b Deflate the cuff if you hear a blood pressure sound. Re-inflate the cuff to 200 mm Hg.

20 Deflate the cuff at an even rate of 2 to 4 millimeters per second. Turn the valve counter-clockwise to deflate the cuff.

21 Note the point where you hear the first sound (Fig. 29-31). This is the systolic reading. It is near the point where the pulse disappeared (Method 1) or returned (Method 2).

22 Continue to deflate the cuff completely. Note the point where the sound disappears. This is the diastolic reading.

23 Deflate the cuff completely. Remove it from the person's arm. Remove the stethoscope ear-pieces from your ears.

24 Note the person's name and blood pressure on your note pad or assignment sheet.

25 Return the cuff to the case or wall holder.

POST-PROCEDURE

26 Provide for comfort. (See the inside of the front cover.)

27 Place the call light and other needed items within reach.

28 Unscreen the person.

29 Complete a safety check of the room. (See the inside of the front cover.)

30 Clean the stethoscope ear-pieces and chest-piece with the wipes.

31 Return the equipment to its proper place.

32 Practice hand hygiene.

33 Report and record the BP (Fig. 29-32). Note which arm was used. Report an abnormal BP at once.

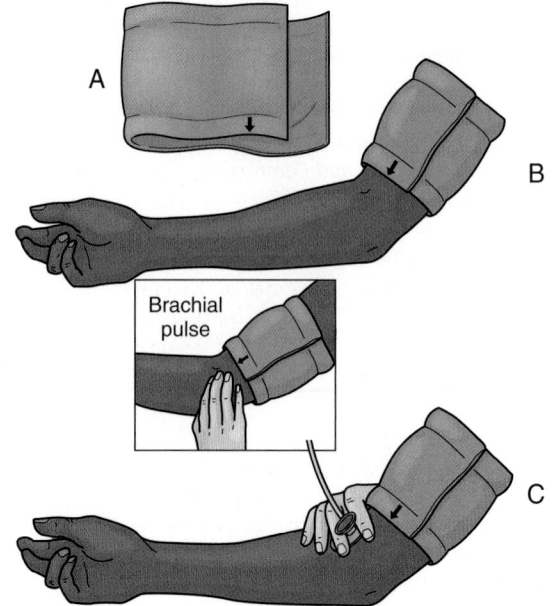

FIGURE 29-30 Measuring blood pressure. **A,** The arrow is used for correct cuff alignment. **B,** The cuff is placed so the arrow is aligned with the brachial artery. **C,** The diaphragm of the stethoscope is over the brachial artery.

Brachial pulse

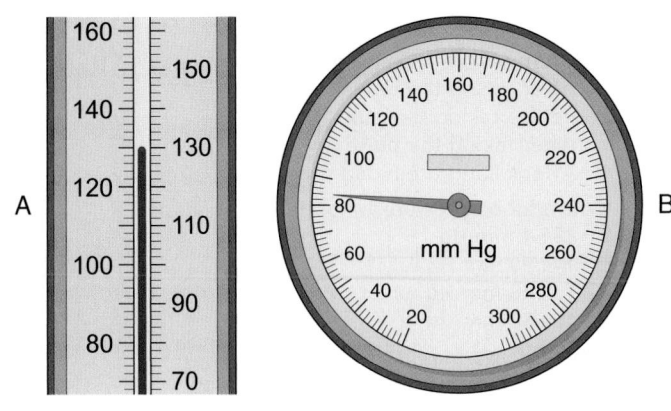

FIGURE 29-31 Manometer readings. **A,** This mercury manometer is at 130 mm Hg. **B,** This aneroid manometer is at 84 mm Hg.

DAILY SUMMARY AND GRAPHIC

DATE		6/12					
HOUR		2400	0400	0800	1200	1600	2000
BP		118/72	124/76	122/78			
BP SITE		R arm	R arm	L arm			
T E M P E R A T U R E 104	40						
102.2	39						
100.4	38						
98.6	37						
96.6	36						
TEMP ROUTE		Oral	Oral	Oral			
PULSE		76	74	78			
RESPIRATION		16	16	18			

FIGURE 29-32 Charting sample.

PAIN

Pain is a warning sign from the body. It signals tissue damage. Therefore many agencies consider it to be a vital sign. See "Pain" in Chapter 31.

FOCUS ON **PRIDE**

The Person, Family, and Yourself

P **ersonal and Professional Responsibility**

Vital sign measurements are important for the nursing process. They help the nurse plan for and evaluate the person's care. You must know normal vital sign ranges.

For an adult:
- Oral temperature—98.6°F (37.0°C). See Table 29-1 for normal temperatures at other sites.
- Pulse—60 to 100 beats per minute.
- Respirations—12 to 20 breaths per minute.
- Blood pressure—90/60 mm Hg or higher but lower than 120/80 mm Hg.

Report abnormal measurements. The person is at risk if you do not. Take pride in safely assisting with the nursing process.

R **ights and Respect**

When you report abnormal vital signs, the nurse may ask you to repeat the measurements. The nurse may ask you to use different equipment, change the person's position, or check a measurement again later. Follow the nurse's directions.

The nurse may re-check the measurements. Do not be offended. Show respect. Avoid negative thoughts or statements about the nurse or yourself. It does not mean the nurse cannot trust you or that you have done something wrong. The nurse needs to check the measurements for safe care.

I **ndependence and Social Interaction**

Personal choice promotes independence. The person may prefer that you use a certain arm for pulses and blood pressures. If safe to do so, use the arm the person prefers. Unless orders direct otherwise, allow the person to choose to sit or lie when vital signs are measured.

D **elegation and Teamwork**

You may care for persons needing Transmission-Based Precautions (Chapter 16). You must prevent the spread of infection from equipment. Some agencies have isolation carts or kits that contain equipment. A stethoscope, blood pressure cuff, and thermometer are common. The equipment is taken into the person's room or home and left there. Use that equipment when measuring vital signs. Do not use your own stethoscope or bring other equipment into the room or home. If equipment must be brought in, it is cleaned after use. Special cleansers may be needed. Follow agency policy to protect others from infection.

E **thics and Laws**

Measurements must be accurate. Tell the nurse if you are unsure of any measurement. For example, you cannot feel a pulse or hear a blood pressure. Never make up a measurement. Reporting or recording false measurements is wrong. The person can be harmed. Take pride in doing the right thing by honest reporting and recording.

FOCUS ON **PRIDE**: *Application*

Learning to measure vital signs requires practice. Do not be upset if you struggle at first. Plan to practice at school and at home. Practice on classmates, family, and friends. Who will you practice with?

Plan when and what you will practice. Use class time wisely. If you do not have equipment to practice temperature and BP at home, practice at school as much as you can. Practice measuring pulse and respirations at home.

Tell your instructor if you need more practice. Never be ashamed to ask for more practice time. Practice builds confidence.

REVIEW QUESTIONS

Circle the BEST answer.

1 Which should you report at once?
   a An oral temperature of 98.4°F
   b A rectal temperature of 101.6°F
   c An axillary temperature of 97.6°F
   d An oral temperature of 99.0°F

2 A rectal temperature is taken when the person
   a Is unconscious
   b Has heart disease
   c Is confused
   d Has diarrhea

3 Which site is used to take an infant's temperature?
   a Oral site
   b Rectal site
   c Axillary site
   d Tympanic membrane site

4 When using an electronic thermometer
   a Shake down the thermometer before each use
   b Leave the thermometer in place for 2 minutes
   c Cover the probe with a probe cover
   d Use the blue probe for a rectal temperature

5 Which is usually used to take an adult's pulse?
   a The radial pulse
   b The apical pulse
   c The carotid pulse
   d The brachial pulse

6 For an adult, which pulse do you report at once?
   a A regular pulse at 64 beats per minute
   b A strong pulse at 78 beats per minute
   c A regular pulse at 90 beats per minute
   d An irregular pulse at 124 beats per minute

7 You count a regular pulse for 30 seconds. Which is *true*?
   a Divide the number of beats by 2 for the pulse rate.
   b If you count 44 beats, you record a pulse rate of 44.
   c If you count 44 beats, you record a pulse rate of 88.
   d Ask the nurse to check a regular pulse.

8 Which statement about the apical-radial pulse is *true*?
   a The radial pulse can be greater than the apical pulse.
   b The apical pulse can be greater than the radial pulse.
   c The apical and radial pulses are always equal.
   d The pulse deficit is always 0.

9 In an adult, normal respirations are
   a Less than 20 per minute
   b More than 20 per minute
   c 10 to 18 per minute
   d 12 to 20 per minute

10 Respirations are usually counted
   a After taking the temperature
   b Before taking the pulse
   c After taking the pulse
   d After taking the blood pressure

11 Which blood pressure is normal for an adult?
   a 88/54 mm Hg
   b 140/90 mm Hg
   c 112/78 mm Hg
   d 100/58 mm Hg

12 When measuring BP
   a Apply the cuff to the bare upper arm
   b Use the arm with an IV infusion
   c Make sure the cuff is loose
   d Place the stethoscope under the cuff

13 The systolic blood pressure is the point
   a Where the pulse is no longer felt
   b 30 mm Hg above where the pulse was felt
   c Where the first sound is heard
   d Where the last sound is heard

14 When taking a BP, the sound disappears at the 1st short line above 70. You record the
   a Systolic pressure as 70
   b Diastolic pressure as 71
   c Systolic pressure as 72
   d Diastolic pressure as 72

15 You are not sure you heard an accurate BP measurement. You should
   a Record what you think you heard
   b Measure the BP again after 60 seconds
   c Repeat the BP using the bell part of the stethoscope
   d Ask another nursing assistant to take the BP

Answers to Chapter 29 questions are on p. 871.

FOCUS ON PRACTICE

Problem Solving

You measure a patient's vital signs. The pulse is 110. The respiratory rate is 24. The oral temperature is 100.8°F. You think you heard the blood pressure at 86/52. You are unsure of the measurement. What will you do? Which, if any, of these vital signs are abnormal? What must you do?

Exercise and Activity

OBJECTIVES

- Define the key terms and key abbreviations in this chapter.
- Describe bedrest.
- Explain how to prevent the complications from bedrest.
- Describe the devices that support and maintain body alignment.
- Explain the purpose of a trapeze.

- Describe range-of-motion exercises.
- Describe 4 walking aids.
- Perform the procedures described in this chapter.
- Explain how to promote PRIDE in the person, the family, and yourself.

KEY TERMS

abduction Moving a body part away from the mid-line of the body
adduction Moving a body part toward the mid-line of the body
ambulation The act of walking
atrophy The decrease in size or wasting away of tissue
contracture The lack of joint mobility caused by abnormal shortening of a muscle
deconditioning The loss of muscle strength from inactivity
dorsiflexion Bending the toes and foot up at the ankle
extension Straightening a body part
external rotation Turning the joint outward
flexion Bending a body part
footdrop The foot falls down at the ankle; permanent plantar flexion
hyperextension Excessive straightening of a body part
internal rotation Turning the joint inward

opposition Touching an opposite finger with the thumb
orthostatic hypotension Abnormally low *(hypo)* blood pressure when the person suddenly stands up *(ortho* and *static)*; postural hypotension
orthotic device A device used to support a muscle, promote a certain motion, or correct a deformity; *ortho* means *to straighten*
plantar flexion The foot *(plantar)* is bent *(flexion);* bending the foot down at the ankle
postural hypotension See "orthostatic hypotension"
pronation Turning the joint downward
range of motion (ROM) The movement of a joint to the extent possible without causing pain
rotation Turning the joint
supination Turning the joint upward
syncope A brief loss of consciousness; fainting

KEY ABBREVIATIONS

ADL	Activities of daily living	**OBRA**	Omnibus Budget Reconciliation Act of 1987
CMS	Centers for Medicare & Medicaid Services	**ROM**	Range of motion
ID	Identification		

Most people move about and function without help. Illness, surgery, injury, pain, and aging cause weakness and some activity limits. Inactivity, whether mild or severe, affects every body system and mental well-being.

You assist the nurse in promoting exercise and activity in all persons to the extent possible. Physical and occupational therapists help the person improve strength and endurance. Care plan goals may be to improve independence so the person can go home. Or the goal may be to attain the highest level of function possible. The care plan and your assignment sheet include the person's activity level and needed exercises.

See *Focus on Children and Older Persons: Exercise and Activity*, p. 514.

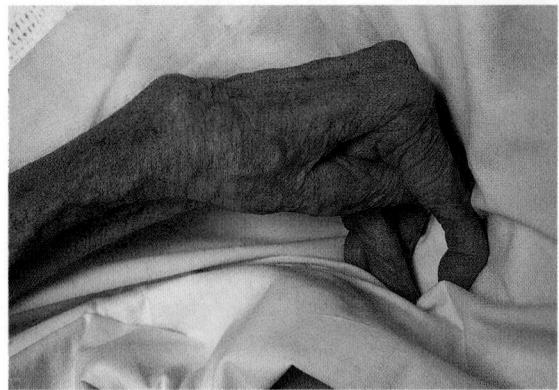

FIGURE 30-1 A contracture.

BEDREST

The doctor orders bedrest to treat a health problem. Or it is a nursing measure if the person's condition changes. Bedrest is ordered to:

- Reduce physical activity.
- Reduce pain.
- Encourage rest.
- Regain strength.
- Promote healing.

  These types of bedrest are common.
- *Strict bedrest.* Everything is done for the person. The person is in bed for all activities of daily living (ADL).
- *Bedrest.* The person performs some ADL. Self-feeding, oral hygiene, bathing, shaving, and hair care are often allowed.
- *Bedrest with commode privileges.* The commode is used for elimination.
- *Bedrest with bathroom privileges (bedrest with BRP).* The bathroom is used for elimination.

The person's care plan and your assignment sheet state the activities allowed. Always ask the nurse what bedrest means for each person. Ask the nurse if you have questions about a person's activity limits.

Complications From Bedrest

Bedrest and lack of exercise and activity can cause serious complications. Every system is affected. Pressure ulcers, constipation, and fecal impaction can result. Urinary tract infections and renal calculi (kidney stones) can occur. So can blood clots (thrombi) and pneumonia (inflammation and infection of the lung).

The musculo-skeletal system is affected too. For normal movement, you must help prevent the following.

- A **contracture** *is the lack of joint mobility caused by abnormal shortening of a muscle.* The contracted muscle is fixed into position, is deformed, and cannot stretch (Fig. 30-1). Common sites are the fingers, wrists, elbows, toes, ankles, knees, and hips. They can also occur in the neck and spine. The site is deformed and stiff.
- *Atrophy is the decrease in size or the wasting away of tissue.* Tissues shrink in size. *Muscle atrophy is a decrease in size or a wasting away of muscle* (Fig. 30-2).

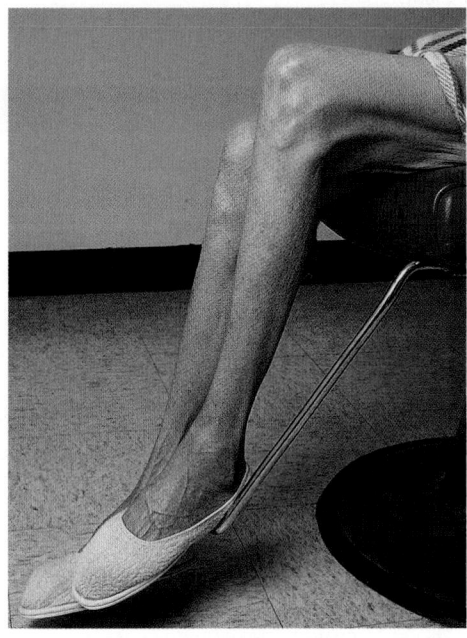

FIGURE 30-2 Muscle atrophy.

Orthostatic hypotension *is abnormally low* (hypo) *blood pressure when the person suddenly stands up* (ortho *and* static). When a person moves from a lying to sitting to standing position, the blood pressure drops. The person is dizzy, weak, and has spots before the eyes. Syncope can occur. *Syncope (fainting) is a brief loss of consciousness.* (The Greek word *synkoptein* means *to cut short.) Orthostatic hypotension also is called* **postural hypotension.** (*Postural* relates to *posture* or *standing.)* Box 30-1 lists measures that prevent orthostatic hypotension. Slowly changing positions is key.

Good nursing care prevents complications from bedrest. Good alignment, range-of-motion exercises (p. 517), and frequent position changes are important measures. These are part of the care plan.

See *Focus on Communication: Complications of Bedrest.*

- Measure blood pressure, pulse, and respirations with the person supine.
- Position the person in Fowler's position. Raise the head of the bed slowly.
  - Ask about weakness, dizziness, or spots before the eyes. Lower the head of the bed if symptoms occur.
  - Measure blood pressure, pulse, and respirations.
  - Keep the person in Fowler's position for a short while. Ask about weakness, dizziness, or spots before the eyes.
- Help the person sit on the side of the bed (Chapter 18).
  - Ask about weakness, dizziness, or spots before the eyes. Help the person to Fowler's position if symptoms occur.
  - Measure blood pressure, pulse, and respirations.
  - Have the person sit on the side of the bed for a short while.
- Help the person stand.
  - Ask about weakness, dizziness, or spots before the eyes. Help the person sit on the side of the bed if symptoms occur.
  - Measure blood pressure, pulse, and respirations.
- Help the person sit in a chair or walk as directed by the nurse.
  - Ask about weakness, dizziness, or spots before the eyes. If the person is walking, help the person sit if symptoms occur.
  - Measure blood pressure, pulse, and respirations.
- Report blood pressure, pulse, and respirations to the nurse. Also report other symptoms or complaints.

FOCUS ON COMMUNICATION

Complications of Bedrest

Orthostatic hypotension can occur when the person moves from lying to sitting or standing. To check for orthostatic hypotension, ask these questions.
- "Do you feel weak?"
- "Do you feel dizzy?"
- "Do you see spots before your eyes?"
- "Do you feel like fainting?"

Positioning

Body alignment and positioning were discussed in Chapter 17. Supportive devices are often used to support and maintain a certain position.
- *Bed-boards*—placed under the mattress to prevent it from sagging (Fig. 30-3). The bed-boards are covered with canvas or other material. Bed boards are used more often in home settings.
- *Foot-board*—prevents plantar flexion that can lead to footdrop. In ***plantar flexion,*** *the foot* (plantar) *is bent* (flexion). ***Footdrop*** *is when the foot falls down at the ankle (permanent plantar flexion).* The foot-board is placed so the soles of the feet are flush against it (Fig. 30-4). Foot-boards also serve as bed cradles by keeping top linens off the feet and toes.

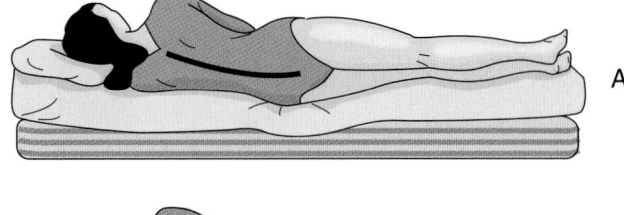
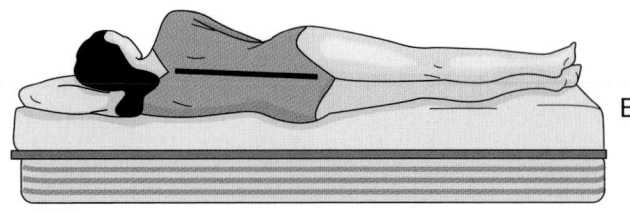

FIGURE 30-3 Bed-boards. **A,** Mattress sagging without bed-boards. **B,** Bed-boards are under the mattress. No sagging occurs.

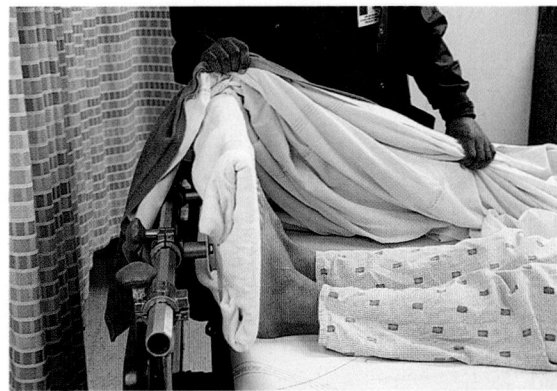

FIGURE 30-4 A foot-board. Feet are flush with the board to keep them in normal alignment.

- *Trochanter roll*—prevents the hips and legs from turning outward (external rotation) (Fig. 30-5, p. 516). A bath blanket is folded to the desired length and rolled up. The loose end is placed under the person from the hip to the knee. Then the roll is tucked alongside the body. Pillows or sandbags also keep the hips and knees in alignment.
- *Hip abduction wedge*—keeps the hips abducted (apart) (Fig. 30-6, p. 516). The wedge is placed between the person's legs. The device is common after hip replacement surgery.
- *Hand roll or hand grip*—prevents contractures of the thumb, fingers, and wrist (Fig. 30-7, p. 516). Foam rubber sponges, rubber balls, and finger cushions (Fig. 30-8, p. 516) also are used.
- *Splints*—keep the elbows, wrists, thumbs, fingers, ankles, or knees in normal position. They are usually secured in place with Velcro (Fig. 30-9, p. 516).
- *Bed cradle*—keeps the weight of top linens off the feet and toes (Fig. 30-10, p. 516). The weight of top linens can cause footdrop and pressure ulcers.

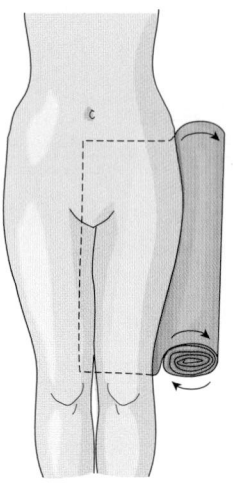

FIGURE 30-5 A trochanter roll is made from a bath blanket. It extends from the hip to the knee.

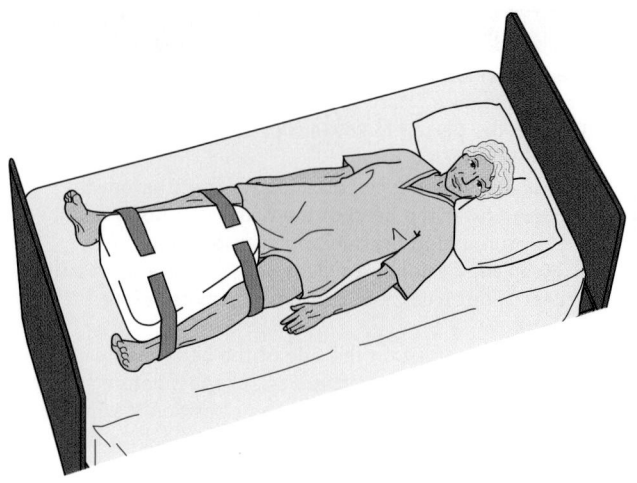

FIGURE 30-6 Hip abduction wedge.

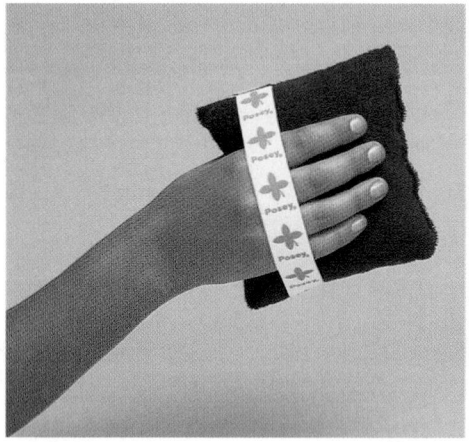

FIGURE 30-7 Hand grip. (Image courtesy Posey Company, Arcadia, Calif.)

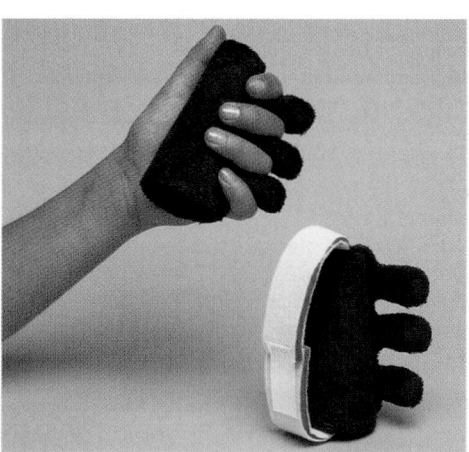

FIGURE 30-8 Finger cushion. (Image courtesy Posey Company, Arcadia, Calif.)

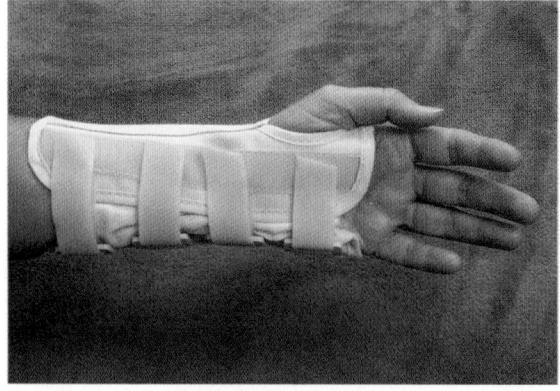

FIGURE 30-9 A splint.

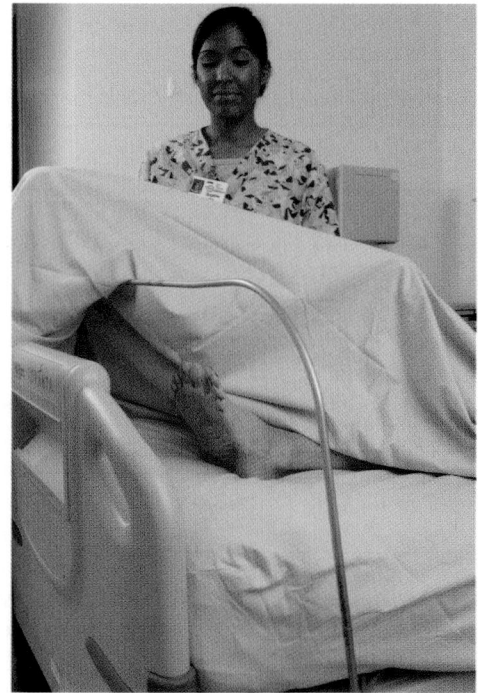

FIGURE 30-10 A bed cradle.

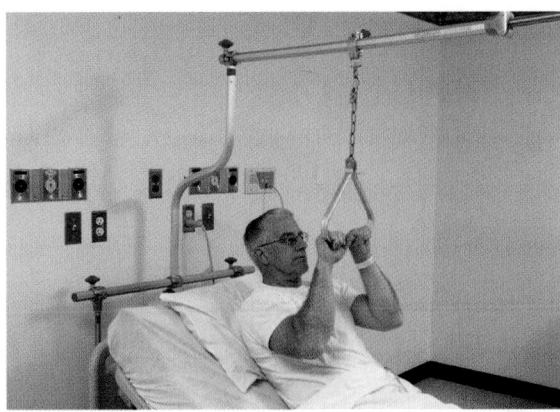

FIGURE 30-11 A trapeze is used to strengthen arm muscles.

Exercise

Exercise helps prevent contractures, muscle atrophy, and other complications from bedrest. Some exercise occurs with ADL. Other exercises are needed for muscles and joints. (See "Range-of-Motion Exercises" and "Ambulation," p. 522.)

A *trapeze* is used for exercises to strengthen arm muscles. The trapeze hangs from an over-bed frame (Fig. 30-11). The person grasps the bar with both hands to lift the trunk off the bed. The trapeze is also used to move up and turn in bed.

▪ RANGE-OF-MOTION EXERCISES

*The movement of a joint to the extent possible without causing pain is the **range of motion (ROM)** of the joint.* Range-of-motion exercises involve moving the joints through their complete range of motion (Box 30-2). They are usually done at least 2 times a day.

- *Active* ROM exercises—are done by the person.
- *Passive* ROM exercises—you move the joints through their range of motion.
- *Active-assistive* ROM exercises—the person does the exercises with some help.

Bathing, hair care, eating, reaching, dressing and undressing, and walking all involve joint movements. Persons on bedrest need more frequent ROM exercises. So do those who cannot walk, turn, or transfer themselves because of illness or injury. The doctor or nurse may order ROM exercises.

See *Focus on Communication: Range-of-Motion Exercises*.
See *Focus on Children and Older Persons: Range-of-Motion Exercises*, p. 518.
See *Focus on Long-Term Care and Home Care: Range-of-Motion Exercises*, p. 518.
See *Delegation Guidelines: Range-of-Motion Exercises*, p. 518.
See *Promoting Safety and Comfort: Range-of-Motion Exercises*, p. 518.
See procedure: *Performing Range-of-Motion Exercises*, p. 519.

Text continued on p. 522.

BOX 30-2 | **Range-of-Motion Exercises**

Joint Movements
- *Abduction*—moving a body part away from the mid-line of the body
- *Adduction*—moving a body part toward the mid-line of the body
- *Opposition*—touching an opposite finger with the thumb
- *Flexion*—bending a body part
- *Extension*—straightening a body part
- *Hyperextension*—excessive straightening of a body part
- *Dorsiflexion*—bending the toes and foot up at the ankle
- *Plantar flexion*—bending the foot down at the ankle
- *Rotation*—turning the joint
- *Internal rotation*—turning the joint inward
- *External rotation*—turning the joint outward
- *Pronation*—turning the joint downward
- *Supination*—turning the joint upward

Safety Measures
- Cover the person with a bath blanket for warmth and privacy.
- Exercise only the joints the nurse tells you to exercise.
- Expose only the body parts being exercised.
- Use good body mechanics.
- Support the part being exercised.
- Move the joint slowly, smoothly, and gently.
- Do not force a joint beyond its present range of motion.
- Do not force a joint to the point of pain.
- Ask the person if he or she has pain or discomfort.

FOCUS ON COMMUNICATION

Range-of-Motion Exercises

Do not force a joint beyond its present range of motion or to the point of pain. Ask if the person:
- Feels that the joint cannot move any farther.
- Feels pain or discomfort in the joint.
- Needs to stop or rest.

The person may not be able to tell you about discomfort or limited joint movement. Observe for signs of pain (Chapter 31). Restlessness and grimacing are examples. Stop if you suspect pain or meet resistance. Tell the nurse.

FOCUS ON CHILDREN AND OLDER PERSONS

Range-of-Motion Exercises

Children

Most play activities promote active ROM exercise. For example:

- Kicking a Mylar balloon or foam ball.
- Touching a Mylar balloon that is held or hung in different places. For example, hang a Mylar balloon from the trapeze for a child in traction.
- Playing basketball with bean-bags, wadded paper, or foam balls. Use a hoop or wastebasket as the target.
- Playing "pat-a-cake" or "Simon Says" (clap, kick, jump, and other motions).
- Having the child act like a bird, butterfly, spider, monkey, horse, or other animal.
- Playing video or computer games for finger and hand movements.
- Playing with finger paints, clay, or play dough.
- Having tricycle or wheelchair races.
- Playing "hide and seek." Hide a toy in the bed or room.
  Check with the nurse and care plan for the child's activity limits. Make sure the nurse approves of the play activity.

Modified from Hockenberry MJ and others: Wong's nursing care of infants and children, *ed 10, St Louis, 2015, Mosby.*

FOCUS ON LONG-TERM CARE AND HOME CARE

Range-of-Motion Exercises

Long-Term Care

The *Omnibus Budget Reconciliation Act of 1987 (OBRA)* and the Centers for Medicare & Medicaid Services (CMS) require an assessment and care plan focused on the person's ROM. The goal may be 1 of the following.

- Prevent loss in range of motion.
- Increase range of motion.
- Prevent further decreases in range of motion.
  During a survey, CMS surveyors may observe you performing ROM activities.

DELEGATION GUIDELINES

Range-of-Motion Exercises

When delegated ROM exercises, you need this information from the nurse and the care plan.

- The ROM exercises ordered—active, passive, active-assistive
- Which joints to exercise
- How often the exercises are done
- How many times to repeat each exercise
- What observations to report and record:
  - The time the exercises were performed
  - The joints exercised
  - The number of times the exercises were performed on each joint
  - Complaints of pain or signs of stiffness or spasm; specify the joint or body part involved
  - The degree to which the person took part in the exercises
  - When to report observations
- What patient or resident concerns to report at once

PROMOTING SAFETY AND COMFORT

Range-of-Motion Exercises

Safety

ROM exercises can cause injury if not done properly. Muscle strain, joint injury, and pain are possible. Practice the measures in Box 30-2. Remind the person to tell you about any pain during the procedure.

ROM exercises to the neck can cause serious injury if not done properly. Some agencies provide nursing assistants with special training before doing such exercises. Other agencies do not let nursing assistants do them. Know your agency's policy. Perform ROM exercises to the neck only if allowed by your agency and if the nurse instructs you to do so. In some agencies, only physical therapists do neck exercises.

Comfort

To promote physical comfort during ROM exercises, see Box 30-2. Provide privacy to promote mental comfort.

Performing Range-of-Motion Exercises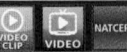

QUALITY OF LIFE

- Knock before entering the person's room.
- Address the person by name.
- Introduce yourself by name and title.

- Explain the procedure before starting and during the procedure.
- Protect the person's rights during the procedure.
- Handle the person gently during the procedure.

PRE-PROCEDURE

1 Follow *Delegation Guidelines: Range-of-Motion Exercises.* See *Promoting Safety and Comfort: Range-of-Motion Exercises.*
2 Practice hand hygiene.
3 Identify the person. Check the ID (identification) bracelet against the assignment sheet. Use 2 identifiers (Chapter 13). Also call the person by name.
4 Obtain a bath blanket.
5 Provide for privacy.
6 Raise the bed for body mechanics. Bed rails are up if used.

PROCEDURE

7 Lower the bed rail near you if up.
8 Position the person supine.
9 Cover the person with the bath blanket. Fan-fold top linens to the foot of the bed.
10 Exercise the neck *if allowed by your agency and if the nurse instructs you to do so* (Fig. 30-12).
  a Place your hands over the person's ears to support the head. Support the jaw with your fingers.
  b Flexion—bring the head forward. The chin touches the chest.
  c Extension—straighten the head.
  d Hyperextension—bring the head backward until the chin points up.
  e Rotation—turn the head from side to side.
  f Lateral flexion—move the head to the right and to the left.
  g Repeat flexion, extension, hyperextension, rotation, and lateral flexion 5 times—or the number of times stated on the care plan.

11 Exercise the shoulder (Fig. 30-13).
  a Grasp the wrist with 1 hand. Grasp the elbow with the other hand.
  b Flexion—raise the arm straight in front and over the head.
  c Extension—bring the arm down to the side.
  d Hyperextension—move the arm behind the body. (Do this if the person sits in a straight-backed chair or is standing.)
  e Abduction—move the straight arm away from the side of the body.
  f Adduction—move the straight arm to the side of the body.
  g Internal rotation—bend the elbow. Place it at the same level as the shoulder. Move the forearm and hand so the fingers point down.
  h External rotation—move the forearm and hand so the fingers point up.
  i Repeat flexion, extension, hyperextension, abduction, adduction, and internal and external rotation 5 times—or the number of times stated on the care plan.

Continued

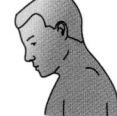 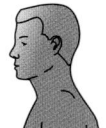 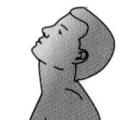 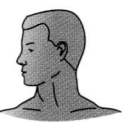 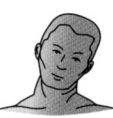

Flexion Extension Hyperextension Rotation Lateral flexion

FIGURE 30-12 Range-of-motion exercises for the neck.

Flexion
Abduction
Adduction
Extension
Hyperextension
External rotation
Internal rotation

FIGURE 30-13 Range-of-motion exercises for the shoulder.

Performing Range-of-Motion Exercise—cont'd

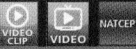

PROCEDURE—cont'd

12 Exercise the elbow (Fig. 30-14).
   a Grasp the person's wrist with 1 hand. Grasp the elbow with your other hand.
   b Flexion—bend the arm so the same-side shoulder is touched.
   c Extension—straighten the arm.
   d Repeat flexion and extension 5 times—or the number of times stated on the care plan.

13 Exercise the forearm (Fig. 30-15).
   a Continue to support the wrist and elbow.
   b Pronation—turn the hand so the palm is down.
   c Supination—turn the hand so the palm is up.
   d Repeat pronation and supination 5 times—or the number of times stated on the care plan.

14 Exercise the wrist (Fig. 30-16).
   a Hold the wrist with both of your hands.
   b Flexion—bend the hand down.
   c Extension—straighten the hand.
   d Hyperextension—bend the hand back.
   e Radial flexion—turn the hand toward the thumb.
   f Ulnar flexion—turn the hand toward the little finger.
   g Repeat flexion, extension, hyperextension, radial flexion, and ulnar flexion 5 times—or the number of times stated on the care plan.

15 Exercise the thumb (Fig. 30-17).
   a Hold the person's hand with 1 hand. Hold the thumb with your other hand.
   b Abduction—move the thumb out from the inner part of the index finger.
   c Adduction—move the thumb back next to the index finger.
   d Opposition—touch each fingertip with the thumb.
   e Flexion—bend the thumb into the hand.
   f Extension—move the thumb out to the side of the fingers.
   g Repeat abduction, adduction, opposition, flexion, and extension 5 times—or the number of times stated on the care plan.

16 Exercise the fingers (Fig. 30-18).
   a Abduction—spread the fingers and thumb apart.
   b Adduction—bring the fingers and thumb together.
   c Flexion—make a fist.
   d Extension—straighten the fingers so the fingers, hand, and arm are straight.
   e Repeat abduction, adduction, flexion, and extension 5 times—or the number of times stated on the care plan.

17 Exercise the hip (Fig. 30-19).
   a Support the leg. Place 1 hand under the knee. Place your other hand under the ankle.
   b Flexion—raise the leg.
   c Extension—straighten the leg.
   d Hyperextension—move the leg behind the body. (Do this if the person is standing.)
   e Abduction—move the leg away from the body.
   f Adduction—move the leg toward the other leg.
   g Internal rotation—turn the leg inward.
   h External rotation—turn the leg outward.
   i Repeat flexion, extension, hyperextension, abduction, adduction, and internal and external rotation 5 times—or the number of times stated on the care plan.

18 Exercise the knee (Fig. 30-20).
   a Support the knee. Place 1 hand under the knee. Place your other hand under the ankle.
   b Flexion—bend the knee.
   c Extension—straighten the knee.
   d Repeat flexion and extension 5 times—or the number of times stated on the care plan.

19 Exercise the ankle (Fig. 30-21, p. 522).
   a Support the foot and ankle. Place 1 hand under the foot. Place your other hand under the ankle.
   b Dorsiflexion—pull the foot upward. Push down on the heel at the same time.
   c Plantar flexion—turn the foot down. Or point the toes.
   d Repeat dorsiflexion and plantar flexion 5 times—or the number of times stated on the care plan.

20 Exercise the foot (Fig. 30-22, p. 522).
   a Continue to support the foot and ankle.
   b Pronation—turn the outside of the foot up and the inside down.
   c Supination—turn the inside of the foot up and the outside down.
   d Repeat pronation and supination 5 times—or the number of times stated on the care plan.

21 Exercise the toes (Fig. 30-23, p. 522).
   a Flexion—curl the toes.
   b Extension—straighten the toes.
   c Abduction—spread the toes.
   d Adduction—put the toes together.
   e Repeat flexion, extension, abduction, and adduction 5 times—or the number of times stated on the care plan.

22 Cover the leg. Raise the bed rail if used.

23 Go to the other side. Lower the bed rail near you if up.

24 Repeat steps 11 through 21. Cover the leg when done.

POST-PROCEDURE

25 Provide for comfort. (See inside of the front cover.)

26 Cover the person with the top linens. Remove the bath blanket.

27 Place the call light and other needed items within reach.

28 Lower the bed to a safe and comfortable level for the person. Follow the care plan.

29 Raise or lower bed rails. Follow the care plan.

30 Fold and return the bath blanket to its proper place. Or follow agency policy for used linens.

31 Unscreen the person.

32 Complete a safety check of the room. (See the inside of the front cover.)

33 Practice hand hygiene.

34 Report and record your observations.

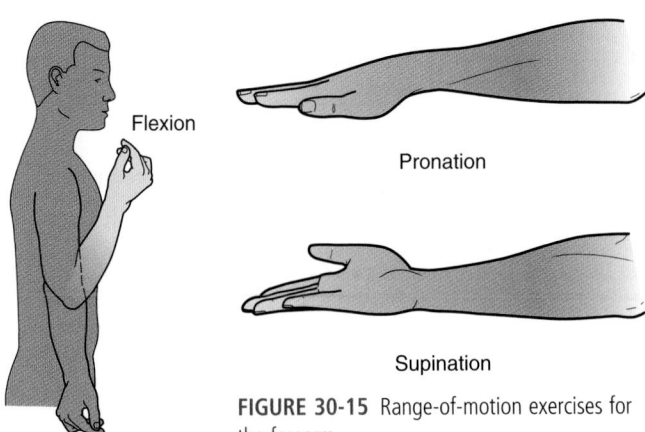

FIGURE 30-15 Range-of-motion exercises for the forearm.

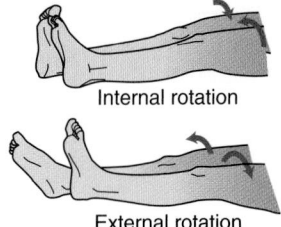

FIGURE 30-14 Range-of-motion exercises for the elbow.

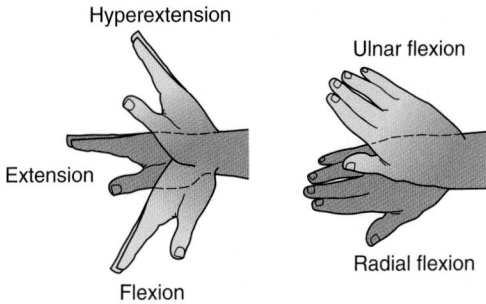

FIGURE 30-16 Range-of-motion exercises for the wrist.

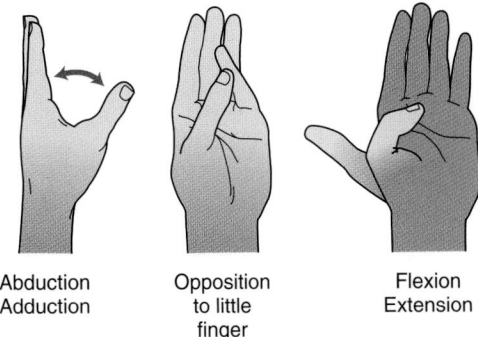

FIGURE 30-17 Range-of-motion exercises for the thumb.

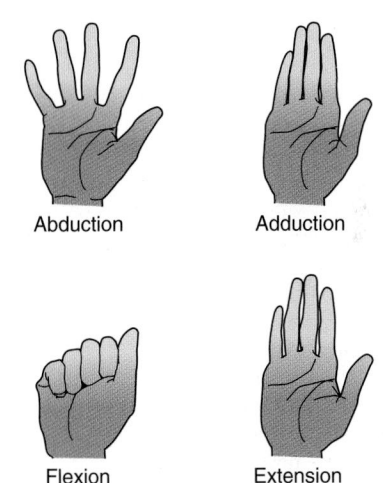

FIGURE 30-18 Range-of-motion exercises for the fingers.

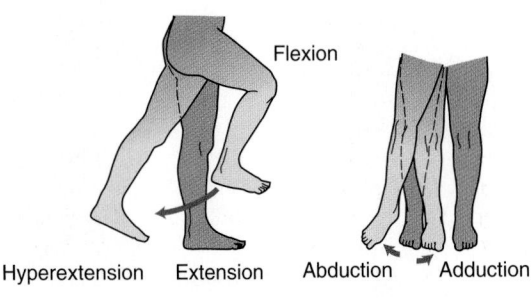

FIGURE 30-19 Range-of-motion exercises for the hip.

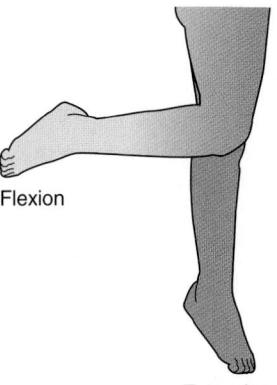

FIGURE 30-20 Range-of-motion exercises for the knee.

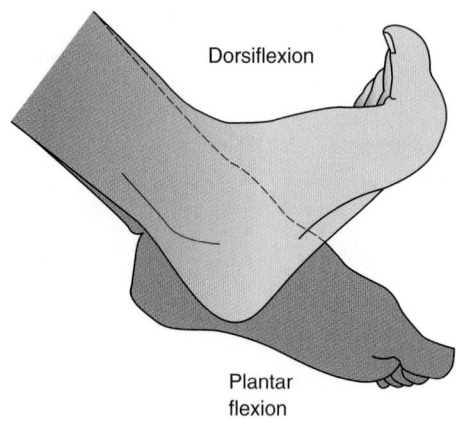

FIGURE 30-21 Range-of-motion exercises for the ankle.

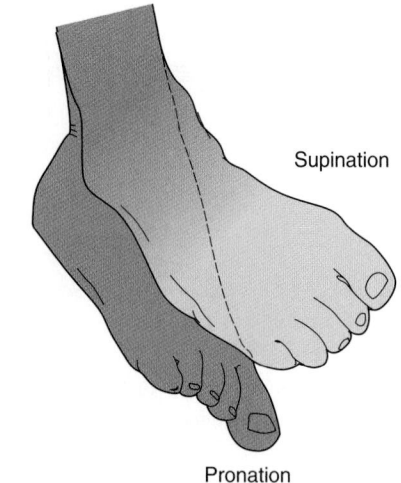

FIGURE 30-22 Range-of-motion exercises for the foot.

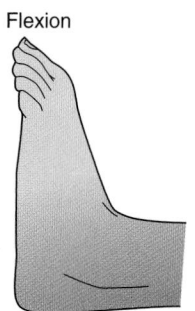 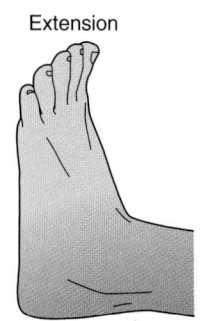 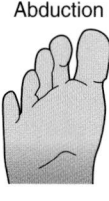 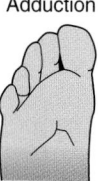

FIGURE 30-23 Range-of-motion exercises for the toes.

AMBULATION

Ambulation is the act of walking. Some people are weak and unsteady from bedrest, illness, surgery, or injury. They need help walking. Some become strong enough to walk alone. Others will always need help. Walkers and canes are commonly used for safety. Sometimes other walking aids—crutches and orthotic devices are needed (p. 526).

Canes and Walkers

Canes and walkers provide support when walking. The doctor, nurse, or physical therapist (PT) orders them. The need may be temporary or permanent. The type ordered depends on the person's condition, the support needed, and the type of disability. The PT measures and teaches the person to use the device.

Canes. Canes are used for weakness on 1 side of the body. They help provide balance and support. Single-tip and 4-point (quad) canes are common (Fig. 30-24). A cane is held on the *strong side* of the body. (If the left leg is weak, the cane is held in the right hand.) A 4-point cane gives more support than a single-tip cane. However, 4-point canes are harder to move.

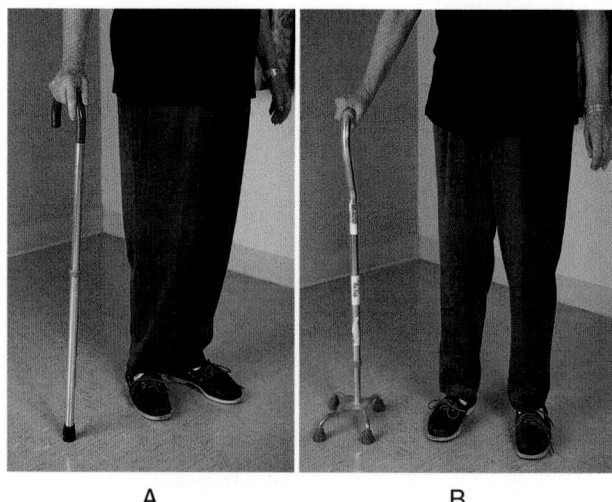

A   B

FIGURE 30-24 **A,** Single-tip cane. **B,** Four-point cane.

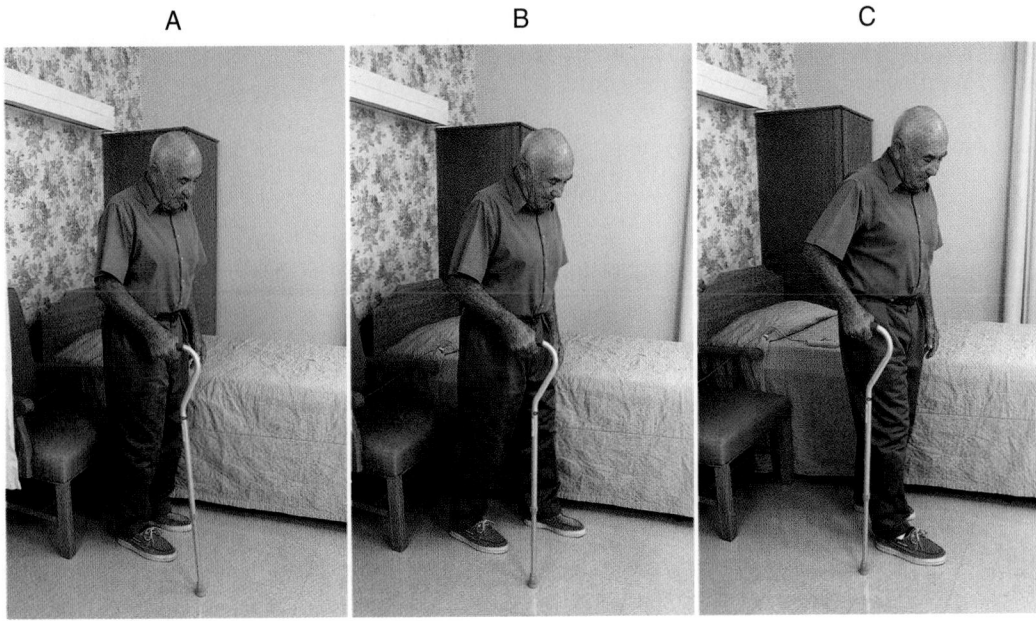

FIGURE 30-25 Walking with a cane. **A,** The cane (on the strong side) is moved forward about 6 to 10 inches. **B,** The leg opposite the cane (weak leg) is brought forward even with the cane. **C,** The leg on the cane side (strong side) is moved ahead of the cane and the weak leg.

For proper cane position, the cane is held to the side and in front of the *strong foot.*

- Side—the cane tip is about 6 to 10 inches to the side of the foot.
- Front—the cane tip is about 6 to 10 inches in front of the foot.

The grip is level with the hip on the strong side. The person walks as follows.

- *Step A:* The cane (on the strong side) is moved forward 6 to 10 inches (Fig. 30-25, *A*).
- *Step B:* The weak leg (opposite the cane) is moved forward even with the cane (Fig. 30-25, *B*).
- *Step C:* The strong leg is moved forward and ahead of the cane and the weak leg (Fig. 30-25, *C*).

Walkers. A walker gives more support than a cane. Wheeled walkers have wheels on the front legs and rubber tips on the back legs (Fig. 30-26). Rubber tips on the back legs prevent the walker from moving while the person is standing. Some walkers have a braking action when weight is applied to the back legs. To walk, the person pushes the walker about 6 to 8 inches in front of the feet.

Baskets, pouches, and trays attach to the walker for needed items. This allows more independence. The hands are free to grip the walker.

See *Promoting Safety and Comfort: Walkers.*

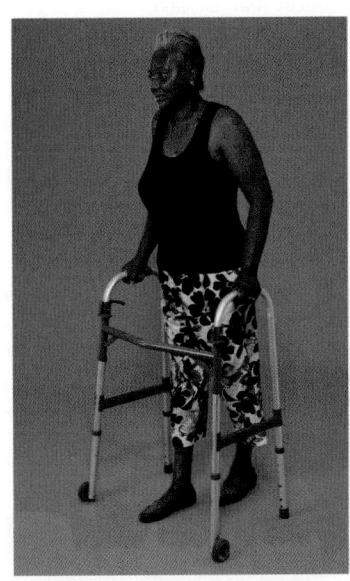

FIGURE 30-26 Wheeled walker.

PROMOTING SAFETY AND COMFORT

Walkers

Safety

Wheels are usually on the outside of the walker (see Fig. 30-26). With the wheels on the outside, the walker may be too wide for some doorways. Moving the wheels to the inside of the walker reduces the width. It will be easier for the person to go through some doorways.

Some walkers have seats. The person sits to rest. Never push the walker when the person is seated.

Helping the Person Walk

To walk, contractures and muscle atrophy must be prevented. Proper positioning and exercises are needed during bedrest.

After bedrest, activity increases slowly and in steps. First the person sits on the side of the bed (dangles). Sitting in a chair follows. Next the person walks in the room and then in the hallway.

Regular walking helps prevent deconditioning. Follow the care plan when helping a person walk. Use a gait (transfer) belt if the person is weak or unsteady. The person also uses hand rails along the wall or a cane or walker. Always check for orthostatic hypotension (p. 514).

See *Focus on Communication: Helping the Person Walk.*

See *Delegation Guidelines: Helping the Person Walk.*

See *Promoting Safety and Comfort: Helping the Person Walk.*

See procedure: *Helping the Person Walk.*

DELEGATION GUIDELINES

Helping the Person Walk

Before helping with ambulation, you need this information from the nurse and the care plan.

- How much help the person needs
- If the person uses a cane, walker, crutches (p. 526), or an orthotic device (p. 528)
- Areas of weakness—right arm or leg, left arm or leg
- How far to walk the person
- What observations to report and record:
  - How well the person tolerated the activity
  - Shuffling, sliding, limping, or walking on tip-toes
  - Complaints of pain or discomfort
  - Complaints of orthostatic hypotension—weakness, dizziness, spots before the eyes, feeling faint
  - The distance walked
- When to report observations
- What patient or resident concerns to report at once

FOCUS ON COMMUNICATION

Helping the Person Walk

Before ambulating, explain the activity. This promotes comfort and reduces fear. Explain:
- How far to walk
- What assistive (adaptive) devices are used
- That you will use a gait belt
- How you will assist
- What the person is to report to you
- How you will help if the person begins to fall
  For example, you can say:

  Mr. Owens, I am going to help you walk from your bed to the doorway and back. This belt helps support you while you walk. I will be at your side and hold the belt at all times. Tell me right away if you feel unsteady, dizzy, weak, or faint. Also tell me if you feel any pain or discomfort. If you begin to fall, I will use the belt to pull you close to me and gently lower you to the floor. Do you have any questions?

PROMOTING SAFETY AND COMFORT

Helping the Person Walk

Safety

Practice the safety measures to prevent falls (Chapter 14). Use a gait belt to help the person stand. Also use it during ambulation.

Remind the person to walk normally. Encourage the person to stand erect with the head up and the back straight. Discourage shuffling, sliding, and walking on tip-toes.

Comfort

The fear of falling affects mental comfort. Explain the purpose of the gait belt. Also explain how you will help the person if he or she starts to fall (Chapter 14).

Helping the Person Walk

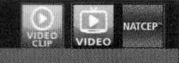

QUALITY OF LIFE

- Knock before entering the person's room.
- Address the person by name.
- Introduce yourself by name and title.

- Explain the procedure before starting and during the procedure.
- Protect the person's rights during the procedure.
- Handle the person gently during the procedure.

PRE-PROCEDURE

1 Follow *Delegation Guidelines: Helping the Person Walk.* See *Promoting Safety and Comfort: Helping the Person Walk.*
2 Practice hand hygiene.
3 Collect the following.
   - Robe and non-skid footwear
   - Paper or towel to protect bottom linens

- Gait (transfer) belt
- Walker or cane (if needed)

4 Identify the person. Check the ID bracelet against the assignment sheet. Use 2 identifiers (Chapter 13). Also call the person by name.
5 Provide for privacy.

Helping the Person Walk—cont'd

PROCEDURE

6 Lower the bed to a safe and comfortable level for the person. Follow the care plan. Lock (brake) the bed wheels. Lower the bed rail if up.

7 Fan-fold top linens to the foot of the bed.

8 Place the paper or towel under the person's feet. Put the shoes on the person. Fasten the shoes.

9 Help the person sit on the side of the bed. (See procedure: *Sitting on the Side of the Bed [Dangling]* in Chapter 18.)

10 Make sure the person's feet are flat on the floor.

11 Help the person put on the robe.

12 Apply the gait belt at the waist over clothing. (See procedure: *Using a Transfer/Gait Belt* in Chapter 14.)

13 Position the walker (if used) in front of the person. Or have the person hold the cane (if used) on his or her strong side.

14 Help the person stand. (See procedure: *Transferring the Person to a Chair or Wheelchair* in Chapter 19.) Grasp the gait belt at each side.

15 Stand at the person's weak side while he or she gains balance. Hold the belt at the side and back.

16 Encourage the person to stand erect with the head up and the back straight.

17 *If using a walker or cane:*
   a Walker—the walker is 6 to 8 inches in front of the person.
   b Cane—the cane is held on the strong side.
      1) The cane tip is 6 to 10 inches to the side of the strong foot.
      2) The cane tip is 6 to 10 inches in front of the strong foot.

18 Help the person walk. Walk to the side and slightly behind the person on the person's weak side. Provide support with the gait belt (Fig. 30-27). Encourage the person to use the hand rail on his or her strong side (unless using a walker or cane).

19 *If using a walker or cane:*
   a Walker—with both hands, the person pushes the walker 6 to 8 inches in front of the feet.
   b Cane:
      1) The cane is moved forward 6 to 10 inches (see Fig. 30-25, *A*).
      2) The weak leg (opposite the cane) is moved forward even with the cane (see Fig. 30-25, *B*).
      3) The strong leg is moved forward and ahead of the cane and the weak leg (see Fig. 30-25, *C*).

20 Encourage the person to walk normally. The heel strikes the floor first. Discourage shuffling, sliding, or walking on tip-toes.

21 Walk the required distance if the person tolerates the activity. Do not rush the person.

22 Help the person return to bed. Remove the gait belt. (See procedure: *Transferring the Person From a Chair or Wheelchair to Bed* in Chapter 19.)

23 Lower the head of the bed. Help the person to the center of the bed.

24 Remove the shoes. Remove the paper or sheet over the bottom sheet.

POST-PROCEDURE

25 Provide for comfort. (See the inside of the front cover.)

26 Place the call light and other needed items within reach.

27 Raise or lower bed rails. Follow the care plan.

28 Return the robe and shoes to their proper place.

29 Unscreen the person.

30 Complete a safety check of the room. (See the inside of the front cover.)

31 Practice hand hygiene.

32 Report and record your observations (Fig. 30-28, p. 526).

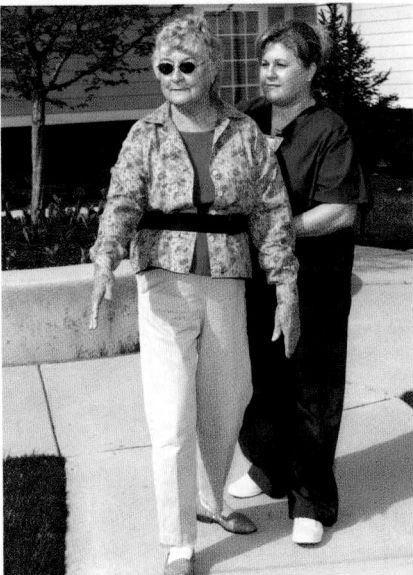

FIGURE 30-27 Assisting with ambulation. The nursing assistant walks at the person's side and slightly behind her. A gait belt is used for safety.

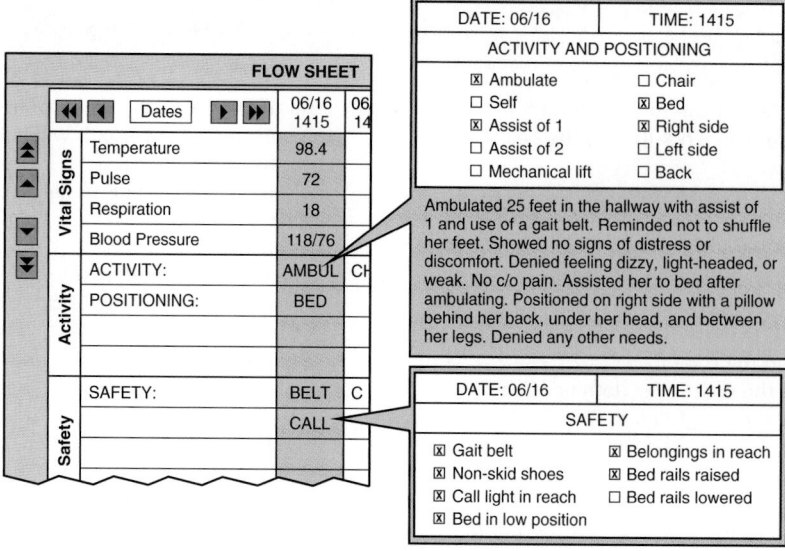

FIGURE 30-28 Charting sample.

Other Walking Aids

Injury, surgery, and deformity are some reasons for crutches or orthotic devices. The need may be temporary or permanent.

Crutches Crutches are used when the person cannot use 1 leg or when 1 or both legs need to gain strength. Some persons with permanent leg weakness can use crutches. They usually use forearm crutches (Fig. 30-29). Underarm crutches extend from the underarm to the ground (Fig. 30-30).

The person learns to crutch walk, use stairs, and sit and stand. The person on crutches is at risk for falls. Follow these safety measures.

- Check the crutch tips. They must not be worn down, torn, or wet. Replace worn or torn crutch tips. Dry wet tips with a towel or paper towels.
- Check crutches for flaws. Check wooden crutches for cracks and metal crutches for bends.
- Tighten all bolts.
- Have the person wear street shoes. They must be flat and have non-skid soles.
- Make sure clothes fit well. Loose clothes may get caught between the crutches and underarms. Loose clothes and long skirts can hang forward and block the person's view of the feet and crutch tips.
- Practice safety rules to prevent falls (Chapter 14).
- Keep crutches within the person's reach. Put them by the person's chair or against a wall.
- Know which crutch gait the person uses.
  - 4-point gait (Fig. 30-31)
  - 3-point gait (Fig. 30-32)
  - 2-point gait (Fig. 30-33)
  - Swing-to gait (Fig. 30-34)
  - Swing-through gait (Fig. 30-35, p. 528)

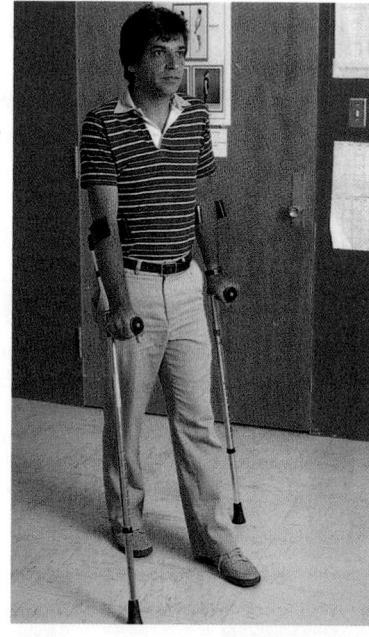

FIGURE 30-29 Forearm crutches. (From Elkin MK, Perry AG, Potter PA: *Nursing interventions & clinical skills,* ed 2, St Louis, 2000, Mosby.)

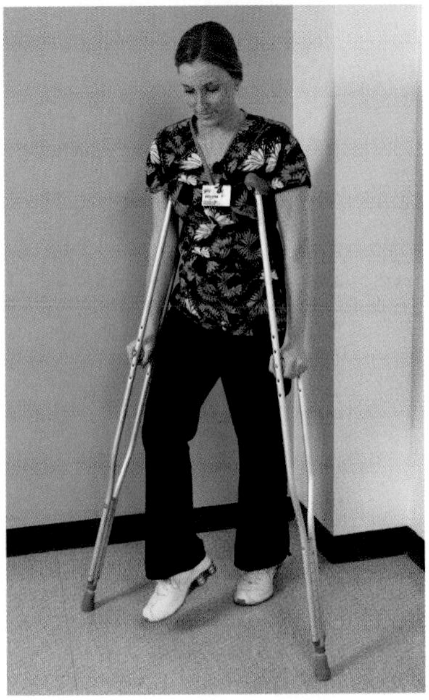

FIGURE 30-30 Underarm crutches.

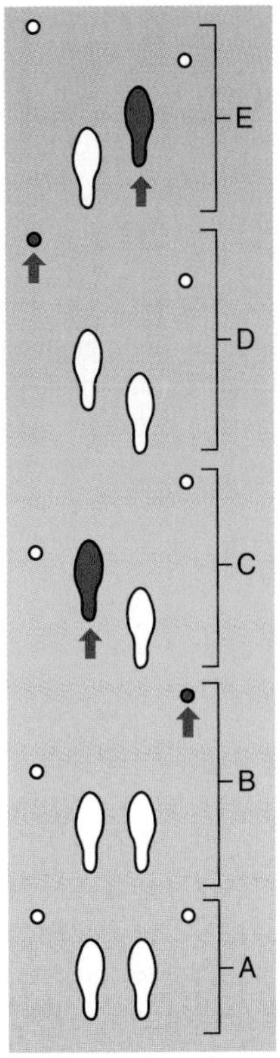

FIGURE 30-31 The 4-point gait. The person uses both legs. The right crutch is moved forward and then the left foot. Then the left crutch is moved forward followed by the right foot.

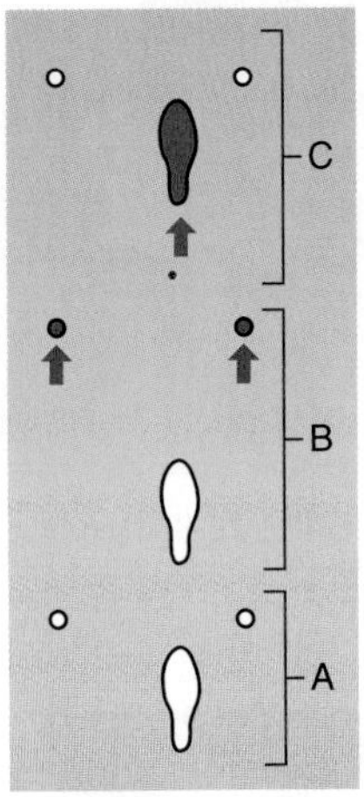

FIGURE 30-32 The 3-point gait. One leg is used. Both crutches are moved forward. Then the good foot is moved forward.

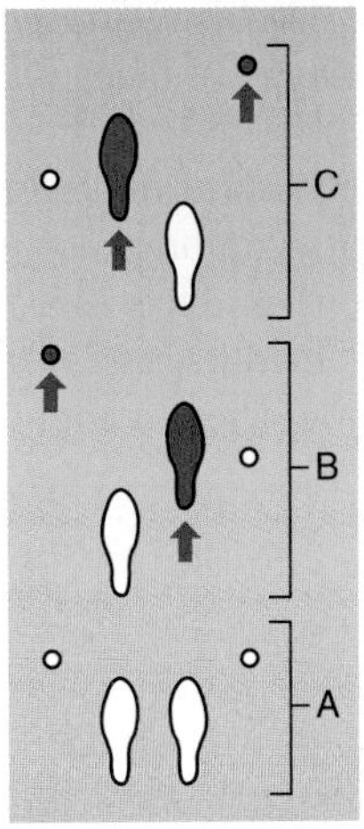

FIGURE 30-33 The 2-point gait. The person bears some weight on each foot. The left crutch and right foot are moved forward at the same time. Then the right crutch and left foot are moved forward.

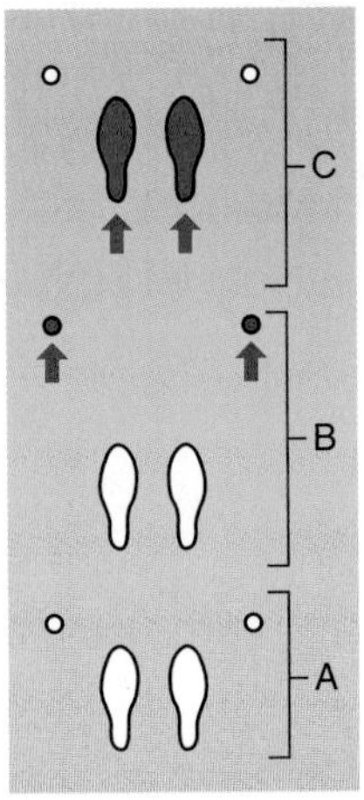

FIGURE 30-34 Swing-to gait. The person bears some weight on each leg. Both crutches are moved forward. Then the person lifts both legs and *swings to* the crutches.

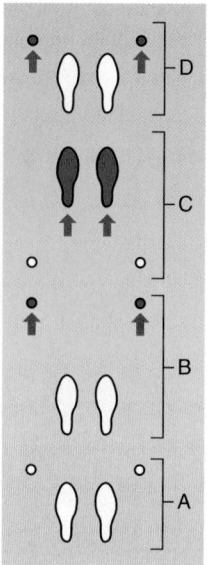

FIGURE 30-35 Swing-through gait. The person bears some weight on each leg. Both crutches are moved forward. Then the person lifts both legs and *swings through* the crutches.

Orthotic Devices. An ***orthotic device*** *is used to support a muscle, promote a certain motion, or correct a deformity.* (Ortho *means* to straighten.) Paralysis and muscle weakness are common reasons for orthotic devices.

- *Braces.* Braces support weak body parts. They also prevent or correct deformities or prevent joint movement. Metal, plastic, or leather is used for braces. A brace is applied over the ankle, knee, or back (Fig. 30-36).
- An ankle-foot orthosis (AFO) is worn with a shoe (Fig. 30-37). The AFO is secured in place with a Velcro strap. This type of brace is common after a stroke.

Keep skin and bony points under orthotic devices clean and dry. This prevents skin breakdown. Report redness or signs of skin breakdown at once. Also report complaints of pain or discomfort. The nurse assesses the skin every shift. The care plan tells you when to apply and remove a brace or AFO.

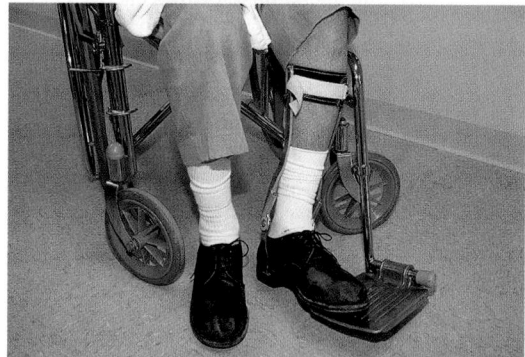

FIGURE 30-36 Leg brace.

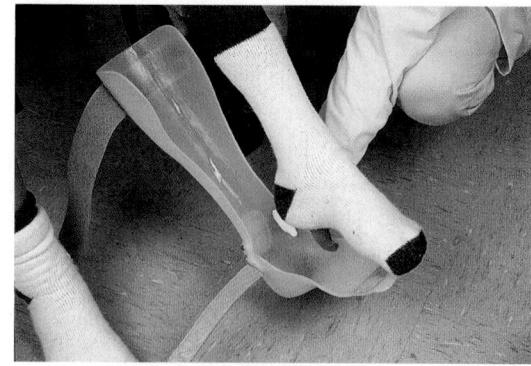

FIGURE 30-37 Ankle-foot orthosis (AFO).

FOCUS ON **PRIDE**

The Person, Family, and Yourself

P ersonal and Professional Responsibility

Exercise and activity promote normal function of all body systems. Good conditioning has long-term effects. The more active a person is now, the more likely he or she will remain active in the future.

Every person has a responsibility to do his or her best to be active. Disease, injury, pain, and aging affect a person's ability to do daily activities. Even with such limits, you can promote activity, exercise, and well-being. You can:

- Encourage the person to be as active as possible.
- Resist the urge to do things for the person that he or she can safely do alone or with some assistance.
- Focus on the person's abilities.
- Tell the person when you notice he or she is doing well or making progress.
- Tell the person you are proud of what he or she did or tried to do.

R ights and Respect

Make sure the person's garments provide needed privacy during exercise and activity. When ambulating, the person must not walk in the room or hallway with a gown open in the back. During range-of-motion exercises, cover the person with a bath blanket. Expose only the body part being exercised. Protect the person's right to privacy. Privacy promotes dignity and mental comfort.

I ndependence and Social Interaction

OBRA requires activity programs for nursing center residents. The programs are important for physical and mental well-being. Joints and muscles are exercised. Circulation is stimulated. Social interaction is mentally stimulating.

Activities must meet the interests and physical, mental, and social needs of each resident. Bingo, movies, dances, exercise groups, shopping and museum trips, concerts, and guest speakers are often arranged. Some centers have gardening activities. Residents may share ideas with you or tell you about favorite pastimes. Or you may have ideas. Share these with the health team. They are given to the resident group that plans activities.

Encourage residents to be involved. Listen to the person's interests. Suggest options that the person may like. Allow personal choice in selecting activities. Independence and well-being are promoted when the person attends activities that he or she chooses. Do not force the person to take part in activities that are not of interest.

D elegation and Teamwork

You must know the person's activity limits. The person's care plan and your assignment sheet tell you the activities allowed. Always ask the nurse what bedrest means for each person. Ask the nurse if you have questions about a person's activity limits. Take pride in providing safe care by following the person's activity level.

E thics and Laws

Persons with contractures must be moved slowly and carefully. Pain and injury occur if the person is moved carelessly. The following case shows the result of a nursing assistant's disregard for safe care.

A licensed nursing assistant (LNA) cared for a person with Alzheimer's disease. The resident was severely contracted. Her ability to communicate was poor. And she could not make decisions. The LNA admitted to:

- *Being observed pulling the resident's arms away from her body and allowing them to snap back*
- *Being observed pulling the resident's legs upward from the bed and allowing them to fall back down*
- *Failing to remove a bowel movement while cleaning the resident*

The Board found that the LNA abused and improperly cared for the resident. The unprofessional conduct violated the Administrative Rules of the Board of Nursing because of:

- *Abusing or improperly caring for a patient*
- *Performing unsafe or unacceptable patient care*
- *Failing to conform to acceptable standards of practice*
- *Engaging in conduct likely to harm the public*

The LNA's license was suspended indefinitely. (State of Vermont Board of Nursing, 2000.)

Suspend indefinitely means that the LNA:

- Had to give her license to the Board.
- Could ask the Board to re-instate her license but had to prove that:
  - She posed no danger to the public or practice of nursing.
  - She would safely and competently perform an LNA's duties.
  - She meets the requirements for license renewal and re-instatement.

You can lose your ability to work as a nursing assistant for handling persons in ways that cause harm. Always work carefully. Move patients and residents in a way that shows you care for their comfort, safety, and well-being.

FOCUS ON **PRIDE**: *Application*

Emotional responses to activity limits vary. What emotional changes might you expect? Promoting mental well-being is an important part of the person's care. How can you encourage independence and self-worth in persons needing help with exercise and activity?

REVIEW QUESTIONS

*Circle **T** if the statement is TRUE or **F** if it is FALSE.*

1   T   F   You must know the person's activity level.

2   T   F   A hip abduction wedge keeps the legs together.

3   T   F   A person is dizzy when walking. Help the person to sit.

4   T   F   A walker and a cane give the same support.

5   T   F   When using a cane, the feet move first.

6   T   F   When using a wheeled walker, the walker is pushed 6 to 8 inches in front of the person's feet.

7   T   F   An orthotic device is used to support a muscle or promote a certain motion.

8   T   F   A person has a brace. Bony areas need protection from skin breakdown.

Circle the BEST answer.

9   The purpose of bedrest is to
   a   Prevent orthostatic hypotension
   b   Reduce pain and promote healing
   c   Prevent pressure ulcers, constipation, and blood clots
   d   Cause contractures and muscle atrophy

10   Which helps prevent plantar flexion?
   a   Bed-boards
   b   A foot-board
   c   A trochanter roll
   d   Hand rolls

11   Which prevents the hip from turning outward?
   a   A cane
   b   A foot-board
   c   A trochanter roll
   d   A leg brace

12   A contracture is
   a   The loss of muscle strength from inactivity
   b   A decrease in the size of a muscle
   c   A blood clot in the muscle
   d   The lack of joint mobility from shortening of a muscle

13   A trapeze is used to
   a   Prevent footdrop
   b   Prevent contractures
   c   Strengthen arm muscles
   d   Strengthen leg muscles

14   Active ROM exercises are performed by
   a   The person
   b   The physical therapist
   c   You
   d   The person with the help of another

15   When performing ROM exercises, which may cause injury?
   a   Supporting the part being exercised
   b   Moving the joint slowly, smoothly, and gently
   c   Forcing the joint through its full range of motion
   d   Exercising only the joints indicated by the nurse

16   Flexion involves
   a   Bending the body part
   b   Straightening the body part
   c   Moving the body part toward the body
   d   Moving the body part away from the body

17   Turning the joint downward is called
   a   Dorsiflexion
   b   Rotation
   c   Supination
   d   Pronation

18   When ambulating a person
   a   A gait belt is used if the person is weak or unsteady
   b   The person can shuffle or slide when walking after bedrest
   c   Encourage the person to walk quickly
   d   You walk on the person's strong side

19   A cane is held
   a   At waist level
   b   On the strong side
   c   On the weak side
   d   On either side

20   A person uses crutches. Which is a safety problem?
   a   Crutch tips are wet.
   b   The person is wearing non-skid shoes.
   c   Crutches are kept within the person's reach.
   d   Crutch bolts are tight.

Answers to Chapter 30 questions are on p. 871.

FOCUS ON PRACTICE

Problem Solving

You are ambulating a resident in the hallway with a walker and gait belt. The resident says: "I feel dizzy." A chair is not nearby. You see a wheelchair at the nurses' station at the end of the hallway. What will you do? How might you use planning and teamwork to avoid this in the future?

Comfort, Rest, and Sleep

OBJECTIVES

- Define the key terms and key abbreviations in this chapter.
- Explain why comfort, rest, and sleep are important.
- List the OBRA room requirements for comfort, rest, and sleep.
- Describe 4 types of pain and the factors affecting pain.
- Explain why pain is personal.
- List the signs and symptoms of pain.
- List the nursing measures that relieve pain.
- Explain the purposes of a back massage.
- Explain why meeting basic needs is important for rest.
- Identify when rest is needed.

- Explain how circadian rhythm affects sleep.
- Describe the stages of sleep.
- Know the sleep requirements for each age-group.
- Describe the factors affecting sleep.
- Describe the common sleep disorders.
- List the nursing measures that promote rest and sleep.
- Explain how dementia affects sleep.
- Perform the procedure described in this chapter.
- Explain how to promote PRIDE in the person, the family, and yourself.

KEY TERMS

acute pain Pain that is felt suddenly from injury, disease, trauma, or surgery

chronic pain Pain that continues for a long time (months or years) or occurs off and on; persistent pain

circadian rhythm Daily rhythm based on a 24-hour cycle; the day-night cycle or body rhythm

comfort A state of well-being; the person has no physical or emotional pain and is calm and at peace

discomfort See "pain"

distraction To change the person's center of attention

enuresis Urinary incontinence in bed at night

guided imagery Creating and focusing on an image

insomnia A chronic condition in which the person cannot sleep or stay asleep all night

NREM sleep The phase of sleep with "no rapid eye movement;" non-REM sleep

pain To ache, hurt, or be sore; discomfort

persistent pain See "chronic pain"

phantom pain Pain felt in a body part that is no longer there

radiating pain Pain felt at the site of tissue damage and in nearby areas

relaxation To be free from mental and physical stress

REM sleep The phase of sleep with "rapid eye movement"

rest To be calm, at ease, and relaxed with no anxiety or stress

sleep A state of unconsciousness, reduced voluntary muscle activity, and lowered metabolism

sleep deprivation The amount and quality of sleep are reduced

sleepwalking When the person leaves the bed and walks about

KEY ABBREVIATIONS

CMS	Centers for Medicare & Medicaid Services	**OBRA**	Omnibus Budget Reconciliation Act of 1987
NREM	No rapid eye movement	**REM**	Rapid eye movement

Comfort, rest, and sleep are needed for well-being. The total person—the physical, emotional, social, and spiritual—is affected by comfort, rest, and sleep problems. Discomfort and pain can be physical or emotional. Whatever the cause, they affect rest, sleep, function, and quality of life.

Rest and sleep restore energy and well-being. Illness and injury increase the need for rest and sleep. The body needs more energy for healing, repair, and daily functions.

See *Focus on Long-Term Care and Home Care: Comfort, Rest, and Sleep.*

COMFORT

Comfort is a state of well-being. The person has no physical or emotional pain. He or she is calm and at peace. Age, illness, and activity affect comfort. So do temperature, ventilation, noise, odors, and lighting. Such factors are controlled to the meet the person's needs (Chapter 20).

See *Focus on Communication: Comfort.*

FOCUS ON LONG-TERM CARE AND HOME CARE

Comfort, Rest, and Sleep

Long-Term Care
The *Omnibus Budget Reconciliation Act of 1987 (OBRA)* and the Centers for Medicare & Medicaid Services (CMS) require care that promotes well-being. Therefore nursing center rooms are designed and equipped for comfort.
- No more than 4 persons in a room
- A suspended curtain that goes around the bed for privacy
- A bed of proper height and size for the person
- A clean, comfortable mattress
- Linens (sheets, blankets, spreads) for the weather and climate
- A clean and orderly room
- An odor-free room
- A room temperature between 71°F and 81°F (Fahrenheit)
- A comfortable sound level
- Adequate ventilation and room humidity
- Adequate and comfortable lighting

FOCUS ON COMMUNICATION

Comfort

Do not assume the person is comfortable. Ask the following.
- "Are you comfortable?"
- "How can I help you be more comfortable?"
- "Are you warm enough?"
- "Do you need another blanket?"
- "Do you need another pillow?"
- "Should I adjust your pillow?"

PAIN

Pain or *discomfort means to ache, hurt, or be sore. It is unpleasant.* Comfort and discomfort are subjective (Chapter 8). That is, you cannot see, hear, touch, or smell pain or discomfort. You must rely on what the person says. Report complaints to the nurse for the nursing process.

Pain differs for each person. What *hurts* to one person may *ache* to another. What one person calls *sore*, another may call *aching*. If a person complains of pain or discomfort, the person has pain or discomfort. Believe the person.

Pain is a warning sign from the body. Often called the fifth vital sign (Chapter 29), it signals tissue damage. Pain often causes the person to seek health care.

See *Focus on Communication: Pain.*
See *Focus on Surveys: Pain.*

FOCUS ON COMMUNICATION

Pain

Communicating with persons about pain promotes comfort. You can say:
- "I want you to be comfortable. Please tell me if you are having any pain."
- "I will tell the nurse about your pain."

If a person complains of pain, the person has pain. You must rely on what the person tells you. Promptly report any complaints of pain to the nurse.

FOCUS ON SURVEYS

Pain

Pain interferes with well-being. Pain affects function, mobility, mood, sleep, and quality of life. The agency must:
- Recognize when a person has pain.
- Identify when pain might occur.
- Evaluate pain and its causes.
- Manage or prevent pain.

You may be the first to notice signs and symptoms of pain. You must recognize a change in the person's behavior and function. And you must report such changes to the nurse.

You provide pain-relief measures according to the care plan. Therefore a surveyor may ask you questions about pain. Examples are:
- What are the signs and symptoms of pain?
- How do you ask a person to rate the intensity of pain?
- What factors can cause pain or make it worse?
- When and how do you report observations about pain?
- How do you assist the nurse with pain-relief measures?

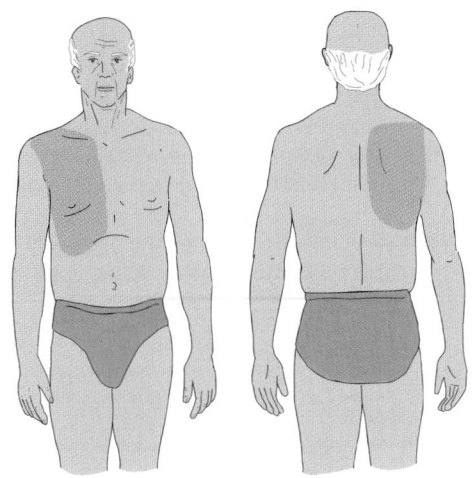

FIGURE 31-1 Gallbladder pain may radiate to the right upper abdomen, the back, and the right shoulder.

Types of Pain

Doctors use the type of pain for diagnosing. Nurses use the type for the nursing process.

- *Acute pain is felt suddenly from injury, disease, trauma, or surgery.* It may signal a new injury or a life-threatening event. There is tissue damage. Acute pain lasts a short time and lessens with healing.
- *Chronic pain (persistent pain) continues for a long time (months or years) or occurs off and on.* There is no longer tissue damage. Chronic pain remains long after healing. Arthritis is a common cause.
- *Radiating pain is felt at the site of tissue damage and in nearby areas.* Pain from a heart attack is often felt in the left chest, left jaw, left shoulder, and left arm. Gallbladder disease can cause pain in the right upper abdomen, the back, and the right shoulder (Fig. 31-1).
- *Phantom pain is felt in a body part that is no longer there.* For example, a person with an amputated leg may still sense leg pain.

Factors Affecting Pain

A person may handle pain well one time and poorly the next time. Many factors affect reactions to pain.

Past Experience. Past experiences help us learn what to do or expect. Whether it is going to school, driving, taking a test, shopping, having a baby, or caring for children, the past prepares us for like events at another time. We also learn from the experiences of others.

The severity of pain, its cause, how long it lasted, and if relief occurred all affect the current response to pain. Knowing what to expect can help or hinder the person's response.

Some people have not had pain. When it occurs, pain can cause fear and anxiety. They can make pain worse.

Anxiety. Anxiety relates to feelings of fear, dread, worry, and concern. The person is uneasy, tense, and feels troubled or threatened. Sensing danger, the person does not know what is wrong or why.

Pain and anxiety are related. Pain can cause anxiety. Anxiety worsens pain. Reducing anxiety helps lessen pain. For example, the nurse explains about pain after surgery and about pain-relief drugs. The person knows the cause of pain and what to expect. This helps lessen anxiety and therefore the amount of pain.

Rest and Sleep. Rest and sleep restore energy and reduce body demands. The body repairs itself. Without needed rest and sleep, thinking and coping with daily life are affected. Pain seems worse. Rest and sleep needs increase with illness and injury.

Attention. Thinking about pain makes it seem worse. Pain may be all that the person thinks about. Even mild pain can seem worse if it is the person's main focus.

Pain often seems worse at night. Activity is less, music and TV are off, and it is quiet. There are no visitors. Others are asleep. When unable to sleep, the person has time to think about pain.

Personal and Family Duties. Often pain is ignored when there are children to care for. Some people go to work with pain. Others deny pain, fearing a serious illness. Illness can interfere with a job, going to school, or caring for children, a partner, or ill parents.

The Value or Meaning of Pain. To some people, pain is a sign of weakness. It may mean a serious illness with painful tests and treatments. Therefore pain is ignored or denied. Pain can bring pleasure. The pain of childbirth is an example.

For some persons, pain means not having to work or assume daily routines. Pain is used to avoid certain people or things. The pain is useful. Some people like to be doted on and pampered. The person values and wants the attention.

Support From Others. Dealing with pain is often easier when family and friends offer comfort and support. The pain of childbirth is easier with support and encouragement from a loving father. A child bears pain better when comforted by a parent or family member. The use of touch by a valued person is comforting. Just being nearby also helps.

With no family or friends, some people deal with pain alone. Being alone can increase anxiety. The person has more time to think about the pain. Facing pain alone is hard, especially for children and older persons.

Culture. Culture affects pain responses. In some cultures, the person in pain is stoic. To be *stoic* means *to show no reaction to joy, sorrow, pleasure, or pain.* Strong verbal and nonverbal pain reactions are seen in other cultures. See *Caring About Culture: Pain Reactions.*

Non-English-speaking persons may have problems describing pain in English. The agency must identify these persons. The agency uses interpreters to communicate with the person. All persons have the right to be comfortable and as pain-free as possible.

Illness. Some diseases affect pain sensations. Central nervous system disorders are examples. The person may not feel pain. Or it may be severe. Pain signals illness or injury. If pain is not felt, the person does not know to seek health care. The person is at risk for undetected disease or injury.

Age. See *Focus on Children and Older Persons: Factors Affecting Pain.*

Signs and Symptoms

You cannot see, hear, feel, or smell the person's pain. Rely on what the person tells you. Promptly report any information you collect about pain. Write down what the person says. Use the person's exact words to report and record. The nurse needs the following information.

- *Location.* Where is the pain? Ask the person to point to the area of pain. Pain can radiate. Ask the person if the pain is anywhere else and to point to those areas.
- *Onset and duration.* When did the pain start? How long has it lasted?
- *Intensity.* Does the person complain of mild, moderate, or severe pain? Ask the person to rate the pain on a scale of 0 to 10, with 10 as the most severe (Fig. 31-2). Or use the *Wong-Baker FACES® Pain Rating Scale* (Fig. 31-3). Designed for children, the scale is useful for all age-groups. To use the scale, tell the person that each face shows how a person feels. Read the description for each face. Then ask the person to choose the face best describing how he or she feels.
- *Description.* Ask the person to describe the pain. If necessary, offer some of the words listed in Box 31-1.
- *Factors causing pain.* These are called *precipitating factors.* To *precipitate* means *to cause.* Such factors include moving or turning in bed, coughing or deep breathing, and exercise. Ask what the person was doing before the pain started and when it started.
- *Factors affecting pain.* Ask what makes the pain better. Also ask what makes it worse.
- *Vital signs.* Measure pulse, respirations, and blood pressure (Chapter 29). Increases in these vital signs often occur with acute pain. Vital signs may be normal with chronic pain.
- *Other signs and symptoms.* Does the person have other symptoms—dizziness, nausea, vomiting, weakness, numbness or tingling, or others? Box 31-2 lists the signs and symptoms that often occur with pain. See *Focus on Communication: Signs and Symptoms.*

FOCUS ON **CHILDREN AND OLDER PERSONS**

Factors Affecting Pain

Children

Children know that pain feels bad. They have fewer pain experiences. They do not understand pain or know what to expect.

Children rely on adults to help relieve their pain. They may restrict play, school, and sports to lessen pain. Children cannot manage pain like adults do. Adults can buy some pain-relief drugs. They can go to a doctor. They apply heat or cold applications. They can distract attention away from pain with music, work, reading, and hobbies.

You must be alert to behaviors that signal a child's pain. Infants cry, fuss, and are restless. Such behaviors also mean hunger and needing a diaper changed. Toddlers and pre-schoolers may not have the words to express pain.

Older Persons

Some older persons have many painful health problems. Chronic pain may mask new pain. Older persons may ignore or deny new pain. They may think it relates to a known problem. Or they deny or ignore pain because of what it may mean.

Thinking and reasoning are affected in some older persons. Some cannot tell you about pain. Behavior changes may signal pain. Increased confusion, grimacing, restlessness, and loss of appetite are examples. A person who normally moans and groans may become quiet and withdraw. A friendly and outgoing person may become agitated and aggressive. One who is nonverbal and quiet may become restless and cry easily.

Always report changes in the person's behavior. All persons have the right to correct pain management. The nurse does a pain assessment when behavior changes.

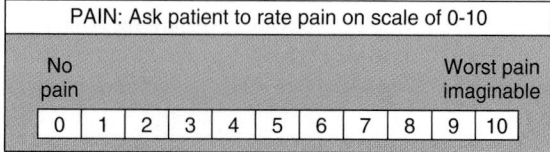

FIGURE 31-2 Pain rating scale. (From deWit SC: *Fundamental concepts and skills for nursing,* ed 3, St Louis, 2009, Saunders.)

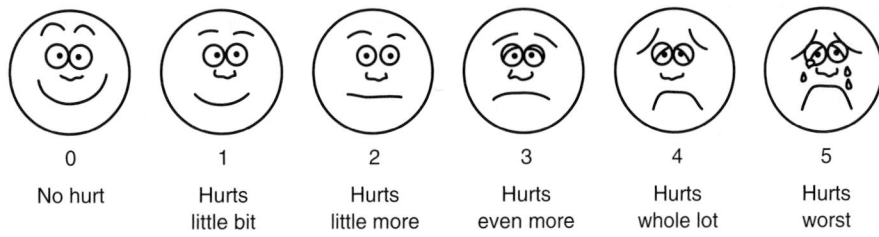

0	1	2	3	4	5
No hurt	Hurts little bit	Hurts little more	Hurts even more	Hurts whole lot	Hurts worst

FIGURE 31-3 Wong-Baker FACES® Pain Rating Scale. (From Hockenberry MJ and others: *Wong's nursing care of infants and children*, ed 10, St Louis, 2015, Mosby.)

BOX 31-1	**Words Used to Describe Pain**

- Aching
- Burning
- Cramping
- Crushing
- Discomfort
- Dull
- Gnawing
- Heaviness
- Hurting
- Knife-like
- Numbness
- Piercing
- Pins and needles
- Pressure
- Radiating
- Ripping
- Sharp
- Shooting
- Soreness
- Spasms
- Squeezing
- Stabbing
- Tearing
- Tenderness
- Throbbing
- Tingling
- Vise-like

FOCUS ON COMMUNICATION

Signs and Symptoms

A person may use words like "hurt" or "discomfort" instead of "pain." Children may use "owie" or "boo boo." Use words that the person uses.

Some persons have trouble rating pain intensity on a 0 to 10 scale. Instead, ask if the pain is mild, moderate, or severe.

BOX 31-2	Pain—Signs and Symptoms

Body Responses
- Appetite: changes in
- Dizziness
- Nausea
- Numbness
- Skin: pale *(pallor)*
- Sleep: difficulty with
- Sweating *(diaphoresis)*
- Tingling
- Vital signs (pulse, respirations, and blood pressure): increased
- Vomiting
- Weakness
- Weight loss

Behaviors
- Clenching the jaw
- Crying
- Frowning
- Gait: changes in; limping
- Gasping
- Grimacing
- Groaning
- Grunting
- Holding the affected body part (splinting; guarding)
- Irritability
- Moaning
- Mood: changes in; depressed
- Pacing
- Positioning: maintaining 1 position; refusing to move; frequent position changes
- Pulling away when touched
- Quietness
- Resisting care
- Restlessness
- Rubbing a body part or area
- Screaming
- Speech: slow or rapid; loud or quiet
- Whimpering

Nursing Measures

The nurse uses the nursing process to promote comfort and relieve pain. The care plan may include the measures in Box 31-3. See Figure 31-4.

Sometimes distraction, relaxation, and guided imagery are needed. If asked to assist, the nurse tells you what to do.

Distraction means to change the person's center of attention. Attention is moved away from the pain. Music, games, singing, praying, TV, and needlework can distract attention (Fig. 31-5).

BOX 31-3   Comfort and Pain-Relief Measures

- Position the person in good alignment. Use pillows for support.
- Keep bed linens tight and wrinkle-free.
- Make sure the person is not lying on tubes.
- Assist with elimination needs.
- Adjust the room temperature to meet the person's needs.
- Provide blankets for warmth and to prevent chilling.
- Use correct moving and turning procedures.
- Wait 30 minutes after pain-relief drugs are given before giving care or starting activities.
- Give a back massage.
- Provide soft music to distract the person.
- Talk softly and gently.
- Use touch to provide comfort.
- Allow family and friends at the bedside as requested by the person.
- Avoid sudden or jarring movements of the bed or chair.
- Handle the person gently.
- Practice safety measures if the person takes strong pain-relief drugs or sedatives.
  - Keep the bed in a low position that is safe and comfortable for the person. Follow the care plan.
  - Raise bed rails as directed. Follow the care plan.
  - Check on the person every 10 to 15 minutes.
  - Provide help when the person needs to get up and when he or she is up and about.
- Apply warm or cold applications as directed by the nurse (Chapter 38).
- Provide a calm, quiet, darkened setting.

Relaxation means to be free from mental and physical stress. This state reduces pain and anxiety. The person is taught to breathe deeply and slowly and to contract and relax muscle groups. A comfortable position is important. So is a quiet room.

Guided imagery is creating and focusing on an image. The person is asked to create a pleasant scene. This is noted on the care plan so all staff use the same image. A calm, soft voice is used to help the person focus on the image. Soft music, a blanket for warmth, and a darkened room may help. The person is coached to focus on the image and to practice relaxation exercises.

Doctors often order pain-relief drugs. Nurses give these drugs. Such drugs can cause orthostatic hypotension (Chapter 30), drowsiness, dizziness, and coordination problems. Protect the person from injury, falls, and fractures. The nurse and care plan alert you to needed safety measures.

See *Focus on Children and Older Persons: Nursing Measures.*

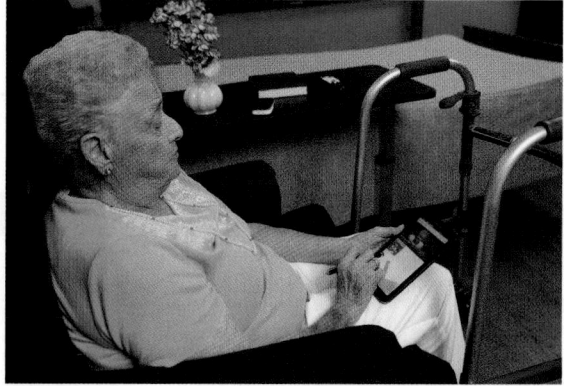

FIGURE 31-5 For distraction, this woman views family photos on an electronic device.

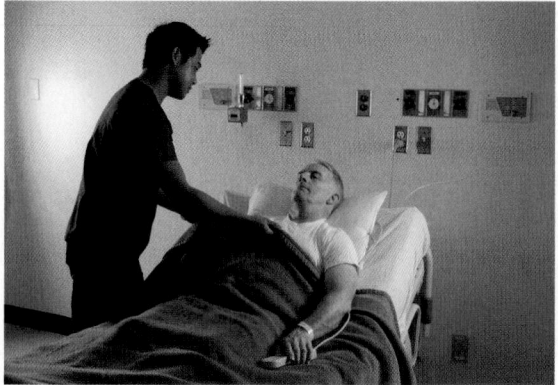

FIGURE 31-4 Measures are implemented to relieve pain. The person is in good alignment with pillows used for comfort. The room is darkened. Blankets provide warmth.

FOCUS ON CHILDREN AND OLDER PERSONS

Nursing Measures

Children
Pacifiers and favorite toys and blankets can comfort infants and young children. So can holding, rocking, touching, and talking or singing to them. Check with the nurse before you pick up and hold a child. Sometimes children are not held for treatment reasons.

The Back Massage

The back massage (back rub) can promote comfort and help relieve pain. It relaxes muscles and stimulates circulation. A good time to give back massages is after re-positioning. You also give them after baths and showers and with evening care. Back massages last 3 to 5 minutes. Observe the skin before the massage. Look for breaks in the skin, bruises, reddened areas, and other signs of skin breakdown.

Lotion reduces friction during the massage and keeps the skin soft. Warm the lotion before applying it. Do 1 of the following.
- Rub some lotion between your hands.
- Place the bottle in the bath water.
- Hold the bottle under warm water.

Use firm strokes. Also keep your hands in contact with the person's skin. After the massage, apply lotion to the elbows, knees, and heels. Those bony areas are at risk for skin breakdown.

See *Delegation Guidelines: The Back Massage.*
See *Promoting Safety and Comfort: The Back Massage.*
See procedure: *Giving a Back Massage.*

DELEGATION GUIDELINES
The Back Massage

Before giving a back massage, you need this information from the nurse and the care plan.
- If the person can have a back massage (see *Promoting Safety and Comfort: The Back Massage*).
- How to position the person.
- If the person has position limits. If yes, what are they?
- When to give a back massage.
- If the person needs back massages often for comfort and to relax.
- What observations to report and record:
  - Breaks in the skin
  - Bruising
  - Reddened areas
  - Signs of skin breakdown
- When to report observations.
- What patient or resident concerns to report at once.

PROMOTING SAFETY AND COMFORT
The Back Massage

Safety
Back massages can harm persons with certain heart diseases, back injuries and surgeries, skin diseases, and lung disorders. Check with the nurse and the care plan before giving back massages.

Do not massage reddened bony areas. Reddened areas signal skin breakdown and pressure ulcers. Massage can cause more tissue damage.

Wear gloves if the person's skin is not intact. Do not massage areas of non-intact skin. Always follow Standard Precautions and the Bloodborne Pathogen Standard.

Comfort
The prone position is best for a massage. The side-lying position is often used. Older and disabled persons usually find the side-lying position more comfortable.

Giving a Back Massage

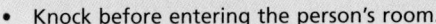

QUALITY OF LIFE

- Knock before entering the person's room.
- Address the person by name.
- Introduce yourself by name and title.

- Explain the procedure before starting and during the procedure.
- Protect the person's rights during the procedure.
- Handle the person gently during the procedure.

PRE-PROCEDURE

1 Follow *Delegation Guidelines: The Back Massage.* See *Promoting Safety and Comfort: The Back Massage.*
2 Practice hand hygiene.
3 Identify the person. Check the ID (identification) bracelet against the assignment sheet. Use 2 identifiers (Chapter 13). Also call the person by name.

4 Collect the following.
  - Bath blanket
  - Bath towel
  - Lotion
5 Provide for privacy.
6 Raise the bed for body mechanics. Bed rails are up if used.

Continued

Giving a Back Massage—cont'd

PROCEDURE

7   Lower the bed rail near you if up.
8   Position the person in the prone or side-lying position. The back is toward you.
9   Cover the person with a bath blanket. Expose the back, shoulders, and upper arms.
10 Lay the towel on the bed along the back. Do this if the person is in a side-lying position.
11 Warm the lotion.
12 Explain that the lotion may feel cool and wet.
13 Apply lotion to the lower back area.
14 Stroke up from the lower back to the shoulders. Then stroke down over the upper arms. Stroke up the upper arms, across the shoulders, and down the back (Fig. 31-6). Use firm strokes. Keep your hands in contact with the person's skin.
15 Repeat step 14 for at least 3 minutes.

16 Knead the back (Fig. 31-7).
    a   Grasp the skin between your thumb and fingers.
    b   Knead half of the back. Start at the lower back and move up to the shoulder. Then knead down from the shoulder to the lower back.
    c   Repeat on the other half of the back.
17 Apply lotion to bony areas. Use circular motions with the tips of your index and middle fingers. *(Do not massage reddened bony areas.)*
18 Use fast movements to stimulate. Use slow movements to relax the person.
19 Stroke with long, firm movements to end the massage. Tell the person when you are finishing.
20 Straighten and secure clothing or sleepwear.
21 Cover the person. Remove the towel and bath blanket.

POST-PROCEDURE

22 Provide for comfort. (See the inside of the front cover.)
23 Place the call light and other needed items within reach.
24 Lower the bed to a safe and comfortable level for the person. Follow the care plan.
25 Raise or lower bed rails. Follow the care plan.
26 Return lotion to its proper place.

27 Unscreen the person.
28 Complete a safety check of the room. (See the inside of the front cover.)
29 Follow agency policy for used linens.
30 Practice hand hygiene.
31 Report and record your observations.

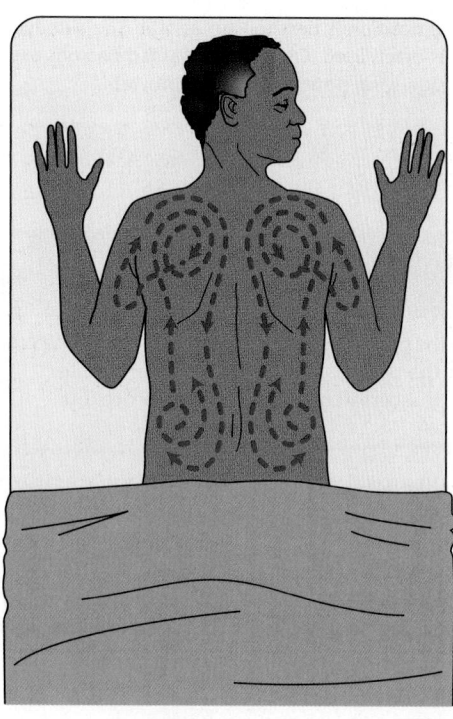

FIGURE 31-6 The person lies in the prone position for a back massage. Stroke upward from the lower back to the shoulders, down over the upper arms, back up the upper arms, across the shoulders, and down to the lower back.

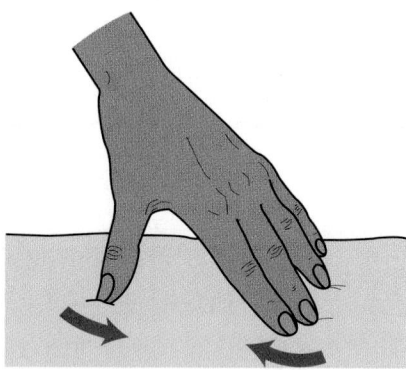

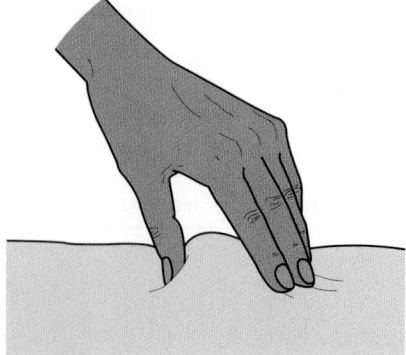

FIGURE 31-7 Kneading is done by picking up tissue between the thumb and fingers.

REST

Rest means to be calm, at ease, and relaxed with no anxiety or stress. Rest may involve no activity. Or the person does calming and relaxing things. Reading, music, TV, needlework, and prayer are examples. Some people garden, bake, golf, walk, or do woodworking.

To promote rest, meet basic needs.

- *Physical needs.* Thirst, hunger, and elimination needs can affect rest. So can pain or discomfort. A comfortable position and good alignment are important. So is a quiet setting with a clean, dry, and wrinkle-free bed. Some people rest easier in a clean, neat, and uncluttered room.
- *Safety and security needs.*
  - The person must feel safe from falling or other injuries. Keep the call light within reach.
  - Understanding the reason for care helps the person feel safe. So does knowing how care is given. Always explain procedures before doing them.
  - Many people have rituals or routines before resting. Going to the bathroom, brushing teeth, and washing the face and hands are examples. Some people pray. Some have a snack, lock doors, or make sure loved ones are safe at home. The person may want a certain blanket or afghan. Follow routines and rituals whenever possible.
- *Love and belonging needs.* Visits or calls from family and friends may relax the person. The person knows that others care. Reading cards and letters may be relaxing and restful (Fig. 31-8).
- *Self-esteem needs.* Patient gowns embarrass some people. Others fear exposure. Many persons rest better in their own sleepwear. Hygiene and grooming are important. This includes hair care and being clean and odor-free.

A 15- or 20-minute rest refreshes some people. Others need more time. Health care routines usually allow for afternoon rest.

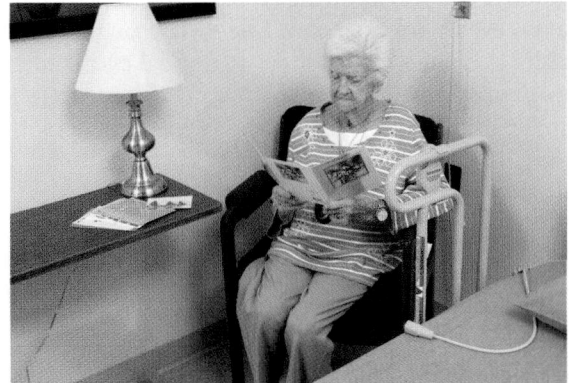

FIGURE 31-8 The resident reads cards and letters from family and friends.

Ill or injured persons need to rest often. Some rest during or after a procedure. For example, a bath tires a person. So does getting dressed. The person needs to rest before you make the bed. Some people need to rest after meals. Do not push the person beyond his or her limits. Allow rest when needed.

Distraction, relaxation, and guided imagery also promote rest. So does a back massage. Plan and organize care to allow uninterrupted rest.

The doctor may order bedrest for a person. Bedrest is presented in Chapter 30.

SLEEP

Sleep is a state of unconsciousness, reduced voluntary muscle activity, and lowered metabolism. An unconscious person cannot respond to people and things. There are no voluntary arm or leg movements. *Metabolism* is the burning of food to produce energy for the body. Less energy is needed during sleep. Thus metabolism is reduced during sleep. People wake up from sleep.

Sleep is a basic physical need. The mind and body rest. The body saves energy. Body functions slow. Vital signs are lower than when awake. Tissue healing and repair occur. Sleep lowers stress, tension, and anxiety. It refreshes and renews the person. The person regains energy and mental alertness. The person thinks and functions better after sleep.

Circadian Rhythm

Sleep is part of circadian rhythm. (*Circa* means *about*. *Dies* means *day*.) *Circadian rhythm is a daily rhythm based on a 24-hour cycle.* Called the *day-night cycle* or *body rhythm*, circadian rhythm affects functioning. Some people function, think, and react better in the morning. They are more alert and active. Others do better in the evening.

Circadian rhythm includes a sleep-wake cycle. The person's *biological clock* signals when to sleep and when to wake up. You sleep and wake up at certain times. You may awaken before the alarm clock goes off. That is part of your biological clock. Health care often interferes with a person's circadian rhythm and the sleep-wake cycle. Sleep problems easily occur.

Many people work evening and night shifts. Their bodies must adjust to changes in the sleep-wake cycle.

Sleep Cycle

Sleep has 2 phases (Box 31-4, p. 540). *NREM sleep (non-REM sleep) is the phase of sleep with "no rapid eye movement."* NREM sleep has 4 stages. Sleep goes from light to deep as the person moves through the 4 stages.

The phase of sleep with "rapid eye movement" is REM sleep. The person is hard to arouse. Mental restoration occurs. Events and problems of the day are thought to be reviewed. The person prepares for the next day.

There are usually 4 to 6 cycles of NREM and REM sleep during 7 to 8 hours of sleep. Stage 1 of NREM is usually not repeated (Fig. 31-9, p. 540).

BOX 31-4	Sleep Cycle

Stage 1: NREM Sleep—Lightest Sleep Level
- Lasts a few minutes
- Gradual decrease in vital signs
- Gradual lowering of metabolism
- Person feels drowsy and relaxed
- Person is easily aroused
- Daydreaming feeling after being aroused

Stage 2: NREM Sleep—Sound Sleep
- Relaxation increases
- Still easy to arouse
- Lasts 10 to 20 minutes
- Body functions continue to slow

Stage 3: NREM Sleep—First Stage of Deep Sleep
- Hard to arouse the person
- Person rarely moves
- Muscles relax completely
- Vital signs decrease
- Lasts 15 to 30 minutes

Stage 4: NREM Sleep—Deepest Stage of Sleep
- Hard to arouse the person
- Body rests and is restored
- Vital signs much lower than when awake
- Lasts about 15 to 20 minutes
- Sleepwalking may occur
- *Enuresis (urinary incontinence in bed at night)* may occur

REM Sleep—Vivid, Full-Color Dreaming
- Usually lasts 50 to 90 minutes after sleep has begun
- Rapid eye movements
- Blood pressure, pulse, and respirations may fluctuate (increase and decrease)
- Voluntary muscles are relaxed
- Mental restoration occurs
- Hard to arouse the person
- Lasts about 20 minutes

Modified from Potter PA, Perry AG, Stockert PA, Hall AM: Fundamentals of nursing, ed 8, St Louis, 2013, Mosby.

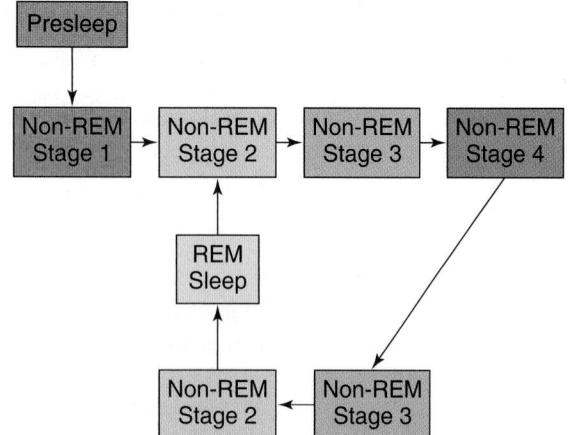

FIGURE 31-9 Adult sleep cycle.

Factors Affecting Sleep

Many factors affect the amount and quality of sleep. Quality relates to how well the person slept. It also involves getting needed amounts of NREM and REM sleep.

- *Age.* Sleep needs vary for each age-group. The amount needed decreases with age (Table 31-1).
- *Illness.* Illness increases the need for sleep. However pain, nausea, vomiting, coughing, difficulty breathing, diarrhea, frequent voiding, and itching can interfere with sleep. So can treatments and therapies and being awakened for treatments or drugs. Care devices can cause uncomfortable positions.
- *Nutrition.* Sleep needs increase with weight gain. They decrease with weight loss. Foods with caffeine (chocolate, coffee, tea, or colas) prevent sleep. The protein *tryptophan* tends to help sleep. It is found in protein sources—milk, cheese, red meat, fish, poultry, and peanuts.
- *Exercise.* People usually feel good after exercising. Eventually they tire, which helps them sleep well. Exercise causes the release of substances into the bloodstream that stimulate the body. Exercise is avoided 2 hours before bedtime.
- *Environment.* People adjust to their usual sleep settings. They get used to the bed, pillows, noises, lighting, and a sleeping partner. Any change in the usual setting can affect sleep.
- *Drugs and other substances.* Sleeping pills promote sleep. Drugs for anxiety, depression, and pain may cause sleep. However, these drugs and sleeping pills reduce the length of REM sleep. Behavior problems and sleep deprivation can occur. Alcohol causes drowsiness and sleep. However, it interferes with REM sleep. After drinking alcohol, the person may awaken and have difficulty returning to sleep. Caffeine is a stimulant and prevents sleep. Caffeine is found in drugs, coffee, tea, chocolate, and colas. The side effects of some drugs cause frequent voiding and nightmares.
- *Life-style changes.* Life-style relates to a person's daily routines and way of living. Work, school, play, and social events are examples. Life-style changes can affect sleep. Travel, vacation, and social events often affect usual sleep and wake times. Children are usually up longer and sleep later during school holidays. If work hours change, so may sleep hours. Normal sleep-wake cycles and the circadian rhythm are affected.
- *Emotional problems.* Fear, worry, depression, and anxiety affect sleep. Causes include illness and work, personal, family, or money problems. Loss of a loved one or friend is another cause. People may have problems falling asleep or they awaken often. Some have problems getting back to sleep.

TABLE 31-1	Sleep Guidelines
Age-Group	Hours per Day
Newborns (birth to 4 weeks)	16-18
Pre-schoolers (3 to 6 years)	11-12
School-age	At least 10
Teenagers	9-10
Adults (including older persons)	7-8

Modified from Centers for Disease Control and Prevention: How much sleep do I need, updated July 1, 2013, as reported in National Heart, Lung, and Blood Institute: How much sleep is enough, February 22, 2012.

BOX 31-5	Sleep Disorders—Signs and Symptoms

- Agitation
- Attention: decreased
- Coordination: problems with
- Disorientation
- Eyes: red, puffy, dark circles under the eyes
- Fatigue
- Hallucinations (Chapters 48 and 49)
- Irritability
- Memory: reduced word memory; problems finding the right word
- Mood: moodiness; mood swings
- Pulse: irregular
- Reasoning and judgment: decreased
- Responses to questions, conversations, or situations: slowed
- Restlessness
- Sleepiness
- Speech: slurred
- Tremors: in the hands

Sleep Disorders

Sleep disorders involve repeated sleep problems. The amount and quality of sleep are affected. See Box 31-5 for the signs and symptoms of sleep disorders.

Insomnia. *Insomnia is a chronic condition in which the person cannot sleep or stay asleep all night.* There are 3 forms of insomnia.
- Cannot fall asleep
- Cannot stay asleep
- Early awakening and cannot fall back asleep
  Common causes are:
- Emotional problems.
- The fear of dying during sleep. Some people are afraid of not waking up. This may occur with heart disease or when told of a terminal illness.
- The fear of not being able to sleep.
- Physical and emotional discomforts from illness, injury, or surgery.

TEAMWORK AND TIME MANAGEMENT
Sleepwalking
You may find a person sleepwalking. Help him or her back to bed even if not assigned to provide the person's care. Provide for comfort. Then tell the nurse what happened and what you did.

Sleep Deprivation. With *sleep deprivation, the amount and quality of sleep are decreased.* Sleep is interrupted. NREM and REM sleep stages are not completed. Illness, pain, and hospital care are common causes. Factors that affect sleep can also lead to sleep deprivation. The signs and symptoms in Box 31-5 may occur.

Sleepwalking. *Sleepwalking is when the person leaves the bed and walks about.* The person is not aware of sleepwalking and has no memory of the event. Children sleepwalk more than adults. The event lasts 3 to 4 minutes or longer.

Stress, fatigue, and some drugs are common causes. Protect the person from injury. Falling is a risk. Care tubings (intravenous, catheters, naso-gastric) can cause injury if pulled out of the body when the person gets out of bed. Guide sleepwalkers back to bed. They startle easily. Awaken them gently.

See *Teamwork and Time Management: Sleepwalking.*

Promoting Sleep

The nurse assesses the person's sleep patterns. Report any of the signs and symptoms listed in Box 31-5 and your observations about how the person slept. Measures are planned to promote sleep (Box 31-6, p. 542). Follow the care plan.

Bedtime rituals and routines are important to many people. They are allowed if safe. The person may have a bedtime snack or perform hygiene in a certain order. Some watch TV in bed. Others read religious writings, pray, or say a rosary before going to sleep.

The person is involved in planning care. The person chooses when to nap or go to bed. The person chooses the measures that promote comfort, rest, and sleep. Follow the care plan and the person's wishes.

See *Focus on Children and Older Persons: Promoting Sleep,* p. 542.

See *Focus on Long-Term Care and Home Care: Promoting Sleep,* p. 542.

BOX 31-6   Promoting Sleep

- Plan care for uninterrupted rest.
- Avoid physical activity before bedtime.
- Encourage the person to avoid business or family matters before bedtime.
- Allow a flexible bedtime. Bedtime is when the person is tired, not a certain time.
- Provide a comfortable room temperature.
- Let the person take a warm bath or shower.
- Provide a bedtime snack.
- Avoid caffeine (coffee, tea, colas, chocolate).
- Avoid alcoholic beverages.
- Have the person void before going to bed.
- Make sure incontinent persons are clean and dry. Change a baby's diaper.
- Follow bedtime routines.
- Have the person wear loose-fitting sleepwear.
- Provide for warmth (blankets, socks) for those who tend to be cold.
- Reduce noise.
- Darken the room—close window coverings and the privacy curtain. Shut off or dim lights.
- Dim lights in hallways and the nursing unit.
- Make sure linens are clean, dry, and wrinkle-free.
- Position the person in good alignment and in a comfortable position.
- Support body parts as ordered.
- Give a back massage.
- Provide measures to relieve pain.
- Let the person read. Read to children. You can read to an adult if he or she prefers.
- Let the person listen to music or watch TV.
- Assist with relaxation exercises as ordered.
- Sit and talk with the person.

FOCUS ON CHILDREN AND OLDER PERSONS

Promoting Sleep

Older Persons

Older persons have less energy than younger people. They may nap during the day. You need to let the person sleep. Plan care to allow uninterrupted naps.

Sleep problems are common with Alzheimer's disease and other dementias. Night wandering is common. Restlessness and confusion often increase at night. This increases the risk of falls. Quietly and calmly directing the person to his or her room may help. Night-time wandering in a safe and supervised setting is the best approach for some persons. The measures listed in Box 31-6 are tried. Follow the care plan.

FOCUS ON LONG-TERM CARE AND HOME CARE

Promoting Sleep

Long-Term Care

Some persons like to check on other residents before going to bed. Some have the duty of turning off lights at bedtime. These actions promote the person's dignity and mental comfort.

FOCUS ON **PRIDE**

The Person, Family, and Yourself

Personal and Professional Responsibility

Unmanaged pain decreases quality of life. You have an important role in assisting the nurse with pain control. You spend a lot of time with patients and residents. You observe them. You talk with them and listen to their needs.

You must report signs and symptoms of pain. Report what the person said and what you observed. The nurse uses this information to assess, plan, and evaluate pain relief.

Rights and Respect

OBRA and the CMS protect the right to quality of life. Measures that promote comfort, rest, and sleep are required. They relate to the bed, mattress, room temperature, noise level, lighting, linens, odors, and the number of persons in each room (Chapter 20). Respecting personal choice and taking part in planning care also promote comfort.

Your care of the person and setting affects quality of life and well-being. You can either promote comfort and relaxation or cause stress, discomfort, and worry. Take pride in providing comfort and peace of mind.

Independence and Social Interaction

A person's comfort involves more than physical needs. Emotional, spiritual, and social needs must also be met. Try not to focus only on physical needs. Consider the person's thoughts, feelings, values, and beliefs.

Time spent with friends and family often provides comfort. For some, religious ceremonies or rituals promote peace and healing. Allow time and privacy for those needs. Small gestures show that you care. You can:

- Ask: "How are you feeling today?"
- Give the person time to pray before meals or at bedtime if this is something he or she values.
- While giving care, ask about the person's friends and family.

Emotional, spiritual, and social needs all interact and affect the person's well-being. Focus on the person as a whole.

Delegation and Teamwork

You work with other staff to promote comfort and rest. The health team coordinates care and therapies with pain-relief measures and rest periods. It is common to wait about 30 minutes after a pain-relief drug is given to perform procedures and provide care. The nurse tells you how long to wait. The person is allowed to rest after tiring activities, procedures, and therapies. Planning and communication are needed for effective teamwork and quality care.

Ethics and Laws

You may question what the person tells you about his or her pain. For example, Mrs. Watson rates her headache pain as 9 on the 0 to 10 pain rating scale. She is working a crossword puzzle and listening to music. When you have a headache that severe, you need to rest in a dark, quiet room. You doubt that her pain is really a 9 on the scale. You decide not to tell the nurse.

Mrs. Watson's pain really was severe. She was trying to distract herself from the pain. She did not receive prompt pain relief because the pain was not reported to the nurse.

Pain is personal. It is handled in different ways. Ignoring a person's pain is wrong. Reporting a different pain rating is wrong. Avoid making judgments about the person's pain. Accurate reporting is needed for proper pain management.

FOCUS ON **PRIDE**: *Application*

Family and visitors often provide comfort. How will you welcome the person's visitors? How will you show you value them and their time with the patient or resident?

REVIEW QUESTIONS

Circle T if the statement is TRUE or F if it is FALSE.

1 T F   Pain is a warning from the body.

2 T F   Pain differs for each person.

3 T F   Pain can be seen.

4 T F   Doctors use the type of pain to make diagnoses.

5 T F   Changes in usual behavior may signal pain.

6 T F   A person's culture may affect how he or she reacts to pain.

7 T F   A back massage relaxes muscles and stimulates circulation.

8 T F   After lunch, Mrs. Bell asks for a back massage. You must wait until evening to give the massage.

9 T F   Persons with dementia usually sleep well at night.

10 T F   Tissue healing and repair occur during sleep.

11 T F   Voluntary muscle activity increases during sleep.

12 T F   Sleep refreshes and renews the person.

13 T F   Sleep increases stress, tension, and anxiety.

14 T F   Sleep deprivation affects NREM and REM sleep.

15 T F   Sleep deprivation can affect functioning.

Circle the BEST answer.

16 A person has pain in the left chest, the left jaw, and the left shoulder and arm. This is
a Gallbladder pain
b Chronic pain
c Radiating pain
d Phantom pain

17 A person is restless and complains of pain. You should
a Rate the intensity based on the person's behavior
b Give a pain-relief drug and tell the nurse
c Tell the nurse only if you think the person has pain
d Report the person's exact words

18 The nurse gave a person a drug for pain relief. When should you give scheduled care?
a Before the drug is given
b Right after the drug is given
c 30 minutes after the drug is given
d The next day

19 A drug was given for pain relief. To promote safety
a Keep the bed in the high position
b Quickly change positions to avoid dizziness
c Check on the person every hour
d Provide help if the person needs to get up

20 Which measure promotes comfort and pain relief?
a Providing a blanket
b Speaking loudly
c Keeping the lights on in the room
d Asking about comfort every 5 minutes

21 When giving a back massage
a Massage for 15 to 20 minutes
b Warm the lotion before applying it
c Massage reddened areas
d Position the person in Fowler's position

22 A person tires easily. You are giving morning care. When should the person rest?
a After you complete morning care
b After the bath and before hair care
c After you make the bed
d When the person needs to

23 A healthy 70-year-old person needs about
a 11 to 12 hours of sleep per day
b 9 to 10 hours of sleep per day
c 7 to 8 hours of sleep per day
d 5 to 6 hours of sleep per day

24 Which prevents sleep?
a Cheese
b Chocolate
c Milk
d Beef

25 Which measure before bedtime promotes sleep?
a Having the person void
b Having the person walk
c Providing hot tea
d Leaving the hallway light on

Answers to Chapter 31 questions are on p. 871.

FOCUS ON PRACTICE

Problem Solving

Prioritize the following comfort needs. What do you need to do and in what order?
- Mrs. Harper asked for a blanket.
- Mr. Williams says his chest suddenly began hurting.
- Mrs. Ivy received a strong pain-relief drug 1 hour ago. She needs help to the bathroom.
- Ms. Lopez needs a back massage before bedtime.

Admissions, Transfers, and Discharges

KEY TERMS

admission Official entry of a person into a health care setting

discharge Official departure of a person from a health care setting

transfer Moving the person to another health care setting; moving the person to a new room

KEY ABBREVIATIONS

ft	Feet	**in**	Inch; inches
ID	Identification	**lb**	Pound

*A*dmission *is the official entry of a person into a health care setting.* It causes anxiety and fear in patients, residents, and families. Worries and fears about serious health problems, treatments, surgeries, and pain are common.

Patients, residents, and families are in a new, strange setting. They may have concerns and fears about:
- Where to go, what to do, and what to expect
- Never returning home
- Who gives care, how care is given, and if the correct care is given
- Getting meals
- Finding the bathroom
- How to get help
- Being abused
- Strange sights and sounds
- Being apart from family and friends
- Making new friends
- Leaving homes and possessions behind

Moving to another room may cause similar concerns. So may transfer to another health care setting—hospital or nursing center. Discharge to a home setting is usually a happy time. However, the person may need home care.

Discharge and transfer are defined as follows.
- *Discharge is the official departure of a person from a health care setting.*
- *Transfer is moving the person to another health care setting. In some agencies it also means moving the person to a new room within the agency.*

Admission, transfer, and discharge are critical events. So is moving to a new room. The new room may be on another nursing unit. These events involve:
- Privacy and confidentiality
- Reporting and recording
- Understanding and communicating with the person
- Communicating with the health team
- Respect for the person and the person's property
- Being kind, courteous, and respectful

See *Focus on Long-Term Care and Home Care: Admissions, Transfers, and Discharges*, p. 546.

See *Teamwork and Time Management: Admissions, Transfers, and Discharges*, p. 546.

See *Delegation Guidelines: Admissions, Transfers, and Discharges*, p. 546.

See *Promoting Safety and Comfort: Admissions, Transfers, and Discharges*, p. 546.

FOCUS ON LONG-TERM CARE AND HOME CARE

Admissions, Transfers, and Discharges

Long-Term Care

The *Omnibus Budget Reconciliation Act of 1987 (OBRA)* and the Centers for Medicare & Medicaid Services (CMS) have standards for nursing center transfers and discharges. The person's rights are protected. Reasons for the transfer or discharge are part of the person's medical record. The person and family are informed in advance of the transfer or discharge plans. A procedure is followed if the person objects. An ombudsman protects the person's interests.

Reasons for a transfer or discharge include:
- The measure is needed to meet the person's welfare. The person's welfare cannot be met in the center.
- The person's health has improved. The person no longer needs the center's services.
- The health or safety of others is in danger.
- The person has failed to pay to stay in the center.
- The center closes.

The person and family are told of the date and time of the transfer or discharge. They are given the name and location where the person will be going.

TEAMWORK AND TIME MANAGEMENT

Admissions, Transfers, and Discharges

Transfers, discharges, and changing rooms are easier if a co-worker helps you. When asking for help, politely tell your co-worker:
- The procedure you need help with
- When you plan to do the procedure
- What you need the person to do
- How much time it will take

Remember to thank the person for helping you.

DELEGATION GUIDELINES

Admissions, Transfers, and Discharges

To admit, transfer, or discharge a person, you need this information from the nurse. You also need this information when moving a person to a new room.
- If you need to admit, transfer, or discharge the person or move the person to a new room
- If moving to a new room, the person's new room and bed number
- The transportation method to or from the agency—car, ambulance, or wheelchair van
- How the person will move about within the agency—walking, wheelchair, stretcher, or bed
- The person's room and bed number
- What equipment and supplies are needed
- If the person stays dressed or needs to wear a patient gown or sleepwear
- If the person stays in bed or can be in a chair
- When to report observations
- What patient or resident concerns to report at once

PROMOTING SAFETY AND COMFORT

Admissions, Transfers, and Discharges

Safety

The person may develop pain or become distressed during admission, transfer, discharge, or when moving to a new room. If so, call for the nurse at once. Stay with the person. When the nurse arrives, assist as needed.

Follow agency policies for transporting persons requiring Transmission-Based Precautions. See Chapter 16.

Comfort

Admission, transfer, or discharge may be stressful for the person. So may moving to a new room. Some persons are happy. Others are sad and fearful. Some anxiety is normal. To provide mental comfort:
- Explain what you are doing and why.
- Do not rush the person.
- Be sensitive to the person's needs and feelings.

ADMISSIONS

The admission process usually starts in the admitting office. In hospitals, it may start in the emergency room (ER). Admitting staff or a nurse obtains information for the admission record. This includes the person's identifying information—full name, age, birth date, and so on.

The person is given an identification (ID) number and ID bracelet (Chapter 13). The person or legal representative signs admitting papers and a general consent for treatment.

The admitting office tells the nursing unit when to expect a new patient or resident. The person's room and bed number are given. In some agencies, the person can walk to the room if able. Most persons require transport by wheelchair or stretcher.

See *Focus on Long-Term Care and Home Care: Admissions.*

Admissions

Long-Term Care

Nursing centers' admission coordinators ease the admission process. Often admission procedures are done 2 or 3 days before the person enters the center. Needed information is obtained from the person or family member.

The room assignment is made before the person arrives. Some residents arrive by ambulance or wheelchair van. The attendants take them to their rooms. Some arrive by car. Nurses or nursing assistants take them to their rooms. Often a family member is present.

A nurse or social worker explains the resident's rights to the person and family. They also get a booklet explaining them.

The person's photo is taken. The person may receive an ID bracelet. Photos or ID bracelets are used to identify the person (Chapter 13).

Persons with dementia and their families may need extra help during the admission process. Often confusion increases in a new setting. Fear, agitation, and wanting to leave are common. The family also is fearful. Many feel guilty about the need for nursing center care. The health team helps the person and family feel safe and welcome.

Admission is often a hard time for the person and family. They do not part until ready to do so. Remember, the center is now the person's home.

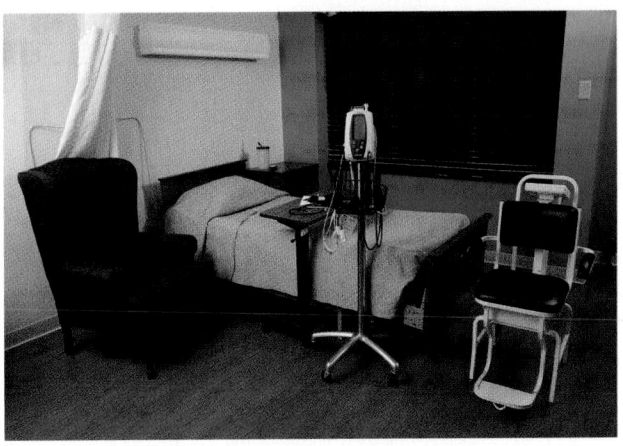

FIGURE 32-1 The room is ready for a new resident.

PREPARING THE ROOM

You prepare the room before the person arrives. Figure 32-1 shows a room ready for a new resident.

See procedure: *Preparing the Person's Room.*

Text continued on p. 550.

Preparing the Person's Room

PROCEDURE

1 Follow *Delegation Guidelines: Admissions, Transfers, and Discharges.*
2 Practice hand hygiene.
3 Collect the following.
   - Admission kit—wash basin, soap, toothpaste, toothbrush, water mug, and so on
   - Bedpan and urinal (for a man)
   - Admission form (Fig. 32-2, p. 548)
   - Thermometer
   - Stethoscope and blood pressure cuff
   - Patient gown or pajamas (if needed)
   - Towels and washcloth
   - IV (intravenous) pole (if needed)
   - Other items requested by the nurse
4 Place the following on the over-bed table.
   - Thermometer
   - Stethoscope and blood pressure cuff
   - Admission form

5 Place the water mug on the bedside stand or over-bed table.
6 Place the following in the bedside stand.
   - Admission kit
   - Bedpan and urinal
   - Patient gown or pajamas
   - Towels and washcloth
7 *If the person arrives by stretcher:*
   a Make a surgical bed (Chapter 21).
   b Raise the bed for a transfer from a stretcher.
8 *If the person is ambulatory or arrives by wheelchair:*
   a Leave the bed closed.
   b Lower the bed to a safe and comfortable level as directed by the nurse.
9 Attach the call light to the bed linens.
10 Practice hand hygiene.

ADMISSION NURSING ASSESSMENT
STATUS UPON ADMISSION

Admission Notes

Date of admission ____/____/____   Time _____ a.m.
                                                     p.m.

Transported by _____

Accompanied by _____

Age _____ Sex _____ Weight _____ Height: _____ Ft. _____ In.

Vitals: T _____ P _____ (☐ Reg ☐ Irreg) R _____ B/P _____/_____

Attending physician notified? ☐ No ☐ Yes, date/time ____/____/____ _____ a.m.
                                                                              p.m.

Diagnosis: _____ Date last chest x-ray or PPD ____/____/____

Allergies

Meds _____

Food _____

_____

Other _____

Skin Condition

Using the diagrams provided, indicate all body marks such as old/recent scars (surgical and other), bruises, discolorations, abrasions, pressure ulcers, or questionable markings. Indicate size, depth (in cms), color and drainage.

PAIN
(As described by resident/representative)

Frequency:
☐ No pain   ☐ Daily, but not
☐ Less than daily   constant
                   ☐ Constant

Location: _____

Intensity:
☐ No pain   ☐ Severe pain
☐ Mild pain   ☐ Horrible pain
☐ Distressing pain ☐ Excruciating
                       pain

Pain on admission:
☐ No ☐ Yes, describe _____
_____

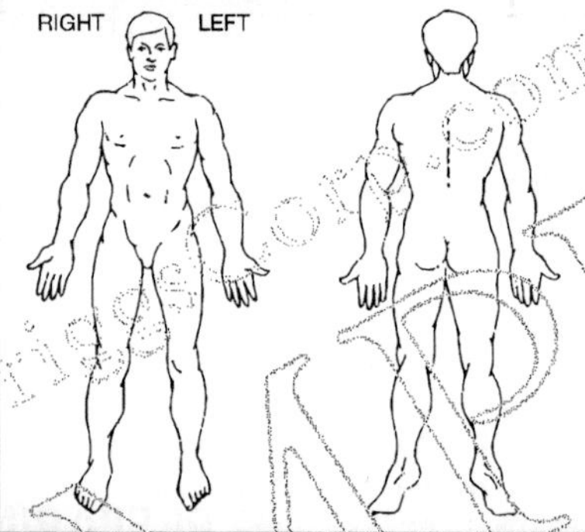

RIGHT   LEFT

COMMENTS: _____
_____
_____
_____

SPECIAL TREATMENTS & PROCEDURES:
_____
_____

CURRENT STATUS

General Skin Condition

Check all that apply.
☐ Reddened ☐ Pale ☐ Jaundiced
  ☐ Cyanotic ☐ Ashen
☐ Dry ☐ Moist ☐ Oily ☐ Warm ☐ Cold
☐ Edema, site _____

Physical Status (describe if applicable otherwise indicate NA)

Paralysis/paresis-site, degree _____
Contracture(s)-site, degree _____
Congenital anomalies _____
Prosthesis: _____
Other _____

Functional Status

TRANSFERS-ABLE TO TRANSFER
☐ Independently
☐ 1 person assist
☐ 2 person assist
☐ Total assist

WEIGHT BEARING-ABLE TO BEAR
☐ Full weight
☐ Partial weight
☐ Non-weight bearing

AMBULATION-ABLE TO AMBULATE
☐ Independently
☐ 1 person assist
☐ 2 person assist
☐ With device
   Type _____
☐ Wheelchair only
☐ Wheelchair/propels self
☐ Bedrest

SUPPORTIVE DEVICES USED:
☐ Elastic hose   ☐ Footboard
☐ Bed cradle   ☐ Air mattress
☐ Sheepskin   ☐ Eggcrate
☐ Hand rolls ☐ Sling ☐ Trapeze
☐ Other _____
_____
☐ Other _____
_____

Drug Therapy

DRUG	DOSE/FREQUENCY		DRUG	DOSE/FREQUENCY
1		6		
2		7		
3		8		
4		9		
5		10		

NAME–Last	First	Middle	Attending Physician	Record No.	Room/Bed

CFS 5-3HH   © 1992 Briggs Corporation, Des Moines, IA 50306 (800) 247-2343
R1001   PRINTED IN U.S.A.

ADMISSION NURSING ASSESSMENT
☐ Continued on Reverse

FIGURE 32-2 A sample admission form. (Courtesy Briggs Corp., Des Moines, Iowa.)

CURRENT STATUS - CONTINUED

Hearing	Right	Left	R & L	Vision	Right	Left	R & L	Communication
Adequate				Adequate				❏ Clear
Adequate w/aid				Adequate w/glasses				❏ Aphasic ❏ Dysphasic
Poor				Poor				Language(s) Spoken:
Deaf				Blind				

Oral Assessment | Eating/Nutrition

Oral Assessment	Eating/Nutrition

Complete oral cavity exam: ❏ Yes ❏ No
  If yes, condition _____
  _____
Own teeth: ❏ Yes ❏ No
  If yes, condition _____
 	
Dentures: Upper ❏ Comp ❏ Part
           Lower ❏ Comp ❏ Part
Do dentures fit? ❏ Yes ❏ No
	❏ Dependent ❏ Independent ❏ Needs assist
	❏ Dysphagic; reason _____
	❏ Adaptive equipment (specify) _____
	_____
	Type/consistency of diet _____ | Food likes _____
	_____
	Food dislikes _____
	
	Bev. preference _____
	HS snack preferred: ❏ Yes ❏ No

Sleep Patterns | Bathing/Oral Hyg. | General Grooming

Sleep Patterns	Bathing/Oral Hyg.	Indep.	Assist	Dep.	General Grooming	Indep.	Assist	Dep.
Usual bed time _____ a.m./p.m.	Tub				Shave			
Usual arising time _____ a.m./p.m.	Shower				Grooming			
Usual nap time _____ a.m./p.m.	Bed bath				Dressing			
Other _____	Oral hygiene				Shampoo			

Psychosocial Functioning

FAMILY RELATIONSHIPS:

Members visit (frequency) _____

_____

_____

Closest relationship with _____

_____

ORIENTED: ❏ Yes ❏ No, if No,

DISORIENTED TO: ❏ Time ❏ Place

❏ Person

RESIDENT GIVEN EXPLANATION OF/OR INVOLVED IN PLAN OF CARE? ❏ Yes ❏ No

RESIDENT ORIENTED TO FACILITY? ❏ Call light ❏ Bathroom ❏ Mealtime ❏ Activities

WHICH WORDS BEST DESCRIBE RESIDENT? ❏ Alert ❏ Angry ❏ Fearful ❏ Noisy ❏ Friendly ❏ Cooperative ❏ Lethargic ❏ _____ ❏ Non-questioning ❏ Combative

ANSWERS QUESTIONS: ❏ Readily ❏ Reluctantly ❏ Inappropriately

MOOD: ❏ Passive ❏ Depressed ❏ Elated ❏ Quiet ❏ Secure ❏ Questioning ❏ Talkative ❏ Homesick ❏ Wanders mentally ❏ Hyperactive ❏ _____

COMPREHENSION: ❏ Slow ❏ Quick ❏ Unable to understand

MOTIVATION: ❏ Good ❏ Fair ❏ Poor

PERSONAL HABITS: Smokes? ❏ Yes ❏ No Uses alcohol? ❏ Yes ❏ No

Bowel and Bladder Evaluation

Uses: ❏ Toilet ❏ Urinal ❏ Bedpan ❏ Bedside commode

BOWEL HABITS: Continent? ❏ Yes ❏ No Constipated? ❏ Yes ❏ No Laxative used? ❏ Yes ❏ No

Enemas used? ❏ Yes ❏ No Last bowel movement _____ a.m./p.m.

BLADDER HABITS: Continent? ❏ Yes ❏ No Dribbles? ❏ Yes ❏ No Catheter? ❏ Yes, type _____ ❏ No

Urine color _____ Consistency _____ Time last voiding _____ a.m./p.m.

Restorative Programs Indicated | Therapy Indicated

Restorative Programs Indicated	Therapy Indicated
Based on the foregoing assessment, check all that apply. ❏ ROM ❏ Splint or brace assistance ❏ Bed mobility training & skill practice ❏ Transfer training & skill practice ❏ Walking training & skill practice ❏ Dressing/grooming training & skill practice ❏ Eating/swallowing training & skill practice ❏ Appliance/prosthesis training & skill practice ❏ Communication training & skill practice ❏ Scheduled toileting ❏ Bladder retraining Comments: _____ _____	❏ Physical ❏ Occupational ❏ Speech Comments: _____ _____ _____ _____ _____ _____

Completed by: Signature/Title _____				Date _____	
NAME–Last	First	Middle	Attending Physician	Record No.	Room/Bed

ADMISSION NURSING ASSESSMENT

FIGURE 32-2, cont'd

Admitting the Person

A nurse usually greets and escorts the person and family to the room. The nurse may ask you to do so if the person has no discomfort or distress.

Admission is your first chance to make a good impression. You must:
- Greet the person by name and title. Use the admission form to find out the person's name.
- Introduce yourself by name and title to the person, family, and friends (Fig. 32-3).
- Make roommate introductions.
- Act in a professional manner.
- Treat the person with dignity and respect.
  See *Focus on Long-Term Care and Home Care: Admitting the Person.*

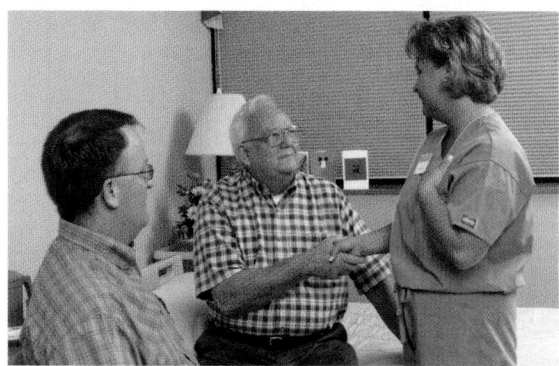

FIGURE 32-3 The nursing assistant introduces herself to the person and family member.

The Admission Procedure. During the admission procedure the nurse may ask you to:
- Collect some information for the admission form.
- Measure the person's weight and height.
- Measure the person's vital signs.
- Obtain a urine specimen.
- Complete a clothing and personal belongings list.
- Orient the person to the room, the nursing unit, and the agency.
  See procedure: *Admitting the Person.*

Admitting the Person

QUALITY OF LIFE

- Knock before entering the person's room.
- Address the person by name.
- Introduce yourself by name and title.

- Explain the procedure before starting and during the procedure.
- Protect the person's rights during the procedure.
- Handle the person gently during the procedure.

PRE-PROCEDURE

1 Follow *Delegation Guidelines: Admissions, Transfers, and Discharges*, p. 546. See *Promoting Safety and Comfort: Admissions, Transfers, and Discharges*, p. 546.

2 Practice hand hygiene.
3 Prepare the room. See procedure: *Preparing the Person's Room*, p. 547.

PROCEDURE

4 Identify the person. Use 2 identifiers (Chapter 13). Check the information on the admission form and ID bracelet.
5 Greet the person by name. Ask if he or she prefers a certain name.
6 Introduce yourself to the person and others present. Give your name and title. Explain that you assist the nurses in giving care.
7 Introduce the roommate.
8 Provide for privacy. Ask family or friends to leave the room. Tell them how much time you need and direct them to the waiting area. Let a family member or friend stay if the person prefers.

9 Let the person stay dressed if his or her condition permits. Or help the person change into a patient gown or pajamas.
10 Provide for comfort. The person is in bed or in a chair as directed by the nurse.
11 Assist the nurse with assessment.
   a Measure vital signs (Chapter 29).
   b Measure weight and height (p. 552).
   c Collect information for the admission form as requested by the nurse.

Admitting the Person—cont'd

PROCEDURE—cont'd

12 Orient the person and family to the area.
  a Give names of the nurses and nursing assistants (Fig. 32-4).
  b Identify items in the bedside stand. Explain the purpose of each.
  c Explain how to use the over-bed table.
  d Show how to use the call light.
  e Show how to use the bed, TV, and light controls.
  f Explain how to make phone calls. Place the phone within reach.
  g Show the person the bathroom. Explain how to use the call light in the bathroom.
  h Explain visiting hours and policies.
  i Explain where to find the nurses' station, lounge, chapel, dining room, and other areas.
  j Identify staff—housekeeping, dietary, physical therapy, and others. Also identify students who are in the agency.
  k Explain when meals and snacks are served.

13 Fill the water mug if oral fluids are allowed.
14 Place the call light within reach.
15 Place other controls and needed items within reach.
16 Provide a denture cup if needed. Label it with the person's name and room and bed number.
17 Label the person's property and personal care items with his or her name (if not done by the family). Follow agency policy for how to label items.
18 Complete a clothing and personal belongings list (Chapter 13). Follow agency policy for how to label clothing.
19 Help the person put away clothes and personal items. Put them in the closet, drawers, and bedside stand. (The family may help with this step.)

POST-PROCEDURE

20 Provide for comfort. (See the inside of the front cover.)
21 Lower the bed to a safe and comfortable level for the person. Follow the nurse's directions.
22 Raise or lower bed rails as directed by the nurse.

23 Complete a safety check of the room. (See the inside of the front cover.)
24 Practice hand hygiene.
25 Report and record your observations.

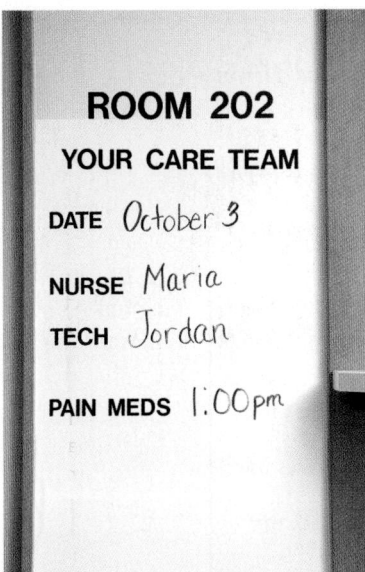

FIGURE 32-4 The names of nursing team members are posted on a marker board.

Weight and Height

Weight and height are measured on admission to the agency. Then the person is weighed daily, weekly, or monthly. This is done to measure weight gain or loss.

Standing, chair, wheelchair, bed, and lift scales are used (Fig. 32-5). A standing scale is used for ambulatory patients or residents—those able to stand and walk. Chair, wheelchair, bed, and lift scales are used for persons who cannot stand. Follow the manufacturer's instructions and agency procedures.

To measure weight and height, follow these guidelines.

- The person wears only a patient gown or pajamas. Clothes add weight. No footwear is worn. Footwear adds to the weight and height measurements.
- The person voids before being weighed. A full bladder adds weight.
- A dry incontinence product is worn. A wet product adds weight.
- Weigh the person at the same time of day. Before breakfast is the best time. Food and fluids add weight.
- Use the same scale for daily, weekly, and monthly weights. Scales weigh differently.
- Balance the scale at zero (0) before weighing the person. For balance scales, move the weights to zero. A digital scale should read at zero.

See *Focus on Communication: Weight and Height.*
See *Focus on Math: Weight and Height.*
See *Teamwork and Time Management: Weight and Height,* p. 554.
See *Delegation Guidelines: Weight and Height,* p. 554.
See *Promoting Safety and Comfort: Weight and Height,* p. 554.
See procedure: *Measuring Weight and Height,* p. 555.
See procedure: *Measuring Height—The Person Is in Bed,* p. 556.

Text continued on p. 557.

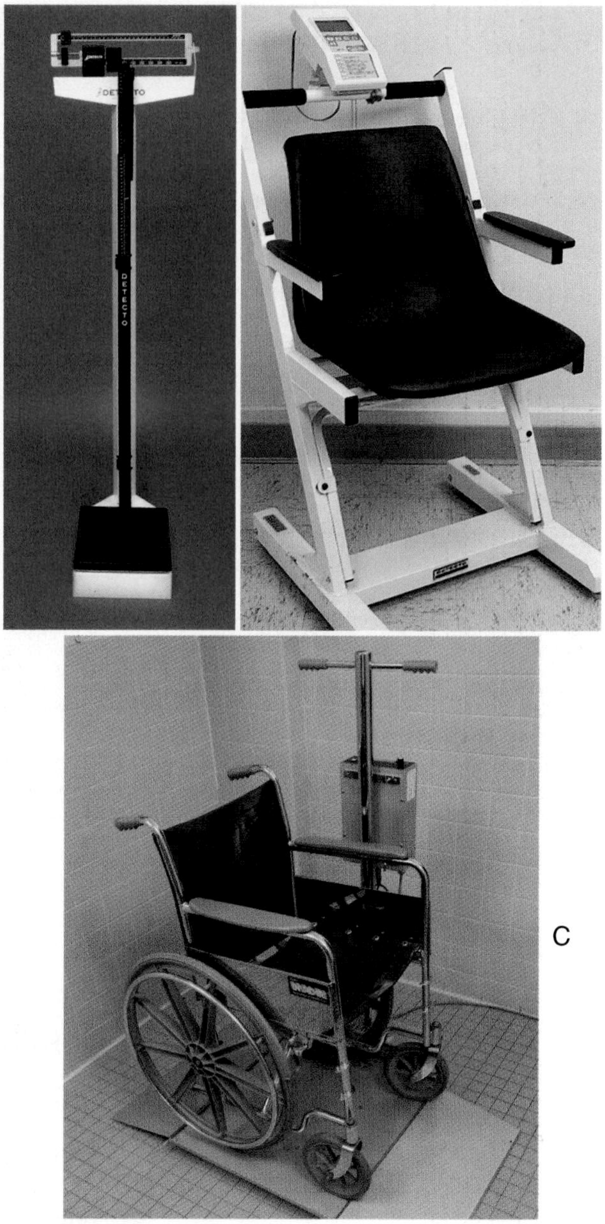

FIGURE 32-5 Types of scales. **A,** Standing scale. **B,** Chair scale. **C,** Wheelchair scale.

FOCUS ON COMMUNICATION

Weight and Height

Accurate reporting and recording are needed for safe care. Some agencies use pounds (lb) for weight. Others use kilograms (kg) (2.2 lb = 1 kg). For height, some agencies use feet and inches. Others only use inches.

If you do not know what measurements to use, ask the nurse. Follow agency policy for reporting and recording height and weight.

FOCUS ON MATH

Weight and Height

Weight—Reading the Scale

Standing scales (balance scales) have 2 bars with measurements (Fig. 32-6).

- The lower bar is divided into 50 lb values.
- The upper bar has long and short lines.
  - Long lines are 1 lb values.
  - Short lines are ¼, ½, and ¾ lb values.

The lower and upper bar values are added for the weight. For example, the lower bar is at 150 lb and the upper bar is at 22½ lb. The person's weight is 172½ lb.

$$150\ lb + 22\tfrac{1}{2}\ lb = 172\tfrac{1}{2}\ lb$$

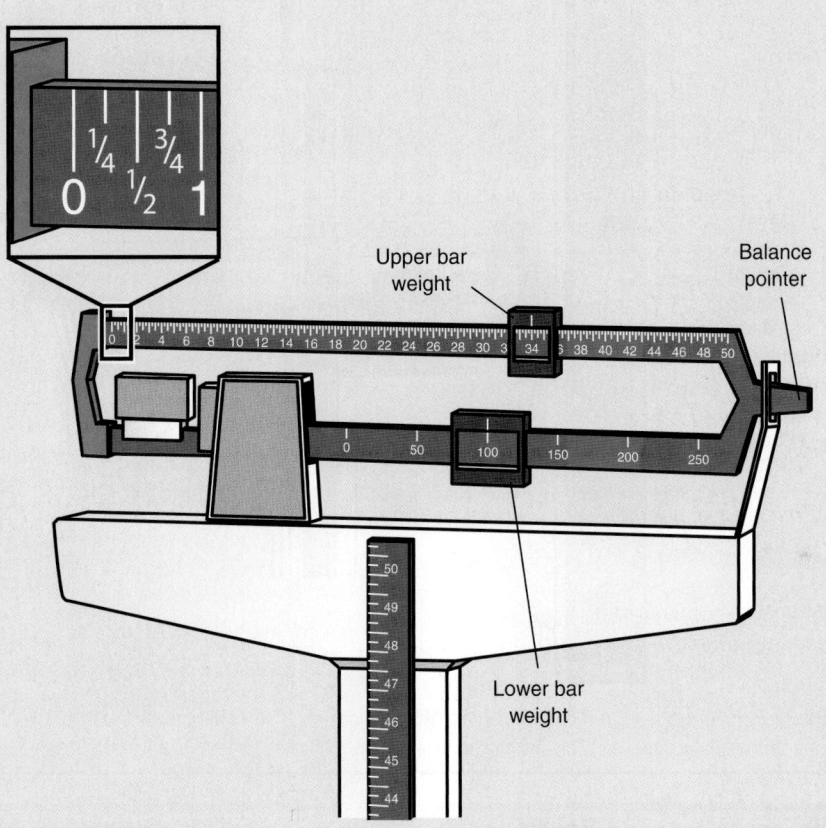

FIGURE 32-6 Reading a balance scale. On this scale the lower bar weight is at 100 lb. The upper bar weight is at 34 lb. The weight is 134 lb (100 lb + 34 lb = 134 lb).

Continued

FOCUS ON MATH—cont'd

Weight and Height—cont'd

Height—Reading the Height Rod

The height rod has 2 sections—upper and lower. You raise or lower the upper section to adjust to the person's height. If the person is taller than the lower section, read the height at the movable part of the height rod.

The rod is marked with 1 inch (in) and ¼ inch values (¼, ½, ¾). Read height to the nearest ¼ inch. The numbers on the lower section increase moving up the rod. The numbers on the upper section increase moving down the rod. See Figure 32-7.

Height—Converting Inches into Feet and Inches

There are 12 inches (in) in 1 foot (ft) (1 ft = 12 in). To convert inches into feet and inches, divide the number of inches by 12. If it does not divide evenly by 12, the number left over is the number of inches.

For example: Convert 64 inches into feet and inches.

$$\begin{array}{r} 5 \text{ Number of feet} \\ 12 \text{ Inches per foot} \overline{\smash{\big)}\ 64 \ \text{Inches}} \\ \underline{-60} \\ 4 \ \text{Number of inches} \end{array}$$

64 inches = 5 ft 4 in

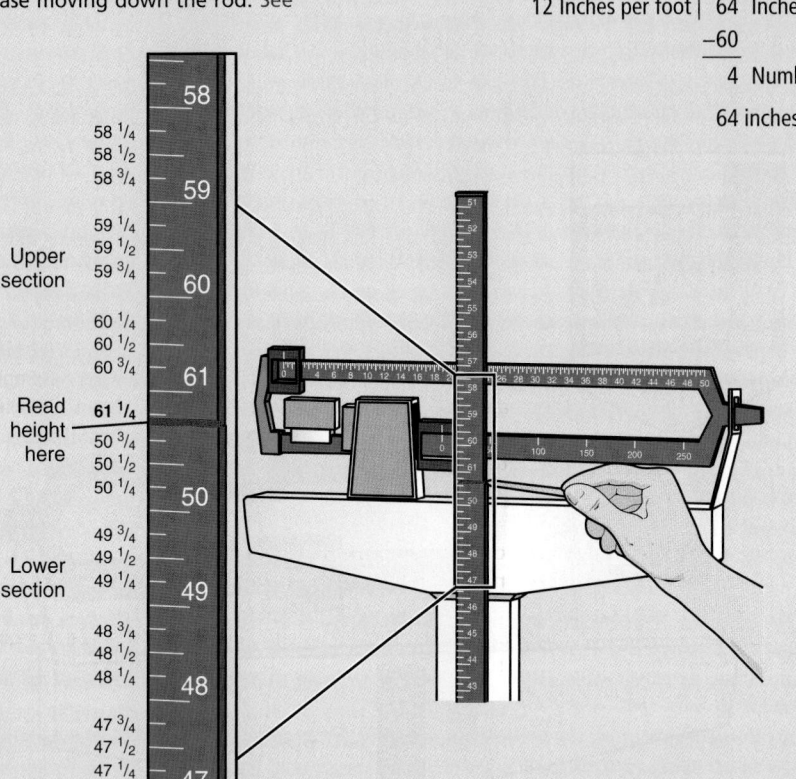

FIGURE 32-7 Height is read at the movable part of the height rod. (NOTE: The movable part of the height rod is marked with a yellow line.) This height rod measures 61¼ inches (5 feet 1¼ inches).

TEAMWORK AND TIME MANAGEMENT

Weight and Height

Nursing units usually have just 1 standing scale. In some agencies, chair, wheelchair, and lift scales are shared with other nursing units. Return the device to the storage area as quickly as possible. Do not have your co-workers wait or look for the scale.

DELEGATION GUIDELINES

Weight and Height

To measure weight and height, you need this information from the nurse and the care plan.
- When to measure weight and height
- What scale to use
- If height is measured with the person in bed
- When to report the measurements
- What patient or resident concerns to report at once

PROMOTING SAFETY AND COMFORT

Weight and Height

Safety

Follow the manufacturer's instructions to use chair, wheelchair, bed, or lift scales. Also follow the agency's procedures. Practice safety measures to prevent falls.

Comfort

The person wears only a patient gown or pajamas for the weight measurement. Prevent chilling and drafts (Chapter 20).

Measuring Weight and Height

QUALITY OF LIFE

- Knock before entering the person's room.
- Address the person by name.
- Introduce yourself by name and title.
- Explain the procedure before starting and during the procedure.
- Protect the person's rights during the procedure.
- Handle the person gently during the procedure.

PRE-PROCEDURE

1 Follow *Delegation Guidelines: Weight and Height*. See *Promoting Safety and Comfort: Weight and Height*.
2 Ask the person to void.
3 Practice hand hygiene.
4 Bring the scale and paper towels (for a standing scale) to the person's room.
5 Practice hand hygiene.
6 Identify the person. Check the ID bracelet against the assignment sheet. Use 2 identifiers (Chapter 13). Also call the person by name.
7 Provide for privacy.

PROCEDURE

8 Place the paper towels on the scale platform.
9 Raise the height rod.
10 Move the weights to zero (0). The pointer is in the middle.
11 Have the person remove the robe and footwear. Assist as needed. (NOTE: For some state competency tests, shoes are worn.)
12 Help the person stand on the scale. The person stands in the center of the scale. Arms are at the sides. The person does not hold on to anyone or any thing. See Figure 32-8.
13 Move the lower and upper weights until the balance pointer is in the middle (see Fig. 32-6).
14 Note the weight on your note pad or assignment sheet.
15 Ask the person to stand very straight.
16 Lower the height rod until it rests on the person's head (Fig. 32-9).
17 Read the height at the movable part of the height rod. Record the height in inches (or in feet and inches) to the nearest $\frac{1}{4}$ inch. See Figure 32-7.
18 Note the height on your note pad or assignment sheet.
19 Raise the height rod. Help the person step off of the scale.
20 Help the person put on a robe and non-skid footwear if he or she will be up. Or help the person back to bed.
21 Lower the height rod. Adjust the weights to zero (0) if this is your agency's policy.

POST-PROCEDURE

22 Provide for comfort. (See the inside of the front cover.)
23 Place the call light and other needed items within reach.
24 Raise or lower bed rails. Follow the care plan.
25 Unscreen the person.
26 Complete a safety check of the room. (See the inside of the front cover.)
27 Discard the paper towels.
28 Return the scale to its proper place.
29 Practice hand hygiene.
30 Report and record the measurements.

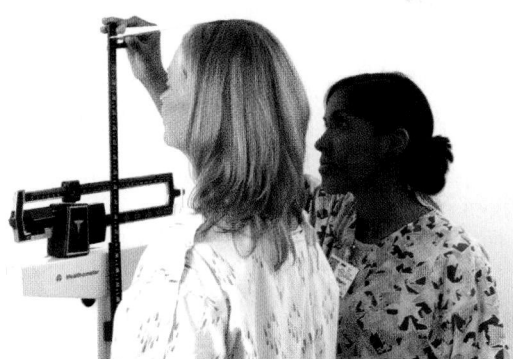

FIGURE 32-9 The height rod rests on the person's head.

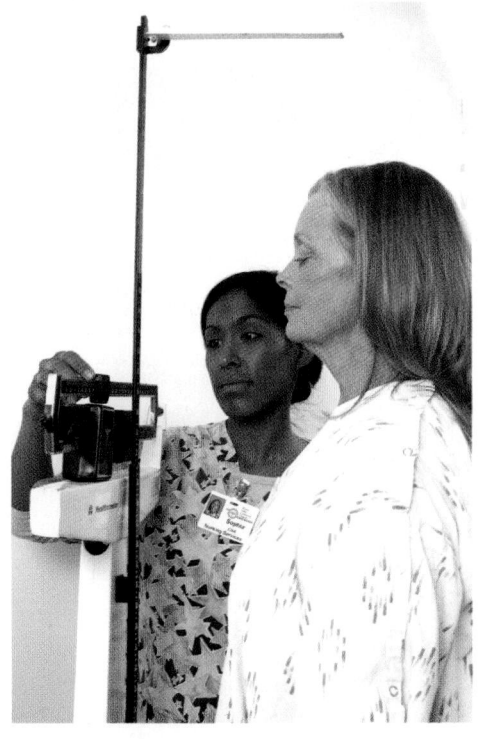

FIGURE 32-8 The person is weighed.

Measuring Height—The Person Is in Bed

QUALITY OF LIFE

- Knock before entering the person's room.
- Address the person by name.
- Introduce yourself by name and title.

- Explain the procedure before starting and during the procedure.
- Protect the person's rights during the procedure.
- Handle the person gently during the procedure.

PRE-PROCEDURE

1 Follow *Delegation Guidelines: Weight and Height*, p. 554. See *Promoting Safety and Comfort: Weight and Height*, p. 554.
2 Practice hand hygiene.
3 Ask a co-worker to help you.
4 Collect a measuring tape and ruler.

5 Practice hand hygiene.
6 Identify the person. Check the ID bracelet against the assignment sheet. Use 2 identifiers (Chapter 13). Also call the person by name.
7 Provide for privacy.
8 Raise the bed for body mechanics. Bed rails are up if used.

PROCEDURE

9 Lower the bed rails (if up).
10 Position the person supine if the position is allowed.
11 Have your co-worker place and hold the beginning of the tape measure at the person's heel.
12 Pull the other end of the tape measure along the person's body. Pull it until it extends a few inches past the head.

13 Place the ruler flat across the top of the person's head (Fig. 32-10). The ruler extends from the person's head to over the tape measure. Make sure the ruler is level.
14 Read the height measurement. This is the point where the lower edge of the ruler touches the tape measure.
15 Note the height measurement on your note pad or assignment sheet.

POST-PROCEDURE

16 Provide for comfort. (See the inside of the front cover.)
17 Place the call light and other needed items within reach.
18 Lower the bed to a safe and comfortable level for the person. Follow the care plan.
19 Raise or lower bed rails. Follow the care plan.

20 Complete a safety check of the room. (See the inside of the front cover.)
21 Return equipment to its proper place.
22 Practice hand hygiene.
23 Report and record the height.

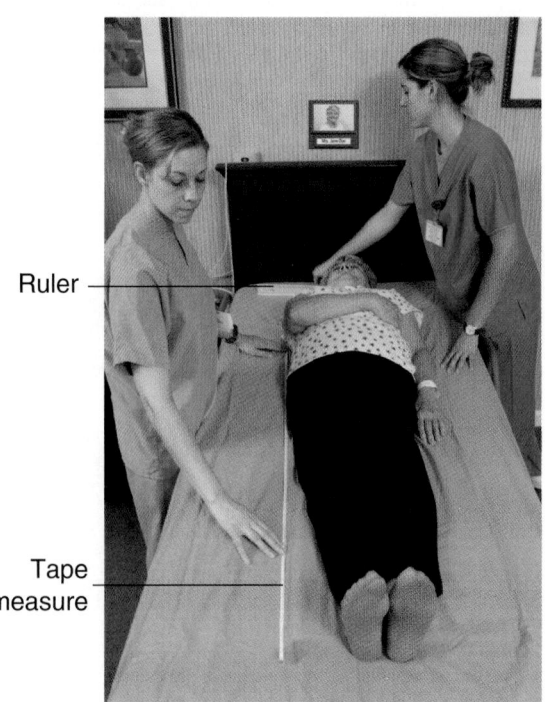

FIGURE 32-10 Height is measured in bed. The tape measure extends from the heel to the top of the head. The ruler is flat across the top of the person's head.

Ruler

Tape measure

MOVING THE PERSON TO A NEW ROOM

Sometimes a person is moved to a new room. Reasons include:

- A change in condition.
- The person requests a room change.
- Roommates do not get along.
- Changes in care needs.

The doctor, nurse, or social worker explains the reasons for the move. The family and business office are told. You assist with the move or perform the entire procedure. The person is transported by wheelchair, stretcher, or the bed.

Support and reassure the person. If the new room is on another nursing unit, the person does not know the staff. Use good communication skills.

- Avoid pat answers. "It will be okay" is an example.
- Use touch to provide comfort.
- Introduce the person to the staff and roommate.
- Wish the person well as you leave him or her.
  See procedure: *Moving the Person to a New Room.*

Moving the Person to a New Room

QUALITY OF LIFE

- Knock before entering the person's room.
- Address the person by name.
- Introduce yourself by name and title.

- Explain the procedure before starting and during the procedure.
- Protect the person's rights during the procedure.
- Handle the person gently during the procedure.

PRE-PROCEDURE

1 Follow *Delegation Guidelines: Admissions, Transfers, and Discharges*, p. 546. See *Promoting Safety and Comfort: Admissions, Transfers, and Discharges*, p. 546.
2 Ask a co-worker to help you.
3 Practice hand hygiene.
4 Collect the following.
   - Wheelchair or stretcher
   - Utility cart
   - Bath blanket

5 Practice hand hygiene.
6 Identify the person. Check the ID bracelet against the assignment sheet. Use 2 identifiers (Chapter 13). Call the person by name.
7 Provide for privacy.

PROCEDURE

8 Collect the person's belongings and care equipment. Place them on the cart.
9 Transfer the person to a wheelchair or stretcher (Chapter 19). Cover him or her with the bath blanket.
10 Transport the person to the new room. Your co-worker brings the cart.
11 Help transfer the person to the bed or chair. Help position the person (Chapters 17, 18, and 19).

12 Help arrange the person's belongings and equipment.
13 Report the following to the receiving nurse.
   - How the person tolerated the transfer
   - Any observations made during the transfer
   - That the nurse will bring the person's drugs and written documents—medical record, care plan, Kardex, and so on.

POST-PROCEDURE

14 Return the wheelchair or stretcher and the cart to the storage area.
15 Practice hand hygiene.
16 Report and record the following.
   - The time of the transfer
   - Who helped you with the transfer
   - Where the person was taken
   - How the person was transferred (bed, wheelchair, or stretcher)
   - How the person tolerated the transfer
   - Who received the person
   - Any other observations

17 Strip the bed and clean the unit. Practice hand hygiene and put on gloves for this step. (The housekeeping staff may do this step.)
18 Remove and discard the gloves. Practice hand hygiene.
19 Follow agency policy for used linens.
20 Make a closed bed.
21 Practice hand hygiene.

TRANSFERS AND DISCHARGES

When transferred or discharged, the person leaves the agency. He or she goes home or to another health care setting. Discharge is a happy time if the person is going home. Some persons need home care.

Transfers and discharges are usually planned in advance. If being discharged, the health team teaches the person and family about diet, exercise, drugs, procedures, and treatments. Home care, equipment, and therapies are arranged as needed. A doctor's appointment is given.

The nurse tells you when to start the transfer or discharge procedure. The doctor must give the order before the person can leave. The nurse tells you when the person is ready to leave. Usually a wheelchair is used. If leaving by ambulance, a stretcher is used.

Use good communication skills when assisting with a transfer or discharge. Wish the person and family well as they leave the agency.

A person may want to leave the agency without the doctor's permission. Tell the nurse at once. The nurse or social worker handles the matter.

See procedure: *Transferring or Discharging the Person*.

Transferring or Discharging the Person

QUALITY OF LIFE

- Knock before entering the person's room.
- Address the person by name.
- Introduce yourself by name and title.

- Explain the procedure before starting and during the procedure.
- Protect the person's rights during the procedure.
- Handle the person gently during the procedure.

PRE-PROCEDURE

1 Follow *Delegation Guidelines: Admissions, Transfers, and Discharges*, p. 546. See *Promoting Safety and Comfort: Admissions, Transfers, and Discharges*, p. 546.
2 Ask a co-worker to help you.
3 Practice hand hygiene.

4 Identify the person. Check the ID bracelet against the assignment sheet. Use 2 identifiers (Chapter 13). Also call the person by name.
5 Provide for privacy.

PROCEDURE

6 Help the person dress as needed.
7 Help the person pack. Check the bathroom and all drawers and closets. Make sure all items are collected.
8 Check off the clothing list and personal belongings list. Give the lists to the nurse.
9 Tell the nurse that the person is ready for the final visit. The nurse:
  a Gives prescriptions written by the doctor.
  b Provides discharge instructions.
  c Returns valuables from the safe.
  d Has the person sign the clothing and personal belongings lists.

10 *If the person will leave by wheelchair:*
  a Get a wheelchair and a utility cart for the person's items. Ask a co-worker to help you.
  b Help the person into the wheelchair.
  c Take the person to the exit area.
  d Lock (brake) the wheelchair wheels.
  e Help the person out of the wheelchair and into the car (Fig. 32-11).
  f Help put the person's items into the car.
11 *If the person will leave by ambulance:*
  a Raise the bed rails.
  b Place the call light within reach.
  c Wait for the ambulance attendants.
  d Raise the bed for a transfer to the stretcher when the ambulance attendants arrive.

POST-PROCEDURE

12 Return the wheelchair and cart to the storage area.
13 Practice hand hygiene.
14 Report and record the following.
  - The time of the discharge
  - Who helped you with the procedure
  - How the person was transported
  - Who was with the person
  - The person's destination
  - Any other observations

15 Strip the bed and clean the unit. Practice hand hygiene and put on gloves for this step. (The housekeeping staff may do this step.)
16 Remove and discard the gloves. Practice hand hygiene.
17 Follow agency policy for used linens.
18 Make a closed bed.
19 Practice hand hygiene.

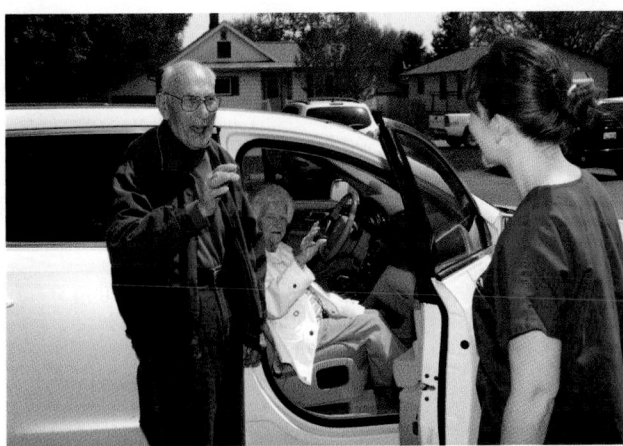

FIGURE 32-11 This resident is being discharged.

FOCUS ON PRIDE

The Person, Family, and Yourself

Personal and Professional Responsibility
Admission to a hospital or nursing center is often hard for the person and family. Transfers and discharges also can cause fear and worry. Discharge is usually a pleasant event. However, it may cause worry if more care and treatment are needed. To help the person adjust:
- Be courteous, caring, efficient, and competent.
- Be sensitive to fears and concerns.
- Handle the person's property and valuables carefully and with respect. Protect them from loss or damage.
- Focus on the person and family. Do not rush. Do not discuss other work you need to do.
- Treat the person and family like you want your loved ones treated.

Rights and Respect
Visitor policies provide rules for who can visit the person and when. Policies vary by agency or unit. For example, psychiatric, intensive care, and pediatric units often have special rules.

The person has the right to decide who can visit. Staff must respect the person's wishes. Tell the nurse about the person's requests.

Know your agency's rules for visitors. Do not assume that all units or agencies have the same rules. Give the person and visitors correct information. If you do not know, ask the nurse.

Independence and Social Interaction
A new setting brings social challenges. A person admitted to a private hospital room may be lonely. A person with a roommate may not like sharing the room. Others like having a roommate. In a nursing center, the first hours and days can be lonely. The person can feel isolated and depressed.

You can help with these social challenges. In a nursing center, visit new residents and introduce them to other residents. Encourage them to take part in activities. In a hospital or nursing center, observe for social isolation or roommate troubles. Tell the nurse what you observe. Be kind and caring. Make sure your interactions are pleasant.

Delegation and Teamwork
The family often wants to be present during admissions, transfers, and discharges. They care about the person. They want to be sure staff are caring, competent, and safe. The family may have questions or need to answer questions. If the person consents, the family may be present.

Sometimes privacy is needed. For example, the nurse may need to ask about personal or embarrassing topics. Or the person needs to undress. The nurse may ask you to manage and assist the family. The family is important. Treat them well. To show care and concern:
- Take them to the waiting area.
- Offer coffee or water while they wait.
- Show where they can get food and drinks.
- Tell them where they can use a phone. Give any special instructions for using the phone.
- Ask if there is anything they need.

Ethics and Laws
Before discharge, the person receives discharge instructions. The doctor tells the nurse what information the person needs. Common information includes drugs to continue or stop, new prescriptions, activity, diet, appointments with the doctor, and special care instructions. The nurse explains the information, provides teaching, and answers questions. The information is given orally and in writing.

You may become familiar with common discharge instructions. You may be tempted to give the person the information. Giving discharge teaching is beyond the scope of your role. You may provide wrong information. The person can be harmed.

If a person asks you about discharge instructions, you can say: "The nurse will give you information and answer your questions before you leave." Take pride in following the limits of your role.

FOCUS ON PRIDE: Application
Admissions, transfers, and discharges take time. You may be busy and have other tasks to do. How will you make the person feel that he or she is most important at the time?

REVIEW QUESTIONS

*Circle **T** if the statement is TRUE or **F** if it is FALSE.*

1 T F You are admitting a new resident. You must introduce yourself by name and title.

2 T F A person arrives at the center by ambulance. You transport the person to his or her room.

3 T F The person is greeted by name and title during the admission process.

4 T F A person complains of pain. Report the complaint after completing the admission form.

5 T F The person is to arrive by stretcher. You make an occupied bed.

6 T F You help orient the person to the new setting.

7 T F Clothing and personal belongings lists are made during the admission process.

8 T F A person's condition may require a transfer to another nursing unit.

9 T F The nurse writes the order for discharge from the center.

10 T F Starting with admission, the person's rights are protected.

11 T F Persons with dementia adjust well to new settings.

12 T F A person objects to a transfer. An ombudsman makes sure the person's rights are protected.

Circle the BEST answer.

13 When the person arrives in the room, you
   a Record the person's identifying information
   b Measure vital signs
   c Explain the person's rights
   d Review the doctor's orders

14 You are about to measure weight with a standing scale. Which should you correct before weighing the person?
   a The person is wearing footwear.
   b The scale is balanced at zero (0).
   c There is a paper towel on the scale platform.
   d The person is in the center of the scale with arms at the sides.

15 When measuring height with a standing scale
   a Balance the height rod at zero (0)
   b Be sure footwear is worn
   c Read the height at the movable part of the rod
   d Record height to the nearest inch

16 What is 68 inches in feet and inches?
   a 4 ft 0 in
   b 5 ft 6 in
   c 5 ft 8 in
   d 6 ft 8 in

17 Before a person is transferred to another nursing unit, you
   a Gather the person's belongings
   b Explain the reason for the move
   c Tell the staff on the new unit to come get the person
   d Reassure the person by saying: "You'll be fine."

18 When discharging a person, you can
   a Teach the person about diet and drugs
   b Arrange for home care
   c Let the person leave when he or she is ready
   d Help the person into the car

Answers to Chapter 32 questions are on p. 871.

FOCUS ON PRACTICE

Problem Solving

Mr. Fuller is waiting to move to a new room on another nursing unit. The room is not yet ready. He is ready to move and is becoming anxious. How can you provide comfort and ease his anxiety? What can you do to ensure a quick move when the room is ready?

Assisting With the Physical Examination

KEY TERMS

dorsal recumbent position The supine position with the legs together (*dorsal* means *the back of something; recumbent* means *to lie down)*; horizontal recumbent position

genupectoral position See "knee-chest position" (*genu* means *knee; pectoral* refers to the *chest*)

horizontal recumbent position See "dorsal recumbent position"

knee-chest position The person kneels and rests the body on the knees and chest; the head is turned to 1 side, the arms are above the head or flexed at the elbows, the back is straight, and the body is flexed about 90 degrees at the hips; genupectoral position

laryngeal mirror An instrument used to examine the mouth, teeth, and throat

lithotomy position The woman lies on her back with the hips at the edge of the exam table, her knees are flexed, her hips are externally rotated, and her feet are in stirrups

nasal speculum An instrument (*speculum* means *mirror*) used to examine the inside of the nose (*nasal*)

ophthalmoscope A lighted instrument (*scope*) used to examine the internal eye (*ophthalmo*) structures

otoscope A lighted instrument (*scope*) used to examine the external ear (*oto*) and the eardrum (tympanic membrane)

percussion hammer An instrument used to tap body parts to test reflexes (*percussion* means *to strike hard);* reflex hammer

tuning fork An instrument vibrated to test hearing

vaginal speculum An instrument (*speculum*) used to open the vagina (*vaginal*) to examine it and the cervix

Doctors and many registered nurses (RNs) perform physical exams. Exams are done to:
- Promote health.
- Determine fitness for work.
- Diagnose disease.

YOUR ROLE

Your role depends on agency policies and on what the examiner prefers. You may be asked to:
- Collect needed linens, equipment, and supplies.
- Prepare the room for the exam.
- Cover the exam table with a clean drawsheet or paper.
- Provide for lighting.
- Transport the person to and from the exam room.
- Measure vital signs, weight, and height.
- Position and drape the person.
- Hand equipment and supplies to the examiner.
- Label specimen containers.
- Discard used supplies and clean equipment.
- Help the person dress or to a comfortable position after the exam.
- Follow agency policy for used linens.

EQUIPMENT

The instruments in Figure 33-1, p. 562 are used in the exam.
- *Laryngeal mirror*—*used to examine the mouth, teeth, and throat.*
- *Nasal speculum*—*used to examine the inside of the nose.* Speculum *means* mirror; nasal *means* nose.
- *Ophthalmoscope*—*a lighted instrument* (scope) *used to examine the internal eye* (ophthalmo) *structures.*
- *Otoscope*—*a lighted instrument* (scope) *used to examine the external ear* (oto) *and the eardrum (tympanic membrane).* Some scopes can be changed into an ophthalmoscope.
- *Percussion hammer* (reflex hammer)—*used to tap body parts to test reflexes.* Percussion *means* to strike hard.
- *Tuning fork*—*vibrated to test hearing.*
- *Vaginal speculum*—*used to open the vagina* (vaginal) *to examine it and the cervix.* Speculum *means* mirror.

Some agencies supply exam trays. If not, collect the items listed in the procedure: *Preparing the Person for an Examination*, p. 563. Arrange them on a tray or table.

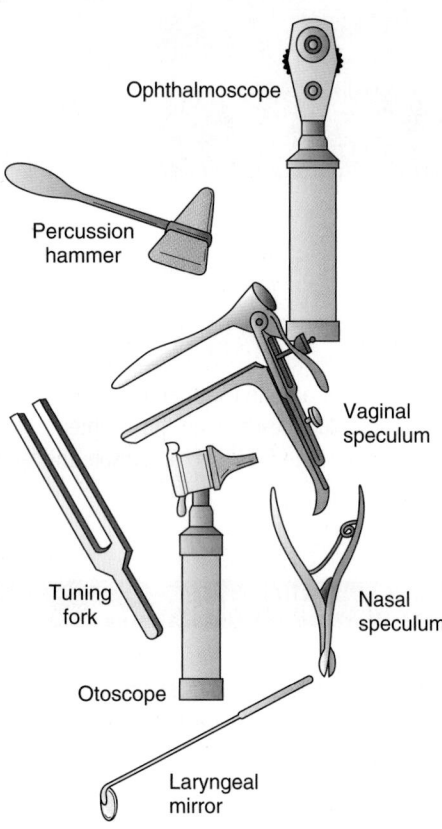

Ophthalmoscope

Percussion hammer

Vaginal speculum

Tuning fork

Nasal speculum

Otoscope

Laryngeal mirror

FIGURE 33-1 Physical exam instruments.

PREPARING THE PERSON

The physical exam can cause concerns. People may worry about findings. Some are confused or fearful about the procedure. Discomfort, embarrassment, exposure, and not knowing the procedure cause anxiety. Respect the person's feelings and concerns.

The person must give informed consent for the exam. The nurse explains the exam's purpose and what to expect. To assist the nurse:

- Provide for privacy.
  - Screen the person and close the room door.
  - Help the person put on a patient gown. Usually all clothes are removed for the exam. The gown reduces the naked feeling and the fear of exposure.
- Have the person void to empty the bladder. This lets the examiner feel the abdominal organs. A full bladder can change the normal position and shape of organs. It also causes discomfort, especially when feeling the abdominal organs.
- Obtain a urine specimen if one is needed. Explain how to collect the specimen (Chapter 34). Label the container.
- Measure vital signs, weight, height, and oxygen concentration (Chapters 29, 32, and 39). Record the measurements on the exam form.
- Drape the person. Use a paper drape, bath blanket, sheet, or drawsheet.
- Position the person for the exam.
  See *Focus on Communication: Preparing the Person.*
  See *Focus on Children and Older Persons: Preparing the Person.*
  See *Delegation Guidelines: Preparing the Person.*
  See *Promoting Safety and Comfort: Preparing the Person.*
  See procedure: *Preparing the Person for an Examination.*

FOCUS ON COMMUNICATION

Preparing the Person

When preparing a person for an exam, do not assume the person knows what to do. Tell the person what clothing to remove, how to put on the gown (opening to the front or to the back), and where to sit. For example:

Mrs. Tucker, you need to remove your clothes and put on this gown. The gown opens in the back. You may leave your under-garments on. Here is a blanket to cover yourself. Please have a seat on the exam table after you change. Do you have any questions?

FOCUS ON CHILDREN AND OLDER PERSONS

Preparing the Person

Children
Babies are undressed for a physical exam. Leave diapers on. Toddlers, pre-school children, and school-age children can wear underpants. Diapers or pants are removed or lowered as needed during the exam.

Older Persons
Nursing center residents have an exam at least once a year. The person has the right to personal choice. The doctor or nurse explains the reason for the exam. The person is told who will do the exam and when and how it will be done.

The exam is done only with the person's consent. The person may want a different examiner. Or the person may want a family member present for the exam and when the results are explained.

DELEGATION GUIDELINES

Preparing the Person

To prepare a person for an exam, you need this information from the nurse and the care plan.
- When to prepare the person
- Where it will be done—an exam room or the person's room
- How to position the person
- What equipment and supplies are needed
- If a urine specimen is needed
- What patient or resident concerns to report at once

PROMOTING SAFETY AND COMFORT

Preparing the Person

Safety
Protect the person from falls and injuries. Do not leave the person unattended.

Comfort
Warmth is important during an exam. Protect the person from chilling. Have an extra bath blanket nearby. Also, take measures to prevent drafts.

The physical exam often involves exposing and touching private areas—breasts, perineum, rectum. Sexual abuse has occurred in health care settings. The person may feel threatened or actually may be abused. He or she needs to call for help. Keep the call light within the person's reach at all times. And always act in a professional manner.

Preparing the Person for an Examination

QUALITY OF LIFE

- Knock before entering the person's room.
- Address the person by name.
- Introduce yourself by name and title.

- Explain the procedure before starting and during the procedure.
- Protect the person's rights during the procedure.
- Handle the person gently during the procedure.

PRE-PROCEDURE

1. Follow *Delegation Guidelines: Preparing the Person*. See *Promoting Safety and Comfort: Preparing the Person*.
2. Practice hand hygiene.
3. Collect the following.
   - Exam form
   - Flashlight
   - Blood pressure cuff
   - Stethoscope
   - Thermometer
   - Pulse oximeter (Chapter 39)
   - Scale
   - Tongue depressors (blades)
   - Laryngeal mirror
   - Ophthalmoscope
   - Otoscope
   - Nasal speculum
   - Percussion (reflex) hammer
   - Tuning fork
   - Vaginal speculum
   - Tape measure
   - Gloves
   - Water-soluble lubricant
   - Cotton-tipped applicators
   - Specimen containers and labels
   - Disposable bag
   - Kidney basin
   - Towel
   - Bath blanket
   - Tissues
   - Drape (sheet, bath blanket, drawsheet, or paper drape)
   - Paper towels
   - Cotton balls
   - Waterproof under-pad
   - Eye chart (Snellen chart)
   - Slides
   - Patient gown
   - Alcohol wipes
   - Wastebasket
   - Container for soiled instruments
   - Marking pencils or pens
4. Practice hand hygiene.
5. Identify the person. Check the ID (identification) bracelet against the assignment sheet. Use 2 identifiers (Chapter 13). Also call the person by name.
6. Provide for privacy.

PROCEDURE

7. Have the person put on the gown. Tell him or her what clothes to remove. Assist as needed.
8. Ask the person to void. Collect a urine specimen if needed. Provide for privacy.
9. Transport the person to the exam room. (Omit this step for an exam in the person's room.)
10. Measure weight and height (Chapter 32). Record the measurements on the exam form.
11. Help the person onto the exam table. Provide a step stool if necessary. (Omit this step for an exam in the person's room.)
12. Raise the far bed rail (if used). Raise the bed to a safe and comfortable working height. (Omit this step if an exam table is used.)
13. Measure vital signs and oxygen concentration (Chapter 39). Record them on the exam form.
14. Position the person as directed.
15. Drape the person.
16. Place a waterproof under-pad under the buttocks.
17. Raise the bed rail near you (if used).
18. Provide for adequate lighting.
19. Put the call light on for the examiner. Do not leave the person alone.

POSITIONING AND DRAPING

The examiner tells you how to position the person. Some positions are uncomfortable and embarrassing. Before helping the person assume and maintain the position, explain:

- Why the position is needed
- How to assume the position
- How you will drape the person for warmth and privacy
- How long to expect to stay in the position

Exam Positions

The examiner may request 1 of the following exam positions.

- *Dorsal recumbent position (horizontal recumbent position)—the person is supine with the legs together.* (Dorsal *means* the back of something; recumbent *means* to lie down.) The position is used to examine the abdomen, chest, and breasts. To examine the perineal area, the knees are flexed and hips externally rotated. Drape the person as in Figure 33-2, *A.*
- *Lithotomy position—the woman lies on her back. Hips are at the edge of the exam table. Knees are flexed and hips externally rotated. Feet are in stirrups.* (See Fig. 33-2, *B.*) The position is used to examine the vagina and cervix. Drape her as for perineal care (Chapter 22). Some agencies provide socks for the feet and calves.
- *Knee-chest position—the person kneels and rests the body on the knees and chest. The head is turned to 1 side. The arms are above the head or flexed at the elbows. The back is straight. The body is flexed about 90 degrees at the hips.* (See Fig. 33-2, *C.*) The position is also called the *genupectoral position.* (Genu *means* knee. Pectoral *refers to the* chest.) The position is used to examine the rectum. Apply the drape in a diamond shape to cover the back, buttocks, and thighs.
- The *Sims' position—*is sometimes used to examine the rectum or vagina (Chapter 17). (See Fig. 33-2, *D.*) Apply the drape in a diamond shape. The examiner folds back the near corner to expose the rectum or vagina.

See *Focus on Children and Older Persons: Positioning and Draping.*

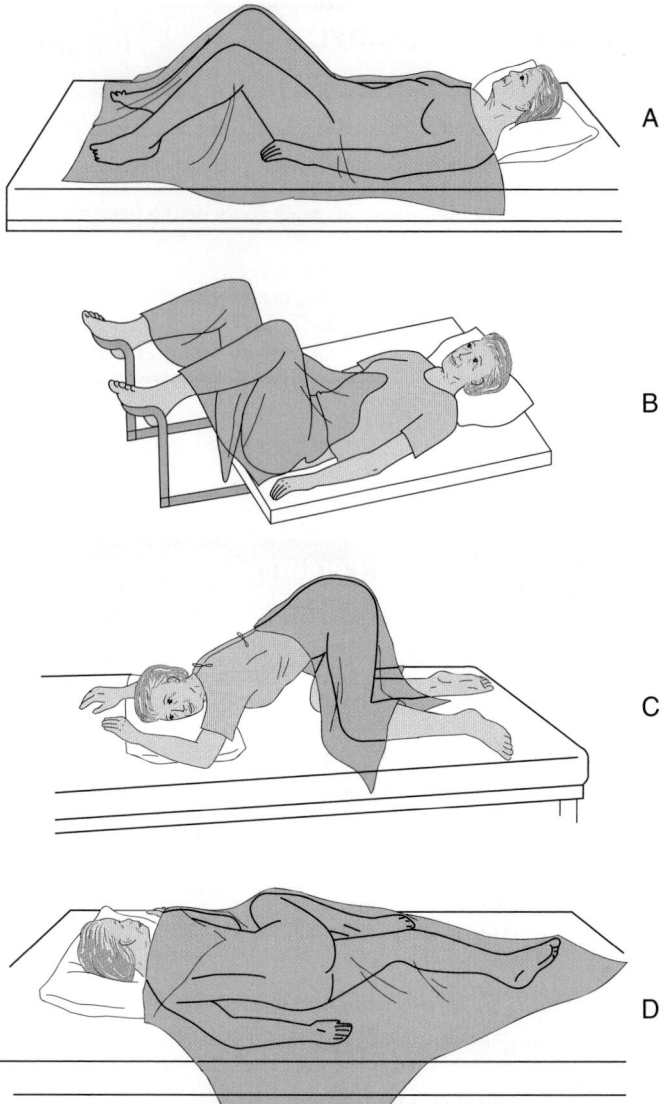

FIGURE 33-2 Positioning and draping for the physical exam. **A,** Dorsal recumbent position. **B,** Lithotomy position. **C,** Knee-chest position. **D,** Sims' position.

FOCUS ON CHILDREN AND OLDER PERSONS

Positioning and Draping

Older Persons

The knee-chest position is rarely used for older persons. For them, the side-lying position is used to examine the rectum.

ASSISTING WITH THE EXAM

You may be asked to prepare, position, and drape the person. If assisting with the exam, follow the rules in Box 33-1.

See *Focus on Communication: Assisting With the Exam.*

See *Focus on Children and Older Persons: Assisting With the Exam.*

After the Exam

After the exam, the person dresses or returns to bed. First, the vagina or rectum is wiped or cleaned if lubricant was used to examine those structures. Assist as needed. You also need to:

- Discard disposable items.
- Replace supplies on the exam tray.
- Clean re-usable items. This includes the otoscope and ophthalmoscope tips and stethoscope. Follow agency policy. Return items to the tray or storage area. Send a re-usable speculum to the supply department. It needs to be sterilized.
- Cover the exam table with a clean drawsheet or paper.
- Label specimens. Take them to the correct area with a requisition slip. See Chapter 34.
- Clean and straighten the person's unit or exam room.
- Follow agency policy for used linens.

See *Teamwork and Time Management: After the Exam.*

BOX 33-1   Assisting With the Physical Exam

- Practice hand hygiene before and after the exam.
- Provide for privacy.
  - Close doors and window coverings.
  - Screen and drape the person.
  - Expose only the body part being examined.
- Position the person as directed by the examiner.
- Place instruments and equipment near the examiner.
- Stay in the room for the legal protection of the person and examiner if:
  - You are a female and a female is being examined by a man.
  - You are a male and a male is being examined by a man.
  - A female examiner wants a male attendant present when examining a male.
- Protect the person from falling.
- Re-assure the person throughout the exam.
- Anticipate the examiner's need for equipment and supplies.
- Place paper or paper towels on the floor if the person is asked to stand.
- Follow Standard Precautions and the Bloodborne Pathogen Standard.
- Keep the call light within the person's reach.

FOCUS ON **PRIDE**

The Person, Family, and Yourself

P ersonal and Professional Responsibility

Physical, mental, and social discomfort are common during an exam. Often only a patient gown is worn. An uncomfortable position may be required. Private body parts (breasts, vagina, penis, and rectum) may be examined. Anxiety and fear are common.

The person needs to feel safe and secure. The person should feel comfortable with the examiner and the assistant. Be professional and courteous. Provide care in a way that promotes dignity, self-esteem, and well-being.

R ights and Respect

The person has the right to privacy. Protect the person from exposure. Only the examiner and the assistant should see the person's body. The person must consent for others to be present. This includes family. Keep the person properly draped and screened. Expose only the body part being examined.

I ndependence and Social Interaction

Fears about the exam are common.
- Who will perform the exam? How will the exam be done?
- Why is the exam needed?
- Will an illness be found? Is it cancer?
- Will surgery be needed? Will more drugs be needed? Will I die?

  To ease the person's fears:
- Greet the person. Introduce yourself by name and title.
- Talk with the person. Be pleasant.
- Tell the person good things about the examiner or agency. For example: "Dr. Foster will examine you today. She is very kind and thorough."

  Your interactions affect the person's mental comfort. Caring, kindness, and a positive attitude ease worries.

D elegation and Teamwork

Good teamwork involves being helpful, prepared, and knowledgeable. When you begin a job, become familiar with supplies and equipment used for exams. Know where to find them. Know where to find items like extra batteries and light bulbs. When you need an item, you can get it quickly.

Plan ahead. Test equipment before each use. For example, check that the ophthalmoscope and otoscope lights work. If not, correct the issue. Ask a co-worker for help if needed. Thank your co-worker for helping you.

E thics and Laws

You must keep the person's information confidential. Talking about an exam with family, friends, or staff not involved in the person's care violates the *Health Insurance Portability and Accountability Act of 1996* (HIPAA). HIPAA protects the privacy and security of the person's health information. Failure to follow HIPAA rules can result in fines, penalties, and criminal action.

FOCUS ON **PRIDE**: *Application*

Explain the importance of your role before, during, and after the physical exam. How do you prevent delays and promote comfort?

REVIEW QUESTIONS

Circle the BEST answer.

1 The otoscope is used to examine
   a Internal eye structures
   b The external ear and the eardrum
   c Reflexes
   d The vagina

2 When preparing for an exam, you
   a Explain the purpose of the exam
   b Leave to tell the nurse the person is ready
   c Position and drape the person
   d Obtain consent for the exam

3 Which part of an exam can you do?
   a Test reflexes.
   b Inspect the mouth, teeth, and throat.
   c Measure weight, height, and vital signs.
   d Observe the perineum and rectum.

4 A person is supine. The hips are flexed and externally rotated. The feet are supported in stirrups. The person is in the
   a Dorsal recumbent position
   b Knee-chest position
   c Sims' position
   d Lithotomy position

5 You will assist with Mrs. Janz's exam. Which is *true*?
   a Hand hygiene is practiced before and after the exam.
   b A male nursing team member stays in the room.
   c You may restrain her for the exam if needed.
   d A family member is not allowed in the room.

Answers to Chapter 33 questions are on p. 871.

FOCUS ON **PRACTICE**

Problem Solving

During an exam, you must leave the room several times for supplies. What problems does this cause? How could this have been prevented?

Collecting and Testing Specimens

OBJECTIVES

- Define the key terms and key abbreviations in this chapter.
- Explain why specimens are collected.
- Explain the rules for collecting specimens.
- Describe the different types of urine specimens.
- Describe the equipment used for blood glucose testing.

- Identify the skin puncture sites.
- Perform the procedures described in this chapter.
- Explain how to promote PRIDE in the person, the family, and yourself.

KEY TERMS

acetone See "ketone"

glucometer A device for measuring *(meter)* blood glucose *(gluco)*; glucose meter

glucosuria Sugar *(glucose)* in the urine *(uria)*; glycosuria

glycosuria Sugar *(glycos)* in the urine *(uria)*; glucosuria

hematoma A swelling *(oma)* that contains blood *(hemat)*

hematuria Blood *(hemat)* in the urine *(uria)*

hemoptysis Bloody *(hemo)* sputum *(ptysis* means *to spit)*

ketone A substance appearing in urine from the rapid breakdown of fat for energy; acetone, ketone body

ketone body See "ketone"

melena A black, tarry stool

sputum Mucus from the respiratory system that is expectorated (expelled) through the mouth

KEY ABBREVIATIONS

BM	Bowel movement		**oz**	Ounce
ID	Identification		**SDS**	Safety data sheet
I&O	Intake and output		**U/A**	Urinalysis
mL	Milliliter			

Specimens *(samples)* are collected and tested to prevent, detect, and treat disease. Most specimens are tested in the laboratory. All laboratory specimens require requisition slips. The slip has the person's identifying information and the test ordered. The specimen container is labeled following agency policy. Some tests are done at the bedside. To collect specimens, follow the rules in Box 34-1.

See *Teamwork and Time Management: Collecting and Testing Specimens*, p. 568.

See *Promoting Safety and Comfort: Collecting and Testing Specimens*, p. 568.

BOX 34-1 Collecting Specimens

- Follow the rules for medical asepsis.
- Follow Standard Precautions and the Bloodborne Pathogen Standard.
- Use a clean container for each specimen.
- Use the correct container.
- Do not touch the inside of the container or the inside of the lid.
- Identify the person. Check the ID (identification) bracelet against the laboratory requisition slip or assignment sheet. Compare all information. Then ask the person to state his or her first and last name and state his or her birthdate.
- Label the container in the person's presence. Provide clear, accurate information.
- Collect the specimen at the correct time.
- Ask a female if she is having a menstrual period. Tell the nurse. Menstruating may cause blood to be in the urine specimen.

- Ask the person not to have a bowel movement (BM) when collecting a urine specimen. Urine specimens must not contain stools.
- Ask the person to void before collecting a stool specimen. Stool specimens must not contain urine.
- Ask the person to put toilet tissue in the toilet or wastebasket. Urine and stool specimens must not contain tissue.
- Secure the lid on the specimen container tightly.
- Place the specimen container in a labeled *BIOHAZARD* plastic bag. Do not let the container touch the outside of the bag. Seal the bag.
- Take the specimen and requisition slip to the laboratory or storage area.

TEAMWORK AND TIME MANAGEMENT
Collecting and Testing Specimens

Nursing centers have storage areas for specimens. A driver picks up specimens at a certain time and transports them to a laboratory.

Have specimens collected and in the storage area by the pick-up time. If a specimen is not collected, results are delayed at least 1 day. This can harm the person. If not collected in time, a specimen may need to be discarded. Another is collected the next day. This also results in a delay and can harm the person. Using more supplies and equipment costs more money.

PROMOTING SAFETY AND COMFORT
Collecting and Testing Specimens

Safety
Correct identification is important when collecting and testing specimens. To identify the person, check the ID bracelet against all information on the requisition slip. Agency policy may require that you ask the person to identify himself or herself by both of the following.
- Stating or spelling his or her first and last name
- Stating his or her birthdate

Blood, body fluids, secretions, and excretions may contain microbes and blood. This includes urine, stool, and sputum specimens. Follow Standard Precautions and the Bloodborne Pathogen Standard when collecting, testing, and handling specimens.

DELEGATION GUIDELINES
Urine Specimens

To collect a urine specimen, you need this information from the nurse and the care plan.
- Voiding device used—bedpan, urinal, commode, or toilet with specimen pan
- The type of specimen needed
- What time to collect the specimen
- What special measures are needed
- If you need to test the specimen
- If measuring intake and output (I&O) is ordered (Chapter 27)
- What observations to report and record:
  - Problems obtaining the specimen
  - Color, clarity, and odor of urine
  - Blood in the urine
  - Particles in the urine
  - Complaints of pain, burning, urgency, difficulty voiding, or other problems
  - The time the specimen was collected
- When to report observations
- What patient or resident concerns to report at once

PROMOTING SAFETY AND COMFORT
Urine Specimens

Comfort
Urine specimens may embarrass some people, including children. They do not like clear specimen containers that show urine. It may be helpful to place the specimen container in a paper bag. Or provide a paper towel or washcloth to wrap around the container.

URINE SPECIMENS

Urine specimens are collected for urine tests. Follow the rules in Box 34-1.

See *Delegation Guidelines: Urine Specimens.*
See *Promoting Safety and Comfort: Urine Specimens.*

The Random Urine Specimen

The random urine specimen is used for a routine urinalysis (U/A). No special measures are needed. It is collected any time in a 24-hour period. Many people can collect the specimen themselves. Weak and very ill persons need help.

See procedure: *Collecting a Random Urine Specimen.*

Collecting a Random Urine Specimen

QUALITY OF LIFE

- Knock before entering the person's room.
- Address the person by name.
- Introduce yourself by name and title.
- Explain the procedure before starting and during the procedure.
- Protect the person's rights during the procedure.
- Handle the person gently during the procedure.

PRE-PROCEDURE

1 Follow *Delegation Guidelines: Urine Specimens.* See *Promoting Safety and Comfort:*
   a *Collecting and Testing Specimens*
   b *Urine Specimens*
2 Practice hand hygiene.
3 Collect the following before going to the person's room.
   - Laboratory requisition slip
   - Specimen container and lid
   - Voiding device—bedpan and cover, urinal, commode, or specimen pan (Fig. 34-1)
   - Specimen label
   - Plastic bag
   - *BIOHAZARD* label (if needed)
   - Gloves

4 Arrange collected items in the person's bathroom.
5 Practice hand hygiene.
6 Identify the person. Check the ID bracelet against the requisition slip. Compare all information. Also call the person by name. Ask the person to state his or her first and last name and state his or her birthdate.
7 Label the container in the person's presence.
8 Put on gloves
9 Collect a graduate to measure output.
10 Provide for privacy.

PROCEDURE

11 Ask the person to void into the device. Remind him or her to put toilet tissue into the wastebasket or toilet. Toilet tissue is not put in the bedpan or specimen pan.
12 Take the voiding device to the bathroom.
13 Pour about 120 mL (milliliters) (4 oz [ounces]) into the specimen container.
14 Place the lid on the specimen container. Put the container in the plastic bag. Do not let the container touch the outside of the bag. Apply a *BIOHAZARD* label.

15 Measure urine if I&O are ordered. Include the specimen amount.
16 Empty, rinse, clean, disinfect, and dry equipment. Return equipment to its proper place.
17 Remove and discard the gloves. Practice hand hygiene. Put on clean gloves.
18 Assist with hand-washing.
19 Remove and discard the gloves. Practice hand hygiene.

POST-PROCEDURE

20 Provide for comfort. (See the inside of the front cover.)
21 Place the call light and other needed items within reach.
22 Raise or lower bed rails. Follow the care plan.
23 Unscreen the person.
24 Complete a safety check of the room. (See the inside of the front cover.)

25 Practice hand hygiene.
26 Take the specimen and requisition slip to the laboratory or storage area. Wear gloves if that is agency policy.
27 Remove and discard the gloves. Practice hand hygiene.
28 Report and record your observations.

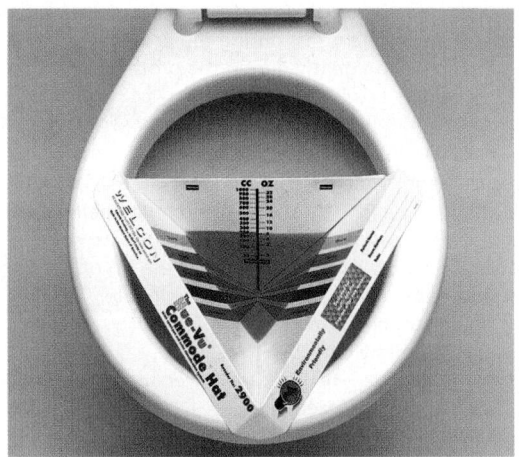

FIGURE 34-1 The specimen pan is placed at the front of the toilet on the toilet rim. This pan has a color chart for urine. (Courtesy Weldon, Inc., Fort Worth, Tex.)

The Midstream Specimen

The midstream specimen is also called a *clean-voided specimen* or *clean-catch specimen*. The perineal area is cleaned first to reduce the number of microbes in the urethral area. The person starts to void into a device. Then the person stops the urine stream and a sterile specimen container is positioned. The person voids into the container until the specimen is obtained.

Stopping the urine stream is hard for many people. You may need to position and hold the specimen container in place after the person starts to void (Fig. 34-2).

See *Focus on Communication: The Midstream Specimen.*

See *Promoting Safety and Comfort: The Midstream Specimen.*

See procedure: *Collecting a Midstream Specimen.*

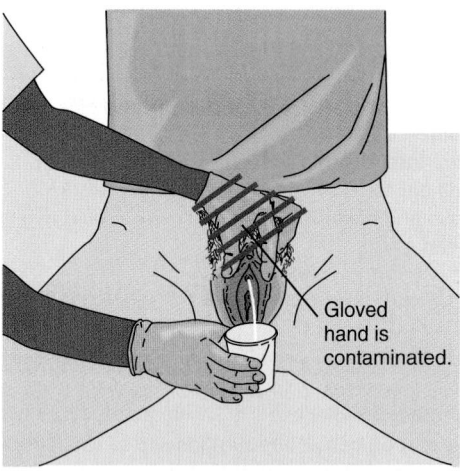

FIGURE 34-2 The labia are separated to collect a midstream specimen.

Gloved hand is contaminated.

Collecting a Midstream Specimen

QUALITY OF LIFE

- Knock before entering the person's room.
- Address the person by name.
- Introduce yourself by name and title.

- Explain the procedure before starting and during the procedure.
- Protect the person's rights during the procedure.
- Handle the person gently during the procedure.

PRE-PROCEDURE

1 Follow *Delegation Guidelines: Urine Specimens,* p. 568. See *Promoting Safety and Comfort:*
   a *Collecting and Testing Specimens,* p. 568
   b *Urine Specimens,* p. 568
   c *The Midstream Specimen*
2 Practice hand hygiene.
3 Collect the following before going to the person's room.
   - Laboratory requisition slip
   - Midstream specimen kit—specimen container, label, towelettes, sterile gloves
   - Plastic bag
   - Sterile gloves, if not part of the kit
   - Disposable gloves
   - *BIOHAZARD* label (if needed)

4 Arrange your work area.
5 Practice hand hygiene.
6 Identify the person. Check the ID bracelet against the requisition slip. Compare all information. Also call the person by name. Ask the person to state his or her first and last name and state his or her birthdate.
7 Put on disposable gloves.
8 Collect the following.
   - Voiding device—bedpan and cover, urinal, commode, or specimen pan if needed
   - Supplies for perineal care (Chapter 22)
   - Graduate to measure output
   - Paper towels
9 Provide for privacy.

Collecting a Midstream Specimen—cont'd

PROCEDURE

10 Provide perineal care (Chapter 22). (Wear gloves for this step. Practice hand hygiene after removing and discarding them.)
11 Open the sterile kit.
12 Put on the sterile gloves.
13 Open the packet of towelettes.
14 Open the sterile specimen container. Do not touch the inside of the container or lid. Set the lid down so the inside is up.
15 *For a female*—clean the perineal area with towelettes.
   a Spread the labia with your thumb and index finger. Use your non-dominant hand. (This hand is now contaminated. It must not touch anything sterile.)
   b Clean down the urethral area from front to back (top to bottom). Use a clean towelette for each stroke.
   c Keep the labia separated to collect the urine specimen (steps 17 through 20).
16 *For a male*—clean the penis with towelettes.
   a Hold the penis with your non-dominant hand. (This hand is now contaminated. It must not touch anything sterile.)
   b Clean the penis starting at the meatus. (Retract the foreskin if the male is uncircumcised.) Clean in a circular motion. Start at the center and work outward.
   c Hold the penis (and keep the foreskin retracted in the uncircumcised male) until the specimen is collected (steps 17 through 20).

17 Ask the person to void into a device.
18 Pass the specimen container into the urine stream. Keep the labia separated (see Fig. 34-2).
19 Collect about 30 to 60 mL (1 to 2 oz) of urine.
20 Remove the specimen container before the person stops voiding. Release the foreskin of the uncircumcised male.
21 Release the labia or penis. Let the person finish voiding into the device.
22 Put the lid on the specimen container. Touch only the outside of the container and lid. Wipe the outside of the container. Set the container on a paper towel.
23 Provide toilet tissue when the person is done voiding.
24 Take the voiding device to the bathroom.
25 Measure urine if I&O are ordered. Include the specimen amount.
26 Empty, rinse, clean, disinfect, and dry equipment. Return equipment to its proper place.
27 Remove and discard the gloves. Practice hand hygiene. Put on clean disposable gloves.
28 Label the specimen container in the person's presence. Place the container in the plastic bag. Do not let the container touch the outside of the bag. Apply a *BIOHAZARD* label.
29 Assist with hand-washing.
30 Remove and discard the gloves. Practice hand hygiene.

POST-PROCEDURE

31 Provide for comfort. (See the inside of the front cover.)
32 Place the call light and other needed items within reach.
33 Raise or lower the bed rails. Follow the care plan.
34 Unscreen the person.
35 Complete a safety check of the room. (See the inside of the front cover.)

36 Practice hand hygiene.
37 Take the specimen and requisition slip to the laboratory or storage area. Wear gloves if that is agency policy.
38 Remove and discard the gloves. Practice hand hygiene.
39 Report and record your observations.

The 24-Hour Urine Specimen

All urine voided during 24 hours is collected for a 24-hour urine specimen. To prevent the growth of microbes, the urine is chilled on ice or refrigerated. Sometimes a preservative is added to the collection container.

The person voids to start the test with an empty bladder. Discard this voiding. Save *all voidings* for the next 24 hours. The person and staff must clearly understand the procedure and the test period. This test is re-started if:

* A voiding was not saved.
* Toilet tissue was discarded into the specimen.
* The specimen contains stools.

See *Promoting Safety and Comfort: The 24-Hour Urine Specimen.*

See procedure: *Collecting a 24-Hour Urine Specimen*, p. 572.

PROMOTING SAFETY AND COMFORT

The 24-Hour Urine Specimen

Safety

The urine container or preservative may contain an acid. Pour urine into the container carefully and avoid splashes and splatters. Do not get the preservative or urine from the container on your skin or in your eyes. If you do, flush your skin or eyes with a large amount of water. Tell the nurse what happened and check the safety data sheet (SDS) (Chapter 13). Also complete an incident report.

Keep the specimen chilled to prevent the growth of microbes. If not refrigerated, place the urine container in a bucket with ice. Add ice to the bucket as needed.

Assist the person with hand-washing after every voiding. This prevents the spread of microbes that may be in the urine.

Collecting a 24-Hour Urine Specimen

QUALITY OF LIFE

- Knock before entering the person's room.
- Address the person by name.
- Introduce yourself by name and title.

- Explain the procedure before starting and during the procedure.
- Protect the person's rights during the procedure.
- Handle the person gently during the procedure.

PRE-PROCEDURE

1 Follow *Delegation Guidelines: Urine Specimens,* p. 568. See *Promoting Safety and Comfort:*
   a *Collecting and Testing Specimens,* p. 568
   b *Urine Specimens,* p. 568
   c *The 24-Hour Urine Specimen,* p. 571
2 Practice hand hygiene.
3 Collect the following before going to the person's room.
   - Laboratory requisition slip
   - Urine container for a 24-hour collection
   - Specimen label
   - Preservative if needed
   - Bucket with ice if needed
   - Two 24-HOUR URINE labels
   - Funnel
   - *BIOHAZARD* label
   - Gloves
4 Arrange collected items in the person's bathroom.

5 Place one 24-HOUR URINE label in the bathroom. Place the other near the bed.
6 Practice hand hygiene.
7 Identify the person. Check the ID bracelet against the requisition slip. Compare all information. Also call the person by name. Ask the person to state his or her first and last name and state his or her birthdate.
8 Label the urine container in the person's presence. Apply the *BIOHAZARD* label. Place the labeled container in the bathroom.
9 Put on gloves.
10 Collect the following.
   - Voiding device—bedpan and cover, urinal, commode, or specimen pan
   - Graduate to measure output
11 Provide for privacy.

PROCEDURE

12 Ask the person to void. Provide a voiding device.
13 Measure and discard the urine. Note the time. This starts the 24-hour period.
14 Mark the time on the urine container.
15 Empty, rinse, clean, disinfect, and dry equipment. Return equipment to its proper place.
16 Remove and discard the gloves. Practice hand hygiene. Put on clean gloves.
17 Assist with hand-washing.
18 Remove and discard the gloves. Practice hand hygiene.
19 Mark the time the test began and the time it ends on the room and bathroom labels.
20 Remind the person to:
   a Use the voiding device during the next 24 hours.
   b Not have a BM when voiding.
   c Put toilet tissue in the toilet or wastebasket.
   d Put on the call light after voiding.

21 Return to the room when the person signals for you. Knock before entering the room.
22 Do the following after every voiding.
   a Practice hand hygiene. Put on clean gloves.
   b Measure urine if I&O are ordered.
   c Use the funnel to pour urine into the urine container. Do not spill any urine. Re-start the test if you spill or discard the urine.
   d Empty, rinse, clean, disinfect, and dry equipment. Return equipment to its proper place.
   e Remove and discard the gloves. Practice hand hygiene. Put on clean gloves.
   f Assist with hand-washing.
   g Remove and discard the gloves. Practice hand hygiene.
   h Follow "Post-Procedure" steps except for steps 28 and 33.
23 Ask the person to void at the end of the 24-hour period. Follow steps 22, a–g.

POST-PROCEDURE

24 Provide for comfort. (See the inside of the front cover.)
25 Place the call light and other needed items within reach.
26 Raise or lower bed rails. Follow the care plan.
27 Put on gloves.
28 Remove the labels from the room and bathroom.
29 Clean, rinse, dry, and return equipment to its proper place. Discard disposable items.
30 Remove and discard the gloves. Practice hand hygiene.

31 Unscreen the person.
32 Complete a safety check of the room. (See the inside of the front cover.)
33 Take the specimen (labeled urine container) and requisition slip to the laboratory or storage area. Wear gloves if that is agency policy.
34 Remove and discard the gloves. Practice hand hygiene.
35 Report and record your observations.

Collecting a Urine Specimen From an Infant or Child

Sometimes urine specimens are needed from infants and children who are not toilet-trained. A collection bag ("wee bag") is applied over the urethra (Fig. 34-3). A parent or another staff member assists if the child is upset.

Voiding on request is hard for toilet-trained toddlers and young children. Potty chairs and specimen pans are useful. Remember to use terms the child understands. "Pee pee," "wee wee," "potty," and "tinkle" are examples. Or ask the parent what term the child uses and understands.

The nurse may have you give the child water or other fluids when a urine specimen is needed. Usually the child can void about 30 minutes after drinking fluids.

See procedure: *Collecting a Urine Specimen From an Infant or Child.*

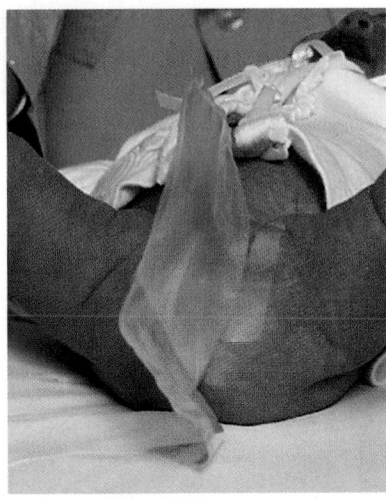

FIGURE 34-3 A urine collection bag applied to a baby girl's perineum.

Collecting a Urine Specimen From an Infant or Child

QUALITY OF LIFE

- Knock before entering the child's room.
- Address the child by name.
- Introduce yourself by name and title.

- Explain the procedure to the child and parents before starting and during the procedure.
- Protect the child's rights during the procedure.
- Handle the child gently during the procedure.

PRE-PROCEDURE

1 Follow *Delegation Guidelines: Urine Specimens*, p. 568. See *Promoting Safety and Comfort:*
   a *Collecting and Testing Specimens*, p. 568
   b *Urine Specimens*, p. 568
2 Practice hand hygiene.
3 Collect the following before going to the child's room.
   - Laboratory requisition slip
   - Collection bag ("wee bag")
   - *BIOHAZARD* label (if needed)
   - Specimen container
   - Plastic bag
   - Scissors

   - Wash basin
   - Bath towel
   - 2 diapers
   - Gloves
4 Arrange your work area.
5 Practice hand hygiene.
6 Identify the child. Check the ID bracelet against the requisition slip. Compare all information. Also call the child by name. Ask the parent to state the child's first and last name and state the child's birthdate.
7 Provide for privacy.

PROCEDURE

8 Practice hand hygiene. Put on gloves.
9 Position the child on his or her back.
10 Remove and set aside the diaper.
11 Clean the perineal area with cotton balls. Use a new cotton ball for each stroke. Rinse and dry the area.
12 Remove and discard the gloves. Practice hand hygiene.
13 Put on clean gloves.
14 Flex the child's knees. Spread the legs.
15 Remove the adhesive backing from the collection bag.
16 Apply the bag to the perineum (see Fig. 34-3).
17 Cut a slit in the bottom of a new diaper.
18 Diaper the child.

19 Pull the collection bag through the slit in the diaper.
20 Remove and discard the gloves. Practice hand hygiene.
21 Raise the head of the crib if allowed. This helps urine collect in the bottom of the bag.
22 Check for crib safety. Medical crib rails are raised and locked before leaving the bedside.
23 Unscreen the child.
24 Dispose of the removed diaper. Follow agency policy. (Wear gloves for this step.)
25 Practice hand hygiene.
26 Check the child often. Check the bag for urine. (Provide for privacy and wear gloves for this step.)

Continued

Collecting a Urine Specimen From an Infant or Child—cont'd

PROCEDURE—cont'd

27 Do the following if the child has voided.
  a Provide for privacy.
  b Practice hand hygiene. Put on clean gloves.
  c Remove the diaper.
  d Remove the collection bag gently.
  e Press the adhesive surfaces of the bag together. Make sure the seal is tight and there are no leaks. Or transfer the urine to the specimen container using the drainage tab.
  f Clean the perineal area. Rinse and dry well.
  g Diaper the child.
  h Remove and discard the gloves. Practice hand hygiene.

28 Put on clean gloves.
29 Label the collection bag or specimen container in the child's presence. Then place it in the plastic bag. Apply the BIOHAZARD label (if needed).

POST-PROCEDURE

30 Provide for comfort. (See the inside of the front cover.)
31 Check for crib safety. Medical crib rails are raised and locked before leaving the bedside.
32 Make sure the call light and other needed items are within reach for the parent.
33 Unscreen the child.
34 Clean, rinse, dry, and return equipment to its proper place. Discard disposable items. (Wear gloves for this step.)

35 Complete a safety check of the room. (See the inside of the front cover.)
36 Remove and discard the gloves. Practice hand hygiene.
37 Take the specimen and requisition slip to the laboratory or storage area. Wear gloves if that is agency policy.
38 Remove and discard the gloves. Practice hand hygiene.
39 Report and record your observations.

Testing Urine

The doctor orders the type and frequency of urine tests. Random urine specimens are needed. The nurse may ask you to do these simple tests.

- *Testing for pH*—Urine pH measures if urine is acidic or alkaline. Changes in normal pH (4.6 to 8.0) occur from illness, food, and drugs.
- *Testing for blood*—Injury and disease can cause hematuria. **Hematuria** *means blood* (hemat) *in the urine* (uria). Sometimes blood is seen in the urine. At other times it is unseen (occult).
- *Testing for glucose and ketones*—In diabetes, the pancreas does not secrete enough insulin (Chapter 46). The body needs insulin to use sugar for energy. If not used, sugar builds up in the blood. Some sugar appears in the urine. **Glucosuria (glycosuria)** *means sugar* (glucose, glycos) *in the urine* (uria). Diabetes may cause ketones in the urine. **Ketones (ketone bodies, acetone)** *are substances appearing in urine from the rapid breakdown of fat for energy.* The body uses fat for energy if it cannot use sugar. Tests for glucose and ketones are usually done 4 times a day—30 minutes before meals and at bedtime. Test results are used for drug and diet decisions.
- *Testing for infection*—The presence of certain white blood cells can signal a urinary tract infection.
- *Testing for protein*—Protein in the urine can signal kidney and other diseases.

Using Reagent Strips. Reagent strips (test strips) have sections that change color when reacting with urine. To use a reagent (test) strip:
- Do not touch the test area on the strip.
- Dip the strip into urine.
- Compare the strip with the color chart on the bottle (Fig. 34-4).
  See *Teamwork and Time Management: Testing Urine.*
  See *Delegation Guidelines: Testing Urine.*
  See *Promoting Safety and Comfort: Testing Urine.*
  See procedure: *Testing Urine With Reagent Strips.*

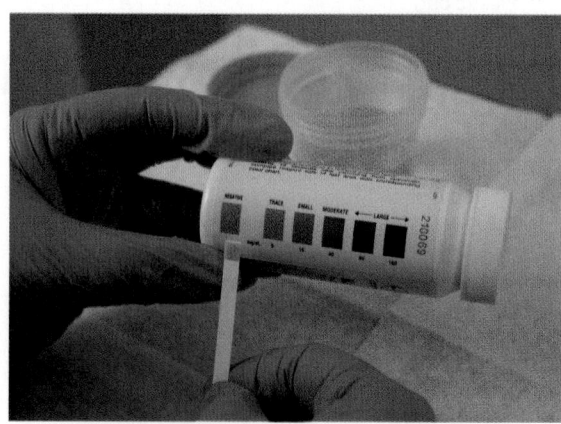

FIGURE 34-4 Reagent (test) strip for sugar and ketones.

TEAMWORK AND TIME MANAGEMENT

Testing Urine

Blood glucose testing is common for persons with diabetes (p. 582). Sometimes urine is tested for glucose and ketones. The nurse uses the test results to give the person diabetic drugs. The drugs are given at a certain time. The nurse needs the results before giving the drugs.

PROMOTING SAFETY AND COMFORT

Testing Urine

Safety

Accuracy is important. Promptly report the results to the nurse. Ordered drugs may depend on the results.

When using reagent (test) strips:

- Check the color of the strips. Do not use discolored strips.
- Check the expiration date on the bottle. Do not use the strips if the date has passed.
- Follow the manufacturer's instructions. Otherwise you could get the wrong result. The doctor uses the test results for diagnosis and treatment. A wrong result can cause serious harm.

DELEGATION GUIDELINES

Testing Urine

When testing urine is delegated to you, you need this information from the nurse and the care plan.

- What test is needed
- What equipment to use
- When to test urine
- Instructions for the test ordered
- If the nurse wants to observe the results of each test
- What observations to report and record:
  - The time you collected and tested the specimen
  - Test results
  - Problems obtaining the specimen
  - Color, clarity, and odor of urine
  - Blood in the urine
  - Particles in the urine
  - Complaints of pain, burning, urgency, difficulty voiding, or other problems
- When to report test results and observations
- What patient or resident concerns to report at once

Testing Urine With Reagent Strips

QUALITY OF LIFE

- Knock before entering the person's room.
- Address the person by name.
- Introduce yourself by name and title.
- Explain the procedure before starting and during the procedure.
- Protect the person's rights during the procedure.
- Handle the person gently during the procedure.

PRE-PROCEDURE

1 Follow *Delegation Guidelines: Testing Urine.* See *Promoting Safety and Comfort:*
  a *Collecting and Testing Specimens,* p. 568
  b *Testing Urine*
2 Practice hand hygiene.
3 Collect gloves and the reagent (test) strips ordered.
4 Practice hand hygiene.

5 Identify the person. Check the ID bracelet against the assignment sheet. Use 2 identifiers (Chapter 13). Also call the person by name. Ask the person to state his or her first and last name and state his or her birthdate.
6 Put on gloves.
7 Collect equipment for the urine specimen. (See procedure: *Collecting a Random Urine Specimen,* p. 569.)
8 Provide for privacy.

PROCEDURE

9 Collect the urine specimen. (See procedure: *Collecting a Random Urine Specimen,* p. 569.)
10 Remove a strip from the bottle. Put the cap on the bottle at once. It must be on tight.
11 Dip the strip test area into the urine.
12 Remove the strip after the correct amount of time. See the manufacturer's instructions.
13 Tap the strip gently against the urine container. This removes excess urine.

14 Wait the required amount of time. See the manufacturer's instructions.
15 Compare the strip with the color chart on the bottle (see Fig. 34-4). Read the results.
16 Discard disposable items and the specimen.
17 Empty, rinse, clean, disinfect, and dry equipment. Return equipment to its proper place.
18 Remove and discard the gloves. Practice hand hygiene.

POST-PROCEDURE

19 Provide for comfort. (See the inside of the front cover.)
20 Place the call light and other needed items within reach.
21 Raise or lower bed rails. Follow the care plan.
22 Unscreen the person.

23 Complete a safety check of the room. (See the inside of the front cover.)
24 Practice hand hygiene.
25 Report and record the test results and other observations.

Straining Urine

A stone (*calculus*) can develop in a kidney, a ureter, or the bladder. Stones (*calculi*) vary in size (Chapter 47). They can be as small as grains of sand, pearl-sized, or larger. Some stones are removed by medical or surgical procedures. Others pass through urine. Therefore all urine is strained. Passed stones are sent to the laboratory.

The person drinks 8 to 12 glasses of water a day to help pass the stone. Expect the person to void in large amounts.

See procedure: *Straining Urine*.

Straining Urine

QUALITY OF LIFE

- Knock before entering the person's room.
- Address the person by name.
- Introduce yourself by name and title.

- Explain the procedure before starting and during the procedure.
- Protect the person's rights during the procedure.
- Handle the person gently during the procedure.

PRE-PROCEDURE

1 Follow *Delegation Guidelines: Urine Specimens*, p. 568. See *Promoting Safety and Comfort*:
   a *Collecting and Testing Specimens*, p. 568
   b *Urine Specimens*, p. 568
2 Practice hand hygiene.
3 Collect the following before going to the person's room.
   - Laboratory requisition slip
   - Urine strainer
   - Specimen container
   - Specimen label
   - 2 STRAIN ALL URINE labels
   - Plastic bag
   - BIOHAZARD label (if needed)
   - Gloves

4 Arrange collected items in the person's bathroom.
5 Place 1 STRAIN ALL URINE label in the bathroom. Place the other near the bed.
6 Practice hand hygiene.
7 Identify the person. Check the ID bracelet against the requisition slip. Compare all information. Also call the person by name. Ask the person to state his or her first and last name and state his or her birthdate.
8 Label the specimen container in the person's presence.
9 Put on gloves.
10 Collect the following.
   - Voiding device—bedpan and cover, urinal, commode, or specimen pan
   - Graduate
11 Provide for privacy.

PROCEDURE

12 Ask the person to use the voiding device for urinating. Ask the person to put on the call light after voiding.
13 Remove and discard the gloves. Practice hand hygiene.
14 Return to the room when the person signals for you. Knock before entering the room.
15 Practice hand hygiene. Put on clean gloves.
16 Place the strainer in the graduate.
17 Pour urine into the graduate. Urine passes through the strainer (Fig. 34-5).
18 Place the strainer in the specimen container if any crystals, stones, or particles appear.

19 Place the specimen container in the plastic bag. Do not let the container touch the outside of the bag. Apply a BIOHAZARD label.
20 Measure urine if I&O are ordered.
21 Empty, rinse, clean, disinfect, and dry equipment. Return equipment to its proper place.
22 Remove and discard the gloves. Practice hand hygiene. Put on clean gloves.
23 Assist with hand-washing.
24 Remove and discard the gloves. Practice hand hygiene.

POST-PROCEDURE

25 Provide for comfort. (See the inside of the front cover.)
26 Place the call light and other needed items within reach.
27 Raise or lower bed rails. Follow the care plan.
28 Unscreen the person.
29 Complete a safety check of the room. (See the inside of the front cover.)

30 Practice hand hygiene.
31 Take the specimen container and requisition slip to the laboratory or storage area. Wear gloves if that is agency policy.
32 Remove and discard the gloves. Practice hand hygiene.
33 Report and record your observations.

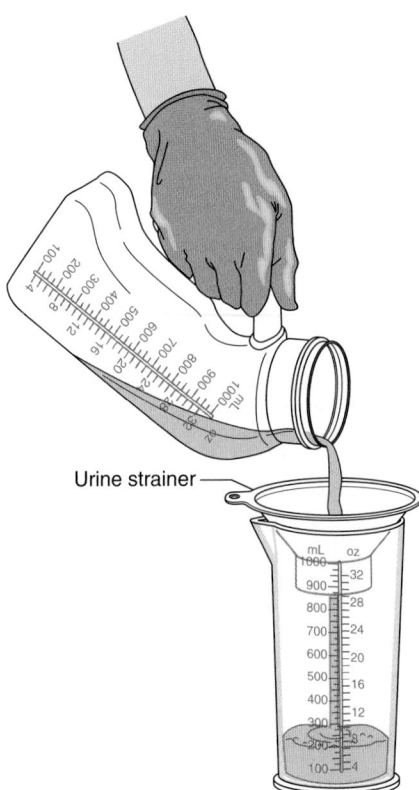

Urine strainer

FIGURE 34-5 The strainer is placed in the graduate. Urine is poured through the strainer into the graduate.

▐ STOOL SPECIMENS

Stools are studied for fat, microbes, worms, blood, and other abnormal contents. Ulcers, colon cancer, and hemorrhoids are common causes of bleeding. Often blood is seen if bleeding is low in the bowels. Stools are black and tarry from bleeding in the stomach or upper gastrointestinal tract. *Melena is a black, tarry stool.*

Bleeding may be in very small amounts. Then stools are tested for *occult blood. Occult* means *hidden* or *not seen.* The test screens for colon cancer and other digestive disorders. Occult blood test kits vary. Follow the manufacturer's instructions.

Urine must not contaminate the stool specimen. The person uses 1 device for voiding and another for a BM. Some tests require a warm stool. The specimen is taken at once to the laboratory or storage area. Follow the rules in Box 34-1.

See *Focus on Communication: Stool Specimens.*
See *Focus on Children and Older Persons: Stool Specimens.*
See *Delegation Guidelines: Stool Specimens.*
See *Promoting Safety and Comfort: Stool Specimens.*
See procedure: *Collecting and Testing a Stool Specimen,* p. 578.

Text continued on p. 580.

FOCUS ON **COMMUNICATION**

Stool Specimens

Explain the procedure before you begin. Explain what the person needs to do and what you will do. Also show the equipment and supplies and how to use them. For example:

> *The doctor wants your stools tested. So we need a specimen from a bowel movement. I'm going to place the specimen pan (show specimen pan) at the back of the toilet bowl. You will urinate into the toilet. Your bowel movement will collect in the specimen pan. Please put toilet tissue in the toilet, not in the specimen pan. After your bowel movement, put your call light on right away. I'll put some stool in this specimen container (show the specimen container).*

After explaining the procedure, ask if the person has questions. If you do not know the answer, tell the nurse.

Also make sure the person understands what to do. You can say: "Mrs. Clark, please tell me what you're going to do so I know that you understand what I said."

FOCUS ON **CHILDREN AND OLDER PERSONS**

Stool Specimens

Children

If the child wears a diaper, you can obtain stool from the diaper. You may need to scrape the diaper.

DELEGATION GUIDELINES

Stool Specimens

Before collecting and testing a stool specimen, you need this information from the nurse.
* What time to collect and test the specimen
* What test is needed (if any)
* What equipment and special measures are needed
* Instructions for the test ordered
* If the nurse wants to observe the stool or test results
* What observations to report and record:
    * The time you collected and tested the specimen
    * Test results
    * Problems obtaining the specimen
    * Color, amount, consistency, and odor of stools
    * Complaints of pain or discomfort
* When to report observations
* What patient or resident concerns to report at once

PROMOTING SAFETY AND COMFORT

Stool Specimens

Safety

You must be accurate when testing stools. Follow the manufacturer's instructions for the test used. Promptly report the results to the nurse.

Comfort

Stools normally have an odor. A person may be embarrassed that you need to collect a specimen. Complete the task quickly and carefully. Act in a professional manner.

Collecting and Testing a Stool Specimen

QUALITY OF LIFE

- Knock before entering the person's room.
- Address the person by name.
- Introduce yourself by name and title.

- Explain the procedure before starting and during the procedure.
- Protect the person's rights during the procedure.
- Handle the person gently during the procedure.

PRE-PROCEDURE

1 Follow *Delegation Guidelines: Stool Specimens,* p. 577. See *Promoting Safety and Comfort:*
  a *Collecting and Testing Specimens,* p. 568
  b *Stool Specimens,* p. 577
2 Practice hand hygiene.
3 Collect the following before going to the person's room.
  - Laboratory requisition slip
  - Occult blood test kit (if needed)
  - Specimen pan for the toilet
  - Stool specimen container and lid (Fig. 34-6)
  - Specimen label
  - Tongue blades (if needed)
  - Disposable bag
  - Plastic bag
  - *BIOHAZARD* label (if needed)
  - Gloves

4 Arrange collected items in the person's bathroom.
5 Practice hand hygiene.
6 Identify the person. Check the ID bracelet against the requisition slip. Compare all information. Also call the person by name. Ask the person to state his or her first and last name and state his or her birthdate.
7 Label the specimen container in the person's presence.
8 Put on gloves.
9 Collect the following.
  - Device for voiding—bedpan and cover, urinal, commode, or specimen pan
  - Toilet tissue
10 Provide for privacy.

PROCEDURE

11 Ask the person to void. Provide the voiding device if the person does not use the bathroom. Empty, rinse, clean, disinfect, and dry the device. Return it to its proper place.
12 Put the specimen pan on the toilet if the person will use the bathroom. Place it at the back of the toilet (Fig. 34-7). Or provide the bedpan or commode.
13 Ask the person not to put toilet tissue into the bedpan, commode, or specimen pan. Provide a bag for toilet tissue.
14 Place the call light and toilet tissue within reach. Raise or lower bed rails. Follow the care plan.
15 Remove and discard the gloves. Practice hand hygiene. Leave the room if the person can be left alone.
16 Return when the person signals. Or check on the person every 5 minutes. Knock before entering.
17 Practice hand hygiene. Put on clean gloves.
18 Lower the bed rail near you if up. Remove the bedpan (if used). Or assist the person off the toilet or commode (if used). Provide perineal care if needed.
19 Note the color, amount, consistency, and odor of stools.
20 Collect the specimen.
  a Use the spoon attached to the lid to pick up several spoonfuls of stool. Or use a tongue blade to take about 2 tablespoons of stool to the specimen container (Fig. 34-8). Take the sample from:
    1) The middle of a formed stool
    2) Areas of pus, mucus, or blood and watery areas
    3) The middle and both ends of a hard stool
  b Put the lid on the specimen container.
  c Place the container in the plastic bag. Do not let the container touch the outside of the bag. Apply a *BIOHAZARD* label according to agency policy.
  d Wrap the tongue blade in toilet tissue. Discard it in the disposable bag.

21 Remove and discard the gloves. Practice hand hygiene. Put on clean gloves.
22 Test the specimen (if needed).
  a Open the test kit.
  b Use a tongue blade to obtain a small amount of stool.
  c Apply a thin smear of stool on *box A* on the test paper (Fig. 34-9, *A*).
  d Use another tongue blade to obtain stool from another part of the specimen.
  e Apply a thin smear of stool on *box B* on the test paper (Fig. 34-9, *B*).
  f Close the packet.
  g Turn the test packet to the other side. Open the flap. Apply developer (from the kit) to *boxes A* and *B*. Follow the manufacturer's instructions (Fig. 34-9, *C*).
  h Wait 10 to 60 seconds as required by the manufacturer.
  i Note the color changes on your assignment sheet (Fig. 34-9, *D*).
  j Dispose of the test packet.
  k Wrap the tongue blades with toilet tissue. Then discard them.
23 Empty, rinse, clean, disinfect, and dry equipment. Return equipment to its proper place.
24 Remove and discard the gloves. Practice hand hygiene. Put on clean gloves.
25 Assist with hand-washing.
26 Remove and discard the gloves. Practice hand hygiene.

Collecting and Testing a Stool Specimen—cont'd

POST-PROCEDURE

27 Provide for comfort. (See the inside of the front cover.)
28 Place the call light and other needed items within reach.
29 Raise or lower bed rails. Follow the care plan.
30 Unscreen the person.
31 Complete a safety check of the room. (See the inside of the front cover.)

32 Deliver the specimen and requisition slip to the laboratory or storage area. Follow agency policy. Wear gloves if that is agency policy.
33 Remove and discard the gloves. Practice hand hygiene.
34 Report and record your observations and the test results.

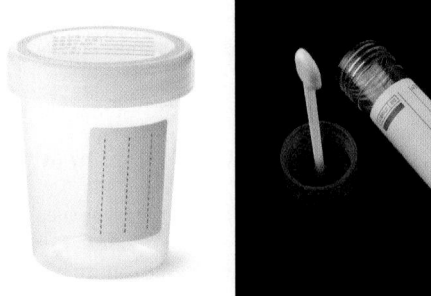

FIGURE 34-6 A, Stool specimen container. **B,** Stool specimen container with attached spoon. (**A,** © Fotofermer/Getty Images. **B,** From Healthlaw Medical Limited, Henso [Hangzhou] Co., Ltd. Hangzhou, China.)

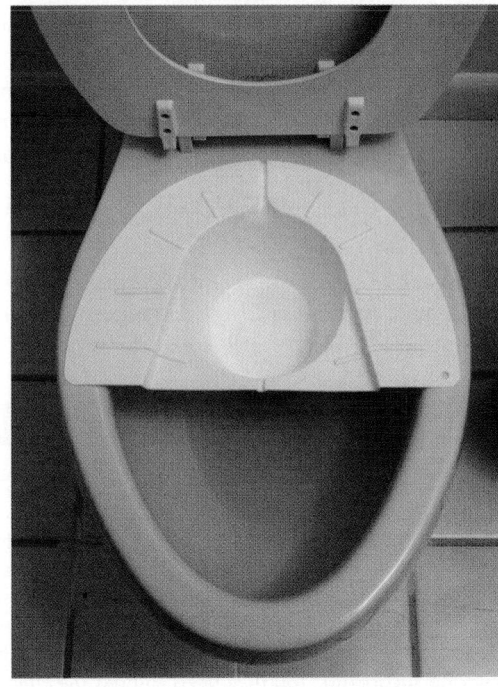

FIGURE 34-7 The specimen pan is placed at the back of the toilet for a stool specimen.

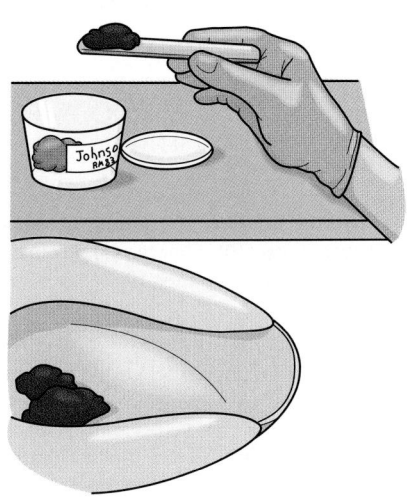

FIGURE 34-8 A tongue blade is used to transfer a small amount of stool from the bedpan to the specimen container.

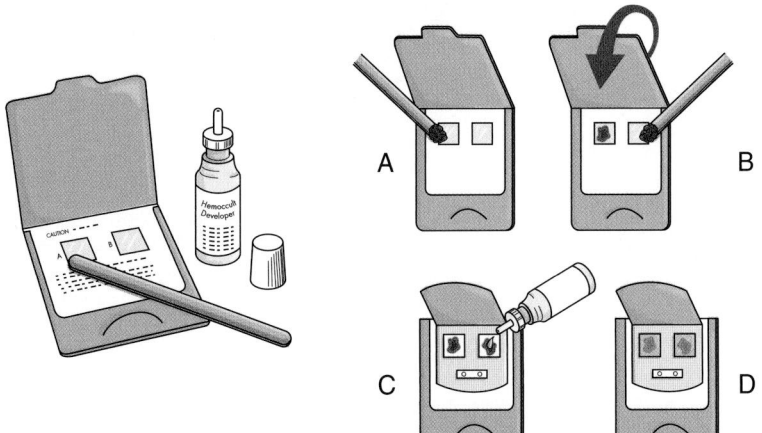

FIGURE 34-9 Testing for occult blood. A, Stool is smeared on *box A.* **B,** Stool is smeared on *box B* and then the flap is closed. **C,** Developer is applied to *boxes A* and *B* on the back side of the test packet. **D,** Color changes are noted.

SPUTUM SPECIMENS

Respiratory disorders cause the lungs, bronchi, and trachea to secrete mucus. *Mucus from the respiratory system is called* **sputum** *when expectorated (expelled) through the mouth.* Sputum is not saliva. Saliva ("spit") is a thin, clear liquid produced by the salivary glands in the mouth.

Sputum specimens are studied for blood, microbes, and abnormal cells. Sputum is coughed up from the bronchi and trachea. This is often painful and hard to do. It is easier to collect a specimen in the morning. Secretions collect in the trachea and bronchi during sleep. They are coughed up on awakening.

Follow the rules in Box 34-1. Also have the person rinse the mouth with water. Rinsing decreases saliva and removes food particles. Mouthwash is not used. It destroys some of the microbes in the mouth.

See *Focus on Children and Older Persons: Sputum Specimens.*

See *Delegation Guidelines: Sputum Specimens.*

See *Promoting Safety and Comfort: Sputum Specimens.*

See procedure: *Collecting a Sputum Specimen.*

FOCUS ON CHILDREN AND OLDER PERSONS

Sputum Specimens

Children

Breathing treatments and suctioning (Chapter 40) are often needed to produce sputum specimens in infants and small children. The RN (registered nurse) or respiratory therapist gives the breathing treatment. The nurse suctions the trachea for the specimen. The infant or child is likely to be upset during suctioning. You may need to hold the child's head and arms still.

Older Persons

Older persons may lack the strength to cough up sputum. Coughing is easier after postural drainage. It drains secretions by gravity. Gravity causes fluids to flow down. The person is positioned so a lung part is higher than the airway (Fig. 34-10). The nurse or respiratory therapist does postural drainage. Assist as directed.

DELEGATION GUIDELINES

Sputum Specimens

To collect a sputum specimen, you need this information from the nurse.

- When to collect the specimen
- How much sputum is needed—usually 1 to 2 teaspoons
- If the person uses the bathroom
- If the person can hold the sputum container
- What observations to report and record:
  - The time the specimen was collected
  - The amount of sputum collected
  - How easily the person raised the sputum
  - Sputum color—clear, white, yellow, green, brown, or red
  - Sputum odor—none or foul odor
  - Sputum consistency—thick, watery, or frothy (with bubbles or foam)
  - *Hemoptysis*—*bloody* (hemo) *sputum* (ptysis *means to* spit)
  - If the person was not able to produce sputum
  - Any other observations
- When to report observations
- What patient or resident concerns to report at once

PROMOTING SAFETY AND COMFORT

Sputum Specimens

Safety

The doctor may order isolation precautions if the person has or may have tuberculosis (TB) (Chapter 45). Protect yourself by wearing a TB respirator (Chapter 16).

Comfort

The procedure can embarrass the person. Coughing and expectorating sounds can disturb others. Also, sputum is not pleasant to look at. Privacy is important. Cover the specimen container and place it in a bag. Some sputum specimen containers are cloudy in color to hide the contents.

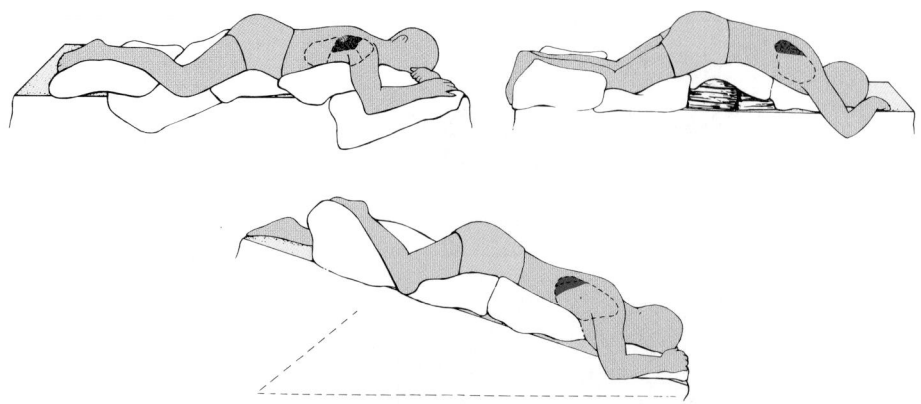

FIGURE 34-10 Some positions for postural drainage. (From Potter PA, Perry AG, Stockert PA, Hall AM: *Fundamentals of nursing*, ed 8, St Louis, 2013, Mosby.)

Collecting a Sputum Specimen

QUALITY OF LIFE

- Knock before entering the person's room.
- Address the person by name.
- Introduce yourself by name and title.

- Explain the procedure before starting and during the procedure.
- Protect the person's rights during the procedure.
- Handle the person gently during the procedure.

PRE-PROCEDURE

1 Follow *Delegation Guidelines: Sputum Specimens.* See *Promoting Safety and Comfort:*
    a *Collecting and Testing Specimens,* p. 568
    b *Sputum Specimens*
2 Practice hand hygiene.
3 Collect the following before going to the person's room.
    - Laboratory requisition slip
    - Sputum specimen container and lid
    - Specimen label
    - Plastic bag
    - *BIOHAZARD* label (if needed)

4 Arrange collected items in the person's bathroom.
5 Practice hand hygiene.
6 Identify the person. Check the ID bracelet against the requisition slip. Compare all information. Also call the person by name. Ask the person to state his or her first and last name and state his or her birthdate.
7 Label the specimen container in the person's presence.
8 Collect gloves and tissues.
9 Provide for privacy. If able, the person uses the bathroom for the procedure.

PROCEDURE

10 Put on gloves.
11 Ask the person to rinse the mouth out with clear water.
12 Have the person hold the container. Only the outside is touched.
13 Ask the person to cover the mouth and nose with tissues when coughing. Follow agency policy for used tissues.
14 Ask him or her to take 2 or 3 breaths and cough up the sputum.
15 Have the person expectorate directly into the container (Fig. 34-11). Sputum should not touch the outside of the container.

16 Collect 1 to 2 teaspoons of sputum unless told to collect more.
17 Put the lid on the container.
18 Place the container in the plastic bag. Do not let the container touch the outside of the bag. Apply a *BIOHAZARD* label according to agency policy.
19 Remove and discard the gloves. Practice hand hygiene. Put on clean gloves.
20 Assist with hand-washing.
21 Remove and discard the gloves. Practice hand hygiene.

POST-PROCEDURE

22 Provide for comfort. (See the inside of the front cover.)
23 Place the call light and other needed items within reach.
24 Raise or lower bed rails. Follow the care plan.
25 Unscreen the person.
26 Complete a safety check of the room. (See the inside of the front cover.)

27 Practice hand hygiene.
28 Deliver the specimen and the requisition slip to the laboratory or storage area. Follow agency policy. Wear gloves if that is agency policy.
29 Remove and discard the gloves. Practice hand hygiene.
30 Report and record your observations.

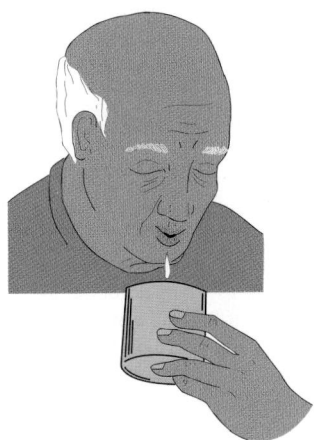

FIGURE 34-11 The person expectorates into the center of the specimen container.

BLOOD GLUCOSE TESTING

Blood glucose testing is used for persons with diabetes. The doctor uses the results to regulate drugs and diet.

A drop of capillary blood is collected through a skin puncture. A fingertip is the most common site for skin punctures.

Inspect the puncture site for trauma and skin breaks. Do not use swollen, bruised, cyanotic (bluish color), scarred, or calloused sites. Such areas have poor blood flow. A *callus* is a thick, hardened area on the skin. Calluses often form over frequently used areas, such as the tips of the thumbs and index fingers. Therefore thumbs and index fingers are not good skin puncture sites.

Use the side toward the tip of the middle or ring finger (Fig. 34-12). Do not use the center, fleshy part of the fingertip. The site has many nerve endings making punctures painful.

You use a sterile, disposable lancet to puncture the skin (Fig. 34-13). The person feels a brief, sharp pinch. A *lancet* is a short, pointed blade that punctures but does not cut the skin. The lancet is inside a protective cover. Do not touch the blade. Discard the blade into the sharps container after use.

A **glucometer** *(glucose meter) is a device for measuring* (meter) *blood glucose* (gluco). Reagent strips (test strips) are used. You apply a drop of blood to the reagent strip. The blood glucose level appears on the screen. How fast results are displayed depends on the type of glucometer. Some take 5 seconds.

You will learn to use your agency's device. Always follow the manufacturer's instructions.

See *Teamwork and Time Management: Blood Glucose Testing.*

See *Delegation Guidelines: Blood Glucose Testing.*

See *Promoting Safety and Comfort: Blood Glucose Testing.*

See procedure: *Measuring Blood Glucose,* p. 584.

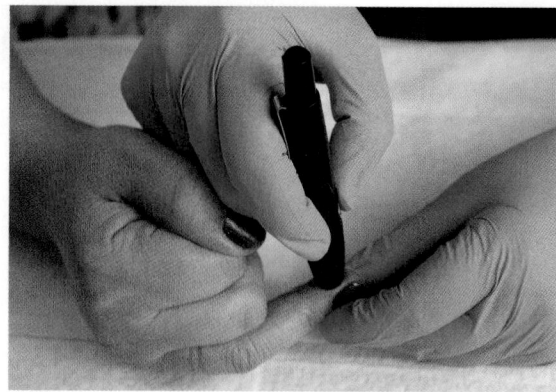

FIGURE 34-13 A lancet in a lancing device used to puncture the skin.

TEAMWORK AND TIME MANAGEMENT
Blood Glucose Testing

Perform blood glucose testing at times directed by the nurse and the care plan. Drugs are given at a certain time. The nurse needs the person's blood glucose results before giving the drugs.

Glucometers are shared with other staff. Tell your co-workers when you have one. Work quickly but carefully. Return the device to the storage area in a timely manner.

DELEGATION GUIDELINES
Blood Glucose Testing

If testing blood glucose is delegated to you, make sure that:
- Your state and agency allow you to perform the procedure.
- The procedure is in your job description.
- You have the necessary training.
- You know how to use the agency's equipment.
- You review the procedure with a nurse.
- The nurse is available to answer questions and to supervise you.

If the above conditions are met, you need this information from the nurse and the care plan.
- What sites to avoid for a skin puncture
- When to collect and test the specimen—usually before meals
- If the person receives drugs that affect blood clotting (NOTE: If yes, it may take a longer time to stop bleeding. Apply pressure until bleeding stops.)
- What to report and record:
  - The time the specimen was collected
  - The blood glucose test result
  - The site used for the skin puncture
  - The amount of bleeding at the skin puncture site
  - Any signs of a **hematoma** *(a swelling* [oma] *that contains blood* [hemat])
  - How the person tolerated the procedure
  - Complaints of pain at the skin puncture site
  - Other observations or patient or resident complaints
- When to report observations and the test result
- What patient or resident concerns to report at once

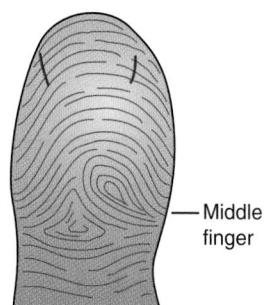

Middle finger

FIGURE 34-12 Site for skin punctures.

PROMOTING SAFETY AND COMFORT

Blood Glucose Testing

Safety

Accurate results are important. Inaccurate results can harm the person. Follow the rules in Box 34-2.

You must know how to use the equipment. Use only the type of reagent strip specified by the manufacturer. Otherwise you will get inaccurate results.

Disinfect the glucometer after testing a patient or resident. Follow the manufacturer's instructions for the disinfectant used. For example, if the instructions say to wait 2 minutes, you must wait 2 minutes. Always follow the time set by the manufacturer.

Comfort

The heel is used for skin punctures in infants who are not walking. The third finger (ring finger) is used for children. See Figure 34-14.

Older persons often have poor circulation in their fingers. To increase blood flow, apply a warm washcloth or wash the hands in warm water.

BOX 34-2	**Blood Glucose Testing**

- Follow the manufacturer's instructions for the glucometer and disinfectant.
- Know how to use the equipment. Request any necessary training.
- Make sure the glucometer was tested for accuracy. Check the testing log.
- Enter a code or user-ID if required by the glucometer. This is provided by the agency. Do not share your user-ID with others.
- Make sure you have the correct reagent (test) strips for the glucometer you are using.
- Scan the bar code on the bottle of reagent strips if needed. Or compare the code on the bottle of reagent strips to the code on the glucometer (Fig. 34-15).
- Check the color of the reagent strips. Do not use discolored strips.
- Check the expiration date on the reagent strips. Do not use them if the date has passed.
- Report the result to the nurse at once.
- Record the result following agency policy.

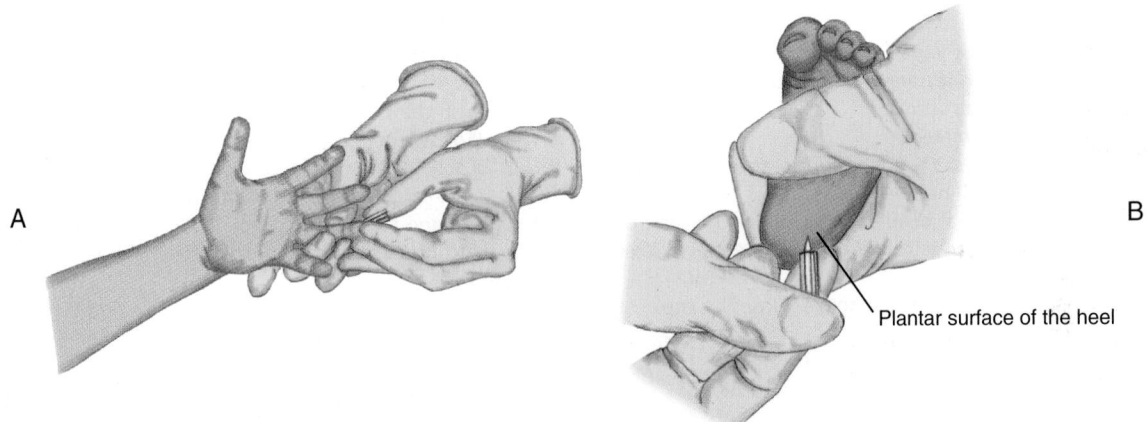

A   B

Plantar surface of the heel

FIGURE 34-14 A, The third finger (ring finger) is used for skin punctures in children. **B,** Heel site is used for skin punctures in infants. (From James SR, Ashwill JW, Droske SC: *Nursing care of children: principles and practice,* ed 3, Philadelphia, 2007, Saunders.)

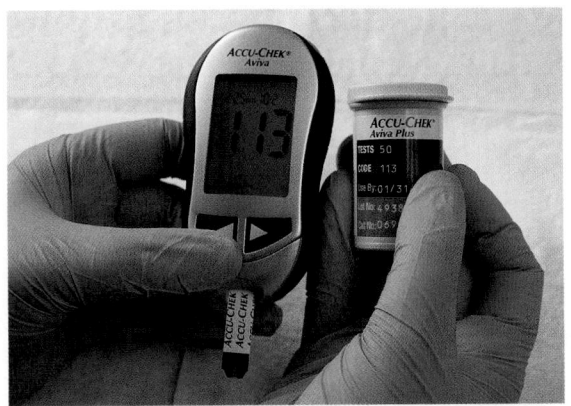

FIGURE 34-15 The code on the bottle of reagent (test) strips is compared to the code on the glucometer.

Measuring Blood Glucose

QUALITY OF LIFE

- Knock before entering the person's room.
- Address the person by name.
- Introduce yourself by name and title.

- Explain the procedure before starting and during the procedure.
- Protect the person's rights during the procedure.
- Handle the person gently during the procedure.

PRE-PROCEDURE

1 Follow *Delegation Guidelines: Blood Glucose Testing*, p. 582. See *Promoting Safety and Comfort:*
   a *Collecting and Testing Specimens*, p. 568
   b *Blood Glucose Testing*, p. 583
2 Practice hand hygiene.
3 Collect the following.
   - Sterile lancet
   - Lancing device (if used)
   - Antiseptic wipes
   - Gloves
   - 2 × 2 gauze squares
   - Glucometer
   - Reagent (test) strips (Use the correct ones for the glucometer. Check the expiration date.)
   - Disinfectant

   - Paper towels
   - Warm washcloth
4 Read the manufacturer's instructions for the lancet and glucometer.
5 Disinfect the glucometer. Follow the manufacturer's instructions for the disinfectant.
6 Arrange your work area.
7 Identify the person. Check the ID bracelet against the assignment sheet. Use 2 identifiers (Chapter 13). Also call the person by name. Ask the person to state his or her first and last name and state his or her birthdate.
8 Provide for privacy.
9 Raise the bed for body mechanics. The far bed rail is up if used.

PROCEDURE

10 Help the person to a comfortable position.
11 Put on the gloves.
12 Prepare the supplies.
   a Open the antiseptic wipes.
   b Prepare the lancet. If using a lancing device, follow the manufacturer's instructions.
   c Turn on the glucometer.
   d Follow the prompts. You may need to enter a user-ID and the person's ID number. Scan the bar code on the bottle of test strips if needed. Or compare the code on the bottle of test strips to the code on the glucometer. See Fig. 34-15.
   e Remove a test strip from the bottle. Close the cap tightly.
   f Insert a test strip into the glucometer (Fig. 34-16).
13 Perform a skin puncture to obtain a drop of blood.
   a Inspect the person's fingers. Select a puncture site.
   b Do the following to increase blood flow to the puncture site.
      1) Warm the finger. Rub it gently or apply a warm washcloth.
      2) Massage the hand and finger toward the puncture site.
      3) Lower the finger below the person's waist.
   c Hold the finger with your thumb and index finger. Use your non-dominant hand. Hold the finger until step 14, b.

   d Clean the site with an antiseptic wipe. *Do not touch the site after cleaning.*
   e Let the site dry.
   f Place the lancet or lancing device against the puncture site.
   g Push the button on the device to puncture the skin. (Follow the manufacturer's instructions.)
   h Apply gentle pressure below the puncture site.
   i Let a large drop of blood form.
14 Collect and test the specimen. Follow the manufacturer's instructions and agency procedures for the glucometer used.
   a Touch the test strip to the drop of blood (Fig. 34-17). The glucometer will test the sample when enough blood is applied.
   b Apply pressure to the puncture site until bleeding stops. Use a gauze square. If able, let the person apply pressure to the site.
   c Read the result on the display (Fig. 34-18). Note the result on your note pad or assignment sheet. Tell the person the result.
   d Turn off the glucometer.
15 Discard the lancet in the sharps container.
16 Discard the gauze square and test strip. Follow agency policy.
17 Remove and discard the gloves. Practice hand hygiene.

Measuring Blood Glucose—cont'd
POST-PROCEDURE

18 Provide for comfort. (See the inside of the front cover.)
19 Place the call light and other needed items within reach.
20 Lower the bed to a safe and comfortable level for the person. Follow the care plan.
21 Raise or lower bed rails. Follow the care plan.
22 Unscreen the person.
23 Discard used supplies.

24 Complete a safety check of the room. (See the inside of the front cover.)
25 Follow agency policy for used linens.
26 Disinfect the glucometer. (Wear gloves.) Follow the manufacturer's instructions. Return the device to its proper place.
27 Remove and discard the gloves. Practice hand hygiene.
28 Report and record the test result and your observations (Fig. 34-19, p. 586).

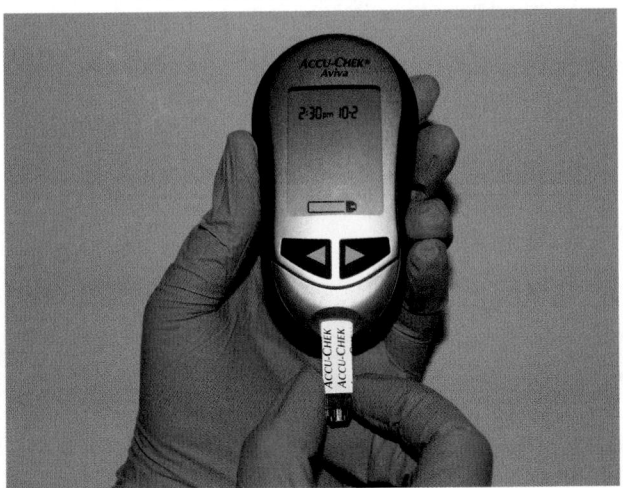
FIGURE 34-16 A reagent (test) strip is in the glucometer.

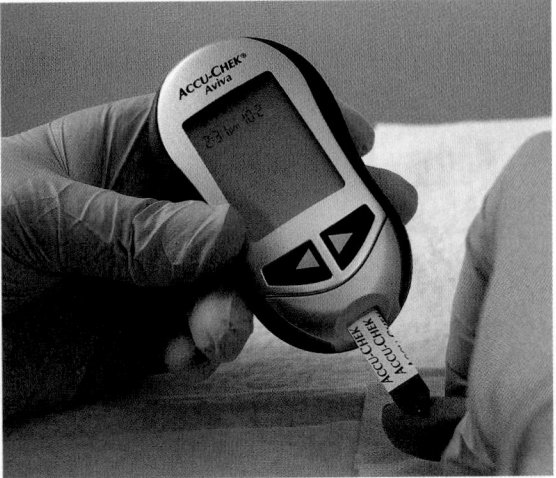
FIGURE 34-17 A drop of blood is applied to the reagent (test) strip.

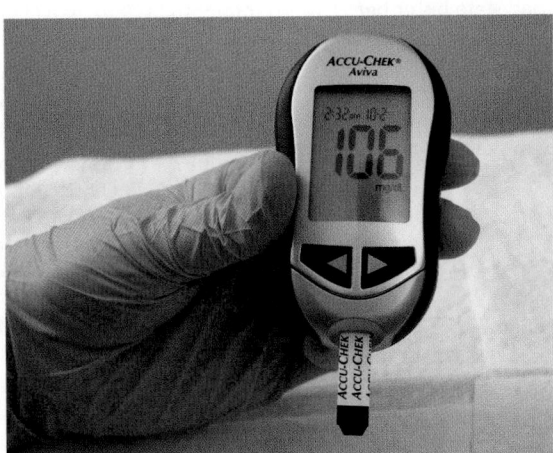
FIGURE 34-18 The result is displayed on the glucometer.

HINDS, DEBRA	DOB: 4/7/1959	GENDER: Female	ID#: 0005718955	Room: 112-A

DATE: May 7   **TIME:** 0730   **USERNAME:** Martina Rivera, CNA

BLOOD GLUCOSE TESTING

Puncture Site	Observations

Click to mark puncture site.

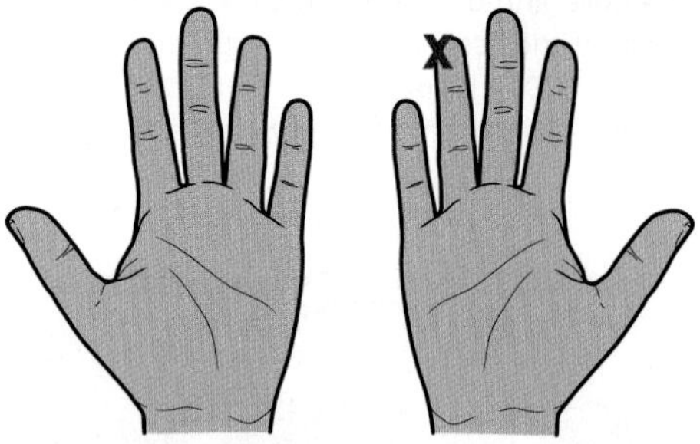

Left hand   Right hand

Observations

☒ Skin intact   ☐ Bruising
☐ Pain   ☐ Cyanosis
☐ Swelling   ☐ Hematoma

Bleeding amount

☒ Small (stopped with brief pressure)
☐ Moderate to large   ☒ Pressure applied to site

Test Result and Reporting

Result: 82   mg/dL

☒ Nurse notified of result and observations

Nurse notified: Phillip Young, RN

FIGURE 34-19 Charting sample.

FOCUS ON PRIDE

The Person, Family, and Yourself

Personal and Professional Responsibility

You must collect specimens on the right person. Otherwise, one or both persons could be harmed. Before collecting a specimen, carefully identify the person. Check the ID bracelet against the laboratory requisition slip. Compare all information, not just the person's name. Also ask the person to state his or her first and last name and state his or her birthdate.

In some agencies collection information is written on the specimen container. Collection date and time and the collector's name or initials are examples. Follow agency policy to label specimens. Take pride in properly collecting and labeling specimens.

Rights and Respect

Specimen collection can embarrass the person. To respect the person's right to privacy:

- Politely ask visitors to leave the room.
- Close doors, privacy curtains, and window coverings.
- Leave the room if it is safe to do so. If you cannot leave, explain this to the person.
- Place the specimen container in a paper bag or wrap it in a paper towel or washcloth so others do not see the specimen.

Independence and Social Interaction

Some persons can collect their own urine and sputum specimens. Doing so promotes independence and reduces embarrassment.

Explain the procedure so the person knows how to collect the specimen correctly. Show the person the specimen container and how it is used. Also, ask the person where to place the container. When ready to collect the specimen, the person knows where to find the container.

Delegation and Teamwork

You may need to take a specimen to the laboratory. Before you go, tell the nurse and your co-workers. Ask if other staff need specimens taken to the laboratory. Doing so saves staff time. This also prevents having too many staff members off the unit at the same time. Return from the laboratory promptly.

Ethics and Laws

Ethics is concerned with right and wrong behavior. If you did not collect a specimen correctly, do not send it to the laboratory. Tell the nurse what happened. Then collect the specimen at the next opportunity. Test results must be accurate for correct diagnosis and treatment. Take pride in honestly reporting mistakes.

FOCUS ON PRIDE: Application

What mistakes could occur in specimen collection? What can you do to prevent such mistakes? Explain why failing to report a mistake can be harmful.

REVIEW QUESTIONS

Circle the BEST answer.

1 A random urine specimen is collected
a After sleep
b Before meals
c After meals
d Any time

2 Perineal care is given before collecting a
a Random specimen
b Midstream specimen
c 24-hour specimen
d Stool specimen

3 A 24-hour urine specimen involves
a Collecting all urine voided during a 24-hour period
b Collecting a random specimen every hour for 24 hours
c Testing urine for ketones every day
d Measuring output every 24 hours

4 To collect a midstream specimen on a female
a Spread the labia to expose the urethral area
b Clean the urethral area from back to front
c Collect urine at the start of the urine stream
d Collect about 10 mL of urine

5 Urine is tested for glucose
a To measure the pH
b To check for blood
c To check for sugar
d To check for ketones

6 You need to strain a person's urine. Straining is done to find
a Blood
b Stones
c Ketones
d Acetone

7 You note a black, tarry stool. This is called
a Melena
b Feces
c Hemostat
d Occult blood

8 A warm stool specimen is needed. After collecting the specimen
a Put it in an oven
b Put it in a paper bag
c Cover it with a towel
d Take it to the laboratory or storage area

9 The best time to collect a sputum specimen is
a On awakening
b After meals
c At bedtime
d After oral hygiene

10 A sputum specimen is needed. You should ask the person to
a Use mouthwash
b Rinse the mouth with clear water
c Brush the teeth
d Remove dentures

11 Which is the *best* site for a skin puncture?
a The thumb
b The index finger
c The ring finger
d The little finger

12 Which is needed to measure blood glucose?
a Glucometer
b Sterile specimen container
c Color-changing reagent strip
d Sphygmomanometer

13 Before using reagent strips for blood glucose testing
a Make sure they are discolored
b Label each strip with the person's name
c Check the size of the test area
d Check the expiration date

14 Which statement about reporting a blood glucose result is *true*?
a Only report an abnormal result.
b Report the result to the nurse at once.
c Report the result after the person's meal.
d Report the result any time before the person's next meal.

Answers to Chapter 34 questions are on p. 871.

FOCUS ON **PRACTICE**

Problem Solving

You need a midstream urine specimen from Mrs. Parker. She can collect the specimen herself. You give her the specimen cup and pack of towelettes and ask: "Do you know what to do?" She says: "Yes, I've done this before." You tell her to leave the specimen cup in the bathroom and signal for you when she is done.

You return to get the specimen and notice the towelettes are unopened. What do you do? Should you send the specimen to the laboratory? How could this have been prevented?

OBJECTIVES

- Define the key terms and key abbreviations in this chapter.
- Describe the common fears and concerns of surgical patients.
- Describe pre-operative and post-operative care.

- List the signs and symptoms to report after surgery.
- Perform the procedures described in this chapter.
- Explain how to promote PRIDE in the person, the family, and yourself.

KEY TERMS

anesthesia The loss of all sensation, especially pain, produced by a drug

elective surgery Surgery done by choice to improve life or well-being

embolus A blood clot that travels through the vascular system until it lodges in a blood vessel

emergency surgery Surgery done at once to save life or function

general anesthesia A treatment with certain drugs that produces a deep sleep and the absence of all sensation, especially pain

local anesthesia The loss of sensation, produced by a drug, in a small area

post-operative After surgery

pre-operative Before surgery

regional anesthesia The loss of sensation, produced by a drug, in a large area

sedation A state of quiet, calmness, or sleep produced by a drug

thrombus A blood clot

urgent surgery Surgery needed for the person's health; it can be delayed for a few days

KEY ABBREVIATIONS

AE	Anti-embolism; anti-embolic		**NPO**	Non per os; nothing by mouth
CBC	Complete blood count		**OR**	Operating room
ECG	Electrocardiogram		**PACU**	Post-anesthesia care unit
EKG	Electrocardiogram		**post-op**	Post-operative
ID	Identification		**pre-op**	Pre-operative
IV	Intravenous		**SCD**	Sequential compression device
NG	Naso-gastric		**TED**	Thrombo-embolic disease

The many reasons for surgery include to:

- Remove, repair, or replace a diseased or injured body part.
- Remove a tumor.
- Make a diagnosis.
- Relieve symptoms.
- Restore or improve function or appearance.

Surgery may require a hospital stay. *In-patients* are admitted the morning of surgery or 1 or 2 days before surgery. Some patients go to surgery from the emergency room. Patients stay for 1 or more days after surgery.

Same-day surgery (out-patient, 1-day, or ambulatory surgery) is common. The surgeries are done in hospitals and *surgi-centers (surgery centers)*. Surgi-centers are designed and equipped for certain surgical and diagnostic procedures. The person goes home the same day or the next day.

Surgeries are described as:
- *Elective surgery—done by choice to improve life or well-being.* It is not life-saving. Joint replacement surgery and cosmetic surgery are examples. The surgery is scheduled in advance.
- *Urgent surgery—needed for the person's health. It can be delayed for a few days.* Sometimes cancer surgery and coronary artery bypass surgery can be delayed for a few days.
- *Emergency surgery—done at once to save life or function.* The need is sudden and not expected. Vehicle crashes, stabbings, and bullet wounds often require emergency surgery.

The person is prepared for what happens before, during, and after surgery. *Pre-operative (pre-op) refers to before surgery. Post-operative (post-op) refers to after surgery.* Some people recover in nursing centers or rehabilitation centers. Some need home care.

PSYCHOLOGICAL CARE

Surgery causes many fears and concerns (Box 35-1). Past experiences affect feelings. Some persons had surgery before. Others have not. Patients are affected when family and friends talk about their own surgeries. Most people know about tragic events—surgery on the wrong person or body part, instruments left in the body, death during or after surgery. Some people do not share fears and concerns. They may cry, be quiet or withdrawn, or talk about other things. Some pace. Others are very cheerful.

Mental preparation is important. Respect the person's fears and concerns. Show warmth, sensitivity, and caring.

BOX 35-1	Surgery Fears and Concerns

The Fear of ...
- Anesthesia and its effects
- Cancer
- Complications from surgery
- Disability
- Disfigurement and scarring
- Dying during or after surgery
- Exposure
- Not waking up after surgery
- Pain: during surgery, after surgery
- Prolonged recovery
- Separation from family and friends
- Surgery on the wrong body part
- Tubes, needles, and other care equipment
- Waking up during surgery
- What happens after surgery—more surgery, treatments, care, and so on

Concerns about ...
- Caring for children and other family members
- Finances—monthly bills, loan payments, mortgages, hospital bills, doctor bills
- House, lawn, and garden
- Pets
- Plants

FOCUS ON COMMUNICATION

Patient Information

Patients and families are eager to know the results. They may ask you about reports. Refer their questions to the nurse. Never tell any results or diagnoses. You can say:
- "The doctor will tell you about the surgery and the results. I'll tell the nurse that you're asking."
- "I'll get the nurse to answer your questions."

Patient Information

The doctor explains the need for surgery to the patient and family. They are told about:
- The surgery, risks, and possible complications
- The risks from not having surgery
- Who will do the surgery
- The date and time of the surgery
- How long the surgery will take

Questions are answered. Misunderstandings are cleared up. Care instructions are given.

After surgery, the doctor talks to the patient and family. Often the health team knows the results before the person.

See *Focus on Communication: Patient Information.*

Your Role

You can assist in the person's psychological care before and after surgery.
- Listen. The person may talk about fears and concerns.
- Refer questions to the nurse.
- Explain the care you will give and its need.
- Follow communication rules (Chapters 7 and 9).
- Use verbal and nonverbal communication (Chapter 9).
- Provide care with skill and ease.
- Report signs of fear or anxiety (Chapter 48).
- Report a request to see a member of the clergy.

PRE-OPERATIVE CARE

The pre-operative (pre-op) period may be many days or a few minutes. If time allows, the person is prepared mentally and physically for anesthesia and surgery. The goal is to prevent complications before, during, and after surgery.

See *Teamwork and Time Management: Pre-Operative Care.*

TEAMWORK AND TIME MANAGEMENT

Pre-Operative Care

The nurse has a limited amount of time for pre-op care. Assist as directed. You must understand what to do and when to complete care.

You may be delegated several tasks. Tell the nurse when you complete each task. For example, you provide personal care (p. 591). Tell the nurse about your progress.

Pre-Operative Teaching

The nurse explains what to expect before, during, and after surgery. Teaching includes:

- *Pre-op care*—includes tests and their purpose, skin preparation, personal care, and the purpose and effects of pre-op drugs.
- *Deep breathing, coughing, and incentive spirometry*—are practiced. Post-op, they are done every 1 to 2 hours when the person is awake. See Chapter 39.
- *Post-anesthesia care unit (PACU)*—commonly called the *recovery room*, this is where the person wakes up after surgery (Fig. 35-1). The care given is explained.
- *Vital signs*—are taken often until they are stable.
- *Food and fluids*—post-op, the person is NPO (non per os; nothing by mouth) and has an IV (intravenous). Food and fluids are allowed when the person's condition is stable.
- *Turning and re-positioning*—are done at least every 1 to 2 hours post-op.
- *Early ambulation*—is done as soon as possible post-op.
- *Pain*—relates to the type and amount of pain to expect and how pain-relief drugs are given.
- *Treatments and equipment*—may involve a urine catheter, NG (naso-gastric) tube, oxygen, wound suction, a cast, or traction.
- *Position restrictions*—are common after some surgeries. For example, the hip is abducted after hip replacement surgery (Chapter 44).

See *Focus on Children and Older Persons: Pre-Operative Care.*

Special Tests

Pre-op, the doctor evaluates the person's health status. These tests are common.

- Chest x-ray.
- Complete blood count (CBC).
- Urinalysis (U/A).
- Electrocardiogram (ECG, EKG). See Figure 35-2.

Other tests depend on the person's condition and surgery. For expected blood loss, the person's blood is tested for blood type and compatible blood. This is called *type and crossmatch*.

The person is prepared for the tests as needed. Test results must be on the chart before surgery.

Nutrition and Fluids

A light meal usually is allowed. Then the person is NPO for 6 to 8 hours before surgery. These measures reduce the risk of vomiting and aspiration during anesthesia and after surgery. An NPO sign is placed in the person's room. The water mug is removed.

Bowel Elimination

Bowel surgeries may require a *bowel prep*—cleansing the bowel of feces. Feces contain microbes. When the intestine is opened, feces can spill into the sterile abdominal cavity. The bowel prep prevents this contamination.

For the bowel prep, the doctor orders special fluids for the person to drink. Or the doctor orders what enemas to give and when.

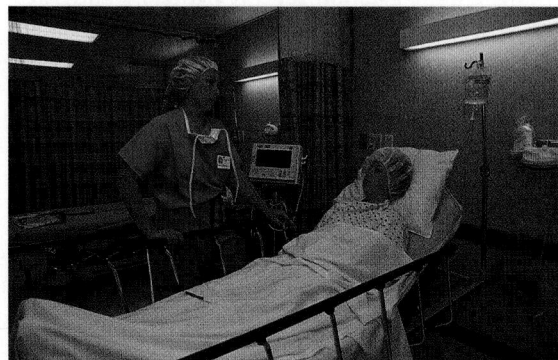

FIGURE 35-1 The post-anesthesia care unit (PACU).

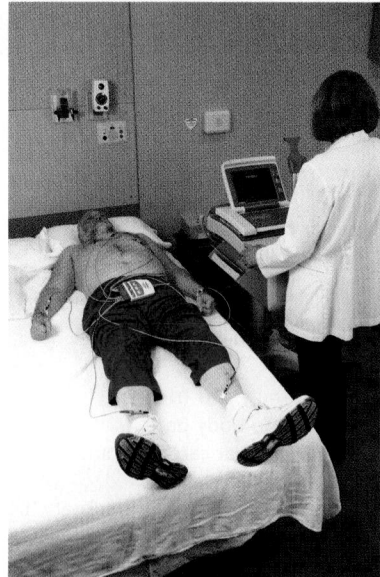

FIGURE 35-2 An electrocardiogram is taken.

Urinary Elimination

The person voids before the nurse gives pre-op drugs. If the person has a catheter, the drainage bag is emptied. The output is measured and recorded.

Often catheters are inserted in the OR. For pelvic and abdominal surgeries, the bladder must be empty. A full bladder is easily injured during surgery. Catheters also allow accurate output measurements during and after surgery.

Personal Care

Personal care before surgery involves:
- *A complete bath, shower, or tub bath and shampoo.* A special soap or cleanser and shampoo may be ordered. The bath and shampoo reduce the number of microbes present. This reduces the risk of a wound infection. A patient gown is worn after bathing.
- *Make-up, nail polish, and fake nail removal.* The skin, lips, and nail beds are observed for color and circulation during and after surgery.
- *Hair care.* All hairpins, clips, combs, and other items are removed. So are wigs and hairpieces. A surgical cap keeps hair out of the face and the operative site.
- *Oral hygiene.* Being NPO causes thirst and a dry mouth. The person must not swallow any water during oral hygiene.
- *Dentures.* Provide denture care and store dentures following agency policy. Some people do not like to be without their dentures. Let them wear dentures as long as possible. This promotes dignity and self-esteem.
- *Prostheses.* Eyeglasses, contact lenses, hearing aids, artificial eyes, and artificial limbs are removed. Hearing aids may be left in if the surgeon needs to talk to or instruct the patient during surgery. Follow agency policy for storage and safe-keeping.
- *Other.* Often elastic stockings (p. 598) are put on before transport to the OR. So are sequential compression devices (p. 601).

See *Promoting Safety and Comfort: Personal Care.*

Jewelry

Jewelry is easily lost or broken in the OR and PACU. Transfers to and from the OR, PACU, and the person's room also present safety risks. And jewelry can cause pressure injuries (Chapter 37). Therefore all jewelry is removed and stored for safe-keeping. This includes body-piercing jewelry. Record jewelry removal and storage according to agency policy.

The person may want to wear a wedding ring or religious medal. Secure the item in place with gauze and tape according to agency policy. Hand, arm, shoulder, and breast surgeries can cause swelling of the fingers. Wedding rings are removed for such surgeries.

Skin Preparation

Microbes from skin and hair can enter the body through the surgical incision. To reduce the risk of infection, a *skin prep* is done. For the skin prep, the doctor orders 1 or more of the following.
- Cleansing with an anti-microbial soap. *Anti* means *against.*
- Clipping the hair at and around the site.
- Removing hair at and around the site.

The incision site and a large area around it are *prepped* (Fig. 35-3, p. 592). The prep is done in the person's room or in the OR. To remove hair, a hair cream remover is used. Or the skin is shaved.

A *skin prep kit* is used for shaving. The kit has a razor, a sponge filled with soap, a basin (tray), a drape, and a towel (Fig. 35-4, p. 593). Lather the skin with soap. Then shave in the direction of hair growth (Fig. 35-5, p. 593).

See *Delegation Guidelines: Skin Preparation*, p. 593.
See *Promoting Safety and Comfort: Skin Preparation*, p. 593.
See procedure: *The Surgical Skin Prep—Shaving the Skin*, p. 593.

Text continued on p. 594.

PROMOTING SAFETY AND COMFORT

Personal Care

Safety
Check for loose teeth. Loose teeth are common in children. Adults may have loose teeth from periodontal disease (Chapter 22). Report loose teeth to the nurse. The nurse notes this on the pre-op checklist and tells the surgery staff. A loose tooth can fall out during anesthesia. The person can aspirate the tooth.

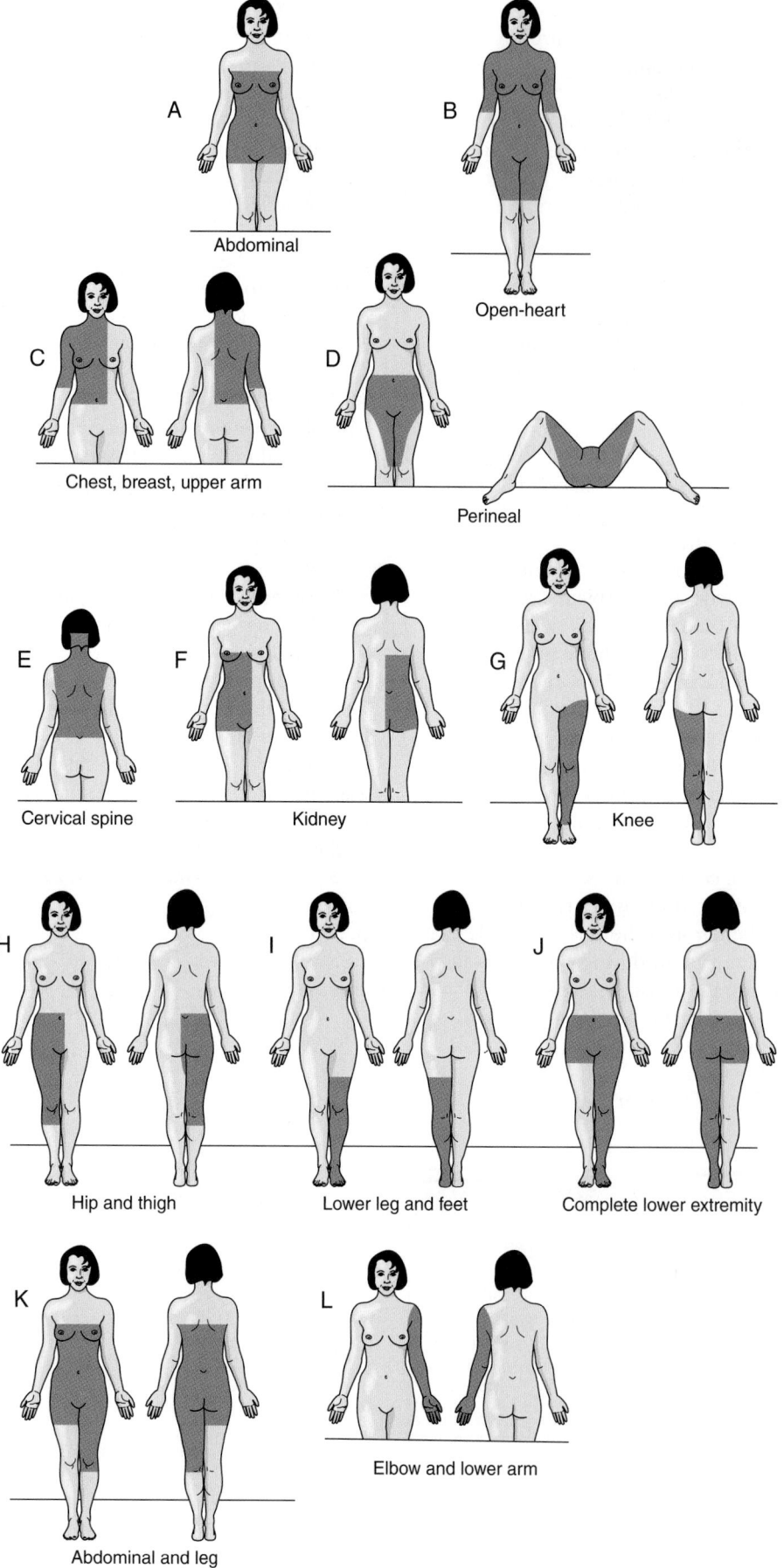

FIGURE 35-3 Skin prep sites. The *shaded area* shows the area to prep for the type of surgery.

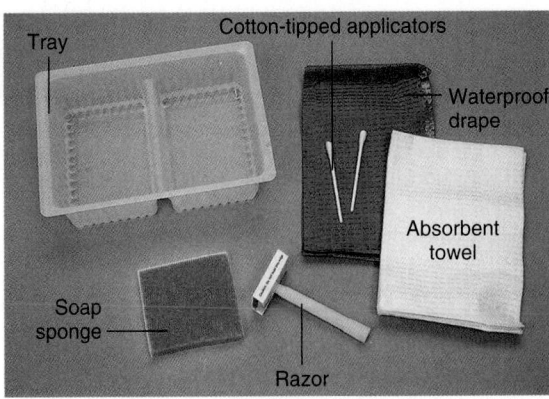

FIGURE 35-4 Skin prep kit.

Tray
Cotton-tipped applicators
Waterproof drape
Absorbent towel
Soap sponge
Razor

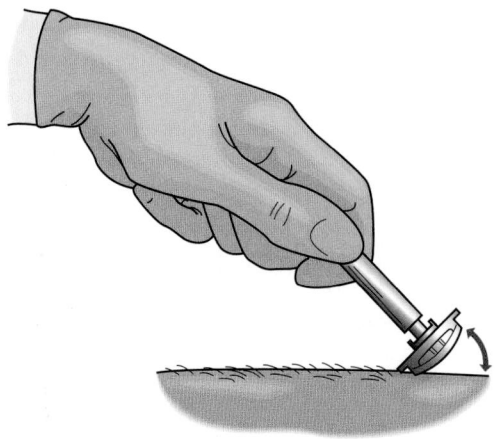

FIGURE 35-5 Shave in the direction of hair growth.

DELEGATION GUIDELINES
Skin Preparation

When reviewing the skin prep procedure with the nurse, you need this information.
- What type of skin prep to do—cleanse the skin, clip hair, shave the skin, or use a hair cream remover
- What site to prep
- What observations to report and record:
  - The area prepped
  - Any cuts, nicks, or scratches
  - Bleeding
  - Sites of non-intact skin
- When to report observations
- What patient concerns to report at once

PROMOTING SAFETY AND COMFORT
Skin Preparation

Safety
Any break in the skin is a possible infection site. Be very careful not to cut, scratch, or nick the skin. Follow Standard Precautions and the Bloodborne Pathogen Standard.

The Surgical Skin Prep—Shaving the Skin

QUALITY OF LIFE

- Knock before entering the person's room.
- Address the person by name.
- Introduce yourself by name and title.
- Explain the procedure before starting and during the procedure.
- Protect the person's rights during the procedure.
- Handle the person gently during the procedure.

PRE-PROCEDURE

1 Follow *Delegation Guidelines: Skin Preparation*. See *Promoting Safety and Comfort: Skin Preparation*.
2 Practice hand hygiene.
3 Collect the following.
  - Skin prep kit
  - Bath blanket
  - Warm water
  - Gloves
  - Waterproof under-pad
  - Bath towel
4 Identify the person. Check the identification (ID) bracelet against the assignment sheet. Use 2 identifiers (Chapter 13). Also call the person by name.
5 Provide for privacy.

Continued

The Surgical Skin Prep—Shaving the Skin—cont'd

PROCEDURE

6 Provide for good lighting.
7 Raise the bed for body mechanics. Lower the bed rail near you (if up).
8 Cover the person with a bath blanket. Fan-fold top linens to the foot of the bed.
9 Position the person for the skin prep.
10 Place the waterproof under-pad under the area you will shave.
11 Open the skin prep kit.
12 Drape him or her with the drape.
13 Add warm water to the basin. Bed rails (if used) are up before you leave the bedside.

14 Put on the gloves.
15 Lather the skin with the sponge.
16 Hold the skin taut. Shave in the direction of hair growth (see Fig. 35-5).
17 Shave outward from the center with short strokes.
18 Rinse the razor often.
19 Make sure the entire area is free of hair. Check for cuts, scratches, or nicks.
20 Rinse the skin thoroughly. Pat dry.
21 Remove the drape and waterproof under-pad.
22 Remove and discard the gloves. Practice hand hygiene.
23 Return top linens. Remove the bath blanket.

POST-PROCEDURE

24 Provide for comfort. (See the inside of the front cover.)
25 Place the call light and other needed items within reach.
26 Lower the bed to a safe and comfortable level for the person. Follow the care plan. Lock (brake) the bed wheels.
27 Raise or lower bed rails. Follow the care plan.
28 Unscreen the person.
29 Return equipment to its proper place.

30 Discard supplies.
31 Complete a safety check of the room. (See the inside of the front cover.)
32 Follow agency policy for used linens.
33 Practice hand hygiene.
34 Tell the nurse that the skin prep is done. Report your observations.

The Surgery Consent

The person's consent is needed for surgery. A surgical consent is signed when the person understands the information given by the doctor. The person's spouse or nearest relative may be required to sign the consent. A parent or legal representative signs for a minor child. The legal representative signs for a person not mentally competent to sign.

The doctor is responsible for securing the written consent. Often this is delegated to a nurse. *You do not obtain the person's written consent for surgery.*

The Pre-Operative Checklist

The pre-operative checklist (Fig. 35-6) is completed before surgery. You may be delegated some things on the list. Promptly report when you complete each task and any observations. The checklist is completed before the nurse gives pre-op drugs.

Marking the Surgical Site.
The doctor marks the surgical site before the surgery. Sometimes the person marks the surgical site. Marking the site prevents surgery on the wrong part.

Site markings may be part of the pre-op checklist. It is done before pre-op drugs are given.

SURGICAL CHECK LIST

Patient's Name   Room

PATIENT STICKER

I.D. Band on	
Surgical Permit Signed	
History & Physical	
Allergies	
Operative Area Prepped	
Pre-op Enema (if ordered)	
NPO after midnight	
Blood Work Done	
Urinalysis	
UCG on females age 12-50	
BP and TRP taken	
Voided and catheterized	
Jewelry removed and secured	
Hairpins, make up and nail polish removed	
Contact lenses and glasses removed	
Dentures removed	
Head cap and gown	
Premedication of _____	
Time given _____	
Date _____ Nurse _____	

IV20064   ©2005 133090 LKCS • www.lk-cs.com

FIGURE 35-6 Pre-operative checklist. (Courtesy Illinois Valley Community Hospital, Peru, Ill.)

Pre-Operative Drugs

Pre-operative drugs are given before transport to the OR. They are given to:
* Help the person relax and feel drowsy.
* Reduce respiratory secretions to prevent aspiration. A dry mouth also results.
* Prevent nausea and vomiting.

The person feels sleepy and light-headed from the drugs. Therefore the person is not allowed out of bed. To help prevent falls, accidents, and damaged equipment:
* Have the person void before the drugs are given. Then have the person use the bedpan or urinal to void.
* Raise the bed rails after the drugs are given.
* Move furniture to make room for the stretcher.
* Clean off the over-bed table and the bedside stand.

Transport to the Operating Room

An OR staff member brings a stretcher to the room. Identification checks are made. Then the patient is transferred to the stretcher and covered with a bath blanket. To prevent falls, safety straps are secured and the side rails raised. If allowed, a pillow is placed under the person's head for comfort.

The person's chart is given to the OR staff member. The person is transported to the OR. The family may be allowed to go as far as the OR entrance.

See *Focus on Children and Older Persons: Transport to the Operating Room.*

FOCUS ON CHILDREN AND OLDER PERSONS

Transport to the Operating Room

Children
Some agencies allow a parent to be with the child while anesthesia is given. The parent stays in the OR until the child is asleep.

SEDATION AND ANESTHESIA

Some procedures only require sedation. *Sedation is a state of quiet, calmness, or sleep produced by a drug.* Levels of sedation are minimal, moderate (conscious), and deep.

Produced by a drug, *anesthesia is the loss of all sensation, especially pain.*
* *General anesthesia is a treatment with certain drugs that produces a deep sleep and the absence of all sensation, especially pain.* Drugs are given IV or inhaled through a gas.
* *Regional anesthesia is the loss of sensation, produced by a drug, in a large area.* The person is awake. A drug is injected into a body part.
* *Local anesthesia is the loss of sensation, produced by a drug, in a small area.* A drug is injected at the site.

An *anesthesiologist* is a doctor who specializes in giving sedation and anesthetics. An *anesthetist* is an RN (registered nurse) with advanced study in giving sedation and anesthetics.

POST-OPERATIVE CARE

After surgery the person is taken to the PACU to begin post-op (post-surgical) care. Recovery from sedation or anesthesia takes 1 to 2 hours. Vital signs are taken and observations are made often. The doctor orders transport to the person's room when:
* Vital signs are stable.
* Respiratory function is good.
* The person can respond and call for help.

Preparing the Person's Room

The person's room must be ready. After the person is taken to the OR, you can:
* Make a surgical bed. Lower the bed rails and raise the bed for a transfer from a stretcher.
* Place equipment and supplies in the room.
  * Thermometer
  * Stethoscope and sphygmomanometer
  * Kidney basin
  * Tissues
  * Waterproof under-pad
  * Vital signs flow sheet
  * I&O (intake and output) record
  * IV pole
  * Other items as directed by the nurse
* Move furniture out of the way for the stretcher.

Return From the PACU

PACU nurses transport the person and a unit nurse meets them in the person's room. Assist as needed with the stretcher-to-bed transfer. Also help position the person.

Vital signs are measured and observations made. They are compared with those taken in the PACU. The nurse checks the surgical site for bleeding. Catheter, IV, and other tube placements and functions are checked. Bed rails are raised. The call light and other needed items are placed within the person's reach. Necessary care and treatments are given. Then the family can be with the person.

Measurements and Observations

Your role in post-op care depends on the person's condition. Often you will measure vital signs and pulse oximetry (Chapter 39) and make post-op observations. These are done:

- Every 15 minutes until the person's condition is stable
- Every 30 minutes for 1 to 2 hours
- Every hour for 4 hours
- Then every 4 hours

The nurse tells you how often to check the person. Many serious complications can result from surgery (Box 35-2). Be alert for the signs and symptoms in Box 35-2. Report them at once.

BOX 35-2   Post-Op Complications and Observations

Complications

- Respiratory System
  - Pneumonia—an inflammation and infection of lung tissue
  - Atelectasis—the collapse of a portion of the lung
  - Pulmonary embolism—a blood clot from a vein that travels (embolus) in the bloodstream until it lodges in a lung
- Circulatory System
  - Hypovolemia—inadequate (hypo) amount (vol) of blood (emia)
  - Hemorrhage—the excessive loss (rrhage) of blood (hemo) in a short time
  - Hypovolemic shock—when organs and tissues do not get enough blood (shock) because of an inadequate (hypo) amount (vol) of blood (emia)
  - Thrombophlebitis—a blood clot (thrombo) causing inflammation (itis) of a vein (phleb)
  - Thrombus—a blood clot
  - Embolus—a blood clot that travels through the vascular system until it lodges in a blood vessel
- Urinary System
  - Urinary retention—urine collects (retention) in the bladder from being unable to void
  - Urinary tract infection—inflammation and infection of the urinary structures (bladder, ureters, urethra)
- Gastro-Intestinal System
  - Nausea
  - Vomiting
  - Constipation
  - Flatulence
  - Post-operative ileus—the absence of normal intestinal (ileus) function from the lack of peristalsis after surgery
- Wound (Chapter 36)
  - Infection
  - Dehiscence—the separation of wound layers
  - Evisceration—the separation of the wound along with the protrusion of abdominal organs

Observations

- Abdominal: distention (swelling); pain; cramping
- Aching
- Anxiety
- Bleeding: from the incision, drainage tubes, suction tubes, or other sites
- Blood pressure: increase or decrease
- Chest pain
- Choking
- Condition: any change in

Observations—cont'd

- Confusion
- Cough: weak
- Discomfort in a leg
- Disorientation
- Drainage:
  - From wound (Chapter 36)
  - On or under dressings
  - On bed linens (including bottom linens and pillowcases)
  - Appearance from urinary catheter, NG tube, wound suction, and other tubes
- Hypoxia (Chapter 39)
- Intake and output
- IV flow rate
- Nausea
- Pain
- Pulse:
  - More than 100 beats per minute
  - Less than 60 beats per minute
  - Weak
  - Irregular
- Pulse oximetry measurement (Chapter 39)
- Respirations:
  - Shallow, slow breathing
  - Rapid
  - Gasping
  - Difficult (dyspnea)
  - Shortness of breath
  - Moist-sounding
  - Gurgling
- Restlessness
- Skin:
  - Moist or clammy
  - Pale (pallor)
  - Cyanosis (bluish color)
  - Cool
  - Warm or hot
- Sputum: clear, white, yellow, green, brown, or red; thick, watery, or frothy (with bubbles)
- Swelling in affected area
- Temperature: increase or decrease
- Thirst
- Urinary complaints: cannot void, burning, urgency, lower abdominal pain
- Urine: amount, character, and time of first voiding after surgery
- Vomiting

Positioning

The person is positioned for comfort and to prevent complications. Position restrictions may be ordered after some surgeries. The person is usually positioned:

- For easy and comfortable breathing
- To prevent stress on the incision
- To prevent aspiration

When supine, the head of the bed is usually raised slightly. The person's head may be turned to the side.

The person is re-positioned at least every 1 to 2 hours. This prevents respiratory and circulatory complications. Turning may be painful. Provide support. Use smooth, gentle motions. Place pillows and positioning devices as the nurse directs (Chapters 17 and 30).

The nurse tells you when to re-position the person and the positions allowed. Usually you assist the nurse. The nurse may delegate these tasks when the person is stable and care is simple.

See *Focus on Children and Older Persons: Positioning.*

Preventing Respiratory and Circulatory Complications

Coughing and deep-breathing exercises help prevent respiratory complications, including post-operative pneumonia (see Box 35-2). So does incentive spirometry. See Chapter 39.

Circulation must be stimulated for blood flow in the legs. If blood flow is sluggish, blood clots may form. They can form in the deep leg veins in the lower leg or thigh (Fig. 35-7, *A*). Many people do not have signs or symptoms. Report the following at once.

- Swollen area of a leg.
- Pain or tenderness in a leg. This may occur only when standing or walking.
- Warmth in the part of the leg that is swollen or painful.
- Red or discolored skin.

A *blood clot* (**thrombus**) can break loose and travel through the bloodstream. It then becomes an embolus. An **embolus** *is a blood clot that travels through the vascular system until it lodges in a blood vessel* (Fig. 35-7, *B*). An embolus from a vein lodges in the lungs (pulmonary embolism) and can cause severe respiratory problems and death. Report chest pain or shortness of breath at once.

Circulation is stimulated and thrombi prevented by:

- Leg exercises
- Ambulation as soon as possible
- Elastic stockings (p. 598)
- Elastic bandages (p. 600)
- Sequential compression devices (p. 601)
- No prolonged standing or sitting

See *Focus on Children and Older Persons: Preventing Respiratory and Circulatory Complications.*

See *Promoting Safety and Comfort: Preventing Respiratory and Circulatory Complications.*

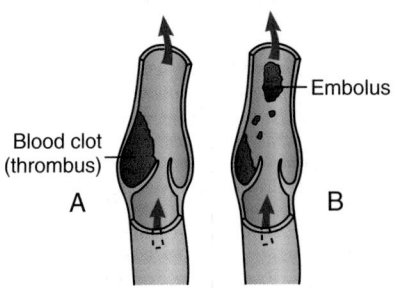

FIGURE 35-7 A, A blood clot is attached to the wall of a vein. The *arrows* show the direction of blood flow. **B,** Part of the thrombus breaks off and becomes an embolus. The embolus travels through the vascular system until it lodges in a distant blood vessel.

Leg Exercises. Leg exercises increase venous blood flow and help prevent thrombi. After leg surgery, the doctor orders needed exercises.

The nurse tells you when to do the exercises. They are done at least every 1 or 2 hours while the person is awake. Assist if the person is weak. These exercises are done 5 times.

- Make circles with the toes. This rotates the ankles.
- Dorsiflex and plantar flex the feet (Chapter 30).
- Flex and extend 1 knee and then the other (Fig. 35-8, *A*).
- Raise and lower the leg off the bed (Fig. 35-8, *B*). Repeat with the other leg.

Elastic Stockings. Elastic stockings exert pressure on the veins. The pressure promotes venous blood return to the heart. The stockings help prevent blood clots in leg veins. Elastic stockings also are called AE stockings (AE means *anti-embolism* or *anti-embolic*). They also are called TED hose (TED means *thrombo-embolic disease*). Persons at risk for thrombi include those who:

- Have heart and circulatory disorders.
- Are on bedrest.
- Have had surgery.
- Are older.
- Are pregnant.

Stockings come in thigh-high and knee-high lengths. The nurse measures the person for the correct size. The opening near the toes is used to check circulation, skin color, and skin temperature.

The person usually has 2 pairs of stockings. Wash 1 pair while the other pair is worn. Wash them by hand with a mild soap. Hang them to dry.

See *Delegation Guidelines: Elastic Stockings.*
See *Promoting Safety and Comfort: Elastic Stockings.*
See procedure: *Applying Elastic Stockings.*

DELEGATION GUIDELINES

Elastic Stockings

To apply elastic stockings, you need this information from the nurse and the care plan.

- What size to use—small, medium, large, extra-large, or bariatric
- What length to use—thigh-high or knee-high
- When to remove them and for how long—usually every 8 hours for 30 minutes
- What observations to report and record:
  - The size and length of stockings applied
  - When you applied the stockings
  - Skin color and temperature
  - Leg and foot swelling
  - Skin tears, wounds, or signs of skin breakdown
  - Complaints of pain, tingling, or numbness
  - When you removed the stockings and for how long
  - When you re-applied the stockings
  - When you washed the stockings
- When to report observations
- What patient or resident concerns to report at once

PROMOTING SAFETY AND COMFORT

Elastic Stockings

Safety

Apply the stocking so the toe opening is over the top of the toes or under the toes. Follow the manufacturer's instructions. Use the opening to check circulation, skin color, and skin temperature in the toes.

Stockings should not have twists, creases, or wrinkles after you apply them. Twists can affect circulation. So can stockings that roll or bunch up. Creases and wrinkles can cause skin breakdown.

Loose stockings do not promote venous blood return to the heart. Stockings that are too tight can affect circulation. Tell the nurse if the stockings are too loose or too tight.

Comfort

Apply stockings before the person gets out of bed. Otherwise the person's legs can swell from sitting or standing. Stockings are hard to put on when the legs are swollen. The person lies in bed while they are off. This prevents the legs from swelling.

Gently handle and move the person's foot and leg. Do not force the joints (toes, foot, ankle, knee, and hip) beyond their range of motion or to the point of pain.

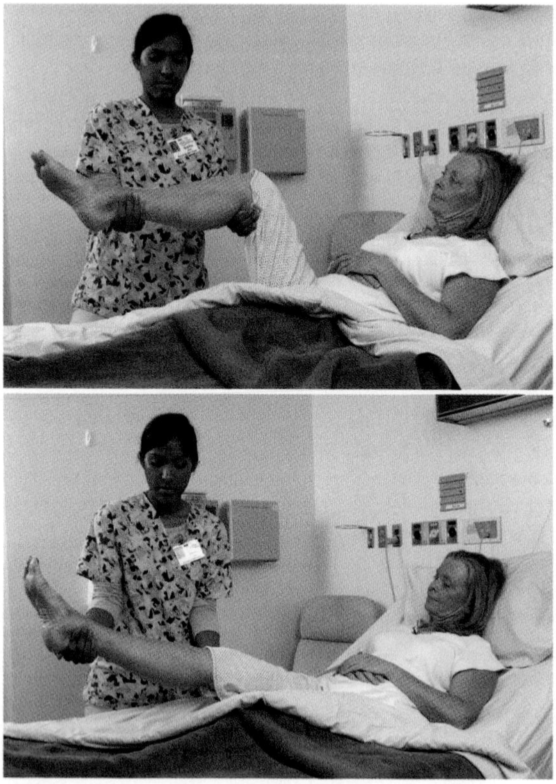

FIGURE 35-8 Leg exercises to stimulate circulation. **A,** The knee is flexed and then extended. **B,** The leg is raised and lowered.

Applying Elastic Stockings

QUALITY OF LIFE

- Knock before entering the person's room.
- Address the person by name.
- Introduce yourself by name and title.

- Explain the procedure before starting and during the procedure.
- Protect the person's rights during the procedure.
- Handle the person gently during the procedure.

PRE-PROCEDURE

1 Follow *Delegation Guidelines: Elastic Stockings.* See *Promoting Safety and Comfort: Elastic Stockings.*
2 Practice hand hygiene.
3 Obtain elastic stockings in the correct size and length. Note the location of the toe opening.

4 Identify the person. Check the ID bracelet against the assignment sheet. Use 2 identifiers (Chapter 13). Also call the person by name.
5 Provide for privacy.
6 Raise the bed for body mechanics. Bed rails are up if used.

PROCEDURE

7 Lower the bed rail.
8 Position the person supine.
9 Expose 1 leg. Fan-fold top linens toward the other leg.
10 Gather or turn the stocking inside out down to the heel.
11 Slip the foot of the stocking over the toes, foot, and heel (Fig. 35-9, *A*). Make sure the heel pocket is properly positioned on the person's heel. The toe opening is over or under the toes.
12 Grasp the stocking top. Roll or pull the stocking up the leg. It turns right side out as it is rolled or pulled up.

13 Make sure the stocking does not cause pressure on the toes. Adjust the stocking as needed.
14 Remove twists, creases, or wrinkles. Make sure the stocking is even, snug, smooth, and wrinkle-free (Fig. 35-9, *B*).
15 Cover the leg. Repeat steps 9 through 14 for the other leg.
16 Cover the person.

POST-PROCEDURE

17 Provide for comfort. (See the inside of the front cover.)
18 Place the call light and other needed items within reach.
19 Lower the bed to a safe and comfortable level for the person. Follow the care plan.
20 Raise or lower bed rails. Follow the care plan.

21 Unscreen the person.
22 Complete a safety check of the room. (See the inside of the front cover.)
23 Practice hand hygiene.
24 Report and record your observations.

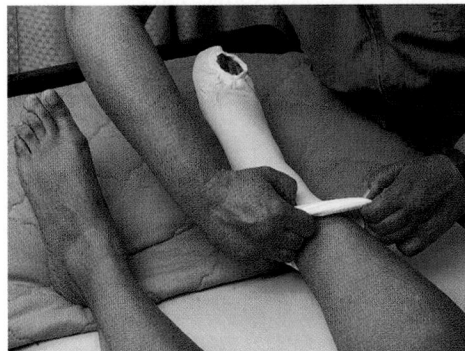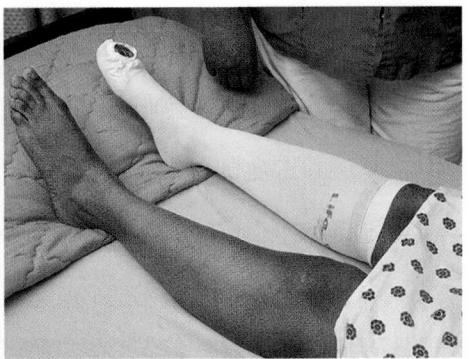

A   B

FIGURE 35-9 Applying elastic stockings. **A,** The stocking is slipped over the toes, foot, and heel. **B,** The stocking turns right side out as it is pulled up over the leg. The heel is positioned in the heel pocket of the stocking.

Elastic Bandages. Elastic bandages have the same purposes as elastic stockings. They also provide support and reduce swelling from injuries. Sometimes they are used to hold dressings in place. They are applied to arms and legs. When applying bandages:

- Use the correct size—length and width.
- Position the person in good alignment.
- Face the person during the procedure.
- Start at the lower (*distal*) part of the extremity. Work upward to the top (*proximal*) part.
- Expose the fingers or toes if possible. This allows circulation checks.
- Apply the bandage with firm, even pressure.
- Check the color and temperature of the extremity every hour.
- Re-apply a loose or wrinkled bandage.
- Replace a moist or soiled bandage.
  See *Focus on Communication: Elastic Bandages.*
  See *Delegation Guidelines: Elastic Bandages.*
  See *Promoting Safety and Comfort: Elastic Bandages.*
  See procedure: *Applying an Elastic Bandage.*

DELEGATION GUIDELINES
Elastic Bandages

To apply elastic bandages, you need this information from the nurse and the care plan.
- Where to apply the bandage
- What width and length to use
- When to remove the bandage and for how long—usually every 8 hours for 30 minutes
- What to do if the bandage is wet or soiled
- What observations to report and record:
  - The width and length applied
  - When you applied the bandage
  - Skin color and temperature
  - Swelling of the part
  - Skin tears, wounds, or signs of skin breakdown
  - Complaints of pain, itching, tingling, or numbness
  - When you removed the bandage and for how long
  - When you re-applied the bandage
- When to report observations
- What patient or resident concerns to report at once

FOCUS ON COMMUNICATION
Elastic Bandages

Elastic bandages should promote comfort. To check for comfort, you can ask:
- "Does the bandage feel too tight?"
- "Do you feel pain, itching, or numbness?" If yes: "What do you feel?" "Where do you feel it?"

PROMOTING SAFETY AND COMFORT
Elastic Bandages

Safety
Elastic bandages must be firm and snug but not tight. A tight bandage can affect circulation.

Bandages are secured in place with clips, tape, or Velcro. Clips are made of metal or plastic. Clips can injure the skin if they become loose, fall off, or cause pressure. Use clips only if the nurse tells you to. Check the bandage often to make sure the clips are correctly in place.

Some agencies do not allow you to apply elastic bandages. Know your agency's policy.

Comfort
A tight bandage can cause pain and discomfort. Apply it with firm, even pressure. If the person complains of pain, tingling, or numbness, remove the bandage. Tell the nurse at once.

Applying an Elastic Bandage

QUALITY OF LIFE

- Knock before entering the person's room.
- Address the person by name.
- Introduce yourself by name and title.

- Explain the procedure before starting and during the procedure.
- Protect the person's rights during the procedure.
- Handle the person gently during the procedure.

PRE-PROCEDURE

1 Follow *Delegation Guidelines: Elastic Bandages.* See *Promoting Safety and Comfort: Elastic Bandages.*
2 Practice hand hygiene.
3 Collect the following.
   - Elastic bandage as directed by the nurse
   - Tape or clips (unless the bandage has Velcro)

4 Identify the person. Check the ID bracelet against the assignment sheet. Use 2 identifiers (Chapter 13). Also call the person by name.
5 Provide for privacy.
6 Raise the bed for body mechanics. Bed rails are up if used.

Applying an Elastic Bandage—cont'd

PROCEDURE

7 Lower the bed rail near you if up.
8 Help the person to a comfortable position. Expose the part you will bandage.
9 Make sure the area is clean and dry.
10 Hold the bandage so the roll is up. The loose end is on the bottom (Fig. 35-10, A).
11 Apply the bandage to the smallest part of the wrist, foot, ankle, or knee.
12 Make 2 circular turns around the part (Fig. 35-10, B).
13 Make over-lapping spiral turns in an upward direction. Each turn over-laps ½ to ¾ of the previous turn (Fig. 35-10, C). Each over-lap is equal.

14 Apply the bandage smoothly with firm, even pressure. It is not tight.
15 End the bandage with 2 circular turns.
16 Secure the bandage in place with Velcro, tape, or clips. Clips are not under the body part.
17 Check the fingers or toes for coldness or cyanosis (bluish color). Ask about pain, itching, numbness, or tingling. Remove the bandage if any are noted. Report your observations.

POST-PROCEDURE

18 Provide for comfort. (See the inside of the front cover.)
19 Place the call light and other needed items within reach.
20 Lower the bed to a safe and comfortable level for the person. Follow the care plan.
21 Raise or lower bed rails. Follow the care plan.

22 Unscreen the person.
23 Complete a safety check of the room. (See the inside of the front cover.)
24 Practice hand hygiene.
25 Report and record your observations.

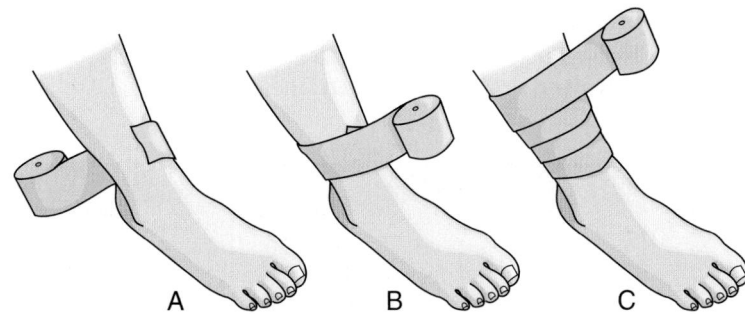

FIGURE 35-10 Applying an elastic bandage. **A,** The bandage roll is up. The loose end is at the bottom. **B,** The bandage is applied to the smallest part with 2 circular turns. **C,** The bandage is applied with spiral turns in an upward direction.

Sequential Compression Devices. A sequential compression device (SCD) is a sleeve that straps around the leg (Fig. 35-11). Made of cloth or plastic, the SCD is secured in place with Velcro. Elastic stockings are often worn under SCDs.

A pump inflates the device with air. This promotes venous blood flow to the heart by causing pressure on the veins. Then the pump deflates the device.

SCDs are applied to both legs. After 1 side deflates, the other inflates. Applied pre-op, SCDs are worn post-op until the doctor orders removal.

Early Ambulation

Early ambulation prevents complications such as thrombi, pneumonia, atelectasis, constipation, and urinary tract infections. The person usually walks in the room or hallway the day of surgery. The person dangles (sits on the side of the bed) first. Blood pressure and pulse are measured. If they are stable, the person is assisted out of bed.

The nurse tells you when the person can walk and how far to go. Distance increases as the person gains strength. Usually you assist the nurse the first time.

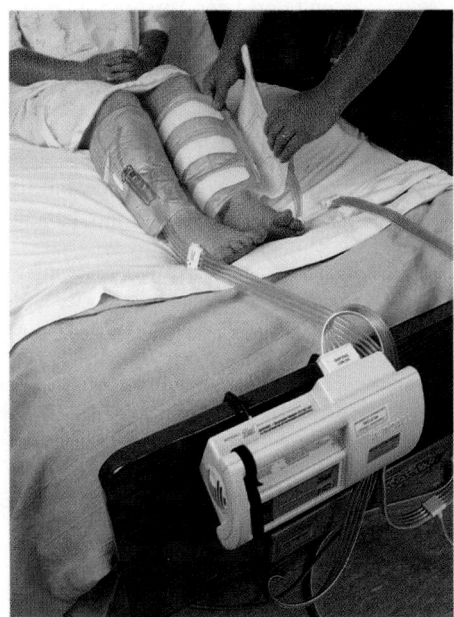

FIGURE 35-11 Sequential compression device. (From deWit SC: *Fundamental concepts and skills for nursing,* Philadelphia, 2001, Saunders.)

Wound Healing

The incision needs protection to promote healing and prevent infection. A dressing may be over the incision. Sterile dressing changes are done by the doctor or nurse. Your agency may let you do simple dressing changes. See Chapter 36 for wound care.

Nutrition and Fluids. The person returns from the OR with an IV. Continued IV therapy depends on the type of surgery and the person's condition. Anesthesia may cause nausea and vomiting. Diet progresses from NPO to clear liquids, to full liquids, to a regular diet. Frequent oral hygiene is important while NPO.

Some patients have NG tubes (Chapter 28). Often the NG tube is attached to suction to keep the stomach empty. The person is NPO and has an IV.

Elimination

Anesthesia, the surgery, and being NPO affect bowel and urinary elimination. Pain-relief drugs can cause constipation. Provide measures to promote elimination as directed by the nurse and the care plan (Chapters 24 and 26).

Intake and output are measured. The person must void within 8 hours after surgery. Report the time and amount of the first voiding. If the person does not void within 8 hours, a catheter may be needed. Some patients have a catheter after surgery. See Chapter 25.

Fluid intake and a regular diet are needed for bowel elimination. Suppositories or enemas may be ordered for constipation.

Comfort and Rest

Pain is common after surgery. The degree of pain depends on:
- The extent of surgery.
- The incision site and size.
- If drainage tubes, casts, or other devices are present.
- Positioning during surgery. The position can cause muscle strains and discomfort.

The doctor orders pain-relief drugs. The nurse uses the nursing process to promote comfort and rest. Many of the measures listed in Chapter 31 are part of the person's care plan.

Personal Hygiene

Personal hygiene is important for well-being. Wound drainage and skin prep solutions can irritate the skin and cause discomfort. NPO causes a dry mouth and breath odors. Moist, clammy skin from blood pressure changes or fever also cause discomfort.

Frequent oral hygiene, hair care, and a complete bed bath after surgery help refresh and renew the person. The gown and linens are changed when wet or soiled.

FOCUS ON **PRIDE**

The Person, Family, and Yourself

Personal and Professional Responsibility

Worries and fears about surgery are common. What worries would you have—pain, loss of function, death, caring for your children and home, supporting your family? Imagine having an accident. You wake up hours later. You are told that your right leg was amputated.

The person's fears and concerns are important. Take time to listen. Avoid seeming rushed. Act professionally. Take pride in showing that you care.

Rights and Respect

Before surgery, the doctor and nurse explain what to expect. The person or family may forget to ask a question. Or they need something explained again.

The person has the right to accurate and complete information. The person's questions are important. The person or family may ask you questions. You can answer questions that relate to the care you provide. If you do not know or are unsure of an answer, explain that you will ask the nurse. Some questions are best answered by the nurse. For example: "How long will the surgery last?" or "What will be done for pain after surgery?" Even if you know the answer, say that you will ask the nurse to answer the question. Show good judgment. Only answer questions within the scope of your role.

Independence and Social Interaction

Some people prefer to be alone before and after surgery. Peace and quiet help them relax. Others want family and friends around. They like the support and the conversation distracts from worries and pain. Each person is different. Ask what the person prefers. Tell the nurse. The nurse can talk with the family about the person's wishes and needs.

Delegation and Teamwork

Post-op observation is a critical time. You may be delegated parts of the post-op care. For example, you are asked to monitor vital signs. Vital signs must be checked and reported or recorded promptly, as ordered. Delays risk missing critical changes early.

The patient and nurse rely on you. Complete post-op vital signs on time. Report abnormal values, sudden changes, and any concerns at once. Take pride in your role in post-op care. You can make a difference in the safety and quality of the person's care.

Ethics and Laws

The pre-op checklist has items to be completed before surgery. Some tasks are done by the nurse. Others you can do. See Figure 35-6. Know the tasks you are responsible for and what the nurse must do. For example, you do not obtain written consent for surgery or mark the surgical site.

Always follow agency policy and the limits of your role. Never accept a task outside those limits. You can lose your job or your ability to work as a nursing assistant. Only perform the tasks you are trained and allowed to do.

FOCUS ON **PRIDE**: *Application*

Surgery is stressful. Your attitude and conduct affect the person's experience. You can either ease worries or increase stress. Explain how your behavior affects the person's outlook and comfort.

REVIEW QUESTIONS

Circle **T** *if the statement is TRUE or* **F** *if it is FALSE.*

1 **T F** Pins, clips, or combs are used to keep the hair out of the face during surgery.

2 **T F** Nail polish is removed before surgery.

3 **T F** Make-up can be worn to the OR.

4 **T F** Pajamas are worn to the OR.

5 **T F** Contact lenses are removed in the OR.

6 **T F** A surgical bed is made for the return from the PACU.

7 **T F** A decrease in blood pressure is reported at once.

8 **T F** The person walks for the first time 2 days after surgery.

9 **T F** Intake and output are measured after surgery.

10 **T F** The person should void within 8 hours after surgery.

Circle the BEST answer.

11 Which is true of elective surgery?
  a It is done at once.
  b The need is sudden and not expected.
  c It is scheduled at a later date.
  d General anesthesia is always used.

12 A person states: "I'm afraid of surgery." What should you do?
  a Call a member of the clergy.
  b Listen and use touch.
  c Change the subject.
  d Tell the family.

13 You assist with pre-op care by explaining
  a The reason for the surgery
  b The procedures you are doing
  c The risks and possible complications
  d What to expect during and after surgery

14 Before surgery, a person is
  a NPO
  b Allowed only water
  c Given breakfast
  d Given a tube feeding

15 A bowel prep is ordered to
  a Prevent bleeding
  b Relieve flatus
  c Prevent pain
  d Clean the intestines of feces

16 A skin prep is done to
  a Bathe the body completely
  b Sterilize the skin
  c Reduce the amount of microbes on the skin
  d Destroy non-pathogens and pathogens

17 When shaving the skin
  a Shave in the direction opposite of hair growth
  b Shave toward the center of the operative site
  c Do not cut, scratch, or nick the skin
  d Keep the skin loose

18 Pre-op drugs were given. The patient
  a Must stay in bed
  b Can use the bathroom
  c Can use the commode to void
  d Can have sips of water

19 General anesthesia is
  a A specially educated nurse
  b A treatment causing deep sleep and absence of sensation
  c A treatment causing loss of sensation in a body part
  d A specially educated doctor

20 Coughing and deep breathing after surgery prevent
  a Bleeding
  b A pulmonary embolus
  c Respiratory complications
  d Pain and discomfort

21 Leg exercises
  a Stimulate circulation and prevent thrombi
  b Are done only for leg surgery
  c Are done every 4 hours
  d Are not done if elastic stockings are worn

22 Post-op, a person's position is changed at least
  a Every 2 hours
  b Every 3 hours
  c Every 4 hours
  d Every shift

23 Elastic stockings
  a Hold dressings in place
  b Reduce swelling after injury
  c Prevent pressure ulcers
  d Prevent blood clots

24 Elastic stockings are applied
  a When the person is standing
  b Before the person gets out of bed
  c After the person's shower or bath
  d For 30 minutes and then removed

25 The purpose of an elastic bandage is to
  a Prevent infection
  b Absorb drainage
  c Provide moisture for wound healing
  d Reduce swelling

26 When applying an elastic bandage
  a Position the part in good alignment
  b Cover the fingers or toes if possible
  c Apply it from the large to small part of the extremity
  d Apply it from the upper to lower part of the extremity

Answers to Chapter 35 questions are on p. 871.

FOCUS ON **PRACTICE**

Problem Solving

You are measuring a post-op patient's vital signs. The person is restless. The vital signs are similar to previous measurements. What do you do? Is there anything you need to report? If so, when?

OBJECTIVES

- Define the key terms and key abbreviations in this chapter.
- Describe skin tears, circulatory ulcers, and diabetic foot ulcers and the persons at risk.
- Explain how to help prevent skin tears, circulatory ulcers, and diabetic foot ulcers.
- Describe the process and complications of wound healing.
- Describe what to observe about wounds.
- Explain how to secure dressings.

- Explain the rules for applying dressings.
- Explain the purpose of binders and compression garments and how to apply them.
- Describe how to meet the basic needs of persons with wounds.
- Perform the procedure described in this chapter.
- Explain how to promote PRIDE in the person, the family, and yourself.

KEY TERMS

abrasion A partial-thickness wound caused by the scraping away or rubbing of the skin

arterial ulcer An open wound on the lower legs or feet caused by poor arterial blood flow

chronic wound A wound that does not heal easily

circulatory ulcer An open sore on the lower legs or feet caused by decreased blood flow through the arteries or veins; vascular ulcer

clean-contaminated wound Occurs from the surgical entry of the reproductive, urinary, respiratory, or gastro-intestinal system

clean wound A wound that is not infected

closed wound Tissues are injured but the skin is not broken

contaminated wound A wound with a high risk of infection

contusion A closed wound caused by a blow to the body; a bruise

dehiscence The separation of wound layers

diabetic foot ulcer An open wound on the foot caused by complications from diabetes

dirty wound See "infected wound"

edema Swelling caused by fluid collecting in tissues

evisceration The separation of the wound along with the protrusion of abdominal organs

excoriation Loss of the epidermis (top skin layer) caused by scratching or when skin rubs against skin, clothing, or other material

full-thickness wound The dermis, epidermis, and subcutaneous tissue are penetrated; muscle and bone may be involved

gangrene A condition in which there is death of tissue

hematoma A swelling *(oma)* that contains blood *(hemat)*

hemorrhage The excessive loss *(rrhage)* of blood *(hemo)* in a short time

incision A cut produced surgically by a sharp instrument; it creates an opening into an organ or body space

infected wound A wound containing large amounts of microbes that shows signs of infection; dirty wound

intentional wound A wound created for therapy

laceration An open wound with torn tissues and jagged edges

open wound The skin or mucous membrane is broken

partial-thickness wound The dermis and epidermis of the skin are broken

penetrating wound An open wound that breaks the skin and enters a body area, organ, or cavity

phlebitis Inflammation *(itis)* of a vein *(phleb)*

puncture wound An open wound made by a sharp object

purulent drainage Thick green, yellow, or brown drainage

sanguineous drainage Bloody *(sanguis)* drainage

serosanguineous drainage Thin, watery drainage *(sero)* that is blood-tinged *(sanguineous)*

serous drainage Clear, watery fluid *(serum)*

shock Results when tissues and organs do not get enough blood

skin tear A break or rip in the outer layers of the skin; the epidermis (top skin layer) separates from the underlying tissues

stasis ulcer See "venous ulcer"

trauma An accident or violent act that injures the skin, mucous membranes, bones, and organs

ulcer A shallow or deep crater-like sore of the skin or mucous membrane

unintentional wound A wound resulting from trauma

vascular ulcer See "circulatory ulcer"

venous ulcer An open sore on the lower legs or feet caused by poor venous blood flow; stasis ulcer

wound A break in the skin or mucous membrane

KEY ABBREVIATIONS

GI	Gastro-intestinal	**PPE**	Personal protective equipment

A *wound* is a break in the skin or mucous membrane. Wounds commonly result from:

- Surgery.
- *Trauma*—*an accident or violent act that injures the skin, mucous membranes, bones, and organs.* Falls, vehicle crashes, gunshots, stabbings, bites, burns, and frostbite are examples.
- Unrelieved pressure or friction (Chapter 37).
- Decreased blood flow through the arteries or veins.
- Nerve damage.

Wounds are portals of entry for microbes. Infection is a major threat. Wound care includes preventing infection and further injury to the wound and nearby tissues. Blood loss and pain also are prevented. Box 36-1 describes wound types and causes.

The nurse uses the nursing process to keep the person's skin healthy. Some agencies have wound therapists or skin care teams to manage all skin problems. The team includes an RN (registered nurse), physical therapist, and dietitian.

See *Promoting Safety and Comfort: Wound Care.*

PROMOTING SAFETY AND COMFORT

Wound Care

Safety

Wound care may involve contact with blood, body fluids, secretions, or excretions. Follow Standard Precautions and the Bloodborne Pathogen Standard. Wear personal protective equipment (PPE) as needed. Gloves, gowns, masks, and eye protection are necessary when blood splashes and splatters are likely.

BOX 36-1	**Wound Causes and Types**

Causes

- *Abrasion*—*a partial-thickness wound caused by the scraping away or rubbing of the skin* (Fig. 36-1, p. 606).
- *Excoriation*—*loss of the epidermis (top skin layer) caused by scratching or when skin rubs against skin, clothing, or other material* (Fig. 36-2, p. 606).
- *Contusion*—*a closed wound caused by a blow to the body (a bruise)* (Fig. 36-3, p. 606).
- *Incision*—*a cut produced surgically by a sharp instrument. It creates an opening into an organ or body space* (Fig. 36-4, p. 606).
- *Laceration*—*an open wound with torn tissues and jagged edges* (Fig. 36-5, p. 606).
- *Penetrating wound*—*an open wound that breaks the skin and enters a body area, organ, or cavity* (Fig. 36-6, p. 606).
- *Puncture wound*—*an open wound made by a sharp object (knife, nail, metal, wood, glass).* See Figure 36-7, p. 606.
- *Ulcer*—*a shallow or deep crater-like sore of the skin or mucous membrane* (p. 608).

Types

- Intentional and unintentional wounds
  - *Intentional wound*—*is created for therapy.* Surgical incisions are examples. So are venipunctures for starting intravenous therapy and drawing blood specimens.
  - *Unintentional wound*—*results from trauma.*
- Open and closed wounds
  - *Open wound*—*the skin or mucous membrane is broken.* Intentional and most unintentional wounds are open.
  - *Closed wound*—*tissues are injured but the skin is not broken.* Bruises, twists, and sprains are examples.

- Clean and dirty wounds
  - *Clean wound*—*is not infected.* Microbes have not entered the wound. Closed wounds are usually clean. So are intentional wounds made into sterile body areas. The reproductive, urinary, respiratory, and gastro-intestinal (GI) systems are not entered.
  - *Clean-contaminated wound*—*occurs from the surgical entry of the reproductive, urinary, respiratory, or GI system.* Some or all parts of these systems are not sterile and contain normal flora.
  - *Contaminated wound*—*has a high risk of infection.* Unintentional wounds are usually contaminated. Contamination occurs from breaks in surgical asepsis, spillage of intestinal contents, and trauma. Tissues may show signs of inflammation.
  - *Infected wound (dirty wound)*—*contains large amounts of microbes and shows signs of infection.* Examples include old wounds, surgical incisions into infected areas, and trauma that ruptures the bowel.
  - *Chronic wound*—*does not heal easily.* Pressure ulcers and circulatory ulcers are examples.
- Partial- and full-thickness wounds (describe wound depth)
  - *Partial-thickness wound*—*the dermis and epidermis of the skin are broken.*
  - *Full-thickness wound*—*the dermis, epidermis, and subcutaneous tissue are penetrated.* Muscle and bone may be involved.

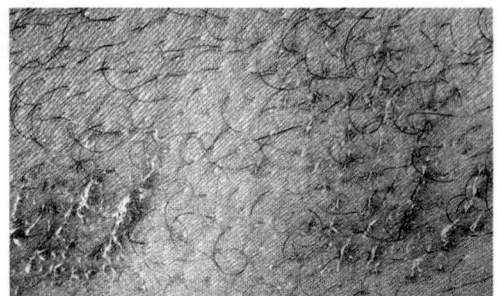

FIGURE 36-1 An abrasion. (From Kumar V, Abbas AK, Fausto N: *Robbins and Cotran pathologic basis of disease*, ed 7, Philadelphia, 2005, Saunders.)

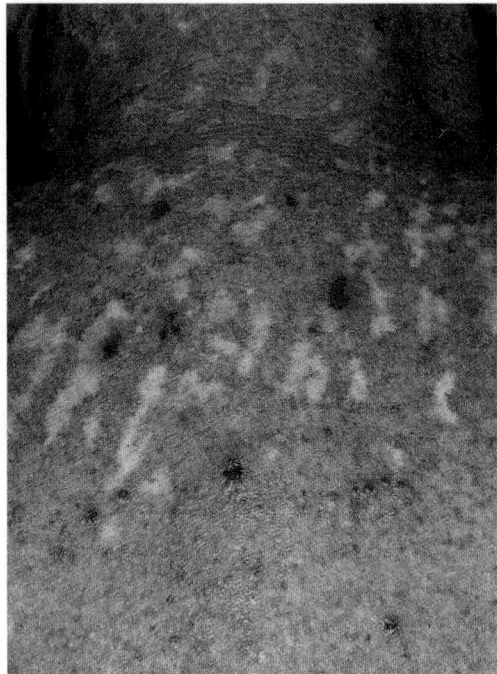

FIGURE 36-2 Excoriation. (From Habif TP: *Clinical dermatology: a color guide to diagnosis and therapy*, ed 4, St Louis, 2004, Mosby.)

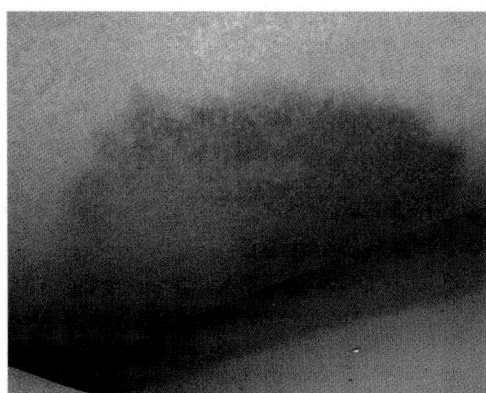

FIGURE 36-3 Contusion. (From Finkbeiner W, Ursell P, Davis R: *Autopsy pathology: a manual and atlas*, London, 2004, Churchill Livingstone.)

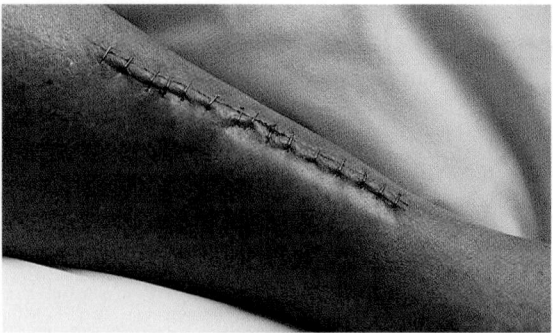

FIGURE 36-4 A surgical incision closed with staples. (From Perry AG, Potter PA, Ostendorf WR: *Nursing intervention and clinical skills*, ed 6, St Louis, 2016, Mosby.)

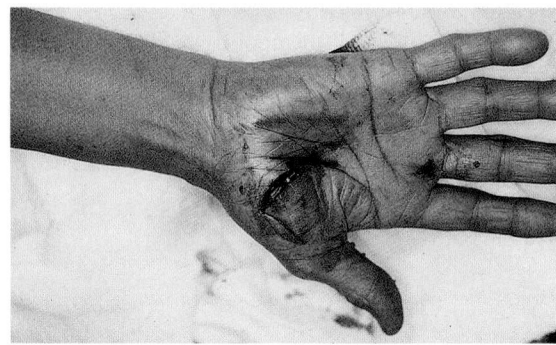

FIGURE 36-5 Laceration. (From Roberts JR, Hedges JR: *Clinical procedures in emergency medicine*, ed 5, St Louis, 2009, Saunders.)

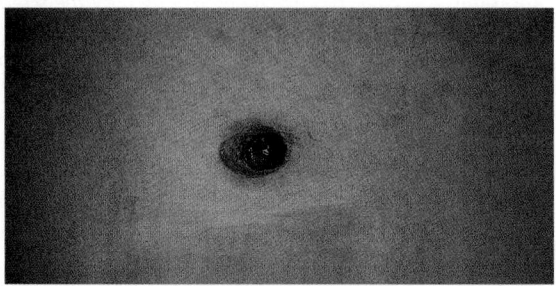

FIGURE 36-6 Penetrating wound. (From McCance KL, Huether SE: *Pathophysiology: the biologic basis for disease in adults and children*, ed 6, St Louis, 2010, Mosby.)

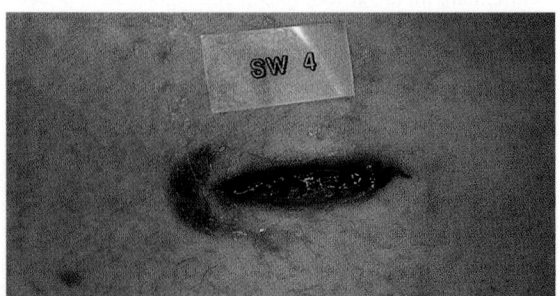

FIGURE 36-7 Puncture wound. (From McCance KL, Huether SE: *Pathophysiology: the biologic basis for disease in adults and children*, ed 6, St Louis, 2010, Mosby.)

SKIN TEARS

A *skin tear* is a break or rip in the outer layers of the skin (Fig. 36-8). *The epidermis (top skin layer) separates from the underlying tissues* (Chapter 10). The skin is "peeled back." The hands, arms, and lower legs are common sites for skin tears. Very thin and fragile skin is common in older persons. Slight pressure can cause a skin tear.

Causes

Skin tears are caused by:
- Friction, shearing (Chapter 18), pulling, or pressure on the skin.
- Falls or bumping a hand, arm, or leg on any hard surface. Beds, bed rails, chairs, wheelchair parts, walkers, and tables are dangers.
- Holding an arm or leg too tight.
- Removing tape or adhesives.
- Bathing, dressing, and other tasks.
- Pulling buttons and zippers across fragile skin.
- Jewelry—yours or the person's. Rings, watches, and bracelets are examples.
- Long or jagged fingernails (yours or the person's) and long or jagged toenails.

Skin tears are painful. They are portals of entry for microbes. Infection is a risk. Tell the nurse at once if you cause or find a skin tear.

Persons at Risk

Persons at risk for skin tears:
- Need help moving.
- Have poor nutrition.
- Have poor hydration.
- Have altered mental awareness.
- Are very thin.

See *Focus on Children and Older Persons: Persons at Risk (Skin Tears).*

Prevention and Treatment

Careful and safe care helps prevent skin tears and further injury. Follow the measures in Box 36-2. Also follow the care plan and the nurse's directions. They may include dressings (p. 614) and elastic bandages (Chapter 35) to protect the skin and promote healing.

FOCUS ON CHILDREN AND OLDER PERSONS

Persons at Risk (Skin Tears)

Older Persons

Persons who are confused may resist care. They often move quickly and without warning. Or they pull away during care. Some try to hit or kick. These sudden movements can cause skin tears.

Never force care on a person. Chapter 49 describes how to care for persons who are confused and resist care. Always follow the care plan.

BOX 36-2   Preventing Skin Tears

- Follow the care plan and safety rules to:
  - Move, turn, position, or transfer the person.
    - Prevent shearing and friction.
    - Use an assist device to move and turn the person in bed.
    - Use pillows to support arms and legs.
  - Pad bed rails and wheelchair arms, footplates, and leg supports.
  - Bathe the person.
  - Keep the skin moisturized and apply lotion.
  - Offer fluids.
- Keep your fingernails short and smoothly filed.
- Keep the person's fingernails short and smoothly filed. Report long, tough, or jagged toenails.
- Do not wear rings with large or raised stones. Do not wear bracelets.
- Be patient and calm when the person is confused, agitated, or resists care.
- Dress and undress the person carefully.
- Dress the person in soft clothes with long sleeves and long pants.
- Apply arm or leg protectors as ordered (Fig. 36-9).
- Provide good lighting so the person can see. The person needs to avoid bumping into furniture, walls, and equipment.
- Provide a safe area for wandering (Chapter 49).
- Remove tape carefully (p. 616).
- Do not apply adhesive tape (p. 615).

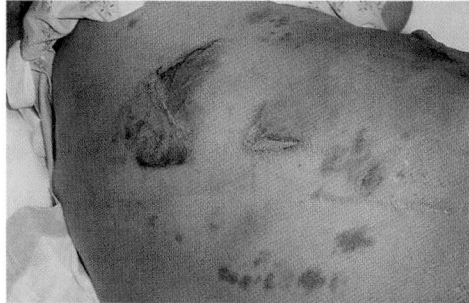

FIGURE 36-8 Skin tear. (Used with permission from Rosemary Kohr, RN, PhD, ACNP (cert), www.lhsc.on.ca/wound, Rosemary.Kohr@Lhasa.on.ca.)

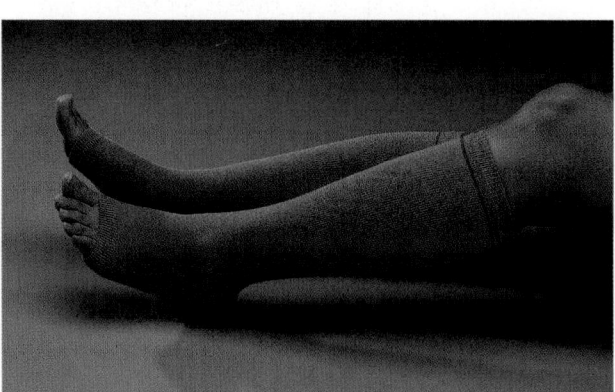

FIGURE 36-9 Skin protector. (Image courtesy Posey Company, Arcadia, Calif.)

CIRCULATORY ULCERS

Some diseases affect blood flow to and from the legs and feet. Poor circulation can cause pain, open wounds, and edema. *Edema* is *swelling caused by fluid collecting in tissues.* Open wounds and poor circulation can lead to infection and gangrene. *Gangrene* is *a condition in which there is death of tissue* (Chapter 44).

Circulatory ulcers (vascular ulcers) are *open sores on the lower legs or feet. They are caused by decreased blood flow through the arteries or veins.* These wounds are painful and hard to heal. Persons with diseases affecting the blood vessels are at risk.

Drugs and treatments are ordered. The nurse uses the nursing process to meet the person's needs (Box 36-3). You must help prevent skin breakdown on the legs and feet.

Venous Ulcers

Venous ulcers (stasis ulcers) are *open sores on the lower legs or feet caused by poor venous blood flow* (Fig. 36-10). *Stasis* means *stopped or slowed fluid flow.*

Venous ulcers can develop when valves in the leg veins do not close well. The veins do not pump blood back to the heart in a normal way. Blood and fluid collect in the legs and feet. Small skin veins rupture. This allows hemoglobin to enter the tissues, causing the skin to turn brown. (Hemoglobin gives blood its red color). The skin is dry, leathery, and hard. Itching is common.

The heels and inner part of the ankles are common sites for venous ulcers. They can occur from skin injury. Scratching and trauma are examples.

Venous ulcers are painful and walking is difficult. Fluid may seep from the wound. Infection is a risk. Healing is slow.

Risk Factors. Risk factors for venous ulcers include:
- History of blood clots (Chapter 35)
- History of varicose veins (Fig. 36-11)
- Decreased mobility
- Obesity
- Surgery: leg, foot, bones, joints
- Advanced age
- *Phlebitis* (*inflammation* [itis] *of a vein* [phleb])

Prevention and Treatment. To prevent venous ulcers:
- Prevent skin breakdown. Follow the measures in Box 36-3.
- Prevent injury. Do not bump the legs and feet.
- Move and transfer the person carefully and gently.

Persons at risk need professional foot care. Attention is given to toenails, corns, calluses, and other toe and foot problems. *You do not cut the toenails of persons with diseases affecting circulation.*

Venous ulcers are hard to heal. The doctor may order:
- Drugs for infection and to decrease swelling
- Medicated bandages and other wound care products
- Devices used for pressure ulcers (Chapter 37)
- Elastic stockings or elastic bandages (Chapter 35)

BOX 36-3 **Preventing Circulatory Ulcers**

- Remind the person not to sit with the legs crossed.
- Re-position the person according to the care plan—at least every 2 hours.
- Do not use elastic or rubber band–type garters to hold socks or hose in place.
- Do not dress the person in tight clothes.
- Provide good skin care daily. Keep the feet clean and dry. Clean and dry between the toes.
- Do not scrub or rub the skin during bathing and drying.
- Keep linens clean, dry, and wrinkle-free.
- Avoid injury to the legs and feet.
- Make sure shoes fit well.
- Keep pressure off the heels and other bony areas. Use pillows or other devices as directed.
- Check the person's legs and feet. Report skin breaks or changes in skin color.
- Do not massage over pressure points (Chapter 37). *Never rub or massage reddened areas.*
- Use protective devices as directed.
- Follow the care plan for walking and exercises.

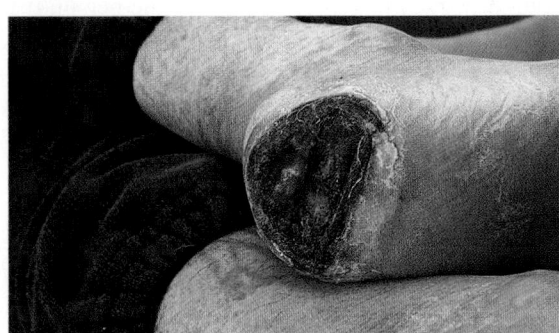

FIGURE 36-10 Venous ulcer.

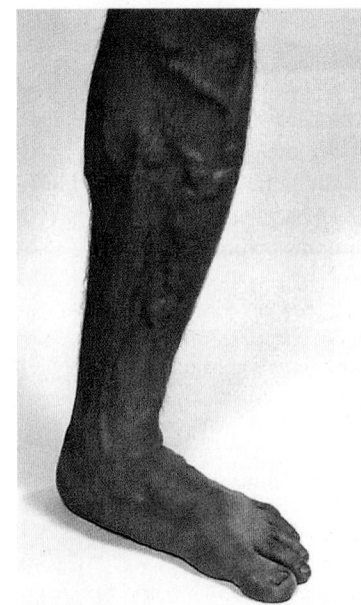

FIGURE 36-11 Varicose veins. Veins under the skin are dilated (wide) and bulging. (From Belch J and others: *Color atlas of peripheral vascular diseases*, ed 2, London, 1996, Wolfe Medical Publishers.)

Arterial Ulcers

Arterial ulcers are open wounds on the lower legs or feet caused by poor arterial blood flow. They are found between the toes, on top of the toes, and on the outer side of the ankle (Fig. 36-12). The leg and foot may feel cold and look blue or shiny. The ulcer is very painful.

These ulcers are caused by decreased arterial blood flow to the legs and feet. High blood pressure, diabetes, injuries, and narrowed arteries from aging are causes. Smoking is a risk factor.

The problem causing the ulcer is treated. Drugs, wound care, and a walking and exercise program are ordered. Professional foot care is important. Follow the care plan (see Box 36-3) and prevent further injury.

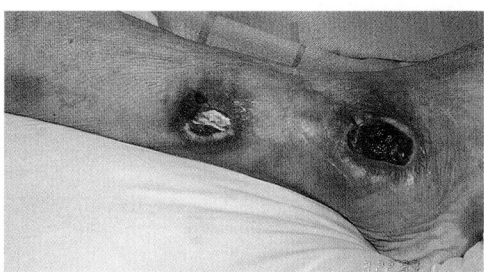

FIGURE 36-12 Arterial ulcer. (From Black JM, Hawks JH: *Medical-surgical nursing: clinical management for positive outcomes,* ed 7, St Louis, 2005, Saunders.)

Diabetic Foot Ulcers

A *diabetic foot ulcer is an open wound on the foot caused by complications from diabetes.* Often painless, diabetic foot ulcers can take several weeks or months to heal. Some never heal.

Diabetes (Chapter 46) can affect the nerves and blood vessels.

- *Nerves.* Nerve damage can cause loss of sensation in a foot or leg. The person may not feel a cut, blister, burn, or other trauma to the foot. Infection and a large sore can develop.
- *Blood vessels.* Blood flow decreases. Tissues and cells do not get needed oxygen and nutrients. Sores heal poorly. Infection and tissue death (gangrene) can occur. If the person smokes, he or she must stop smoking. Smoking decreases blood flow to the feet.

Some persons have both nerve and blood vessel damage. Infection and gangrene are risks. Sometimes the affected part is amputated to prevent the spread of gangrene.

Check the person's feet every day. Look for the foot problems described in Box 36-4 (Fig. 36-13, p. 610). Report any sign of a foot problem at once. Follow the care plan to prevent and treat diabetic foot ulcers. The measures in Box 36-4 may be part of the person's care plan.

See *Focus on Long-Term Care and Home Care: Diabetic Foot Ulcers,* p. 610.

BOX 36-4	Diabetes Foot Care

Common Problems
- *Corns and calluses* (see Fig. 36-13, *A*). These are thick layers of skin caused by too much rubbing or pressure on the same spot. They occur over bony areas.
- *Blisters* (see Fig. 36-13, *B*). These form when shoes rub on the same spot. Ill-fitting shoes and wearing shoes without socks are causes.
- *Ingrown toenails* (see Fig. 36-13, *C*). An edge of a toenail grows into the skin. This occurs when the skin is cut while trimming toenails or from tight shoes.
- *Bunions* (see Fig. 36-13, *D*). A bunion is a bump on the outside edge of the big toe. The big toe slants toward the small toes. Heredity is a factor. Shoes that fit poorly (too tight or narrow), high heels, and pointy shoes are causes. Bunions are removed by surgery.
- *Plantar warts* (see Fig. 36-13, *E*). *Plantar* means *sole.* Plantar warts occur on the soles (bottoms) of the feet. Caused by a virus, plantar warts are painful.
- *Hammer toes* (see Fig. 36-13, *F*). One or more toes are flexed. Diabetic nerve damage can weaken foot muscles. Because of deformed toes, the person has problems walking. Shoes do not fit well. Sores can develop on the tops of the toes and on the bottoms of the feet. High heels and pointy shoes are avoided.
- *Dry and cracked skin* (see Fig. 36-13, *G*). Dry skin can occur from nerve damage or poor blood flow in the legs and feet. The dry skin can crack, causing portals of entry for microbes. Infection can occur.

Common Problems—cont'd
- *Athlete's foot* (see Fig. 36-13, *H*). This is a fungus causing itching, burning, redness, and cracked skin between the toes and on the soles of the feet. The cracks are portals of entry for microbes.
- *Fungal infection of the toenails* (see Figure 36-13, *I*). The toenails become thick and hard to cut. They may be yellow, brown, or black. A nail may fall off.

Care Measures
- Check the feet daily for:
  - Cuts
  - Sores
  - Blisters
  - Redness
  - Calluses
  - Infected toenails
  - Pus
  - Warm skin
- Wash the feet every day in warm water with mild soap.
  - Do not use hot water.
  - Test the water temperature with your elbow or use a bath thermometer. Because the person has diabetes and burns are a risk, water temperature should be 90°F to 95°F (Fahrenheit).
  - Do not allow the feet to soak in water. The skin could dry out.
  - Dry the feet well, especially between the toes.

Continued

BOX 36-4 Diabetes Foot Care—cont'd

Care Measures—cont'd
- Apply talcum powder or cornstarch between the toes. This keeps the skin between the toes dry.
- Apply a thick layer of lotion, cream, or petroleum jelly on the tops and bottoms of the feet (not between the toes). Do so after washing and drying them. This keeps the skin soft and smooth.
- Have the person wear closed-toed shoes and clean socks, stockings, or nylons. This prevents blisters and sores.
  - Socks, stockings, and nylons should not have holes or seams.
  - Lightly padded socks are best.
  - Tight socks or knee-high stockings are avoided.
  - Athletic and walking shoes are best. Shoes should have laces, Velcro, or buckles for easy adjustment.
  - Open-toed shoes, sandals, flip-flops, pointy shoes, and high-heels are not worn.
  - Shoes are made of canvas, leather, or suede. Vinyl and plastic shoes are not worn. They do not stretch and do not allow air movement inside the shoes.

Care Measures—cont'd
- Check the insides of shoes before they are put on. Look for sharp edges or objects in the shoes. Make sure the lining is smooth.
- Do not allow the person to walk barefoot. The person could step on something and hurt the foot.
- Provide socks at night for cold feet.
- Promote blood flow to the feet. Have the person:
  - Elevate the feet when sitting.
  - Wiggle the toes for 5 minutes 2 or 3 times a day.
  - Move the ankles up and down and in and out.
  - Avoid crossing the legs.
- Do not trim or cut toenails or cut corns or calluses or try to smooth them. Professional foot care is needed.

(Modified from National Diabetes Information Clearinghouse: Prevent diabetes problems: keep your feet healthy, NIH Publication No. 14-4282, Bethesda, Md, February 2014, U.S. Department of Health and Human Services.)

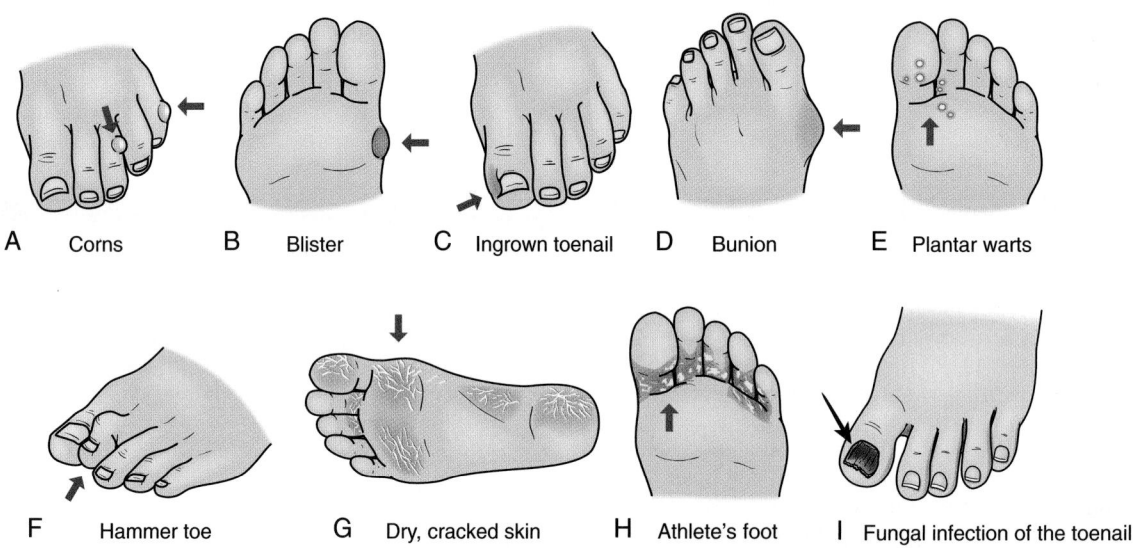

A Corns   B Blister   C Ingrown toenail   D Bunion   E Plantar warts

F Hammer toe   G Dry, cracked skin   H Athlete's foot   I Fungal infection of the toenail

FIGURE 36-13 Foot problems common with diabetes. (Redrawn from National Diabetes Information Clearinghouse [NDICH]: *Prevent diabetes problems: keep your feet healthy,* NIH Publication No. 14-4282, Bethesda, Md, February 2014, U.S. Department of Health and Human Services.)

FOCUS ON LONG-TERM CARE AND HOME CARE

Diabetic Foot Ulcers

Home Care

The measures in Box 36-4 also apply in the home setting. The person with diabetes should also:
- Break in new shoes slowly. The shoes are worn for 1 to 2 hours a day for the first few weeks.
- Wear warm socks in cold weather.
- Limit the time outside in cold weather.
- Wear lined boots in the winter.

- Wear shoes on hot pavements or at the beach.
- Apply sunscreen to the tops of the feet to prevent sunburn.
- Keep the feet away from radiators, fireplaces, and open fires.
- Avoid placing hot water bottles or heating pads on the feet.
- Choose activities that are easy on the feet. Walking, dancing, swimming, and bicycling are examples. Running and jumping are hard on the feet.

WOUND HEALING

The healing process has 3 phases.

- *Inflammatory phase* (3 days). Bleeding stops. A scab forms, preventing microbes from entering the wound. An increased blood supply to the wound brings nutrients and healing substances. Because blood supply increases, signs and symptoms of inflammation appear—redness, swelling, heat or warmth, and pain. Loss of function may occur.
- *Proliferative phase* (day 3 to 21). *Proliferate* means *to multiply rapidly.* Cells multiply to repair the wound.
- *Maturation phase* (day 21 to 2 years). The scar gains strength. The red, raised scar becomes thin and pale.

Types of Wound Healing

Healing occurs in 3 ways (Fig. 36-14).

- *First intention (primary intention, primary closure).* The wound is closed. Sutures (stitches), staples, clips, special glue, or adhesive strips hold the wound edges together.
- *Second intention (secondary intention).* Contaminated and infected wounds are cleaned and dead tissue removed. Wound edges are not brought together. The wound gaps. Healing takes longer, leaving a larger scar. Infection is a great risk.
- *Third intention (delayed intention, tertiary intention).* The wound is left open and closed later. It combines first and second intention. Infection and poor circulation are reasons for third intention.

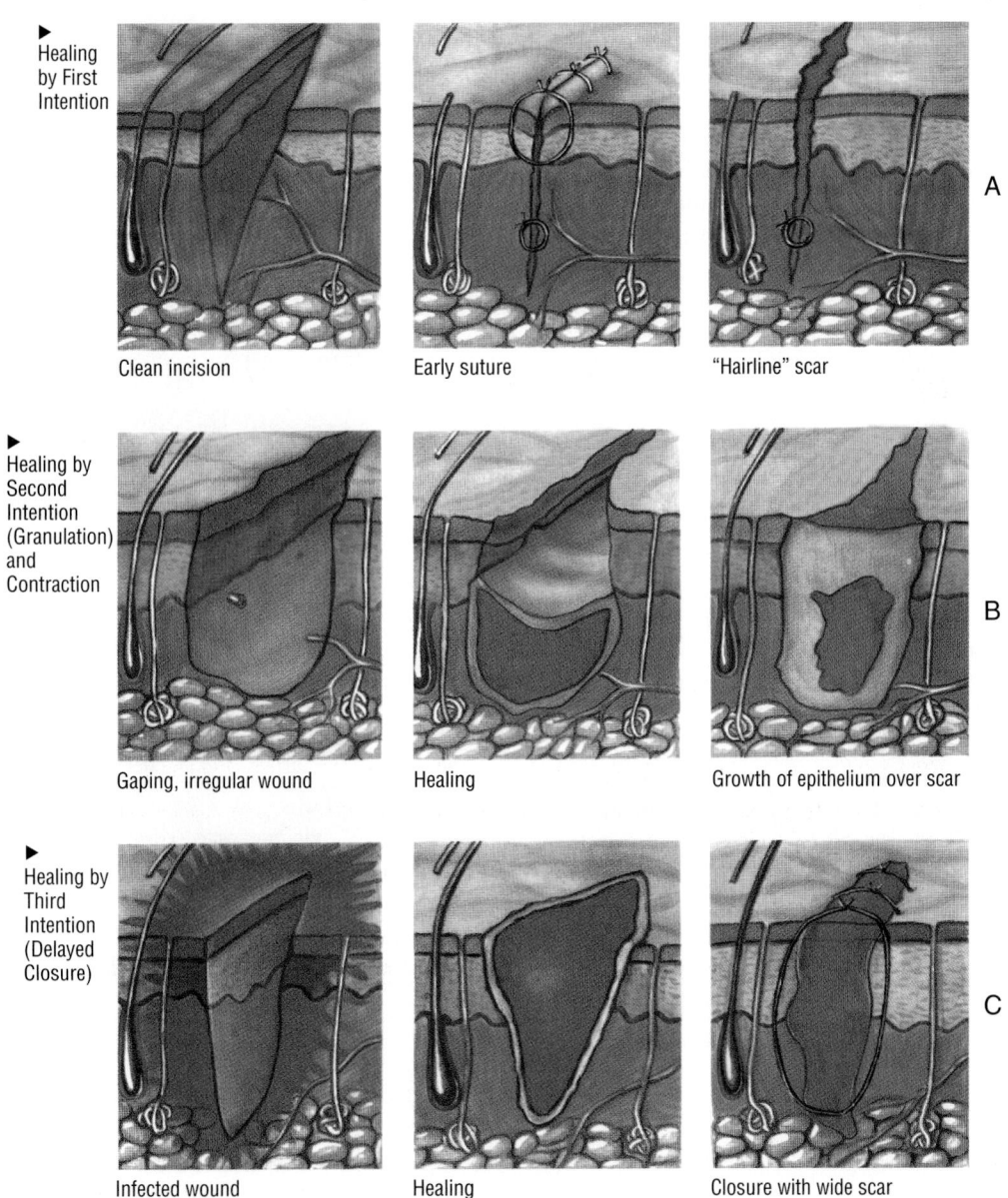

▶ Healing by First Intention

Clean incision   Early suture   "Hairline" scar

▶ Healing by Second Intention (Granulation) and Contraction

Gaping, irregular wound   Healing   Growth of epithelium over scar

▶ Healing by Third Intention (Delayed Closure)

Infected wound   Healing   Closure with wide scar

A

B

C

FIGURE 36-14 Wound healing. **A,** First intention. **B,** Second intention. **C,** Third intention. (Modified from Ignatavicius DD, Workman ML: *Medical-surgical nursing: critical thinking for collaborative care,* ed 5, St Louis, 2006, Saunders.)

Complications of Wound Healing

Many factors affect healing and the risk for complications. They include wound type, age, health, nutrition, and lifestyle. Age, smoking, circulatory disease, and diabetes affect circulation. Certain drugs (Coumadin, aspirin, and heparin) prolong bleeding.

Good nutrition is needed. Protein is needed for tissue growth and repair.

Immune system changes and antibiotics increase the risk of infection. Specific antibiotics kill specific pathogens. In doing so, other pathogens may grow and multiply.

Hemorrhage and Shock. *Hemorrhage is the excessive loss* (rrhage) *of blood* (hemo) *in a short time* (Chapter 54). *Shock results when tissues and organs do not get enough blood* (Chapter 54). The person can die from hemorrhage or shock.

- *Internal hemorrhage.* You cannot see internal hemorrhage. Bleeding occurs inside the body into tissues and body cavities. A hematoma may form. A *hematoma is a swelling* (oma) *that contains blood* (hemat). The area is swollen and reddish blue in color. Shock, vomiting blood, coughing up blood, and loss of consciousness signal internal hemorrhage.
- *External hemorrhage.* You can see external hemorrhage. Common signs are bloody drainage and dressings soaked with blood. Gravity causes fluid to flow down. Check under the body part for pooling of blood. Signs and symptoms of shock include:
- Blood pressure: low
- Pulse: rapid and weak
- Respirations: rapid
- Skin: cold, moist, pale
- Restlessness
- Thirst
- Confusion
- Consciousness: loss of

Hemorrhage and shock are emergencies. Alert the nurse at once. Assist as requested.

Infection. Contamination can occur during or after injury or surgery. An infected wound appears inflamed (reddened) and has drainage. The wound is painful and tender. The person has a fever.

Dehiscence and Evisceration. *Dehiscence is the separation of wound layers* (Fig. 36-15). *(Dehiscence is from the Latin word meaning to gap.)* It may involve the skin layer or underlying tissues. Abdominal wounds are commonly affected. *Evisceration is the separation of the wound along with the protrusion of abdominal organs* (Fig. 36-16). *(E means out from. Viscera relates to the internal organs.)* Coughing, vomiting, and abdominal distention (swelling) place stress on the wound. The person often describes the sensation of the wound "popping open."

Dehiscence and evisceration are surgical emergencies. Tell the nurse at once. The nurse covers the wound with large sterile dressings saturated with saline. Help prepare the person for surgery as directed.

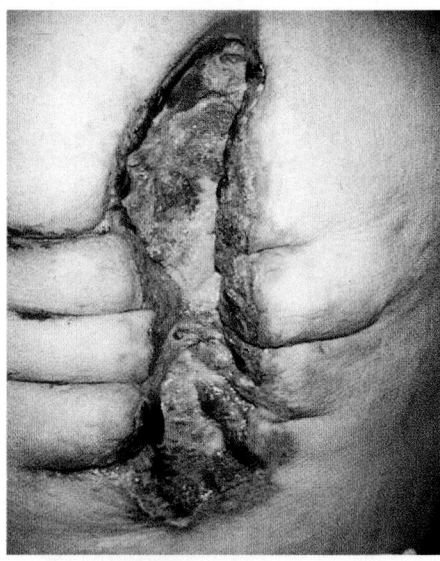

FIGURE 36-15 Wound dehiscence. (Courtesy KCI Licensing, Inc., San Antonio, Tex.)

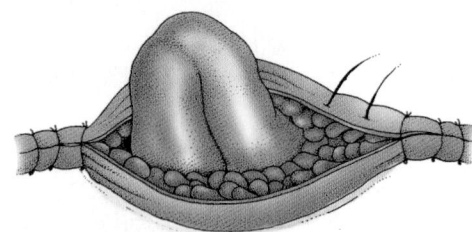

FIGURE 36-16 Wound evisceration. (Modified from Ignatavicius DD, Workman ML: *Medical-surgical nursing: critical thinking for collaborative care,* ed 5, St Louis, 2006, Saunders.)

Wound Appearance

The wound and any drainage are observed for healing and complications. See Box 36-5 for observations to make when assisting with wound care. Report and record your observations according to agency policy.

See *Focus on Long-Term Care and Home Care: Wound Appearance.*

- Wound site:
  - Surgery or trauma may result in multiple wounds.
- Wound size and depth are measured in centimeters (cm). The nurse uses a disposable ruler.
  - Size. The nurse measures from the top to the bottom and side to side (Fig. 36-17).
  - Depth. The nurse:
    - Inserts a sterile swab inside the deepest part of the wound.
    - Removes the swab.
    - Measures the distance on the swab.
- Wound appearance:
  - Is the wound red and swollen?
  - Is the area around the wound warm to touch?
  - Are sutures, staples, or clips intact or broken?
  - Are wound edges closed or separated?
  - Did the wound break open?
- Drainage:
  - Is the drainage serous, sanguineous, serosanguineous, or purulent?
  - What is the amount of drainage?
- Odor:
  - Does the wound or drainage have an odor?
- Surrounding skin:
  - Is surrounding skin intact?
  - What is the color of surrounding skin?
  - Are surrounding tissues swollen?

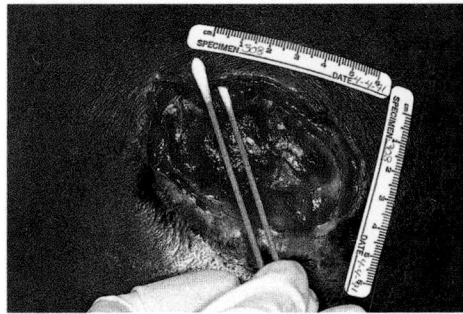

FIGURE 36-17 The size and depth of the wound are measured. (From Potter PA, Perry AG, Stockert PA, Hall AM: *Fundamentals of nursing,* ed 8, St Louis, 2013, Mosby.)

Wound Drainage

During injury and wound healing, fluid and cells escape from tissues. The amount and kind of drainage depends on wound size and site, bleeding, and infection. Wound drainage is observed and measured. See Figure 36-18, p. 614.

- *Serous drainage—clear, watery fluid* (serum). *Serous* comes from the word *serum.* Serum is the clear, thin, fluid portion of blood. Serum does not contain blood cells or platelets. Fluid in a blister is serous.
- *Sanguineous drainage—bloody* (sanguis) *drainage.* The Latin word *sanguis* means *blood.* Hemorrhage is suspected when large amounts are present. Bright drainage means fresh bleeding. Older bleeding is darker.
- *Serosanguineous drainage—thin, watery drainage* (sero) *that is blood-tinged* (sanguineous).
- *Purulent drainage—thick green, yellow, or brown drainage.*

Drainage must leave the wound for healing. Trapped drainage causes swelling of underlying tissues. The wound may heal at the skin level but underlying tissues do not close. Infection and complications can occur.

When large amounts of drainage are expected, the doctor inserts a drain. A *Penrose drain* is a rubber tube that opens and drains onto a dressing (Fig. 36-19, p. 614). An open drain, microbes can enter the drain and wound.

Closed drainage systems prevent microbes from entering the wound. A drain is attached to suction. The *Hemovac* (Fig. 36-20, p. 614) and *Jackson-Pratt* (Fig. 36-21, p. 614) systems are examples. Other systems are used depending on the wound type, size, and site.

Drainage is measured in 3 ways.

- Weighing dressings before applying them. The weight of each new dressing is noted. Dressings are weighed after removal. The dry dressing weight is subtracted from the wet dressing weight. (Wet dressings weigh more.)
- Noting the number and size of dressings with drainage. What is the amount and kind of drainage? Are dressings saturated? Is drainage on just part of the dressing? If so, which part? Is drainage through some or all layers?
- Measuring the amount of drainage in the collection container. This is done for closed drainage.

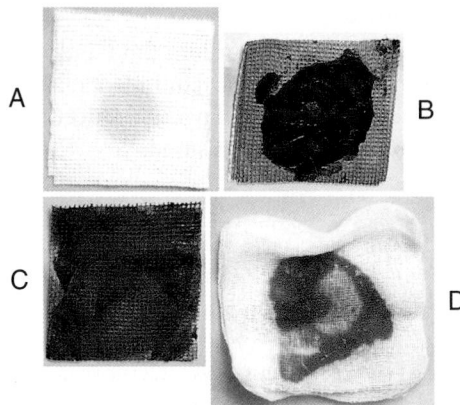

FIGURE 36-18 Wound drainage. **A,** Serous drainage. **B,** Sanguineous drainage. **C,** Serosanguineous drainage. **D,** Purulent drainage. (From Potter PA, Perry AG, Stockert PA, Hall AM: *Fundamentals of nursing,* ed 8, St Louis, 2013, Mosby.)

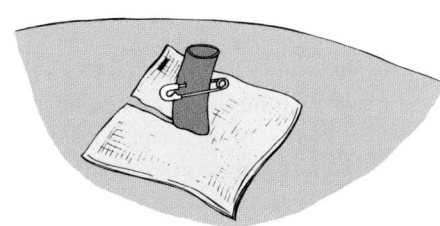

FIGURE 36-19 Penrose drain. (From Potter PA, Perry AG, Stockert PA, Hall AM: *Fundamentals of nursing,* ed 8, St Louis, 2013, Mosby.)

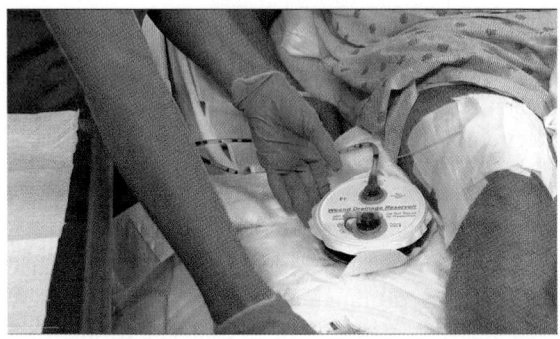

FIGURE 36-20 Hemovac. Drains are sutured to the wound and connected to a reservoir. (From Mosby's Nursing Video Skills 4.0, St. Louis, Basic Intermediate and Advanced Skills, St. Louis, 2014, Mosby.)

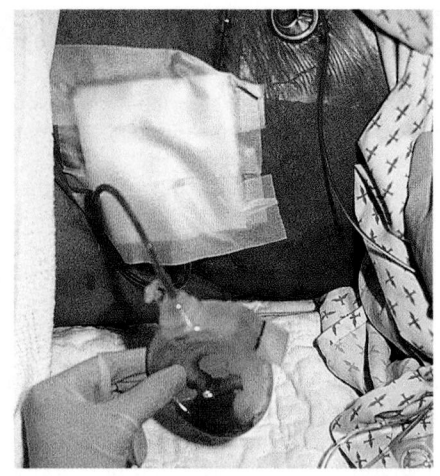

FIGURE 36-21 Jackson-Pratt drainage system. (From Potter PA, Perry AG, Stockert PA, Hall AM: *Fundamentals of nursing,* ed 8, St Louis, 2013, Mosby.)

DRESSINGS

Wound dressings have many functions. They:
- Protect wounds from injury and microbes.
- Absorb drainage.
- Remove dead tissue.
- Promote comfort.
- Cover unsightly wounds.
- Provide a moist environment for wound healing.
- Apply pressure (pressure dressings) to help control bleeding.

Dressing type and size depend on the type of wound, its size and site, and the amount of drainage. Infection is a factor. The dressing's function and the frequency of dressing changes are other factors. The doctor and nurse choose the dressing for each wound.

Types of Dressings

Dressings are described by the material used and application. The following dressing products are common (Fig. 36-22).
- *Gauze.* It comes in squares, rectangles, pads, and rolls. Gauze dressings absorb drainage and moisture.
- *Non-adherent gauze.* This gauze dressing has a non-stick surface. It removes easily without sticking to or injuring tissue.
- *Transparent adhesive film.* Air can reach the wound but fluids and microbes cannot. The wound is kept moist. Drainage is not absorbed. The transparent film allows for wound observation.

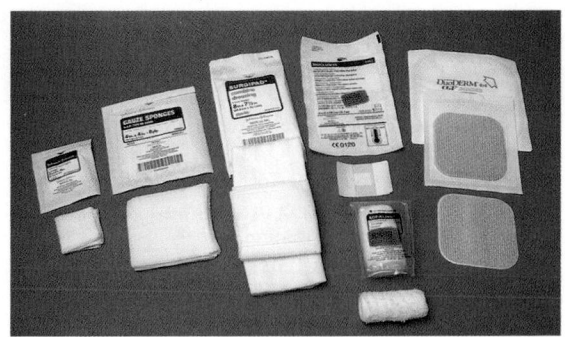

FIGURE 36-22 Types of dressings. (From deWit SC: *Fundamental concepts and skills for nursing*, ed 3, St Louis, 2000, Saunders.)

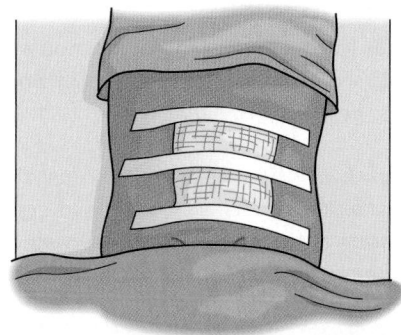

FIGURE 36-23 Tape is applied at the top, middle, and bottom of the dressing. The tape extends several inches beyond both sides of the dressing.

Some dressings have special agents for wound healing. If you assist with a dressing change, the nurse explains its use to you.

Dressings are dry or wet.

- *Dry dressing.* A dry gauze dressing is placed over the wound. More dressings are added to the first dressing as needed. Absorbed drainage is removed with the dressing. A dry dressing can stick to the wound. The dressing is removed carefully to prevent tissue injury and discomfort.
- *Wet dressing.* The wound is filled with gauze saturated with a solution. The moist gauze is covered with a dry dressing. The gauze absorbs drainage and provides a moist environment for wound healing. The frequency of dressing changes determines if the gauze is wet, damp, or dry on removal.

Securing Dressings

Dressings must be secured over wounds. Microbes can enter the wound and drainage can escape if the dressing is dislodged. Tape and Montgomery ties are used to secure dressings. Binders (p. 618) hold dressings in place.

Tape. Adhesive, paper, plastic, cloth, and elastic tapes are common. Adhesive tape sticks well. However, problems with adhesive include:

- It is hard to remove from the skin.
- It can irritate the skin.
- Skin tears or abrasions occur if skin is removed with tape.
- Many people are allergic to adhesive tape.

Paper, plastic, and cloth tapes usually do not cause allergic reactions. Elastic tape allows movement of the body part.

Tape comes in different sizes—½, ¾, 1, 2, and 3 inch widths. Tape is applied to the top, middle, and bottom of the dressing. The tape extends several inches beyond each side of the dressing (Fig. 36-23). *Do not apply tape to circle the entire body part. If swelling occurs, circulation to the part is impaired.*

See *Focus on Communication: Tape.*

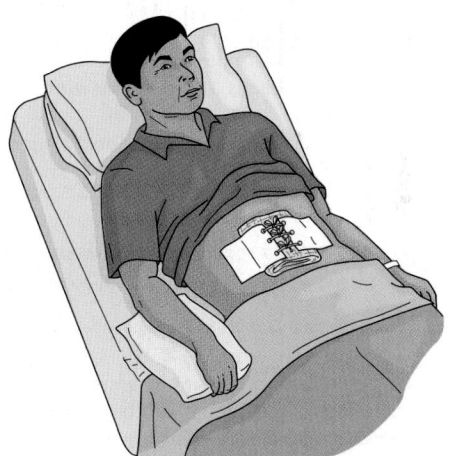

FIGURE 36-24 Montgomery ties.

Montgomery Ties. Montgomery ties (Fig. 36-24) are used for large dressings and frequent dressing changes. A Montgomery tie has an adhesive strip and cloth tie. With the dressing in place, the adhesive strips are placed on both sides of the dressing. Then the cloth ties are secured over the dressing.

A wound may need 2 or 3 Montgomery ties on each side. The ties are undone for the dressing change. The adhesive strips stay in place. They are not removed unless soiled. Montgomery ties protect the skin from frequent tape application and removal.

Applying Dressings

Some agencies let you apply simple, dry, non-sterile dressings to simple wounds. Follow the rules in Box 36-6.

See *Focus on Children and Older Persons: Applying Dressings.*

See *Teamwork and Time Management: Applying Dressings.*
See *Delegation Guidelines: Applying Dressings.*
See *Promoting Safety and Comfort: Applying Dressings.*
See procedure: *Applying a Dry, Non-Sterile Dressing.*

BOX 36-6   Applying Dressings

- Let pain-relief drugs take effect, usually 30 minutes. The dressing change can cause discomfort. The nurse gives the drug and tells you how long to wait.
- Meet fluid and elimination needs before you begin.
- Collect equipment and supplies before you begin.
- Do not bend or reach over your work area.
- Control your nonverbal communication. Wound odors, appearance, and drainage may be unpleasant. Do not communicate your thoughts or reaction to the person.
- Remove soiled dressings so the person cannot see the soiled side. The drainage and its color may upset the person.
- Do not force the person to look at the wound. A wound can affect body image and self-esteem. The nurse helps the person deal with the wound.
- Remove tape by pulling it toward the wound.
- Remove dressings gently. They may stick to the wound, drain, or surrounding skin. If the dressing sticks, the nurse may have you wet the dressing with a saline solution. A wet dressing is easier to remove.
- Touch only the outer edges of old and new dressings (Chapter 16).
- Report and record your observations. See *Delegation Guidelines: Applying Dressings.*

FOCUS ON CHILDREN AND OLDER PERSONS

Applying Dressings

Children

Children are often afraid of dressing changes. Tape removal can be painful. Wound appearance can be frightening. A calm, cooperative child helps prevent contamination of the sterile field. A parent or caregiver holds the child so the wound can be reached easily. Holding or playing with a toy can comfort the child.

Older Persons

Older persons have thin, fragile skin. Prevent skin tears. Use extreme care to remove tape.

TEAMWORK AND TIME MANAGEMENT

Applying Dressings

Collect all needed items before starting the procedure. Have extra dressings, tape, and other supplies on hand. Leave un-used items in the room for the next dressing change. Wound contamination can occur if you need to leave the room during the procedure.

DELEGATION GUIDELINES

Applying Dressings

When applying a dressing is delegated to you, make sure that:

- Your state allows you to perform the procedure.
- The procedure is in your job description.
- You have the necessary training.
- You know how to use the equipment.
- You review the procedure with the nurse.
- A nurse is available to answer questions and to supervise you.

  If the above conditions are met, you need this information from the nurse.
- When to change the dressing
- When the person received a pain-relief drug; when it will take effect
- What to do if the dressing sticks to the wound
- How to clean the wound
- What dressings to use
- How to secure the dressing—tape or Montgomery ties
- What kind of tape to use—adhesive, paper, plastic, cloth, or elastic
- What size tape to use—½, ¾, 1, 2, or 3 inch width
- What observations to report and record:
  - What you used to dress the wound and secure the dressing
  - A red or swollen wound
  - An area around the wound that is warm to touch
  - If wound edges are closed or separated
  - A wound that has broken open
  - Drainage appearance—clear, bloody, or watery and blood-tinged; thick and green, yellow, or brown
  - The amount of drainage
  - Wound or drainage odor
  - Intactness and color of surrounding tissues
  - Possible dressing contamination—urine; feces; other body fluids, secretions, or excretions; dislodged dressing
  - Pain
  - Fever
- When to report observations
- What patient or resident concerns to report at once

PROMOTING SAFETY AND COMFORT

Applying Dressings

Safety

Do not apply tape to irritated, injured, or non-intact skin. Tape can further damage the skin.

Comfort

Wounds and dressing changes can cause discomfort or pain. The nurse may give a pain-relief drug before the dressing change. Allow time for the drug to take effect. Gently apply and remove tape and dressings.

The person may not report discomfort from a dressing. You should ask:

- "Is the dressing comfortable?"
- "Does the tape cause pain or itching?"

Applying a Dry, Non-Sterile Dressing

QUALITY OF LIFE

- Knock before entering the person's room.
- Address the person by name.
- Introduce yourself by name and title.
- Explain the procedure before starting and during the procedure.
- Protect the person's rights during the procedure.
- Handle the person gently during the procedure.

PRE-PROCEDURE

1 Follow *Delegation Guidelines: Applying Dressings.* See *Promoting Safety and Comfort:*
   a *Wound Care,* p. 605
   b *Applying Dressings*
2 Practice hand hygiene.
3 Collect the following.
   - Gloves
   - PPE (personal protective equipment) as needed
   - Tape or Montgomery ties
   - Dressings as directed by the nurse
   - 4 × 4 gauze
   - Saline solution as directed by the nurse
   - Cleaning solution as directed by the nurse

   - Adhesive remover
   - Dressing set with scissors and forceps
   - Plastic bag
   - Bath blanket
4 Practice hand hygiene.
5 Identify the person. Check the ID (identification) bracelet against the assignment sheet. Use 2 identifiers (Chapter 13). Also call the person by name.
6 Provide for privacy.
7 Arrange your work area. You should not have to reach over or turn your back on your work area.
8 Raise the bed for body mechanics. Bed rails are up if used.

PROCEDURE

9 Lower the bed rail near you if up.
10 Help the person to a comfortable position.
11 Cover the person with a bath blanket. Fan-fold top linens to the foot of the bed.
12 Expose the affected body part.
13 Make a cuff on the plastic bag. Place the bag within reach.
14 Practice hand hygiene.
15 Put on needed PPE. Put on gloves.
16 Remove tape or undo Montgomery ties.
   a *Tape:* hold the skin down. Gently pull the tape toward the wound.
   b *Montgomery ties:* fold ties away from the wound.
17 Remove any adhesive from the skin. Pick up a gauze square with the forceps. Wet a 4 × 4 gauze dressing with adhesive remover. Clean away from the wound.
18 Remove gauze dressings. Start with the top dressing and remove each layer. Keep the soiled side away from the person's sight. Put dressings in the plastic bag. They must not touch the outside of the bag.

19 Remove the dressing over the wound very gently. It may stick to the wound or drain site. Moisten the dressing with saline if it sticks to the wound. Discard the dressing as in step 18.
20 Observe the wound, drain site, and wound drainage.
21 Remove the gloves and put them in the bag. Practice hand hygiene.
22 Open the new dressings.
23 Put on clean gloves.
24 Clean the wound with saline as directed by the nurse. See Figure 36-25.
25 Apply dressings as directed by the nurse.
26 Secure the dressings. Use tape or Montgomery ties.
27 Remove the gloves. Put them in the bag.
28 Remove and discard PPE.
29 Practice hand hygiene.
30 Cover the person. Remove the bath blanket.

POST-PROCEDURE

31 Provide for comfort. (See the inside of the front cover.)
32 Place the call light and other needed items within reach.
33 Lower the bed to a safe and comfortable level for the person. Follow the care plan.
34 Raise or lower bed rails. Follow the care plan.
35 Return equipment and supplies to their proper place. Leave extra dressings and tape in the room.
36 Discard used supplies in the bag. Tie the bag closed. Discard the bag following agency policy. (Wear gloves for this step.)

37 Clean your work area. Follow the Bloodborne Pathogen Standard.
38 Unscreen the person.
39 Complete a safety check of the room. (See the inside of the front cover.)
40 Remove and discard the gloves. Practice hand hygiene.
41 Report and record your observations.

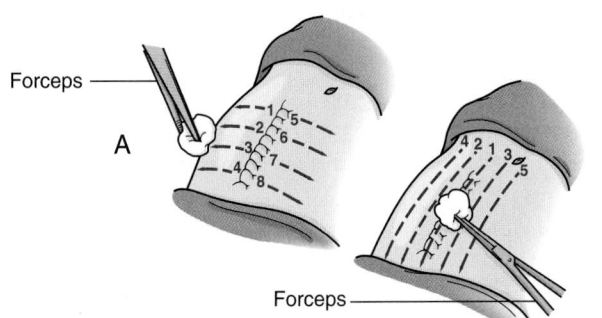

FIGURE 36-25 Cleaning a wound. A, Clean starting at the wound and stroking out to the surrounding skin. Use new gauze for each stroke. **B,** Clean the wound from the top to the bottom. Start at the wound. Then clean the surrounding areas. Use new gauze for each stroke. (From Potter PA, Perry AG, Stockert PA, Hall AM: *Fundamentals of nursing,* ed 8, St Louis, 2013, Mosby.)

BINDERS AND COMPRESSION GARMENTS

Binders are wide bands of elastic fabric. They are applied to the abdomen, chest, or perineal area. Binders promote healing because they support wounds and hold dressings in place. They also prevent or reduce swelling, promote comfort, and prevent injury. These binders are common.

- *Abdominal binder*—provides abdominal support and holds dressings in place (Fig. 36-26). The top part is at the waist. The lower part is over the hips. Binders are secured in place with Velcro or with hook and loop closures.
- *Breast binder*—supports the breasts after surgery (Fig. 36-27). It is secured in place with Velcro or padded zippers.

Compression garments are made of a tight, stretchy fabric (Fig. 36-28). They are commonly worn after plastic surgery. They help:

- Reduce swelling.
- Prevent fluid buildup at the surgical site.
- Hold the skin against the body.
- Achieve the desired shape.

Box 36-7 lists the rules for applying binders and compression garments.

See *Focus on Communication: Binders and Compression Garments*.

See *Promoting Safety and Comfort: Binders and Compression Garments*.

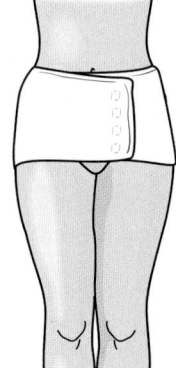

FIGURE 36-26 Abdominal binder.

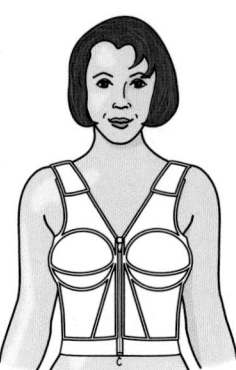

FIGURE 36-27 Breast binder.

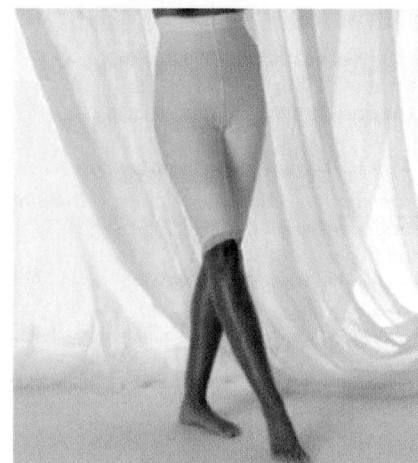

FIGURE 36-28 Compression garment. (Courtesy Rainey Compression Essentials, Atlanta, Ga.)

BOX 36-7	Applying Binders and Compression Garments

- Follow the manufacturer's instructions.
- Position the person in good alignment.
- Apply the device so there is firm, even pressure over the area.
- Apply the device so it is snug. It must not interfere with breathing or circulation.
- Re-apply the device if it is out of position or causes discomfort.
- Secure safety pins, if used, pointing away from the wound.
- Change the device if it is moist or soiled. This prevents the growth of microbes.
- Tell the nurse at once if the person's breathing changes.
- Check the skin under and around the device. Tell the nurse at once if there is redness, irritation, or other signs of a skin problem.

FOCUS ON **COMMUNICATION**

Binders and Compression Garments

The person may not tell you about pain or discomfort. You need to ask:

- "Is the binder (or garment) too tight or too loose?"
- "Does the binder (or garment) cause pain?"
- "Do you feel pressure from the binder (or garment)?" If yes: "Where? Please show me."

PROMOTING SAFETY AND COMFORT

Binders and Compression Garments

Safety
Apply binders and compression garments properly. Otherwise, severe discomfort, skin irritation, and circulatory and respiratory problems can occur. Correct application is needed for safety and for the device to work properly.

Comfort
A binder or compression garment should promote comfort. Tell the nurse if the device causes pain or discomfort.

HEAT AND COLD APPLICATIONS

Heat and cold applications promote healing and comfort. They also reduce tissue swelling. See Chapter 38.

MEETING BASIC NEEDS

The wound can affect basic needs. However, it is only part of the person's care. Remember, the *person* has the wound.

The wound causes pain and discomfort. These may affect breathing and moving. Turning, re-positioning, and walking may be painful. Handle the person gently. Allow pain-relief drugs to take effect before giving care.

Good nutrition is needed for healing. However, pain, discomfort, and odors from wound drainage can affect appetite. Promptly remove soiled dressings from the room. Use room deodorizers as directed. Also keep drainage containers out of the person's sight. Tell the nurse if the person wants certain foods or drinks.

Infection is always a threat. Follow Standard Precautions and the Bloodborne Pathogen Standard. Carefully observe the wound for signs and symptoms of infection.

Delayed healing is a risk for persons who are older, obese, or have poor nutrition. Protein is needed for tissue growth and repair. Poor circulation and diabetes also affect healing, increasing the risk of infection.

Safety and security needs are affected. The person fears scarring, disfigurement, delayed healing, and infection. Fears about the wound "popping open" are common. Medical bills are other concerns. The person may need care for a long time.

Victims of violence have many other concerns. Future attacks, finding and convicting the attacker, and fears for family are common concerns. Victims of intimate partner, child, and elder abuse often hide the source of their injuries.

Wounds may be large or small. Others can see wounds on the face, arms, or legs. Clothing can hide some wounds. Wound drainage may have odors. Some wounds are disfiguring. They can affect sexual performance or feelings of sexual attraction. Amputation can affect function, everyday activities, and job. Eye injuries can affect vision. Abdominal trauma and surgery can affect eating and elimination.

Wounds affect body image. Love and belonging and self-esteem needs are affected. The person may be sad and tearful or angry and hostile. Adjustment may be hard and require rehabilitation. Be gentle and kind, give thoughtful care, and practice good communication.

FOCUS ON **PRIDE**

The Person, Family, and Yourself

Personal and Professional Responsibility

You assist with hygiene and grooming, dressing and undressing, and transfers and positioning. Those roles bring responsibilities for wound care.

If you are careless during a transfer, you can cause a skin tear. If you rush during a bath, you may not notice a wound between skin folds. If you do not apply shoes properly, a foot ulcer can develop.

The way you provide care affects the person's health, safety, and quality of life. Take pride in working safely and carefully.

Rights and Respect

A person may ask about a wound care measure. Avoid answers like: "It's to help you get better" or "The doctor (nurse) says you need it." The person has the right to be informed.

Be kind, caring, and patient when the person asks questions. Tell the person that you will ask the nurse to explain reasons for care. Wait until the person's questions are answered before performing the care measure.

Independence and Social Interaction

Wounds, dressings, drainage and drainage devices, and wound odors may disturb patients, residents, and visitors. Visitors may feel uncomfortable. To promote comfort and interaction with family and friends:

- Keep the wound or dressing covered if able.
- Ask visitors to leave the room during dressing changes or when exposing the wound or dressing.
- Remove soiled dressings from the room promptly.
- Keep drainage containers out of sight if able. Some large containers can be covered with a towel as directed by the nurse.
- Use a room deodorizer for odors as directed.

Delegation and Teamwork

Wound care can be painful and tiring. The team coordinates care to promote comfort and rest. To assist:

- Plan care with the nurse. Ask when drugs for pain will be given and when they will take effect. Allow rest periods before and after care that is tiring.
- Be prepared. Gather supplies. Leaving to get supplies causes delays. Care and procedures take longer than planned.
- Work with the nurse as instructed. You may need to position the person or raise a body part while the nurse changes a dressing. Teamwork reduces the amount of energy the person must use.

Ethics and Laws

Agency practices vary for charging supplies. Some are stored in a room or cart. Stickers on the items are removed and saved or a log is kept. The person's name and the type and amount of items removed are recorded. Some agencies use an electronic cabinet. A code is used to open the cabinet. The person's name is chosen from a list on a screen. Then a button is pressed to select the type and amount of supplies needed.

Ethical practice involves honestly following agency rules. Not charging supplies correctly costs the nursing unit and agency money. Taking supplies home for your own use is unethical. This is stealing. Take pride in following agency rules and being an honest and reliable member of the nursing team.

FOCUS ON **PRIDE**: Application

Define body image. Is body image the same for all persons? Is it the same throughout a person's life? Explain. How can a wound affect body image?

REVIEW QUESTIONS

Circle the BEST answer.

1 A person has a laceration from a fall. The wound is
a Open, unintentional, and contaminated
b Open, unintentional, and infected
c Closed, intentional, and clean
d Closed, intentional, and chronic

2 A person had rectal surgery. The person has a
a Clean wound
b Dirty wound
c Clean-contaminated wound
d Contaminated wound

3 The skin and underlying tissues are pierced. This is
a A penetrating wound
b An incision
c A contusion
d An abrasion

4 Which can cause skin tears?
a Keeping your nails trimmed and smooth
b Dressing the person in soft clothing
c Wearing rings
d Padding wheelchair footplates

5 A person has a circulatory ulcer. Which measure should you question?
a Do not cut or trim toenails.
b Hold socks in place with elastic garters.
c Apply elastic stockings.
d Re-position the person every hour.

6 Diabetic foot ulcers are caused by
a Gangrene
b Amputation
c Infection
d Nerve and blood vessel damage

7 A person has diabetes. The person's feet are checked every
a 2 hours
b Day
c Week
d Month

8 A person with diabetes wears socks with shoes to prevent
a Corns
b Bunions
c Blisters
d Plantar warts

9 A wound is separating. This is called
a Primary intention
b Third intention
c Dehiscence
d Evisceration

10 Clear, watery drainage from a wound is called
a Purulent drainage
b Serous drainage
c Sero-purulent drainage
d Serosanguineous drainage

11 Dressings
a Protect the wound from injury
b Prevent drainage
c Provide a dry environment for healing
d Support the wound and reduce swelling

12 To secure a dressing, apply tape
a Around the entire part
b Along the sides of the dressing
c To the top, middle, and bottom of the dressing
d As the person prefers

13 A person has frequent dressing changes. The nurse will likely have the dressings secured with
a A binder
b Montgomery ties
c Paper or cloth tape
d An elastic bandage

14 A pain-relief drug is given before a dressing change. How long should you wait for the drug to take effect?
a 5 minutes
b 10 minutes
c 15 minutes
d 30 minutes

15 To remove tape
a Pull it toward the wound
b Pull it away from the wound
c Use forceps
d Use a saline solution

16 An abdominal binder is used to
a Prevent blood clots
b Prevent wound infection
c Provide support and hold dressings in place
d Decrease swelling and circulation

Answers to Chapter 36 questions are on p. 871.

FOCUS ON PRACTICE

Problem Solving

You are dressing an older resident with thin, fragile skin. You notice a new skin tear on the person's arm. What do you do? How can you prevent skin tears?

Pressure Ulcers

OBJECTIVES

- Define the key terms and key abbreviations in this chapter.
- Describe the causes and risk factors for pressure ulcers.
- Identify the persons at risk for pressure ulcers.
- Describe the stages of pressure ulcers and the Kennedy terminal ulcer.
- Identify the sites for pressure ulcers.
- Explain how to prevent pressure ulcers.
- Identify the complications from pressure ulcers.
- Explain how to promote PRIDE in the person, the family, and yourself.

KEY TERMS

avoidable pressure ulcer A pressure ulcer that develops from the improper use of the nursing process

bedfast Confined to bed

bony prominence An area where the bone sticks out or projects from the flat surface of the body; pressure point

chairfast Confined to a chair

colonized The presence of bacteria on the wound surface or in wound tissue; the person does not have signs and symptoms of an infection

epidermal stripping Removing the epidermis (outer skin layer) as tape is removed from the skin

eschar Thick, leathery dead tissue that may be loose or adhered to the skin; it is often black or brown

friction The rubbing of 1 surface against another

intact skin Normal skin and skin layers without damage or breaks

pressure point See "bony prominence"

pressure ulcer A localized injury to the skin and/or underlying tissue, usually over a bony prominence, resulting from pressure or pressure in combination with shear; any lesion caused by unrelieved pressure that results in damage to underlying tissues

shear When layers of the skin rub against each other; when the skin remains in place and underlying tissues move and stretch, tearing underlying capillaries and blood vessels and causing tissue damage

skin breakdown Changes or damage to intact skin—normal skin and skin layers

slough Dead tissue that is shed from the skin; it is usually light colored, soft, and moist; may be stringy at times

unavoidable pressure ulcer A pressure ulcer that occurs despite efforts to prevent one through proper use of the nursing process

KEY ABBREVIATIONS

CMS	Centers for Medicare & Medicaid Services	**TJC**	The Joint Commission
NPUAP	National Pressure Ulcer Advisory Panel		

Before defining pressure ulcer, you need to understand these terms.

- *Bony prominence (pressure point)—an area where the bone sticks out or projects from the flat surface of the body*. The back of the hand, shoulder blades, elbows, hips, spine, sacrum, knees, ankles, heels, and toes are bony prominences (Fig. 37-1, p. 622).

- *Shear—when layers of the skin rub against each other. Or shear is when the skin remains in place and underlying tissues move and stretch, tearing underlying capillaries and blood vessels. Tissue damage occurs.* See Chapter 18.
- *Friction—the rubbing of 1 surface against another*. The skin is dragged across a surface. Friction is always present with shearing.

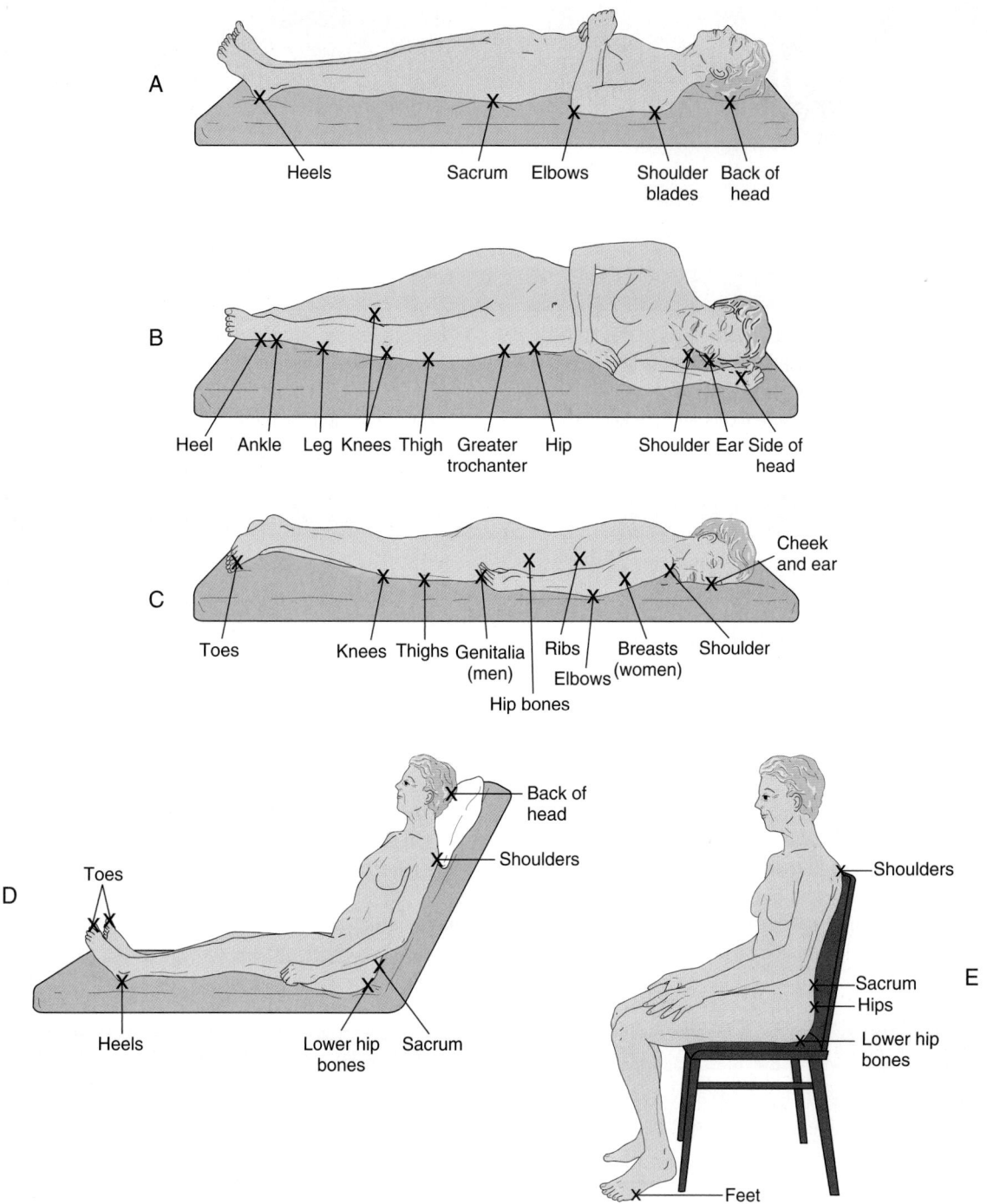

FIGURE 37-1 Bony prominences (pressure points). **A,** The supine position. **B,** The lateral position. **C,** The prone position. **D,** Fowler's position. **E,** Sitting position.

PRESSURE ULCER DEFINITIONS

The National Pressure Ulcer Advisory Panel (NPUAP) defines ***pressure ulcer*** *as a localized injury to the skin and/or underlying tissue, usually over a bony prominence* (Fig. 37-2). *It is the result of pressure or pressure in combination with shear.* Decubitus ulcer, bed sore, and pressure sore are other terms for pressure ulcer.

The Centers for Medicare & Medicaid Services (CMS) defines ***pressure ulcer*** *as any lesion caused by unrelieved pressure that results in damage to underlying tissues.* According to the CMS, friction and shear are factors but not the main causes of pressure ulcers.

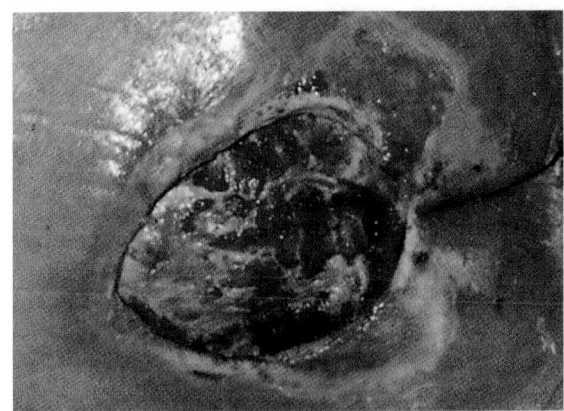

FIGURE 37-2 A pressure ulcer. (From Ostomy Wound Management, *Proceedings from the November National V.A.C. ® 51[2A, supp]: 7S, Feb 2005,* HMP Communications. Used with permission.)

Avoidable and Unavoidable Pressure Ulcers

An *unavoidable pressure ulcer occurs despite efforts to prevent one through proper use of the nursing process.* Such ulcers can develop in hospitals, nursing centers, and home settings. The Kennedy terminal ulcer is unavoidable (p. 626). An *avoidable pressure ulcer develops from the improper use of the nursing process.*

Agencies must:

- Evaluate the person's condition and pressure ulcer risk factors.
- Identify and implement measures to meet the person's needs and goals.
- Monitor and evaluate the effect of such measures.
- Revise the measures as needed.
- Provide the necessary treatment and services to promote healing, prevent infection, and prevent new ulcers from developing.

Agencies must identify persons at risk for pressure ulcers. A person's risk may increase during an illness (cold, flu) or from condition changes. The person's care plan must include measures to reduce or remove risk factors.

See *Focus on Long-Term Care and Home Care: Avoidable and Unavoidable Pressure Ulcers.*

FOCUS ON LONG-TERM CARE AND HOME CARE

Avoidable and Unavoidable Pressure Ulcers

Long-Term Care

The CMS requires that nursing centers identify persons at risk for pressure ulcers. Many pressure ulcers occur within the first 4 weeks of admission to a nursing center. A person can develop a pressure ulcer within 2 to 6 hours after the onset of pressure.

RISK FACTORS

Pressure, friction, and shearing are the major causes of pressure ulcers. They also cause skin breakdown (Box 37-1) that can lead to pressure ulcers. *Skin breakdown involves changes or damage to intact skin. Intact skin is normal skin and skin layers without damage or breaks* (Fig. 37-3, p. 624).

Unrelieved pressure squeezes tiny blood vessels. For example, pressure occurs when the skin over a bony area is squeezed between hard surfaces (Fig. 37-4, p. 624). The bone is 1 hard surface. The other is usually the mattress or chair seat. Squeezing or pressure prevents blood flow to the skin and underlying tissues. Oxygen and nutrients cannot get to the cells. Skin and tissues die.

Friction scrapes the skin, causing an open area. A good blood supply is needed for the open area to heal. A poor blood supply or an infection can lead to a pressure ulcer.

Shear occurs when the person slides down in the bed or chair. Blood vessels and tissues are damaged. Blood flow to the area is reduced.

Other pressure ulcer risk factors include breaks in the skin, poor circulation to an area, moisture, dry skin, and skin irritation by urine and feces.

See *Teamwork and Time Management: Risk Factors,* p. 624.

BOX 37-1   Skin Breakdown—Common Causes

- Age-related skin changes
- Breaks in the skin
- Dry skin
- Fragile and weak capillaries
- General thinning of the skin
- Loss of the fatty layer under the skin
- Decreased sensation to touch, heat, and cold
- Decreased mobility
- Sitting in a chair or lying in bed most or all of the day
- Chronic diseases (diabetes, high blood pressure)
- Diseases that decrease circulation; poor circulation to an area
- Poor nutrition
- Poor hydration
- Incontinence: urinary, fecal
- Moisture in dark body areas: skin folds, under breasts, perineal area
- Pressure on bony parts
- Poor fingernail and toenail care
- Friction and shearing
- Edema

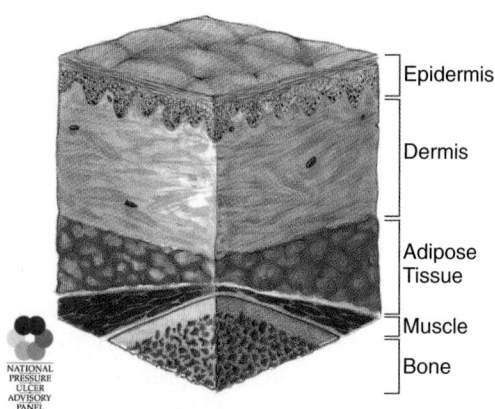

FIGURE 37-3 Intact skin. (From National Pressure Ulcer Advisory Panel.)

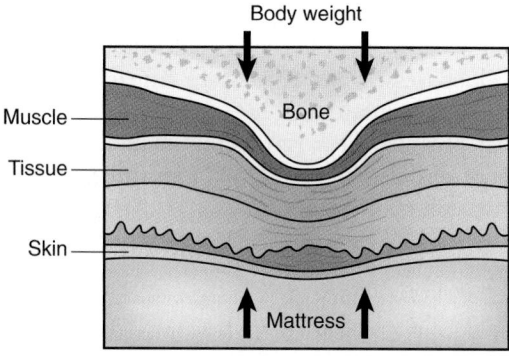

FIGURE 37-4 Tissue under pressure. The skin is squeezed between 2 hard surfaces—the bone and the mattress. (Redrawn from Agency for Healthcare Research and Quality: *Understanding your body: what are pressure ulcers?* Rockville, Md, November 2007, U.S. Department of Health and Human Services.)

TEAMWORK AND TIME MANAGEMENT

Risk Factors

You must help prevent pressure ulcers. As you walk in hallways, look to see if a person has slid down in bed or in a chair. Do the same when people are in dining and lounge areas. Help re-position the person. Ask a co-worker to help you as needed. Report the re-positioning to the nurse.

PERSONS AT RISK

Persons at risk for pressure ulcers are those who:

- Are *bedfast (confined to bed)* or *chairfast (confined to a chair).* Pressure occurs from lying or sitting in the same position too long.
- Need some or total help in moving. Coma, paralysis, and hip fracture are examples of conditions affecting the ability to move.
- Are agitated, have muscle spasms, or have involuntary muscle movements. The movements cause rubbing (friction) against linens and other surfaces.
- Are incontinent. Urine and feces irritate the skin and lead to skin breakdown. They are also sources of moisture.
- Are exposed to moisture. Urine, feces, wound drainage, sweat, and saliva are sources of moisture. Moisture irritates the skin. It also increases the risk of friction and shearing during re-positioning.
- Have poor nutrition or poor fluid balance. A balanced diet is needed to nourish the skin. Fluid balance is needed for healthy skin.
- Have limited awareness. The person does not know to move or change positions. Drugs and health problems affect awareness.
- Have problems sensing pain or pressure. The person does not know to alert the staff to these symptoms of tissue damage.
- Have circulatory problems. Cells and tissues die when starved of oxygen and nutrients.
- Have weight loss or are very thin. Loss of muscle and fat reduces padding between bones and surfaces. Mattresses, chairs, and wheelchairs are such surfaces.
- Are obese. Friction can damage the skin. Persons with bariatric needs are at great risk.
- Have medical devices. A pressure ulcer can develop where medical devices cause pressure on the skin.
- Have a healed pressure ulcer. Healed Stage 3 or 4 pressure ulcers are more likely to recur. See "Pressure Ulcer Stages."

See *Focus on Children and Older Persons: Persons at Risk.*

FOCUS ON CHILDREN AND OLDER PERSONS

Persons at Risk

Children

Ill infants and children and those with mobility problems are at risk for pressure ulcers. The back of the head is the most common site. According to the NPUAP, spina bifida (Chapter 50), cerebral palsy (Chapter 50), open-heart surgery, and respiratory support (Chapter 40) are risk factors. So is incontinence (urine and fecal).

Children—cont'd

Pressure, friction, shearing, poor nutrition, infection, and epidermal stripping are causes. *Epidermal stripping is removing the epidermis (outer skin layer) as tape is removed from the skin.* Newborns are at risk because of their fragile skin.

Older Persons

Older persons have thin and fragile skin that is easily injured. Some have chronic diseases affecting mobility, nutrition, circulation, and awareness.

PRESSURE ULCER STAGES

In persons with light skin, a reddened bony area is the first sign of a pressure ulcer. In persons with dark skin, skin color may differ from surrounding areas. The color change remains after the pressure is relieved. The area may feel warm or cool. The person may complain of pain, burning, tingling, or itching. Or the person may not feel anything unusual. Box 37-2 describes pressure ulcer stages.

See *Focus on Communication: Pressure Ulcer Stages.*

See *Focus on Long-Term Care and Home Care: Pressure Ulcer Stages,* p. 626.

BOX 37-2	Pressure Ulcer Stages

Stage 1: **Intact skin with redness over a bony prominence.** The color does not fade with pressure. In persons with dark skin, skin color may differ from surrounding areas. It may appear pale, blue, or purple. See Figure 37-5, *A.*

Stage 2: **Partial-thickness skin loss** (Fig. 37-5, *B*). The wound may involve a blister or shallow ulcer. An ulcer may appear to be reddish-pink. A blister may be intact or open.

Stage 3: **Full-thickness tissue loss** (Fig. 37-5, *C*). The skin is gone. Subcutaneous fat may be exposed. Slough may be present. *Slough is dead tissue that is shed from the skin. It is usually light colored, soft, and moist. It may be stringy at times.*

Stage 4: **Full-thickness tissue loss with muscle, tendon, and bone exposure** (Fig. 37-5, *D*). Slough and eschar may be present. *Eschar is thick, leathery dead tissue that may be loose or adhered to the skin. It is often black or brown.*

Unstageable: **Full-thickness tissue loss with the ulcer covered by slough and/or eschar** (Fig. 37-5, *E*). Slough is yellow, tan, gray, green, or brown. Eschar is tan, brown, or black. This stage (Stage 3 or 4) cannot be determined until enough slough and eschar are removed.

Suspected deep tissue injury: **A purple or maroon area of intact skin or a blood-filled blister.** Pressure or shear has damaged underlying soft tissue. Involved tissue may be painful, firm, soft, warm, or cool. Skin changes may be hard to see in persons with dark skin. See Figure 37-5, *F.*

(Modified from National Pressure Ulcer Advisory Panel, European Pressure Ulcer Advisory Panel and Pan Pacific Pressure Injury Alliance. Prevention and Treatment of Pressure Ulcers: Quick Reference Guide. Emily Haesler (Ed.). Cambridge Media: Perth, Australia; 2014.)

FOCUS ON COMMUNICATION

Pressure Ulcer Stages

Tell the nurse if you see areas of redness, skin color changes, blisters, or skin or tissue loss. Describe what you observe as best as you can. Tell the nurse the site. The nurse needs to assess the area. For example, you can say:

- "I saw a reddened area on Mr. Drake's left heel. It was about the size of a quarter. The skin looked intact. Please look at it."
- "I just gave Ms. Richards a bath. I noticed a red area with a blister on her left buttock. I didn't see any drainage. Please look at it. I'll help you turn her."

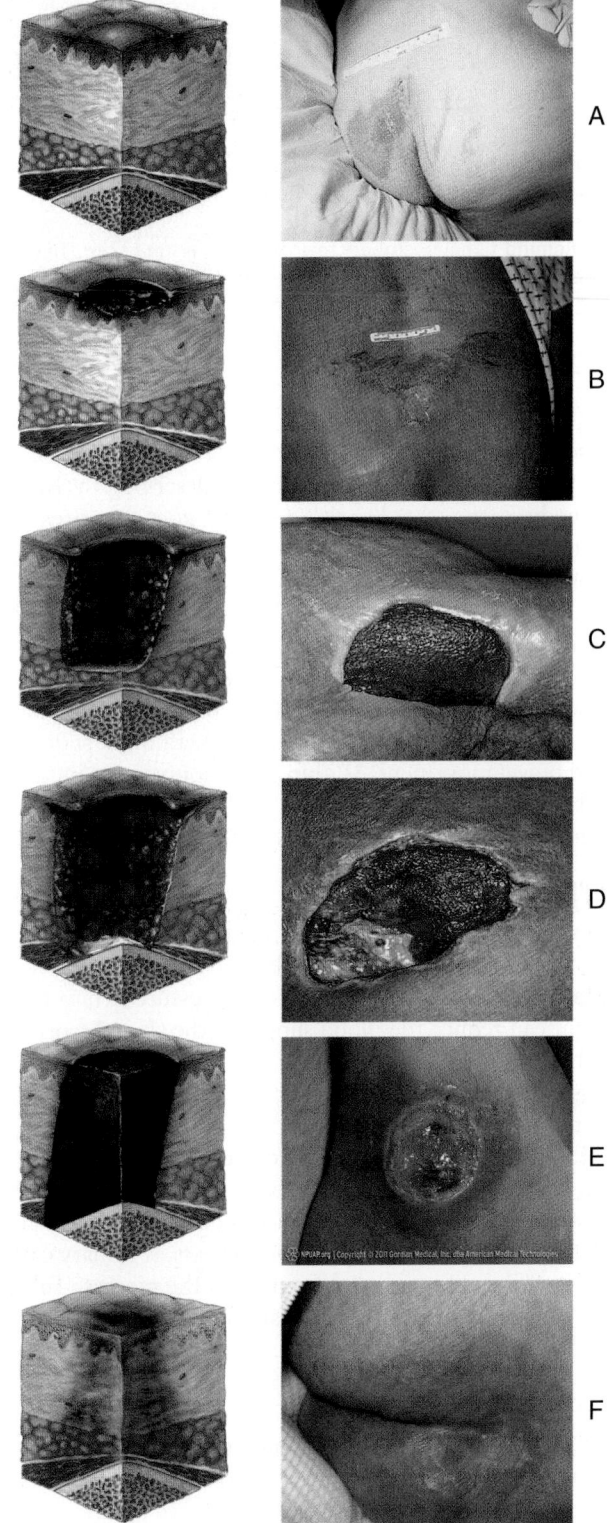

FIGURE 37-5 Pressure ulcer stages. **A,** Stage 1. **B,** Stage 2. **C,** Stage 3. **D,** Stage 4. **E,** Unstageable. **F,** Suspected deep tissue injury. (A, B, C, D, E [part 1], and F [parts 1 & 2] from National Pressure Ulcer Advisory Panel, European Pressure Ulcer Advisory Panel and Pan Pacific Pressure Injury Alliance. *Prevention and Treatment of Pressure Ulcers: Quick Reference Guide.* Emily Haesler (Ed.). Cambridge Media: Perth, Australia; 2014. A, B, C, and D [part 2] courtesy Laurel Wieresma-Bryant, RN, MSN, Clinical Nurse Specialist, Barnes-Jewish Hospital, St. Louis. E [part 2] from Byrant RA, Nix DP: *Acute & chronic wounds: current management concepts,* ed 3, St Louis, 2007, Mosby.)

Kennedy Terminal Ulcer

Persons receiving end-of-life care (Chapter 55) are at risk for unavoidable pressure ulcers. Described by Karen Kennedy-Evans, the *Kennedy terminal ulcer* is a pressure ulcer over a bony prominence that develops 2 to 3 days before death. The sacrum is the most common site. The cause is thought to be *skin failure*—the skin (along with other body organs) shuts down 10 to 14 days before death.

The onset is sudden. Shaped like a pear, butterfly, or horseshoe, the ulcer can be red, yellow, purple, or black (Fig. 37-6). At first it may look like a small black spot or a dried bowel movement. Within a few hours it can increase to the size of a quarter or larger. Usually Stage 2 with a blister at first, it rapidly progresses to Stage 3 or 4.

SITES

Pressure ulcers usually occur over bony prominences (pressure points). These areas bear the body's weight in certain positions (see Fig. 37-1). Pressure from body weight can reduce the blood supply to the skin. According to the CMS, the sacrum is the most common site for a pressure ulcer. However, pressure ulcers on the heels often occur.

The ears also are pressure ulcer sites. This is from pressure on the ear from the mattress when in the side-lying position. Eyeglasses and oxygen tubing (Chapter 39) also can cause pressure and friction on the ears. A urinary catheter can cause pressure and friction on the meatus. Tubes, casts, braces, and other devices can cause pressure on arms, hands, legs, and feet. A pressure ulcer can develop where medical equipment attaches to the skin.

Pressure ulcers can occur from friction in areas where skin has contact with skin. Common sites are between abdominal folds, the legs, the buttocks, the thighs, and under the breasts.

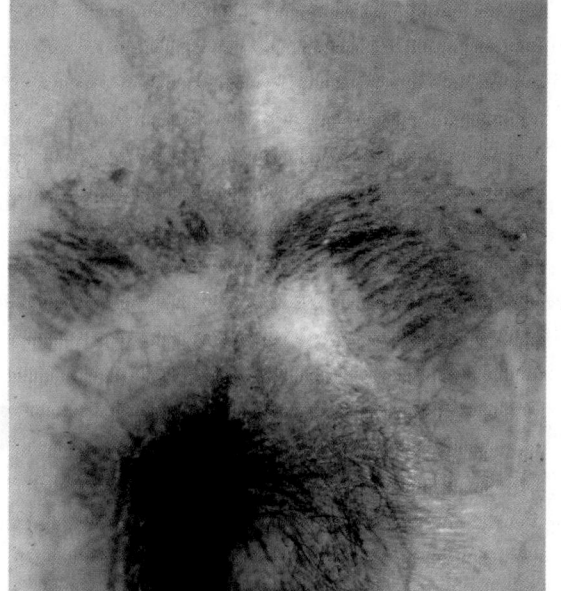

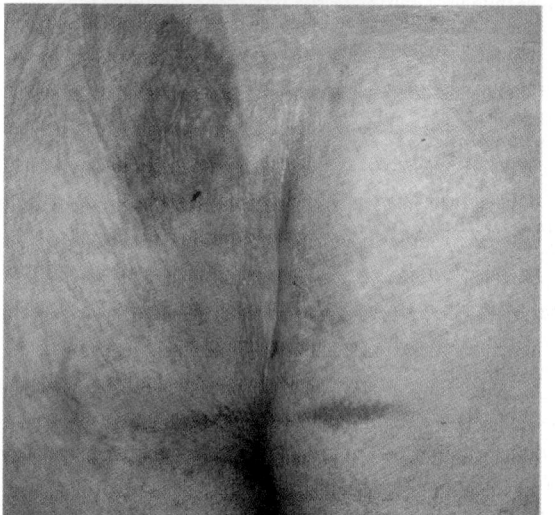

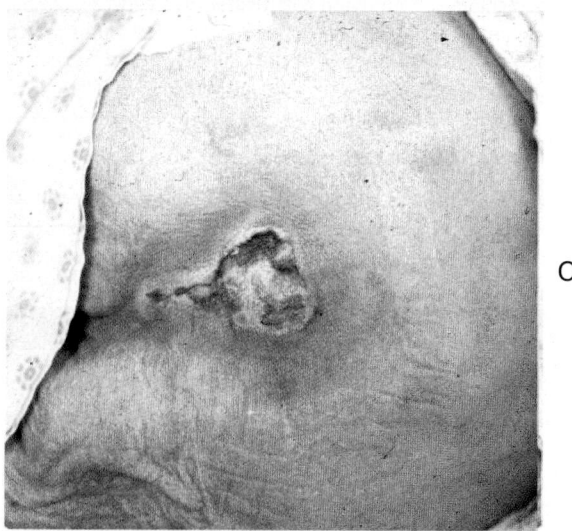

FIGURE 37-6 Kennedy terminal ulcer. **A and B,** First 4 to 8 hours. **C,** After 8 hours. (From Kennedy KL: *Understanding the Kennedy terminal ulcer*, Tucson, 2014.)

PREVENTION AND TREATMENT

Preventing pressure ulcers is much easier than trying to heal them. Good nursing care, cleanliness, and skin care are essential. The Joint Commission (TJC) and the CMS require pressure ulcer prevention programs. Pressure ulcer prevention involves:

- Identifying persons at risk. The nurse assesses the person's risk factors and skin condition (p. 623).
- Prevention measures for those at risk. Managing moisture, good nutrition and fluid balance, and relieving pressure are key measures. Box 37-3 lists common measures used to prevent skin breakdown and pressure ulcers. Always follow the care plan.

Some agencies use symbols or colored stickers as pressure ulcer alerts. Placed on the person's door or medical record, the alerts remind the staff that the person is at risk.

See *Focus on Surveys: Prevention and Treatment.*

FOCUS ON SURVEYS

Prevention and Treatment

Because pressure ulcers are very serious, they are a focus of surveys. You may be interviewed during a site survey. You might be asked about:

- How you are involved in the person's care
- What measures the agency uses to prevent pressure ulcers
- What skin changes you should report and when
- To whom you should report skin changes
- Your knowledge of measures in the person's care plan

BOX 37-3   Preventing Pressure Ulcers

Moving and Positioning

- Follow the person's re-positioning schedule (Fig. 37-7, p. 628). Re-position bedfast persons at least every 1 to 2 hours. Re-position chairfast persons at least every hour. Some persons are re-positioned every 15 minutes.
- Remind persons sitting in chairs to shift positions every 15 minutes.
- Position the person according to the care plan. Use pillows for support as directed. The 30-degree lateral position is recommended (Fig. 37-8, p. 628).
- Do not position the person:
  - On a pressure ulcer
  - On a reddened area
  - On tubes or other medical devices
- Do not leave a person on a bedpan longer than needed.
- Do not let the person sit on donut-shaped cushions.
- Prevent shearing and friction during moving and transfer procedures. Do not drag the person. Use assist devices as directed. See Chapters 18 and 19.
- Prevent friction in bed. Powder sheets lightly to prevent friction if directed to do so by the nurse.
- Prevent shearing. Do not raise the head of the bed more than 30 degrees. Follow the care plan for:
  - When to raise the head of the bed
  - How far to raise the head of the bed
  - How long (in minutes) to raise the head of the bed
- Use pillows, foam wedges, or other devices to prevent bony areas from contact with bony areas. The ankles, knees, hips, and sacrum are examples.
- Keep the heels and ankles off the bed. Use pillows or other devices as directed. Place the pillows or devices under the lower legs from mid-calf to the ankles.
- Use protective devices as directed (p. 628).
- Support the feet properly. Use a footstool if the person's feet do not touch the floor when he or she is sitting in a chair. The body slides forward when the feet do not touch the floor. For the person in a wheelchair, position the feet on the footrests.

Skin Care

- Inspect the skin every time you give care. This includes during or after transfers, re-positioning, bathing, and elimination procedures. Report any concern at once.
- Follow the person's bathing schedule. Some persons do not need a bath every day.
- Do not use hot water to bathe or clean the skin. Hot water can irritate the skin.
- Use a cleansing agent as directed. Soap can dry and irritate the skin.
- Provide good skin care.
  - The skin is clean and dry after bathing.
  - The skin is free of moisture from a bath, urine, feces, perspiration, wound drainage, and other secretions.
  - Areas under the breasts and in the groin area are clean and dry.
- Follow measures to prevent incontinence.
- Prevent skin exposure to moisture. Check persons who are incontinent of urine or feces often. Provide good skin care and change linens and garments at the time of soiling. Use incontinence products as directed.
- Apply an ointment or moisture barrier if the person is incontinent of urine or feces. Follow the care plan.
- Check persons often who perspire heavily or have wound drainage. Change linens and garments as needed. Provide good skin care.
- Apply moisturizer to dry areas—hands, elbows, hips, ankles, heels, and so on. The nurse tells you what to use and what areas need attention.
- Give a back massage when re-positioning the person. Do not massage bony areas.
- Do not massage over pressure points. *Never rub or massage reddened areas.*
- Keep linens clean, dry, and wrinkle-free.
- Make sure the bed or chair is free of objects. Crumbs, pins, pencils, pens, and coins are examples.
- Do not irritate the skin. Avoid scrubbing or vigorous rubbing when bathing or drying the person.
- Use pillows and blankets to prevent skin from being in contact with skin. They also reduce moisture and friction.

Continued

BOX 37-3	Preventing Pressure Ulcers—cont'd

Skin Care—cont'd
- Make sure clothes do not increase the risk for pressure ulcers.
  - Avoid seams, buttons, or zippers that press against the skin.
  - Avoid tight clothes.
  - Keep clothes from bunching up or wrinkling.
- Make sure socks and shoes are in good repair. Socks should not have holes, wrinkles, or creases. Make sure there is nothing in the shoes before the person puts them on.

Skin Care—cont'd
- Do not apply heat or cold (Chapter 38) directly on a pressure ulcer.
- See "Diabetic Foot Ulcers" in Chapter 36.

Medical Devices
- Check the skin under a medical device for edema and signs of skin breakdown or a pressure ulcer (see Box 37-2).
- Protect the skin under the device as directed by the nurse.
- Do not position the person on top of a medical device.
- Tell the nurse if the device is too loose or too tight.

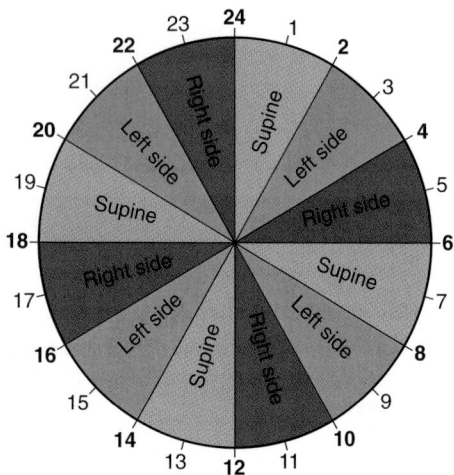

FIGURE 37-7 Turn clock. The clock shows the times to turn the person and to what position.

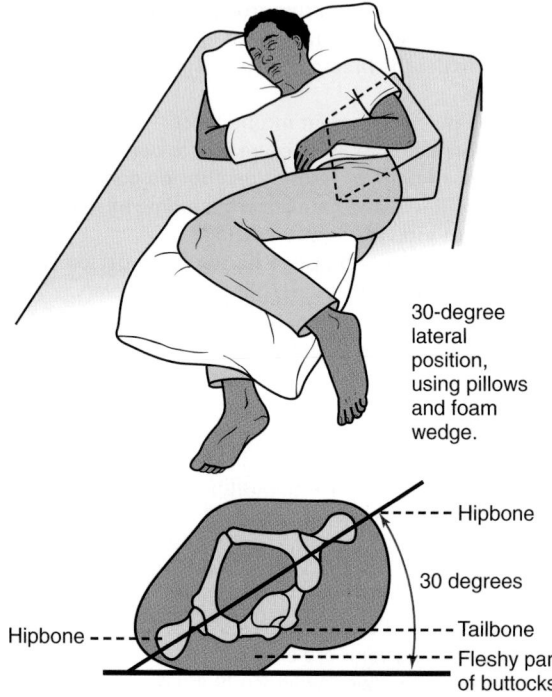

FIGURE 37-8 The 30-degree lateral position. Pillows are placed under the head, shoulder, and leg. This position inclines (lifts up) the hip to avoid pressure on the hip. The person does not lie on the hip as in the side-lying position.

Protective Devices

The doctor orders wound care products, drugs, treatments, and equipment to promote healing. Support surfaces relieve or reduce pressure. Such surfaces include foam, air, alternating air, gel, or water mattresses.

Protective devices are often used to prevent and treat skin breakdown and pressure ulcers. These devices are common.

- *Bed cradle.* A bed cradle is a metal frame placed on the bed and over the person (Chapter 30). Top linens are brought over the cradle to prevent pressure on the legs, feet, and toes. Protect against drafts and chilling by tucking and mitering linens under the mattress bottom and sides.
- *Heel and elbow protectors.* These devices are made of foam padding, pressure-relieving gel, sheepskin, and other cushioning materials. They fit the shape of heels and elbows (Fig. 37-9). Some are inside sleeves or mesh. Others are secured in place with straps. The devices promote comfort and reduce shear and friction.
- *Heel and foot elevators.* These raise the heels and feet off of the bed (Fig. 37-10). They prevent pressure. Some also prevent footdrop (Chapter 30).
- *Gel- or fluid-filled pads and cushions.* These devices have a pressure-relieving gel or fluid (Fig. 37-11). They are used for chairs and wheelchairs to prevent pressure. The outer case is vinyl. The device is placed in a fabric cover to protect the skin. Some covers are 2 colors (Fig. 37-12). The colors remind the staff to re-position the person.
- *Special beds.* Some beds have air flowing through the mattresses (Fig. 37-13). Body weight is distributed evenly. There is little pressure on body parts. Some beds allow re-positioning without moving the person. The person is turned to the prone or supine position or the bed is tilted various degrees. Alignment does not change. Pressure points change as the position changes. There is little friction. Some beds constantly rotate from side to side. They are useful for persons with spinal cord injuries.
- *Other equipment.* Pillows, trochanter rolls, foot-boards, and other positioning devices are used (Chapter 30). They maintain good alignment.

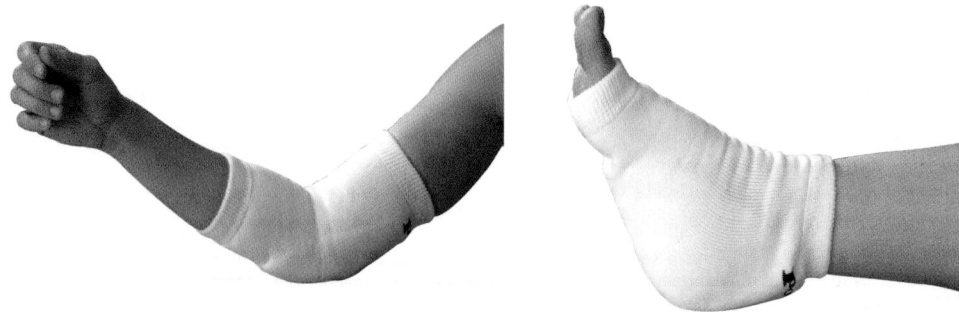

FIGURE 37-9 Heel and elbow protectors. (Images courtesy Posey Company, Arcadia, Calif.)

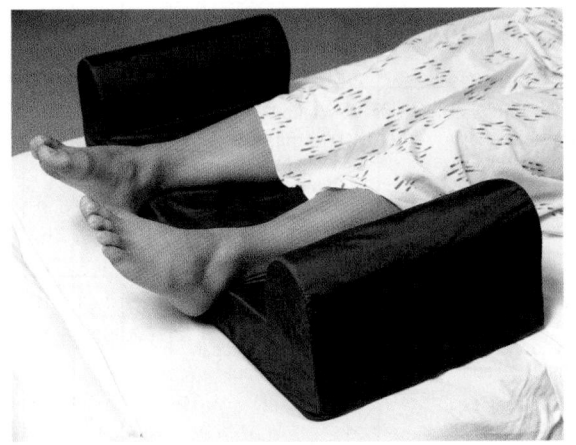

FIGURE 37-10 Heel elevator. (Image courtesy Posey Company, Arcadia, Calif.)

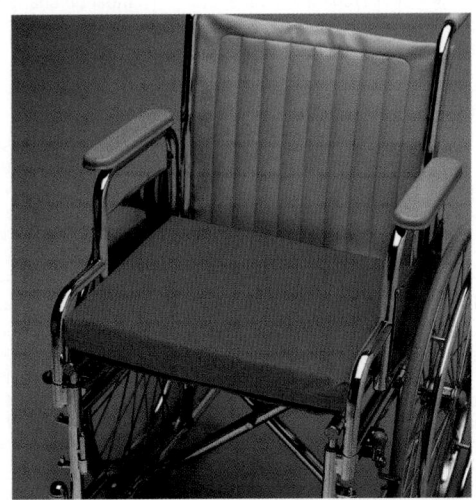

FIGURE 37-11 Gel and foam cushion. (Image courtesy Posey Company, Arcadia, Calif.)

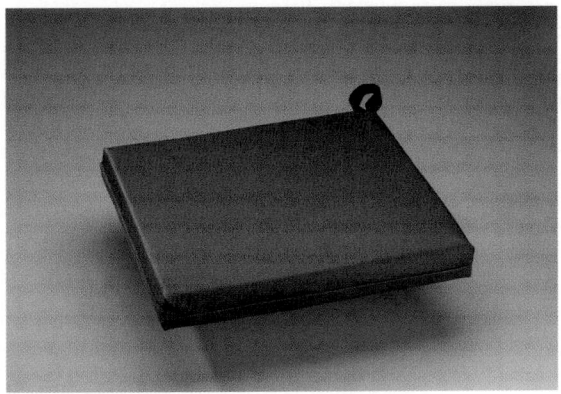

FIGURE 37-12 Two-color foam cushion. (Image courtesy Posey Company, Arcadia, Calif.)

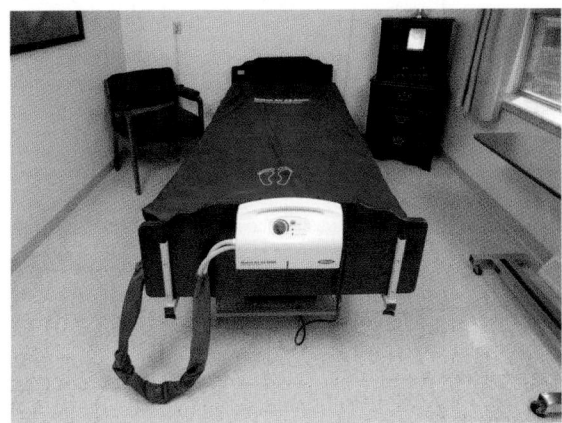

FIGURE 37-13 Air flotation bed.

BRADEN SCALE FOR PREDICTING PRESSURE SORE RISK

Patient's name _____   Evaluator's name _____   Date of assessment

SENSORY PERCEPTION Ability to respond meaningfully to pressure-related discomfort	**1. Completely Limited** Unresponsive (does not moan, flinch, or grasp) to painful stimuli, due to diminished level of consciousness or sedation OR limited ability to feel pain over most of body.	**2. Very Limited** Responds only to painful stimuli. Cannot communicate discomfort except by moaning or restlessness OR has a sensory impairment which limits the ability to feel pain or discomfort over 1/2 of body.	**3. Slightly Limited** Responds to verbal commands, but cannot always communicate discomfort or the need to be turned OR has some sensory impairment which limits ability to feel pain or discomfort in 1 or 2 extremities.	**4. No Impairment** Responds to verbal commands. Has no sensory deficit which would limit ability to feel or voice pain or discomfort.
MOISTURE Degree to which skin is exposed to moisture	**1. Constantly Moist** Skin is kept moist almost constantly by perspiration, urine, etc. Dampness is detected every time patient is moved or turned.	**2. Very Moist** Skin is often, but not always moist. Linen must be changed at least once a shift.	**3. Occasionally Moist** Skin is occasionally moist, requiring an extra linen change approximately once a day.	**4. Rarely Moist** Skin is usually dry, linen only requires changing at routine intervals.
ACTIVITY Degree of physical activity	**1. Bedfast** Confined to bed.	**2. Chairfast** Ability to walk severely limited or non-existent. Cannot bear own weight and/or must be assisted into chair or wheelchair.	**3. Walks Occasionally** Walks occasionally during day, but for very short distances, with or without assistance. Spends majority of each shift in bed or chair.	**4. Walks Frequently** Walks outside room at least twice a day and inside room at least once every two hours during waking hours.
MOBILITY Ability to change and control body position	**1. Completely Immobile** Does not make even slight changes in body or extremity position without assistance.	**2. Very Limited** Makes occasional slight changes in body or extremity position but unable to make frequent or significant changes independently.	**3. Slightly Limited** Makes frequent though slight changes in body or extremity position independently.	**4. No Limitation** Makes major and frequent changes in position without assistance.
NUTRITION Usual food intake pattern	**1. Very Poor** Never eats a complete meal. Rarely eats more than 1/3 of any food offered. Eats 2 servings or less of protein (meat or dairy products) per day. Takes fluids poorly. Does not take a liquid dietary supplement OR is NPO and/or maintained on clear liquids or IVs for more than 5 days.	**2. Probably Inadequate** Rarely eats a complete meal and generally eats only about 1/2 of any food offered. Protein intake includes only 3 servings of meat or dairy products per day. Occasionally will take a dietary supplement OR receives less than optimum amount of liquid diet or tube feeding.	**3. Adequate** Eats over half of most meals. Eats a total of 4 servings of protein (meat, dairy products) per day. Occasionally will refuse a meal, but will usually take a supplement when offered OR is on a tube feeding or TPN regimen which probably meets most of nutritional needs.	**4. Excellent** Eats most of every meal. Never refuses a meal. Usually eats a total of 4 or more servings of meat and dairy products. Occasionally eats between meals. Does not require supplementation.
FRICTION & SHEAR	**1. Problem** Requires moderate to maximum assistance in moving. Complete lifting without sliding against sheets is impossible. Frequently slides down in bed or chair, requiring frequent re-positioning with maximum assistance. Spasticity, contractures or agitation leads to almost constant friction.	**2. Potential Problem** Moves feebly or requires minimum assistance. During a move skin probably slides to some extent against sheets, chair, restraints or other devices. Maintains relatively good position in chair or bed most of the time, but occasionally slides down.	**3. No Apparent Problem** Moves in bed and in chair independently and has sufficient muscle strength to lift up completely during move. Maintains good position in bed or chair.	

Total score

FIGURE 37-14 Braden Scale for Predicting Pressure Sore Risk. (From Braden B. and Bergstrom N. © 1988. All rights reserved. Reprinted with permission.)

Dressings

The nurse decides what dressing to use (Chapter 36). Sometimes wet dressings are used. The wound must be moist enough to promote healing. If too moist, the dressing can interfere with healing.

A pressure ulcer may have drainage. A dressing that absorbs drainage is used. The dressing absorbs slough. The slough is removed when the dressing is removed.

Braden Scale

The *Braden Scale for Predicting Pressure Sore Risk* is a popular tool (Fig. 37-14). Assessment is done daily or weekly depending on the person's condition and risk factors.

You assist the nurse with the assessment step of the nursing process. Report signs and symptoms of a pressure ulcer at once. See Box 37-2.

COMPLICATIONS

Infection is the most common complication. According to the CMS, all Stage 2, 3, and 4 pressure ulcers are colonized with bacteria. ***Colonized*** *refers to the presence of bacteria on the wound surface or in wound tissue. The person does not have signs and symptoms of an infection.* A wound is *infected* when bacteria invade the tissues around or in the pressure ulcer. The person has signs and symptoms of infection (Chapter 16). Pain and delayed healing may signal an infection. For the pressure ulcer to heal, infection must be diagnosed and treated.

Osteomyelitis is a risk if the pressure ulcer is over a bony prominence. The risk is great if the ulcer is not healing. *Osteomyelitis* means inflammation *(itis)* of the bone *(osteo)* and bone marrow *(myel)*. Pain is severe. The person is treated with bedrest and antibiotics. Careful and gentle positioning is needed. Surgery may be needed to remove dead bone and tissue.

Pressure ulcers can cause pain. Pain management is important (Chapter 31). Pain may affect movement and activity. Immobility is a risk factor for pressure ulcers. And it may delay healing of an existing pressure ulcer.

REPORTING AND RECORDING

Report and record any signs of skin breakdown or pressure ulcers at once. See Figure 37-15. See "Wound Appearance" in Chapter 36.

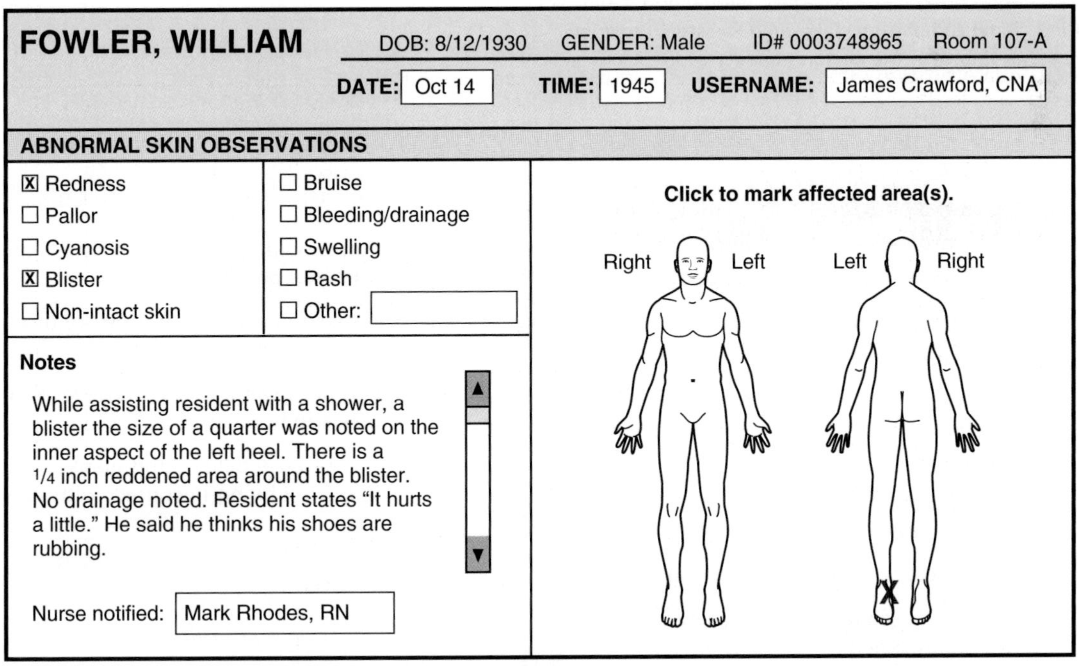
FOWLER, WILLIAM DOB: 8/12/1930 GENDER: Male ID# 0003748965 Room 107-A

DATE: Oct 14 **TIME:** 1945 **USERNAME:** James Crawford, CNA

ABNORMAL SKIN OBSERVATIONS

☒ Redness	☐ Bruise
☐ Pallor	☐ Bleeding/drainage
☐ Cyanosis	☐ Swelling
☒ Blister	☐ Rash
☐ Non-intact skin	☐ Other:

Notes

While assisting resident with a shower, a blister the size of a quarter was noted on the inner aspect of the left heel. There is a 1/4 inch reddened area around the blister. No drainage noted. Resident states "It hurts a little." He said he thinks his shoes are rubbing.

Nurse notified: Mark Rhodes, RN

Click to mark affected area(s).

FIGURE 37-15 Charting sample.

FOCUS ON **PRIDE**

The Person, Family, and Yourself

Personal and Professional Responsibility

You have an important role in preventing and treating pressure ulcers. Tasks like positioning, applying protective devices, and skin care may be delegated to you. You must function in a way that improves the person's quality of life, health, and safety. Your attitude and the quality of your work affect the person. If you take your role seriously and believe you have a positive impact, the person will benefit. If you are careless and lack concern for the person's well-being, harm can result.

You are an important member of the nursing team. Take pride in your role. Work to the best of your ability. The person will benefit and you will find joy in your work.

Rights and Respect

Observing and reporting skin problems can prevent further skin breakdown. You have the right and responsibility to speak for your patients and residents. This is called being an *advocate*. When you see or suspect a problem, tell the nurse. You may be the first to notice a pressure ulcer. Telling the nurse can prevent further harm and result in prompt actions that promote healing. Take pride in being a voice for your patients and residents.

Independence and Social Interaction

A pressure ulcer is a serious matter. Infection, pain, amputation, and longer hospital or nursing center stays are complications. Healing can be a very long process. As time passes, family and friends may not visit as often. Or the person may feel that he or she is a burden to others. Loneliness and depression can occur.

Physical needs are great. Do not neglect mental and social needs. Be kind. Show compassion. Take time to listen. Provide care in a way that improves the person's quality of life.

Delegation and Teamwork

Always report and record the completion of delegated tasks. Be accurate and honest. Never report or record something you did not do. Also, do not report or record before completing a task.

For example, Mrs. Scott was placed on the bedpan at 2250 (10:50 PM). The nursing assistant did not report this to the nurse. The next shift began at 2300 (11:00 PM). At 0700 (7:00 AM), the day shift found Mrs. Scott still on the bedpan. A pressure ulcer had developed. At risk for pressure ulcers, Mrs. Scott was to be re-positioned every 2 hours. Mrs. Scott's chart showed that she had been re-positioned every 2 hours from 2300 (11:00 PM) to 0700 (7:00 AM).

Poor communication, false recording, and negligence will cause harm. You must be thorough, honest, and careful when completing, reporting, and recording delegated tasks.

Ethics and Laws

Agencies must have a plan to predict, prevent, and treat pressure ulcers early. Many agencies use a form or screening tool to identify persons at risk. Assessments are done on admission and regularly. The agency must take action to address risks.

Know your agency's policies and procedures for identifying those at risk for pressure ulcers. Follow the measures in Box 37-3 and the care plan to do your part to prevent pressure ulcers.

FOCUS ON **PRIDE**: *Application*

Describe the physical, mental, and social effects a pressure ulcer can have. How can you help meet the person's needs?

REVIEW QUESTIONS

Circle T if the statement is TRUE or F if it is FALSE.

1 T F   All pressure ulcers are avoidable.

2 T F   Skin breakdown can lead to a pressure ulcer.

3 T F   Unrelieved pressure squeezes tiny blood vessels. Tissues do not receive needed oxygen and nutrients.

4 T F   Persons who are bedfast or chairfast are at risk for pressure ulcers.

5 T F   Pressure ulcers can develop on the ears.

6 T F   Pressure ulcers can develop where medical devices are attached to the skin.

7 T F   You assess the person's risk for pressure ulcers.

8 T F   Pressure ulcers can involve muscles, tendons, and bones.

9 T F   To prevent pressure ulcers, the head of the bed is raised higher than 30 degrees.

10 T F   You should inspect the person's skin every time you provide care.

11 T F   A person is at risk for pressure ulcers. A bath is needed every day.

12 T F   You are giving a back massage. You should massage bony areas.

13 T F   You can use pillows and blankets to prevent skin from being in contact with skin.

Circle the BEST answer.

14 A pressure ulcer is
   a An open wound
   b A localized injury to the skin and/or underlying tissue
   c A bony prominence
   d Dead tissue

15 Pressure ulcers are the result of
   a Moisture
   b Medical devices
   c Aging
   d Unrelieved pressure

16 Which contributes to the development of pressure ulcers?
a Shear and friction
b Slough
c Eschar
d CMS and TJC

17 A pressure ulcer can develop within
a 2 to 6 hours
b 6 to 10 hours
c 10 to 14 hours
d 14 to 18 hours

18 Which is a risk factor for pressure ulcers?
a Balanced diet
b Intact skin
c Incontinence
d Increased circulation

19 Which is the most common site for a Kennedy pressure ulcer?
a Back of the head
b Hip
c Sacrum
d Heel

20 In a light-skinned person, the first sign of a pressure ulcer is
a A blister
b A reddened area
c Drainage
d Gangrene

21 A care plan includes the following. Which should you question?
a Re-position the person every 2 hours.
b Scrub and rub the skin during bathing.
c Apply lotion to dry areas.
d Keep linens clean, dry, and wrinkle-free.

22 You should position the person
a On an existing pressure ulcer
b On a reddened area
c On tubes or other medical devices
d Using assist devices

23 What is the preferred position for preventing pressure ulcers?
a 30-degree lateral position
b Semi-Fowler's position
c Prone position
d Supine position

24 Which keeps the heels and ankles off the bed?
a Bed cradles
b Pillows
c Air flotation bed
d Trochanter rolls

25 Persons sitting in chairs should shift their positions every
a 15 minutes
b 30 minutes
c Hour
d 2 hours

26 A person is sitting in a chair. The feet do not touch the floor. What should you do?
a Have the person slide forward until the feet touch the floor.
b Let the feet dangle.
c Stack pillows under the person's feet.
d Position the feet on a footstool.

27 Which helps treat pressure ulcers?
a Donut-shaped cushions
b Weight loss
c Gel or fluid-filled pads and cushions
d Cleansing with soap and hot water

28 To prevent skin breakdown from moisture
a Avoid using lotion on dry areas
b Check incontinent persons every 4 hours
c Dry under the breasts and the groin area well
d Change linens once daily for persons who perspire heavily

29 You see a reddened area on the person's skin. What should you do?
a Rub or massage the area.
b Apply a moisturizer.
c Apply a moisture barrier.
d Tell the nurse.

30 A pressure ulcer is colonized. This means that
a The wound is infected
b Bacteria are present
c The person has osteomyelitis
d The person has a gauze dressing

Answers to Chapter 37 questions are on p. 871.

FOCUS ON PRACTICE

Problem Solving

Mr. Russell is at risk for pressure ulcers. He is to be re-positioned every 2 hours. He complains when you awaken him to provide care. You and a co-worker enter his room to re-position him. He is asleep. What will you do? What is the risk of waiting to re-position him? How can you provide safe, quality care that avoids causing him frustration?

Heat and Cold Applications

KEY TERMS

compress A soft pad applied over a body area
constrict To narrow
cyanosis Bluish *(cyano)* color
dilate To expand or open wider

hyperthermia A body temperature *(thermia)* that is much higher *(hyper)* than the person's normal range
hypothermia A very low *(hypo)* body temperature *(thermia)*
pack Wrapping a body part with a wet or dry application

KEY ABBREVIATIONS

C   Centigrade

F   Fahrenheit

Heat and cold applications:

- Promote healing.
- Promote comfort.
- Reduce tissue swelling.

Heat and cold have opposite effects on body functions. Severe injuries and changes in body function can occur. The risks are great.

Some agencies do not let nursing assistants apply heat or cold. Before you apply heat or cold, make sure that:

- Your state allows you to perform the procedure.
- The procedure is in your job description.
- You have the necessary training.
- You know how to use the equipment.
- You review the procedure with a nurse.
- A nurse is available to answer questions and to supervise you.

See *Focus on Children and Older Persons: Heat and Cold Applications.*

FOCUS ON **CHILDREN AND OLDER PERSONS**

Heat and Cold Applications

Children
Infants and young children have fragile skin. At risk for burns, they need careful attention. Always respond when a child cries. Crying can communicate pain.

Older Persons
Older persons have thin and fragile skin. Burns are a risk. Changes from aging and health problems increase the risk for burns. They include circulatory and nervous system changes. Some drugs affect the ability to sense pain. Confused persons and those with dementia may not recognize pain. Behavior changes can signal pain.

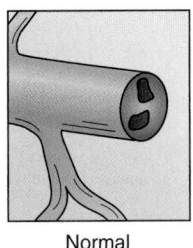 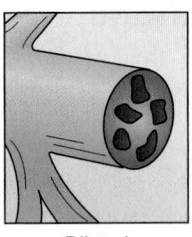 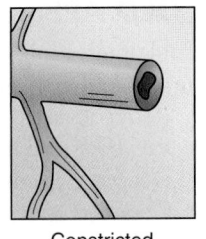

Normal	Dilated	Constricted
A	B	C

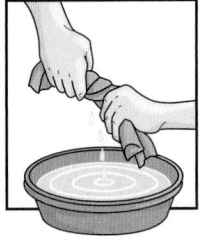 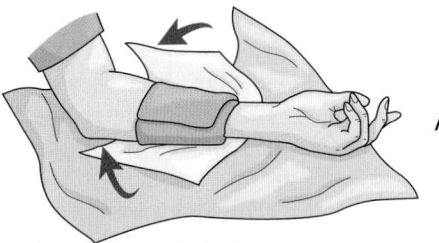

A

FIGURE 38-1 A, A blood vessel under normal conditions. **B,** Dilated blood vessel. **C,** Constricted blood vessel.

HEAT APPLICATIONS

Heat applications can be applied to almost any body part. They are often used for musculo-skeletal injuries or problems (sprains, arthritis). Heat:

- Relieves pain.
- Relaxes muscles.
- Promotes healing.
- Reduces tissue swelling.
- Decreases joint stiffness.

When heat is applied to the skin, blood vessels in the area dilate. ***Dilate*** *means to expand or open wider* (Fig. 38-1). Blood flow increases. Tissues have more oxygen and nutrients for healing. Excess fluid is removed from the area faster. The skin is red and warm.

Complications

High temperatures can cause burns. Report pain, excess redness, and blisters at once. Also observe for pale skin. When heat is applied too long, blood vessels ***constrict*** *(narrow)* (see Fig. 38-1). Blood flow decreases. Tissues receive less blood. Tissue damage occurs and the skin is pale.

Older and fair-skinned persons have fragile skin that is easily burned. Persons with problems sensing heat and pain also are at risk. Nervous system damage, altered awareness, and circulatory disorders affect sensation. So do confusion and some drugs.

Metal implants pose risks. Metal conducts heat. Deep tissues can be burned. Pacemakers (cardiac devices) and joint replacements are made of metal. Do not apply heat to an implant area.

Heat is not applied to a pregnant woman's abdomen. The heat can affect fetal growth.

Moist and Dry Heat Applications

With a *moist heat application,* water is in contact with the skin. Water conducts heat. Moist heat has greater and faster effects than dry heat. Heat penetrates deeper with a moist application. To prevent injury, moist heat applications have lower (cooler) temperatures than dry heat applications. Moist heat applications (Fig. 38-2) include:

- *Hot compress.* A ***compress*** *is a soft pad applied over a body area.* It is usually made of cloth. Sometimes an aquathermia pad (p. 636) is applied over the compress to maintain the temperature of the compress.

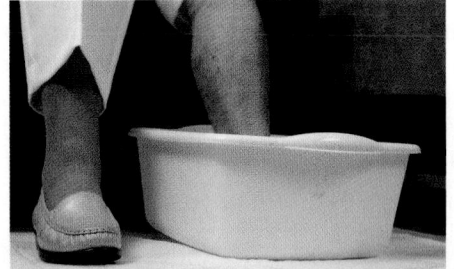

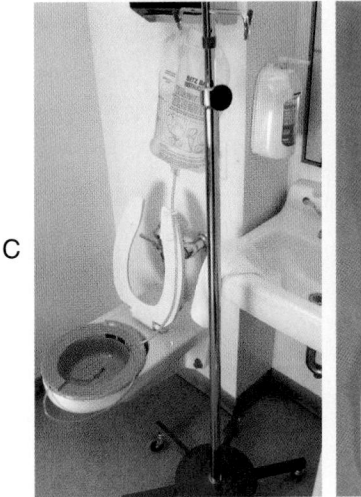 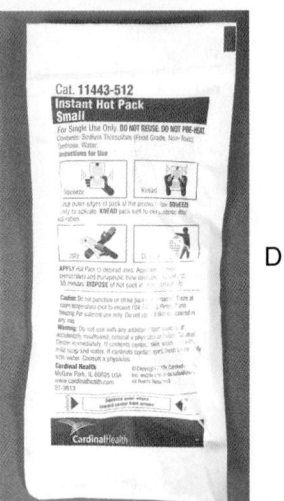

B

C

D

FIGURE 38-2 Moist heat applications. **A,** Compress. **B,** Hot soak. **C,** Disposable sitz bath. **D,** Hot pack. (NOTE: Compresses can be hot or cold. And some hot packs can also be used as cold packs.)

- *Hot soak.* A body part is put into water. This is usually used for smaller parts—a hand, lower arm, foot, or lower leg. A tub is used for larger areas.
- *Sitz bath.* The perineal and rectal areas are immersed in warm or hot water. (*Sitz* means *seat* in German.) Sitz baths are common for hemorrhoids, after rectal or female pelvic surgeries, and after childbirth. They are used to:
  - Clean perineal and anal wounds
  - Promote healing
  - Relieve pain and soreness
  - Increase circulation
  - Stimulate voiding
- *Hot pack.* A ***pack*** *involves wrapping a body part with a wet or dry application.* There are single-use (disposable) and re-usable packs. Some are used for heat or cold. Follow the manufacturer's instructions to activate the heat or cold. To clean re-usable packs, follow agency policy and the manufacturer's instructions.

With *dry heat applications,* water is not in contact with the skin. A dry heat application stays at the desired temperature longer. Dry heat does not penetrate as deep as moist heat. Because water is not used, dry heat needs higher (hotter) temperatures for the desired effect. Therefore burns are still a risk.

Some *hot packs* and warming therapy pads are dry heat applications. The *aquathermia pad* (Aqua-K, K-Pad) is a common therapy pad (Fig. 38-3). Tubes inside the pad are filled with distilled water. Heated water flows to the pad through a hose. Another hose returns water to the electric heating unit. Reheated water flows back into the pad.

See *Focus on Long-Term Care and Home Care: Moist and Dry Heat Applications.*

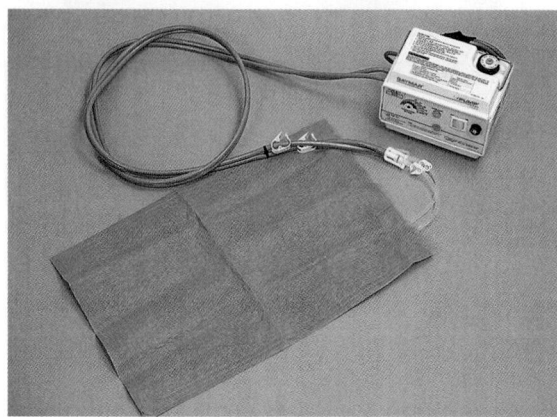

FIGURE 38-3 The aquathermia pad.

FOCUS ON LONG-TERM CARE AND HOME CARE

Moist and Dry Heat Applications

Home Care
Heating pads have electrical coils made of wire. The coils present fire hazards if they break. Always make sure the heating pad is in good repair.

Heating pad temperatures are easy to adjust. Burns are a great risk. Check the temperature often. Make sure the person has not changed it.

Some devices serve as heat and cold applications. They are filled with a special fluid. The pad is kept in the freezer until needed. To use as a heating pad, follow the manufacturer's instructions.

COLD APPLICATIONS

Cold applications are often used to treat sprains and fractures. Cold applications:
- Reduce pain.
- Prevent swelling.
- Decrease circulation and bleeding.
- Cool the body when fever is present.

Cold has the opposite effect of heat. When cold is applied to the skin, blood vessels constrict (see Fig. 38-1). Blood flow decreases. Tissues receive less oxygen and nutrients.

Cold applications are useful right after an injury. Decreased blood flow reduces bleeding. Less fluid collects in the tissues. Cold has a numbing effect on the skin. This helps reduce or relieve pain in the part.

Complications

Complications include pain, burns, blisters, and poor circulation. Burns and blisters occur from intense cold. They also occur when dry cold is in direct contact with the skin.

When cold is applied for a long time, blood vessels dilate. Blood flow increases. Prolonged application of cold has the same effect as heat applications.

Older and fair-skinned persons have fragile skin. They are at great risk for complications. So are persons with sensory impairments.

Moist and Dry Cold Applications

Moist cold applications penetrate deeper than dry ones. Therefore moist cold applications are warmer than dry cold applications.

The cold compress is a moist cold application (see Fig. 38-2, *A*). Dry cold applications include ice bags, ice collars, and ice gloves (Fig. 38-4). The device is filled with crushed ice.

Cold packs can be moist or dry applications (see Fig. 38-2, *D*). Commercial cold packs are single-use (disposable) or re-usable. To activate the cold, follow the manufacturer's instructions. You will strike, knead, or squeeze the pack. Keep re-usable cold packs in the freezer. Clean them after use. Discard single-use cold packs after use.

See *Focus on Long-Term Care and Home Care: Moist and Dry Cold Applications.*

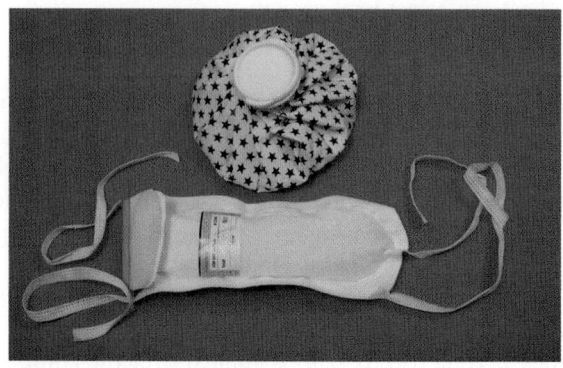

FIGURE 38-4 Ice bags.

◼ Applying Heat and Cold

Protect the person from injury during heat and cold applications. Follow the rules in Box 38-1. See Table 38-1 for heat and cold temperature ranges.

See *Focus on Communication: Applying Heat and Cold.*

See *Teamwork and Time Management: Applying Heat and Cold.*

See *Delegation Guidelines: Applying Heat and Cold*, p. 638.

See *Promoting Safety and Comfort: Applying Heat and Cold*, p. 638.

See procedure: *Applying Heat and Cold Applications*, p. 638.

Text continued on p. 640.

BOX 38-1	Applying Heat and Cold

- Know how to use the equipment. Follow the manufacturer's instructions for commercial devices.
- Measure the temperature of moist applications. Follow agency policy or use a bath thermometer.
- Follow agency policies for safe temperature ranges. See Table 38-1.
- Do not apply *very hot* (above 106°F or 41.1°C) applications. Tissue damage can occur. A nurse applies *very hot* applications.
- Ask the nurse what the temperature should be.
  - Heat—cooler temperatures for persons at risk.
  - Cold—warmer temperatures for persons at risk.
- Know the exact site of the application. Have the nurse show you the site.
- Cover dry heat or cold applications before applying them. Use a flannel cover, towel, or other cover as directed.
- Provide for privacy. Properly screen and drape the person. Expose only the body part involved. Avoid unnecessary exposure.
- Maintain comfort and body alignment during the procedure.
- Observe the skin every 5 minutes during the procedure. See *Delegation Guidelines: Applying Heat and Cold*, p. 638.
- Do not let the person change the temperature of the application.
- Know how long to leave the application in place. Heat and cold are applied no longer than 15 to 20 minutes.
- Follow the rules for electrical safety when using electrical appliances to apply heat. See Chapter 13.
- Place the call light within the person's reach.
- Complete a safety check before leaving the room. (See the inside of the front cover.)

TABLE 38-1	Heat and Cold Temperature Ranges	
Temperature	**Fahrenheit (F) Range**	**Centigrade (C) Range**
Hot	99°F to 106°F	37°C to 41°C
Warm	93°F to 98°F	34°C to 37°C
Tepid	80°F to 92°F	26°C to 34°C
Cool	65°F to 79°F	18°C to 26°C
Cold	50°F to 64°F	10°C to 18°C

From Perry AG, Potter PA, Ostendorf WR: Nursing interventions & clinical skills, ed 6, St Louis, 2016, Mosby.

FOCUS ON **COMMUNICATION**

Applying Heat and Cold

The person may not report pain or discomfort. The person may not know what symptoms to report. For heat and cold applications, you need to ask:
- "Does the application feel too hot or too cold?"
- "Do you feel any pain, numbness, or burning?"
- "Do you feel weak, faint, or drowsy?" If yes: "Tell me how you feel?"

TEAMWORK AND TIME MANAGEMENT

Applying Heat and Cold

After applying heat or cold, check the person and the application every 5 minutes. Plan your work so you can stay in or near the person's room. For example, during the application:
- Make the bed and straighten the person's unit.
- Provide care to the person's roommate if assigned to him or her.
- Help the person complete the daily or weekly menu.
- Read cards and letters to the person, with his or her consent.
- Address envelopes and other correspondence for the person.
- Take time to visit with the person.

DELEGATION GUIDELINES

Applying Heat and Cold

To apply heat or cold, you need this information from the nurse and the care plan.

- The type of application—hot compress or pack, commercial compress, hot soak, sitz bath, or aquathermia pad; ice bag, ice collar, ice glove, cold pack, or cold compress
- How to cover the application
- What temperature to use (see Table 38-1)
- The application site
- How long to leave the application in place
- What observations to report and record:
  - Complaints of pain or discomfort, numbness, or burning
  - Excess redness
  - Blisters
  - Pale, white, or gray skin
  - *Cyanosis*—*bluish* (cyano) *color*
  - Shivering
  - Rapid pulse, weakness, faintness, and drowsiness (sitz bath)
  - Time, site, and length of application
- When to report observations
- What patient or resident concerns to report at once

PROMOTING SAFETY AND COMFORT

Applying Heat and Cold

Safety

Keep the call light within reach and check the person every 5 minutes. Also follow these safety measures.

- *Sitz bath.* Blood flow increases to the perineum and rectum. Therefore less blood flows to other areas. Observe for signs of weakness, fainting, or fatigue. Also protect the person from injury. Prevent chills and burns.
- *Commercial hot and cold packs.* Read warning labels and follow the manufacturer's instructions.
- *Aquathermia pad:*
  - Follow electrical safety precautions (Chapter 13).
  - Check the device for damage or flaws.
  - Follow the manufacturer's instructions.
  - Place the heating unit on an even, uncluttered surface. This prevents it from being knocked over or knocked off the surface.
  - Make sure the hoses do not have kinks or bubbles. Water must flow freely.
  - Use a flannel cover to insulate the pad. It absorbs perspiration at the application site. (Some agencies use towels or pillowcases.)
  - Secure the pad in place with ties, tape, or rolled gauze. Do not use pins. They can puncture the pad and cause leaks.
  - Do not place the pad under a body part. This prevents the escape of heat. Burns can result if heat cannot escape.
  - Give the temperature setting key to the nurse. This prevents anyone from changing the temperature. The temperature is usually set at 105°F (40.5°C) with a key.

Some persons have medicated patches or ointments applied to the skin. Do not apply heat over such areas.

Comfort

Cold applications can cause chills and shivering. Provide for warmth. Use bath blankets or other blankets as needed.

Applying Heat and Cold Applications

QUALITY OF LIFE

- Knock before entering the person's room.
- Address the person by name.
- Introduce yourself by name and title.

- Explain the procedure before starting and during the procedure.
- Protect the person's rights during the procedure.
- Handle the person gently during the procedure.

PRE-PROCEDURE

1 Follow *Delegation Guidelines: Applying Heat and Cold.* See *Promoting Safety and Comfort: Applying Heat and Cold.*
2 Practice hand hygiene.
3 Collect equipment.
  - *For a hot compress:*
    - Basin
    - Bath thermometer
    - Small towel, washcloth, or gauze squares
    - Plastic wrap or aquathermia pad
    - Ties, tape, or rolled gauze
    - Bath towel
    - Waterproof under-pad

  - *For a hot soak:*
    - Water basin or arm or foot bath
    - Bath thermometer
    - Waterproof under-pad
    - Bath blanket
    - Towel
  - *For a sitz bath:*
    - Disposable sitz bath
    - Bath thermometer
    - 2 bath blankets, bath towels, and a clean gown
  - *For an aquathermia pad:*
    - Aquathermia pad and heating unit
    - Distilled water
    - Flannel cover or other cover as directed
    - Ties, tape, or rolled gauze

Applying Heat and Cold Applications—cont'd

PRE-PROCEDURE—cont'd

- *For a hot or cold pack:*
  - Commercial pack
  - Pack cover
  - Ties, tape, or rolled gauze (if needed)
  - Waterproof under-pad
- *For an ice bag, ice collar, ice glove, or dry cold pack:*
  - Ice bag, collar, glove, or cold pack
  - Crushed ice (except for a cold pack)
  - Flannel cover or other cover as directed
  - Paper towels

- *For a cold compress:*
  - Large basin with ice
  - Small basin with cold water
  - Gauze squares, washcloths, or small towels
  - Waterproof under-pad

4 Identify the person. Check the ID (identification) bracelet against the assignment sheet. Use 2 identifiers (Chapter 13). Also call the person by name.

PROCEDURE

5 Provide for privacy.
6 Position the person for the procedure.
7 Place the waterproof under-pad (if needed) under the body part.
8 *For a hot compress:*
  a Fill the basin ½ to ⅔ full with hot water as directed. Measure water temperature.
  b Place the compress in the water and wring out.
  c Apply the compress over the area. Note the time.
  d Cover the compress as directed. Do 1 of the following.
    1) Apply plastic wrap and then a bath towel. Secure the towel in place with ties, tape, or rolled gauze.
    2) Apply an aquathermia pad.
9 *For a hot soak:*
  a Fill the container ½ full with hot water. Measure water temperature.
  b Place the part into the water. Pad the edge of the container with a towel. Note the time.
  c Cover the person with a bath blanket for warmth.
10 *For a sitz bath:*
  a Place the disposable sitz bath on the toilet seat.
  b Fill the sitz bath ⅔ full with water. Measure water temperature.
  c Secure the gown above the waist.
  d Help the person sit on the sitz bath. Note the time.
  e Provide for warmth. Place a bath blanket around the shoulders. Place the other over the legs.
  f Stay with the person if he or she is weak or unsteady.
11 *For an aquathermia pad:*
  a Fill the heating unit to the fill line with distilled water.
  b Remove the bubbles. Place the pad and tubing below the heating unit. Tilt the heating unit from side to side.
  c Set the temperature as the nurse directs (usually 105°F [40.5°C]). Remove the key.
  d Place the pad in the cover.
  e Plug in the unit. Let water warm to the desired temperature.
  f Set the heating unit on the bedside stand. Keep the pad and connecting hoses level with the unit.
  g Apply the pad to the part. Note the time.
  h Secure the pad in place with ties, tape, or rolled gauze.

12 *For a hot or cold pack:*
  a Squeeze, knead, or strike the pack as directed by the manufacturer.
  b Place the pack in the cover.
  c Apply the pack. Note the time.
  d Secure the pack in place with ties, tape, or rolled gauze. Some packs are secured with Velcro straps.
13 *For an ice bag, collar, or glove:*
  a Fill the device with water. Put in the stopper. Turn the device upside down to check for leaks.
  b Empty the device.
  c Fill the device ½ to ⅔ full with crushed ice or ice chips.
  d Remove excess air. Bend, twist, or squeeze the device. Or press it against a firm surface.
  e Place the cap or stopper on securely.
  f Dry the device with paper towels.
  g Place the device in the cover.
  h Apply the device. Note the time.
  i Secure the device with ties, tape, or rolled gauze.
14 *For a cold compress:*
  a Place the small basin with cold water into the large basin with ice.
  b Place the compresses into the cold water.
  c Wring out a compress.
  d Apply the compress to the part. Note the time.
15 Place the call light and other needed items within reach. Unscreen the person if appropriate.
16 Raise or lower bed rails. Follow the care plan.
17 Do the following every 5 minutes.
  a Check the person for signs and symptoms of complications (see *Delegation Guidelines: Applying Heat and Cold*). Remove the application if any occur. Tell the nurse at once.
  b Check the application for cooling (hot application) or warming (cold application).
18 Remove the application at the specified time. Heat and cold applications are left on for 15 to 20 minutes.

POST-PROCEDURE

19 Provide for comfort. (See the inside of the front cover.)
20 Place the call light and other needed items within reach.
21 Raise or lower bed rails. Follow the care plan.
22 Unscreen the person.
23 Clean, rinse, dry, and return re-usable items to their proper place. Follow agency policy for used linens. Wear gloves.

24 Complete a safety check of the room. (See the inside of the front cover.)
25 Remove and discard the gloves. Practice hand hygiene.
26 Report and record your observations.

COOLING AND WARMING BLANKETS

Hyperthermia is a body temperature (thermia) *that is much higher* (hyper) *than the person's normal range.* Body temperature is greater than 103°F (39.4°C). It is often called *heat stroke* when caused by hot weather. Other causes include illness, dehydration, and not being able to perspire. Lowering the person's body temperature is necessary. Otherwise, death can occur. The doctor orders ice packs applied to the head, neck, underarms, and groin. Sometimes cooling blankets are used alone or with ice packs.

Hypothermia is a very low (hypo) *body temperature* (thermia). Body temperature is less than 95°F (35°C). Cold weather is a common cause. The person is warmed to prevent death. Treatment may include a warming blanket. A warming blanket is like a cooling blanket except warm settings are used. Vital signs are checked often to prevent rapid or excess warming.

An electrical device, the blanket is made of rubber or plastic. When used for cooling, the device is called a *hypothermia blanket.* When used for warming, it is called a *hyperthermia blanket.* The device has warm and cool settings. Warm or cool fluid flows through tubes in the blanket. Vital signs are measured often.

See *Focus on Children and Older Persons: Cooling and Warming Blankets.*

FOCUS ON CHILDREN AND OLDER PERSONS

Cooling and Warming Blankets

Children

Rapid temperature changes can occur in infants and children. Observe them closely. Measure temperature as the nurse directs. Report the following at once.
- The temperature measurement and other vital signs
- Changes in vital signs
- Changes in the child's condition

FOCUS ON PRIDE

The Person, Family, and Yourself

Personal and Professional Responsibility

You are responsible for the tasks you perform. If unsure about applying heat or cold, ask the nurse and check your job description. If not familiar with the equipment, tell the nurse. Never perform a task you are not comfortable doing. The person may be harmed. Do not be afraid, embarrassed, or ashamed to ask the nurse about your concerns. Take pride in acting responsibly.

Rights and Respect

Respect the right to privacy. Be sure the person is properly screened and covered. This will vary by application site, method, and personal preference. For example:
- During a sitz bath, ensure the person is covered and no one enters the bathroom during the procedure.
- A resident receiving a hot soak to a foot prefers that the privacy curtain remains pulled.
- A patient has an ice bag on his hand. He enjoys talking to his roommate and would like to be unscreened during the application.

Independence and Social Interaction

Remember to explain procedures to patients and residents. They can plan if they know what will happen. For example, a person wants to make a phone call or finish an activity first. Or a person may want a procedure done by a certain time—before visitors arrive or before an activity. You promote independence when you involve the person in planning.

Delegation and Teamwork

Safety and comfort measures require time and planning. Heat and cold are usually applied for 15 to 20 minutes. The procedure involves:
- Meeting elimination needs before the procedure
- Positioning the person for comfort
- Placing needed items within reach—call light, water mug, reading material, computer, phone, other requested items
- Checking the person often
- Reporting and recording task completion and your observations

With practice and experience you will learn how much time you need for tasks. You can also ask for advice from co-workers who manage their work well.

Ethics and Laws

Complications from heat and cold can be severe. Burns, blisters, circulation problems, and tissue damage are examples. Safety is a priority. Harm and legal action can result if you:
- Apply a heat or cold application without an order.
- Use the equipment without training.
- Apply an application that is too hot or too cold.
- Do not cover an application as directed.
- Neglect to check the person often.
- Leave the application on longer than directed.
- Fail to report complications to the nurse.

Follow the rules in Box 38-1. Take pride in protecting the person from injury.

FOCUS ON PRIDE: *Application*

Providing comfort is an important part of every task. What special considerations are needed for heat and cold applications? How will you know if you have met the person's comfort needs?

REVIEW QUESTIONS

Circle the BEST answer.

1 Heat applications
   a Decrease blood flow
   b Constrict vessels before dilating them
   c Tighten muscles
   d Relieve pain

2 The *greatest* threat from heat applications is
   a Infection
   b Burns
   c Chilling
   d Skin tears

3 Who is at *greatest* risk for complications from heat applications?
   a An older person with dark skin
   b An older person with nerve damage
   c An adult with a circulatory disorder
   d A child with fair skin

4 Which statement about moist and dry heat applications is *true*?
   a With moist applications, water has contact with the skin.
   b Moist heat has fewer effects than dry heat.
   c Dry heat penetrates deeper than moist heat.
   d Lower temperatures are required for dry heat applications.

5 A hot application is usually
   a 80°F to 92°F
   b 93°F to 98°F
   c 99°F to 106°F
   d Above 106°F

6 A nurse asks you to apply a hot pack. Which should you question?
   a Check that the pack's temperature is at least 110°F (43.3°C).
   b Place the pack in a cover.
   c Secure the pack in place with ties.
   d Check the person for complications every 5 minutes.

7 Which statement about sitz baths is *true*?
   a Sitz baths last 25 to 30 minutes.
   b Weakness and fainting can occur.
   c The lower body is immersed in warm water.
   d Sitz baths decrease circulation to the perineum and rectum.

8 When using an aquathermia pad
   a Do not cover the pad
   b Place the pad under the person
   c Check for kinks in the hoses
   d Secure the pad in place with pins

9 Cold applications
   a Prevent swelling and decrease circulation
   b Dilate blood vessels
   c Prevent the spread of microbes
   d Increase bleeding

10 Which signals a complication of a cold application?
   a Cool skin
   b Cyanosis
   c Decreased swelling
   d Fever

11 When applying a cold application
   a Use cooler temperatures for persons at risk
   b Observe the skin every 10 minutes
   c Place the application on a bluish skin area
   d Provide for warmth and privacy

12 Before applying an ice bag
   a Place the bag in the freezer
   b Measure the temperature of the bag
   c Place the bag in a cover
   d Provide perineal care

13 Moist cold compresses are left in place no longer than
   a 20 minutes
   b 30 minutes
   c 45 minutes
   d 60 minutes

14 A cooling blanket is used for
   a Hypothermia
   b Hyperthermia
   c Cyanosis
   d Shivering

Answers to Chapter 38 questions are on p. 872.

FOCUS ON PRACTICE

Problem Solving

You enter Mr. Cooper's room to remove his hot pack. He says: "My knee feels much better with that on. Can I leave it on longer?" What do you do? Is it safe or are there risks to leaving the application in place? Explain.

OBJECTIVES

- Define the key terms and key abbreviations in this chapter.
- Describe the factors affecting oxygen needs.
- List the signs and symptoms of altered respiratory function.
- Describe the tests for respiratory problems.
- Explain the measures that promote oxygenation.

- Describe the devices used to give oxygen.
- Explain how to safely assist with oxygen therapy.
- Perform the procedures described in this chapter.
- Explain how to promote PRIDE in the person, the family, and yourself.

KEY TERMS

allergy A sensitivity to a substance that causes the body to react with signs and symptoms

apnea The lack or absence *(a)* of breathing *(pnea)*

atelectasis The collapse of a portion of a lung

Biot's respirations Rapid and deep respirations followed by 10 to 30 seconds of apnea

bradypnea Slow *(brady)* breathing *(pnea)*; respirations are fewer than 12 per minute

Cheyne-Stokes respirations Respirations gradually increase in rate and depth and then become shallow and slow; breathing may stop *(apnea)* for 10 to 20 seconds

cyanosis Bluish color *(cyano)* to the skin, lips, mucous membranes, and nail beds

dyspnea Difficult, labored, or painful *(dys)* breathing *(pnea)*

hemoptysis Bloody *(hemo)* sputum *(ptysis means to spit)*

hyperventilation Breathing *(ventilation)* is rapid *(hyper)* and deeper than normal

hypoventilation Breathing *(ventilation)* is slow *(hypo)*, shallow, and sometimes irregular

hypoxemia A reduced amount *(hypo)* of oxygen *(ox)* in the blood *(emia)*

hypoxia Cells do not have enough *(hypo)* oxygen *(oxia)*

Kussmaul respirations Very deep and rapid respirations

orthopnea Breathing *(pnea)* deeply and comfortably only when sitting *(ortho)*

orthopneic position Sitting up *(ortho)* and leaning over a table to breathe *(pneic)*

oxygen concentration The amount (percent) of hemoglobin containing oxygen

pollutant A harmful chemical or substance in the air or water

pulse oximetry Measures *(metry)* the oxygen *(oxi)* concentration in arterial blood

respiratory arrest When breathing stops

respiratory depression Slow, weak respirations at a rate of fewer than 12 per minute

sputum Mucus from the respiratory system that is expectorated (expelled) through the mouth

tachypnea Rapid *(tachy)* breathing *(pnea)*; respirations are more than 20 per minute

KEY ABBREVIATIONS

CO_2	Carbon dioxide	O_2	Oxygen
ID	Identification	RBC	Red blood cell
L/min	Liters per minute	SpO_2	Saturation of peripheral oxygen (oxygen concentration)

Oxygen (O_2) is a gas. It has no taste, odor, or color. It is a basic need required for life. Death occurs within minutes if breathing stops. Brain damage and serious illness can occur without enough oxygen. Illness, surgery, and injuries affect the amount of oxygen in the body. Respiratory complications are risks after surgery.

You assist in the care of persons with oxygen needs. You must give safe and effective care.

See *Body Structure and Function Review: The Respiratory System.*

BODY STRUCTURE AND FUNCTION REVIEW
The Respiratory System

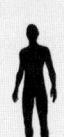

Oxygen is needed to live. Every cell needs oxygen. Air contains about 21 percent (%) oxygen. This meets the body's needs under normal conditions. The respiratory system (Fig. 39-1) brings oxygen (O_2) into the lungs and removes carbon dioxide (CO_2).

Respiration is the process of supplying the cells with O_2 and removing CO_2 from them. Respiration involves breathing in *(inhalation, inspiration)* and breathing out *(exhalation, expiration)*.

Air enters the body through the *nose*. The air then passes into the *pharynx* (throat)—a tube-shaped passage-way for air and food. Air passes from the pharynx into the *larynx* (voice box). Then air passes from the larynx into the *trachea* (windpipe).

The trachea divides at its lower end into the *right bronchus* and *left bronchus*. Each bronchus enters a *lung*. Upon entering the lungs, the bronchi divide many times into smaller branches *(bronchioles)*. Eventually the bronchioles subdivide, ending up in tiny 1-celled air sacs *(alveoli)*.

O_2 and CO_2 are exchanged between the alveoli and capillaries. Blood in the capillaries picks up O_2 from the alveoli. Then the blood is returned to the left side of the heart and pumped to the rest of the body. Alveoli pick up CO_2 from the capillaries for exhalation.

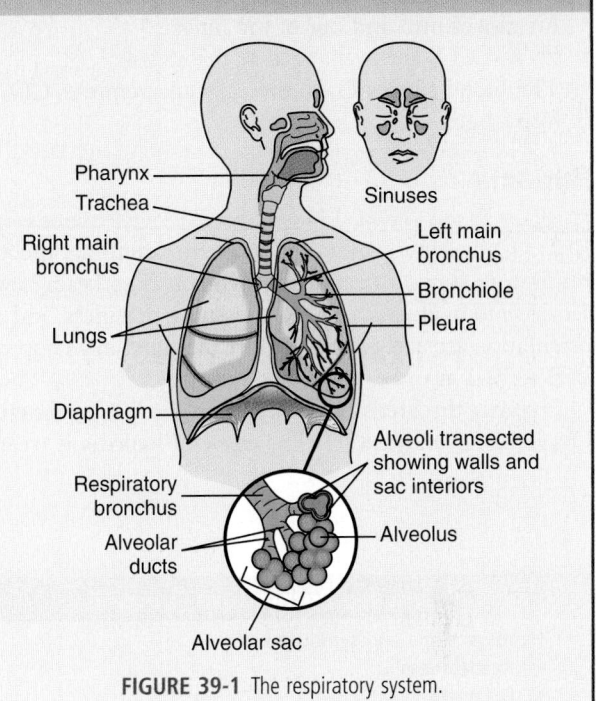

FIGURE 39-1 The respiratory system.

FACTORS AFFECTING OXYGEN NEEDS

Any disease, injury, or surgery involving the respiratory or circulatory systems affects the intake and use of O_2. Body systems depend on each other. Altered function of any system (for example, the nervous, musculo-skeletal, or urinary system) affects oxygen needs. Oxygen needs are affected by:

- *The circulatory system.* Narrowed vessels affect blood flow. Capillaries and cells must exchange O_2 and CO_2.
- *Red blood cell count.* Red blood cells (RBCs) contain hemoglobin. Hemoglobin picks up O_2 in the lungs and carries it to the cells. The bone marrow must produce enough RBCs. Blood loss also reduces the number of RBCs.
- *The nervous system.* Nervous system diseases and injuries can affect respiratory muscles. Narcotics and depressant drugs affect the brain and slow respirations. O_2 and CO_2 blood levels also affect brain function. When O_2 is lacking, respirations increase to bring in more oxygen. When CO_2 increases, respirations increase to rid the body of CO_2.
- *Aging.* Respiratory muscles weaken. Lung tissue is less elastic. Strength for coughing decreases. *Pneumonia* (inflammation and infection of the lungs) can develop.
- *Exercise.* O_2 needs increase with exercise. Respiratory rate and depth increase to bring in O_2. Persons with heart and respiratory diseases may have enough oxygen at rest. However, even slight activity can increase O_2 needs. The doctor may limit activity.
- *Fever.* O_2 needs increase. Respiratory rate and depth increase.
- *Pain.* O_2 needs increase. Respirations increase to meet this need. Chest and abdominal injuries and surgeries often involve respiratory muscles. It hurts to breathe.
- *Drugs.* Some drugs depress the respiratory center in the brain. *Respiratory depression means slow, weak respirations at a rate of fewer than 12 per minute. Respiratory arrest is when breathing stops.* Narcotics (morphine, Demerol, and others) can have these effects. (*Narcotic* comes from the Greek word *narkoun. It means stupor* or *to be numb.*) Substance abusers are at risk for respiratory depression and respiratory arrest.
- *Smoking.* Smoking causes lung cancer and chronic obstructive pulmonary disease (COPD). It is a risk factor for coronary artery disease.
- *Allergies.* An *allergy is a sensitivity to a substance that causes the body to react with signs and symptoms.* Runny nose, wheezing, and congestion are common. Mucous membranes in the upper airway swell. Severe swelling can close the airway. Shock and death are risks. Pollens, dust, foods, drugs, insect bites, powders, flowers, perfumes, sprays, animals, and cigarette smoke often cause allergies.
- *Pollutants.* A *pollutant is a harmful chemical or substance in the air or water.* Examples are dust, fumes, toxins, asbestos, coal dust, and sawdust. They damage the lungs.
- *Nutrition.* The body needs iron and vitamins (vitamin B_{12}, vitamin C, and folate) to produce RBCs.
- *Alcohol.* Alcohol depresses the brain. Excessive amounts reduce the cough reflex and increase the risk of aspiration. Obstructed airway and pneumonia are risks from aspiration.

ALTERED RESPIRATORY FUNCTION

Respiratory function involves 3 processes. Respiratory function is altered if even 1 process is affected.
- Air moves into and out of the lungs.
- O_2 and CO_2 are exchanged at the alveoli.
- The blood carries O_2 to the cells and removes CO_2 from them.

Hypoxia

Hypoxia means that cells do not have enough (hypo) *oxygen* (oxia). Cells cannot function properly. Anything affecting respiratory function can cause hypoxia. The brain is very sensitive to inadequate O_2. Restlessness, dizziness, and disorientation are early signs. Report the signs and symptoms in Box 39-1 at once.

Hypoxia threatens life. All organs need O_2 to function. Oxygen is given (p. 651). The cause of hypoxia is treated.

BOX 39-1   Altered Respiratory Function

- Hypoxia: signs and symptoms of
  - Restlessness
  - Dizziness
  - Disorientation and confusion
  - Behavior and personality changes
  - Concentrating and following directions: problems with
  - Anxiety and apprehension
  - Fatigue
  - Agitation
  - Pulse rate: increased
  - Respirations: increased rate and depth
  - Sitting position—upright, leaning forward, hunched over a table
  - *Cyanosis*—bluish color (cyano) *to the skin, lips, mucous membranes, and nail beds*
  - Dyspnea
- Breathing pattern: abnormal
- Shortness of breath or complaints of being "winded" or "short-winded"
- Cough (note frequency and time of day)
  - Dry and hacking
  - Harsh and barking
  - Productive (produces sputum) or non-productive
- Sputum (mucus from the respiratory system)
  - Color—clear, white, yellow, green, brown, or red
  - Odor—none or foul odor
  - Consistency—thick, watery, or frothy (with bubbles or foam)
  - *Hemoptysis*—bloody (hemo) *sputum* (ptysis *means* to spit); note if the sputum is bright red, dark red, blood-tinged, or streaked with blood
- Respirations—noisy, wheezing, wet-sounding, crowing sounds
- Chest pain (note location)
  - Constant or comes and goes
  - Person's description—stabbing, knife-like, aching
  - What makes it worse—movement, coughing, yawning, sneezing, sighing, deep breathing
- Vital signs: changes in

Abnormal Respirations

Adults normally breathe 12 to 20 times per minute. Infants and children have faster rates. Normal respirations are quiet, effortless, and regular. Both sides of the chest rise and fall equally. These breathing patterns are abnormal (Fig. 39-2).

- *Tachypnea—rapid* (tachy) *breathing* (pnea). *Respirations are more than 20 per minute.* Fever, exercise, pain, pregnancy, airway obstruction, and hypoxemia are causes. *Hypoxemia is a reduced amount* (hypo) *of oxygen* (ox) *in the blood* (emia).
- *Bradypnea—slow* (brady) *breathing* (pnea). *Respirations are fewer than 12 per minute.* Drug over-dose and nervous system disorders are causes.
- *Apnea—lack or absence* (a) *of breathing* (pnea). It occurs in cardiac arrest and respiratory arrest. Sleep apnea is another type of apnea (Chapter 45).
- *Hypoventilation—breathing* (ventilation) *is slow* (hypo), *shallow, and sometimes irregular.* Lung disorders affecting the alveoli are causes. Pneumonia is an example. Other causes include obesity, airway obstruction, and drug side effects. Nervous system and musculo-skeletal disorders affecting the respiratory muscles also are causes.
- *Hyperventilation—breathing* (ventilation) *is rapid* (hyper) *and deeper than normal.* Causes include asthma, emphysema, infection, fever, nervous system disorders, hypoxia, anxiety, pain, and some drugs.
- *Dyspnea—difficult, labored, or painful* (dys) *breathing* (pnea). Heart disease and anxiety are causes.
- *Cheyne-Stokes respirations—respirations gradually increase in rate and depth and then become shallow and slow. Breathing may stop* (apnea) *for 10 to 20 seconds.* Drug over-dose, heart failure, renal failure, and brain disorders are causes. Cheyne-Stokes are common when death is near.
- *Orthopnea—breathing* (pnea) *deeply and comfortably only when sitting* (ortho). Causes are emphysema, asthma, pneumonia, angina, and other heart and respiratory disorders.
- *Biot's respirations—rapid and deep respirations followed by 10 to 30 seconds of apnea.* They occur with nervous system disorders.
- *Kussmaul respirations—very deep and rapid respirations.* They signal diabetic coma.

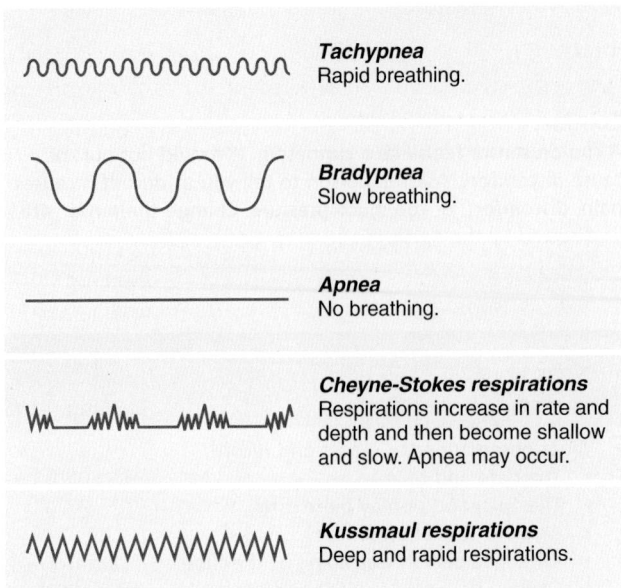

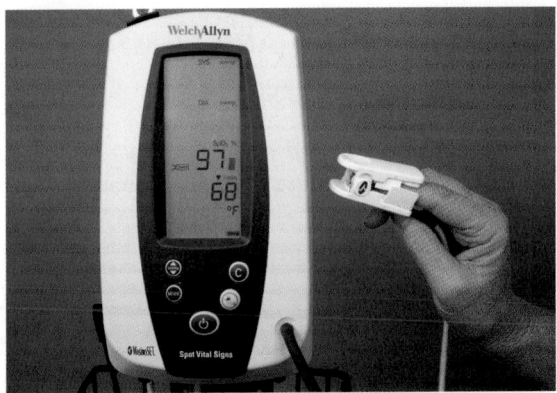

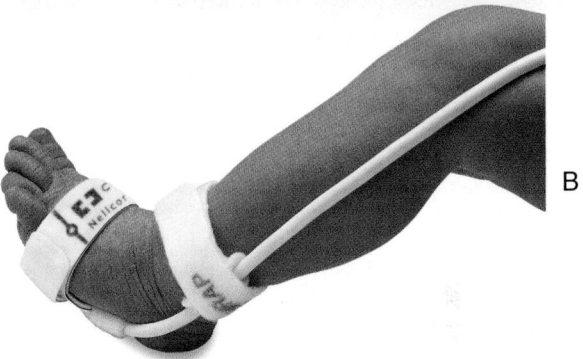

FIGURE 39-2 Some abnormal breathing problems. (Modified from Talbot L, Meyers-Marquardt M: *Pocket guide to critical care assessment,* ed 3, St Louis, 1997, Mosby.)

In the figure:
- **Tachypnea** — Rapid breathing.
- **Bradypnea** — Slow breathing.
- **Apnea** — No breathing.
- **Cheyne-Stokes respirations** — Respirations increase in rate and depth and then become shallow and slow. Apnea may occur.
- **Kussmaul respirations** — Deep and rapid respirations.

FIGURE 39-3 A, A pulse oximetry sensor is attached to a finger. The device displays the O_2 concentration and pulse. **B,** A pulse oximetry sensor for children. (**B,** From Covidien ©2015. All rights reserved. Used with permission of Covidien.)

RESPIRATORY TESTS

Respiratory problems may be acute or chronic. Report your observations promptly and accurately (see Box 39-1). The health team must take quick action to meet oxygen needs. The problem must be corrected and prevented from becoming worse.

The doctor may order a chest x-ray to detect lung changes. If necessary, other complex tests are ordered. You may be involved in pulse oximetry and sputum specimens. Assist with other tests as directed by the nurse.

Pulse Oximetry

Pulse oximetry measures (metry) *the oxygen* (oxi) *concentration in arterial blood.* **Oxygen concentration** *is the amount (percent) of hemoglobin containing O_2.* An agency may use 1 of these terms.

- *Pulse oximetry* or *pulse ox*
- *O_2 saturation* or *O_2 sat*
- *SpO_2* (saturation of peripheral oxygen)

Measurements are used to prevent and treat hypoxia. The normal range is 95 to 100%. For example, if 97% of all hemoglobin (100%) carries O_2, tissues get enough oxygen. If only 90% contains O_2, tissues do not get enough oxygen. As low as 85% may be normal for persons with some chronic diseases.

A sensor attaches to a finger, toe, earlobe, nose, or forehead (Fig. 39-3). Light beams on 1 side of the sensor pass through tissues. A detector on the other side measures the amount of light passing through the tissues. With this information, the oximeter measures the O_2 concentration.

A good sensor site is needed. Avoid swollen sites and sites with skin breaks. If blood flow to fingers or toes is poor, then the earlobe, nose, and forehead sites are used.

Bright light, nail polish, fake nails, and movements affect measurements.

- Place a towel over the sensor to block bright lights.
- Remove nail polish or use another site.
- Do not use a finger site if there are fake nails.
- Use the earlobe if the person has movements from shivering, seizures, or tremors.
- Do not measure blood pressure on the side of a finger site. Blood pressure cuffs affect blood flow.

Oxygen concentration is often measured with vital signs. The pulse rate may be displayed on the pulse oximeter along with the oxygen concentration. Report and record measurements according to agency policy.

Oximeter alarms are set for continuous monitoring. An alarm sounds if:

- O_2 concentration is low.
- The pulse rate is too fast or slow.
- Other problems occur.

See *Focus on Children and Older Persons: Pulse Oximetry.*
See *Delegation Guidelines: Pulse Oximetry,* p. 646.
See *Promoting Safety and Comfort: Pulse Oximetry,* p. 646.
See procedure: *Using a Pulse Oximeter,* p. 646.

> ### FOCUS ON **CHILDREN AND OLDER PERSONS**
>
> #### *Pulse Oximetry*
>
> **Children**
> Different sensors may be used for children (see Fig. 39-3, *B*). The sensor is attached to the sole of the foot, palm of the hand, toe, or earlobe. If the child moves a lot, the earlobe is a better site.

PROMOTING SAFETY AND COMFORT
Pulse Oximetry

Safety

The person's condition can change quickly. Pulse oximetry does not lessen the need for good observations. Observe for signs and symptoms of hypoxia and altered respiratory system function (see Box 39-1).

Comfort

A clip-on sensor feels like a clothespin. It should not hurt or cause discomfort. Ask the person to tell you at once if it causes pain, discomfort, or too much pressure. Change the sensor site as directed by the nurse.

DELEGATION GUIDELINES
Pulse Oximetry

To assist with pulse oximetry, you need this information from the nurse and the care plan.
- What site to use
- How to use the equipment
- What sensor to use
- What type of tape to use (if needed)
- The person's normal range of SpO_2
- Alarm limits for SpO_2 and pulse rate (if set)
- When to do the measurement
- What pulse site to use: apical or radial
- How often to check the site for continuous monitoring (usually every 2 hours)

- What observations to report and record:
  - The date and time
  - The SpO_2 and display pulse rate
  - Apical or radial pulse rate
  - What the person was doing at the time
  - Oxygen flow rate (p. 654) and the device used (p. 653)
  - Reason for the measurement: routine, continuous monitoring, or condition change
- When to report observations
- What patient or resident concerns to report at once:
  - An SpO_2 below the alarm limit (usually 95%)
  - A pulse rate above or below the alarm limit
  - The signs and symptoms listed in Box 39-1

Using a Pulse Oximeter

QUALITY OF LIFE

- Knock before entering the person's room.
- Address the person by name.
- Introduce yourself by name and title.

- Explain the procedure before starting and during the procedure.
- Protect the person's rights during the procedure.
- Handle the person gently during the procedure.

PRE-PROCEDURE

1 Follow *Delegation Guidelines: Pulse Oximetry.* See *Promoting Safety and Comfort: Pulse Oximetry.*
2 Practice hand hygiene.
3 Collect the following before going to the person's room.
   - Oximeter
   - Tape (if needed)
   - Towel

4 Arrange your work area.
5 Practice hand hygiene.
6 Identify the person. Check the identification (ID) bracelet against your assignment sheet. Use 2 identifiers (Chapter 13). Also call the person by name.
7 Provide for privacy.

PROCEDURE

8 Provide for comfort.
9 Dry the site with a towel.
10 Clip or tape the sensor to the site.
11 Turn on the oximeter.
12 *For continuous monitoring:*
   a Set the high and low alarm limits for SpO_2 and pulse rate.
   b Turn on audio and visual alarms.

13 Check the person's pulse (apical or radial) with the pulse on the display. The pulse rates should be about the same. Note both pulses on your assignment sheet.
14 Read the SpO_2 on the display. Note the value on the flow sheet and your assignment sheet.
15 Leave the sensor in place for continuous monitoring. Otherwise, turn off the device and remove the sensor.

POST-PROCEDURE

16 Provide for comfort. (See the inside of the front cover.)
17 Place the call light and other needed items within reach.
18 Unscreen the person.
19 Complete a safety check of the room. (See the inside of the front cover.)

20 Return the device to its proper place (unless monitoring is continuous).
21 Practice hand hygiene.
22 Report and record the SpO_2, the pulse rates, and your other observations.

Sputum Specimens

Respiratory disorders cause the lungs, bronchi, and trachea to secrete mucus. *Mucus from the respiratory system is called* **sputum** *when expectorated (expelled) through the mouth.* Sputum specimens are studied for blood, microbes, and abnormal cells. See Chapter 34.

MEETING OXYGEN NEEDS

Air must move deep into the lungs to alveoli where O_2 and CO_2 are exchanged. Disease, injury, and surgery can prevent air from reaching the alveoli. Pain, immobility, and some drugs interfere with deep breathing and coughing. Therefore secretions collect in the airway and lungs. They interfere with air movement and lung function. Microbes can grow and multiply in the secretions. Infection is a threat.

Oxygen needs must be met. The following measures are common in care plans.

- Positioning
- Deep breathing and coughing
- Incentive spirometry (p. 650)

See *Focus on Communication: Meeting Oxygen Needs.*

FOCUS ON **COMMUNICATION**

Meeting Oxygen Needs

The questions you ask the person assist the nurse with the nursing process. For example:

- "Do you need more pillows?"
- "Do you want the head of your bed raised more?"
- "How often are you coughing?"
- "Are you coughing anything up?"
- "Are you coughing up any mucus? Please use a tissue when you cough up mucus, then put on your call light. The nurse needs to observe the mucus."

Positioning

Breathing is usually easier in the semi-Fowler's and Fowler's positions. Persons with difficulty breathing often prefer the **orthopneic position**—*sitting up and leaning over a table to breathe.* (Ortho *means* sitting *or* standing. Pneic *means* breathing.) Place a pillow on the table to increase comfort (Fig. 39-4).

Frequent position changes are needed. Unless the doctor limits positioning, the person must not lie on 1 side for a long time. Secretions pool. The lungs cannot expand on that side. Position changes are needed at least every 2 hours. Follow the care plan.

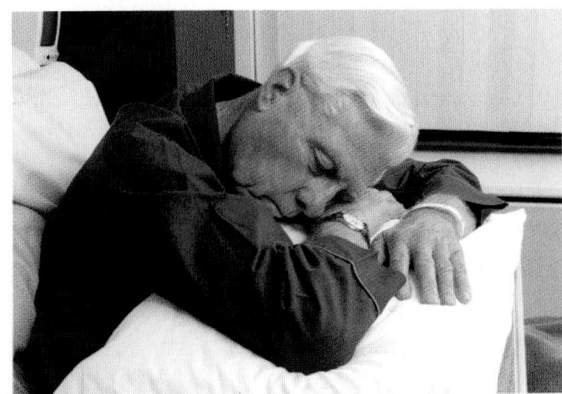

FIGURE 39-4 The person is in the orthopneic position. A pillow is on the over-bed table for the person's comfort.

Deep Breathing and Coughing

Deep breathing moves air into most parts of the lungs. Coughing removes mucus. Deep-breathing and coughing exercises promote oxygenation. They are done after surgery or injury and during bedrest. The exercises are painful after surgery or injury. Breaking an incision open while coughing is a fear.

Deep breathing and coughing are usually done every 1 to 2 hours while awake. They help prevent pneumonia and atelectasis. *Atelectasis is the collapse of a portion of a lung.* It occurs when mucus collects in the airway. Air cannot get to a part of the lung. The lung collapses. Surgery, bedrest, lung diseases, and paralysis are risk factors.

See *Focus on Communication: Deep Breathing and Coughing.*

See *Focus on Children and Older Persons: Deep Breathing and Coughing.*

See *Delegation Guidelines: Deep Breathing and Coughing.*

See *Promoting Safety and Comfort: Deep Breathing and Coughing.*

See procedure: *Assisting with Deep-Breathing and Coughing Exercises.*

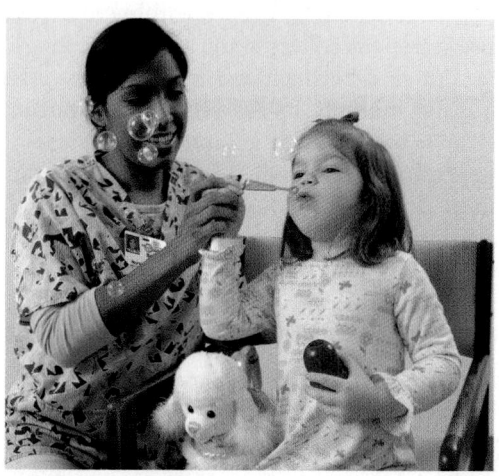

FIGURE 39-5 The child blows bubbles for a deep-breathing exercise.

Assisting With Deep-Breathing and Coughing Exercises

QUALITY OF LIFE

- Knock before entering the person's room.
- Address the person by name.
- Introduce yourself by name and title.

- Explain the procedure before starting and during the procedure.
- Protect the person's rights during the procedure.
- Handle the person gently during the procedure.

PRE-PROCEDURE

1 Follow *Delegation Guidelines: Deep Breathing and Coughing.* See *Promoting Safety and Comfort: Deep Breathing and Coughing.*
2 Practice hand hygiene.

3 Identify the person. Check the ID bracelet against the assignment sheet. Use 2 identifiers (Chapter 13). Also call the person by name.
4 Provide for privacy.

PROCEDURE

5 Lower the bed rail if up.
6 Help the person to a comfortable sitting position.
  - Sitting on the side of the bed
  - Semi-Fowler's
  - Fowler's
7 Have the person deep breathe.
  a Have the person place the hands over the rib cage (Fig. 39-6).
  b Have the person breathe as deeply as possible. Remind the person to inhale through the nose.
  c Ask the person to hold the breath for 2 to 3 seconds.
  d Ask the person to exhale slowly through pursed lips (Fig. 39-7). Ask the person to exhale until the ribs move as far down as possible.
  e Repeat this step 4 more times.

8 Ask the person to cough.
  a Have the person place both hands over the incision. One hand is on top of the other (Fig. 39-8, *A*, p. 650). The person holds a pillow or folded towel over the incision (Fig. 39-8, *B*, p. 650). If the person is covering the nose and mouth for respiratory etiquette, splint the incision with your hands or pillow. Wear gloves.
  b Have the person take in a deep breath as in step 7.
  c Ask the person to cough strongly 2 times with the mouth open.

POST-PROCEDURE

9 Provide for comfort. (See the inside of the front cover.)
10 Place the call light and other needed items within reach.
11 Raise or lower bed rails. Follow the care plan.
12 Unscreen the person.

13 Complete a safety check of the room. (See the inside of the front cover.)
14 Practice hand hygiene.
15 Report and record your observations (Fig. 39-9, p. 650).

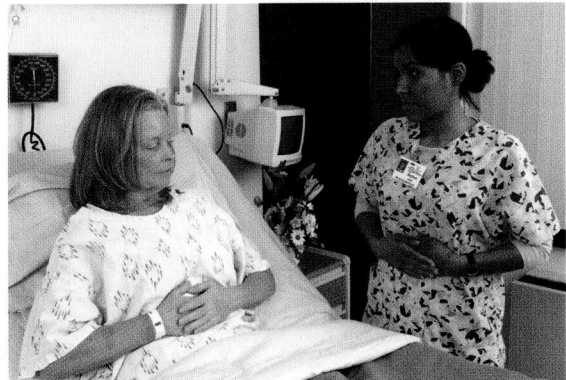

FIGURE 39-6 The hands are over the rib cage for deep breathing.

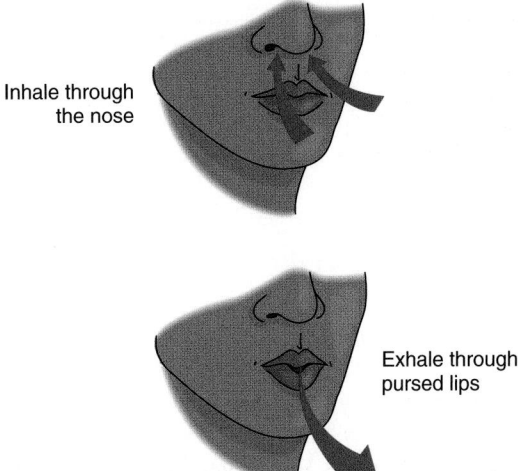

Inhale through the nose

Exhale through pursed lips

FIGURE 39-7 The person inhales through the nose and exhales through pursed lips during the deep-breathing exercise.

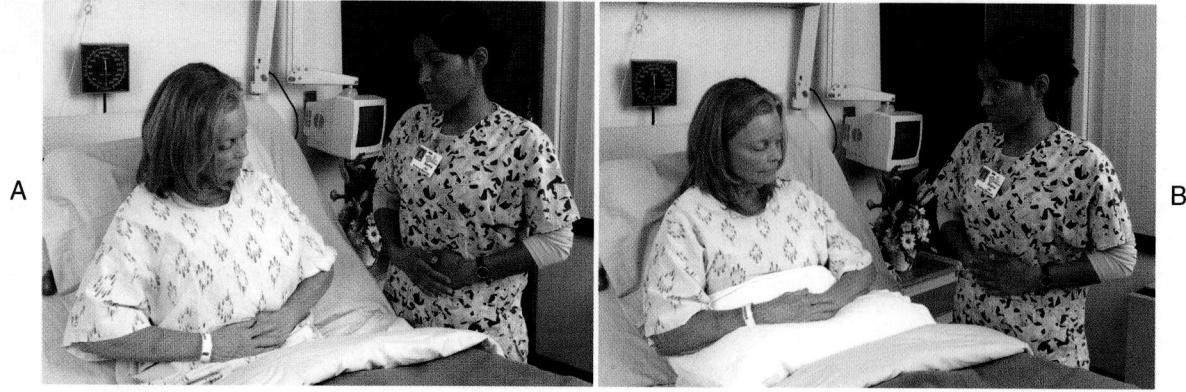

FIGURE 39-8 The incision is supported for the coughing exercise. **A,** The hands are over the incision. **B,** A pillow is held over the incision.

FLOWSHEET		
◀◀ ◀ Date Time ▶ ▶▶	04/19 1530	
Vital Signs	Temperature	98.2
	Pulse	80
	Respiration	18
	Blood Pressure	110/68
	SpO_2	98
	O_2 L/MIN	2
Oxygen Needs	OBSERVATIONS:	REGULAR
	POSITION:	FOWLER'S
	CARE MEASURES:	DEEP BREATHE/ COUGH
	OXYGEN DEVICE:	CANNULA

DATE: 04/19	TIME: 1530
OXYGEN NEEDS: CARE MEASURES	

☒ Deep breathe   ☐ Turn
   5 Times   ☒ Back
☒ Cough   ☐ Right side
   2 Times   ☐ Left side
☐ Incentive spirometry   ☐ Suction
   ☐ Times
   Volume ☐ mL

Assisted patient with deep-breathing and coughing exercises. Incision splinted with a pillow. He states: "It is getting easier." Denied pain or discomfort. Over-bed table with water mug and tissues in reach. Call light in reach.

Nurse notified: Karyl Somers, RN

FIGURE 39-9 Charting sample.

Incentive Spirometry

Incentive means *to encourage.* A *spirometer* is a machine that measures the amount *(volume)* of air inhaled (Fig. 39-10). Incentive spirometry also is called *sustained maximal inspiration (SMI). Sustained* means *constant. Maximal* means *the most* or *the greatest.* And *inspiration* relates to *breathing in.* The person inhales as deeply as possible and holds the breath for a certain time—usually 3 to 5 seconds.

The goal is to improve lung function and prevent complications. Like yawning or sighing, breathing is long, slow, and deep. This moves air deep into the lungs. Secretions loosen. O_2 and CO_2 exchange occurs between the alveoli and capillaries.

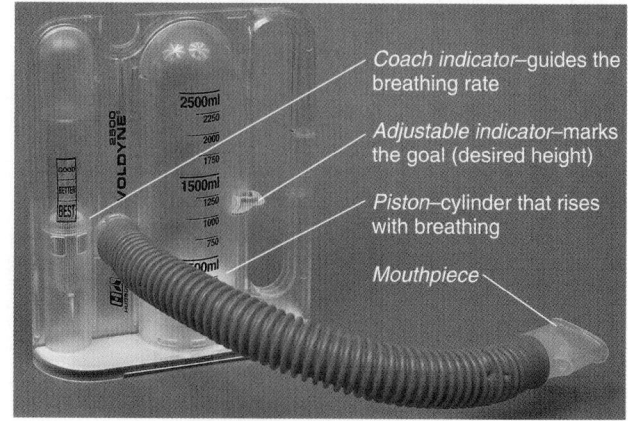

Coach indicator–guides the breathing rate

Adjustable indicator–marks the goal (desired height)

Piston–cylinder that rises with breathing

Mouthpiece

FIGURE 39-10 Parts of a spirometer.

The incentive spirometer is used as follows. The person:

1. Sits on the side of the bed, in Fowler's position, or in a chair.
2. Places the spirometer upright.
3. Exhales normally.
4. Seals the lips around the mouthpiece.
5. Takes a slow, deep breath until the piston rises to the desired height. A marker on the spirometer shows the desired height.
6. Holds the breath for 3 to 5 seconds to keep the piston floating.
7. Removes the mouthpiece and exhales slowly.
8. Rests for a few seconds.
9. Repeats steps 3 through 8 at least 10 to 15 times. The doctor orders the number of breaths.
10. Coughs after at least 10 breaths.
11. Repeats steps 1 through 10 at least every 1 to 2 hours while awake.

See *Delegation Guidelines: Incentive Spirometry.*

DELEGATION GUIDELINES

Incentive Spirometry

To assist with incentive spirometry, you need this information from the nurse and the care plan.

- How often the person needs incentive spirometry
- How many breaths the person needs to take
- The desired height of the floating piston
- How to clean the mouthpiece
- What observations to report and record:
  - How many breaths the person took
  - The height of the floating piston
  - If the person coughed after the procedure
  - How the person tolerated the procedure
- When to report observations
- What patient or resident concerns to report at once

ASSISTING WITH OXYGEN THERAPY

Disease, injury, and surgery often interfere with breathing. The doctor orders oxygen therapy when the amount of O_2 in the blood is less than normal *(hypoxemia)*.

Oxygen is treated as a drug. The doctor orders when to give O_2, the amount, and the device to use. Oxygen is needed constantly or for symptom relief—chest pain or shortness of breath. Persons with respiratory diseases may have enough oxygen at rest. With mild exercise or activity, they become short of breath. Oxygen helps relieve shortness of breath.

You do not give oxygen. The nurse and respiratory therapist start and maintain oxygen therapy. You help provide safe care.

Oxygen Sources

Oxygen is supplied as follows.

- *Wall outlet.* O_2 is piped into each person's unit (Fig. 39-11).
- *Oxygen tank.* The tank is placed at the bedside. Small tanks are used for emergencies and transfers. They also are used by persons who walk or use wheelchairs (Fig. 39-12). A gauge tells how much O_2 is left (Fig. 39-13, p. 652).
- *Oxygen concentrator.* The machine removes oxygen from the air (Fig. 39-14, p. 652). A power source is needed. If not portable, the person stays near the machine. A small oxygen tank is needed for power failures and mobility.
- *Liquid oxygen system.* A portable unit is filled from a stationary unit. The portable unit has enough O_2 for about 8 hours of use. A dial shows the amount of O_2 in the unit. The portable unit is worn over the shoulder (Fig. 39-15, p. 652).

See *Focus on Long-Term Care and Home Care: Oxygen Sources*, p. 652.

See *Teamwork and Time Management: Oxygen Sources*, p. 652.

See *Promoting Safety and Comfort: Oxygen Sources*, p. 652.

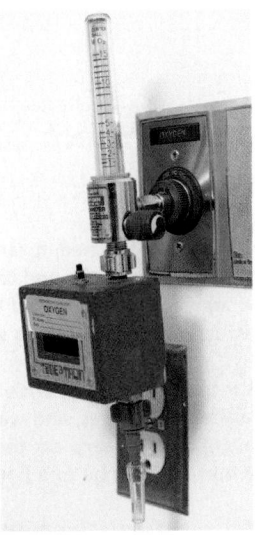

FIGURE 39-11 Wall oxygen outlet.

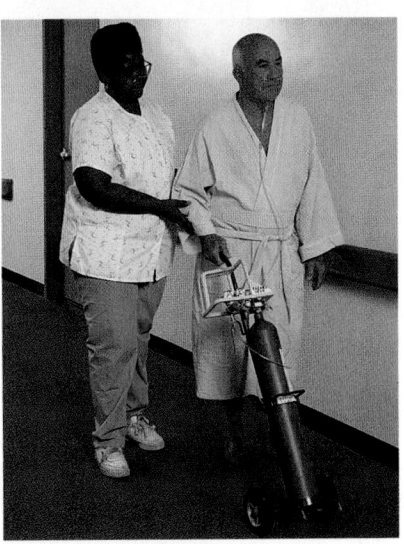

FIGURE 39-12 A portable oxygen tank is used when walking.

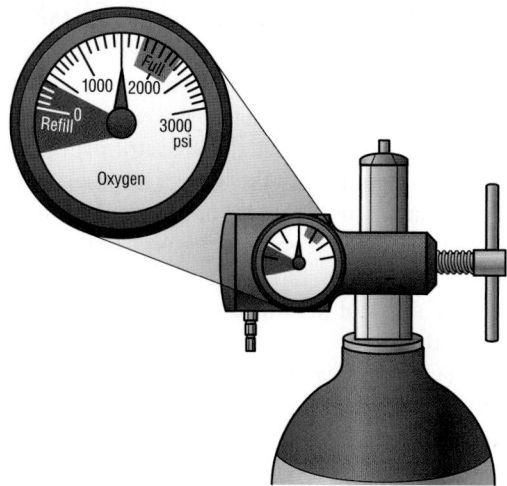

FIGURE 39-13 The gauge shows the amount of oxygen in the tank.

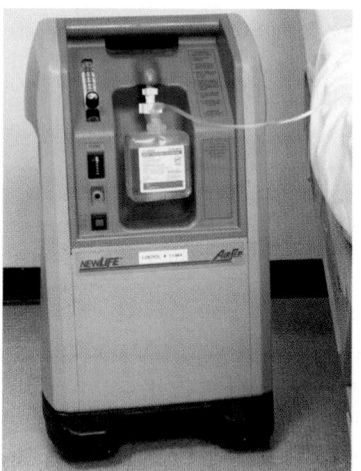

FIGURE 39-14 Oxygen concentrator.

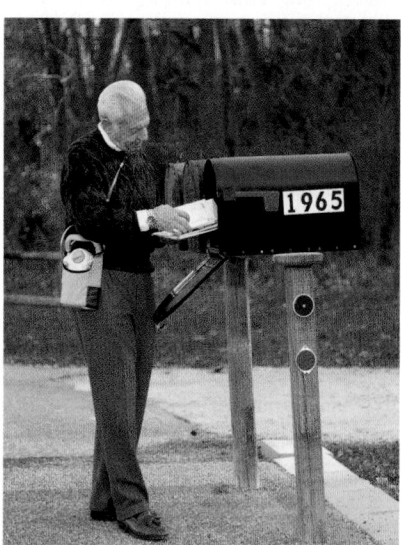

FIGURE 39-15 A portable liquid oxygen unit is worn over the shoulder. This allows the person to be mobile. (Image used by permission from Nellcor Puritan Bennett LLC, Boulder, Colo; part of Covidien.)

FOCUS ON LONG-TERM CARE AND HOME CARE

Oxygen Sources

Home Care
Oxygen tanks, oxygen concentrators, and liquid oxygen systems are used in home care. They are maintained by a medical supply company. Keep the company's name and phone number near the phone.

The patient and family must practice safety measures for using and storing oxygen. This includes measures to prevent fires.

- Practice fire prevention measures. See Chapter 13.
- Keep a fire extinguisher in the room.
- Place NO SMOKING signs in the room and on the room door.
- Remove smoking materials—cigarettes, cigars, pipes, matches, lighters, and so on.
- Remove materials that ignite easily—alcohol, nail polish remover, oils, greases, and so on.
- Keep O_2 sources and O_2 tubing away from heat sources and open flames. These include candles, stoves, heating ducts, radiators, heating pipes, space heaters, oil lamps, and kerosene heaters and lamps.
- Turn off electrical items before unplugging them.
- Use electrical items that are in good repair—shaver, radio, TV, music players, computers, and so on.
- Use only electrical items with 3-prong plugs.
- Do not use materials that cause static electricity (wool and synthetic fabrics).
- Turn off the O_2 if a fire occurs. Get the person and family out of the home. Call 911 to report a fire.

TEAMWORK AND TIME MANAGEMENT

Oxygen Sources

Oxygen tanks and liquid oxygen systems contain a certain amount of O_2. When the O_2 level is low, a new tank is needed or the liquid oxygen system is refilled. Check the O_2 level often. Report a low O_2 level at once.

PROMOTING SAFETY AND COMFORT

Oxygen Sources

Safety
Liquid oxygen is very cold. If touched, it can freeze the skin. Tampering with equipment is unsafe and could damage the equipment. Follow agency procedures and the manufacturer's instructions when working with liquid oxygen.

Many activities increase the need for O_2. This includes moving in bed, transfer procedures, and walking. Do not remove the person's O_2. If necessary, ask the nurse for longer tubing. Or ask the nurse to change to a portable oxygen tank.

Oxygen Devices

The doctor orders the device for giving O_2. These devices are common.

- *Nasal cannula* (Fig. 39-16). The prongs are inserted into the nostrils (Fig. 39-17). A band goes behind the ears and under the chin to keep the device in place. A cannula allows eating and drinking. Tight prongs can irritate the nose. Pressure on the ears and cheekbones is possible.
- *Simple face mask* (Fig. 39-18). It covers the nose and mouth. The mask has small holes in the sides. CO_2 escapes when exhaling.
- *Partial-rebreather mask* (Fig. 39-19). A bag is added to the simple face mask for exhaled air. When breathing in, the person inhales O_2 and some exhaled air. Some room air also is inhaled. The bag should not totally deflate when inhaling.
- *Non-rebreather mask* (Fig. 39-20). Exhaled air and room air cannot enter the bag. Exhaled air leaves through holes in the mask. When inhaling, only O_2 from the bag is inhaled. The bag must not totally collapse during inhalation.
- *Venturi mask* (Fig. 39-21, p. 654). Precise amounts of O_2 are given. Color-coded adapters show the amount of O_2 given.

Talking and eating are hard to do with a mask. Listen carefully. Moisture can build up under the mask. Keep the face clean and dry to help prevent irritation from the mask. For eating, the nurse changes the oxygen mask to a cannula.

See *Focus on Children and Older Persons: Oxygen Devices*, p. 654.

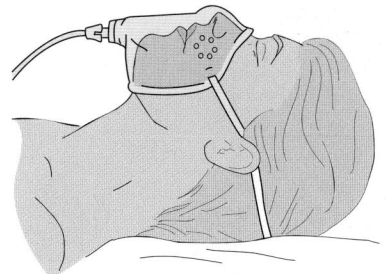

FIGURE 39-18 Simple face mask.

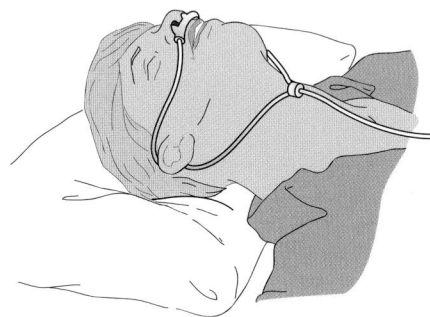

FIGURE 39-16 Nasal cannula.

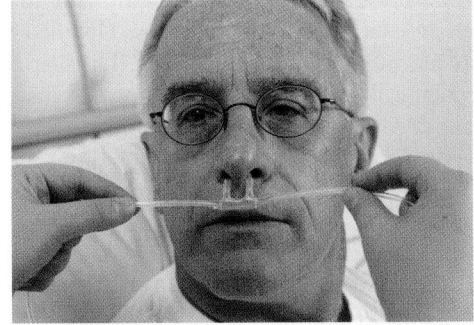

FIGURE 39-17 Cannula prongs are inserted. The prong openings face downward.

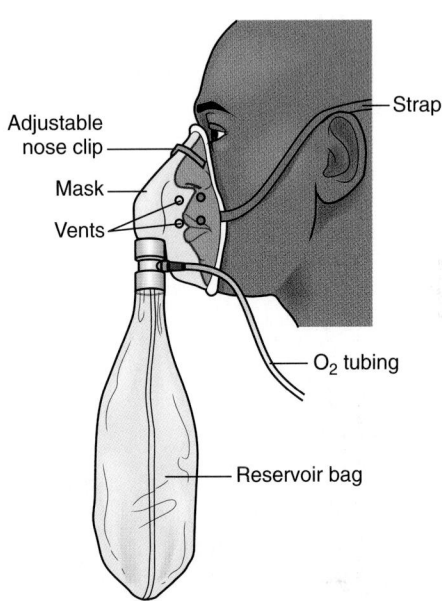

FIGURE 39-19 Partial-rebreather mask.

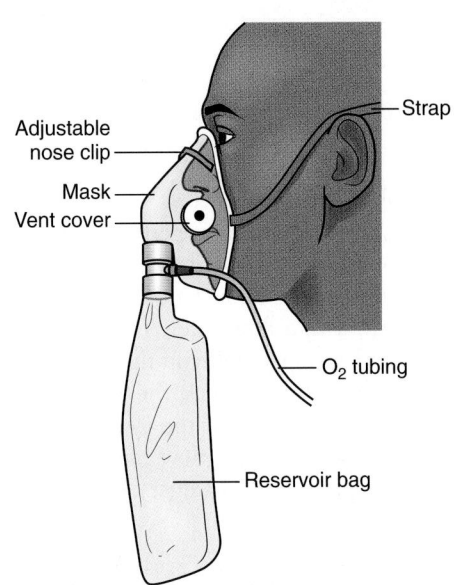

FIGURE 39-20 Non-rebreather mask.

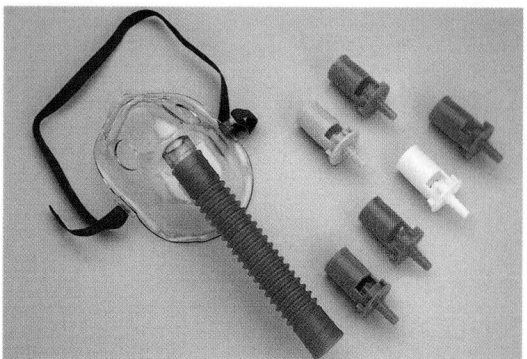

FIGURE 39-21 Venturi mask.

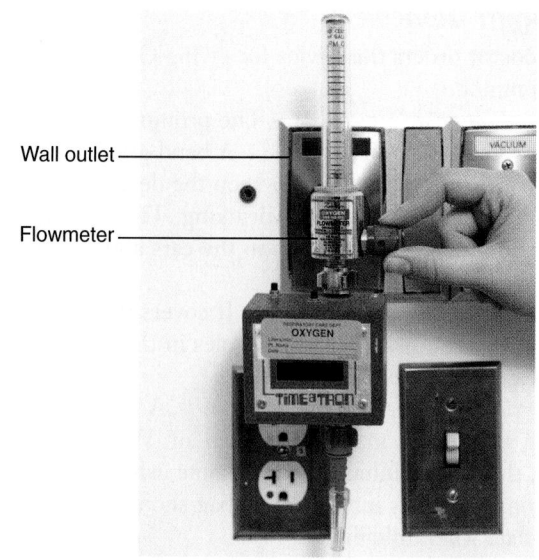

FIGURE 39-23 The flowmeter is used to set the oxygen flow rate.

FOCUS ON CHILDREN AND OLDER PERSONS

Oxygen Devices

Children

Oxygen devices for children include cannulas, face masks, partial- and non-rebreather masks, and Venturi masks. Oxygen hoods are used for infants (Fig. 39-22).

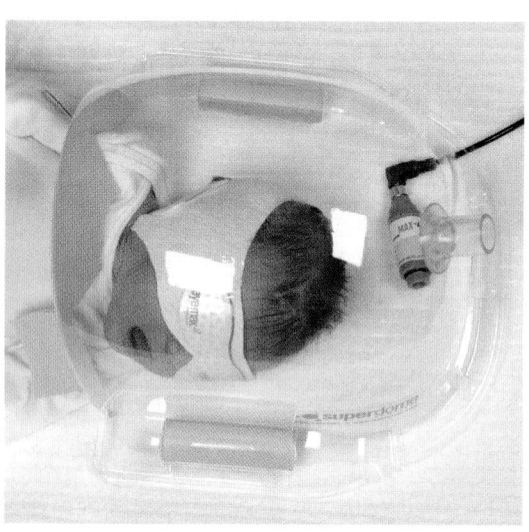

FIGURE 39-22 Oxygen hood. (From Maxtec, West Salt Lake City, Utah.)

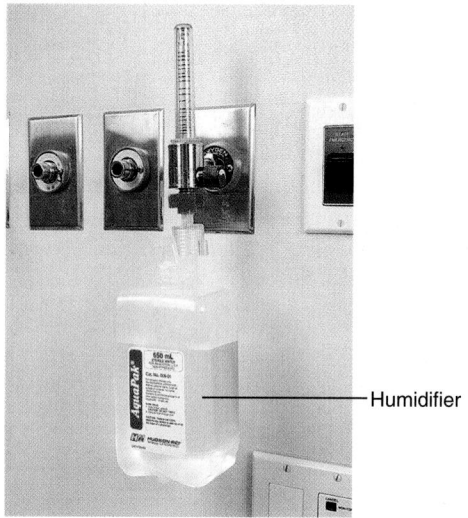

FIGURE 39-24 Oxygen set-up with a humidifier.

Oxygen Flow Rates

The *flow rate* is the amount of oxygen given. It is measured in liters per minute (L/min). The doctor orders 1 to 15 liters of O_2 per minute. The nurse or respiratory therapist sets the flow rate with a flowmeter (Fig. 39-23).

The nurse and care plan tell you the person's flow rate. When giving care, always check the flow rate. Tell the nurse at once if it is too high or too low. A nurse or respiratory therapist will adjust the flow rate. Some states and agencies let nursing assistants adjust O_2 flow rates. Know your agency's policy.

▉ Oxygen Set-Up

Oxygen is a dry gas. If not humidified (made moist), O_2 dries the airway's mucous membranes. Distilled water is added to the humidifier (Fig. 39-24). (Distilled water is pure. A chemical process removes dissolved salts.)

When added to the humidifier, distilled water creates water vapor. Oxygen picks up the water vapor as it flows into the system. Bubbling in the humidifier means water vapor is being produced. Low flow rates (1 to 2 L/min) by cannula are usually not humidified.

See *Teamwork and Time Management: Oxygen Set-Up.*
See *Delegation Guidelines: Oxygen Set-Up.*
See *Promoting Safety and Comfort: Oxygen Set-Up.*
See procedure: *Setting Up Oxygen.*

TEAMWORK AND TIME MANAGEMENT

Oxygen Set-Up

As you walk past the room of any person receiving humidified O_2, always check the humidifier. Check for and tell the nurse if:

- There is no bubbling.
- The water level is low.

PROMOTING SAFETY AND COMFORT

Oxygen Set-Up

Safety

You do not give oxygen. Tell the nurse when the O_2 system is set up. The nurse turns on the O_2, sets the flow rate, and applies the O_2 device.

Practice medical asepsis. Do not let the connecting tubing hang on the floor.

DELEGATION GUIDELINES

Oxygen Set-Up

If setting up O_2 is delegated to you, you need this information from the nurse.

- The person's name and room and bed numbers
- What oxygen device to use
- If you need a humidifier

Setting Up Oxygen

QUALITY OF LIFE

- Knock before entering the person's room.
- Address the person by name.
- Introduce yourself by name and title.

- Explain the procedure before starting and during the procedure.
- Protect the person's rights during the procedure.
- Handle the person gently during the procedure.

PRE-PROCEDURE

1 Follow *Delegation Guidelines: Oxygen Set-Up*. See *Promoting Safety and Comfort: Oxygen Set-Up*.
2 Practice hand hygiene.
3 Collect the following before going to the person's room.
   - Oxygen device with connecting tubing
   - Flowmeter
   - Humidifier (if ordered)
   - Distilled water (if using a humidifier)

4 Arrange your work area.
5 Practice hand hygiene.
6 Identify the person. Check the ID bracelet against the assignment sheet. Use 2 identifiers (Chapter 13). Also call the person by name.

PROCEDURE

7 Make sure the flowmeter is in the OFF position.
8 Attach the flowmeter to the wall outlet or to the tank.
9 Fill the humidifier with distilled water.
10 Attach the humidifier to the bottom of the flowmeter.
11 Attach the oxygen device and connecting tubing to the humidifier. *Do not set the flowmeter. Do not apply the O_2 device on the person.*

12 Place the cap securely on the distilled water. Store the water according to agency policy.
13 Discard the packaging from the O_2 device and connecting tubing.

POST-PROCEDURE

14 Provide for comfort. (See the inside of the front cover.)
15 Place the call light and other needed items within reach.
16 Complete a safety check of the room. (See the inside of the front cover.)

17 Practice hand hygiene.
18 Tell the nurse when you are done. The nurse will:
   - Turn on the O_2 and set the flow rate.
   - Apply the O_2 device on the person.

Oxygen Safety

You assist the nurse with oxygen therapy. You do not give oxygen. *You do not adjust the flow rate unless allowed by your state and agency.* However, you must give safe care. Follow the rules in Box 39-2, p. 656. Also follow the rules for fire and the use of oxygen (Chapter 13).

BOX 39-2   Oxygen Safety

- Do not remove the oxygen device.
- Make sure the oxygen device is secure but not tight.
- Check for irritation from the device. Check:
  - Behind the ears
  - Under the nose (cannula)
  - Around the face (mask)
  - The cheekbones
- Keep the face clean and dry when a mask is used.
- Do not shut off the O_2 flow. *However, turn off the O_2 flow if there is a fire. Remove the oxygen device.*
- Do not adjust the flow rate unless allowed by your state and agency.
- Tell the nurse at once if the:
  - Flow rate is too high or too low
  - Humidifier is not bubbling
- Maintain an adequate water level in the humidifier.
- Secure tubing in place. Tape or pin it to the person's garment following agency policy. Do not puncture the tubing.
- Make sure there are no kinks in the tubing.
- Make sure the person does not lie on any part of the tubing.
- Make sure the oxygen tank is secure in its holder.
- Report at once signs and symptoms of altered respiratory function or abnormal breathing patterns (see Box 39-1).
- Follow the care plan for oral hygiene.
- Make sure the oxygen device is clean and free of mucus.
- See "Fire and Oxygen" in Chapter 13.

FOCUS ON PRIDE

The Person, Family, and Yourself

Personal and Professional Responsibility

You are responsible for reporting the person's complaints. A person may say: "I can't breathe" or "I'm not getting enough air." Yet you see the person breathing. Do not dismiss the complaint. Tell the nurse at once. You cannot feel what the person does. Trust what the person tells you.

Rights and Respect

People have the right to a safe setting. For safety, smoking is not allowed where oxygen is used and stored. NO SMOKING signs are common in rooms and hallways. You may need to remind the person or visitors not to smoke. Be polite and respectful. Show the person where smoking is allowed.

Independence and Social Interaction

Needing long-term oxygen therapy changes a person's life. Work, daily activities, and hobbies can be a challenge. The person may feel alone and depressed. Social support from family and friends is important.

Portable oxygen sources increase independence. Small oxygen tanks and portable liquid oxygen units are examples. Such devices allow freedom and promote quality of life.

Delegation and Teamwork

Oxygen is treated as a drug. You assist with oxygen therapy. You do not give oxygen. You do not adjust the flow rate unless allowed by your state and agency and instructed to do so by the nurse.

If asked to give oxygen or adjust a flow rate, politely refuse. Remember, refusing to perform a task is your right and duty when the task is beyond the legal limits of your role. Do not ignore the request. Tell the nurse that you can assist. Gathering and setting up the supplies are examples. Or ask if you can help with another task instead.

Ethics and Laws

Safe use of oxygen is a serious issue. The following case shows how harm resulted from unsafe use of oxygen by a certified nursing assistant (CNA) who was not trained or qualified to handle oxygen.

Ethics and Laws—cont'd

A CNA took a group of residents outside to smoke. One resident, who used oxygen, was taken outside with her oxygen tank. Center policy stated that oxygen was to be used and handled only by nurses. The CNA tried to turn off the oxygen so the resident could smoke but she did not turn it off completely. The resident's cigarette set fire to the oxygen and caused severe facial burns.

The CNA lost her job at the center. The state's board of nursing asked the CNA to provide a written response to complaints against her. The CNA did not respond.

The CNA's conduct provided grounds for disciplinary action. The CNA was charged with:

- *Committing an act that deceives, defrauds, or harms the public*
- *Conduct or practice that is or may be harmful to the health of a patient or the public*
- *Failing to follow policies and procedures designed to protect the patient or resident*
- *Violating the rights or dignity of a patient or resident*
- *Neglecting or abusing a resident physically, verbally, emotionally, or financially*
- *Accepting patient or resident care tasks that the CNA lacks the education or competence to perform*
- *Failing to cooperate with the board during an investigation by:*
  - *Not providing a complete, written explanation of the matter*
  - *Not completing and returning a board-issued questionnaire within 30 days*

The CNA's certificate was revoked.

(Arizona State Board of Nursing, 2010.)

Performing tasks that you are not trained to do can cause harm. You can lose your job and your ability to work as a nursing assistant. Take pride in following the limits of your role and providing safe care.

FOCUS ON PRIDE: Application

There are limits to your role when assisting with oxygen therapy. Why are these limits important? Explain the value of your role. How do you help the nurse and patient or resident?

REVIEW QUESTIONS

Circle the BEST answer.

1 Alcohol and narcotics affect oxygen needs because they
   a Depress the brain
   b Are pollutants
   c Cause allergies
   d Cause infection

2 Hypoxia is
   a Not enough oxygen in the blood
   b The amount of hemoglobin that affects oxygen
   c Not enough oxygen in the cells
   d The lack of carbon dioxide

3 An early sign of hypoxia is
   a Cyanosis
   b Increased pulse
   c Restlessness
   d Dyspnea

4 A person can breathe deeply and comfortable only while sitting. This is called
   a Biot's respirations
   b Orthopnea
   c Bradypnea
   d Kussmaul respirations

5 Tachypnea means that respirations are
   a Slow
   b Rapid
   c Absent
   d Difficult or painful

6 Which should you report to the nurse at once?
   a A respiratory rate of 18 per minute
   b An SpO_2 of 97%
   c Bubbling in a humidifier
   d Dyspnea

7 A person's SpO_2 is 98%. Which is *true*?
   a The person's pulse oximeter is wrong.
   b The pulse is 98 beats per minute.
   c The measurement is within normal range.
   d The person has respiratory depression.

8 A person has fake nails. Which is a good pulse oximetry sensor site?
   a The wrist
   b A finger
   c The upper arm
   d An earlobe

9 You are assisting with deep breathing and coughing. You need to explain the procedure again if the person
   a Inhales through pursed lips
   b Sits in a comfortable position
   c Inhales deeply through the nose
   d Holds a pillow over an incision

10 A person has a productive cough. You remind the person to
   a Use a face mask
   b Cover the nose and mouth when coughing
   c Cough and deep breathe twice daily
   d Inhale through the mouth

11 Liquid oxygen can freeze the skin.
   a True
   b False

12 Which is useful for deep breathing?
   a Pulse oximeter
   b Incentive spirometer
   c Simple face mask
   d Partial-rebreather mask

13 Which oxygen device allows for eating?
   a Simple face mask
   b Partial-rebreather mask
   c Venturi mask
   d Nasal cannula

14 Oxygen flow rate is measured in
   a mm/Hg
   b Minutes
   c L/min
   d SpO_2

15 When assisting with oxygen therapy, you can
   a Turn the oxygen on and off
   b Start the oxygen
   c Decide what device to use
   d Keep connecting tubing secure and free of kinks

16 A person has humidified oxygen. The water level should move up with inspiration and down with expiration.
   a True
   b False

17 A person is receiving O_2. Which is unsafe?
   a Smoking materials are in the room.
   b Electrical items are turned off, then unplugged.
   c 3-pronged electrical items are used.
   d There is a fire extinguisher in the room.

18 A person is receiving O_2. Which measure should you question?
   a Provide oral hygiene.
   b Check for signs of irritation.
   c Adjust the flow rate if it is too high or too low.
   d Secure tubing in place.

Answers to Chapter 39 questions are on p. 872.

FOCUS ON PRACTICE

Problem Solving

You are a student training in the clinical setting. You are helping a nursing assistant transfer a resident to a wheelchair. The nursing assistant asks you to connect the person's nasal cannula to the portable O_2 tank and turn it on to 2 L/min. Nursing assistants in your state are not allowed to adjust O_2 flow rates. How will you respond? What will you do if the nursing assistant adjusts the flow rate?

Respiratory Support and Therapies

OBJECTIVES

- Define the key terms and key abbreviations in this chapter.
- Explain how to assist in the care of persons with artificial airways.
- Describe the principles and safety measures for suctioning.
- Explain how to assist in the care of persons on mechanical ventilation.

- Explain how to assist in the care of persons with chest tubes.
- Explain how to promote PRIDE in the person, the family, and yourself.

KEY TERMS

hemothorax Blood *(hemo)* in the pleural space *(thorax)*
intubation Inserting an artificial airway
mechanical ventilation Using a machine to move air into and out of the lungs
patent Open and unblocked
pleural effusion The escape and collection of fluid *(effusion)* in the pleural space

pneumothorax Air *(pneumo)* in the pleural space *(thorax)*
suction The process of withdrawing or sucking up fluid (secretions)
tracheostomy A surgically created opening *(stomy)* into the trachea *(tracheo)*

KEY ABBREVIATIONS

CO_2	Carbon dioxide	O_2	Oxygen
ET	Endotracheal	RT	Respiratory therapist

Some persons have serious problems affecting the respiratory system. They need complex procedures and equipment. The nurse may ask you to assist in their care.

See *Body Structure and Function Review: The Respiratory System* (Chapter 39).

See *Promoting Safety and Comfort: Respiratory Support and Therapies.*

PROMOTING SAFETY AND COMFORT

Respiratory Support and Therapies

Safety
Respiratory secretions may contain microbes or blood. Follow Standard Precautions and the Bloodborne Pathogen Standard.

ARTIFICIAL AIRWAYS

Artificial airways keep the airway *patent (open and unblocked)*. They are needed:
- When disease, injury, secretions, or aspiration obstructs the airway.
- For mechanical ventilation (p. 662)
- By some persons who are semi-conscious or unconscious
- During recovery from anesthesia

Intubation means inserting an artificial airway. Such airways are usually plastic and disposable. They come in various sizes.
- *Oro-pharyngeal airway*—inserted through the mouth and into the pharynx (Fig. 40-1, *A*). A nurse or respiratory therapist (RT) inserts the airway.
- *Endotracheal (ET) tube*—inserted through the mouth or nose into the trachea (Fig. 40-1, *B*). A doctor inserts it using a lighted scope. Some registered nurses (RNs) and RTs are trained to insert ET tubes.
- *Tracheostomy tube*—inserted through a surgically created opening *(stomy)* into the trachea *(tracheo)* (Fig. 40-1, *C*). Cuffed tubes are common. Doctors perform tracheostomies.

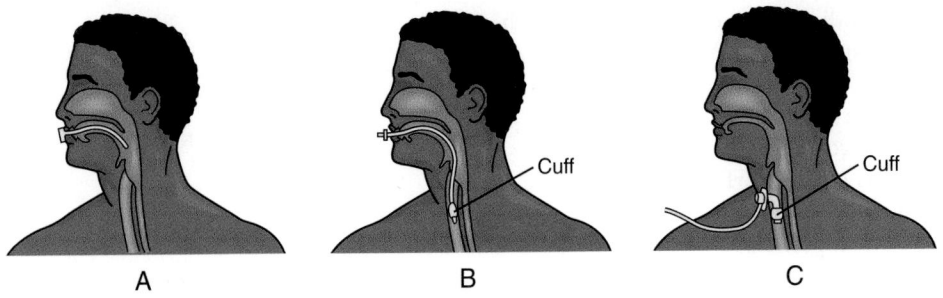

FIGURE 40-1 Artificial airways. **A,** Oro-pharyngeal airway. **B,** Endotracheal tube with cuff. **C,** Tracheostomy tube with cuff. (NOTE: Inflated cuffs keep endotracheal and tracheostomy tubes in place.)

Vital signs and pulse oximetry are measured often. Observe for hypoxia and other signs and symptoms of respiratory distress. If an airway comes out or is dislodged, tell the nurse at once. Frequent oral hygiene is needed. Follow the care plan.

Gagging and choking feelings are common. Imagine something in your mouth, nose, or throat. Comfort and reassure the person. Remind the person that the airway helps breathing. Use touch to show you care.

See *Focus on Communication: Artificial Airways.*

Tracheostomies

A *tracheostomy is a surgically created opening* (stomy) *into the trachea* (tracheo). Tracheostomies are often temporary. When no longer needed, the stoma is allowed to heal or is closed surgically.

Tracheostomies are permanent when the larynx is surgically removed. Cancer, airway injuries, long-term coma, spinal cord injuries, and diseases causing weakness or paralysis of the respiratory muscles may require a permanent tracheostomy.

A tracheostomy tube has 3 parts (Fig. 40-2).

* The *obturator* has a round end. It is used to guide insertion of the outer cannula (tube). Then it is removed. The obturator is kept at the bedside in case the tracheostomy tube falls out and needs insertion. It is taped to the wall or bedside stand.
* The *outer cannula* is secured in place with ties around the neck or a Velcro collar. The outer cannula is not removed. It keeps the tracheostomy patent. *Call for the nurse at once if the outer cannula comes out.*
* The *inner cannula* is inserted into the outer cannula and locked in place. It is removed for cleaning and mucus removal. This keeps the airway patent. Most tracheostomy tubes have inner cannulas.

The cuffed tracheostomy tube provides a seal between the cannula and the trachea (see Fig. 40-1, *C*). This prevents air from leaking around the tube and aspiration. A nurse or RT inflates and deflates the cuff.

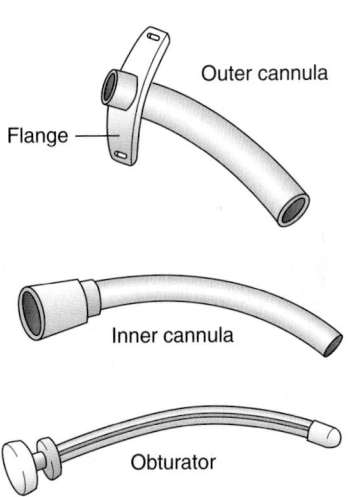

FIGURE 40-2 Parts of a tracheostomy tube.

The tube must not come out (*extubation*). If not secure, it could come out with coughing or if pulled on. A loose tube moves up and down, damaging the trachea. The tube must remain patent. If able, the person coughs up secretions. Otherwise suctioning is needed (p. 660). *Call for the nurse at once if you note signs and symptoms of hypoxia or respiratory distress.*

Safety Measures. Nothing must enter the stoma. Otherwise the person can aspirate. These safety measures are needed.

- Dressings do not have loose gauze or lint.
- The stoma or tube is covered when outdoors. The person wears a stoma cover, scarf, or shirt or blouse that buttons at the neck. The cover prevents dust, insects, and other small particles from entering the stoma.
- The stoma is not covered with plastic, leather, or similar materials. They prevent air from entering the stoma. The person cannot breathe.
- Tub baths are taken. For showers, a shower guard is worn. A hand-held nozzle is used to direct water away from the stoma.
- The person is assisted with shampooing. Water must not enter the stoma.
- The stoma is covered when shaving.
- Swimming is not allowed. Water will enter the tube or stoma.
- Medical-alert jewelry is worn. The person carries a medical-alert ID (identification) card.

Assisting With Tracheostomy Care. The nurse may ask you to assist with tracheostomy care (trach care). Trach care is done daily or every 8 to 12 hours to prevent infection, promote healing, and promote comfort. It also is done as needed for excess secretions, soiled ties or collar, or soiled or moist dressings. The nurse tells you what supplies are needed. Assist as directed.

Trach care involves:

- Cleaning the inner cannula to remove mucus and keep the airway patent. A disposable inner cannula is discarded and new one is inserted. Re-usable cannulas are cleaned with a small bottle brush or a pipe cleaner. The nurse tells you what cleaning agent is needed.
- Cleaning the stoma to prevent infection and skin breakdown.
- Applying clean ties or a Velcro collar. Clean ties are applied before removing the used ones. Hold the outer cannula in place until the nurse secures the new ties or collar. The ties or collar must be secure but not tight. For an adult, a finger should slide under the ties or collar (Fig. 40-3, *A*).

See *Focus on Children and Older Persons: Assisting With Tracheostomy Care.*

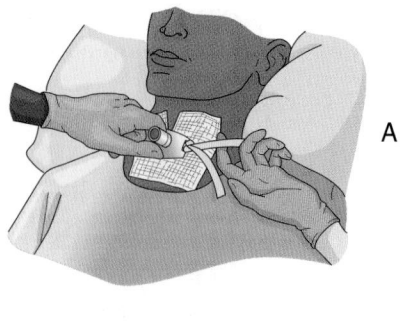

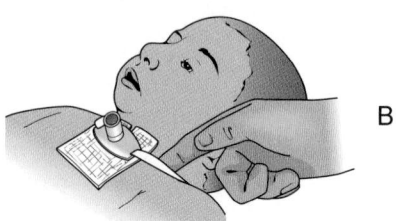

FIGURE 40-3 **A,** For an adult, a finger is inserted under the ties. **B,** For children, only a fingertip is inserted under the ties.

FOCUS ON CHILDREN AND OLDER PERSONS

Assisting With Tracheostomy Care

Children

Some children have congenital defects. (The Latin word *congenitus* means *to be born with*.) Congenital defects are present at birth. Tracheostomies are needed for some congenital defects affecting the neck and airway.

Some infections cause swelling of the airway structures. This obstructs air flow. So does foreign body aspiration. These problems may require emergency tracheostomies.

Tracheostomy ties must be secure but not tight. Only a fingertip should slide under the ties (Fig. 40-3, *B*). Ties are too loose if you can slide your whole finger under them.

Assist the nurse by holding the child still. Position the child's head as the nurse directs.

SUCTIONING

Secretions can collect in the airway. Retained secretions:

- Obstruct air flow into and out of the airway.
- Provide an environment for microbes.
- Interfere with oxygen (O_2) and carbon dioxide (CO_2) exchange.

Hypoxia can occur. Usually coughing removes secretions. Some persons cannot cough or the cough is too weak to remove secretions. They need suctioning.

Suction is the process of withdrawing or sucking up fluid (secretions). A tube connects to a suction source—wall outlet or suction machine—at 1 end and to a suction catheter at the other end. The catheter is inserted into the airway. Secretions are suctioned through the catheter.

The upper airway (nose, mouth, and pharynx) and lower airway (trachea and bronchi) are suctioned. These routes are used to suction the airway.

- *Oro-pharyngeal.* A suction catheter is passed through the mouth *(oro)* into the pharynx *(pharyngeal)*. The Yankauer suction catheter is used to suction the mouth and for thick secretions (Fig. 40-4).
- *Naso-pharyngeal.* The suction catheter is passed through the nose *(naso)* into the pharynx *(pharyngeal)*.
- *Lower airway.* The suction catheter is passed through an ET or tracheostomy tube (Fig. 40-5).

The person's lungs are hyperventilated before suctioning an ET or tracheostomy tube. *Hyperventilate* means to give extra *(hyper)* breaths *(ventilate)*. An Ambu bag (Fig. 40-6) attached to an oxygen source is used. The oxygen delivery device is removed from the ET or tracheostomy tube. Then the Ambu bag is attached to the ET or tracheostomy tube. To give a breath, the bag is squeezed with both hands. The nurse or RT gives 3 to 5 breaths.

Oxygen is treated like a drug. You do not give drugs. Check if your state and agency allow you to use an Ambu bag attached to an oxygen source.

To assist the nurse with suctioning, follow the safety measures in Box 40-1.

See *Focus on Children and Older Persons: Suctioning*, p. 662.
See *Delegation Guidelines: Suctioning*, p. 662.
See *Promoting Safety and Comfort: Suctioning*, p. 662.

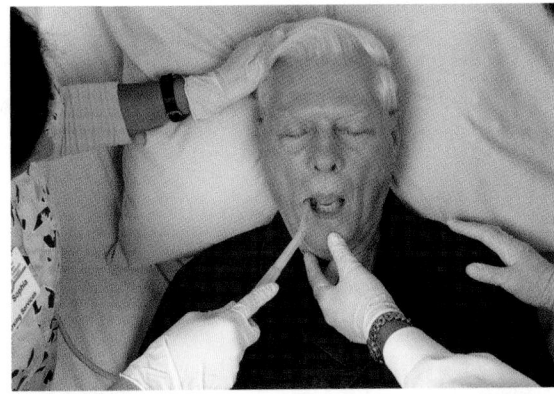

FIGURE 40-4 The Yankauer suction catheter is used to suction the mouth and for large amounts of thick secretions.

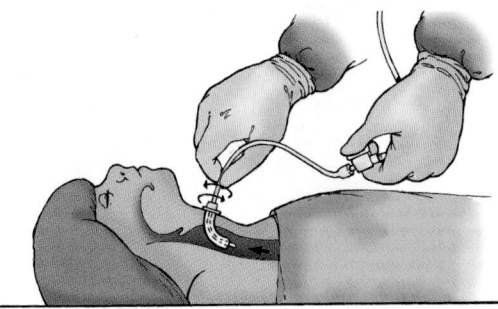

FIGURE 40-5 A tracheostomy tube is suctioned. (Modified from Hockenberry MJ, Wilson D: *Wong's essentials of pediatric nursing*, ed 9, St Louis, 2013, Mosby.)

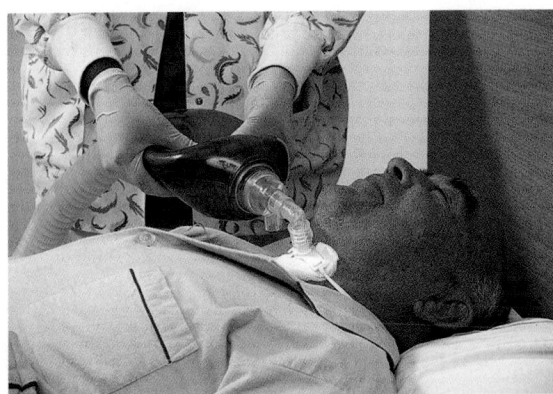

FIGURE 40-6 The Ambu bag is squeezed with 2 hands.

BOX 40-1	**Assisting With Suctioning**

- Review the procedure with the nurse. Know what you are to do.
- Report coughing and the signs and symptoms of respiratory distress (Chapter 39). Suctioning is done as needed, not on a schedule.
- Position the person as directed by the nurse—semi-Fowler's position with the head turned to 1 side or lateral position with the head turned to 1 side.
- Follow Standard Precautions and the Bloodborne Pathogen Standard. Secretions may contain blood and are potentially infectious.
- Sterile technique (Chapter 16) is used for naso-pharyngeal suctioning and to suction ET and tracheostomy tubes. This helps prevent microbes from entering the airway.
- The nurse tells you the catheter type and size needed. If too large, it can injure the airway.
- Keep needed suction supplies and equipment at the bedside. They are ready when the person needs suctioning.
- Suction is *not* applied while inserting the catheter. When suction is applied, air is sucked out of the airway.
- The catheter is inserted smoothly. This helps prevent injury to mucous membranes.
- A suction cycle for adults takes no more than 10 to 15 seconds and involves:
    - Inserting the catheter
    - Suctioning for 5 to 10 seconds
    - Removing the catheter
- The catheter is cleared with sterile water or saline between suction cycles.
- The nurse waits 20 to 30 seconds between each suction cycle. Some agencies require waiting 60 seconds.
- The suction catheter is passed (inserted) no more than 3 times. Injury and hypoxia are risks when the catheter is passed.
- Check the pulse, respirations, and pulse oximeter measurements before, during, and after the procedure. Also observe level of consciousness. Tell the nurse if any of these occur:
    - A decrease in pulse rate or pulse rate less than 60 beats per minute.
    - Irregular pulse rhythm.
    - An increase or decrease in blood pressure.
    - Respiratory distress.
    - A decrease in oxygen saturation. Normal range is 95% to 100%. See Chapter 39.

MECHANICAL VENTILATION

Mechanical ventilation is using a machine to move air into and out of the lungs (Fig. 40-7). An ET or tracheostomy tube is needed.

Problems that interfere with breathing or normal oxygen levels include:

- Weak muscle effort, obstructed airway, and damaged lung tissue
- Nervous system diseases and injuries affecting the respiratory center in the brain
- Nerve damage interfering with messages between the lungs and the brain
- Drug over-dose depressing the brain

Ventilator alarms sound when something is wrong. One alarm means the person is disconnected from the ventilator. The nurse shows you how to reconnect the ET or tracheostomy tube. When any alarm sounds, first check if the tube is attached to the ventilator. If not, re-attach it to the ventilator. The person can die if not attached to the ventilator. Then tell the nurse at once about the alarm. Do not re-set alarms.

Persons needing mechanical ventilation are often very ill. Other problems and injuries are common. Some persons are confused, disoriented, or cannot think clearly. The machine, fear of dying, and needing the machine life-long are concerns. Some are relieved to get enough oxygen. Mechanical ventilation can be painful for those with chest injuries or chest surgery. Tubes and hoses restrict movement, causing more discomfort.

The nurse may have you assist with the person's care. See Box 40-2.

See *Focus on Long-Term Care and Home Care: Mechanical Ventilation*.

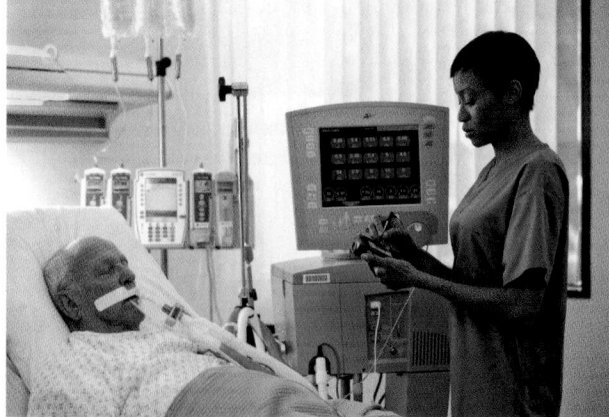

FIGURE 40-7 A mechanical ventilator. (Courtesy and © Becton, Dickinson and Company.)

BOX 40-2	Assisting With Mechanical Ventilation

- Keep the call light and other needed items within reach.
- Answer call lights promptly. The person depends on others for basic needs.
- Make sure hoses and connecting tubes have slack. They must not pull on the artificial airway.
- Explain who you are and what you are going to do. Do this each time you enter the room.
- Give the day, date, and time every time you give care.
- Report signs of respiratory distress or discomfort at once.
- Do not change machine settings or re-set alarms.
- Follow the care plan for communication. The person cannot talk. Use agreed-upon hand or eye signals for "yes" and "no." Everyone must use the same signals. Some persons can use the communication aids described in Chapter 9. Ask questions with simple answers. It may be hard to write long responses.
- Watch what you say and do. This includes when you are near and away from the person and family. They are aware of your verbal and nonverbal communication. Do not say or do anything that could upset the person.
- Use touch to comfort and reassure the person. Also tell the person about the weather, pleasant news events, and gifts and cards.
- Meet basic needs. Follow the care plan.
- Tell the person when you are leaving the room and when you will return.
- Complete a safety check before leaving the room. (See the inside of the front cover.)

FOCUS ON LONG-TERM CARE AND HOME CARE

Mechanical Ventilation

Long-Term Care
Some people need mechanical ventilation for a few hours or days. Others need long-term care or sub-acute care. When possible, the person is weaned from the ventilator. That is, the person needs to breathe without the machine. The RT and RN plan the weaning process. Weaning can take many weeks.

Home Care
Some ventilator-dependent persons receive home care. The nurse teaches you and the family how to care for the person. You must be able to reach the nurse by phone. Make sure delegated tasks are allowed by your state and agency.

CHEST TUBES

Air, blood, or fluid can collect in the pleural space (sac or cavity). This occurs when the chest is entered because of injury or surgery.

- *Pneumothorax is air* (pneumo) *in the pleural space* (thorax).
- *Hemothorax is blood* (hemo) *in the pleural space* (thorax).
- *Pleural effusion is the escape and collection of fluid* (effusion) *in the pleural space.*

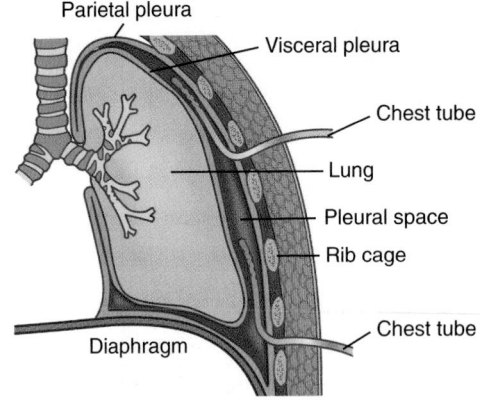

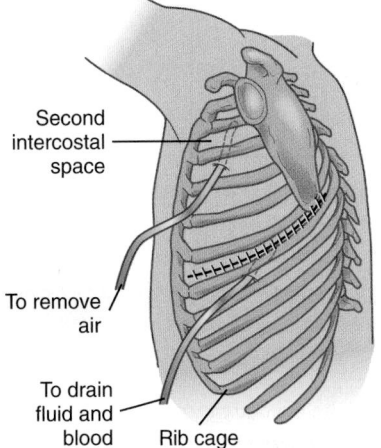

FIGURE 40-8 Chest tubes inserted into the pleural space. (From Lewis SL, Dirksen SR, Heitkemper MM, Bucher LB: *Medical-surgical nursing: assessment and management of clinical problems,* ed 9, St Louis, 2014, Mosby.)

Pressure occurs when air, blood, or fluid collects in the pleural space. The pressure collapses the lung. Air cannot reach affected alveoli for O_2 and CO_2 exchange. Respiratory distress and hypoxia result. Pressure on the heart affects the heart's ability to pump blood.

Hospital care is required. The doctor inserts chest tubes to remove the air, blood, or fluid (Fig. 40-8). The sterile procedure is done in surgery, the emergency room, or at the bedside. A nurse assists.

Chest tubes attach to a drainage system (Fig. 40-9, p. 664). The system must be air-tight so air does not enter the pleural space. Water-seal drainage keeps the system air-tight. The bottles in Figure 40-10, p. 664 show how the system works.

- A chest tube attaches to connecting tubing.
- Connecting tubing attaches to a tube in the drainage container.
- The tube in the drainage container extends under the water. The water prevents air from entering the chest tube and then the pleural space.

See Box 40-3, p. 664 for care of the person with chest tubes.

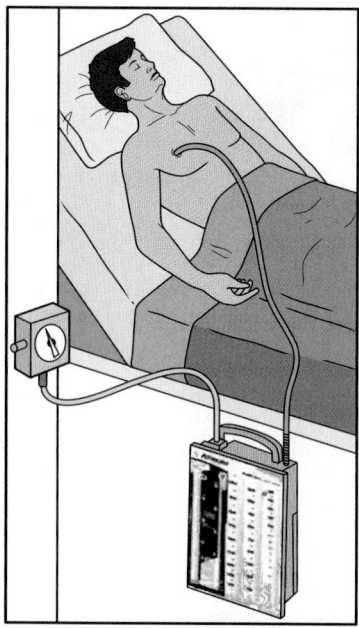

FIGURE 40-9 Chest tube attached to a disposable water-seal drainage system. (Redrawn from Atrium Medical, Maquet Getinge Group, Hudson, NH.)

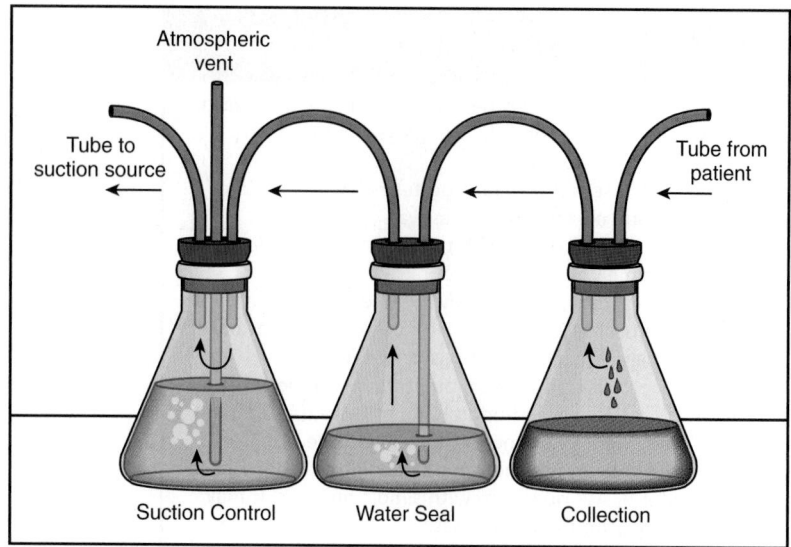

FIGURE 40-10 Water-seal drainage system. (Redrawn from Atrium Medical, Maquet Getinge Group, Hudson, NH.)

BOX 40-3	**Assisting With Chest Tubes**

- Keep the drainage system below the chest.
- Report the following at once.
  - Vital signs and pulse oximetry measurements. The nurse tells you when to take them.
  - Signs and symptoms of hypoxia and respiratory distress. See Chapter 39.
  - Complaints of pain or difficulty breathing.
  - Changes in chest drainage. This includes increases in drainage or the appearance of bright red drainage.
  - If bubbling in the drainage system increases, decreases, or stops.
  - If any part of the drainage system is loose or disconnected.
- Keep connecting tubing coiled on the bed. Allow enough slack so the chest tubes are not dislodged when the person moves. If tubing hangs in loops, drainage collects in the loops.

- Prevent tubing kinks. Kinks obstruct the chest tube. Air, blood, or fluid collects in the pleural space.
- Record chest drainage according to agency policy.
- Turn and position the person as directed. Be careful and gentle to prevent the chest tubes from dislodging.
- Assist with deep breathing and coughing exercises and incentive spirometry as directed.
- Keep sterile petrolatum gauze at the bedside. It is needed if a chest tube comes out.
- Call for help at once if a chest tube comes out. Cover the insertion site with sterile petrolatum gauze. Stay with the person. Follow the nurse's directions.
- Complete a safety check before leaving the room. (See the inside of the front cover.)

FOCUS ON **PRIDE**

The Person, Family, and Yourself

Personal and Professional Responsibility

The person's airway must be clear for survival. You must know the signs and symptoms that signal the need for suctioning (see Box 40-1 and Chapter 39). Tell the nurse at once if you suspect suctioning is needed. Delay can cause harm or death.

Observing the person and reporting concerns are important parts of your role. Take pride in safely assisting with respiratory support and therapies.

Rights and Respect

Persons with ET tubes cannot speak. Many cannot respond in any way. Coma (Chapter 13) and sedation (Chapter 35) are causes. However, the person may hear and understand. Show dignity and respect when providing care.

- Tell the person when he or she will be moved or touched.
- Explain what the person will feel and where it will be felt.
- Talk to the person. Tell about pleasant things.
- Focus on the person. Do not ignore the person or talk with co-workers about personal matters.
- Use touch to show you care.

Every person has the right to dignified care. Take pride in providing care in a way that shows respect for the person.

FOCUS ON **P R I D E—cont'd**

The Person, Family, and Yourself

Independence and Social Interaction

Mechanical ventilation brings fears and worries for the family. How long is the ventilator needed? Will the person die? The doctor and nurse answer the family's questions. You can provide social support. Quality time with the person can bring the family peace and ease stress. You can:

- Encourage the family to talk to the person. If the person cannot respond, tell the family that he or she may hear and understand.
- Allow private time.
- Promote the use of touch. Provide chairs so the family can sit by the person to hold a hand, stroke the hair, and so on.
- Allow family involvement in care measures. Brushing hair, applying lotion, and giving nail care are examples.

Delegation and Teamwork

Some team members have 1 focus of care. For example, an RT provides respiratory treatments and therapies. Develop a good working relationship with the RT. Be polite. Offer to help as needed. The RT is a good source of knowledge and skill for respiratory issues. Ask questions and thank the RT for answering them.

Ethics and Laws

Respiratory support and therapies involve complex care. Many in this chapter are outside the scope of your role. Serious problems can occur from the wrong care. Know your limits. Follow the nurse's directions to assist with care measures. Remember your legal and ethical responsibilities. You have the right to refuse a function or task. Do not function beyond your legal scope, preparation, skill level, and job description.

FOCUS ON **PRIDE**: *Application*

Imagine if your parent, spouse, or child required mechanical ventilation. What concerns and fears would you have? Describe the quality of care you would expect. How would you like the health team to treat you? How will you apply these qualities in your interactions with the person and family?

REVIEW QUESTIONS

Circle the BEST answer.

1 A person has a tracheostomy. Which is *true*?
   a The person must not cough.
   b The obturator is kept at the nurses' station.
   c The tube must remain patent.
   d The nurse removes the outer cannula for cleaning.

2 A person with a tracheostomy *cannot*
   a Shampoo
   b Shave
   c Shower with a hand-held nozzle
   d Swim

3 The nurse is changing tracheostomy ties. You must
   a Remove the inner cannula
   b Clean the stoma
   c Remove the dressing
   d Hold the outer cannula in place

4 You cannot slide a finger under the tracheostomy ties. This means that the ties
   a Are secure   c Need to be replaced
   b Are too tight   d Need to be removed

5 Which signals the need for suctioning?
   a A pulse rate of 90 beats per minute
   b Signs and symptoms of respiratory distress
   c The orthopneic position
   d Being unable to speak

6 Suctioning the lower airway requires
   a Sterile technique
   b Mechanical ventilation
   c A Yankauer catheter
   d Chest tubes

7 You are assisting the nurse with suctioning. Your role involves
   a Inserting the catheter no more than 3 times
   b Suctioning for no more than 10 to 15 seconds
   c Clearing the suction catheter with water
   d Keeping needed supplies at the bedside

8 You note the following while assisting with suctioning. Which should you report at once?
   a A pulse rate of 82 beats per minute
   b A regular heart rhythm
   c Oxygen saturation of 92%
   d Thick secretions

9 A person has an ET tube with mechanical ventilation. Which is *true*?
   a The ET tube must stay attached to the ventilator.
   b You should remove slack from hoses and tubing.
   c The person cannot respond or sense touch.
   d You can re-set alarms on the ventilator.

10 A ventilator alarm sounds. What should you do?
   a Re-set the alarm.
   b Check if the airway is attached to the machine.
   c Do nothing.
   d Ask the person what is wrong.

11 A person has a pneumothorax. This is
   a Fluid in the pleural space
   b Blood in the pleural space
   c Air in the pleural space
   d Secretions in the pleural space

12 Assisting with chest tube care involves
   a Avoiding deep breathing and coughing
   b Making sure tubing is not kinked
   c Keeping the drainage system at chest level
   d Hanging tubing in loops

Answers to Chapter 40 questions are on p. 872.

FOCUS ON PRACTICE

Problem Solving

The nurse suctioned Mr. Patrick's tracheostomy tube 2 hours ago. Now his breathing is noisy and wet-sounding. He tries to cough. His cough sounds harsh. Is this normal? What do you do? How often is suctioning done?

Rehabilitation and Restorative Nursing Care

KEY TERMS

activities of daily living (ADL) The activities usually done during a normal day in a person's life

disability Any lost, absent, or impaired physical or mental function

prosthesis An artificial replacement for a missing body part

rehabilitation The process of restoring the person to his or her highest possible level of physical, psychological, social, and economic function

restorative aide A nursing assistant with special training in restorative nursing and rehabilitation skills

restorative nursing care Care that helps persons regain health, strength, and independence

KEY ABBREVIATIONS

ADL   Activities of daily living

ROM   Range of motion

Disease, injury, and surgery can affect body function. So can birth injuries and birth defects (Chapter 50). Often more than 1 function is lost.

A *disability* is any lost, absent, or impaired physical or mental function. Causes are acute or chronic (Box 41-1).

- An *acute problem* has a short course with complete recovery. A fracture (broken bone) is an example.
- A *chronic problem* has a long course. The problem is controlled—not cured—with treatment. Diabetes and arthritis are chronic health problems. A spinal cord injury is long-term if paralysis results.

Disabilities can affect eating, bathing, dressing, walking, and the ability to work. These daily activities and others are hard or seem impossible. The degree of disability affects how much function is possible. The person may depend totally or in part on others for basic needs.

Rehabilitation is the process of restoring the person to his or her highest possible level of physical, psychological, social, and economic function. The goals of rehabilitation are to:

- Prevent or reduce the degree of disability.
- Improve abilities. This promotes function at the highest level of independence. Returning to work may be a goal. For others, self-care is the goal. If improved function is not possible, the goal is to prevent further loss of function. This helps the person maintain the best possible quality of life.
- Help the person adjust to the disability.

Some persons return home after rehabilitation. The process may continue in home or community settings.

See *Focus on Long-Term Care and Home Care: Rehabilitation and Restorative Nursing Care.*

BOX 41-1	Common Problems Requiring Rehabilitation	
• Amputation	• Chronic obstructive pulmonary disease	• Spinal cord injury
• Birth defects		• Spinal cord tumor
• Brain tumor	• Fractures	• Stroke
• Burns	• Head injury	• Substance abuse—drug, alcohol
• Cerebral palsy	• Myocardial infarction (heart attack)	

RESTORATIVE NURSING

Some persons are weak. Many cannot perform daily functions. *Restorative nursing care is care that helps persons regain health, strength, and independence.* With progressive illnesses, disabilities increase. Restorative nursing:
• Helps maintain the highest level of function.
• Prevents unnecessary decline in function.
  Restorative nursing measures promote:
• Self-care
• Elimination
• Positioning
• Mobility
• Communication
• Cognitive function
  Many persons need restorative nursing and rehabilitation. In many agencies, they mean the same thing. Both focus on the whole person.

Restorative Aides

Some agencies have restorative aides. A *restorative aide is a nursing assistant with special training in restorative nursing and rehabilitation skills.* These aides assist the nursing and health teams as needed. Required training varies among states. If there are no state requirements, the agency provides needed training.

REHABILITATION AND THE WHOLE PERSON

A health problem has physical, psychological, and social effects. So does a disability. Suppose an illness left you paralyzed from the waist down.
• Would you be angry, afraid, or depressed?
• How would you move about?
• How would you care for yourself and your family?
• How would you worship, shop, or visit friends?
• Could you work and support yourself?
  The person needs to adjust physically, psychologically, socially, and economically. Abilities—what the person can do—are stressed. Complications may cause further disability.
  See *Focus on Children and Older Persons: Rehabilitation and the Whole Person.*

Physical Aspects

Rehabilitation starts when the person first seeks health care. Complications are prevented. They can occur from bedrest, a long illness, or recovery from surgery or injury. Bowel and bladder problems are prevented. So are contractures and pressure ulcers. Good alignment, turning and re-positioning, range-of-motion (ROM) exercises, and supportive devices are needed (Chapters 17, 18, and 30). Good skin care also prevents pressure ulcers (Chapters 22 and 37).

Elimination. Some persons need bladder training (Chapter 24). The method depends on the person's problems, abilities, and needs. Some need bowel training (Chapter 26). Control of bowel movements and regular elimination are goals. Fecal impaction, constipation, and fecal incontinence are prevented.

Self-Care. Self-care is a major goal. *Activities of daily living (ADL) are the activities usually done during a normal day in a person's life.* ADL include bathing, oral hygiene, dressing, eating, elimination, and moving about. The health team evaluates the person's ability to perform ADL.
  Sometimes the hands, wrists, and arms are affected. Adaptive (assistive) devices are often needed. Equipment is changed, made, or bought to meet the person's needs.
• Eating devices include glass holders, plate guards, and silverware with curved handles or cuffs (Chapter 27). Some devices attach to splints (Fig. 41-1, p. 668).
• Electric toothbrushes have back-and-forth brushing motions for oral hygiene.
• Adaptive (assistive) devices for hygiene promote independence.
  Adaptive (assistive) devices are useful for cooking, dressing, writing, phone calls, and other tasks. Some are shown in Figure 41-2, p. 668. Also see Chapters 22 and 23.
  See *Focus on Surveys: Self-Care*, p. 668.

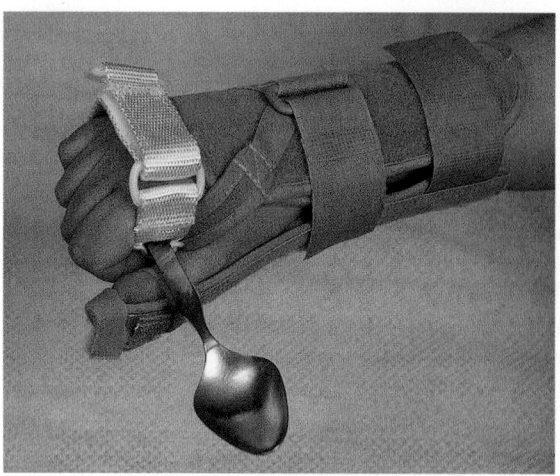

FIGURE 41-1 Eating device attached to a splint.

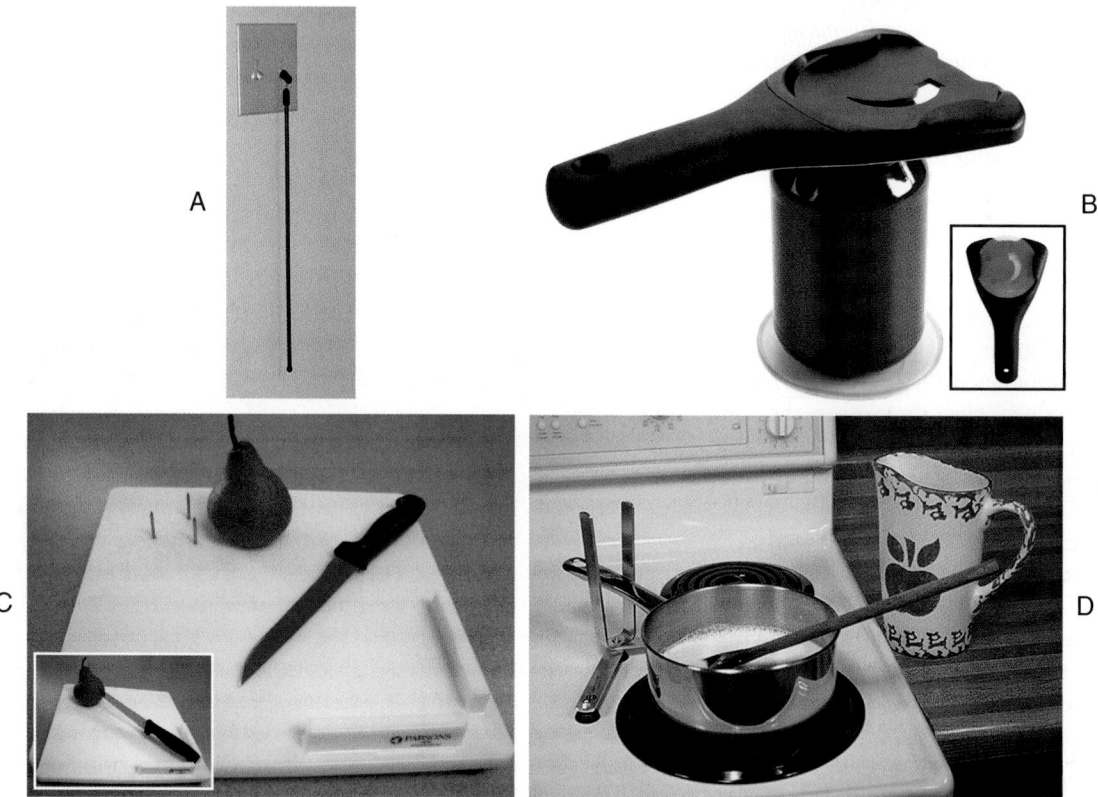

FIGURE 41-2 A, Light switch extender. **B,** Jar opener. **C,** Cutting board. **D,** Pot stabilizer. (A, C, and D, Courtesy Parsons ADL, Inc. Tottenham, Ontario. B, Courtesy OXO International, Inc., New York, NY.)

Mobility. The person may need crutches or a walker, cane, or brace (Chapter 30). Physical and occupational therapies are common for musculo-skeletal and nervous system problems (Fig. 41-3). Some people need wheelchairs. If possible, they learn wheelchair transfers. Such transfers include to and from the bed, toilet, bathtub, sofa, and chair and in and out of vehicles (Figs. 41-4, 41-5, and 41-6, p. 670).

A *prosthesis is an artificial replacement for a missing body part.* The person learns how to use the artificial arm or leg (Chapter 44). The goal is for the device to be like the missing body part in function and appearance.

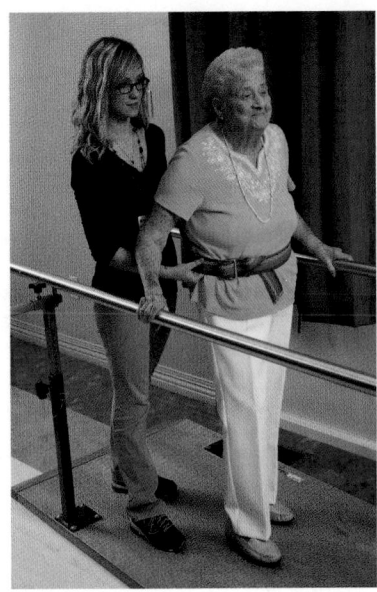

FIGURE 41-3 The person is assisted with walking in physical therapy.

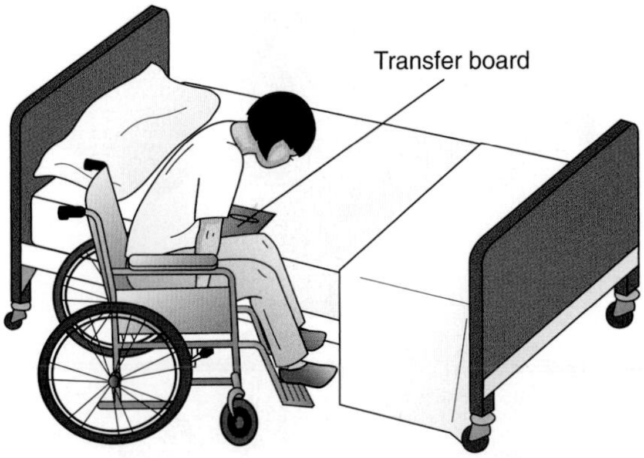

FIGURE 41-4 The person uses a transfer board (sliding board) to transfer from wheelchair to bed.

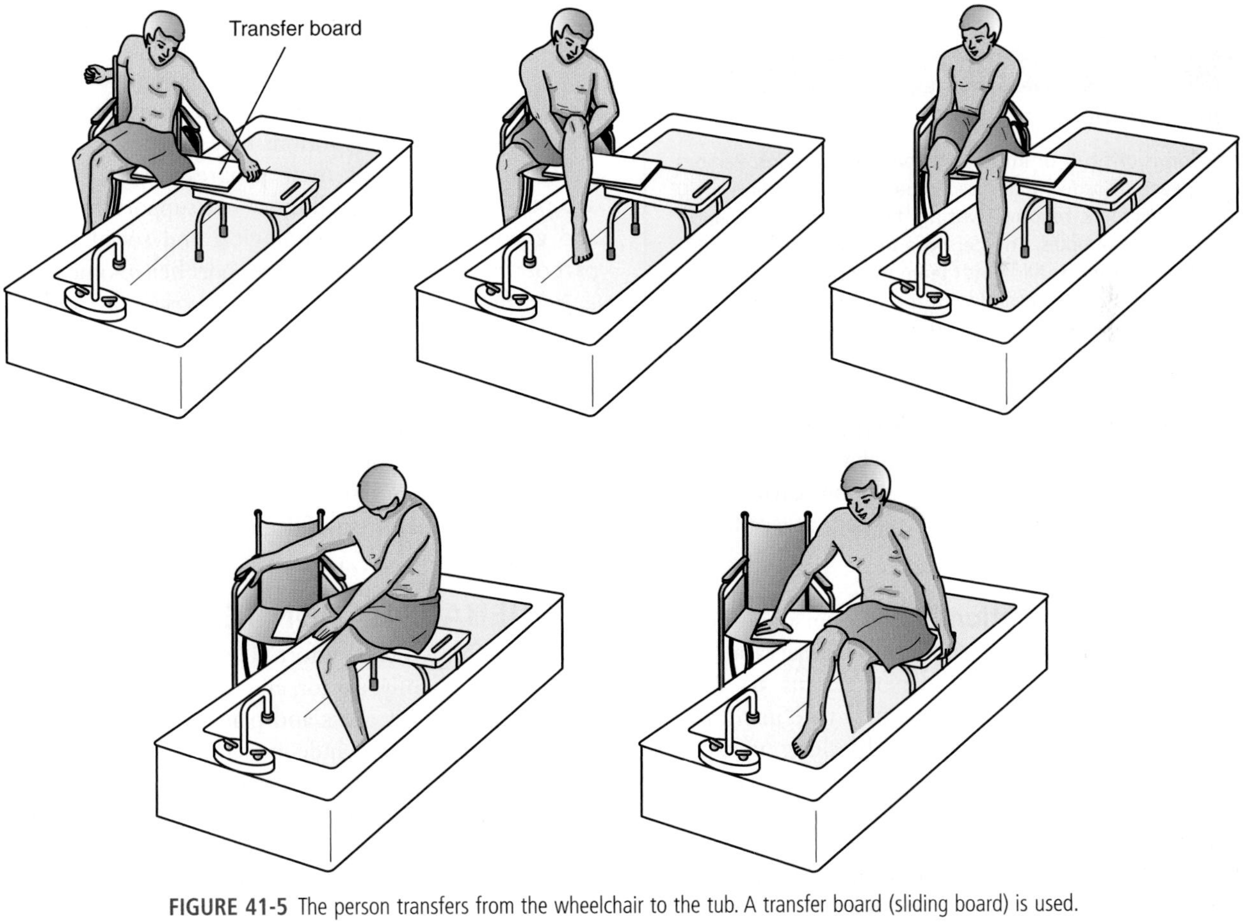

FIGURE 41-5 The person transfers from the wheelchair to the tub. A transfer board (sliding board) is used.

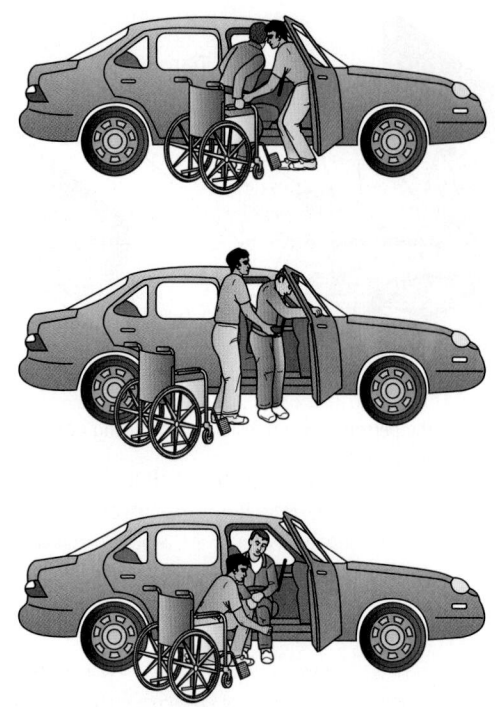

FIGURE 41-6 The person transfers from the wheelchair to the car.

FOCUS ON COMMUNICATION

Communication

Speaking is difficult or impossible for some persons. Persons with speech disorders may need other communication methods. Pictures, reading, writing, facial expressions, and gestures are examples. The person and health team decide on the best method. All health team members and the family use the same method with the person. Changing methods can cause confusion and delay progress.

Nutrition. Difficulty swallowing *(dysphagia)* may occur after a stroke. The person may need a dysphagia diet (Chapter 27). When possible, the person learns exercises to improve swallowing. Persons who cannot swallow need enteral nutrition (Chapter 28).

Mechanical Ventilation. Some persons needing mechanical ventilation (Chapter 40) are weaned from the ventilator. That is, the person learns to breathe without the machine. The process may take many weeks. Other persons learn to live with life-long mechanical ventilation.

Communication

Aphasia (Chapter 42) may occur from a stroke. *Aphasia* is the total or partial loss *(a)* of the ability to use or understand language *(phasia)*. It results from damage to parts of the brain responsible for language and speech. Speech therapy and communication devices are helpful (Chapter 9).

See *Focus on Communication: Communication.*

FOCUS ON COMMUNICATION

Psychological and Social Aspects

Emotional needs are great during rehabilitation. Good communication and support provide encouragement.
- Listen to the person.
- Show concern, not pity.
- Focus on what the person can do. Point out even slight progress.
- Be polite but firm. Do not let the person control you.
- Do not shout at or insult the person. Such behaviors are abuse and mistreatment.
- Do not argue with the person.
- Tell the nurse. The person may need other support measures.

Psychological and Social Aspects

A disability can affect function and appearance. Self-esteem and relationships may suffer. Some persons feel unwhole, useless, unattractive, unclean, or undesirable. They may deny the disability and expect therapy to correct the problem. Some persons are depressed, angry, and hostile.

A good attitude is important. The person must be motivated and accept limits. The focus is on abilities and strengths. Despair and frustration are common. Progress may be slow. Learning a new task is a reminder of the disability. Old fears and emotions may recur.

Remind persons of their progress. They need help accepting disabilities and limits. Give support, reassurance, and encouragement. Psychological and social needs are part of the care plan. Spiritual support helps some persons.

See *Focus on Communication: Psychological and Social Aspects.*

Economic Aspects

Some persons return to their jobs. Others cannot do so. They are assessed for work skills, work history, interests, and talents. A job skill may be restored or a new one learned. The goal is gainful employment. Help is given finding a job.

THE REHABILITATION TEAM

Rehabilitation is a team effort. The person is the key team member. The family, doctor, and nursing and health teams help the person set goals and plan care. The focus is on regaining function and independence.

The team meets often to discuss the person's progress. The rehabilitation plan is changed as needed. The person and family attend the meetings when possible. Families provide support and encouragement. Often they help with home care.

Your Role

You help promote the person's independence. Preventing decline in function also is a goal. The many procedures, care measures, and rules in this book apply. Safety, communication, legal, and ethical aspects apply. So do the measures in Box 41-2.

See *Focus on Communication: Your Role.*

See *Teamwork and Time Management: Your Role.*

TEAMWORK AND TIME MANAGEMENT

Your Role

Rehabilitation can frustrate the person, you, and the health team. Teamwork is about helping with care. But it is also about giving emotional support. Talk about your feelings. The team can help you control or express your feelings. You may need to assist with other patients or residents for a while.

BOX 41-2	Assisting With Rehabilitation and Restorative Care

- Follow the care plan and the nurse's instructions.
- Follow the person's daily routine.
- Provide for safety.
- Protect the person's rights. Privacy and personal choice are very important.
- Report early signs and symptoms of complications. They include pressure ulcers, contractures, and bowel and bladder problems.
- Keep the person in good alignment at all times.
- Turn and re-position the person as directed.
- Use safe transfer methods.
- Practice measures to prevent pressure ulcers.
- Perform ROM exercises as instructed.
- Apply assistive devices as ordered.
- Provide needed assistive (adaptive) devices.
- Do not pity the person or give sympathy.
- Encourage the person to perform ADL to the extent possible.
- Give the person time to complete tasks. Do not rush the person.
- Give praise when even a little progress is made.
- Provide emotional support and reassurance.
- Try to understand and appreciate the person's situation, feelings, and concerns.
- Provide for spiritual needs.
- Practice the methods developed by the rehabilitation team. This helps you better assist the person.
- Practice the task that the person must do. This helps you guide and direct the person.
- Know how to use and apply the person's assistive (adaptive) devices.
- Stress what the person can do. Focus on abilities and strengths. Do not focus on disabilities and weaknesses.
- Remember that muscles will atrophy if not used. And contractures can develop.
- Have a hopeful outlook.

REHABILITATION PROGRAMS AND SERVICES

Common rehabilitation programs include:
- *Cardiac rehabilitation*—for heart disorders
- *Brain injury rehabilitation*—for nervous system disorders including traumatic brain injury
- *Spinal cord rehabilitation*—for spinal cord injuries
- *Stroke rehabilitation*—after a stroke
- *Respiratory rehabilitation*—for respiratory system disorders such as chronic obstructive pulmonary disease, after lung surgery, for respiratory complications from other health problems, and for mechanical ventilation
- *Orthopedic rehabilitation*—for fractures, joint replacement surgery, and other musculo-skeletal problems
- *Amputee rehabilitation*—for amputation of a limb
- *Hearing, speech, and vision rehabilitation*—for persons who are deaf, have speech problems, are blind, or have severe vision problems
- *Drug and alcohol treatment*—for persons addicted to drugs or alcohol
- *Behavioral health treatment*—for those with mental health problems
- *Rehabilitation for complex medical and surgical conditions*—wound care, diabetes, and burns are examples

After hospital discharge, the person may transfer to a nursing center or rehabilitation agency. Some agencies are for certain types of problems. Home care agencies also provide rehabilitation services. So do some assisted living residences (Chapter 53) and adult day-care centers.

See *Focus on Children and Older Persons: Rehabilitation Programs and Services.*

See *Focus on Long-Term Care and Home Care: Rehabilitation Programs and Services*, p. 672.

FOCUS ON COMMUNICATION

Your Role

You may need to guide and direct the person during care. First, listen to how the nurse or therapist guides and directs the person. Use those words. Hearing the same thing helps the person learn and remember what to do.

FOCUS ON CHILDREN AND OLDER PERSONS

Rehabilitation Programs and Services

Children

Federal laws require that schools provide needed therapies. In-school therapy is required to meet the child's learning needs.

FOCUS ON LONG-TERM CARE AND HOME CARE
Rehabilitation Programs and Services

Long-Term Care

The *Omnibus Budget Reconciliation Act of 1987* (OBRA) requires that nursing centers provide rehabilitation services. If not provided by center staff, the service is obtained from another source. For example, a center does not have a speech therapist. The service is obtained from another agency.

Long-Term Care—cont'd

The center must provide services required by a person's care plan. If a person requires physical therapy, it must be provided. If occupational therapy is required, it must be provided. If speech therapy is required, it must be provided.

Home Care

The rehabilitation team assesses the person's home setting (Box 41-3). Changes in the home are made as needed. Some persons require personal attendants 24 hours a day.

BOX 41-3   Home Assessment Checklist

Appliances, Kitchen, and Bathroom
- Cabinet door knobs are easy to use.
- Stove controls are easy to use and clearly marked.
- Faucets are easy to use.
- Grab bars are securely installed where needed.
- Appliances and utensils are in convenient, safe, and easy-to-reach places.
- The oven and refrigerator open easily.
- The person can sit down while in the kitchen or bathroom.
- The person can get in and out of the bathtub or shower easily.
- Kitchen and bathroom counter heights and depths are comfortable for the person.
- The water temperature is regulated to prevent scalds or burns.
- Needed convenience items are available.
  - Hand-held shower nozzle
  - Garbage disposal
  - Trash compactor
  - Dish washer
  - Other

Closets and Storage Areas
- Closets and storage areas are conveniently located.
- Closet shelves are within reach.
- Items in closets are easily reached.
- The person has adequate storage space.
- Closet and storage areas are well-organized with space well-used.

Doors and Windows
- Doors are easy to open and close.
- Door locks and dead-bolts are sturdy and easy to operate.
- Doors have lever handles, not door knobs.
- Doors and hallways are wide enough for walker or wheelchair use.
- Doors have peepholes or view windows.
- Windows are easy to open from the inside. Locks prevent access from the outside.

Driveway and Garage
- The garage door has an automatic opener.
- A parking space is always available.
- The parking space is close to the home or apartment entrance.

Electrical Outlets, Switches, and Safety Devices
- Light and power switches are easy to turn on and off.
- Electrical outlets are easy to reach.
- Electrical outlets are properly grounded to prevent shocks.
- Extension cords are in good condition.
- The doorbell can be heard in every part of the home.
- Smoke alarms and carbon monoxide alarms:
  - Are on every level of the home, in sleeping areas, and inside bedrooms.
  - Are tested and work properly.
  - Have new batteries within the last year.
- There is a home security system.
- Phones are available in each room, including the bedroom, for emergencies. Emergency numbers are by each phone.
- Phones can be reached from the floor in case of a fall.
- Assistive devices for phone use are available.

Floors
- The home is 1 level.
- Floor surfaces are safe and covered with non-slip or non-skid materials.
- Floor coverings are in good repair.
- Scatter rugs and doormats are not used.

Hallways, Steps, and Stairs
- Hallways, steps, and stairs are in good condition with smooth and safe surfaces.
- Steps are big enough for the whole foot.
- Hand rails are securely installed on both sides of stairways and are easy to grasp.
- A ramp replaces stairs or steps inside and outside the home.

Lighting
- Night-lights are placed where needed.
- Lighting in each room meets the person's needs.
- Lighting is bright enough for safety.

Furniture
- Furniture is safely arranged. The person does not need to walk around furniture.
- Chairs and sofas are sturdy and safe.
- Chairs and sofas allow for easy sitting and rising.

BOX 41-3	Home Assessment Checklist—cont'd

Bedroom
- A lamp and flashlight are near the bed.
- A night-light is in the bedroom.
- The person has ample room to walk around the bed.
- The person has a nightstand for phone, glasses, and needed items.
- An arm chair is where the person can sit with ease.

Outside and Entrances
- Porches and entrances are well-lit.
- Light switches are by entrances.
- Outside steps and entrances are in good repair and slip-resistant.
- Outside steps have easy-to-grasp hand rails.

Other
- The building has an elevator.
- Thermostats for heat and air conditioning are within reach.
- Each room is well-ventilated with good air circulation.
- Safety measures in Chapter 13: Safety are followed.
- Safety measures in Chapter 14: Preventing Falls are followed.
- Safety measures in Chapter 39: Oxygen Needs are followed.
- Safety measures in Chapter 49: Confusion and Dementia are followed.

Modified from Eldercarelocator: Home modifications, Washington, DC, last modified July 23, 2012, Administration on Aging, Department of Health and Human Services; and Consumer Product Safety Commission: Safety for older consumers—home safety checklist, publication 701, Bethesda, Md.

QUALITY OF LIFE

Successful rehabilitation and restorative care improves quality of life. A hopeful and winning outlook is needed. The more the person can do alone, the better his or her quality of life. To promote quality of life:
- Protect the right to privacy.
- Encourage personal choice.
- Protect the right to be free from abuse and mistreatment.
- Learn to deal with your anger and frustration.
- Encourage activities.
- Provide a safe setting.
- Show patience, understanding, and sensitivity.

FOCUS ON **PRIDE**

The Person, Family, and Yourself

Personal and Professional Responsibility

Often nursing assistants are promoted to restorative aide positions. Professional behaviors are highly valued when considering who to promote. Restorative aides require patience, kindness, and good communication skills. Staff with a positive attitude, good work ethics, and excellent job performance are considered first.

Becoming a restorative aide is a rewarding option to advance as a nursing assistant. Seek out learning opportunities and practice positive work habits. Take pride in continuing to learn, improve, and grow as a nursing assistant.

Rights and Respect

Rehabilitation is challenging for the person, the family, and the nursing staff. No matter how difficult the situation, the person's rights are protected.
- *Right to privacy*—The person re-learns old skills or practices new skills in private. No one needs to watch. They do not need to see mistakes, falls, spills, or clumsiness. Nor do they need to see anger or tears. Privacy protects dignity and promotes self-respect.

Rights and Respect—cont'd
- *Right to be free from abuse and mistreatment*—Re-learning skills takes time. Simple things are often hard. You, other staff, or the family may become upset and short-tempered. Protect the person from abuse and mistreatment. No one can shout at, scream at, yell at, or call the person names. They cannot hit or strike the person. Unkind remarks are not allowed. Report signs of abuse or mistreatment.
- *Right to a safe setting*—The setting must meet the person's needs. Needed changes are made. The over-bed table, bedside stand, call light, and other needed items are moved to the person's strong (unaffected) side. If unable to use the call light, another communication aid is used. The rehabilitation team suggests these and other changes. They explain the need and purpose to the person and family.

Continued

FOCUS ON **P R I D E—cont'd**

The Person, Family, and Yourself

Independence and Social Interaction

The more the person can do for himself or herself, the better his or her quality of life. To promote independence:

- Stress the person's abilities and strengths.
- Let the person choose activities of interest.
- Remain patient. Avoid rushing the person.
- Resist the urge to do things for the person that he or she can do. This hinders the ability to regain function.
- Offer encouragement and support. The person may worry about how others view the disability. A caring and positive attitude can help motivate them.
- Have the person use assistive (adaptive) devices as needed.
- Encourage personal choice. Not being able to control body movements or functions is very frustrating.

Delegation and Teamwork

Disability affects the whole person. Anger and frustration are common. Many are upset and discouraged. Some persons have trouble controlling such feelings. They may have outbursts.

You may feel short-tempered. You must learn to deal with your anger and frustration. The person does not choose loss of

Delegation and Teamwork—cont'd

function. If the process upsets you, think how the person must feel. You must:

- Show patience, understanding, sensitivity, and respect.
- Be calm and act in a professional manner.
- Control your words and actions.

Managing your feelings can be a challenge. The nurse can suggest ways to help you control or express your feelings. You may need to assist with other persons for a while. Take pride in being a part of a strong, supportive team.

Ethics and Laws

The person may not want to practice rehabilitation procedures or methods. He or she may want you to give care instead. Personal choice is important. However, the person needs to follow the rehabilitation plan. Otherwise, he or she will not make progress. Do not let the person control you. Letting the person control you is the wrong thing to do. Report any problems to the nurse.

FOCUS ON **PRIDE**: *Application*

Explain how a disability affects the whole person. Write a brief scenario describing a person with a disability. Discuss the impact on the whole person and family.

REVIEW QUESTIONS

Circle T if the statement is TRUE and F if it is FALSE.

1. T F You should give praise for even slight progress.

2. T F Speech therapy should be done in private.

3. T F A person is not allowed dessert until exercises are done. This is abuse and mistreatment.

4. T F A person refuses to attend a concert at the nursing center. The person must attend. It is part of the rehabilitation plan.

5. T F Rehabilitation for older persons is usually faster paced than for younger persons.

6. T F You need to stress what the person can do.

7. T F Making changes in the home limits rehabilitation progress.

8. T F You should know how to use and apply assistive (adaptive) devices.

9. T F You need to convey hopefulness to the person.

Circle the BEST answer.

10. Rehabilitation and restorative nursing care focus on
    a What the person cannot do
    b Self-care
    c The whole person
    d Mobility and communication

11. Rehabilitation begins with preventing
    a Angry feelings
    b Contractures tend pressure ulcers
    c Illness and injury
    d Loss of self-esteem

12. A person has weakness on the right side. ADL are
    a Done by the person to the extent possible
    b Done by you
    c Postponed until the right side can be used
    d Supervised by a therapist

13. To provide emotional support during rehabilitation
    a Remind the person of his or her limits
    b Give sympathy and show pity
    c Talk about your feelings
    d Listen and give praise

14. During therapy, a person wants music played. You should
    a Explain that music is not allowed
    b Choose some music
    c Ask the person to choose some music
    d Ask a therapist to choose some music

15. A person's right side is weak. You move the call light to the left side. You promote quality of life by
    a Protecting the person from abuse and mistreatment
    b Allowing personal choice
    c Providing for safety
    d Taking part in activities

Answers to Chapter 41 questions are on p. 872.

FOCUS ON PRACTICE

Problem Solving

Ms. Mills requires rehabilitation after a hip fracture. The care plan includes long-handled devices for dressing and bathing. While helping Ms. Mills bathe, you give her the long-handled sponge. She says: "I don't feel like using that today. Will you wash my feet for me?" What will you say and do? How will your response affect her progress?

Hearing, Speech, and Vision Problems

OBJECTIVES

- Define the key terms and key abbreviations in this chapter.
- Describe the common ear disorders.
- Describe how to communicate with persons who have hearing loss.
- Explain the purpose of a hearing aid.
- Describe how to care for hearing aids.
- Describe the common speech disorders.
- Explain how to communicate with persons who have speech disorders.
- Describe the common eye disorders.
- Explain how to assist persons who are visually impaired or blind.
- Explain how to protect an ocular prosthesis from loss or damage.
- Perform the procedure described in this chapter.
- Explain how to promote PRIDE in the person, the family, and yourself.

KEY TERMS

aphasia The total or partial loss *(a)* of the ability to use or understand language *(phasia);* parts of the brain responsible for language are damaged

blindness The absence of sight

braille A touch reading and writing system that uses raised dots for each letter of the alphabet; the first 10 letters also represent the numbers 0 through 9

Broca's aphasia See "expressive aphasia"

cerumen Earwax

deafness Hearing loss in which it is impossible for the person to understand speech through hearing alone

expressive aphasia Difficulty expressing or sending out thoughts through speech or writing; motor aphasia, Broca's aphasia

global aphasia Difficulty expressing or sending out thoughts and difficulty understanding language; mixed aphasia

hearing loss Not being able to hear the normal range of sounds associated with normal hearing

low vision Vision loss that cannot be corrected with eyeglasses, contact lenses, drugs, or surgery; vision loss interferes with every-day activities

mixed aphasia See "global aphasia"

motor aphasia See "expressive aphasia"

receptive aphasia Difficulty understanding language; Wernicke's aphasia

tinnitus A ringing, roaring, hissing, or buzzing sound in the ears or head

vertigo Dizziness

Wernicke's aphasia See "receptive aphasia"

KEY ABBREVIATIONS

AMD	Age-related macular degeneration	**TRS**	Telecommunications Relay Service
ASL	American Sign Language		

Hearing, speech, and vision allow communication, learning, and moving about. They are important for self-care, work, most activities, and safety and security needs. For example, you see dark clouds and hear tornado warning sirens. You know to seek shelter. With speech, you alert others.

Hearing, speech, and vision disorders occur in all age-groups. Common causes are birth defects, injuries, infections, diseases, and aging.

EAR DISORDERS

The ear functions in hearing and balance.

See *Body Structure and Function Review: The Ear*, p. 676.

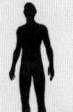

BODY STRUCTURE AND FUNCTION REVIEW
The Ear

A sense organ, the ear (Fig. 42-1) functions in hearing and balance. It has 3 parts: the *external ear, middle ear,* and *inner ear.*

Sound waves are guided through the external ear (outer part) into the *auditory canal.* Glands in the auditory canal secrete a waxy substance called *cerumen.* The auditory canal extends about 1 inch into the *eardrum.* The eardrum *(tympanic membrane)* separates the external and middle ear.

The middle ear contains the *eustachian tube* and 3 small bones called *ossicles.* The eustachian tube connects the middle ear and the throat. Air enters the eustachian tube so there is equal pressure on both sides of the eardrum. The ossicles amplify sound received from the eardrum and transmit the sound to the inner ear. The 3 ossicles are:

- The *malleus*—looks like a hammer.
- The *incus*—looks like an anvil.
- The *stapes*—is shaped like a stirrup.

The inner ear consists of *semicircular canals* and the *cochlea.* The cochlea looks like a snail shell. It contains fluid that carries sound waves from the middle ear to the *acoustic nerve.* The acoustic nerve then carries messages to the brain.

The 3 semicircular canals are involved with balance. They sense the head's position and changes in position. They send messages to the brain.

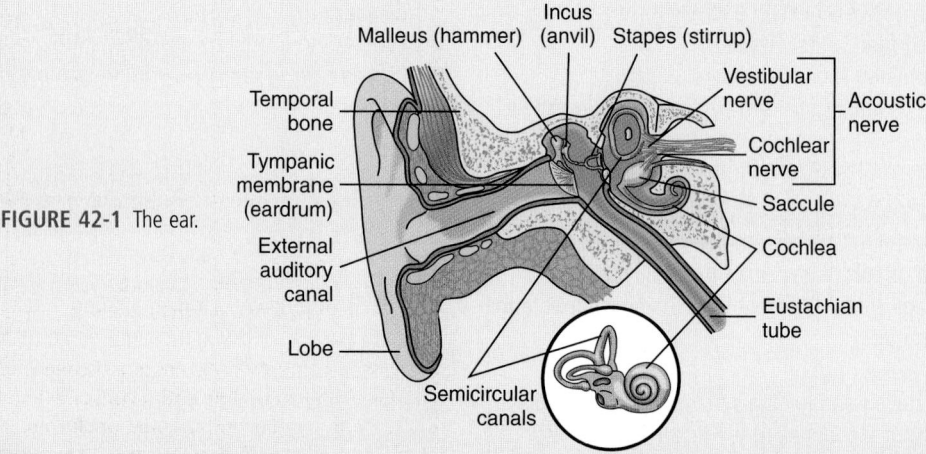

FIGURE 42-1 The ear.

FOCUS ON CHILDREN AND OLDER PERSONS
Otitis Media

Children
Otitis media is common in infants and children. Infants cannot tell you about an earache. The child may:
- Have a fever.
- Tug or pull at the ears.
- Roll the head back.
- Cry a lot.
- Be fussy and irritable.
- Have fluid draining out of the ear.
- Sleep poorly.
- Have problems with balance.
- Have trouble hearing.
- Not respond to quiet sounds.

Older Persons
Persons with dementia cannot tell you about pain or when something is wrong. Be alert for behavior changes. The following may signal otitis media.
- Unusual irritability
- Problems sleeping
- Tugging or pulling at 1 or both ears
- Fever
- Fluid draining from the ear
- Balance problems
- Signs of hearing problems

Otitis Media

Otitis media is an infection *(itis)* of the middle *(media)* ear *(ot).* It often begins with sore throats, colds, or other respiratory infections that spread to the middle ear. Viruses and bacteria are causes.

Otitis media is acute or chronic. Chronic otitis media can damage the structures needed for hearing. Permanent hearing loss can occur.

Fluid builds up in the ear. Pain (earache), hearing loss, fever, and tinnitus occur. *Tinnitus is a ringing, roaring, hissing, or buzzing sound in the ears or head.* An untreated infection can travel to the brain and other structures in the head. The doctor orders antibiotics, pain-relief drugs, or drugs to relieve congestion.

See *Focus on Children and Older Persons: Otitis Media.*

Meniere's Disease

Meniere's disease involves the inner ear. Usually 1 ear is affected. Symptoms include:

- *Vertigo* (dizziness)
- Tinnitus
- Hearing loss
- Feeling of fullness or pressure in the ear

With Meniere's disease, fluid builds up in the inner ear. The increased fluid causes swelling and pressure in the inner ear. Symptoms are sudden.

An attack usually involves vertigo, tinnitus, and hearing loss. Vertigo causes whirling and spinning sensations. The dizziness causes severe nausea and vomiting. An episode can last 20 minutes or 2 to 24 hours.

Drugs and a low-salt diet decrease fluid in the inner ear. Smoking, caffeine, and alcohol are avoided.

Safety is needed during vertigo.

- Have the person lie down.
- Prevent falls. Assist with walking and use bed rails according to the care plan.
- Remind the person to keep the head still. The person avoids turning the head. To talk to the person, stand directly in front of him or her.
- Avoid sudden movements. The person moves slowly.
- Prevent bright or glaring lights.

Hearing Loss

Hearing loss is not being able to hear the normal range of sounds associated with normal hearing. Losses are mild to deafness, the most severe form. *Deafness is hearing loss in which it is impossible for the person to understand speech through hearing alone.*

Common in older persons, hearing loss is more common in men than in women. Causes include damage to the outer, middle, or inner ear or to the acoustic nerve. Risk factors include:

- Aging
- Exposure to loud job-related noises, loud music, loud engines, firearms, and so on
- Drugs—antibiotics, too much aspirin
- Infections
- Reduced blood flow to the ear from high blood pressure, heart and vascular diseases, and diabetes
- Stroke
- Head injuries
- Tumors
- Heredity
- Birth defects

Temporary hearing loss can occur from *earwax (cerumen)*. Hearing improves after the earwax is removed.

Clear speech, responding to others, safety, and awareness of surroundings require hearing.

See *Focus on Communication: Hearing Loss.*
See *Promoting Safety and Comfort: Hearing Loss.*

> ### FOCUS ON **COMMUNICATION**
> #### *Hearing Loss*
>
> The National Association of the Deaf (NAD) uses the terms *deaf* and *hard-of-hearing* to describe persons with hearing loss. Do not use the terms *deaf and dumb, deaf-mute,* or *hearing-impaired.* Such terms offend persons who are hard-of-hearing.

> ### PROMOTING SAFETY AND COMFORT
> #### *Hearing Loss*
>
> **Safety**
> Do not try to remove earwax. This is done by a doctor or a nurse. Do not insert anything, including cotton swabs, into the ear.

> ### BOX 42-1   Hearing Loss—Signs and Symptoms
>
> - Problems:
>   - Hearing on the phone
>   - Hearing with background noise or in noisy areas
>   - Following conversations when 2 or more people are speaking
>   - Understanding women and children
> - Straining to understand a conversation
> - Hearing voices as mumbled or slurred
> - Misunderstanding what others are saying
> - Answering questions or responding inappropriately
> - Asking others to repeat themselves
> - Speaking too loudly
> - Leaning forward to hear
> - Turning and cupping the better ear toward the speaker
> - Turning up the TV, radio, music, or other sound sources so loud that others complain

Effects on the Person. A person may deny hearing loss or not notice gradual hearing loss. Others may see changes in the person's behavior or attitude. They may not relate the changes to hearing loss. See Box 42-1 for signs and symptoms of hearing loss.

Psychological and social changes may occur. People may give wrong answers or responses. Therefore they tend to shun social events to avoid embarrassment. Often they feel lonely, bored, and left out. Only parts of conversations are heard. They may become suspicious. They think others are talking about them or are talking softly on purpose. Some control conversations to avoid responding or being labeled "senile" because of poor answers. Straining and working hard to hear can cause fatigue, frustration, and irritability.

Hearing is needed for speech. Pronouncing words and voice volume depend on hearing yourself. Hearing loss may result in slurred speech or pronouncing words wrong. Some people have monotone speech or drop word endings. It may be hard to understand what the person says. Do not assume or pretend that you understand. Serious problems can result. See "Speech Disorders" on p. 681.

See *Focus on Children and Older Persons: Effects on the Person.*

FOCUS ON CHILDREN AND OLDER PERSONS

Effects on the Person

Children

Some babies are born with hearing problems. Others develop hearing problems as they grow older. Hearing is needed for language development. Children learn to talk by imitating sounds and voices.

Medical attention is needed if a child does not hear well or speak clearly. See Box 42-2. Items checked "No" may signal hearing loss. Report concerns about a child's hearing to the nurse.

Communication. Persons with hearing loss may wear hearing aids or lip-read (speech-read). They watch facial expressions, gestures, and body language. Some people learn American Sign Language (ASL) (Figs. 42-2 and 42-3). ASL uses signs made with the hands and other movements such as facial expressions, gestures, and postures. (Different sign languages are used in different countries. For example, British Sign Language is different from ASL.)

Some people have *hearing assistance dogs* (hearing dogs). The dog alerts the person to sounds. Phones, doorbells, smoke alarms, alarm clocks, babies' cries, sirens, and on-coming cars are examples.

Hearing Aids. *Hearing aids* fit inside or behind the ear (Fig. 42-4, p. 680). They make sounds louder. They do not correct, restore, or cure hearing problems. Hearing ability does not improve. The person hears better because the device makes sounds louder. Background noise and speech are louder. The measures in Box 42-3, p. 680 apply.

BOX 42-2   Hearing Checklist for Children

Items marked "No" may signal hearing loss.

No	Yes	**Birth to 3 Months**
—	—	Reacts to loud sounds.
—	—	Calms down or smiles when spoken to.
—	—	Recognizes your voice and calms down if crying.
—	—	When feeding, starts or stops sucking in response to sound.
—	—	Coos and makes pleasure sounds.
—	—	Has a special way of crying for different needs.
—	—	Smiles when he or she sees you.

No	Yes	**4 to 6 Months**
—	—	Follows sounds with his or her eyes.
—	—	Responds to changes in the tone of your voice.
—	—	Notices toys that make sounds.
—	—	Pays attention to music.
—	—	Babbles in a speech-like way and uses many different sounds, including sounds that begin with *p*, *b*, and *m*.
—	—	Laughs.
—	—	Babbles when excited or unhappy.
—	—	Makes gurgling sounds when alone or playing with you.

No	Yes	**7 Months to 1 Year**
—	—	Enjoys playing peek-a-boo and pat-a-cake.
—	—	Turns and looks in the direction of sounds.
—	—	Listens when spoken to.
—	—	Understands words for common items such as "cup," "shoe," or "juice."
—	—	Responds to requests ("Come here.").
—	—	Babbles using long and short groups of sounds ("tata," "upup," "bibibi").
—	—	Babbles to get and keep attention.
—	—	Communicates using gestures such as waving or holding up arms.
—	—	Imitates different speech sounds.
—	—	Has 1 or 2 words ("Hi," "dog," "Dada," or "Mama") by first birthday.

No	Yes	**1 to 2 Years**
—	—	Knows a few parts of the body and can point to them when asked.
—	—	Follows simple commands ("Roll the ball.") and understands simple questions ("Where's your shoe?").
—	—	Enjoys simple stories, songs, and rhymes.
—	—	Points to pictures, when named, in books.
—	—	Acquires new words on a regular basis.
—	—	Uses some 1- or 2-word questions ("Where kitty?" or "Go bye-bye?").
—	—	Puts 2 words together ("More cookie.").
—	—	Uses many different consonant sounds at the beginning of words.

No	Yes	**2 to 3 Years**
—	—	Has a word for almost everything.
—	—	Uses 2- or 3-word phrases to talk about and ask for things.
—	—	Uses *k*, *g*, *f*, *t*, *d*, and *n* sounds.
—	—	Speaks in a way that is understood by family members and friends.
—	—	Names objects to ask for them or to direct attention to them.

No	Yes	**3 to 4 Years**
—	—	Hears you when you call from another room.
—	—	Hears the TV or radio at the same sound level as other family members.
—	—	Answers simple "Who?" "What?" "Where?" and "Why?" questions.
—	—	Talks about activities at day care, pre-school, or friends' homes.
—	—	Uses sentences with 4 or more words.
—	—	Speaks easily without repeating syllables or words.

BOX 42-2	Hearing Checklist for Children—cont'd			
No	**Yes**	**4 to 5 Years**	**No**	**Yes**	**4 to 5 Years—cont'd**

No	Yes	4 to 5 Years	No	Yes	4 to 5 Years—cont'd
___	___	Pays attention to a short story and answers simple questions about it.	___	___	Communicates easily with other children and adults.
___	___	Hears and understands most of what is said at home and in school.	___	___	Says most sounds correctly except for a few (*l, s, r, v, z, ch, sh,* and *th*).
___	___	Uses sentences that give many details.	___	___	Uses rhyming words.
___	___	Tells stories that stay on topic.	___	___	Names some letters and numbers.
			___	___	Uses adult grammar.

Modified from National Institute on Deafness and Other Communication Disorders: Your baby's hearing and communicative development checklist, *NIH Publication No. 10-4040, Bethesda, Md, updated June 14, 2015, National Institutes of Health.*

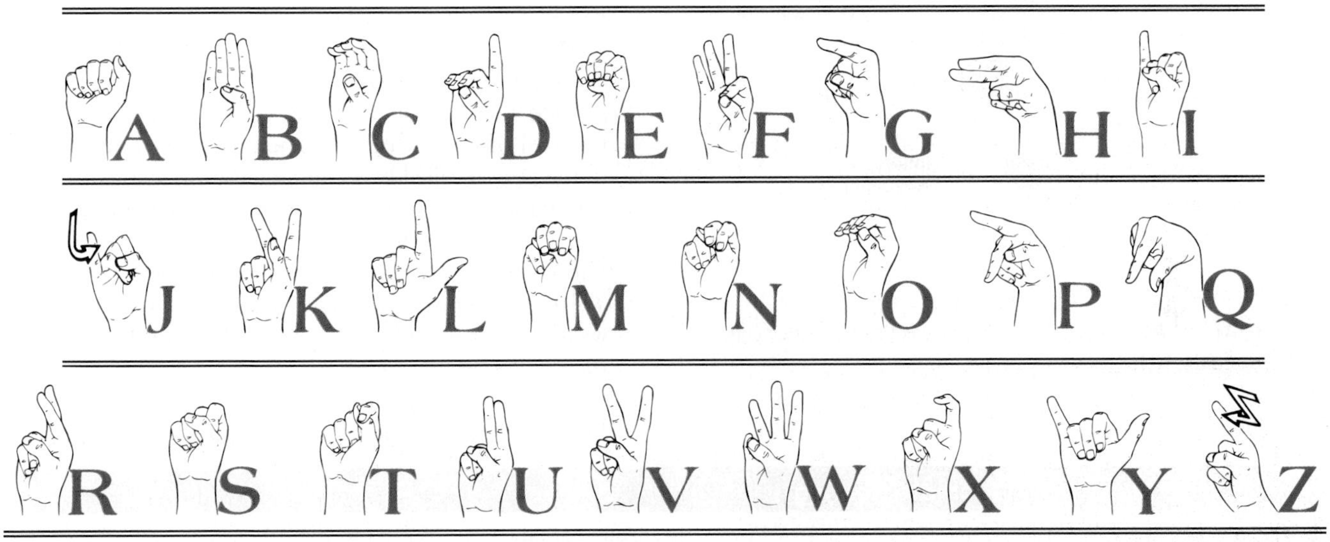

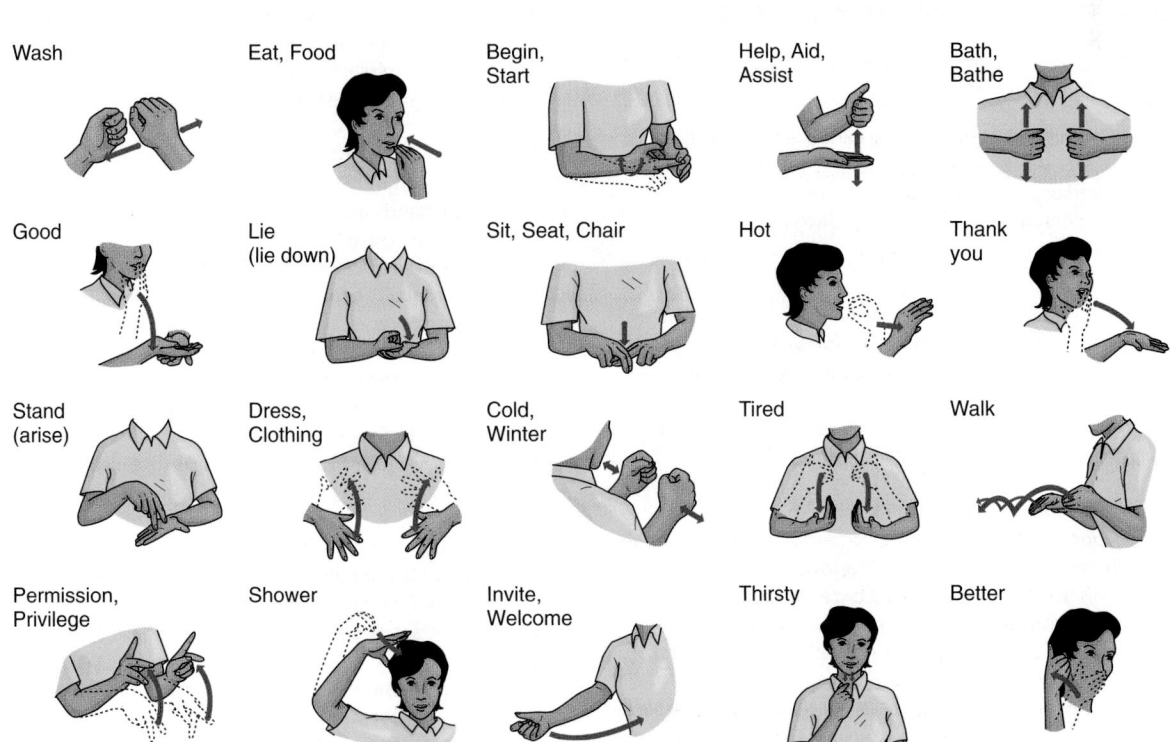

FIGURE 42-2 Manual alphabet. (Courtesy National Association of the Deaf, Silver Spring, Md.)

FIGURE 42-3 American Sign Language examples.

Hearing aids are battery-operated. If the device does not seem to work properly:

- Check if the hearing aid is *on*. It has an *on* and *off* switch.
- Check the battery position.
- Insert a new battery if needed.
- Clean the hearing aid. *Follow the nurse's directions and the manufacturer's instructions.*

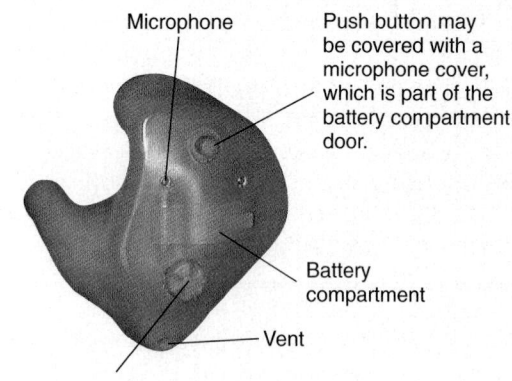

Microphone

Push button may be covered with a microphone cover, which is part of the battery compartment door.

Battery compartment

Vent

On/Off switch/Volume control

FIGURE 42-4 A hearing aid. (Courtesy Siemens Hearing Instruments, Inc., Piscataway, NJ.)

Hearing aids are turned off when not in use. And the battery is removed. These measures prolong battery life. Hair spray and other hair care products are avoided while wearing a hearing aid. They can damage the device.

Hearing aids are costly. Handle and care for them properly. When not in the ear, store a hearing aid in its case. Place the case in the top drawer of the bedside stand. Report lost or damaged hearing aids at once.

Other Hearing Devices. Other devices can help the person with hearing loss.

- *Phone amplifying devices.* Special phone receivers make sounds louder. Some phones work with hearing aids.
- Extension bells that make phones ring louder.
- *Telecommunications Relay Service (TRS)* (Fig. 42-5). The *Americans With Disabilities Act of 1990* requires that states provide access to the TRS. Messages are typed by the hard-of-hearing person. They are relayed orally to the person called by a communications assistant. The communications assistant must relay everything that is said and maintain the confidentiality of all conversations. Various services are available to meet the person's needs.
- *TV and radio listening systems.* These are used with or without hearing aids. The person does not have to turn the volume up high.
- Smoke alarms with strobe lights.
- Doorbells that can be heard throughout the house.

BOX 42-3   Measures to Promote Hearing

The Setting

- Reduce or eliminate background noises. Turn off radios, music players, TVs, air conditioners, fans, and so on.
- Provide a quiet place to talk. Avoid areas with loud sound.
- Have the person sit where he or she hears best.

The Person

- Have the person wear his or her hearing aid. It must be turned on and working.
- Have the person wear needed eyeglasses or contact lenses. The person needs to see your face to lip-read (speech-read).

You

- Gain attention. Alert the person to your presence. Raise an arm or hand or lightly touch the person's hand, arm, or shoulder. Do not startle or approach the person from behind.
- Position yourself at the person's level. Sit if the person is sitting. Stand if the person is standing.
- Face the person when speaking. Do not turn or walk away while you are talking. Do not talk from the doorway or another room.
- Have light shining on your face. Shadows and glares affect the person's ability to see your face clearly.
- Maintain eye contact with the person.
- Speak clearly, distinctly, and at a normal rate. Do not talk too fast or too slow.
- Speak in a normal tone of voice. Do not shout or mumble.
- State the person's name before starting a conversation. This gains the person's attention and focus.

You—cont'd

- Adjust the pitch of your voice as needed. Ask if the person can hear you better.
  - If no hearing aid, lower the pitch if you are a female. Women's voices are higher-pitched and harder to hear than lower-pitched male voices.
  - If the person is wearing a hearing aid, raise the pitch slightly.
- Do not cover your mouth, smoke, eat, or chew gum while talking. Mouth movements are affected.
- Keep your hands away from your face. The person needs to see your face clearly.
- Stand or sit on the side of the better ear.
- State the topic of conversation first.
- Tell the person when you are changing the subject. State the new topic.
- Use short sentences and simple words.
- Pause between sentences. Make sure the person understands before you speak again.
- Use gestures and facial expressions to give useful clues.
- Write out important names, words, numbers, addresses, appointments, and so on.
- Say things in another way if the person does not seem to understand. Do not repeat the same words over and over again. Re-phrase rather than repeat.
- Keep conversations and discussions short. This avoids tiring the person.
- Be alert to messages sent by your facial expressions, gestures, and body language.
- Be alert to the person's nonverbal communication. For example, watch for puzzled looks and expressions of anger, frustration, excitement, fatigue, and so on.

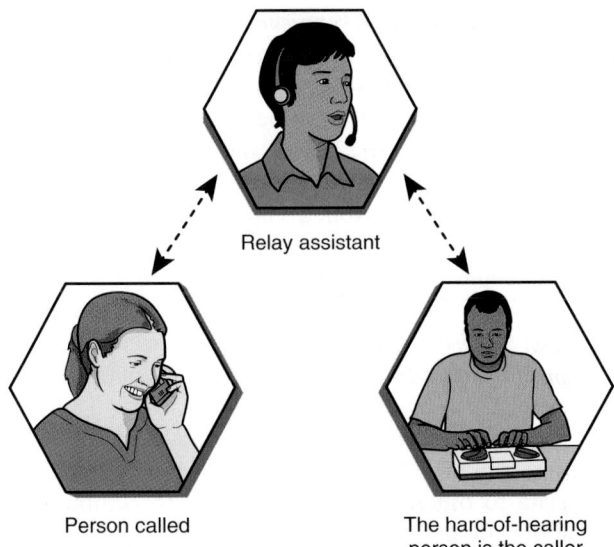

Relay assistant

Person called

The hard-of-hearing person is the caller

FIGURE 42-5 Telecommunications Relay Service (TRS). The person with a hearing disability uses a teletypewriter (TTY) for a TRS call. The communications assistant relays messages between the calling party and the party called.

SPEECH DISORDERS

Speech disorders result in impaired or ineffective oral communication. Hearing loss, developmental disabilities (Chapter 50), and brain injury are common causes. These problems are common.

- *Aphasia.* See "Aphasia" on p. 682.
- *Apraxia* means not *(a)* to act, do, or perform *(praxia)*. The person with *apraxia of speech* cannot use speech muscles for understandable speech. The person understands speech and knows what to say. However, the brain cannot coordinate the speech muscles to make the words. The motor speech area in the brain is damaged.
- *Dysarthria* means difficult or poor *(dys)* speech *(arthria)*. Nervous system damage affects mouth and face muscles. Slurred speech, speaking slowly or softly, hoarseness, and drooling also can occur.

To communicate with the speech-impaired person, practice the measures in Box 42-4.

Some persons need speech rehabilitation. A speech-language pathologist helps the person:

- Use remaining abilities.
- Restore or improve language abilities to the extent possible.
- Learn other communication methods.
- Strengthen speech muscles.

Improvement depends on many factors. They include the cause, amount, and area of brain damage; age; health; and willingness and ability to learn.

BOX 42-4	**Communicating With Speech-Impaired Persons**

The Person
- Ask the person to repeat or re-phrase statements as needed.
- Repeat what the person has said. Ask if you understood correctly.
- Ask the person to write down key words or the message.
- Ask the person to point, gesture, or draw key words.

You
- Follow the care plan. A consistent approach is needed.
- Provide a calm, quiet setting. Turn off the TV, radio, music, and other distractions.
- Include the person in conversations.
- Listen and give the person your full attention.
- Use short, simple sentences.

You—cont'd
- Repeat what you are saying as needed.
- Write down key words as needed.
- Speak in a normal tone. Do not treat or talk to an adult in a babyish or child-like way.
- Ask the person questions to which you know the answers. This helps you learn how the person speaks.
- Allow the person plenty of time to talk.
- Determine the topic being discussed. This helps you understand main points. Watch the person's lip movements.
- Watch facial expressions, gestures, and body language. They give clues about what is being said.
- Do not correct the person's speech.

Aphasia

Aphasia is the total or partial loss (a) *of the ability to use or understand language* (phasia). *Parts of the brain responsible for language are damaged.* Stroke, head injury, brain infections, dementia, and cancer are common causes. Most people who have aphasia are middle-aged or older.

Expressive aphasia (motor aphasia, Broca's aphasia) relates to difficulty expressing or sending out thoughts through speech or writing. The person knows what to say but has problems speaking, spelling, counting, gesturing, or writing. The person may:

- Omit small words such as "is," "and," "of," and "the."
- Speak in single words or short sentences. "Walk dog" can mean "I will take the dog for walk" or "You take the dog for a walk."
- Put words in the wrong order. Instead of "bathroom," the person may say "room bath."
- Think one thing but say another. The person may want food but asks for a book.
- Call people by the wrong names.
- Make up words.
- Produce sounds and no words.
- Cry or swear for no reason.

Receptive aphasia (Wernicke's aphasia) is difficulty understanding language. The person has trouble understanding what is said or written. Words do not make sense. What the person says has no meaning. The person may not be aware of mistakes. People and common objects are not recognized. The person may not know how to use every-day items—fork, toilet, cup, TV, phone, or other items.

Some people have both expressive and receptive aphasia. *Global aphasia (mixed aphasia) involves difficulty expressing or sending out thoughts and difficulty understanding language.* The person has problems speaking and understanding language.

Emotional needs are great. Frustration, depression, and anger are common. Communication is needed to function and relate to others. The person wants to communicate but cannot. Be patient and kind.

EYE DISORDERS

Vision problems range from mild loss to complete blindness. *Blindness is the absence of sight.* Vision loss is sudden or gradual. One or both eyes are affected.

See *Body Structure and Function Review: The Eye.*

BODY STRUCTURE AND FUNCTION REVIEW

The Eye

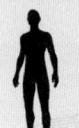

Receptors for vision are in the eyes (Fig. 42-6). Bones of the skull, eyelids and eyelashes, and tears protect the eyes from injury. The eye has 3 layers.

- The *sclera,* the white of the eye, is the outer layer. It is made of tough connective tissue.
- The *choroid* is the second layer. Blood vessels, the *ciliary muscle,* and the *iris* make up the choroid. The iris gives the eye its color. The opening in the middle of the iris is the *pupil.* Pupil size varies with the amount of light entering the eye. The pupil *constricts* (narrows) in bright light. It *dilates* (widens) in dim or dark places.
- The *retina* is the inner layer. It has receptors for vision and the nerve fibers of the *optic nerve.* The *macula* is near the center of the retina. The area contains cells that are sensitive to light, color, and the fine detail needed for central vision (p. 684).

Light enters the eye through the *cornea*—the transparent part of the outer layer that lies over the eye. Light rays pass to the *lens,* which lies behind the pupil. The light is then reflected to the retina. Light is carried to the brain by the optic nerve.

The *aqueous chamber* separates the cornea from the lens. The chamber is filled with a fluid called *aqueous humor.* The fluid helps the cornea keep its shape and position. The *vitreous humor* is behind the lens. It is a gelatin-like substance that supports the retina and maintains the eye's shape.

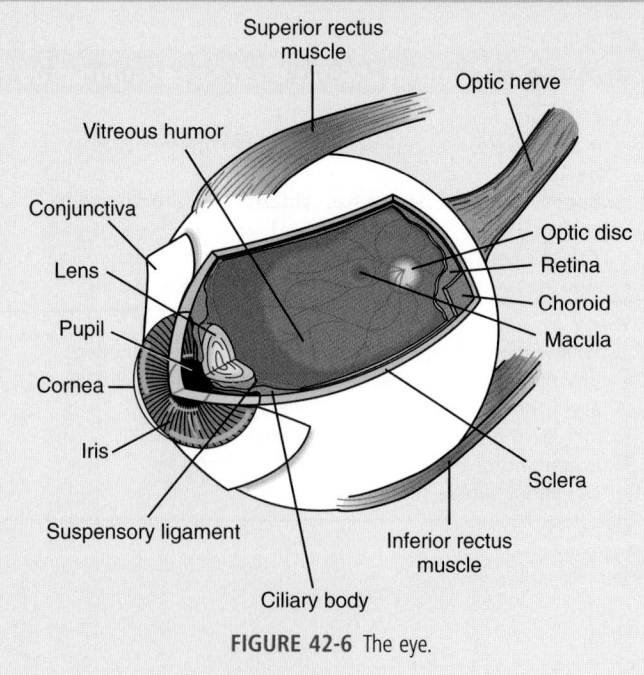

FIGURE 42-6 The eye.

Cataracts

A cataract is clouding of the lens (Fig. 42-7). The normal lens is clear. *Cataract* comes from the Greek word for *waterfall*. Trying to see is like looking through a waterfall. A cataract can occur in 1 or both eyes. Signs and symptoms include:

* Cloudy, blurry, or dimmed vision (Fig. 42-8, *A and B*).
* Colors seem faded and brownish. Blues and purples are hard to see.
* Sensitivity to light and glares.
* Poor vision at night.
* Halos around lights.
* Double vision in the affected eye.

Risk Factors. Most cataracts are caused by aging. A family history, diabetes, smoking, excessive alcohol use, and prolonged exposure to sunlight are risk factors. So are high blood pressure, obesity, and eye injuries and surgeries.

Treatment. Surgery is the only treatment. The lens is removed and a plastic lens is implanted. Surgery is done when the cataract affects daily activities. Driving, reading, and watching TV are examples. Vision improves after surgery.

Post-operative care includes:

* Keep the eye shield in place as directed. If ordered, the shield is worn for sleep, including naps.
* Follow measures for persons who are visually impaired or blind when an eye shield is worn (p. 685). The person may have vision loss in the other eye.
* Remind the person not to rub or press the affected eye.
* Do not bump the eye.
* Place the over-bed table and the bedside stand on the un-operative side.
* Place the call light and other needed items within reach.
* Report eye drainage or complaints of pain at once.
* Remind the person not to bend, stoop, cough, or lift things.

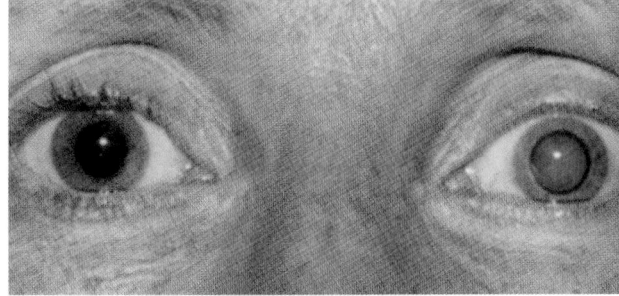

FIGURE 42-7 The right eye is normal. The left eye has a cataract. (From Swartz MH: *Textbook of physical diagnosis,* ed 6, Philadelphia, 2010, Saunders.)

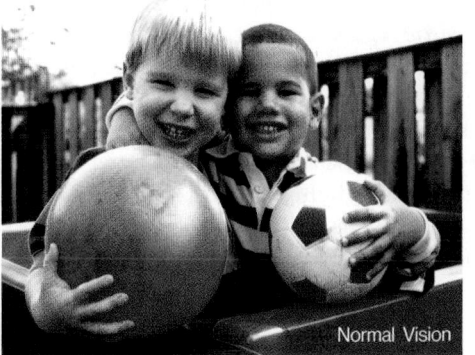

A — Normal Vision

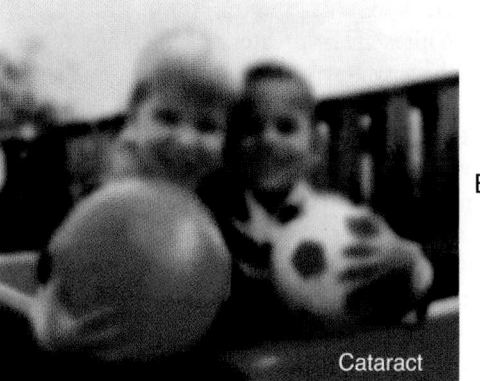

B — Cataract

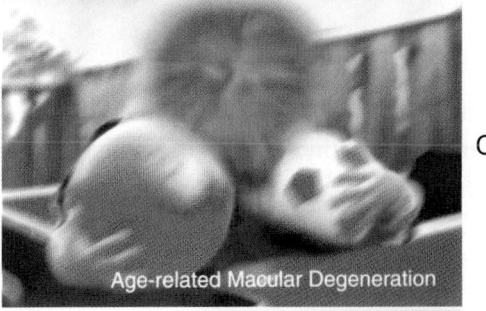

C — Age-related Macular Degeneration

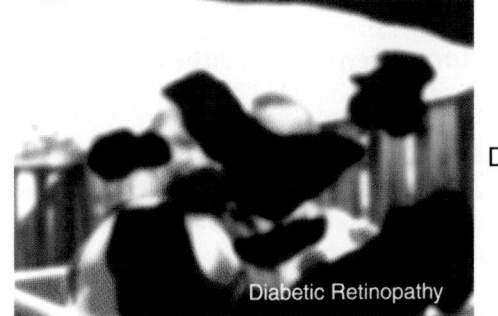

D — Diabetic Retinopathy

FIGURE 42-8 **Vision loss with eye disorders. A,** Normal vision. **B,** Vision loss from a cataract. **C,** Vision loss from macular degeneration. **D,** Vision loss from diabetic retinopathy. (A and B, From National Eye Institute: *Facts about cataract,* Bethesda, Md, September 2009, National Institutes of Health. C, Modified from National Eye Institute: *Don't lose sight of age-related macular degeneration,* Bethesda, Md, NIH Publication No. 12-3251, revised 2012, National Institutes of Health. D, Modified from National Eye Institute: *Facts about diabetic eye disease,* Bethesda, Md, updated June 2012, National Institutes of Health.)

Age-Related Macular Degeneration

Age-related macular degeneration (AMD) blurs central vision. *Central vision* is what you see "straight-ahead." AMD causes a blind spot in the center of vision (see Fig. 42-8, *A and C*). Central vision is needed for reading, sewing, driving, and seeing faces and fine detail.

AMD damages the macula in the center of the retina. The retina receives light and sends messages to the brain through the optic nerve. Normal signals are not sent to the brain. Onset is gradual and painless.

Risk Factors. AMD risk increases after age 60. Besides age, risk factors include:
- Smoking.
- Race. Whites are at greater risk than any other group.
- Family history.

Treatment. For advanced AMD, no treatment can prevent vision loss. Some treatments may stop or slow the disease progress. They may save what is left of central vision. Laser surgery is an example.

The following can reduce the risk of AMD.
- Eating a healthy diet high in green, leafy vegetables and fish
- Not smoking
- Maintaining normal blood pressure and cholesterol levels
- Regular exercise

Diabetic Retinopathy

In diabetic retinopathy, blood vessels in the retina are damaged. A complication of diabetes, it is a leading cause of blindness. Usually both eyes are affected.

Vision blurs (see Fig. 42-8, *A and D*). The person may see spots "floating." Often there are no early warning signs.

Risk Factors. Everyone with diabetes (Chapter 46) is at risk.

Treatment. The person needs to control diabetes, blood pressure, and cholesterol. Laser surgery may help. In another surgery, blood is removed from the center of the eye. The person may need low vision services.

Glaucoma

With glaucoma, fluid builds up in the eye causing pressure on the optic nerve. The optic nerve is damaged. Vision loss with eventual blindness occurs.

Glaucoma can occur in 1 or both eyes. Onset is sudden or gradual. Peripheral vision (side vision) is lost. The person sees through a tunnel (Fig. 42-9), has blurred vision, and sees halos around lights. Severe eye pain, nausea, and vomiting occur with sudden onset.

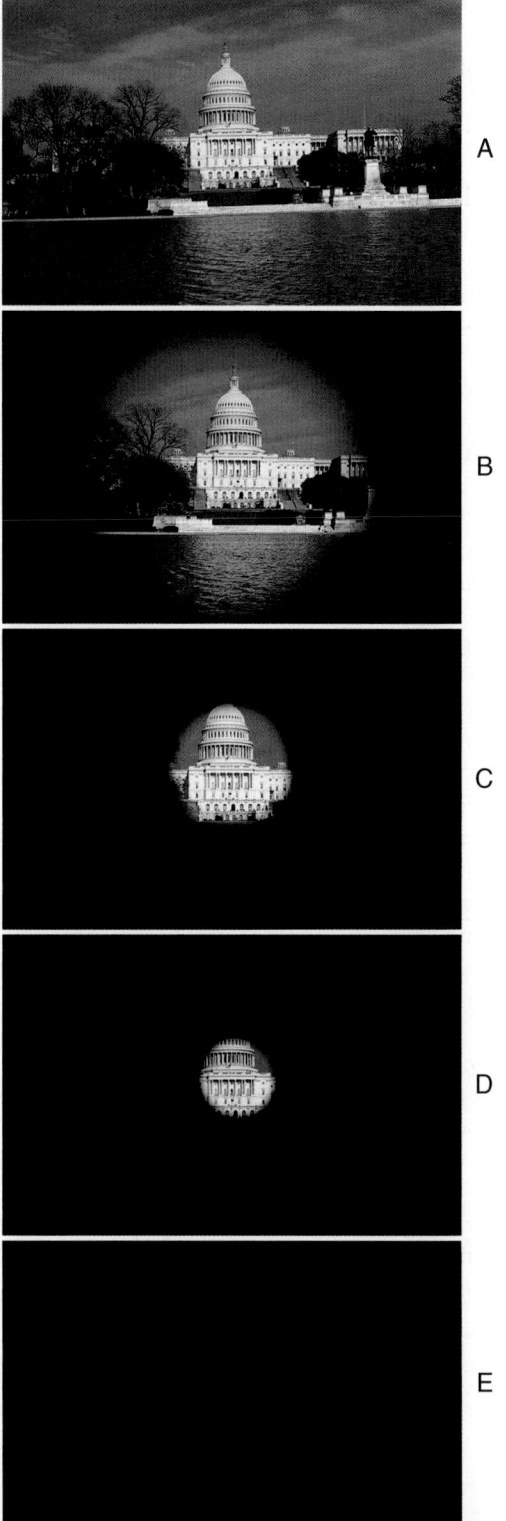

FIGURE 42-9 Vision loss from glaucoma. **A,** Normal vision. **B,** Loss of peripheral vision begins. **C, D,** and **E,** Vision loss continues, with eventual blindness.

Risk Factors. Glaucoma is a leading cause of vision loss in the United States. Persons at risk include:
- African-Americans over 40 years of age
- Everyone over 60 years of age, especially Mexican-Americans
- Those with a family history of the disease

Treatment. Glaucoma has no cure. Prior damage cannot be reversed. Drugs and surgery can control glaucoma and prevent further damage to the optic nerve.

Low Vision

Low vision is vision loss that cannot be corrected with eyeglasses, contact lenses, drugs, or surgery. The vision loss interferes with every-day activities. Reading, shopping, cooking, watching TV, writing, and other tasks are hard to do.

While wearing eyeglasses or contact lenses, the person has problems:
- Recognizing faces of family and friends
- Doing tasks that require close vision—reading, cooking, sewing, and so on
- Picking out and matching clothing colors
- Reading signs (traffic, stores)
- Doing things because lighting seems dimmer

Risk Factors. Low vision risk factors include:
- Eye diseases including glaucoma, cataracts, and AMD
- Diabetes
- Eye injuries
- Birth defects

Treatment. The person learns to use visual and adaptive (assistive) devices. Examples include:
- Prescription reading glasses
- Large-print reading materials
- Hand-held and video magnifiers
- Telescopic aids for far vision
- A black felt-tip marker for writing
- Paper with bold lines for writing
- Audio tapes
- Electronic reading machines
- Computers with large print and speech systems
- Closed-circuit TV
- Phones, clocks, and watches with large numbers and that talk
- Lighting that can be adjusted
- Dark-colored light switches and electrical outlets against light-colored walls
- Motion lights that turn on when the person enters a room

Impaired Vision and Blindness

Some people are totally blind. Others sense some light but have no usable vision. Others have some usable vision but cannot read newsprint. The legally blind person sees at 20 feet what a person with normal vision sees at 200 feet. See Box 42-5 for the signs and symptoms of vision problems.

BOX 42-5	Vision Problems—Signs and Symptoms

The Person Complains Of:
- Halos or rings around lights
- Headaches with blurry vision
- Not being able to see at night
- Spots in front of the eyes
- Eyes hurting
- Seeing flashes of light
- Seeing double
- Things looking distorted
- Needing more light

You Observe the Person:
- Bumping into things
- Hesitating when moving
- Walking close to the wall
- Groping for objects
- Touching things in an uncertain way
- Squinting to see
- Tilting the head to see
- Asking for more or different lighting
- Holding reading materials close to the face
- Dropping food when eating
- Having trouble making out faces
- Having trouble reading signs
- Not seeing stains on clothing
- Wearing clothes that do not match
- Acting disoriented or confused in familiar settings
- Tripping on rugs

Modified from American Foundation for the Blind, Recognizing signs of vision loss, *2015.*

Loss of sight is serious. Adjustments can be hard and long. Special education and training are needed. Rehabilitation programs help the person adjust to the vision loss and learn to be independent. The goal is for the person to be as active as possible and to have quality of life. The person learns to use visual and adaptive (assistive) devices, braille, long canes, and guide dogs. Follow the practices in Box 42-6.

See *Focus on Long-Term Care and Home Care: Impaired Vision and Blindness.*

FOCUS ON LONG-TERM CARE AND HOME CARE

Impaired Vision and Blindness

Home Care

The practices in Box 42-6 apply in the home setting. A safe setting is needed. Outdoor walks and stairs must be free of toys, ice, and snow. Furniture, closets, drawers, shelves, and other items are arranged to meet the person's needs. Always replace items where you found them. Do not re-arrange the person's belongings.

BOX 42-6   Caring for Blind and Visually Impaired Persons

The Setting

- Report worn carpeting and other flooring.
- Keep furniture, equipment, and electrical cords out of areas where the person will walk.
- Keep chairs pushed in under the table or desk.
- Keep doors fully open or fully closed. This includes room, closet, and cabinet doors.
- Keep drawers fully closed.
- Report burnt-out light bulbs.
- Provide lighting as the person prefers. Tell the person when the lights are on or off.
- Adjust window coverings to prevent glares. Sunny days and bright, snowy days cause glares.
- Keep the call light and TV, light, and other controls within reach.
- Turn on night-lights in the person's room and bathroom and in hallways.
- Practice safety measures to prevent falls (Chapter 14).
- Orient the person to the room. Describe the layout. Include the location and purpose of furniture and equipment.
- Let the person move about. Let him or her touch and find furniture and equipment.
- Do not re-arrange furniture and equipment.
- Use colors and contrast. Solid, bright colors (red, orange, yellow) are best. Avoid pastels, patterns, prints, designs, and stripes. White or yellow against black provides strong contrast. Place light-colored objects against dark backgrounds or dark-colored objects against light backgrounds. For example, use a white plate with a dark placemat or tablecloth.
- Provide a consistent meal-time setting.
  - Have the person sit in good light.
  - Keep place settings the same.
    - The knife and spoon are to the right of the plate.
    - The fork and napkin are to the left of the plate.
    - The glass or cup is to the right of the plate if the person is right-handed. It is to the left of the plate if the person is left-handed.
  - Arrange main dishes, side dishes, seasonings, and condiments in a straight line or in a semi-circle just beyond the person's place setting. Arrange things in the same way for each meal.
  - Explain the location of food and beverages. Use the face of a clock (Chapter 27). Or guide the person's hand to each item on the tray or place setting.
  - Cut meat, open containers, butter bread, and perform other tasks as needed.
- Complete a safety check before leaving the room. (See the inside of the front cover.)

The Person

- Have the person use railings to climb stairs.
- Have the person wear comfortable shoes that fit correctly.
- Assist with walking as needed. Offer to guide the person. Ask if he or she would like help. Respect the person's answer. If your help is accepted:
  - Offer your arm. Tell the person which arm is offered. Tap the back of your hand against the person's hand.
  - Have the person hold on to your arm just above the elbow (Fig. 42-10). Do not grab the person's arm.
  - Walk at a normal pace. Walk 1 step ahead of the person. Stand next to the person at the top and bottom of stairs and when crossing streets.
  - Never push, pull, or guide the person in front of you.
  - Pause when changing direction, stepping up, and stepping down.
  - Warn of stairs, elevators, escalators, doors, turns, furniture, and other obstructions. State if steps are up or down.
  - Have the person hold on to a railing, the wall, or other strong surface if you need to leave his or her side. Tell the person that you are leaving and what to hold on to.
- Guide the person to a seat by placing your guiding arm on the seat. The person will move his or her hand down your arm to the seat.
- Let the person do as much as possible. Do not do things that the person can do. Cutting meat, seasoning food, getting dressed, and putting on shoes are examples.
- Provide visual and adaptive devices. Follow the care plan.

You

- Identify yourself when you enter the room. Give your name, title, and reason for being there. Do not touch the person until you have indicated your presence.
- Ask the person how much he or she can see. Do not assume the person is totally blind or that the person has some vision.
- Identify others. Explain where each person is located and what the person is doing.
- Offer to help. Simply say: "May I help you?" Respect the person's answer.
- Leave the person's belongings in the same place that you found them. Do not move or re-arrange things. If you have to move things, tell the person what you moved and where.

BOX 42-6   Caring for Blind and Visually Impaired Persons—cont'd

Communication

- Face the person when speaking. Speak slowly and clearly.
- Use a normal tone of voice. Do not shout or speak loudly. Vision loss does not mean there is hearing loss.
- Address the person by name. This tells the person that you are directing a comment or question to him or her.
- Speak directly to the person. Do not talk just to family and friends who are present.
- Feel free to use words such as "see," "look," "read," or "watch TV." You also can use "blind" and "visually impaired."
- Feel free to refer to colors, sizes, shapes, patterns, designs, and so on.
- Describe people, places, and things thoroughly. Do not leave out a detail because you do not think it is important.
- Warn of dangers. Give a calm and clear warning. You can say "wait" first. Then describe the danger. For example: "Wait, there is ice on the walk."
- Greet the person by name when he or she enters a room. This alerts the person to your presence in the room. Tell the person who you are. Also identify others in the room.

Communication—cont'd

- Listen to the person. Give verbal cues that you are listening. Say: "yes," "okay," "I see," "tell me more," "I don't understand," and so on.
- Answer the person's questions. Provide specific and descriptive responses.
- Give step-by-step explanations of procedures as you perform them. Say when the procedure is over.
- Give specific directions.
  - Say: "right behind you," "on your left," or "in front of you." Avoid phrases like "over here" or "over there."
  - Tell the distance. For example: "Three steps in front of you" or "At the end of the hallway by the nurses' station."
  - Give landmarks if possible. Sounds and scents can serve as "landmarks." "By the kitchen" is an example.
- Tell the person when you are leaving the room or the area. If appropriate, tell the person where you are going. For example: "I'm going to go into your bathroom now."
- Tell the person when you are ending a conversation. For example: "I enjoyed hearing about your children. Thank you for sharing stories with me."

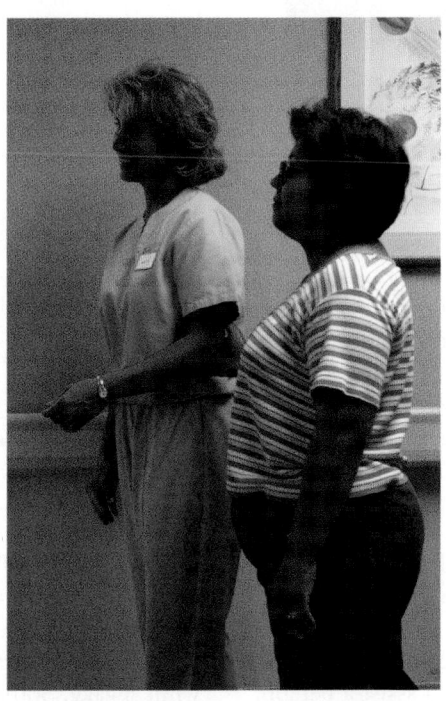

FIGURE 42-10 The blind person walks slightly behind the nursing assistant. She touches the nursing assistant's arm lightly.

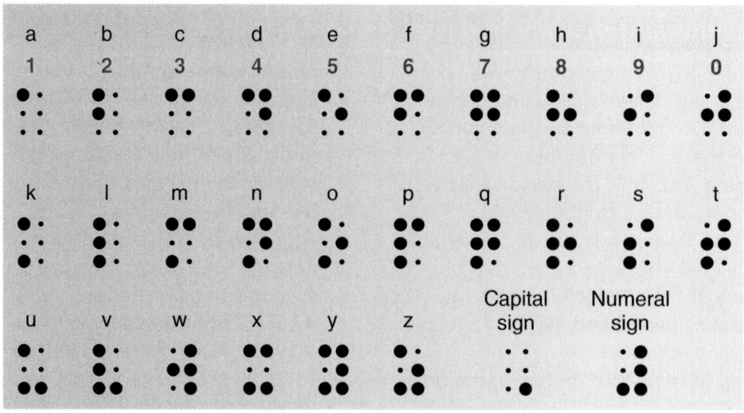

a	b	c	d	e	f	g	h	i	j
1	2	3	4	5	6	7	8	9	0

k	l	m	n	o	p	q	r	s	t

u	v	w	x	y	z	Capital sign	Numeral sign

FIGURE 42-11 Braille.

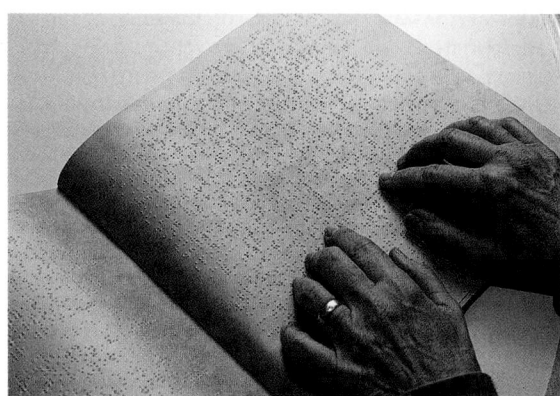

FIGURE 42-12 Braille is read by moving the fingers left to right across the braille lines.

Braille. *Braille is a touch reading and writing system that uses raised dots for each letter of the alphabet* (Fig. 42-11). *The first 10 letters also represent the numbers 0 through 9.* Braille is read by moving the hands from left to right along each line of braille (Fig. 42-12).

Special devices allow computer access—keyboards, displays, and printers. A "braille display" lets the person read the information. Braille printers produce printouts in braille.

Mobility. Blind and visually impaired persons learn to move about using a long cane with a red tip or using a guide dog. Both are used world-wide.

- Long canes are white or silver-gray. Some are 1 piece. Others fold or collapse for storage. To assist a person, announce your presence first. Ask if you can assist before trying to help. Do not interfere with the arm holding the cane. The person stores the cane. If you store it, tell the person where.
- The guide dog sees for the person. The dog moves in response to the master's commands. Commands are disobeyed to avoid danger. For example, the master wants to cross the street. The guide dog disobeys the command if a car is coming. Do not pet, feed, or distract a guide dog. Such actions can place the person in danger.

PROMOTING SAFETY AND COMFORT

Corrective Lenses

Safety

Eyeglasses are costly. Protect them from loss or damage. When not worn, put them in their case. Place the case in the top drawer of the bedside stand.

Some agencies let nursing assistants remove and insert contact lenses. Others do not. Know your agency's policy. If allowed to insert and remove contacts, follow agency procedures.

DELEGATION GUIDELINES

Eyeglasses

Cleaning eyeglasses is a routine care measure. Do not wait until the nurse tells you to clean them. Clean them daily and as needed.

To clean eyeglasses, find out if you need a special cleaning solution. Then follow the manufacturer's instructions.

Corrective Lenses

Eyeglasses and contact lenses correct many vision problems. Eyeglasses are worn for reading, for seeing at a distance, or for all activities. Contact lenses are usually worn while awake. Some contacts can be worn day and night for up to 30 days.

See *Promoting Safety and Comfort: Corrective Lenses.*

Eyeglasses. Lenses are hardened glass or plastic. Clean them daily and as needed. Wash glass lenses with warm water. Dry them with a lens cloth or cotton cloth. Plastic lenses scratch easily. Use special cleaning solutions and cloths.

See *Delegation Guidelines: Eyeglasses.*
See procedure: *Caring for Eyeglasses.*

Caring for Eyeglasses

QUALITY OF LIFE

- Knock before entering the person's room.
- Address the person by name.
- Introduce yourself by name and title.

- Explain the procedure before starting and during the procedure.
- Protect the person's rights during the procedure.
- Handle the person gently during the procedure.

PRE-PROCEDURE

1   Follow *Delegation Guidelines: Eyeglasses.*
    See *Promoting Safety and Comfort: Corrective Lenses.*
2   Practice hand hygiene.

3   Collect the following.
    - Eyeglass case
    - Cleaning solution or warm water
    - Disposable lens cloth or cotton cloth

PROCEDURE

4   Remove the eyeglasses.
    a   Hold the frames in front of the ears (Fig. 42-13, *A*).
    b   Lift the frames from the ears. Bring the eyeglasses down away from the face (Fig. 42-13, *B*).
5   Clean the lenses with a cleaning solution or warm water. Clean in a circular motion. Dry the lenses with the cloth.
6   *If the person will not wear the eyeglasses:*
    a   Open the eyeglass case.
    b   Fold the glasses. Put them in the case. Do not touch the clean lenses.
    c   Place the case in the top drawer of the bedside stand.

7   *If the person wears the eyeglasses:*
    a   Hold the frames at each side. Place them over the ears.
    b   Adjust the eyeglasses so the nose-piece rests on the nose.
    c   Return the case to the top drawer of the bedside stand.

POST-PROCEDURE

8   Provide for comfort. (See the inside of the front cover.)
9   Place the call light and other needed items within reach.
10 Return the cleaning solution to its proper place.
11 Discard the disposable cloth.

12 Complete a safety check of the room. (See the inside of the front cover.)
13 Practice hand hygiene.
14 Report and record your observations.

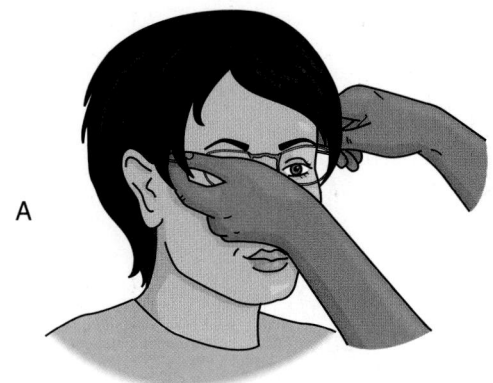
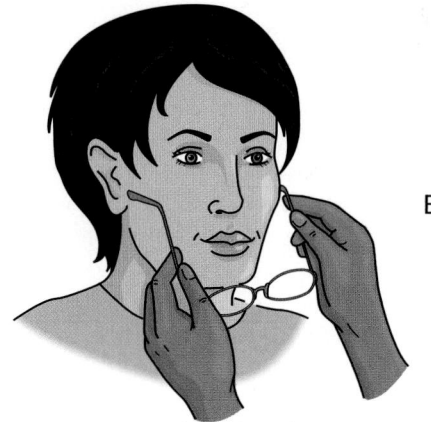

FIGURE 42-13 Removing eyeglasses. A, Hold the frames in front of the ears. **B,** Lift the frames from the ears. Bring the glasses down away from the face.

Contact Lenses. Contact lenses fit on the eye. There are hard and soft contacts. Disposable ones are discarded daily, weekly, or monthly. Contacts are cleaned, removed, and stored according to the manufacturer's instructions.

Report and record the following.

- Eye redness or irritation
- Eye drainage
- Complaints of eye pain, blurred or fuzzy vision, or uncomfortable lenses

Ocular Prostheses

Injury or disease may require removing an eyeball. The person is fitted with an ocular (eye) prosthesis. See Figure 42-14. This artificial eye does not provide vision. It matches the other eye in color and shape. The other eye may have normal, some, or no vision.

Some prostheses are permanent implants. Others are removable. If removed, the person learns to remove, clean, and insert it. If the prosthesis is not inserted after removal:

1. Practice hand hygiene.
2. Collect a kidney basin, denture cup, or other container as directed by the nurse. Line the container with a soft cloth or 4 × 4 gauze. This prevents scratches and damage.
3. Have the person put the eye in the container.
4. Line the sink with a towel.
5. Wash the eye with mild soap and warm water. Rinse well. Do not use a cloth to wash or dry the eye.
6. Line a container with a new soft cloth or 4 × 4 gauze.
7. Fill the container with sterile water or saline (salt) solution.
8. Place the eye in the container. Close the container.
9. Label the container with the person's name and room and bed number.
10. Place the labeled container in the top drawer of the bedside stand.
11. Wash the eye socket with warm water or saline. Use a washcloth or gauze square. Remove excess moisture with a gauze square.
12. Wash the eyelid and eyelashes with warm water. Clean from the inner to the outer aspect of the eye (Chapter 22). Dry the eyelid.
13. Rinse the prosthesis with sterile water before the person inserts the eye.

See *Promoting Safety and Comfort: Ocular Prostheses.*

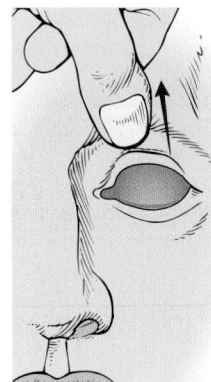 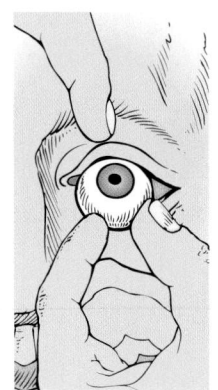 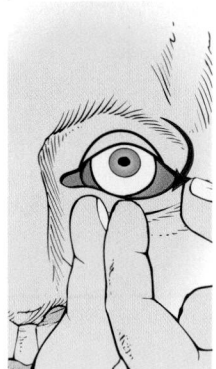

FIGURE 42-14 An ocular prosthesis is inserted. (From Lewis SM, Heitkemper MM, Dirksen SR: *Medical-surgical nursing: assessment and management of clinical problems,* ed 5, St Louis, 2000, Mosby.)

PROMOTING SAFETY AND COMFORT

Ocular Prostheses

Safety

When an ocular prosthesis is removed, you must prevent chips and scratches. It must not fall on the floor or other hard surface. Always hold the eye over a towel or other soft surface.

The prosthesis is the person's property. Protect it from loss or damage.

FOCUS ON **PRIDE**

The Person, Family, and Yourself

Personal and Professional Responsibility

Hearing aids, contact lenses, eyeglasses, and artificial eyes are costly to repair or replace. While the device is fixed or replaced the person is without it. Protect devices from loss or damage. If a device is lost or damaged, tell the nurse. Take pride in being a responsible and honest member of the nursing team.

Rights and Respect

Too often persons are defined by a disability. For example, a person is called "the blind woman" or "the deaf man." Or the person is treated like a child because others think that he or she cannot function.

Many persons with hearing, speech, and vision problems have overcome great challenges. They take pride in how they have adapted. They deserve to be treated with dignity and respect. Do not pity the person. Treat the person like an adult, not like a child. Focus on the person's abilities, not disabilities.

Always refer to the person first. Then state the person's disability if needed. For example, a nurse says: "Please take Mrs. Jones a warm blanket. She is blind, so knock and introduce yourself before entering the room. She will place the blanket as she prefers."

Independence and Social Interaction

Hearing, speech, and vision problems can interfere with quality of life. Adjusting is often long and hard. The person may be frustrated and angry. Take time to listen. Be patient, understanding, and sensitive to the person's needs and feelings. Allow the person to be in control to the extent possible. This helps promote independence to improve quality of life.

Delegation and Teamwork

Communicating with persons with hearing problems requires adjusting the setting and how you talk to the person. See Box 42-3. The health team must provide for the person's needs. Measures are included in the care plan. Using gestures, written notes, or an ASL interpreter are examples.

You must try to communicate with the person. Follow the care plan. These measures take time. Plan ahead. Do not be afraid to ask for help or advice. The nurse and other staff may have ideas for helping you communicate. Take pride in being part of a supportive health team that works together to meet the person's needs.

Ethics and Laws

The *Americans With Disabilities Act (ADA) of 1990* is a federal law. The law protects the rights of persons with disabilities. It includes persons with limited hearing, speech, and vision. The ADA covers rights such as employment, access to services and places, and the use of communication devices.

Agencies comply with the ADA in many ways. Agencies often provide:

- Braille on signs for areas with public access. Offices, lobbies, restrooms, elevators, and cafeterias are examples.
- Communication devices for those with hearing or speech problems. For example, a device with a keyboard and small screen is connected to a phone line. The device is used instead of a phone.
- ASL interpreters. Some agencies have a person on staff or on call. Others use an outside agency.
- Information in a form the person can understand. Large print and braille are examples.

Know your agency's resources for persons with disabilities. Offer to help. If you are unsure how to help, ask the nurse. Take pride in helping others.

FOCUS ON **PRIDE**: *Application*

Hearing, speech, and vision problems do not affect intelligence. Some behaviors insult the person. Treating the person like a child and talking to others but not the person are examples. What are other examples? Identify ways to show dignity and respect.

REVIEW QUESTIONS

Circle the BEST answer.

1 Care of the person with Meniere's disease includes
   a Wearing a hearing aid
   b Preventing falls from vertigo
   c Speech therapy
   d Treating infection

2 Which is a sign of hearing loss?
   a An adult tugs or pulls at the ears.
   b A 5-month-old babbles and makes gurgling sounds.
   c An adult asks others to repeat themselves.
   d A 10-month-old uses gestures to communicate.

3 When talking to a person with hearing loss
   a Shout
   b Change the subject if the person does not seem to understand
   c Avoid using gestures and facial expressions
   d Use short sentences and simple words

4 A hearing aid
   a Corrects a hearing problem
   b Makes sounds louder
   c Makes speech clearer
   d Lowers background noise

5 A hearing aid does not seem to be working. Your *first* action is to
   a See if it is turned on
   b Wash it with soap and water
   c Have it repaired
   d Remove the batteries

6 A person has aphasia. You know that
   a The person cannot hear
   b Mouth and face muscles are affected
   c The person has a language disorder
   d The person cannot speak

7 A person with receptive aphasia has trouble
   a Talking
   b Writing
   c Understanding messages
   d Using gestures

8 A person has a speech disorder. You should
   a Correct the person's speech
   b Discourage the writing of words
   c Leave the TV on while talking
   d Ask the person to repeat as needed

9 A person with a cataract
   a Has cloudy, blurry, or dim vision
   b Loses central vision
   c Has eye pain
   d Is blind

10 A person had cataract surgery. Which measure would you question?
   a Remind the person not to bend or cough.
   b Let the person rub the eye.
   c Place the over-bed table on the un-operative side.
   d Have the person wear an eye shield during naps.

11 A person has AMD. Which is *true*?
   a There is a blind spot in the center of the eye.
   b Lost vision can be restored with surgery.
   c Peripheral (side) vision is lost.
   d Vision is blurry with spots.

12 With low vision
   a There is no usable vision
   b Surgery can correct vision loss
   c Visual and adaptive devices are needed
   d Every-day activities are not affected

13 Who is at risk for low vision?
   a The person with diabetic retinopathy
   b The person with global aphasia
   c The person with Meniere's disease
   d The person who is blind

14 Braille involves
   a A long cane for walking
   b Raised dots arranged for letters of the alphabet
   c A guide dog
   d Corrective lenses

15 Which are dangers to persons who are blind or visually impaired?
   a Drawers that are fully closed
   b Doors that are fully open
   c Burnt-out bulbs
   d Night-lights

16 A person is blind. The meal-time setting should
   a Be the same for every meal
   b Provide variety for mental stimulation
   c Include plates, napkins, and placemats with designs
   d Be at the same time everyday

17 A person is visually impaired. You should
   a Move furniture to provide variety
   b Avoid words such as "see" and "look"
   c Assume that the person has no sight
   d Explain procedures step-by-step

18 A person is blind. To give directions you can say
   a "Over there"
   b "Right here"
   c "Across the room"
   d "On your left"

19 When eyeglasses are not worn they should be
   a Soaked in a cleansing solution
   b Taken to the nurses' station
   c Put in the eyeglass case
   d Placed on the over-bed table

20 To care for an ocular prosthesis
   a Dry the eye with a cloth
   b Wash the eye with mild soap and warm water
   c Scrub the eye with 4 × 4 gauze
   d Store the eye in an empty container

Answers to Chapter 42 questions are on p. 872.

FOCUS ON PRACTICE

Problem Solving

Mr. Tyler is waiting in the dining room for lunch to be served. He asks for help completing his weekly menu. You are to read each option and mark his choices. Mr. Tyler is hard-of-hearing. You repeat the meal options several times. He struggles to hear you. What will you do? What can be done to promote hearing?

Cancer, Immune System, and Skin Disorders

CHAPTER

43

OBJECTIVES

- Define the key terms and key abbreviations in this chapter.
- Explain the differences between benign tumors and cancer.
- Identify cancer risk factors, signs, and symptoms.
- Explain the common cancer treatments.
- Describe the needs of persons with cancer.
- Describe the common immune system disorders.
- Describe the human immunodeficiency virus (HIV) and acquired immunodeficiency syndrome (AIDS).

- Explain how to assist in the care of persons with AIDS.
- Describe the cause, signs and symptoms, and treatment of shingles.
- Explain how to promote PRIDE in the person, the family, and yourself.

KEY TERMS

benign tumor A tumor that does not spread to other body parts
cancer See "malignant tumor"
malignant tumor A tumor that invades and destroys nearby tissues and can spread to other body parts; cancer
metastasis The spread of cancer to other body parts

mole A brown, tan, or black spot on the skin that is flat or raised and round or oval
stomatitis Inflammation (itis) of the mouth (stomat)
tumor A new growth of abnormal cells that is benign or malignant

KEY ABBREVIATIONS

AIDS	Acquired immunodeficiency syndrome	**STD**	Sexually transmitted disease
CDC	Centers for Disease Control and Prevention	**TB**	Tuberculosis
HIV	Human immunodeficiency virus		

Understanding cancer, immune system, and skin disorders gives meaning to the required care. Refer to Chapter 10 while you study this chapter.

CANCER

Cells reproduce for tissue growth and repair. Cells divide in an orderly way. Sometimes cell division and growth are out of control. A mass or clump of cells develops. This *new growth of abnormal cells is called a* **tumor.** *Tumors are benign or malignant* (Fig. 43-1, p. 694).

- *Benign tumors do not spread to other body parts.* They can grow to a large size but rarely threaten life. They usually do not grow back when removed.
- *Malignant tumors (cancer) invade and destroy nearby tissues. They can spread to other body parts* (Fig. 43-2, p. 694). They may be life-threatening. Sometimes they grow back after removal.

Metastasis is the spread of cancer to other body parts (Fig. 43-3, p. 694). Cancer cells break off the tumor and travel to other body parts. New tumors grow at those sites. This occurs if cancer is not treated and controlled.

Cancer can occur almost anywhere. If detected early, cancer can be treated and controlled (Box 43-1, p. 695).

See *Focus on Children and Older Persons: Cancer*, p. 696.

Text continued on p. 697.

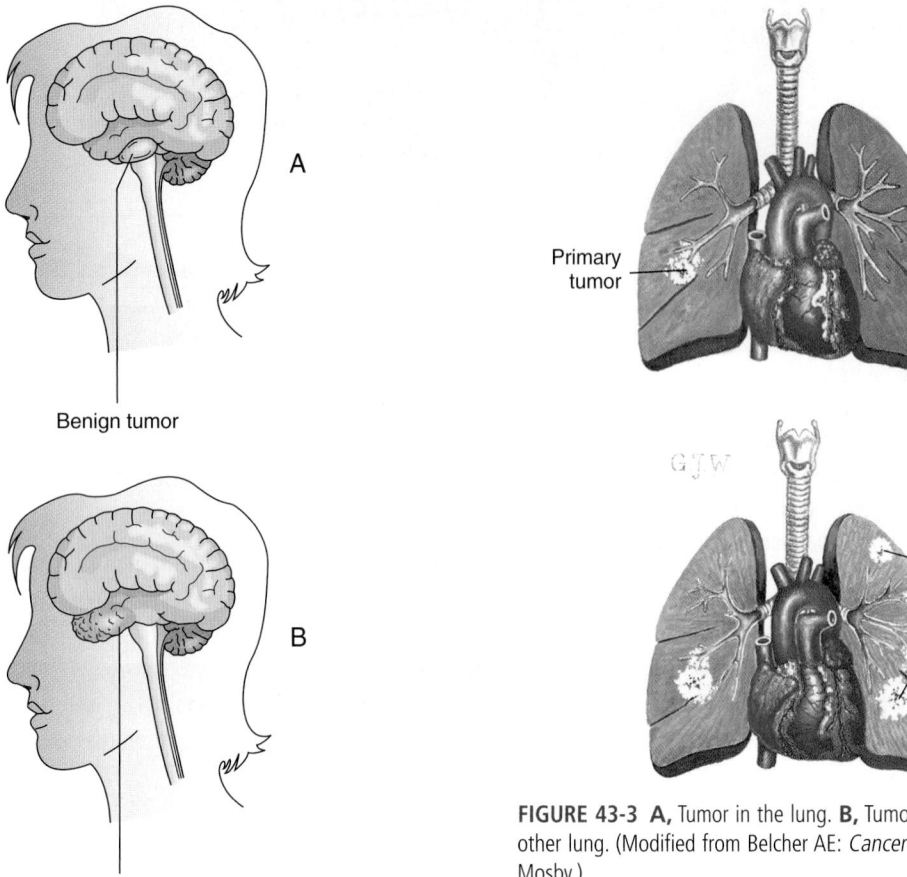

FIGURE 43-3 A, Tumor in the lung. **B,** Tumor has metastasized to the other lung. (Modified from Belcher AE: *Cancer nursing,* St Louis, 1992, Mosby.)

FIGURE 43-1 Tumors. A, A benign tumor grows within a local area. **B,** A malignant tumor invades other tissues.

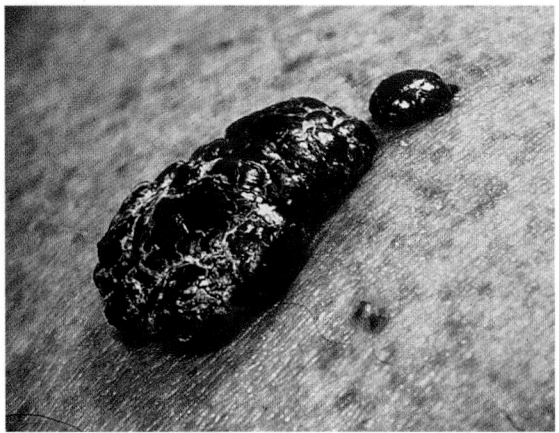

FIGURE 43-2 Malignant tumor on the skin. (From Belcher AE: *Cancer nursing,* St Louis, 1992, Mosby.)

BOX 43-1 Cancer—Signs and Symptoms

General Signs and Symptoms
- Unexplained weight loss
- Fever
- Fatigue
- Pain
- Skin changes—darker looking skin, reddened skin, itching, excessive hair growth
- Jaundice (yellowish skin and eyes)
- Change in bowel habits
- Change in bladder function
- Sores that do not heal
- White patches in the mouth
- White spots on the tongue
- Unusual bleeding or discharge
- Thickening or lump in the breast or any other part of the body
- Indigestion or trouble swallowing
- Change in a wart or mole or new skin change
- Nagging cough or hoarseness

Brain Tumor
- Headaches (usually worse in the morning)
- Nausea and vomiting
- Changes in speech, vision, or hearing
- Problems with balance and walking
- Changes in mood, personality, or ability to concentrate
- Problems with memory
- Seizures or convulsions
- Numbness or tingling in the arms or legs

Cervix
- Abnormal vaginal bleeding
  - Between regular menstrual periods
  - After intercourse, douching, or pelvic exam
  - Longer or heavier menstrual periods
  - After menopause
- Increased vaginal discharge
- Pelvic pain
- Pain during sex

Breast
- Swelling of all or part of a breast
- Irritation or dimpling of the skin
- Pain in a breast or nipple
- A nipple turned inward into the breast
- Discharge (fluid) from the nipple, especially if bloody
- Scaly, red, or thickened nipple or skin

Bladder
- Hematuria (urine looks rusty or dark red)
- Urinary urgency or frequency
- Feeling unable to empty the bladder
- Needing to strain (bear down) to void
- Dysuria

Colon and Rectum
- Change in bowel habits—diarrhea, constipation, narrow stools
- Feeling that the bowel does not empty completely
- Rectal bleeding
- Blood (bright red or very dark) in the stool
- Cramping or abdominal pain
- Weight loss
- Fatigue
- Weakness

Kidney
- Hematuria (urine looks rusty or dark red)
- Pain in the side that does not go away
- An abnormal lump or mass in the side
- Weight loss
- Fever
- Fatigue

Larynx
- A hoarse voice or other voice changes for more than 3 weeks
- A sore throat or trouble swallowing for more than 6 weeks
- A lump in the neck
- Dyspnea
- A cough that does not go away
- An earache that does not go away

Leukemia
- Weight loss
- Painless, swollen lymph nodes in the neck or underarm
- Fevers or night sweats
- Frequent infections
- Fatigue
- Weakness
- Feeling dizzy or light-headed
- Loss of appetite
- Bleeding or bruising (bleeding gums, nose bleeds)
- Abdominal swelling or discomfort
- Weight loss
- Shortness of breath

Lung
- A cough that does not go away
- Changes in a chronic cough
- Dyspnea
- Wheezing
- Shortness of breath
- Chest pain
- Coughing up blood (hemoptysis)
- Hoarse voice
- Weight loss
- Bone pain
- Headache

Lymphoma
- Painless, swollen lymph nodes in the neck, underarm, or groin
- Weight loss
- Fever
- Night sweats
- Coughing, dyspnea, or chest pain
- Weakness or fatigue
- Pain, swelling, or full feeling in the abdomen

Melanoma
- Change in the shape, color, size, or feel of a *mole (a brown, tan, or black spot on the skin that is flat or raised and round or oval)*
- New mole or spot
- A spot that looks different from other spots
- Uneven mole shape—one half does not match the other half
- Mole edges are ragged, notched, or blurred
- Mole color is uneven with shades of black, brown, and tan; areas of pink, red, white, or blue

Continued

BOX 43-1   Cancer—Signs and Symptoms—cont'd

Melanoma—cont'd
- Mole is hard or lumpy or itchy, tender, or painful
- Mole surface is bleeding, scaly, or oozing

Mouth and Lips
- White or red patches inside the mouth or on the lips
- A mouth or lip sore that does not heal
- Bleeding in the mouth
- Loose teeth or problems wearing dentures
- Dysphagia
- A lump in the neck
- Earache that does not go away
- Numbness of the lower lip and chin

Pancreas
- Jaundice—dark urine, pale stools, yellow skin and eyes
- Upper abdominal pain
- Middle back pain not improved with position change
- Nausea and vomiting
- Stools that float in the toilet
- Fatigue
- Anorexia or full feeling
- Weight loss

Skin
- Itching
- Bleeding
- Pain or discomfort

Skin—cont'd
- Flat, firm, or pale area or blue, brown, or black areas
- Pink, red, shiny, or pearly bump
- Oozing, rough, scaly, or crusted areas
- Red-colored patches

Prostate
- Problems urinating
- Slow or weak urine flow
- Frequent urination, especially at night
- Blood in the urine
- Erection problems
- Pain in the back, hips, or chest
- Weakness or numbness in the legs or feet
- Loss of bowel or bladder control

Thyroid
- Lump or swelling in the neck
- Hoarseness or voice changes
- Dysphagia
- Dyspnea
- Pain in the front of the neck and sometimes the ears
- Constant cough

Uterus
- Abnormal vaginal bleeding, spotting, or discharge
- Vaginal bleeding or spotting after menopause
- Vaginal discharge
- Pelvic pain

Modified from National Cancer Institute
- What you need to know about™ brain tumors, *updated May 2009.*
- What you need to know about™ cervical cancer, *revised January 2012.*
- What you need to know about™ bladder cancer, *updated August 2010.*
- What you need to know about™ kidney cancer, *updated August 2010.*
- What you need to know about™ cancer of the larynx, *updated August 2010.*
- What you need to know about™ non-Hodgkin lymphoma, *updated September 2007.*
- What you need to know about™ oral cancer, *updated July 2009.*
- What you need to know about™ cancer of the pancreas, *updated May 2010.*

American Cancer Society
- Signs and symptoms of cancer: what are signs and symptoms? *revised August 11, 2014.*
- Signs and symptoms of breast cancer, *revised June 10, 2015.*
- Signs and symptoms of colorectal cancer, *revised August 13, 2015.*
- Signs and symptoms of acute lymphocytic leukemia, *revised January 12, 2015.*
- Signs and symptoms of melanoma skin cancer, *revised March 20, 2015.*
- Signs and symptoms of basal and squamous cell skin cancers, *revised April 3, 2015.*
- Signs and symptoms of prostate cancer, *revised March 12, 2015.*
- Signs and symptoms of thyroid cancer, *revised March 17, 2015.*
- Signs and symptoms of uterine sarcomas, *revised March 18, 2015.*

Mayo Clinic, Diseases and conditions: lung cancer, *March 19, 2014.*

FOCUS ON CHILDREN AND OLDER PERSONS

Cancer

Children

Sites of cancer in children are the same as for adults. However, some cancers are more common in children. They include:
- Leukemia—a cancer of the blood and bone marrow. The bone marrow is a spongy substance found inside bones. Blood cells are made in the bone marrow. Leukemia is the most common form of childhood cancer.
- Brain tumors.
- Lymphomas—tumors of the lymph tissues.
- Bone cancers.
- Soft tissue cancers.
- Cancer of the eye.
- Kidney cancers.
- Cancer of nerve cells.

Often signs and symptoms are similar to common illnesses and injuries. Children should see a doctor when the following signs and symptoms do not go away.
- Unusual lump or swelling
- Paleness
- Loss of energy
- Easy bruising
- On-going pain in 1 area of the body
- Limping
- Unexplained fever or illness
- Frequent headaches and headaches with vomiting
- Eye or vision changes
- Unexplained weight loss

Childhood cancers often occur suddenly. They have a high cure rate.

Risk Factors

Cancer is the second leading cause of death in the United States. The National Cancer Institute describes these risk factors.

- *Age.* Advancing age is the most important risk factor. However, cancer can occur at any age.
- *Tobacco.* This includes using tobacco (smoking, snuff, and chewing tobacco) and being around tobacco (second-hand smoke). This risk can be avoided.
- *Radiation.* Sources are sun light, x-rays, and radon gas that forms in the soil and some rocks.
- *Infections.* Certain viruses and bacteria increase the risk of cancers—cervix, penis, vagina, anus, mouth, liver, lymphoma, leukemia, Kaposi's sarcoma (associated with AIDS, p. 700), stomach.
- *Immuno-suppressive drugs.* These drugs lower the body's ability to stop cancer from forming. Such drugs are often used for organ transplant patients to prevent rejection of the transplant.
- *Alcohol.* Alcohol is linked to the increased risk of cancers of the mouth, esophagus, breast, colon, and rectum.
- *Diet.* Diet may affect the risk of cancer. Fruits and vegetables may protect against cancers of the mouth, esophagus, and stomach. A diet high in fat, protein, calories, and red meat may increase the risk of colon and rectal cancers.
- *Hormones.* The female hormones estrogen and progesterone are known to increase the risk of breast and endometrial (uterine) cancers.
- *Obesity.* Obesity is linked to post-menopausal breast cancer and cancers of the colon, rectum, uterus, esophagus, kidney, and pancreas.
- *Environment.* Air pollution, second-hand smoke, and asbestos are linked to lung cancer. Drinking water containing large amounts of arsenic is linked to skin, bladder, and lung cancers.

Treatment

Treatment depends on the tumor type, its site and size, and if it has spread. The treatment goal may be to:

- Cure the cancer. Remove cancer from the body and kill cancer cells.
- Control the disease. Help the person live longer.
- Reduce signs and symptoms from the cancer and its treatments.

Some cancers respond to 1 type of treatment. Others require 2 or more types. Cancer treatments also damage healthy cells and tissues. Side effects depend on the type and extent of the treatment.

Surgery. Surgery removes tumors. It is done to cure or control cancer or to relieve pain. See Chapter 35.

Radiation Therapy. Radiation therapy *(radiotherapy)* kills cancer cells. X-ray beams are aimed at the tumor. Sometimes radioactive material is implanted in or near the tumor.

Cancer cells and normal cells receive radiation. Both are destroyed. Radiation therapy:

- Destroys certain tumors.
- Shrinks a tumor before surgery.
- Destroys cancer cells that remain after surgery.
- Controls tumor growth to prevent or relieve pain.

Skin changes occur at the treatment site—dryness, itching, swelling, peeling, redness, blistering. Special skin care measures are ordered. Dry mouth and sore throat can result from radiation to the head and neck. Extra rest is needed for fatigue. Discomfort, nausea, vomiting, diarrhea, and loss of appetite *(anorexia)* are other side effects.

See *Promoting Safety and Comfort: Radiation Therapy.*

Chemotherapy. Chemotherapy involves drugs that kill cancer cells. It is used to:

- Cure the cancer.
- Shrink a tumor before surgery.
- Slow growth of the cancer.
- Prevent the cancer from spreading.
- Kill cells that break off the tumor to prevent metastasis.
- Relieve symptoms caused by the cancer.

PROMOTING SAFETY AND COMFORT

Radiation Therapy

Safety

Radiation implants (seeds, ribbons, capsules) are placed near the tumor. Therefore the person's body gives off radiation. Practice these safety measures.

- Tell the nurse if you are or may be pregnant. The nurse needs to change your assignment.
- Don protective gloves and shoe coverings before entering the person's room.
- Work quickly.
- Stay as far away from the person as possible while still giving effective care.
- Leave trash, linens, and food trays in the room. These items will be removed by staff trained to do so.
- Remove and discard your gloves and shoe coverings before leaving the room.
- Wash your hands after leaving the room.
- Talk to the person from the doorway if you do not need to enter the room. Radiation exposure decreases with distance.

Comfort

The person has a private room to protect others from radiation exposure. A visitor may be limited to 30 minutes or less a day. Visitors may stand at the doorway rather than enter the room. Children under 18 years of age and pregnant women are not allowed to visit.

Therefore the person may feel sad, lonely, and depressed. Assure the person that care needs will be met. Treat the person with caring, kindness, and dignity.

Chemotherapy affects the whole body. Cancer cells and normal cells are affected. Side effects depend on the drug used.

- Hair loss (*alopecia*).
- Gastro-intestinal irritation. Poor appetite, nausea, vomiting, and diarrhea can occur. *Stomatitis, an inflammation* (itis) *of the mouth* (stomat), may occur.
- Decreased blood cell production. Bleeding and infection are risks. The person may be weak and tired.
- Changes in thinking and memory.
- Emotional changes.

The drug usually stays in the person's body for 3 to 7 days. It is excreted through body fluids—urine, feces, vomit, tears, saliva, semen, and vaginal secretions. Safety measures are listed in Box 43-2.

Hormone Therapy.
Some cancers need hormones to grow. Hormone therapy involves blocking or removing hormone sources from the body. Drugs are given to prevent the production of certain hormones. Organs or glands that produce a certain hormone are removed. For example, the ovaries are removed if breast cancer needs estrogen. A prostate cancer may need testosterone. The testicles may be removed.

Side effects include fatigue, fluid retention, weight gain, hot flashes, nausea, vomiting, appetite changes, and blood clots. Fertility is affected in men and women. Men may experience impotence (Chapter 51) and loss of sexual desire.

Biological Therapy.
Biological therapy *(immunotherapy)* helps the immune system fight the cancer. It also protects the body from the side effects of cancer treatments.

Side effects include flu-like symptoms—chills, fever, muscle aches, weakness, loss of appetite, nausea, vomiting, and diarrhea. Bleeding, bruising, swelling, and skin rashes may occur.

Other Therapies.
Other therapies include:

- *Stem cell transplants.* A stem cell is a cell from which new cell types develop. The new cells have certain functions—blood cells, brain cells, bone cells, and so on. High doses of chemotherapy or radiation therapy can kill cancer cells and blood cells in the bone marrow. Fewer blood cells are produced. The person is given blood-forming stem cells. New blood cells develop from the stem cells.
- *Complementary and alternative medicine (CAM). Complementary medicine* is used with standard cancer treatments. *Alternative medicine* is used instead of standard cancer treatments. CAM includes massage therapy, herbal products, vitamins, special diets, spiritual healing, and acupuncture. Acupuncture involves inserting small needles at certain points in the skin to control pain and other symptoms.

The Person's Needs
Persons with cancer have many needs. They include:
- Pain relief or control
- Rest and exercise
- Fluids and nutrition
- Preventing skin breakdown
- Preventing bowel problems—constipation from pain-relief drugs; diarrhea from some cancer treatments
- Dealing with treatment side effects
- Psychological and social needs
- Spiritual needs
- Sexual needs

BOX 43-2 | Safety During Chemotherapy

General Safety
- Wear gloves for any contact with the person's body fluids, secretions, or excretions. Wash your hands after removing and discarding the gloves.
- Wash the hands or any body part or area that has contact with the person's body fluids, secretions, or excretions. Do so at once. Use soap and water. This applies to you, the person, and others.

Elimination and Vomiting
- Wear gloves to handle bedpans, urinals, or kidney basins.
- Empty and rinse bedpans, urinals, and kidney basins after use.
- Flush after the person uses the toilet or you empty a bedpan, urinal, or kidney basin. Put the lid down first to avoid splashing. Flush twice if young children or pets will have contact with the toilet.
- Wash bedpans, urinals, and kidney basins at least once a day with soap and water. Or provide the person with new items. Follow agency policy.

Elimination and Vomiting—cont'd
- Wear gloves when changing and handling diapers, incontinence products, waterproof under-pads, and ostomy pouches.
- Double-bag diapers, incontinence products, waterproof under-pads, and ostomy pouches. Follow agency policy.
- Place ostomy waste in a tied plastic bag or a zip-lock bag. Then double-bag the bag with waste.

Laundry
- Follow agency policy for soiled linens and clothing. In the home setting:
  - Wash soiled linens as soon as possible. Or place them in a plastic bag. Discard the plastic bag in the trash after washing the items.
  - Wash soiled items separately from other linens or garments.
  - Wash soiled items twice.

Modified from UPMC: Patient education: safe handling of chemotherapy waste material, Pittsburgh, Pa, 2015, UPMC.

Psychological and social needs are great. Anger, fear, and depression are common. Some surgeries are disfiguring. The person may feel unwell, unattractive, or unclean. The person and family need support.

Spiritual needs are important. A spiritual leader may provide comfort. To many people, spiritual needs are just as important as physical needs.

Persons dying of cancer often receive hospice care (Chapters 1 and 55). Support is given to the person and family.

See *Focus on Communication: The Person's Needs.*

IMMUNE SYSTEM DISORDERS

The immune system protects the body from microbes, cancer cells, and other harmful substances. It defends against threats inside and outside the body. Immune system disorders occur from problems with the immune response. The response may be inappropriate, too strong, or lacking.

See *Body Structure and Function Review: The Immune System.*

Autoimmune Disorders

Autoimmune disorders occur when the immune system attacks the body's own *(auto)* healthy cells, tissues, or organs. One of these may occur.

- One or more types of body tissues are affected (Fig. 43-4, p. 700).
- An organ grows abnormally.
- There is a change in how an organ functions. Common autoimmune disorders include:
- *Celiac disease.* The person cannot tolerate gluten—a substance in wheat, rye, barley, and some drugs. When gluten is ingested, the immune system causes damage to the small intestines. Signs and symptoms include abdominal bloating and pain, diarrhea or constipation, weight loss or gain, and fatigue.
- *Graves' disease.* The thyroid gland produces excess *(hyper)* amounts of the thyroid hormone. The person has anxiety, problems sleeping, rapid heart rate, weight loss, sweating, muscle weakness, shaky hands, and bulging eyes (Fig. 43-5, p. 700).

- *Hashimoto's disease.* The thyroid gland does not produce enough thyroid hormone. The person has fatigue, weakness, weight gain, sensitivity to cold, muscle aches, stiff joints, facial swelling, and constipation.
- *Lupus.* This disease can damage the joints, skin, kidneys, heart, lungs, and other body parts. A rash across the nose and cheeks is common. See Figure 43-6, p. 700.
- *Multiple sclerosis* (Chapter 44).
- *Rheumatoid arthritis* (Chapter 44).
- *Type 1 diabetes* (Chapter 46).
- *Inflammatory bowel disease* (Chapter 46).

Body Parts That Can Be Affected by Autoimmune Diseases

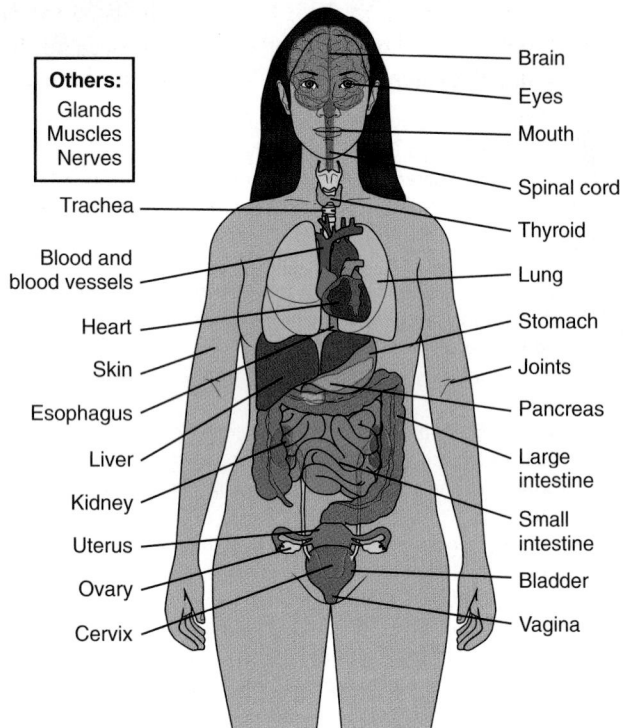

FIGURE 43-4 Body parts affected by autoimmune disorders. (Redrawn from Office on Women's Health, U.S. Department of Health and Human Services: *ePublications: autoimmune diseases fact sheet,* updated July 16, 2012.)

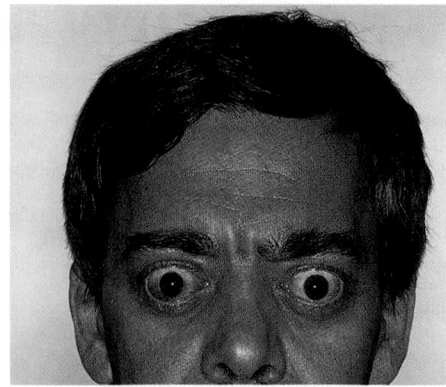

FIGURE 43-5 Bulging eyes occurs in Graves' disease. (From Belchetz PE, Hammond P: *Diabetes and endocrinology,* London, 2003, Mosby.)

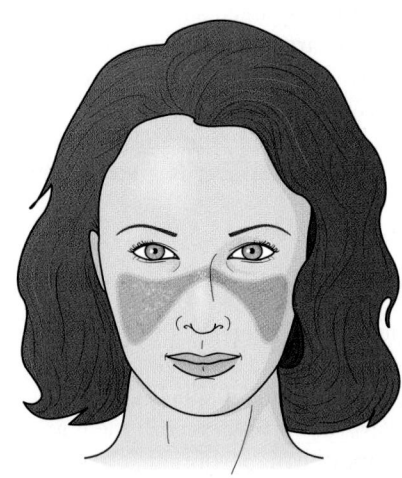

FIGURE 43-6 Called the "butterfly" rash, the rash from lupus is across the nose and cheeks. (Redrawn from National Institute of Arthritis and Musculoskeletal and Skin Diseases: *Do I have lupus?* Bethesda, Md, National Institutes of Health.)

Most autoimmune disorders are chronic. Treatment depends on the disorder and the tissues and organs affected. Treatment is aimed at:

- Relieving symptoms
- Replacing needed hormones
- Suppressing the immune system

HIV/AIDS

Acquired immunodeficiency syndrome (AIDS) is caused by the *human immunodeficiency virus (HIV)*. HIV attacks the immune system. Therefore it destroys the body's ability to fight infections and disease.

According to the Centers for Disease Control and Prevention (CDC), 50,000 people become infected with HIV each year. The CDC reports that there are about 1.2 million people in the United States with HIV.

HIV is spread through certain body fluids—blood, semen, vaginal fluids, rectal fluids, and breast-milk. HIV is not spread by air, water, saliva, tears, sweat, insects, casual contact (shaking hands, hugging, dancing, sharing dishes), closed mouth or social kissing, or toilet seats.

HIV is transmitted *mainly* by:

- Having sex with someone who has HIV.
  - Anal sex
  - Vaginal sex
  - Multiple sex partners
- Sharing needles, syringes, rinse water, or other equipment used to prepare injection drugs.

The CDC reports that HIV *may* be spread by:

- HIV-infected mothers to children during pregnancy, birth, or breast-feeding.
- Being stuck with an HIV-contaminated needle or other sharp object
- Receiving blood transfusions, blood products, or organ or tissue transplants contaminated with HIV
- Eating food pre-chewed by an HIV-infected person if the food mixes with blood
- Being bitten and skin broken by an HIV-infected person
- Oral sex
- Contact between broken skin, wounds, or mucous membranes and HIV-infected blood or blood-contaminated body fluids
- Deep, open-mouth kissing if blood is exchanged when the person with HIV has sores or bleeding gums

Box 43-3 lists the stages and signs and symptoms of HIV and AIDS. HIV can be transmitted to others during any stage. Some HIV-infected persons are symptom-free for more than 10 years. However, they carry HIV and can spread it to others.

Drugs are available to treat or reduce HIV symptoms. They also reduce complications and prolong life. AIDS has no vaccine and no cure at present. It is a life-threatening disease.

You may care for persons who are HIV positive, are HIV carriers, or have AIDS (Box 43-4). You may have contact with the person's blood or body fluids. Protect yourself and others. Follow Standard Precautions and the Bloodborne Pathogen Standard. A person may have the HIV virus but no symptoms. In some persons, HIV or AIDS is not yet diagnosed.

See *Focus on Children and Older Persons: HIV/AIDS.*

See *Promoting Safety and Comfort: HIV/AIDS,* p. 702.

BOX 43-3	AIDS—Stages and Signs and Symptoms

Acute Infection
- May occur within 2 to 4 weeks after HIV infection.
- Flu-like symptoms often described as the "worst flu ever."
  - Fever
  - Swollen glands
  - Sore throat
  - Rash
  - Fatigue
  - Muscle and joint aches and pains
  - Headache
- Symptoms may last a few days to several weeks.

Clinical Latency Stage
- *Latency* means *present and developing but not obvious or visible.*
- The HIV is living and developing without producing symptoms.
- The person has no HIV-related symptoms or only mild ones.
- This stage lasts an average of 10 years. Some people progress to the next stage faster.

AIDS
- The immune system is badly damaged.
- The person is at risk for infections, illnesses, and cancers. They include pneumonia, tuberculosis (TB), Kaposi's sarcoma, nervous system disorders, mental health disorders, and dementia.
- Signs and symptoms:
  - Rapid weight loss
  - Recurring fever
  - Night sweats
  - Fatigue: extreme and unexplained
  - Swollen lymph glands: underarms, groin, neck
  - Diarrhea lasting more than a week
  - Sore throat
  - Sores: mouth, anus, genitals
  - Red, brown, pink, or purple blotches: under the skin; inside the mouth, nose, or eyelids
  - Memory loss
  - Depression
  - Loss of coordination
  - Paralysis

BOX 43-4	Caring for the Person With AIDS

- Follow Standard Precautions and the Bloodborne Pathogen Standard.
- Provide daily hygiene. Avoid irritating soaps.
- Follow the care plan for oral hygiene. A toothbrush with soft bristles is best.
- Provide oral fluids as ordered.
- Measure and record intake and output.
- Measure weight daily.
- Encourage deep-breathing and coughing exercises as ordered.
- Prevent pressure ulcers.
- Assist with range-of-motion exercises and ambulating as ordered.
- Encourage self-care. The person may use assistive devices (walker, commode, eating devices).
- Encourage the person to be as active as possible.
- Change linens and garments when damp or wet.
- Listen and provide emotional support.

FOCUS ON **CHILDREN AND OLDER PERSONS**

HIV/AIDS

Older Persons

In 2015, the CDC reported over 313,200 cases of HIV in persons 55 years and older. In 2013, the CDC reported 8,575 new cases in people aged 55 and older.

Older persons get and spread HIV through sexual contact and intravenous (IV) drug use. Many do not consider themselves at risk. They tend not to practice safe sex. A blood transfusion between 1978 and 1985 increases the HIV risk.

Aging and some diseases mask the signs and symptoms of AIDS. Older persons are less likely to be tested for HIV/AIDS. Often the person dies without the disease being diagnosed. You must follow Standard Precautions and the Bloodborne Pathogen Standard.

HIV Prevention. The CDC recommends the following measures to prevent HIV.

- Choosing less risky sexual behaviors. Anal sex carries the highest risk. Oral sex is less risky than anal or vaginal sex.
- Using condoms consistently and correctly.
- Reducing the number of sexual partners. The greater the number of partners, the greater the risk of a partner with HIV.
- Taking pre-exposure prophylaxis (PrEP) drugs. (*Prophylaxis* means *prevention measures.*) Such drugs are indicated for:
  - HIV-negative persons who have an on-going sexual relationship with an HIV-positive partner.
  - Gay or bi-sexual men who have had anal sex without a condom.
  - Gay or bi-sexual men diagnosed with an STD in the past 6 months.
  - Heterosexual men or women who do not regularly use condoms during sex with partners who are at risk for HIV. Such partners include bi-sexual men and persons who inject drugs.
- Seeing a doctor within 3 days after possible exposure to HIV. The doctor may order post-exposure prophylaxis.
- Testing and treatment for other STDs.
- Encouraging HIV-positive partners to get and continue treatment.

SKIN DISORDERS

There are many types of skin disorders. Alopecia, hirsutism, dandruff, lice, and scabies are discussed in Chapter 23. Skin tears and pressure ulcers are discussed in Chapters 36 and 37. Burns are discussed in Chapter 54.

See *Body Structure and Function Review: The Integumentary System.*

BODY STRUCTURE AND FUNCTION REVIEW

The Integumentary System

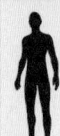

The *integumentary system,* or *skin,* is the largest system. It is the body's natural covering. There are 2 skin layers (Fig. 43-7).

- The *epidermis* is the outer layer. It has living cells and dead cells. Dead cells constantly flake off and are replaced by living cells. Living cells also die and flake off. Living cells of the epidermis contain *pigment.* Pigment gives skin its color. The epidermis has no blood vessels and few nerve endings.
- The *dermis* is the inner layer. It is made up of connective tissue. Blood vessels, nerves, sweat glands, oil glands, and hair roots are found in the dermis.

Sweat glands help regulate body temperature. Sweat is secreted through the skin's pores. The body is cooled as sweat evaporates. *Oil glands* secrete an oily substance into the space near the hair shaft. Oil travels to the skin surface. This helps keep the hair and skin soft and shiny.

The skin has many functions.

- Provides the body's protective covering.
- Prevents microbes and other substances from entering the body.
- Prevents excess amounts of water from leaving the body.
- Protects organs from injury.
- Contains sensory structures. Nerve endings in the skin sense both pleasant and unpleasant stimulation. They sense cold, pain, touch, and pressure to protect the body from injury.
- Helps regulate body temperature. Blood vessels dilate (widen) when the temperature outside the body is high. More blood is brought to the body surface for cooling during evaporation. When blood vessels constrict (narrow), the body retains heat. This is because less blood reaches the skin.
- Stores fat and water.

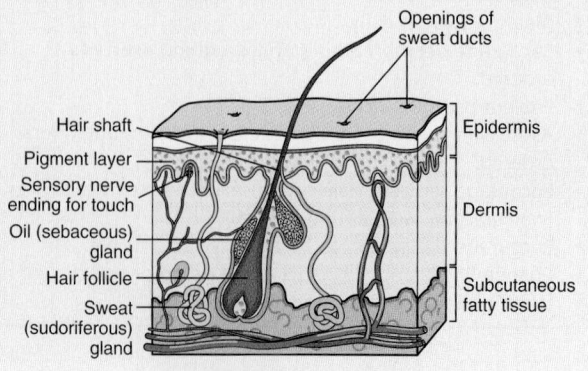

FIGURE 43-7 Structures of the skin.

Shingles

Shingles (herpes zoster) is caused by the same virus that causes chicken pox. The virus lies dormant in nerve tissue. (*Dormant* means *to be inactive.*) The virus can become active years later.

A rash or blisters can occur. At first there is burning or tingling pain, numbness, or itching. This occurs in an area on 1 side of the body or 1 side of the face. After a few days or a week, a rash with fluid-filled blisters appears (Fig. 43-8). Pain is mild to intense. Itching is a common complaint.

Shingles is most common in persons over 50 years of age. Persons who have had chicken pox are at risk. So are persons with weakened immune systems from HIV infections, cancer treatments, transplant surgeries, and stress.

Anti-viral drugs and pain-relief drugs are used. For many healthy people, blisters heal and pain is gone in 3 to 5 weeks. A vaccine is now available to prevent shingles.

According to the CDC, shingles lesions are infectious until they crust over. Avoid contact with an infected person if you:
- Have never had chicken pox or the vaccine to prevent chicken pox.
- Are pregnant and have not had chicken pox or the vaccine to prevent chicken pox.
- Have a weakened immune system.

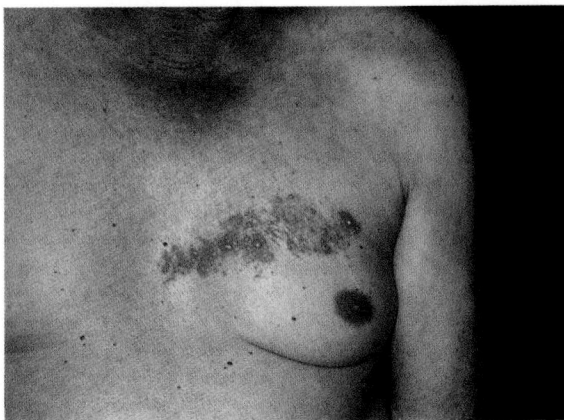

FIGURE 43-8 Shingles. (Courtesy Department of Dermatology, School of Medicine, University of Utah, Salt Lake City, Utah.)

FOCUS ON **PRIDE**

The Person, Family, and Yourself

Personal and Professional Responsibility
Hospital oncology units are for cancer patients. *Oncology* is the study of cancer. Staff are experienced with the care and needs of persons with cancer. Some hospitals have oncology units for children.

Working on an oncology unit is challenging and rewarding. Patients value staff who are kind, caring, patient, and compassionate. Such units want staff with a positive attitude, strong work ethic, and good communication skills. Professional qualities are needed to provide quality care and to work well with the team.

Rights and Respect
People often form opinions about others. Opinions may be based on life-style, appearance, or even a disease. Often this affects how the person is treated. For example, a staff member is more caring toward a person with cancer than a person with AIDS.

You cannot always control your opinions or feelings. However, they must not affect the care you give. Treat all persons with dignity and respect.

Independence and Social Interaction
Any illness affects the family. The person and family have many reactions—fear, anger, worry, guilt. This is especially true for persons with cancer, AIDS, and other immune system disorders. The person may have chronic health problems. Treatments require hospital stays and many appointments. Nursing center care or home care may be needed. Help and support are needed from the family.

Families respond in different ways. A helping and encouraging family provides motivation and support. Family bonds are stronger when the family shares responsibility and relies on each other during stress. The person's health and quality of life also benefit. Some families refuse to help. Or only 1 or 2 members help and support the person. This strains the family and places extra stress on the person.

Delegation and Teamwork
Some disorders are life-threatening. AIDS and some malignant tumors are examples. Caring for dying persons is a challenge. You may have emotions and responses similar to the family. The nursing team can give support. Share your feelings with the nursing team. Listen when others need to talk.

Continued

FOCUS ON **P R I D E**—cont'd

The Person, Family, and Yourself

E thics and Laws

Oncology staff often care for persons many times. Staff get to know the person well. They learn about likes, dislikes, and preferences. Staff learn about the person's family, school or work, hobbies, and so on. Interest in the person adds to quality of care.

However, staff must avoid crossing professional boundaries (Chapter 5). For example, a nursing assistant visits a patient during breaks and after work. She brings the person food from home. She talks badly about care given by other nursing assistants.

E thics and Laws—cont'd

These actions signal the crossing of professional boundaries. Maintaining these boundaries can be hard when caring for persons you see often and get to know well. However, you must protect the person's privacy and rights. Watch your behavior closely to avoid crossing boundaries. Tell the nurse if you suspect a person is crossing boundaries.

FOCUS ON **PRIDE**: *Application*

Many of the disorders in this chapter are life-changing. The disorder does not only affect the person. Choose 1 disorder in this chapter. Discuss the impact on the person and others.

REVIEW QUESTIONS

*Circle **T** if the statement is TRUE and **F** if it is FALSE.*

1 T F Lung cancer is more common in children than adults.

2 T F Cancer treatments damage healthy cells and tissues.

3 T F A person has a radiation implant. You are exposed to radiation when near the person.

4 T F For chemotherapy, agency policy may require double-bagging incontinence products.

5 T F A person has an autoimmune disorder. The person's body has attacked its own cells, tissues, and organs.

6 T F Celiac disease causes the thyroid gland to produce excess thyroid hormone.

7 T F Autoimmune disorders are usually chronic.

8 T F A person infected with HIV does not have signs and symptoms. The person can spread the virus to others.

9 T F Persons who have had chicken pox are at risk for shingles.

10 T F With shingles, a painful rash covers the body.

Circle the BEST answer.

11 A person has cancer. You know that
 a The tumor will not threaten life
 b The tumor can spread to other body parts
 c The tumor is benign
 d The person's mouth is inflamed

12 Who has the greatest risk of cancer?
 a The person who smokes
 b The person who is physically active
 c The person who limits time in the sun
 d The person who is 43 years old

13 Which is a general sign of cancer?
 a Painful, swollen joints   c A rash with blisters
 b Feeling very tired   d Weight gain

14 Care after cancer surgery will likely include
 a Pain-relief measures
 b Mouth care for stomatitis
 c Skin care for burns at the treatment site
 d Measures to prevent hair loss

15 Chemotherapy will likely cause
 a Burns
 b Skin breakdown
 c Nausea and vomiting
 d Weight gain

16 Mrs. Jones has cancer. She is telling you about her treatments and how she feels. You should
 a Change the subject
 b Call for the nurse
 c Ask about her feelings
 d Listen

17 HIV is spread through
 a Body fluids
 b Coughing and sneezing
 c Using public phones and restrooms
 d Hugging or dancing with an infected person

18 Which poses the *lowest* risk for HIV transmission?
 a Sex with an infected person
 b Needle-sharing
 c Sharing dishes with an infected person
 d Being born to an infected mother

19 HIV can be prevented by
 a Taking immuno-suppressive drugs
 b Getting an HIV vaccine
 c Using complementary and alternative medicine
 d Avoiding risky sexual behaviors

20 A person has shingles. You know that
 a Healing occurs in 3 to 5 days
 b Itching and pain are common
 c Lesions are not infectious
 d Antibiotics are used for treatment

Answers to Chapter 43 questions are on p. 872.

FOCUS ON **PRACTICE**

Problem Solving

You work for a home health agency. Your only visit today is a patient with AIDS. You notice that you have a slight cough and fever. Otherwise you feel well. What do you do? Do you go to work or call to say you cannot work today? Explain the reason for your decision.

Nervous System and Musculo-Skeletal Disorders

OBJECTIVES

- Define the key terms and key abbreviations in this chapter.
- Describe the care required for stroke, Parkinson's disease, multiple sclerosis, and amyotrophic lateral sclerosis.
- Describe the care required for traumatic brain injury, spinal cord injury, and autonomic hyperreflexia.
- Describe the care required for arthritis and osteoporosis.
- Explain how to assist in the care of persons after total joint replacement surgery.

- Explain how to assist in the care of persons in casts, in traction, and with hip fractures.
- Describe the effects of amputation.
- Explain how to promote PRIDE in the person, the family, and yourself.

KEY TERMS

amputation The removal of all or part of an extremity
arthritis Joint *(arthr)* inflammation *(itis)*
arthroplasty The surgical replacement *(plasty)* of a joint *(arthro)*
closed fracture The bone is broken but the skin is intact
compound fracture See "open fracture"
fracture A broken bone
gangrene A condition in which there is death of tissue
hemiplegia Paralysis *(plegia)* on 1 side *(hemi)* of the body
open fracture The broken bone has come through the skin; compound fracture

paralysis Loss of muscle function, sensation, or both
paraplegia Paralysis in the legs, lower trunk, and pelvic organs *(para* means *beyond; plegia* means *paralysis)*
quadriplegia Paralysis in the arms, legs, trunk, and pelvic organs *(quad* means *4; plegia* means *paralysis)*; tetraplegia
simple fracture The bone is broken in 1 place
tetraplegia See "quadriplegia" *(tetra* means *4; plegia* means *paralysis)*

KEY ABBREVIATIONS

ADL	Activities of daily living	**RA**	Rheumatoid arthritis
ALS	Amyotrophic lateral sclerosis	**ROM**	Range-of-motion
CVA	Cerebrovascular accident	**TBI**	Traumatic brain injury
JRA	Juvenile rheumatoid arthritis	**TIA**	Transient ischemic attack
MS	Multiple sclerosis		

Understanding nervous and musculo-skeletal disorders gives meaning to the required care. Refer to Chapter 10 while you study this chapter.

NERVOUS SYSTEM DISORDERS

Nervous system disorders can affect mental and physical function. They can affect the ability to speak, understand, feel, see, hear, touch, think, control bowels and bladder, and move.

See *Body Structure and Function Review: The Nervous System*, p. 706.

BODY STRUCTURE AND FUNCTION REVIEW
The Nervous System

The nervous system controls, directs, and coordinates body functions. It consists of the brain and spinal cord (Fig. 44-1) and nerves throughout the body.

Nerves connect to the spinal cord. Nerves carry messages or impulses to and from the brain. A *stimulus* causes a nerve impulse. A stimulus is anything that excites or causes a body part to function, become active, or respond. A *reflex* is the body's response (function or movement) to a stimulus. Reflexes are involuntary, unconscious, and immediate. The person cannot control reflexes.

Some nerve fibers have a protective covering called a *myelin sheath*. Nerve fibers covered with myelin conduct impulses faster than those fibers without it.

The Central Nervous System

The *brain* and *spinal cord* make up the central nervous system. The brain is covered by the skull. The 3 main parts of the brain are the *cerebrum,* the *cerebellum,* and the *brainstem* (Fig. 44-2).

The cerebrum is the center of thought and intelligence. The cerebrum is divided into 2 halves called *right* and *left hemispheres.* The right hemisphere controls movement and activities on the body's left side. The left hemisphere controls the right side.

The outside of the cerebrum is called the *cerebral cortex.* It controls reasoning, memory, consciousness, speech, voluntary muscle movement, vision, hearing, sensation, and other activities.

The cerebellum regulates and coordinates body movements. It controls balance and the smooth movements of voluntary muscles.

The brainstem contains the *midbrain, pons,* and *medulla.* The midbrain and pons relay messages between the medulla and the cerebrum. The medulla controls heart rate, breathing, blood vessel size, swallowing, coughing, and vomiting. The brain connects to the spinal cord at the lower end of the medulla.

The spinal cord lies within the spinal column. It contains pathways that conduct messages to and from the brain. The brain and spinal cord are covered and protected by 3 layers of connective tissue called *meninges.*

Cerebrospinal fluid circulates around the brain and spinal cord. Cerebrospinal fluid cushions shocks that could easily injure brain and spinal cord structures.

The Peripheral Nervous System

The peripheral nervous system has 12 pairs of *cranial nerves* and 31 pairs of *spinal nerves.* The cranial nerves conduct impulses between the brain and the head, neck, chest, and abdomen. They conduct impulses for smell, vision, hearing, pain, touch, temperature, and pressure. They also conduct impulses for voluntary and involuntary muscles. Spinal nerves carry impulses from the skin, extremities, and internal structures not supplied by the cranial nerves.

Some peripheral nerves form the *autonomic nervous system.* This system controls involuntary muscles and certain body functions—heartbeat, blood pressure, intestinal contractions, and glandular secretions.

The autonomic nervous system is divided into the *sympathetic nervous system* and the *parasympathetic nervous system.* They balance each other. The sympathetic nervous system speeds up functions. The parasympathetic nervous system slows functions.

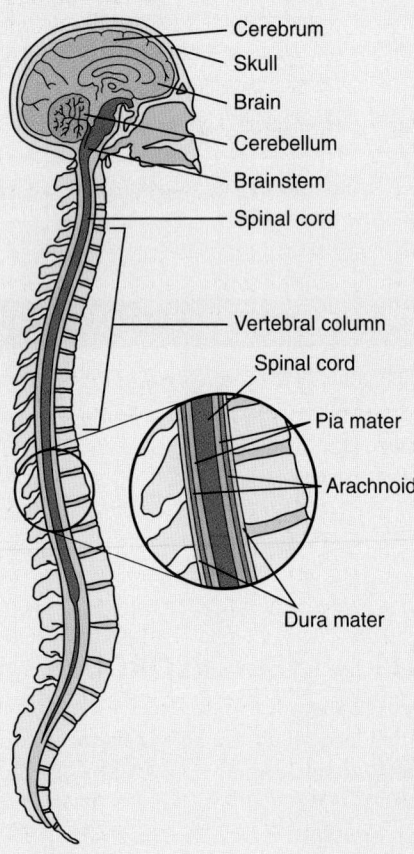

FIGURE 44-1 Central nervous system.

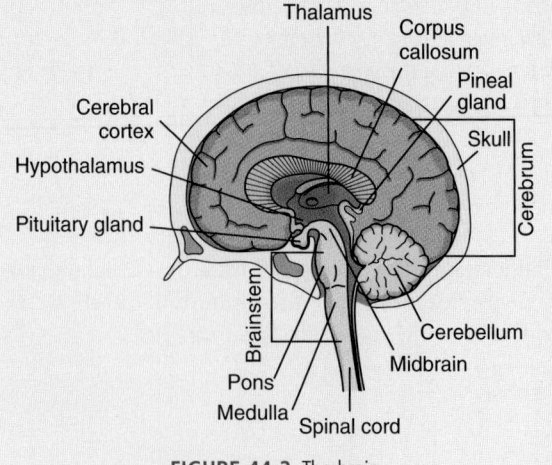

FIGURE 44-2 The brain.

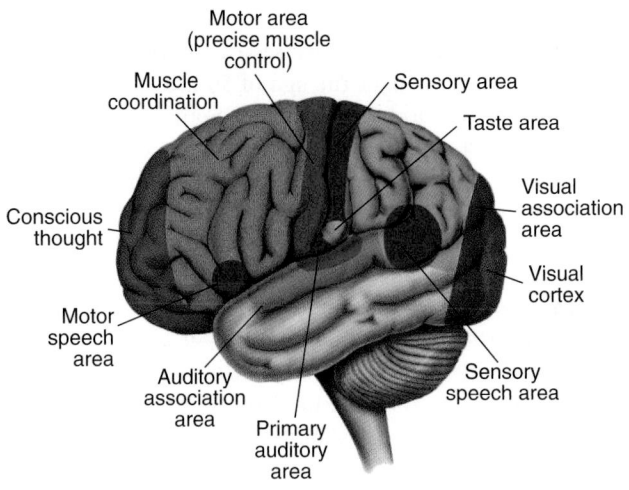

FIGURE 44-3 Functions lost from a stroke depend on the area of brain damage. (Modified from Thibodeau GA, Patton KT: *The human body in health & disease,* ed 6, St Louis, 2014, Mosby.)

| BOX 44-1 | Stroke—Warning Signs |

- Sudden numbness or weakness of the face, arm, or leg, especially on 1 side of the body
- Sudden confusion, trouble speaking or understanding speech
- Sudden trouble seeing in 1 or both eyes
- Sudden trouble walking, dizziness, loss of balance or coordination
- Sudden, severe headache with no known cause

From National Institute of Neurological Disorders and Stroke: Know stroke. Know the signs. Act in time. NIH Publication Number 08-4872, Bethesda, Md, January 2008, updated December 24, 2013, National Institutes of Health.

Stroke

Stroke (*brain attack* or *cerebrovascular accident [CVA]*) occurs when 1 of these happens.

- A blood vessel in the brain bursts and bleeds into the brain (cerebral hemorrhage).
- A blood clot blocks a blood vessel in the brain. Blood flow stops.

Brain cells in the affected area do not get enough oxygen and nutrients. Brain damage occurs. Functions controlled by that part of the brain are lost (Fig. 44-3).

Stroke is a leading cause of death in the United States. It is a leading cause of disability in adults. See Box 44-1 for warning signs. The person needs emergency care. Blood flow to the brain must be restored as soon as possible.

Warning signs may last a few minutes. This is called a *transient ischemic attack (TIA)*. (*Transient* means *temporary* or *short term*. *Ischemic* means *to hold back* [ischein] *blood* [hemic].) Blood supply to the brain is interrupted for a short time. A TIA may occur before a stroke. All stroke-like symptoms signal the need for emergency care.

Risk Factors. Risk factors include:

- High blood pressure
- Smoking
- Heart disease
- Diabetes
- High cholesterol
- TIAs
- Age 55 and older
- Being over-weight
- Lack of physical activity
- Family history of stroke

Signs and Symptoms. Stroke can occur suddenly. The person may have warning signs (see Box 44-1). The person also may have nausea, vomiting, and memory loss. Unconsciousness, noisy breathing, high blood pressure, slow pulse, redness of the face, and seizures may occur. So can *hemiplegia—paralysis* (plegia) *on 1 side* (hemi) *of the body.* The person may lose bowel and bladder control and the ability to speak. (See "Aphasia" in Chapter 42.)

Effects on the Person. If the person survives, some brain damage is likely. The entire body may be affected. Functions lost depend on the area of brain damage (see Figure 44-3). They include:

- Loss of face, hand, arm, leg, or body control
- Hemiplegia
- Changing emotions (crying easily or mood swings sometimes for no reason)
- Difficulty swallowing (dysphagia)
- Aphasia or slowed or slurred speech (Chapter 42)
- Changes in sight, touch, movement, and thought
- Impaired memory
- Urinary frequency, urgency, or incontinence
- Loss of bowel control or constipation
- Depression and frustration
- Behavior changes

The person may forget about or ignore the weaker side. This is called *neglect.* It is from the loss of vision or movement and feeling on that side. Sometimes thinking is affected. The person may not recognize or know how to use common items. Activities of daily living (ADL) and other tasks are hard to do. The person may forget what to do and how to do it. If the person does know, the body may not respond.

Rehabilitation starts at once. The goal is to regain the highest possible level of function (Box 44-2, p. 708).

See *Focus on Long-Term Care and Home Care: Effects on the Person (Stroke),* p. 708.

BOX 44-2   Stroke Care Measures

- Position the person in the lateral (side-lying) position to prevent aspiration.
- Keep the bed in semi-Fowler's position.
- Approach the person from the strong (unaffected) side. Place objects on the strong (unaffected side). The person may have loss of vision on the affected side.
- Turn and re-position the person at least every 2 hours.
- Use assist devices to move, turn, re-position, and transfer the person.
- Encourage incentive spirometry and deep breathing and coughing.
- Prevent contractures. Assist with range-of-motion (ROM) exercises.
- Meet food and fluid needs. The person may need a dysphagia diet.
- Apply elastic stockings to prevent thrombi (blood clots) in the legs.
- Meet elimination needs. Follow the care plan for:
  - Catheter care or bladder training
  - Bowel training
- Practice safety precautions.
  - Keep the call light and other needed items within reach on the strong (unaffected) side.
  - Check the person often if he or she cannot use the call light. Follow the care plan.
  - Use bed rails according to the care plan.
  - Prevent falls and other injuries.
- Have the person do as much self-care as possible. This includes turning, positioning, and transferring. The person uses assistive (adaptive) and walking aids as needed.
- Do not rush the person. Movements are slower after a stroke.
- Follow established communication methods.
- Give support, encouragement, and praise.
- Complete a safety check before leaving the room. (See the inside of the front cover.)

FOCUS ON LONG-TERM CARE AND HOME CARE

Effects on the Person (Stroke)

Long-Term Care
Some persons return home after rehabilitation. For others, long-term care is often permanent. Many measures listed in Box 44-2 are part of the person's care.

Home Care
Many stroke survivors return home. The family assists with care. Home health care is often needed. The measures in Box 44-2 continue. The health team recommends home changes to help the person function.

Parkinson's Disease

Parkinson's disease is a progressive disorder affecting movement. Persons over the age of 50 are at risk. One or both sides of the body are affected. Signs and symptoms are mild at first (Fig. 44-4). They include:

- *Tremors*—often start in the hand. Pill-rolling movements—rubbing the thumb and index finger—may occur. The person may have trembling in the hands, arms, legs, jaw, and face.
- *Rigid, stiff muscles*—in the arms, legs, neck, and trunk.
- *Stooped posture and impaired balance*—it is hard to walk. Falls are a risk.
- *Mask-like expression*—the person cannot blink and smile. A fixed stare is common.

Other signs and symptoms develop over time. They include swallowing and chewing problems, constipation, sleep problems, depression, and emotional changes (fear, insecurity). Memory loss and slow thinking can occur. The person may have slow, monotone, and soft speech.

With no cure, drugs are ordered to control the disease. Exercise and physical therapy help improve strength, posture, balance, and mobility. Therapy is needed for speech and swallowing problems. The person may need help with eating and self-care. Normal elimination is a goal. Safety measures are needed to prevent falls and injuries.

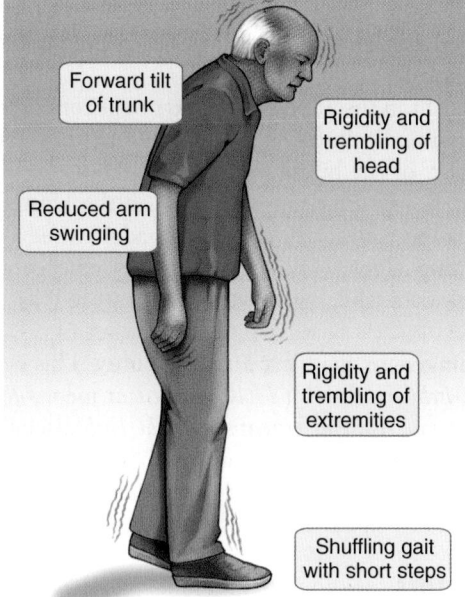

FIGURE 44-4 Signs of Parkinson's disease. (From Thibodeau GA, Patton KT: *The human body in health & disease*, ed 6, St Louis, 2014, Mosby.)

Multiple Sclerosis

Multiple sclerosis (MS) is a central nervous system disease. *Multiple* means *many*. *Sclerosis* means *hardening or scarring*. The myelin (which covers nerve fibers) in the brain and spinal cord is destroyed. Nerve impulses are not sent to and from the brain in a normal way. Functions are impaired or lost.

Symptoms usually start between the ages of 20 and 40. Women and whites are at greater risk than other groups. The risk increases if a family member has MS. Signs and symptoms may include:

- Blurred or double vision; blindness in 1 eye
- Muscle weakness in the arms and legs
- Balance and coordination problems
- Tingling, prickling, or numb sensations
- Partial or complete paralysis
- Pain
- Speech problems
- Tremors
- Dizziness
- Concentration, attention, memory, and judgment problems
- Depression
- Bladder problems
- Problems with sexual function
- Hearing loss
- Fatigue

MS can present in many ways. For example:

- Symptoms appear for a while then seem to go away. The person is in *remission*. Later, symptoms flare up again *(relapse)*.
- More symptoms appear. The person's condition worsens.
- The person has remissions and relapses at first. Eventually symptoms become worse. More symptoms occur with each flare-up. The person's condition declines.

MS has no cure. Some drugs can slow the disease. Persons with MS are kept as active and as independent as possible. The care plan reflects changing needs. Skin care, hygiene, and ROM exercises are important. So are turning, positioning, and deep breathing and coughing. Elimination needs are met. Injuries and complications from bedrest are prevented.

See *Focus on Long-Term Care and Home Care: Multiple Sclerosis*.

FOCUS ON LONG-TERM CARE AND HOME CARE

Multiple Sclerosis

Home Care

The person may need help with housekeeping to avoid fatigue. As mobility decreases, the person depends more on others. Occupational and physical therapists are often involved in the person's care.

Amyotrophic Lateral Sclerosis

Amyotrophic lateral sclerosis (ALS) attacks the nerve cells that control voluntary muscles. Commonly called Lou Gehrig's disease, it is rapidly progressive and fatal. (Lou Gehrig was a New York Yankees baseball player who died of the disease.)

ALS usually strikes persons between 40 and 60 years of age. Most die 2 to 5 years after onset.

The disease attacks the nerve cells responsible for voluntary muscles. Such cells are in the brain, brainstem, and spinal cord. These cells stop sending messages to the muscles. The muscles weaken, waste away (atrophy), and twitch. Over time, the brain cannot start voluntary movements or control them. The person cannot move the arms, legs, and body. Muscles for speaking, chewing and swallowing, and breathing also are affected. Eventually respiratory muscles fail. The person needs a ventilator to breathe (Chapter 40).

The disease usually does not affect the mind, intelligence, or memory. However, some persons develop dementia. Sight, smell, taste, hearing, and touch are not affected. Usually bowel and bladder functions remain intact.

ALS has no cure. Some drugs can slow the disease and improve symptoms. However, damage cannot be reversed. The person is kept active and independent to the extent possible. The care plan reflects changing needs. It may include:

- Physical, occupational, and speech-language therapies
- ROM exercises
- Mobility aides—braces, walker, wheelchair
- Comfort and pain-relief measures
- Communication methods
- Dysphagia diet or feeding tube
- Respiratory support—suctioning, mechanical ventilation
- Safety measures to prevent falls and injuries
- Psychological and social support
- Hospice care

Head Injuries

Head injuries result from trauma to the scalp, skull, or brain. Injuries range from a minor bump to a serious, life-threatening brain injury. Traffic accidents, falls, assaults, and gunshots are common causes. So are home, work, sports, and outdoor accidents.

Head injuries are open or closed. Bleeding may occur.

- Closed—a hard blow to the head did not break the skull.
- Open (penetrating)—an object broke the skull and entered the brain.

Symptoms may develop at the time of the injury. Or they can take several hours or days to develop. Symptoms are from bleeding or swelling inside the skull.

Most head injuries need emergency care. See Chapter 54.

Traumatic Brain Injury. Traumatic brain injury (TBI) occurs from violent injury to the brain—bumps, blows, or jolts to the head or penetrating injuries. Common causes include:

- *Falls.* Older persons and children are at risk for falling out of bed, slipping in the shower or bathtub, falling down steps, and falling from ladders.
- *Traffic accidents.* Cars, motorcycles, and bikes are often involved. Persons who were walking or jogging have been involved.
- *Violence.* Gunshots, intimate partner violence (Chapter 5), and child abuse can result in TBI.
- *Sports.* Many sports increase the risk of TBI—football, soccer, boxing, baseball, hockey, lacrosse, skateboarding, and other high-impact sports.
- *Explosive blasts and combat injuries.* TBI can occur from penetrating injuries, blows to the head, and falls. Military personnel are at risk.

TBI results in bruised or torn brain tissue. Bleeding is in the brain or in nearby tissues. Spinal cord injuries are likely.

Men, infants and children, young adults, and older persons are at risk for TBI. Death can occur at the time of injury or later. See Box 44-3 for the signs and symptoms of TBI.

If the person survives, some permanent damage is likely. Disabilities depend on the severity and site of injury. They include:

- Cognitive problems—thinking, memory, and reasoning.
- Sensory problems—sight, hearing, touch, taste, and smell.
- Communication problems—expressing or understanding language.
- Emotional problems—depression, anxiety, personality changes, aggressive behavior, acting out, socially inappropriate behavior.
- Changes in level of consciousness:
  - Coma—the person is unconscious, does not respond, is unaware, and cannot be aroused.
  - Vegetative state—the person is unconscious and unaware of surroundings. He or she has sleep-wake cycles and may open the eyes, make sounds, or move. The person cannot speak or follow commands.
  - Brain death (Fig. 44-5). Despite complete loss of brain function, the heart continues to beat. Reflex activity, movement, and spontaneous respirations are absent.

Emergency care involves drugs and surgery to limit brain damage. Rehabilitation is required. Physical, occupational, speech-language, and mental health therapies depend on the person's needs. Nursing care depends on the person's needs and abilities.

See *Focus on Children and Older Persons: Traumatic Brain Injury.*

BOX 44-3	Traumatic Brain Injury—Signs and Symptoms

Mild TBI
- Loss of consciousness: a few seconds to a few minutes
- Being dazed, confused, or disoriented
- Headache
- Nausea or vomiting
- Fatigue or drowsiness
- Problems sleeping; sleeping more than usual
- Dizziness
- Loss of balance
- Blurred vision
- Ringing in the ears
- Bad taste in the mouth
- Sensitivity to light and sound
- Memory and concentration problems
- Mood changes or mood swings
- Depression
- Anxiety

Moderate to Severe TBI
- See "Mild TBI"
- Loss of consciousness: several minutes to hours
- Headache: persistent or worsens
- Nausea and vomiting: repeated
- Convulsions or seizures
- Large eye pupil: 1 or both eyes
- Clear fluids draining from the nose or ears
- Inability to wake up
- Weakness or numbness: fingers and toes
- Coordination: loss of
- Confusion
- Behavior: unusual—agitation, combativeness, other
- Speech: slurred

Modified from Mayo Clinic: Diseases and conditions: traumatic brain injury, May 15, 2014.

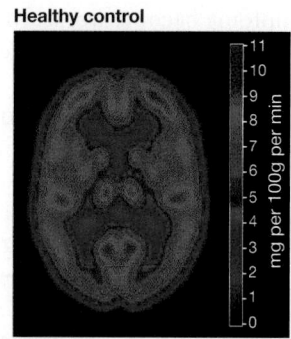

Healthy control

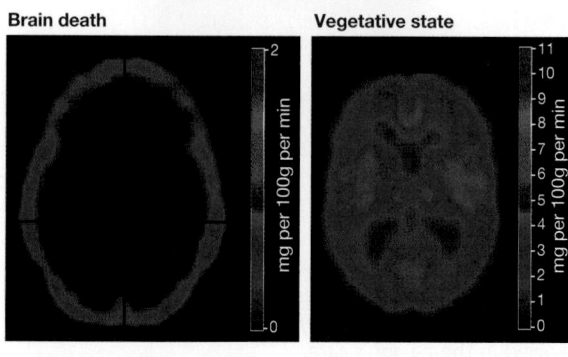

Brain death   **Vegetative state**

FIGURE 44-5 Altered consciousness. (Images courtesy *Nature Reviews Neuroscience*, McMillan Publishers Limited, 2014.)

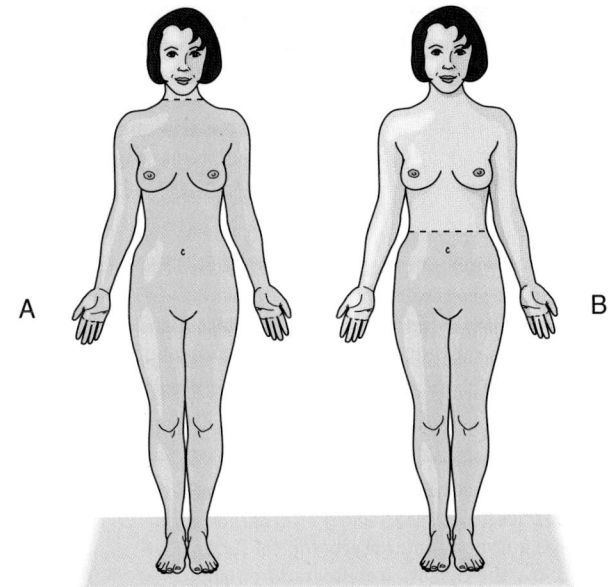

FIGURE 44-6 The *shaded areas* show the area of paralysis. **A,** Quadriplegia (tetraplegia). **B,** Paraplegia.

Spinal Cord Injury

A spinal cord injury usually results from a sudden, traumatic blow to the spine. The trauma fractures or dislocates vertebrae in the spine. Spinal cord tissue is torn or bruised. Spinal cord injuries can seriously damage the nervous system. *Paralysis (loss of muscle function, sensation, or both)* can result. Emergency care is needed.

Young adult men have the highest risk. Common causes are traffic accidents, falls, violence (knife and gunshot wounds), sports injuries, alcohol use, cancer and other diseases.

Problems depend on the amount of damage to the spinal cord and the level of injury. Damage to the spinal cord may be incomplete or complete.

- Incomplete—some sensory (feeling) and muscle (movement) function below the level of the injury remains.
- Complete—no sensory or muscle function below the level of the injury remains.

The higher the level of injury, the more functions lost (Fig. 44-6).

- Lumbar injuries—occur in the low back. Sensory and muscle function in the legs is lost. The person has paraplegia. *Paraplegia is paralysis in the legs, lower trunk, and pelvic organs.* (Para *means* beyond; plegia *means* paralysis).
- Thoracic injuries—occur in the middle and upper back. Sensory and muscle function below the chest is lost. The person has paraplegia.
- Cervical injuries—occur at the neck. Sensory and muscle function of the arms, legs, and trunk is lost. *Paralysis in the arms, legs, trunk, and pelvic organs is called* **quadriplegia** *or* **tetraplegia.** (Quad *and* tetra *mean* 4. Plegia *means* paralysis.)

The person with a spinal cord injury has 1 or more of these signs and symptoms.

- Loss of movement
- Loss of sensation—heat, cold, touch
- Bladder and fecal incontinence
- Problems with balance and walking
- Breathing problems
- Odd position or twisted neck or back

Cervical traction with a special bed may be needed (p. 719). The spine is kept straight at all times. See Box 44-4, p. 712 for care measures. Emotional needs are great. Reactions to paralysis and loss of function are often severe.

If the person lives, rehabilitation is needed. Some agencies focus on spinal cord injuries. The person learns to function at the highest possible level with adaptive (assistive) and other devices. Some persons live independently at home or with home care. Others need long-term care or assisted-living settings.

BOX 44-4   Care of Persons With Paralysis

- Practice safety measures to prevent falls. Use bed rails as directed.
- Keep the bed in a low position. Follow the care plan.
- Keep the call light and other needed items within reach. If unable to use the call light, check the person often.
- Prevent burns. Check bath water, heat applications, and food for proper temperature.
- Turn (logroll) and re-position the person at least every 2 hours.
- Prevent pressure ulcers. Follow the care plan.
- Use supportive devices to maintain good alignment.
- Follow bowel and bladder training programs.
- Keep intake and output records.
- Maintain muscle function and prevent contractures. Assist with ROM exercises.
- Assist with food and fluid needs as needed. Provide adaptive (assistive) devices as ordered.
- Give emotional and psychological support.
- Follow the person's rehabilitation plan.
- Complete a safety check of the room. (See the inside of the front cover.)

BOX 44-5   Preventing Autonomic Hyperreflexia

- Monitor urinary output.
- Follow measures for catheter care. Do not let the drainage bag get too full.
- Prevent urinary tract infections.
- Promote bowel elimination. Prevent constipation and fecal impaction.
- Prevent skin injuries—skin tears, pressure ulcers, cuts, bruises, burns, and so on.
- Check the feet for ingrown toenails, blisters, pressure ulcers, and so on.
- Have the person wear loose and comfortable clothing.
- Remove wrinkles from clothing and linens.
- Re-position the person at least every 2 hours. Avoid prolonged pressure from the bed or chair.
- Report complaints of pain and menstrual cramps.

Autonomic Hyperreflexia. This syndrome occurs with spinal cord injuries above the mid-thoracic (middle back) level. The autonomic nervous system over-reacts to a stimulus. A full bladder, constipation, fecal impaction, and skin disorders are examples. Causing the sudden onset of excessively high blood pressure, stroke, seizures, heart attack, and death are risks. Report any of the following at once.

- High blood pressure
- Headache: throbbing or pounding
- Pulse: slow or rapid; irregular
- Blurred vision
- Sweating
- Skin and face: flushing, reddening
- Cold, clammy skin
- "Goose bumps"
- Nasal congestion
- Nausea
- Anxiety
- Dizziness
- Fainting
- Bowel or bladder problems
- Restlessness

For treatment, the head of the bed is raised or the person sits upright if allowed. Tight clothing is removed. And the cause is treated. See Box 44-5.

See *Promoting Safety and Comfort: Autonomic Hyperreflexia.*

PROMOTING SAFETY AND COMFORT
Autonomic Hyperreflexia

Safety
Constipation and fecal impaction can cause autonomic hyperreflexia. So can checking for an impaction or giving enemas. Do not perform these procedures if the person is at risk for the syndrome. The procedures are best done by a nurse.

MUSCULO-SKELETAL DISORDERS

Musculo-skeletal disorders affect movement. Injury and aging are common causes. Daily living, social activities, and quality of life are affected.

See *Body Structure and Function Review: The Musculo-Skeletal System.*

Arthritis

Arthritis means joint (arthr) *inflammation* (itis). Pain, swelling, stiffness, and reduced range of motion occur in the affected joints. The joints are hard to move.

The 2 main types of arthritis are:
- *Osteoarthritis.* Cartilage covering the ends of bones wears away, allowing the bones to rub together. The hands, knees, hips, and spine are often affected (Fig. 44-8).
- *Rheumatoid arthritis (RA).* An autoimmune disease (Chapter 43), RA attacks the lining of the joint. Wrist and finger joints are commonly affected. RA can also affect the neck, shoulders, elbows, hips, knees, ankles, and feet. RA occurs on both sides of the body. For example, if the right wrist is affected, so is the left wrist. Besides joint symptoms, RA can cause fever and fatigue. Sometimes other body parts are affected—decreased red blood cell production; dry eyes and mouth; and inflammation of the linings of the blood vessels, lungs, and heart.

BODY STRUCTURE AND FUNCTION REVIEW

The Musculo-Skeletal System

Bones

Bones are hard, rigid structures.
- *Long bones* bear the body's weight. Leg bones are long bones.
- *Short bones* allow skill and ease in movement. Bones in the wrists, fingers, ankles, and toes are short bones.
- *Flat bones* protect the organs. They include the ribs, skull, pelvic bones, and shoulder blades.
- *Irregular bones* are the vertebrae in the spinal column. They allow various degrees of movement and flexibility.

Joints

A *joint* is the point at which 2 or more bones meet (Fig. 44-7). Joints allow movement (Chapter 30).
- *Ball-and-socket joint* allows movement in all directions. The rounded end of 1 bone fits into the hollow end of another bone. The hips and shoulders are ball-and-socket joints.
- *Hinge joint* allows movement in 1 direction. The elbow is a hinge joint.
- *Pivot joint* allows turning from side to side. A pivot joint connects the skull to the spine.

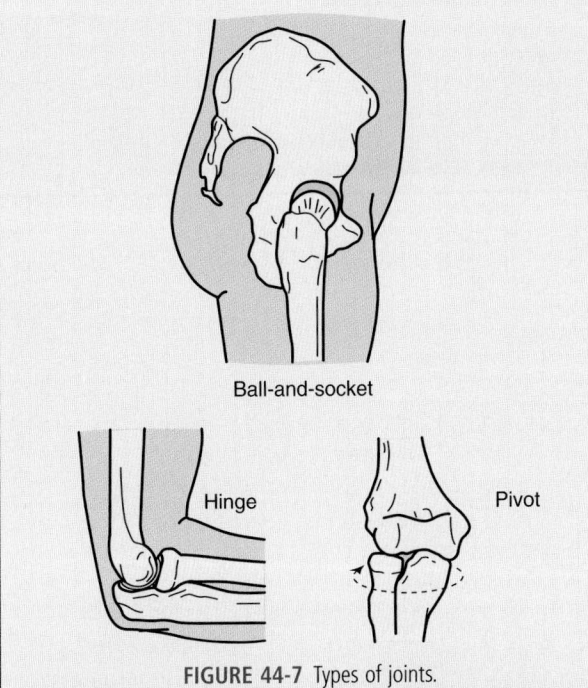

Ball-and-socket

Hinge   Pivot

FIGURE 44-7 Types of joints.

Risk Factors. Arthritis risk factors include:
- *Aging.* The risk increases with age.
- *Being over-weight.* Stress is placed on the weight-bearing joints—knees, hips, and spine.
- *Gender.* RA is more common in women than in men.
- *Joint injury.* A previous joint injury may develop into arthritis.
- *Family history.* Arthritis tends to run in families.

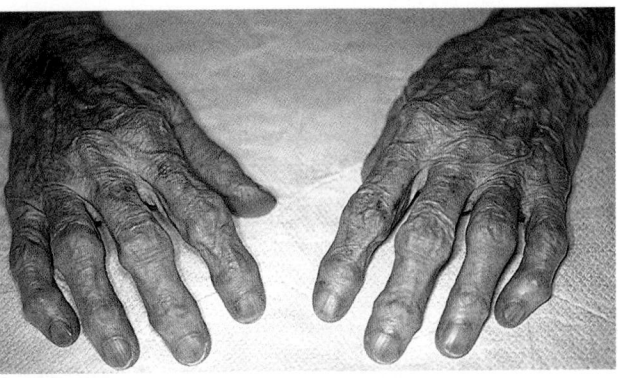

FIGURE 44-8 Bony growths called *Heberden nodes* occur in the finger joints. (From Swartz MH: *Textbook of physical diagnosis,* ed 6, Philadelphia, 2010, Saunders.)

Treatment. Osteoarthritis and RA have no cure. They have similar treatments.
- *Pain control.* Drugs decrease swelling and inflammation and relieve pain.
- *Heat and cold.* Heat relieves pain, increases blood flow, and reduces swelling. Heat applications and water therapy in a heated pool are helpful. Sometimes cold is applied after joint use to reduce swelling and relieve pain.
- *Exercise.* Exercise helps joint flexibility. It helps with weight control and promotes fitness. The person is taught what exercises to do. Swimming and water aerobics reduce stress on the weight-bearing joints.
- *Rest and joint care.* Good body mechanics, posture, and regular rest protect the joints. Relaxation methods are helpful.
- *Assistive (adaptive) devices.* Canes and walkers provide support. Splints support weak joints and promote alignment. Adaptive (assistive) devices for hands and wrists are useful.
- *Weight control.* Weight loss reduces stress on weight-bearing joints. And it helps prevent further joint injury.
- *Healthy life-style.* Arthritis support programs focus on abilities and strengths. Fitness, exercise, rest, managing stress, and good nutrition are stressed.
- *Safety.* Falls are prevented. Help is given with ADL as needed. Toilet seat risers are helpful when hips and knees are affected. So are chairs with higher seats and armrests.
- *Joint replacement surgery.* **Arthroplasty** *is the surgical replacement* (plasty) *of a joint* (arthro). The damaged joint is removed and replaced with an artificial joint (prosthesis). See Figure 44-9, p. 714. Hip and knee replacements are common. Ankle, foot, shoulder, elbow, and finger joints also can be replaced. The surgery is done to relieve pain, restore joint function, or correct a deformed joint. See Box 44-6, p. 714 for care measures following joint replacement surgery. See *Focus on Children and Older Persons: Arthritis,* p. 714.

Text continued on p. 716.

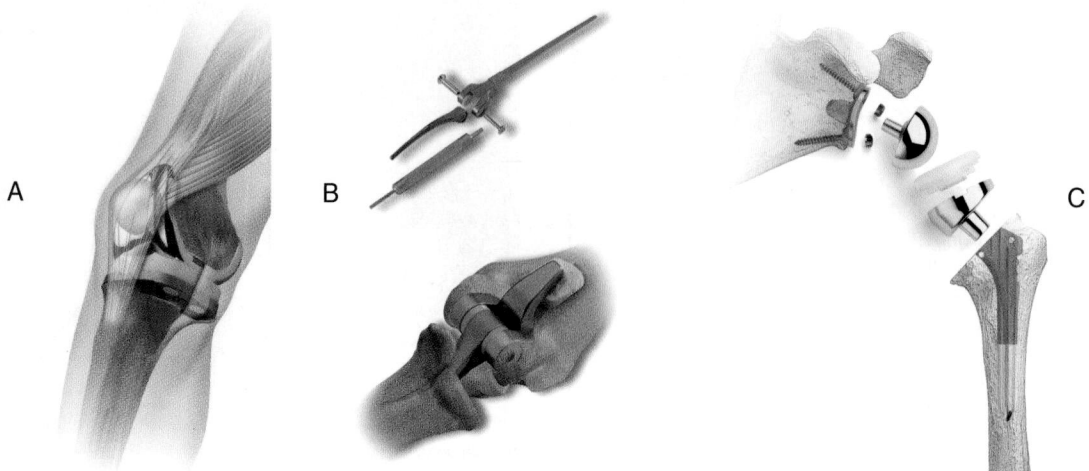

FIGURE 44-9 A, Knee replacement prosthesis. **B,** Elbow replacement prosthesis. **C,** Shoulder replacement prosthesis. (Courtesy Zimmer, Inc., A Bristol-Meyers Squibb Company, Warsaw, Ind.)

BOX 44-6	Care After Total Joint Replacement— Hip and Knee

- Incentive spirometry and deep-breathing and coughing exercises to prevent respiratory complications.
- Elastic stockings to prevent thrombi (blood clots) in the legs.
- Physical therapy and exercises to strengthen the hip or knee.
- Measures to protect the hip as shown in Figure 44-10.
- Food and fluids for tissue healing and to restore strength.
- Safety measures to prevent falls.
- Measures to prevent infection. Wound, urinary tract, and skin infections must be prevented.
- Measures to prevent pressure ulcers.
- Assist devices for moving, turning, re-positioning, and transfers.
- Long-handled device for reaching things.
- Assistance with walking and a walking aid—cane, walker, or crutches.

FOCUS ON CHILDREN AND OLDER PERSONS

Arthritis

Children

RA in children is called juvenile rheumatoid arthritis (JRA). Signs and symptoms include:
- Swollen, painful, and stiff joints
- Fever
- Rash
- Swollen lymph nodes

More common in girls, JRA can affect growth and development. Eye inflammation is a complication.

Do   **Do Not**

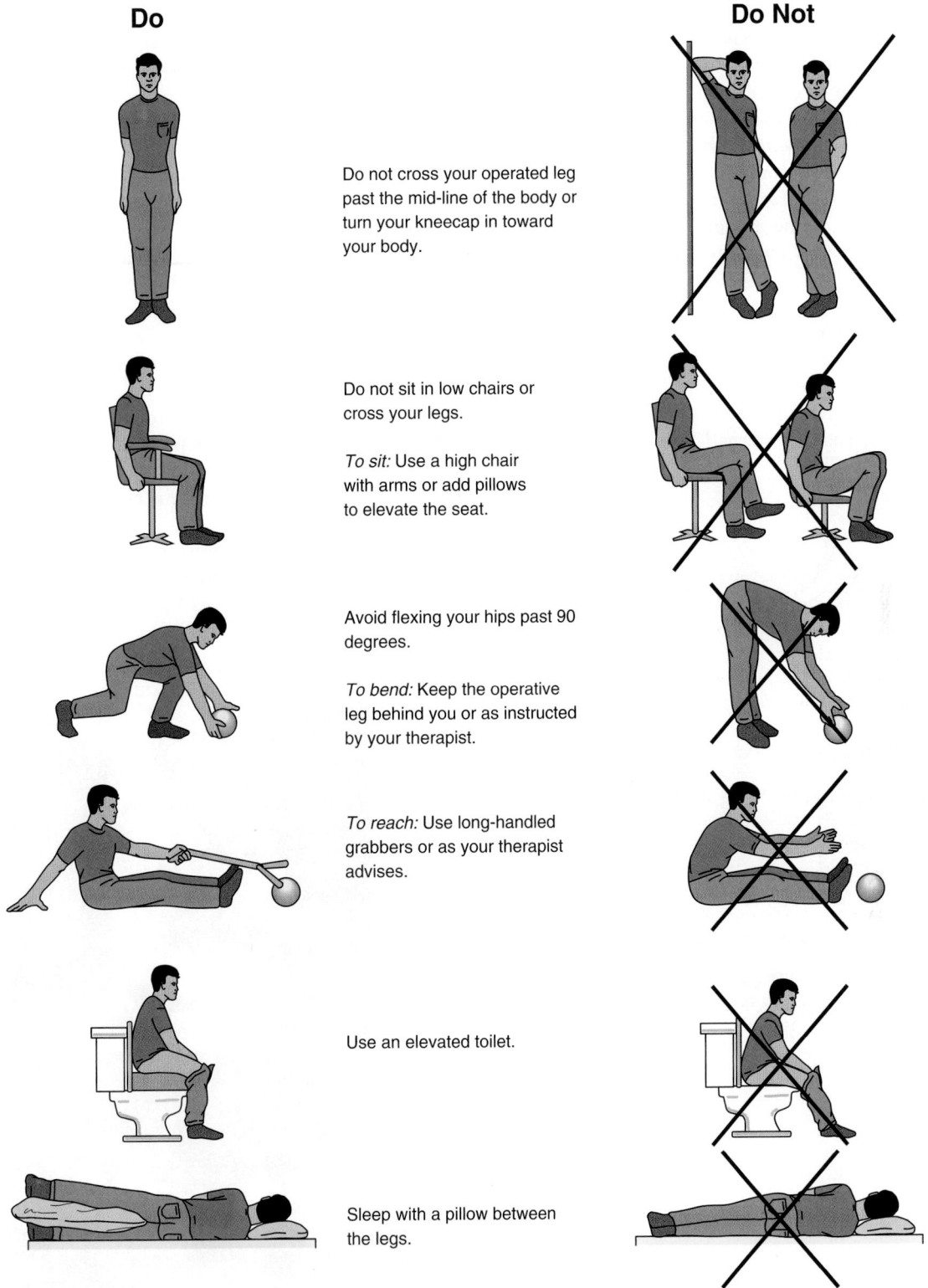

Do not cross your operated leg past the mid-line of the body or turn your kneecap in toward your body.

Do not sit in low chairs or cross your legs.

To sit: Use a high chair with arms or add pillows to elevate the seat.

Avoid flexing your hips past 90 degrees.

To bend: Keep the operative leg behind you or as instructed by your therapist.

To reach: Use long-handled grabbers or as your therapist advises.

Use an elevated toilet.

Sleep with a pillow between the legs.

FIGURE 44-10 Measures to protect the hip after hip replacement surgery. (Modified from Monahan FD and others: *Phipps' medical-surgical nursing: health and illness perspectives,* ed 8, St Louis, 2007, Mosby.)

Fractures

A *fracture* is a broken bone. Tissues around the fracture—muscles, blood vessels, nerves, and tendons—are injured. Fractures are open or closed (Fig. 44-11).

- *Simple fracture*—the bone is broken in 1 place.
- *Open fracture (compound fracture)*—the broken bone has come through the skin.
- *Closed fracture*—the bone is broken but the skin is intact.

Falls, accidents, bone tumors, and osteoporosis are some causes. Signs and symptoms of a fracture are:

- Pain
- Swelling
- Loss of function or movement
- Movement where motion should not occur
- Deformity (abnormal position of the part)
- Bruising and skin color changes at the fracture site
- Bleeding (internal or external)

For healing, bone ends are brought into and held in normal position. This is called *reduction and fixation*.

- Reduction—the bone is moved back into place. Reduction is closed or open.
  - Closed reduction—the bone is not exposed.
  - Open reduction—the bone is surgically exposed and moved into alignment.
- Fixation—the bone is held in place. Fixation is external or internal.
  - External fixation—Pins, screws, or wires are set into the bone above and below the fracture. They are held in place by a ring or bar outside the skin (Fig. 44-12). The device is removed after healing. Or it is used for a short time until the person is healthy enough for surgery.
  - Internal fixation—Nails, rods, pins, screws, plates, or wires are surgically placed to keep the bone in place. The device is under the skin (Fig. 44-13). After healing, the device is either left in place or removed.

Casts, traction, splints, and walking boots also are used. Healing takes 3 to 8 weeks.

See *Focus on Children and Older Persons: Fractures.*

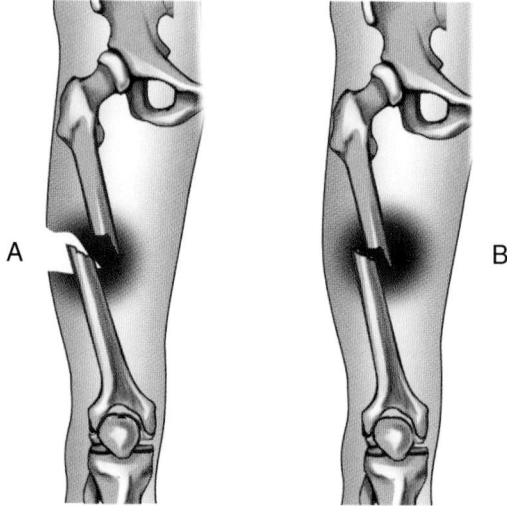

FIGURE 44-11 A, Open fracture. **B,** Closed fracture. (From Thibodeau GA, Patton KT: *The human body in health & disease,* ed 6, St Louis, 2014, Mosby.)

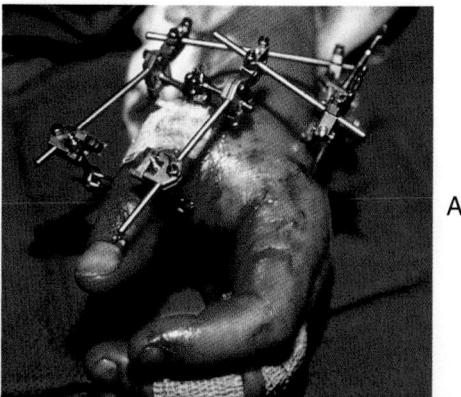

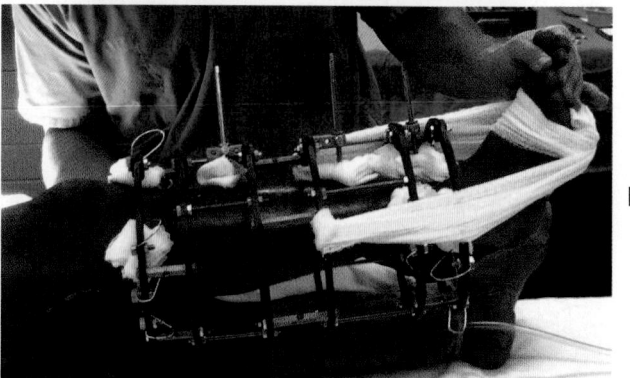

FIGURE 44-12 External fixators. (From Lewis SM and others: *Medical-surgical nursing: assessment and management of clinical problems,* ed 9, St Louis, 2014, Mosby.)

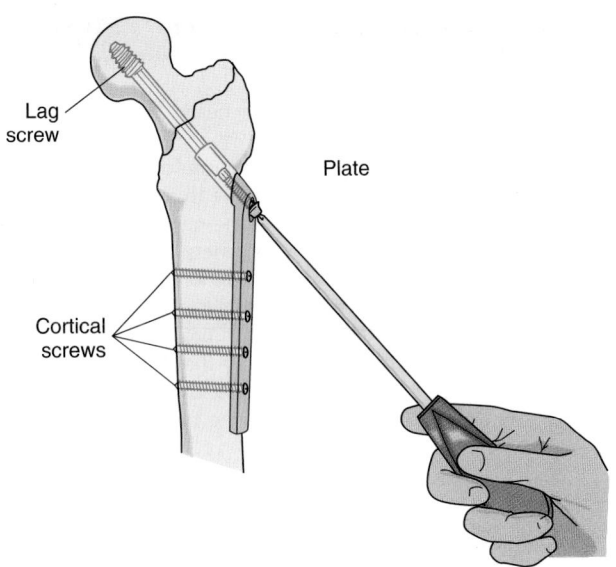

FIGURE 44-13 Devices used for internal fixation of a fracture. (From Monahan FD and others: *Phipps' medical-surgical nursing: health and illness perspectives,* ed 8, St Louis, 2007, Mosby.)

Casts. Casts are made of plaster of Paris, plastic, or fiberglass (Fig. 44-14). Before casting, the part is protected with stockinette and cotton padding. Moistened cast rolls are wrapped around the part. Plastic and fiberglass casts dry quickly. A plaster of Paris cast dries in 24 to 48 hours. It is odorless, white, and shiny when dry. When wet, it is gray and cool and has a musty smell. The nurse may ask you to assist with care (Box 44-7, p. 718).

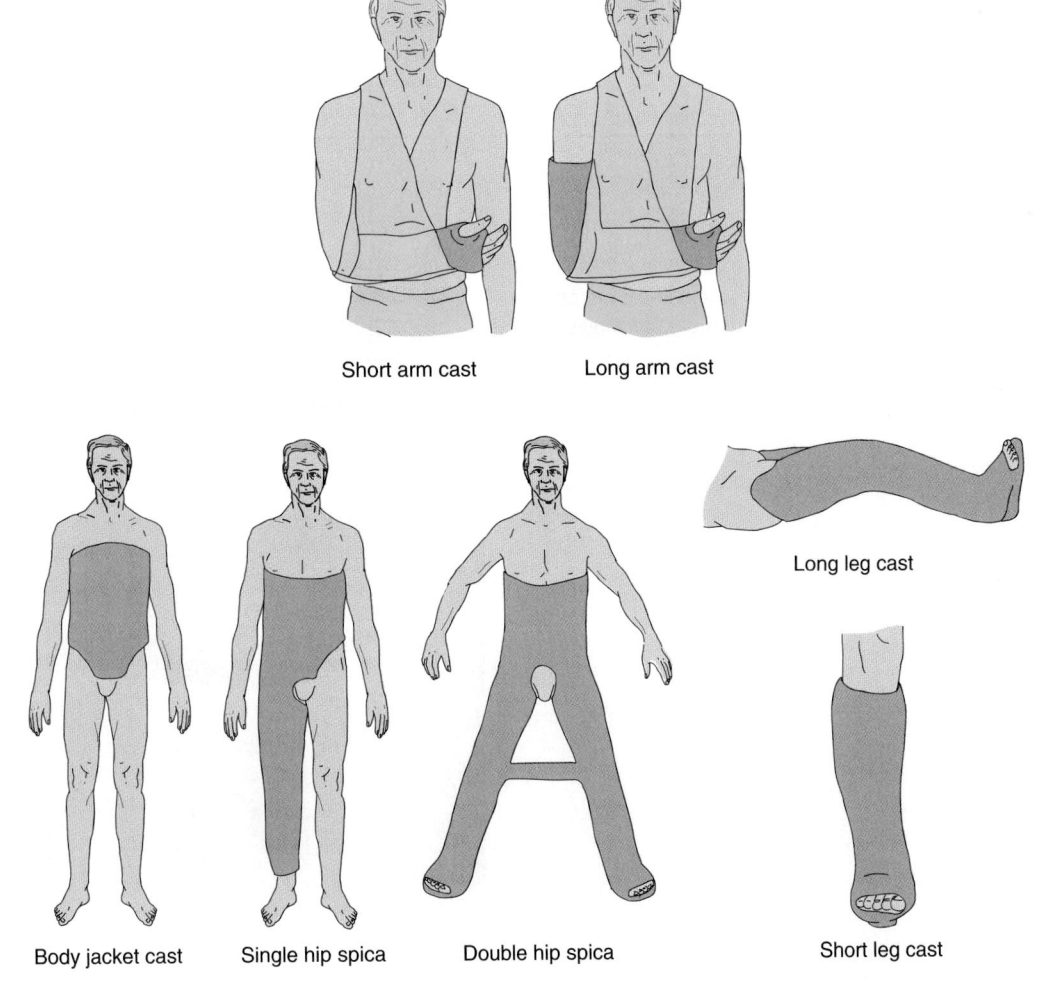

Short arm cast   Long arm cast

Long leg cast

Body jacket cast   Single hip spica   Double hip spica   Short leg cast

FIGURE 44-14 Common casts.

BOX 44-7	Cast Care

The Cast

- Do not cover the cast with blankets, plastic, or other material. A cast gives off heat as it dries. Covers prevent the escape of heat. Burns can occur if heat cannot escape.
- Promote drying of the cast. Turn the person every 2 hours or as directed. All cast surfaces need exposure to air.
- Maintain the shape of the cast.
  - Do not place a wet cast on a hard surface. It flattens the cast.
  - Use pillows to support the entire length of the cast (Fig. 44-15).
  - Support the wet cast with your palms to turn and position the person (Fig. 44-16). Fingertips can dent the cast. The dents can cause pressure areas and skin breakdown.
  - Report rough cast edges. The nurse needs to cover the cast edges with tape.
  - Keep the cast dry. A wet cast loses its shape. For casts near the perineal area, the nurse may apply a waterproof material after the cast dries.
- Do not remove stockinette or padding around the cast edges.

Positioning

- Position the person as directed.
- Elevate a casted arm or leg on pillows to reduce swelling.
- Have enough help to turn and re-position the person. Plaster casts are heavy and awkward. Balance is lost easily.

Safety

- Follow the care plan for elimination needs. Some persons use a fracture pan.
- Do not let the person insert anything into the cast. Itching under the cast causes an intense desire to scratch. Items used for scratching can open the skin—pencils, coat hangers, knitting needles, back scratchers, and so on. Infection is a risk. Scratching items can wrinkle the stockinette or cotton padding. Or they can be lost into the cast. Both can cause pressure and skin breakdown.
- Do not put powder on the skin under the cast.
- Do not let the person put rings on the fingers or toes.
- Complete a safety check before leaving the room. (See the inside of the front cover.)

Reporting and Recording

- Report these signs and symptoms at once.
  - *Pain*—pressure ulcer, poor circulation, nerve damage
  - *Swelling and a tight cast*—reduced blood flow to the part
  - *Pale skin*—reduced blood flow to the part
  - *Cyanosis (bluish skin color)*—reduced blood flow to the part
  - *Odor*—infection
  - *Inability to move the fingers or toes*—pressure on a nerve
  - *Numbness*—pressure on a nerve, reduced blood flow to the part
  - *Temperature changes*—cool skin means poor circulation; hot skin means inflammation
  - *Drainage on or under the cast*—infection or bleeding
  - *Chills, fever, nausea, and vomiting*—infection

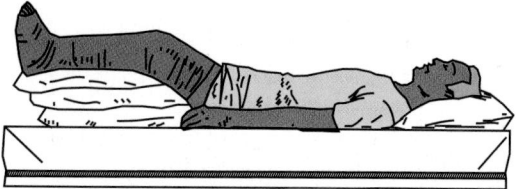

FIGURE 44-15 Pillows support the entire length of the wet cast. (Modified from Harkness GA, Dincher JR: *Medical-surgical nursing: total patient care,* ed 10, St Louis, 1999, Mosby.)

FIGURE 44-16 The cast is supported with the palms.

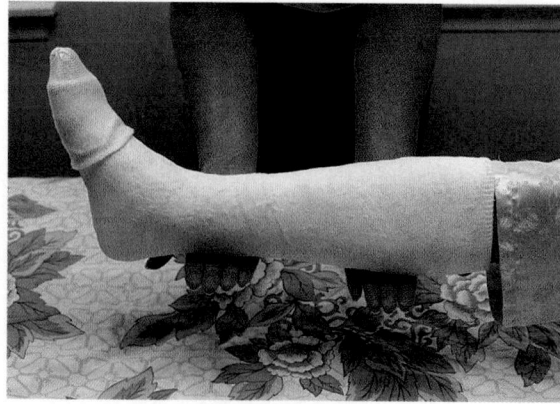

Traction. With traction, a steady pull from 2 directions keeps the bone in place. Traction also is used for muscle spasms and to correct deformities or contractures. Weights, ropes, and pulleys are used (Fig. 44-17). Traction is applied to the neck, arms, legs, or pelvis.

Skin traction is applied to the skin. Boots, wraps, tape, or splints are used.

Weights are attached to the device (see Fig. 44-17). For *skeletal traction*, wires or pins are inserted through the bone (Fig. 44-18). For cervical traction, tongs are applied to the skull (Fig. 44-19). Weights are attached to the bone.

To assist with the person's care, see Box 44-8.

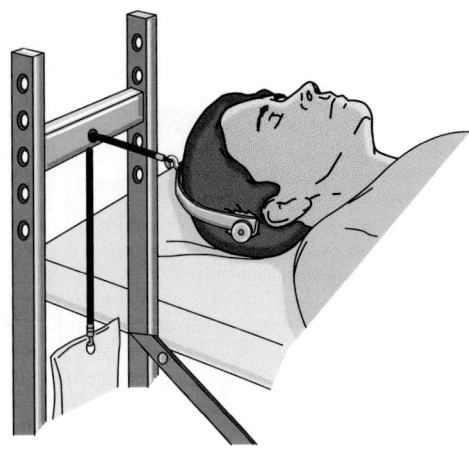

FIGURE 44-19 Tongs are inserted into the skull for cervical traction. (From Monahan FD and others: *Phipps' medical-surgical nursing: health and illness perspectives,* ed 8, St Louis, 2007, Mosby.)

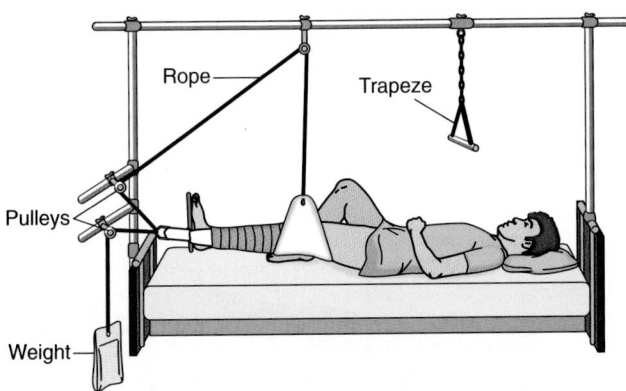

FIGURE 44-17 Traction set-up. Note the weight, pulleys, and ropes. A trapeze is used to raise the upper body off the bed. (Modified from Monahan FD and others: *Phipps' medical-surgical nursing: health and illness perspectives,* ed 8, St Louis, 2007, Mosby.)

BOX 44-8	**Caring for Persons in Traction**

- Keep the person in good alignment.
- Do not remove the traction.
- Keep the weights off the floor. Weights must hang freely from the traction set-up (see Fig. 44-17).
- Do not add or remove weights.
- Check for frayed ropes. Report fraying at once.
- Perform ROM exercises for the uninvolved joints as directed.
- Position the person as directed. Usually only the supine position is allowed. Slight turning may be allowed.
- Provide the fracture pan for elimination.
- Give skin care as directed.
- Put bottom linens on the bed from the top down. The person uses a trapeze to raise the body off the bed (see Fig. 44-17).
- Check pin, nail, wire, or tong sites for redness, drainage, and odors. Report observations at once.
- Observe for the signs and symptoms listed under cast care (see Box 44-7). Report them at once.
- Complete a safety check before leaving the room. (See the inside of the front cover.)

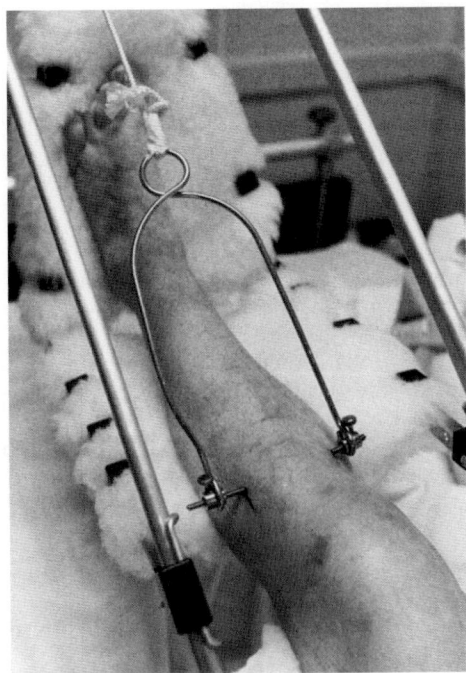

FIGURE 44-18 Skeletal traction is attached to the bone. (From Christensen BL, Kockrow EO: *Adult health nursing,* ed 6, St Louis, 2011, Mosby.)

Hip Fractures. Common in older persons, hip fractures require surgical repair or a hip replacement (Fig. 44-20, p. 720). Risk factors include:
- *Age.* Persons older than 65 years are at risk.
- *Gender.* Hip fractures are more common in women.
- *Osteoporosis.* See p. 721.
- *Drugs.* Some drugs can weaken bones or have dizziness as a side effect.
- *Nutrition.* Calcium and vitamin D are needed for healthy bones.
- *Inactivity.* Weight-bearing exercise and activities are needed to strengthen bones.
- *Smoking and alcohol use.* These can cause bone loss.

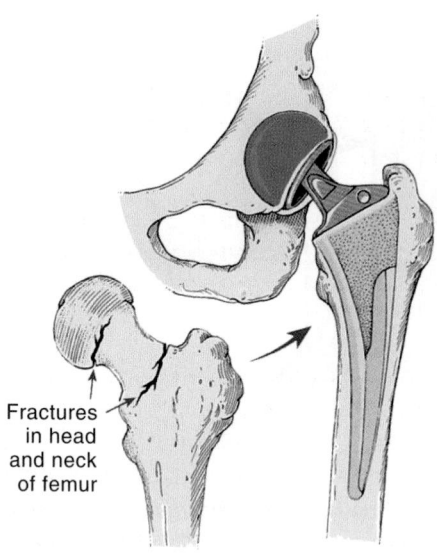

FIGURE 44-20 Hip fracture repaired with a prosthesis. (Modified from Christensen BL, Kockrow EO: *Adult health nursing,* ed 6, St Louis, 2011, Mosby.)

Falls are the most common cause of hip fractures. However, fractures have occurred upon standing or twisting. Signs and symptoms include:

- Being unable to move after falling
- Severe hip or groin pain
- Shorter leg on the injured side
- Turning the leg outward on the injured side
- Not being able to stand on the injured side

Post-operative problems present life-threatening risks. They include pneumonia, urinary tract infections, and thrombi (blood clots) in the leg veins or lungs. Pressure ulcers, constipation, and confusion are other problems.

Adduction, internal rotation, external rotation, and severe hip flexion are avoided after surgery. Rehabilitation is usually needed at home or in long-term care. Recovery can take 6 months. See Box 44-9 for the care required for a hip fracture.

See *Focus on Long-Term Care and Home Care: Hip Fractures.*

BOX 44-9	Care of the Person With a Hip Fracture

- Give good skin care. Skin breakdown can be rapid.
- Prevent pressure ulcers.
- Prevent wound, skin, and urinary tract infections.
- Encourage incentive spirometry and deep-breathing and coughing exercises as directed.
- Turn and position the person as directed. Usually the person is not positioned on the operative side.
- Prevent external rotation of the hip. Use trochanter rolls, pillows, or sandbags.
- Keep the leg abducted at all times. Use pillows (Fig. 44-21) or a hip abduction wedge (abductor splint). Do not exercise the affected leg.
- Provide a straight-back chair with armrests. The person needs a high, firm seat.
- Place the chair on the unaffected side.
- Use assist devices to move, turn, re-position, and transfer the person.
- Do not let the person stand on the operated leg unless allowed by the doctor.
- Elevate the leg following the care plan. With an internal fixation device, the leg is not elevated when the person sits in a chair. Elevating the leg puts strain on the device.
- Apply elastic stockings to prevent thrombi (blood clots) in the legs.
- Remind the person not to cross his or her legs.
- Assist with walking according to the care plan. The person uses a walker or crutches.
- Follow measures to protect the hip. See Box 44-6 and Figure 44-10.
- Practice safety measures to prevent falls.
- Complete a safety check before leaving the room. (See the inside of the front cover.)

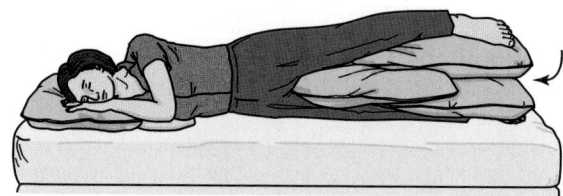

FIGURE 44-21 Pillows are used to keep the hip in abduction. (From Monahan FD and others: *Phipps' medical-surgical nursing: health and illness perspectives,* ed 8, St Louis, 2007, Mosby.)

FOCUS ON LONG-TERM CARE AND HOME CARE

Hip Fractures

Home Care

The prosthesis can dislocate (move out of place) with adduction, internal rotation, and severe hip flexion. Such movements are avoided. See Box 44-9.

Occupational therapy helps the person learn self-care activities. Assistive (adaptive) devices are used for dressing and bathing. Physical therapy helps the person learn muscle-strengthening exercises. A walker is usually needed.

The measures in Box 44-9 are followed.

Osteoporosis

With osteoporosis, the bone (*osteo*) becomes porous and brittle (*porosis*). Bones are fragile and break easily. Spine, hip, and wrist fractures are common.

Older people are at risk. For women, the risk increases after menopause from the lack of estrogen. Low levels of dietary calcium and vitamin D cause bone changes.

All ethnic groups are at risk. Other risk factors include a family history of the disease, being thin or having a small frame, eating disorders (Chapter 48), tobacco use, alcoholism, lack of exercise, bedrest, and immobility. Exercise and activity are needed for bone strength. Bone must bear weight to form properly. If not, calcium is lost from the bone. The bone becomes porous and brittle.

Back pain, loss of height, and stooped posture occur. Fractures are a major threat. Even slight activity can cause fractures. They can occur from turning in bed, getting up from a chair, or coughing. Fractures are great risks from falls and accidents.

Prevention is important. Doctors often order calcium and vitamin supplements. Estrogen is ordered for some women. Other preventive measures include:

- Exercising weight-bearing joints—walking, jogging, stair climbing, weight lifting, dancing
- No smoking and limited alcohol
- Back supports or corsets for good posture
- Walking aids
- Safety measures to prevent falls and accidents
- Good body mechanics
- Safe moving, transfer, and turning and positioning procedures

Loss of Limb

An **amputation** *is the removal of all or part of an extremity.* Severe injuries, tumors, severe infection, gangrene, and vascular disorders are common causes. Diabetes can cause vascular changes leading to amputation.

Gangrene *is a condition in which there is death of tissue.* Causes include infection, injuries, and vascular disorders. Blood flow is affected. Tissues do not get enough oxygen and nutrients. Tissue death results. Tissues become black, cold, and shriveled (Fig. 44-22). Surgery is needed to remove dead tissue. If untreated, gangrene spreads throughout the body. For example, in diabetes the toes are often affected first. If the toes are not removed, gangrene spreads up the foot and leg. Gangrene can cause death.

Much support is needed. The amputation affects the person's life. Body image, appearance, daily activities, moving about, and work are some areas affected. Fear, shock, anger, denial, and depression are common emotions.

The person is fitted with a *prosthesis*—an artificial replacement for a missing body part (Fig. 44-23, p. 722). The stump is conditioned for a proper fit. This involves shrinking and shaping the stump into a cone shape with bandages (Fig. 44-24, p. 722). Exercises are done to strengthen other limbs. The person learns to use the prosthesis.

The person may feel that the limb is still there. Aching, tingling, and itching are common sensations. Or the person complains of pain in the amputated part (*phantom pain*). This is a normal reaction. It may occur for a short time or for many years.

Because of other health problems, many older persons cannot use a leg prosthesis. They need to use wheelchairs. After amputation, most older persons need long-term care.

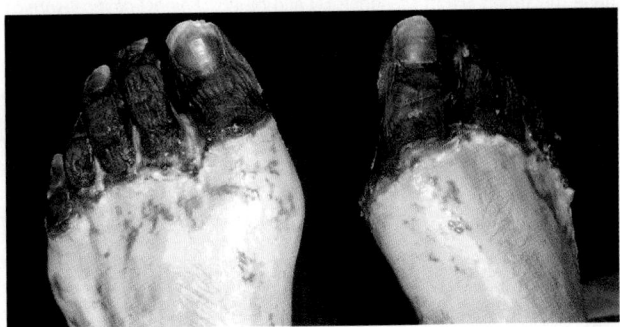

FIGURE 44-22 Gangrene. (From Centers for Disease Control and Prevention/Christina Nelson, MD, MPH, 2012.)

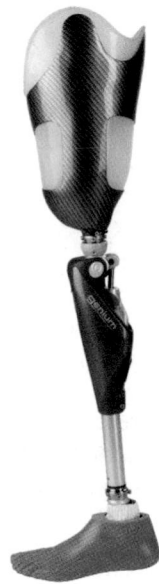

FIGURE 44-23 Above-the-knee prosthesis. (Courtesy Otto Bock Health Care, Minneapolis, Minn.)

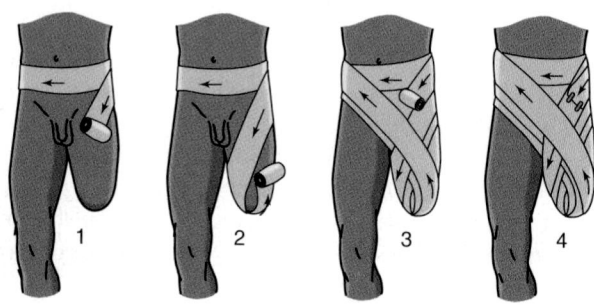

FIGURE 44-24 A mid-thigh amputation is bandaged to shrink and shape the stump. (From Monahan FD and others: *Phipps' medical-surgical nursing: health and illness perspectives*, ed 8, St Louis, 2007, Mosby.)

FOCUS ON **PRIDE**

The Person, Family, and Yourself

P ersonal and Professional Responsibility
Nervous system and musculo-skeletal system disorders affect the whole person. Social, psychological, physical, and spiritual needs must be met. Provide care that focuses on the person as a whole.

R ights and Respect
With some disorders, the person does not improve. For some, function declines over time. The family watches the person struggle to move, perform ADL, or live. The person, family, and caregivers need support and encouragement. Treat the person and family with dignity, respect, and kindness.

I ndependence and Social Interaction
The disorders in this chapter affect independence. The person relies on family and caregivers for support and daily needs. The person may feel useless, angry, and depressed. To promote independence:
- Focus on the person's abilities, not disabilities.
- Tell the person when you notice progress.
- Allow personal choice.
- Encourage the person to try.

D elegation and Teamwork
Providing care often requires teamwork for safety and efficiency. Value your team members. Thank them for helping. Offer to help others. Take pride in being a good team member.

E thics and Laws
Accidents happen. Mistakes do not always mean negligence. To be found negligent, evidence must show that you did not act in a reasonable and careful manner. And as a result, the person or the person's property was harmed.

   Always work carefully. If an accident occurs, tell the nurse. Take pride in being honest and accountable.

FOCUS ON **PRIDE**: *Application*

Many disorders in this chapter have no cure. Problems remain or worsen. Describe the impact on the person and family. How does this differ from disorders that heal?

REVIEW QUESTIONS

Circle the BEST answer.

1 A stroke also is called
   a A cerebrovascular accident
   b Aphasia
   c Hemiplegia
   d A transient ischemic attack

2 Warning signs of stroke occur
   a With exertion
   b Suddenly
   c Between the ages of 20 and 40
   d At rest

3 A person had a stroke. Which should you question?
   a Leave the bed in semi-Fowler's position.
   b Perform ROM exercises every 2 hours.
   c Turn and re-position the person every 2 hours.
   d Place needed items on the weak (affected) side.

4 Which statement about Parkinson's disease is *true*?
   a There is a cure.
   b Mental function is affected first.
   c Tremors, slow movements, and a shuffling gait occur.
   d Paralysis occurs but mental function is intact.

5 Which statement about multiple sclerosis is *true*?
   a There is a cure.
   b Only voluntary muscles are affected.
   c Persons older than 65 are at risk.
   d Women are at greater risk than men.

6 Amyotrophic lateral sclerosis affects nerve cells that control
   a Involuntary muscles
   b Voluntary muscles
   c The brain
   d The lungs

REVIEW QUESTIONS—cont'd

7 A person has amyotrophic lateral sclerosis. Which can you perform?
   a Range-of-motion exercises
   b Tracheostomy suctioning
   c Feeding tube insertion
   d Fall risk assessment

8 Persons with head or spinal cord injuries require
   a Rehabilitation
   b Speech therapy
   c Long-term care
   d Chemotherapy

9 Which carries the *lowest* risk for traumatic brain injury?
   a Falling in the bathroom
   b Motorcycle accident
   c Transferring with a mechanical lift
   d Child abuse

10 A person has tetraplegia from a spinal cord injury. Which should you question?
   a Keep the bed in a low position.
   b Assist with active ROM exercises.
   c Follow the bowel training program.
   d Turn and re-position every hour.

11 Autonomic hyperreflexia occurs
   a After spinal cord injuries
   b In Parkinson's disease
   c With Lou Gehrig's disease
   d Following stroke

12 Autonomic hyperreflexia is usually triggered by
   a High blood sugar
   b High blood pressure
   c A full bladder
   d A virus

13 Arthritis affects the
   a Joints
   b Bones
   c Voluntary muscles
   d Involuntary muscles

14 A person has arthritis. Care includes
   a Keeping joints abducted
   b Applying traction to affected areas
   c Wearing a cast to prevent movement
   d Rest balanced with exercise

15 A person had hip replacement surgery. Which should you question?
   a Do not cross the legs.
   b Provide a chair with a low seat.
   c Keep a hip abduction wedge between the legs.
   d Provide a long-handled brush for bathing.

16 A person with osteoporosis is at risk for
   a Fractures
   b An amputation
   c Phantom pain
   d Paralysis

17 A cast needs to dry. Which should you question?
   a Turn the person so the cast dries evenly.
   b Cover the cast with blankets and plastic.
   c Elevate the cast on pillows.
   d Support the cast by the palms when lifting.

18 A person has an arm cast. Which is normal?
   a Numbness and inability to move the fingers
   b Chills and nausea
   c Cool skin and cyanosis
   d Pulse rate of 76 and a respiratory rate of 18

19 A person is in traction. Care includes
   a Avoiding ROM exercises
   b Keeping the weights on the floor
   c Removing the weights if the person is uncomfortable
   d Giving skin care at frequent intervals

20 After hip surgery the operated leg is kept
   a Abducted
   b Adducted
   c Externally rotated
   d Flexed

21 After an amputation, the person
   a Needs a wheelchair
   b Has quadriplegia
   c Is fitted with a prosthesis
   d Needs arthroplasty

Answers to Chapter 44 questions are on p. 872.

FOCUS ON **PRACTICE**

Problem Solving

Mr. Avery had a stroke. He has hemiplegia, aphasia, and dysphagia. Explain how you will modify the care measures listed below. Apply learning from this and other chapters.
- Transferring from the bed to the wheelchair
- Dressing and undressing
- Assisting with food and fluids
- Explaining a procedure
- Performing a safety check of the room

CHAPTER 45

Cardiovascular, Respiratory, and Lymphatic Disorders

OBJECTIVES

- Define the key terms and key abbreviations in this chapter.
- Describe congenital heart defects.
- Identify cardiovascular disorder risk factors and complications.
- Describe the care required for hypertension, coronary artery disease, angina, myocardial infarction, heart failure, and dysrhythmias.
- Describe the care required for Ebola.

- Describe the care required for chronic obstructive pulmonary disease, asthma, and sleep apnea.
- Explain the differences between a cold and influenza and the care required.
- Describe the care required for enterovirus D68.
- Describe the care required for pneumonia and tuberculosis.
- Describe the care required for lymphedema and lymphoma.
- Explain how to promote PRIDE in the person, the family, and yourself.

KEY TERMS

apnea The lack or absence *(a)* of breathing *(pnea)*
arrhythmia See "dysrhythmia"
congenital To be born with
dysrhythmia An abnormal *(dys)* heart rhythm *(rhythmia);* arrhythmia
hemorrhage The excessive loss of blood in a short time
high blood pressure See "hypertension"
hypertension The systolic pressure is 140 mm Hg or higher *(hyper)* or the diastolic pressure is 90 mm Hg or higher; high blood pressure

lymphedema A buildup of lymph in the tissues causing edema (swelling)
pneumonia Inflammation and infection of lung tissue
pre-hypertension When the systolic pressure is between 120 and 139 mm Hg or the diastolic pressure is between 80 and 89 mm Hg
sleep apnea Pauses *(a)* in breathing *(pnea)* that occur during sleep

KEY ABBREVIATIONS

CAD	Coronary artery disease	MI	Myocardial infarction
CDC	Centers for Disease Control and Prevention	mm Hg	Millimeters of mercury
CHF	Congestive heart failure	O_2	Oxygen
CO_2	Carbon dioxide	RBC	Red blood cell
COPD	Chronic obstructive pulmonary disease	TB	Tuberculosis
EV-D68	Enterovirus D68	VHF	Viral hemorrhagic fever
IV	Intravenous	WBC	White blood cell

Cardiovascular and respiratory system disorders are leading causes of death in the United States. Many people have these disorders. Disorders also occur in the lymphatic system. Understanding these disorders gives meaning to the care you give.

CARDIOVASCULAR DISORDERS

The circulatory (cardiovascular) system delivers blood to the body's cells. Problems occur in the heart or blood vessels. See Chapter 36 for circulatory ulcers.

See *Body Structure and Function Review: The Circulatory System.*

See *Focus on Children and Older Persons: Cardiovascular Disorders*, p. 726.

BODY STRUCTURE AND FUNCTION REVIEW

The Circulatory System

The circulatory system is made up of the *blood, heart,* and *blood vessels.* The heart pumps blood through the blood vessels.

The Blood

The blood consists of blood cells and *plasma.* Plasma is mostly water. It carries blood cells to other body cells. Plasma also carries substances (food, hormones, and chemicals) that cells need to function.

Red blood cells (RBCs) are called *erythrocytes. Hemoglobin* in the RBCs gives blood its red color. As RBCs circulate through the lungs, hemoglobin picks up oxygen (O_2). Hemoglobin carries O_2 to the cells. When blood is bright red, hemoglobin in the RBCs is filled with O_2. As blood circulates through the body, O_2 is given to the cells. Cells release carbon dioxide (CO_2) (a waste product). It is picked up by the hemoglobin. RBCs filled with CO_2 make the blood look dark red.

Blood also contains *white blood cells (WBCs)* and *platelets (thrombocytes).* WBCs are called *leukocytes.* They protect the body against infection. Platelets are needed for blood clotting.

The Heart

The heart is a muscle. It pumps blood through the blood vessels to the tissues and cells. The heart has 4 chambers (Fig. 45-1). Upper chambers receive blood and are called *atria.* The *right atrium* receives blood from body tissues. The *left atrium* receives blood from the lungs. Lower chambers are called *ventricles.* Ventricles pump blood. The *right ventricle* pumps blood to the lungs for O_2. The *left ventricle* pumps blood to all parts of the body.

Valves are between the atria and ventricles (see Fig. 45-1). The valves allow blood flow in 1 direction. They prevent blood from flowing back into the atria from the ventricles. The *tricuspid valve* is between the right atrium and the right ventricle. The *mitral valve (bicuspid valve)* is between the left atrium and the left ventricle.

Heart action has 2 phases.

- *Diastole.* It is the resting phase. Heart chambers fill with blood.
- *Systole.* It is the working phase. The heart contracts. Blood is pumped through the blood vessels when the heart contracts.

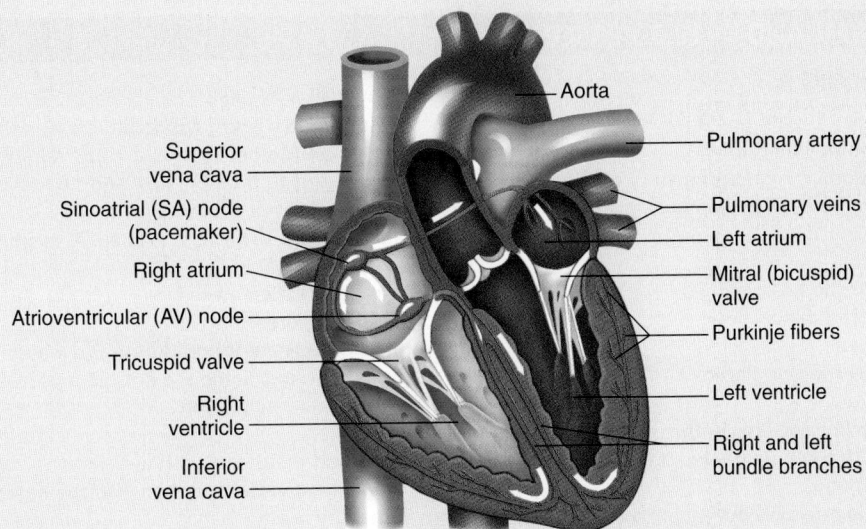

FIGURE 45-1 Structures of the heart. Chambers and major vessels that carry blood full of O_2 are shown in red. Chambers and major vessels that carry blood low in O_2 are shown in blue. Valves are white. The heart's electrical system is yellow. (Modified from Patton KT, Thibodeau GA: *The human body in health & disease,* ed 6, St Louis, 2014, Mosby.)

Continued

BODY STRUCTURE AND FUNCTION REVIEW—cont'd

The Circulatory System—cont'd

The heart has its own electrical system that stimulates the heart to contract. The electrical signal begins in the *sinoatrial (SA) node* (see Fig. 45-1). The SA node sets the pace of the heart. It stimulates the heart to beat at 60 to 100 beats per minute. The electrical signal spreads through the heart, causing the heart to contract.

The Blood Vessels

Blood flows to body tissues and cells through the blood vessels. There are 3 groups of blood vessels: arteries, capillaries, and veins (Fig. 45-2).

Arteries carry blood away from the heart. Arterial blood is rich in O_2. The *aorta* (see Fig. 45-2) is the largest artery. It receives blood directly from the left ventricle. The aorta branches into other arteries that carry blood to all parts of the body. These arteries branch into smaller parts within the tissues. The smallest branch of an artery is an *arteriole*.

Arterioles connect to *capillaries.* Capillaries are very tiny blood vessels. Food, O_2, and other substances pass from capillaries into the cells. The capillaries pick up waste products (including CO_2) from the cells. Veins carry waste products back to the heart.

Veins return blood to the heart. They connect to the capillaries by *venules.* Venules are small veins. Venules branch together to form veins. The many veins also branch together as they near the heart to form 2 main veins—the *inferior vena cava* and the *superior vena cava* (see Fig. 45-2). Both empty into the right atrium. The inferior vena cava carries blood from the legs and trunk. The superior vena cava carries blood from the head and arms. Venous blood is dark red. It has little O_2 and a lot of CO_2.

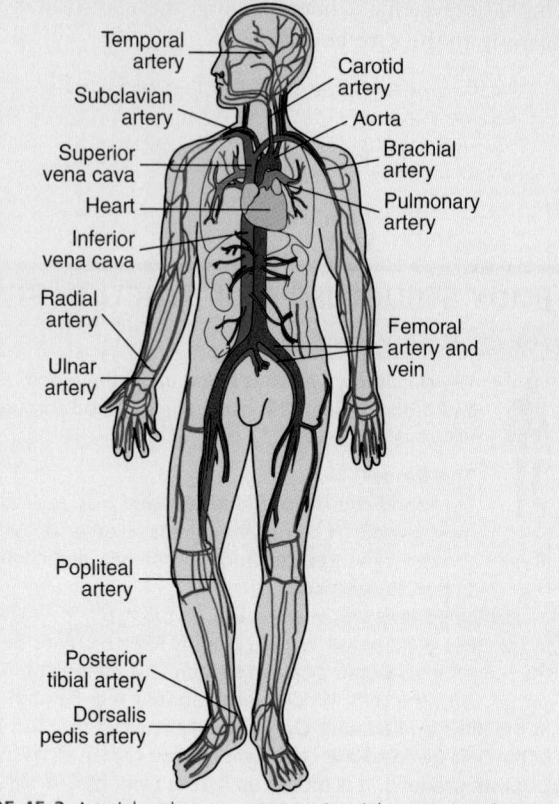

FIGURE 45-2 Arterial and venous systems. Arterial system is red. Venous system is blue.

FOCUS ON CHILDREN AND OLDER PERSONS

Cardiovascular Disorders

Children

Some babies have congenital heart defects. *Congenital means to be born with.* Defects occur during pregnancy as the baby's heart develops. One or more defects can occur in:
- A part of the heart
- The heart valves
- The blood vessels near the heart
  Depending on the defect, blood flow:
- Slows down.
- Goes in the wrong direction or place.
- Is blocked completely.
  Usually the cause is unknown. Risk factors include:
- Heredity. A parent with a congenital heart defect is at risk of having a child with one.
- The mother had a viral infection during pregnancy. German measles (rubella) is a common cause.
- The mother has diabetes.
- The mother took some types of drugs during pregnancy.
- The mother had repeated exposure to some chemicals or x-rays during pregnancy.
- The mother used alcohol or street drugs during pregnancy.

The common signs of congenital heart defects are:
- Heart sounds other than "lub-dub" during an apical pulse.
- A bluish tint to the skin, lips, and fingernails.
- Fast breathing or shortness of breath.
- Poor feeding. The infant tires easily while nursing.
- Poor weight gain.
- Tiring easily during exercise or activity. Be alert for this sign in older children.

Heart defects are found during pregnancy or when the child is very young. Some are not diagnosed until the child is older. Treatment may involve:
- Drugs.
- Correcting the defect with a catheter. A catheter is inserted into a blood vessel and then into the heart.
- Surgery.
- A heart transplant.

With successful treatment, many children with heart defects grow into healthy adults. Some need life-long treatment.

BOX 45-1	Cardiovascular Disorders— Risk Factors

Factors You *Cannot* Change
- Age—45 years or older for men; 55 years or older for women
- Gender—men are at greater risk than women; risk increases for women after menopause
- Race—African-Americans are at greater risk
- Family history—tends to run in families

Factors You *Can* Change
- Being over-weight
- Stress
- Smoking and tobacco use
- Poor diet—high in fat, salt, sugar, and cholesterol
- Excessive alcohol
- Lack of exercise
- Blood pressure
- High blood cholesterol
- Diabetes

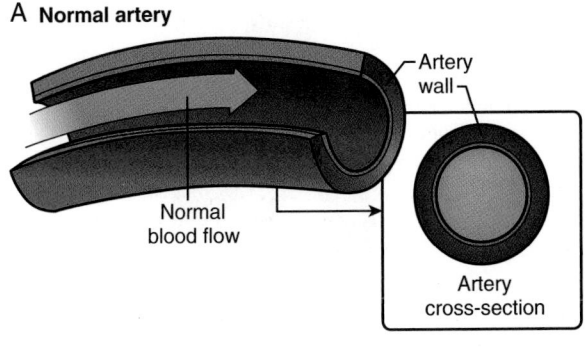

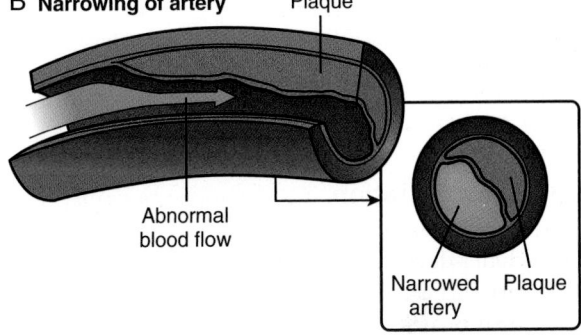

FIGURE 45-3 A, Normal artery. **B,** Plaque on the artery wall in atherosclerosis.

Hypertension

With ***hypertension (high blood pressure),*** *the systolic pressure is 140 mm Hg (millimeters of mercury) or higher* (hyper). *Or the diastolic pressure is 90 mm Hg or higher.* The resting blood pressure is too high. Such measurements must occur several times. ***Pre-hypertension*** *is when the systolic pressure is between 120 and 139 mm Hg or the diastolic pressure is between 80 and 89 mm Hg.* Pre-hypertension eventually develops into hypertension. Most people have hypertension some time during their lives. See Box 45-1 for risk factors.

Narrowed blood vessels are a common cause. The heart pumps with more force to move blood through narrowed vessels. Kidney disorders, head injuries, some pregnancy problems, and adrenal gland tumors are causes.

Known as the "silent killer," hypertension can go unnoticed for many years. Signs and symptoms develop over time. Headache, blurred vision, dizziness, and nose bleeds occur. Hypertension can lead to stroke, hardening of the arteries, heart attack, heart failure, kidney failure, and blindness.

Life-style changes can lower blood pressure. A diet low in fat and salt, a healthy weight, and regular exercise are needed. No smoking is allowed. Alcohol and caffeine are limited. Managing stress and sleeping well also lower blood pressure. Certain drugs lower blood pressure.

Coronary Artery Disease

The *coronary arteries* are the arteries that supply the heart muscle with blood. In coronary artery disease (CAD) (coronary heart disease, heart disease), the coronary arteries become hardened and narrow. One or all are affected. The heart muscle gets less blood and O_2.

The most common cause is atherosclerosis (Fig. 45-3). Plaque—made up of cholesterol, fat, and other substances—collects on artery walls. The narrowed arteries block some or all of blood flow. Blood clots can form along the plaque and block blood flow.

Major complications of CAD are angina, myocardial infarction (heart attack), irregular heartbeats, and sudden death. The more risk factors (see Box 45-1), the greater the chance of CAD and its complications.

CAD can be treated. Treatment goals are to:
- Relieve symptoms (see "Angina," p. 728)
- Slow or stop atherosclerosis
- Lower the risk of blood clots
- Widen or bypass clogged arteries
- Reduce cardiac events (see "Angina" and "Myocardial Infarction," p. 729)

CAD requires life-style changes. The person must quit smoking, exercise, and reduce stress. A healthy diet is needed to lower blood pressure, lower blood cholesterol, and maintain a healthy weight. If over-weight, the person must lose weight.

Some drugs decrease the heart's workload and relieve symptoms. Other drugs prevent a heart attack or sudden death. Drugs can delay medical and surgical procedures that open or bypass diseased arteries (Fig. 45-4, p. 728).

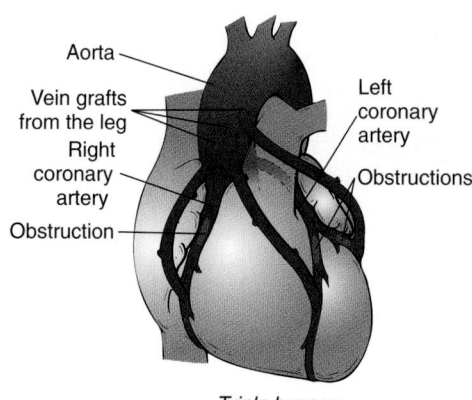

Triple bypass

FIGURE 45-4 Coronary artery bypass surgery. (Modified from Patton KT, Thibodeau GA: *The human body in health & disease*, ed 6, St Louis, 2014, Mosby.)

Cardiac Rehabilitation. CAD complications may require cardiac rehabilitation (cardiac rehab). The cardiac rehab team includes doctors (the person's doctor, a heart specialist, a heart surgeon), nurses, exercise specialists, physical and occupational therapists, dietitians, and mental health professionals.

Cardiac rehab has 2 parts.

- Exercise training. The person learns to exercise safely. The exercises strengthen muscles and improve stamina (staying power, endurance). The exercise plan is based on the person's abilities, needs, and interests.
- Education, counseling, and training. The person learns about:
  - His or her heart condition
  - Reducing the risk of future problems
  - Adjusting to a new life-style
  - Dealing with fears about the future

Angina

Angina is chest pain from reduced blood flow to part of the heart muscle (myocardium). (*Angina* comes from the Latin word *angor* that means *strangling*.) It occurs when the heart needs more O_2. Normally blood flow to the heart increases when O_2 needs increase. Exertion, a heavy meal, stress, and excitement increase the heart's need for O_2. So does smoking and very hot or cold temperatures. In CAD, narrowed vessels prevent increased blood flow.

Chest pain is described as a tightness, pressure, squeezing, or burning in the chest. Pain can occur in the shoulders, arms, neck, jaw, or back (Fig. 45-5). Pain in the jaw, neck, and down 1 or both arms is common. The person may be pale, feel faint, and perspire. Dyspnea is common. Nausea, fatigue, and weakness may occur. Some persons complain of "gas" or indigestion. Rest often relieves symptoms in 3 to 15 minutes. Because rest reduces the heart's need for O_2, normal blood flow is achieved. Heart damage is prevented.

Besides rest, a nitroglycerin tablet is taken when angina occurs. A tablet is placed under the tongue, where it dissolves and is rapidly absorbed into the bloodstream. Kept within the person's reach, the person takes a tablet and then tells the nurse. For some persons, the nurse applies and removes nitroglycerin patches.

Things that cause angina are avoided—over-exertion, heavy meals and over-eating, emotional stress, cold weather, hot and humid weather. Doctor-supervised programs are helpful.

See "Coronary Artery Disease" (p. 727) for the treatment of angina. The goal is increased blood flow to the heart. This prevents or lowers the risk of heart attack and death. Chest pain lasting longer than a few minutes and not relieved by rest and nitroglycerin may signal a heart attack. Emergency care is needed.

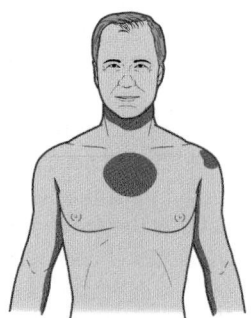
- Mid sternum
- Left shoulder and down both arms
- Neck and arms

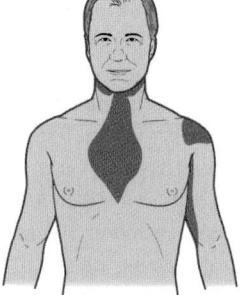
- Substernal radiating to neck and jaw
- Substernal radiating down left arm

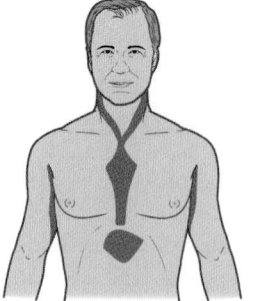
- Epigastric
- Epigastric radiating to neck, jaw, and arms

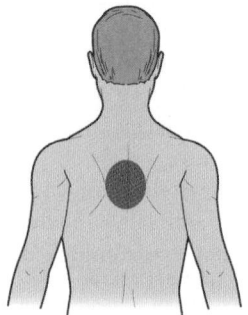
- Intrascapular

FIGURE 45-5 *Shaded areas* show the common locations and patterns of angina. (From Lewis SL, Dirksen SR, Heitkemper MM, Bucher L: *Medical-surgical nursing: assessment and management of clinical problems*, ed 9, St Louis, 2014, Mosby.)

Myocardial Infarction

Myocardial refers to the *heart muscle. Infarction* means *tissue death.* With myocardial infarction (MI) part of the heart muscle dies from sudden blockage of blood flow in a coronary artery. A thrombus (blood clot) in an artery with atherosclerosis blocks blood flow. The damaged area may be small or large (Fig. 45-6).

MI also is called:

- Heart attack
- Acute myocardial infarction (AMI)
- Acute coronary syndrome (ACS)
- Coronary
- Coronary thrombosis
- Coronary occlusion

CAD, angina, and previous MI are risk factors. See Box 45-2 for signs and symptoms. MI is an emergency. Efforts are made to:

- Relieve pain.
- Restore blood flow to the heart.
- Stabilize vital signs.
- Give O_2.
- Calm the person.
- Prevent death and life-threatening problems.

The person may need medical or surgical procedures to open or bypass the diseased artery. Cardiac rehabilitation is needed. The goals are to:

- Recover and resume normal activities.
- Prevent another MI.
- Prevent complications such as heart failure or sudden cardiac arrest (sudden cardiac death) (Chapter 54).

See *Focus on Long-Term Care and Home Care: Myocardial Infarction.*

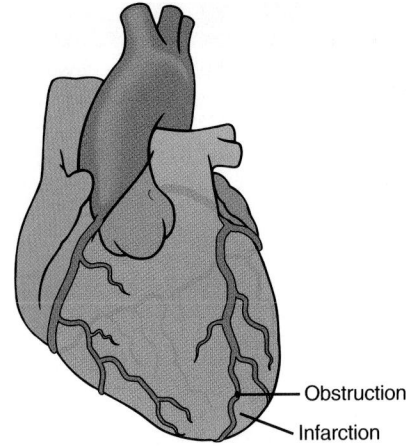

FIGURE 45-6 Myocardial infarction. (Modified from Lewis SL, Dirksen SR, Heitkemper MM, Bucher L: *Medical-surgical nursing: assessment and management of clinical problems,* ed 9, St Louis, 2014, Mosby.)

FOCUS ON LONG-TERM CARE AND HOME CARE

Myocardial Infarction

Home Care
Cardiac rehabilitation continues. The person may go to a gym, health club, or hospital fitness center. Some persons like indoor malls for walking. Normal activities are increased slowly. The person returns to work with the doctor's approval.

BOX 45-2	Myocardial Infarction—Signs and Symptoms

- Chest pain
  - Sudden, severe; usually in the center or on the left side
  - Described as pressure, tightness, fullness, squeezing, or aching
  - More severe and lasts longer than angina
  - Not relieved by rest or nitroglycerin
- Pain or numbness in 1 or both arms, the back, neck, jaw, or stomach
- Indigestion or "heartburn"
- Dyspnea
- Nausea, vomiting
- Dizziness
- Fainting
- Perspiration and cold, clammy skin
- *Pallor* (pale skin) or *cyanosis* (bluish color)
- Pulse: fast, irregular
- Fear, apprehension, and a feeling of doom

Heart Failure

Heart failure or congestive heart failure (CHF) occurs when the weakened heart cannot pump normally. Blood backs up. Tissue congestion occurs.

When the left side of the heart cannot pump blood normally, blood backs up into the lungs. Respiratory congestion occurs. When the right side of the heart cannot pump blood normally, blood backs up into the venous system. Swelling occurs. With both left-sided and right-sided failure, the body does not get enough blood. Signs and symptoms occur from the effects on other organs. See Box 45-3, p. 730. Pulmonary edema (fluid in the lungs) can result from heart failure. It is an emergency. The person can die.

A damaged or weak heart usually causes heart failure. CAD, MI, hypertension, diabetes, age, and irregular heart rhythms (p. 730) are common causes. So are damaged heart valves and kidney disease.

The goals of treatment are to:

- Treat the cause of heart failure.
- Reduce symptoms.
- Prevent worsening heart failure.
- Improve quality of life.
- Prolong life.

BOX 45-3	Heart Failure—Signs and Symptoms

- *Dyspnea* (worse with exertion or lying down)
- Sputum: white, pink, blood-tinged, foamy
- Cough
- Lung sounds: gurgling, wheezing
- Confusion
- Dizziness
- Fainting
- Fatigue
- Weakness
- *Pallor* (pale skin)
- Nocturia
- Nausea
- Appetite: decreased
- Swelling: feet, ankles, legs, abdomen, neck veins
- Weight gain
- Pulse: rapid, irregular

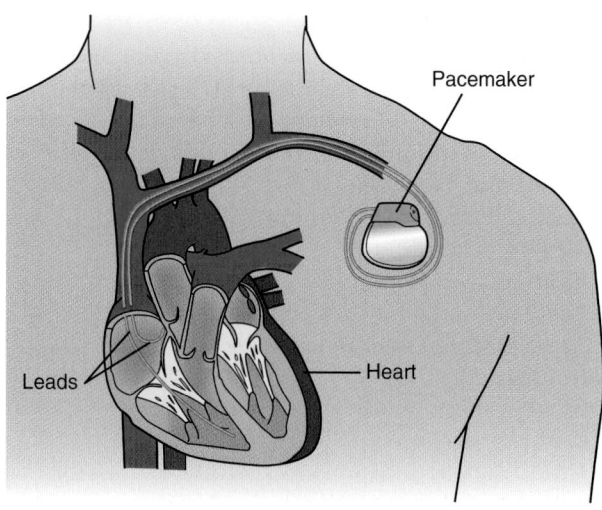

FIGURE 45-7 Pacemaker.

Drugs strengthen the heart, decrease strain on the heart, and reduce fluid buildup. A sodium-controlled diet is ordered. Oxygen is given. Semi-Fowler's position is preferred for breathing. The person must reduce CAD risk factors. If acutely ill, the person needs hospital care.

You assist with these aspects of the person's care.

- Promoting rest and activity as ordered
- Measuring intake and output
- Measuring weight daily
- Assisting with pulse oximetry
- Restricting fluids as ordered
- Promoting a low sodium, fat, and cholesterol diet
- Preventing skin breakdown and pressure ulcers
- Assisting with range-of-motion and other exercises
- Assisting with transfers and ambulation
- Assisting with self-care activities
- Maintaining good alignment
- Applying elastic stockings

Many older persons have heart failure. Skin breakdown is a risk. Tissue swelling, poor circulation, and fragile skin increase the risk of pressure ulcers. Good skin care and regular position changes are needed.

Dysrhythmias

A *dysrhythmia (arrhythmia) is an abnormal* (dys) *heart rhythm* (rhythmia). The rhythm may be too fast, too slow, or irregular. Dysrhythmias are caused by changes in the heart's electrical system. Changes may result from hypertension, CAD, MI, or heart failure. Weakening and changes in the heart muscle are other causes. So are drug and alcohol abuse, excess caffeine intake, and thyroid problems. Some drugs can cause dysrhythmias.

The person may feel dizzy or light-headed and have fluttering in the chest, chest pain, or dyspnea. The person may faint (Chapter 54). Some dysrhythmias are minor. Others are life-threatening.

FOCUS ON LONG-TERM CARE AND HOME CARE

Dysrhythmias

Home Care
The pacemaker's function and battery life are checked regularly. This can be done at home using a telephone. Telephone checks are often done every 3 months or as directed by the doctor. The call is placed by a nurse or the person at a scheduled time.

A transmitter connects to a phone line. Some transmitters work by placing wristbands on both arms. Others work by placing a device over the pacemaker. Some pacemaker checks require placing a special magnet over the site to check the pacemaker settings and battery. The person follows the nurse's instructions.

Newer pacemakers may be monitored using the Internet. The manufacturer's instructions are followed.

Treatment depends on the type of dysrhythmia. Drugs may be given. A procedure may be needed.

- *Defibrillation* (Chapter 54) or *cardioversion*—an electrical shock is given to stop an abnormal rhythm.
- *Ablation*—areas of tissue in the heart sending abnormal electrical signals are destroyed.

Some abnormal rhythms are treated with a pacemaker (Fig. 45-7). This device monitors and regulates the heart's rhythm. The device is inserted under the skin near the heart. One or more wires (leads) are placed in the heart muscle and connected to the pacemaker. The pacemaker sends signals through the leads to stimulate the heart to beat normally.

For life-threatening dysrhythmias, an implantable cardioverter defibrillator (ICD) may be placed. The ICD delivers a shock when the heart is in a life-threatening rhythm. The shock restores a regular heart rhythm. Some devices are both a pacemaker and an ICD.

See *Focus on Long-Term Care and Home Care: Dysrhythmias.*

Viral Hemorrhagic Fevers

Viral hemorrhagic fevers (VHFs) are a group of illnesses caused by viruses. Some VHFs cause mild illnesses. Others are severe and life-threatening. VHFs:

- Affect many organs.
- Damage blood vessels.
- Impair the body's ability to regulate itself.
- May cause hemorrhage. ***Hemorrhage*** *is the excessive loss of blood in a short time.*

The natural reservoir (host) for these viruses is an animal or insect. Rats, mice, and mosquitoes are examples. The viruses are usually only found in areas where the host lives. Humans are infected from contact with an infected host. With some VHFs, the person can then spread the virus to others and cause outbreaks. There is no cure or drug treatment for most VHFs.

Ebola. Ebola virus disease (previously called Ebola hemorrhagic fever) is a severe and deadly VHF caused by the *Ebolavirus.* Ebola was first discovered in Africa in 1976.

Signs and symptoms of Ebola can appear 2 to 21 days after exposure. Usually symptoms appear within 8 to 10 days. Signs and symptoms include:

- Fever
- Severe headache
- Muscle pain
- Weakness and fatigue
- Diarrhea and vomiting
- Abdominal pain
- Hemorrhage—bleeding from the eyes, ears, nose, mouth, and rectum; raised and bleeding rash that covers the body

Ebola is contagious once symptoms appear. The virus is spread through direct contact with:

- Blood or body fluids—including but not limited to saliva, mucus, vomit, urine, feces, sweat, breast-milk, semen
- Contaminated objects—needles and syringes
- Infected animals, their blood or body fluids, or their meat

The virus enters the body through non-intact skin or mucous membranes. The eyes, nose, and mouth are examples. Ebola is not spread through air, water, food, or insects.

Ebola has no cure or vaccine. Treatment involves IV (intravenous) fluids, oxygen, and treatment of complications. Blood or platelet transfusions may be needed.

The health team must prevent the spread of infection. Hand hygiene, Standard Precautions, Transmission-Based Precautions, and the Bloodborne Pathogen Standard are followed. The person has a private room. Special personal protective equipment (PPE) is required to enter the person's room—full face shield, helmet, or headpiece; coveralls with socks or special gowns; double gloving; boot or shoe covers; and aprons. Special training is needed to care for such patients and for donning and removing the PPE.

RESPIRATORY DISORDERS

The respiratory system brings O_2 into the lungs and removes CO_2 from the body. Respiratory disorders interfere with this function and threaten life.

See *Body Structure and Function Review: The Respiratory System.*

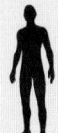

BODY STRUCTURE AND FUNCTION REVIEW

The Respiratory System

Oxygen is needed to live. Every cell needs O_2. The respiratory system (Fig. 45-8) brings O_2 into the lungs and removes CO_2. *Respiration* is the process of supplying the cells with O_2 and removing CO_2 from them. Respiration involves breathing in *(inhalation, inspiration)* and breathing out *(exhalation, expiration).*

Air enters the body through the *nose.* Then the air passes into the *pharynx* (throat). It is a tube-shaped passage-way for air and food. Air passes from the pharynx into the *larynx* (voice box) and then into the *trachea* (windpipe).

The trachea divides at its lower end into the *right bronchus* and the *left bronchus.* Each bronchus enters a *lung.* Upon entering the lungs, the bronchi divide many times into smaller branches *(bronchioles).* Eventually the bronchioles subdivide. They end up in tiny one-celled air sacs called *alveoli.*

O_2 and CO_2 are exchanged between the alveoli and capillaries. Blood in the capillaries picks up O_2 from the alveoli. Then the blood is returned to the left side of the heart and pumped to the rest of the body. Alveoli pick up CO_2 from the capillaries for exhalation.

Each lung is divided into lobes. The right lung has 3 lobes; the left lung has 2. The lungs are separated from the abdominal cavity by a muscle called the *diaphragm.* A bony framework made up of the ribs, sternum, and vertebrae protects the lungs.

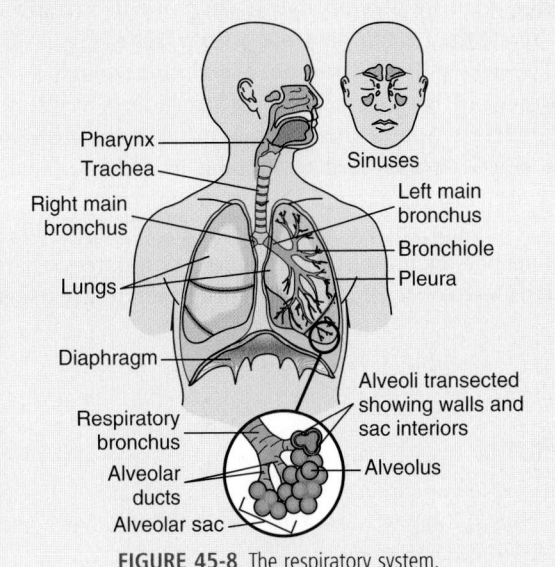

FIGURE 45-8 The respiratory system.

Chronic Obstructive Pulmonary Disease

Chronic obstructive pulmonary disease (COPD) involves 2 disorders—chronic bronchitis and emphysema. These disorders interfere with O_2 and CO_2 exchange in the lungs. They obstruct airflow. Lung function is gradually lost.

Cigarette smoking is the most important risk factor. Pipe, cigar, and other smoking tobaccos are also risk factors. So is exposure to second-hand smoke. Not smoking is the best way to prevent COPD. COPD has no cure. Air pollution and industrial dusts are other risk factors.

COPD affects the airways and alveoli. Less air gets into the lungs; less air leaves the lungs. These changes occur.

* The airways and alveoli (air sacs) become less elastic. They are like old rubber bands.
* The walls between many alveoli are destroyed.
* Airway walls become thick, inflamed, and swollen.
* The airways secrete more mucus than usual. Excess mucus clogs the airways.

Chronic Bronchitis. Chronic bronchitis occurs after repeated episodes of bronchitis. *Bronchitis* means *inflammation* (itis) *of the bronchi* (bronch).

Smoker's cough in the morning is often the first symptom. At first the cough is dry. Over time, the person coughs up mucus. Mucus may contain pus. The cough becomes more frequent. The person has difficulty breathing and tires easily. Mucus and inflamed breathing passages obstruct airflow. The body cannot get enough O_2.

The person must stop smoking. Oxygen therapy and breathing exercises are often ordered. Respiratory tract infections are prevented. If one occurs, prompt treatment is needed.

Emphysema. In emphysema, the alveoli enlarge. They become less elastic. They do not expand and shrink normally with breathing in and out. As a result, some air is trapped in the alveoli. Trapped air is not exhaled. Over time, more alveoli are involved. O_2 and CO_2 exchange cannot occur in affected alveoli. As more air is trapped in the lungs, the person develops a *barrel chest* (Fig. 45-9).

The person has shortness of breath and a cough. At first, shortness of breath occurs with exertion. Over time, it occurs at rest. Sputum may contain pus. Fatigue is common. The person works hard to breathe in and out. And the body does not get enough O_2. Breathing is easier when the person sits upright and slightly forward (Chapter 39).

The person must stop smoking. Respiratory therapy, breathing exercises, oxygen, and drug therapy are ordered.

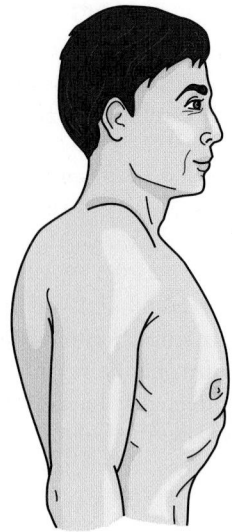

FIGURE 45-9 Barrel chest from emphysema.

Asthma

Asthma comes from the Greek word for *panting*. With asthma, the airway becomes inflamed and narrow. Extra mucus is produced. Dyspnea results. Wheezing and coughing are common. So are pain and tightness in the chest. Symptoms are mild to severe.

Asthma usually is triggered by allergies. Other triggers include air pollutants and irritants, smoking and second-hand smoke, respiratory infections, exertion, and cold air. Sudden attacks *(asthma attacks)* can occur. There is shortness of breath, wheezing, coughing, rapid pulse, sweating, and cyanosis. The person gasps for air and is very frightened. Fear makes the attack worse.

Asthma is treated with drugs. Severe attacks may require emergency care. The person and family learn how to prevent asthma attacks. Repeated attacks can damage the respiratory system.

Sleep Apnea

Apnea is the lack or absence (a) *of breathing* (pnea). In **sleep apnea,** *pauses in breathing occur during sleep.* Pauses last a few seconds to over a minute and can occur many times during sleep.

The most common cause is blockage of the airway. During sleep, muscles in the throat relax and soft tissues collapse, closing the airway.

Signs and symptoms of sleep apnea include:

* Pauses in breathing during sleep
* Loud snoring
* Waking during sleep with a gasp or shortness of breath
* Difficulty staying asleep
* Day-time sleepiness
* Headache in the morning
* Dry mouth or sore throat after sleeping

Life-style changes may help. Weight loss, no smoking, side-lying position for sleep, and avoiding alcohol and sedatives before sleep are examples. For more severe sleep apnea, surgery or 1 of the following devices may be needed.

- *Continuous positive airway pressure (CPAP).* A mask is attached to a pump. Air pressure is forced through the mask. The air keeps the airway open. The same amount of pressure goes through the mask when the person inhales and exhales.
- *Bilevel positive airway pressure (BiPAP).* This works like a CPAP except more pressure is given when breathing in. Less pressure is given when breathing out. The change in pressure is more comfortable for some persons.

Influenza

Influenza *(flu)* is a respiratory infection caused by viruses. Table 45-1 contrasts *cold* and the *flu.* The flu season is October through March. Children and older persons are at great risk. Pneumonia is a common complication.

Treatment involves fluids and rest. Drugs are ordered for symptom relief and to shorten the flu episode. Most people are better in about 1 week.

Coughing and sneezing spread flu viruses. The virus is also spread when a person touches a contaminated surface or object and then touches the mouth, eyes, or nose. Follow Standard Precautions.

The flu vaccine is the best prevention. The Centers for Disease Control and Prevention (CDC) recommends the flu vaccine for all persons 6 months old and older unless the person has a severe, life-threatening allergy to the flu vaccine.

See *Focus on Children and Older Persons: Influenza.*

FOCUS ON CHILDREN AND OLDER PERSONS

Influenza

Older Persons

Older persons may not have the signs and symptoms listed in Table 45-1. The following may signal flu in older persons.

- Changes in mental status or behavior
- Worsening of other health problems
- A body temperature below the normal range
- Fatigue
- Decreased appetite and fluid intake

Enterovirus D68

Enterovirus D68 (EV-D68) can cause mild to severe respiratory illness. In August 2014, the CDC reported that EV-D68 caused the most respiratory illnesses in children in all 50 states. The virus is found in saliva, mucus, and sputum. Coughing, sneezing, and touching contaminated surfaces and then touching the eyes, nose, or mouth can spread infection. Signs and symptoms include:

- Fever
- Runny nose, sneezing, cough
- Skin rash and mouth blisters
- Body and muscle aches

Infants, children, and teenagers are at highest risk for illness from EV-D68 infection. Children with asthma can become very ill.

There is no vaccine to prevent EV-D68. Treatment involves drugs for symptom relief. To protect yourself and others from infection:

- Wash the hands often with soap and water.
- Avoid close contact with sick people.
- Cover coughs and sneezes.
- Avoid touching the face with unwashed hands.
- Clean and disinfect surfaces.
- Stay home when ill.

Pneumonia

Pneumonia means inflammation and infection of lung tissue. (Pneumo means *lungs.)* Affected tissues fill with fluid. O_2 and CO_2 exchange is affected.

Bacteria, viruses, and other microbes are causes. Microbes reach the lungs by being inhaled, aspirated, or carried in the blood to the lungs from an infection in the body. Children under 2 years of age and adults over 65 years of age are at risk. Smoking, aging, stroke, bedrest, immobility, chronic diseases, and tube feedings increase the risk of pneumonia.

TABLE 45-1	Cold Versus the Flu	
Symptoms	**Cold**	**Flu**
Fever	Rare	Usual; high—100°F (Fahrenheit) to 102°F; lasts 3 to 4 days
Headache	Rare	Common
General aches and pains	Slight	Usual; often severe
Fatigue; weakness	Sometimes	Usual; can last 2 to 3 weeks
Extreme exhaustion	Never	Usual; at the beginning of the illness
Stuffy nose	Common	Sometimes
Sneezing	Usual	Sometimes
Sore throat	Common	Sometimes
Chest discomfort; cough	Mild to moderate; hacking cough	Common; can be severe
Complications	Sinus infection; middle ear infection (otitis media); asthma	Bronchitis; pneumonia; can worsen chronic conditions; can be life-threatening

Modified from National Institute of Allergy and Infectious Diseases: Is it a cold or the flu? Bethesda, Md, August 2014, National Institutes of Health.

Onset may be sudden. The person is very ill. Signs and symptoms are listed in Box 45-4.

Drugs are ordered for infection and pain. Fluid intake is increased because of fever and to thin secretions. Thin secretions are easier to cough up. IV therapy and oxygen may be needed. Semi-Fowler's position eases breathing. Rest is important. Standard Precautions are followed. Transmission-Based Precautions are used depending on the cause. Mouth care is important. Frequent linen changes are needed because of fever.

See *Focus on Children and Older Persons: Pneumonia.*

BOX 45-4	Pneumonia—Signs and Symptoms

- Fever
- Chills
- Painful cough
- Chest pain on breathing
- Pulse: rapid
- Breathing: rapid, shortness of breath
- Cyanosis
- Sputum: thick and white, green, yellow, or rust-colored
- Nausea and vomiting
- Headache
- Tiredness
- Muscle aches

FOCUS ON CHILDREN AND OLDER PERSONS

Pneumonia

Children
Pneumonia occurs in children of all ages. It is more common in infants and toddlers.

Older Persons
Changes from aging, diseases, and decreased mobility increase the risk of pneumonia in older persons. Decreased mobility after surgery is a risk factor. Aspiration pneumonia is common in older persons. Dysphagia, decreased cough and gag reflexes, and nervous system disorders are risk factors. So are substances that depress the brain—narcotics, sedatives, alcohol, and drugs for anesthesia. For older adults, pneumonia can be life-threatening.

Older persons may not have the signs and symptoms listed in Box 45-4. Drugs and other diseases can mask signs and symptoms. Older persons may show signs of confusion, dehydration, and rapid respirations.

Tuberculosis

Tuberculosis (TB) is a bacterial infection in the lungs. It also can occur in the kidneys, bones, joints, nervous system (including the spine), muscles, and other parts of the body. If not treated, the person can die.

TB is spread by airborne droplets with coughing, sneezing, speaking, singing, or laughing (Chapter 16). Nearby persons can inhale the bacteria. Those with close, frequent contact with an infected person are at risk. TB is more likely to occur in close, crowded areas. Age, poor nutrition, and HIV (human immunodeficiency virus) infection are other risk factors.

TB can be present in the body but not cause signs and symptoms (latent TB [*latent* means *present but not active*]). An active infection may not occur for many years. Only persons with an active infection can spread the disease to others.

Chest x-rays and TB testing can detect the disease. Signs and symptoms are tiredness, loss of appetite, weight loss, fever, chills, and night sweats. Cough and sputum increase over time. Sputum may contain blood. Chest pain occurs.

Drugs for TB are given. Standard Precautions and airborne precautions are needed (Chapter 16). The person must cover the mouth and nose with tissues when sneezing, coughing, or producing sputum. Tissues are discarded in a no-touch waste container. Hand-washing after contact with sputum is essential.

See *Focus on Children and Older Persons: Tuberculosis.*
See *Focus on Long-Term Care and Home Care: Tuberculosis.*

FOCUS ON CHILDREN AND OLDER PERSONS

Tuberculosis

Older Persons
With aging, persons infected long ago can develop active TB from declining general health. Other older people with extended contact with those infected risk becoming infected. Nursing center residents are examples.

FOCUS ON LONG-TERM CARE AND HOME CARE

Tuberculosis

Long-Term Care
According to the CDC, persons with suspected or confirmed TB should not be treated in long-term care settings. Such settings include skilled nursing facilities and hospices. Persons with suspected or confirmed TB can be treated in long-term care settings if:
- Administrative and environmental controls are in place.
- The agency has a respiratory-protection program.

Cough-inducing procedures are not done unless needed infection controls are in place. Or such procedures are done outside.

Standard Precautions and airborne precautions are followed. See Chapter 16. The person wears a mask during transport to other areas, in waiting areas, and when others are present.

Home Care
The nurse teaches the person and household members about taking drugs, respiratory hygiene and cough etiquette, and the need for medical care. The person may have to stay at home until TB tests are negative or the person is no longer infectious.

Wear a TB respirator to enter the home of a person with suspected or confirmed TB. Also wear a TB respirator to transport the person in a vehicle. The person wears a mask during transport to other areas, in waiting areas, and when others are present.

Cough-inducing procedures are not done unless needed infection controls are in place. Or such procedures are done outdoors.

LYMPHATIC DISORDERS

The lymphatic system drains extra fluid from the tissues, helps fight infection, and absorbs and transports fats. Lymphatic disorders affect these functions.

See *Body Structure and Function Review: The Lymphatic System.*

BODY STRUCTURE AND FUNCTION REVIEW

The Lymphatic System

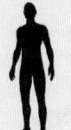

The lymphatic (lymph) system transports lymph throughout the body (Fig. 45-10). *Lymph* is a clear, thin, watery fluid. Lymph contains WBCs, proteins, and fats from the intestines.

The lymphatic system:

- Collects extra lymph from the tissues and returns it to the blood. Water, proteins, and other substances normally leak out of the capillaries into surrounding tissues. The lymphatic system drains the extra fluid from the tissues. Otherwise, the tissues swell.
- Defends the body against infection by producing lymphocytes. *Lymphocytes* are a type of WBC that defends the body against microbes that cause infection.
- Absorbs fats from the intestines and transports them to the blood.

Lymph is formed in the tissues. Lymph is transported by *lymphatic vessels.*

Lymph nodes are shaped like beans. They are found in the neck, underarm, groin area, chest, abdomen, and pelvis. Usually, you cannot see or feel lymph nodes. They swell when producing more lymphocytes to fight infection.

Lymph enters lymph nodes through the lymphatic vessels. The lymph nodes filter bacteria, cancer cells, and damaged cells from the lymph. This prevents such substances from entering the blood and circulating throughout the body.

See Figure 45-10 for the location of the *thymus (thymus gland).* Certain lymphocytes—T lymphocytes (T cells)—develop in the thymus. Such lymphocytes are important for immune system function.

The *tonsils* are in the back of the throat. *Adenoids* are behind the nose. These structures trap microbes in the mouth and nose to help prevent infection.

The *spleen* is the largest structure in the lymphatic system. The spleen:

- Filters and removes bacteria and other substances.
- Destroys old RBCs.
- Saves the iron found in hemoglobin when RBCs are destroyed.
- Stores blood. When needed, the blood is returned to the circulatory system.

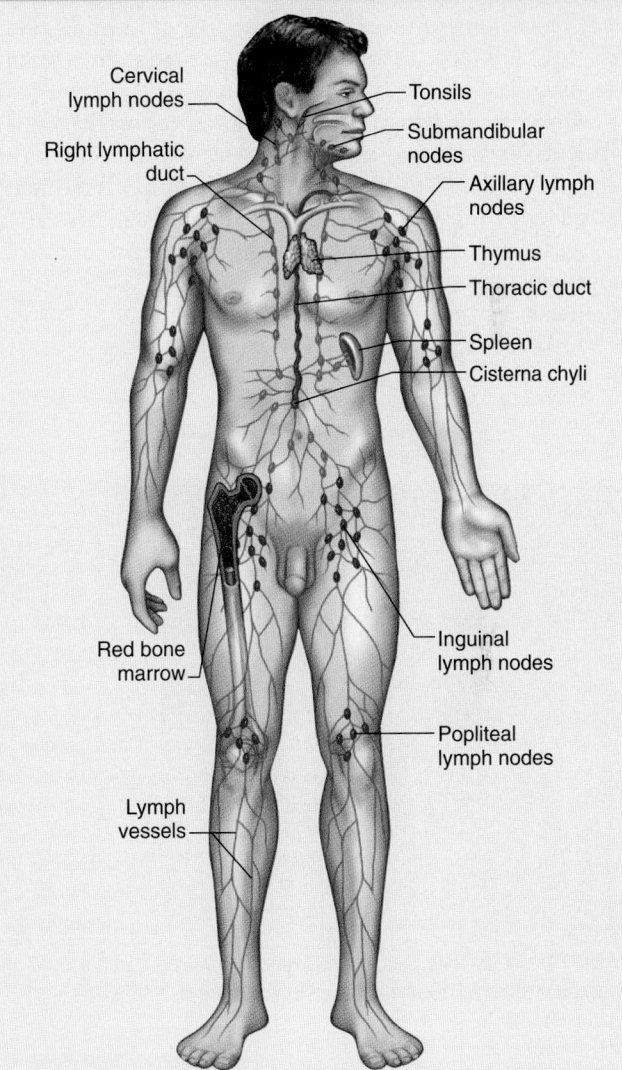

FIGURE 45-10 The lymphatic system. (From Thibodeau GA, Patton KT: *Structure & function of the body,* ed 14, St Louis, 2012, Mosby.)

Lymphedema

Lymphedema is a buildup of lymph in the tissues causing edema (swelling). It occurs with blockage or damage to the lymph system. Causes include:

- Cancer
- Infection
- Surgical removal of lymph nodes
- Scar tissue from radiation therapy or surgery
- Absent or abnormal lymph nodes present at birth

Lymphedema usually affects an arm or leg (Fig. 45-11). Other body parts can be involved. The person may have a tight or heavy feeling and have trouble moving the body part. Thickening of the skin, pain, itching or burning, and hair loss are also common. Daily activities are often affected.

Damage to the lymph system cannot be reversed. Elastic garments or bandages apply pressure to the area. This helps move fluid and prevents fluid buildup. Treatment also includes exercise, good skin care, and massage therapy. The goals are to control swelling, decrease pain, improve movement and use of the body part, and allow daily activities.

See *Promoting Safety and Comfort: Lymphedema.*

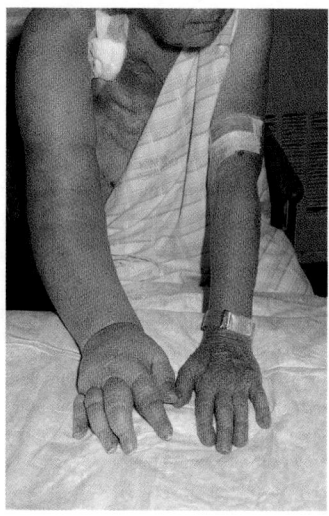

FIGURE 45-11 Lymphedema. (From Swartz MH: *Textbook of physical diagnosis: history and examination,* ed 6, Philadelphia, 2010, Saunders.)

PROMOTING SAFETY AND COMFORT

Lymphedema

Safety

In persons at risk, actions that block fluid flow or increase fluid buildup can cause lymphedema or make it worse. Never apply a blood pressure cuff to an arm with or at risk for lymphedema. For example, lymph nodes are often removed during breast cancer surgery. Do not use the arm on the surgery side to check blood pressure.

If not sure which arm to use, ask the nurse. Also, ask the person if he or she has an arm that must not be used.

Comfort

Lymphedema can be painful and affect movement. Handle the person gently. Tell the person before you move the body part. Ask the person to tell you if he or she feels pain. Stop movements that cause pain.

Lymphoma

Lymphoma is cancer involving cells in the immune system (lymphocytes). Lymphocytes are a type of WBC that protects the body from infection. They are found in lymph nodes and other lymph tissues. In lymphoma, these cells do not function normally.

There are 2 main types of lymphoma—Hodgkin lymphoma and non-Hodgkin lymphoma. They differ in the types of cells involved, how they spread, and how they respond to treatment.

Lymphoma begins with an abnormal lymphocyte. The abnormal cell divides and makes more abnormal cells. These cells cannot protect the body. They also live longer than normal. A mass of abnormal cells develops into a tumor (Chapter 43).

Signs and symptoms of lymphoma (Chapter 43) are also caused by other health problems or infections. Treatment may include chemotherapy, radiation, or both (Chapter 43). Psychological, social, and spiritual support are needed.

FOCUS ON **PRIDE**

The Person, Family, and Yourself

Personal and Professional Responsibility

Heart disease is a major concern in the United States. Life-style factors play an important role. See Box 45-1 to identify your risk factors.

Apply the information in this chapter to your own life. Take pride in making changes to promote a healthy life. A healthy life-style benefits you personally and professionally. You must be healthy and strong to care for others.

Rights and Respect

The right to personal choice promotes independence. Some choices are unhealthy. For example, a person with COPD continues to smoke. Or a person with CAD refuses to exercise or make diet changes. The health team teaches the person the risks and encourages healthy changes. The health team cannot force changes. However, they must be sure the person understands the risks.

Some persons believe that unhealthy choices improve their quality of life. They are aware of the risks but choose not to change. Although you may not respect the person's decision, you must respect the person. Treat the person with dignity and respect.

Independence and Social Interaction

Infections like Ebola, the flu, pneumonia, and TB can spread to others. You must follow Standard Precautions and the Bloodborne Pathogen Standard. Follow Transmission-Based Precautions as directed. These measures protect you and others from contamination.

The infection and the precautions may cause the person to feel unclean. Family and friends may avoid visiting. Feelings of loneliness, sadness, and depression can result.

Social and emotional needs are important. As you provide care, talk with the person. Be polite. Treat the person with kindness and respect. Explain that some precautions are used for all persons. For Transmission-Based Precautions, explain that they are for the safety of the person and others. The person should not feel ashamed or dirty. Tell the nurse about any concerns.

Delegation and Teamwork

A person's condition can change quickly. A person with angina may have an MI. Hypertension may lead to a stroke. A person may have a severe asthma attack.

Sudden condition changes require the nurse's attention. Assist the nurse as directed. You may need to help other patients or residents while the nurse provides care. Always help willingly. The entire nursing team must give "extra effort" during an emergency.

Ethics and Laws

Ethical practice involves performing your job safely and carefully. Some agencies use color-coded wristbands to promote safety and prevent harm (Chapter 13). They communicate alerts or warnings. "Limb alert" or "forbidden extremity" wristbands communicate that an arm must not be used for blood pressures, intravenous infusions, or blood draws. These are useful for lymphedema.

Learn the reason for each wristband used in your agency. Check for wristbands when providing care. Take pride in using such safety measures to prevent harm.

FOCUS ON **PRIDE**: *Application*

List the risk factors for cardiovascular disorders. Circle those that apply to you. Which factors can you change? Do you plan to make changes to lower your risk? Explain. What would help you make changes?

REVIEW QUESTIONS

Circle the BEST answer.

1 A person with a congenital heart defect
   a Needs heart surgery
   b Has damaged heart valves
   c Has blocked coronary arteries
   d Was born with the defect

2 In hypertension, the systolic blood pressure is
   a 140 mm Hg or higher
   b 120 mm Hg or higher
   c 90 mm Hg or higher
   d 80 mm Hg or higher

3 Which is a complication of hypertension?
   a COPD
   b Heart attack
   c Lymphedema
   d Diabetes

4 A person is being treated for hypertension. Which would you question?
   a No smoking
   b A high-sodium diet
   c Regular exercise
   d A low-fat diet

5 A person has angina. Which is *true?*
   a There is heart muscle damage.
   b Pain is described as crushing or stabbing.
   c Pain is relieved with rest and nitroglycerin.
   d Pain is always on the left side of the chest.

6 A person complains of sudden squeezing chest pain. You should
   a Report the pain if it is not relieved in 15 minutes
   b Report the pain at once
   c Give the person a nitroglycerin tablet
   d Give the person oxygen

Continued

REVIEW QUESTIONS—cont'd

7 Cardiac rehabilitation involves
  a Exercise
  b Surgery
  c Catheter procedures
  d A vaccine

8 A person is having an MI. Which is *true?*
  a Pain is relieved by rest.
  b There is no treatment.
  c This is an emergency.
  d The person does not have enough blood.

9 The pain of MI is usually
  a In the center or on the left side of the chest
  b On the right side of the chest
  c In the upper abdomen
  d In the mid-back region

10 A person has heart failure. Which measure should you question?
  a Encourage fluids
  b Measure intake and output
  c Measure weight daily
  d Perform range-of-motion exercises

11 A person has a dysrhythmia. Tell the nurse at once if
  a You notice a hard, round lump under the skin on the chest
  b The person is dizzy
  c The heart rate is 80
  d The person has a barrel chest

12 These statements are about Ebola. Which is *true?*
  a It is spread through the air.
  b It is contagious before symptoms appear.
  c There is a cure.
  d It is spread through blood and body fluids.

13 The most common cause of COPD is
  a Smoking
  b Allergies
  c Being over-weight
  d A high-sodium diet

14 A person has emphysema. Which is *true?*
  a The person has an infection.
  b Breathing is usually easier lying down.
  c The person has dyspnea and a cough.
  d There is swelling in an arm or leg.

15 Which is least likely to help the person with sleep apnea?
  a Weight loss
  b Quitting smoking
  c Avoiding alcohol before sleep
  d Sleeping on the back

16 Who is at highest risk for illness from EV-D68?
  a Infants and children
  b Health care workers
  c The elderly
  d Persons who smoke

17 The flu virus is spread by
  a Coughing and sneezing
  b The fecal-oral route
  c Blood
  d Needle sharing

18 Pneumonia is
  a An inflammation of the airway
  b Narrowing of the airway
  c Inflammation and infection of lung tissue
  d A bacterial infection in the lungs

19 Which position eases breathing in the person with pneumonia?
  a Supine
  b Prone
  c Semi-Fowler's
  d Trendelenberg's

20 Tuberculosis is spread by
  a Coughing and sneezing
  b Contaminated drinking water
  c Contact with wound drainage
  d The fecal-oral route

21 A person has TB. You had contact with the person's sputum. What should you do?
  a Wash your hands.
  b Put on gloves.
  c Use an alcohol-based hand rub.
  d Tell the nurse.

22 When checking blood pressure
  a Apply the cuff to the arm that is easy to reach
  b Deflate the cuff slowly when using an arm that is swollen
  c Report a blood pressure of 110/70 mm Hg at once
  d Ask if the person has an arm that should not be used for blood pressure

Answers to Chapter 45 questions are on p. 872.

FOCUS ON PRACTICE

Problem Solving

Mrs. Uma is 82 years old and lives in a nursing center. Today she seems irritable and does not recall your name. This is not normal for her. She says she is tired and does not want to eat breakfast. When should you report these changes? Why is it important to monitor for such changes in the elderly?

Digestive and Endocrine Disorders

- Define the key terms and key abbreviations in this chapter.
- Describe the care required for gastro-esophageal reflux disease, vomiting, and inflammatory bowel disease.
- Describe the care required for diverticular disease.
- Describe the care required for gallstones.

- Describe the care required for hepatitis and cirrhosis.
- Describe the care required for diabetes.
- Explain how to promote PRIDE in the person, the family, and yourself.

KEY TERMS

emesis See "vomitus"
heartburn A burning sensation in the chest or throat
hyperglycemia High *(hyper)* sugar *(glyc)* in the blood *(emia)*
hypoglycemia Low *(hypo)* sugar *(glyc)* in the blood *(emia)*

jaundice Yellowish color of the skin or whites of the eyes
vomitus Food and fluids expelled from the stomach through the mouth; emesis

KEY ABBREVIATIONS

BMs	Bowel movements		**IBD**	Inflammatory bowel disease
GERD	Gastro-esophageal reflux disease		**I&O**	Intake and output
GI	Gastro-intestinal		**IV**	Intravenous
HBV	Hepatitis B virus			

Problems can develop in any part of the digestive system. This includes the accessory organs of digestion—liver, gallbladder, and pancreas. The pancreas also is part of the endocrine system.

DIGESTIVE DISORDERS

The digestive system breaks down food for the body to absorb. Solid wastes are eliminated. See Chapter 26 for diarrhea, constipation, flatulence, fecal incontinence, and ostomy care.

See *Body Structure and Function Review: The Digestive System*, p. 740.

BODY STRUCTURE AND FUNCTION REVIEW

The Digestive System

The digestive system (*gastro-intestinal [GI] system*) involves the *alimentary canal (GI tract)* and the accessory organs of digestion (Fig. 46-1). The alimentary canal extends from the mouth to the anus.

Digestion begins in the *mouth (oral cavity)*. Using chewing motions, the *teeth* cut, chop, and grind food into small particles for digestion and swallowing. The *tongue* aids in chewing and swallowing. *Salivary glands* in the mouth secrete *saliva*. Saliva moistens food particles to ease swallowing and begin digestion. During swallowing, the tongue pushes food into the *pharynx* (throat).

Contraction of the pharynx pushes food into the *esophagus*. The esophagus extends from the pharynx to the *stomach*. Involuntary muscle contractions *(peristalsis)* move food down the esophagus through the alimentary canal.

The stomach is a muscular, pouch-like sac. The mucous membrane lining the stomach contains glands that secrete *gastric juices*. Food is mixed and churned with the gastric juices to form a semi-liquid substance called *chyme*. Peristalsis pushes chyme from the stomach into the small intestine.

The first part of the *small intestine* is the *duodenum*. More digestive juices are added to the chyme. One is called *bile*—a greenish liquid made in the *liver*. Bile is stored in the *gallbladder*. Juices from the *pancreas* and small intestine are added to the chyme. Digestive juices chemically break down food for absorption.

Peristalsis moves the chyme through the 2 other parts of the small intestine: the *jejunum* and the *ileum*. Most food absorption takes place in the jejunum and the ileum.

Undigested chyme passes from the small intestine into the *large intestine (large bowel* or *colon)*. The colon absorbs most of the water from the chyme. The remaining semi-solid material is called *feces*. Feces contain a small amount of water, solid wastes, and some mucus and germs. These are the waste products of digestion. Feces pass through the colon into the *rectum* by peristalsis. Feces pass out of the body through the *anus*.

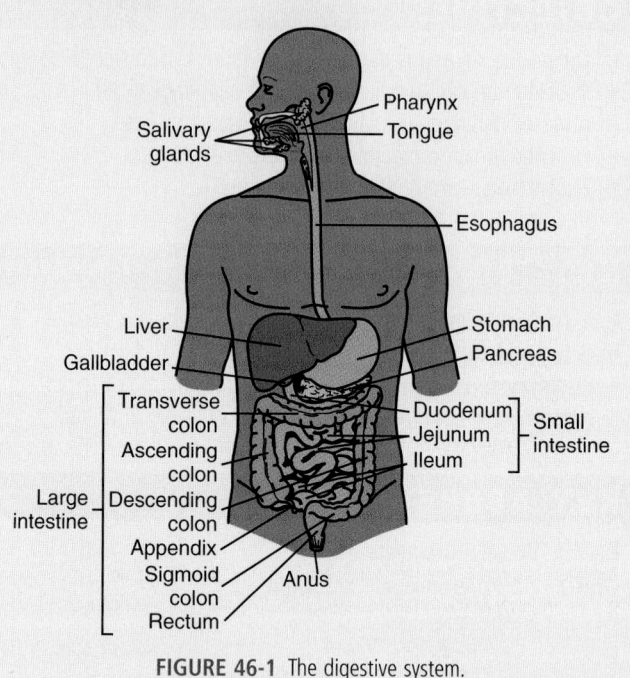

FIGURE 46-1 The digestive system.

Gastro-Esophageal Reflux Disease

Gastro-esophageal reflux disease (GERD) occurs when stomach *(gastro)* contents flow back up *(reflux)* into the esophagus *(esophageal)*. Stomach contents contain acid that can irritate and inflame the esophagus lining. This is called *esophagitis*—inflammation *(itis)* of the esophagus.

Heartburn is the most common symptom. *Heartburn is a burning sensation in the chest or throat.* The person may taste stomach fluid in the back of the mouth. Besides heartburn, other signs and symptoms of GERD include:

- Pain in the chest or upper abdomen
- Hoarseness or sore throat
- Dysphagia
- Dry cough
- Bad breath
- Nausea and vomiting

Risk factors include being over-weight, alcohol use, pregnancy, and smoking. Hiatal hernia is a risk factor. With hiatal hernia, the upper part of the stomach is above the diaphragm (Fig. 46-2). Large meals and lying down after eating can cause gastric reflux. So can chocolate, caffeine drinks, fried and fatty foods, garlic, onions, spicy foods, and tomato sauce.

The doctor may order drugs to prevent stomach acid production or to promote stomach emptying. Surgery may be needed. Life-style changes include:

- No smoking or drinking alcohol
- Losing weight
- Eating small meals
- Wearing loose belts and loose-fitting clothes
- Sitting upright for 3 hours after meals

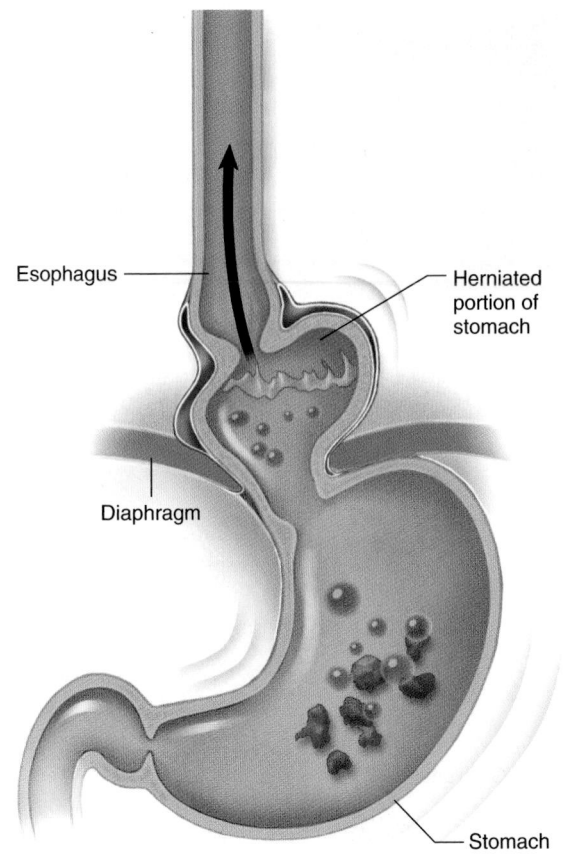

FIGURE 46-2 Hiatal hernia. (Modified from Patton KT, Thibodeau GA: *The human body in health & disease*, ed 6, St Louis, 2014, Mosby.)

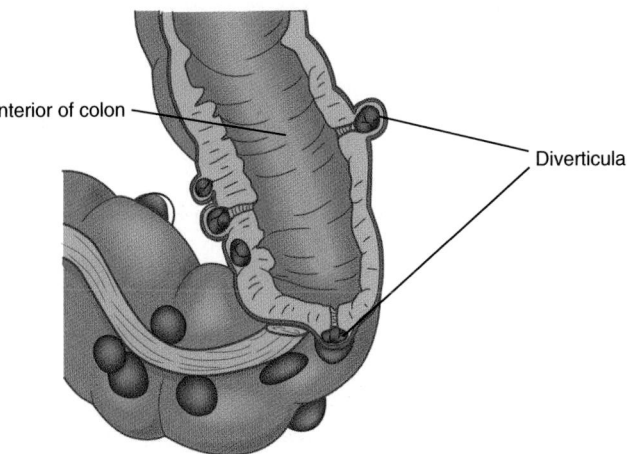

FIGURE 46-3 Diverticulosis. (From Lewis SM and others: *Medical-surgical nursing: assessment and management of clinical problems*, ed 9, St Louis, 2014, Mosby.)

Vomiting

Vomitus (emesis) is the food and fluids expelled from the stomach through the mouth. Vomiting signals illness or injury. Aspirated vomitus can obstruct the airway. Vomiting large amounts of blood can lead to shock (Chapter 54). These measures are needed.

- Follow Standard Precautions and the Bloodborne Pathogen Standard.
- Turn the person's head well to 1 side if the person is supine. This prevents aspiration.
- Place a kidney basin under the person's chin.
- Move vomitus away from the person.
- Provide oral hygiene. This helps remove the bitter taste of vomitus.
- Observe vomitus for blood, color, odor, and undigested food. If it looks like coffee grounds, it contains undigested blood. This signals bleeding. Report your observations.
- Measure, report, and record the amount of vomitus.
- Save a specimen for laboratory study.
- Dispose of vomitus after the nurse observes it.
- Eliminate odors.
- Provide for comfort. (See the inside of the front cover.)

Diverticular Disease

Small pouches can develop in the colon. The pouches bulge outward through weak spots in the colon wall (Fig. 46-3). A pouch is called a *diverticulum*. (*Diverticulare* means *to turn inside out*). *Diverticulosis* is the condition of having these pouches. (*Osis* means *condition of.*) The pouches can become infected or inflamed—*diverticulitis*. (*Itis* means *inflammation.*)

Many people over 50 years of age have diverticulosis. Aging, obesity, smoking, lack of exercise, low-fiber diet, a diet high in animal fat, and some drugs are risk factors.

When feces enter the pouches, they can become inflamed and infected. The person has abdominal pain and tenderness in the lower left abdomen. Fever, nausea and vomiting, chills, cramping, and constipation or diarrhea are likely.

A ruptured pouch is rare. Feces spill into the abdomen. This causes a severe, life-threatening infection. A pouch also can cause a blockage in the intestine (intestinal obstruction). Feces and gas cannot move past the blocked part.

Diet changes are ordered. Sometimes antibiotics and probiotics are ordered. *Probiotics*—found in dietary supplements and some foods—are live bacteria normally found in the colon. Surgery is done for severe disease, obstruction, and ruptured pouches. The diseased part of the bowel is removed. A colostomy may be needed (Chapter 26).

Inflammatory Bowel Disease

Thought to be an autoimmune disorder (Chapter 43), inflammatory bowel disease (IBD) involves a chronic inflammation of the digestive tract. Two types of IBD are:

- *Crohn's disease.* The lining of the large intestine, small intestine, or both is inflamed.
- *Ulcerative colitis.* The lining of the large intestine and rectum is inflamed and has ulcers.
  Signs and symptoms include:
- Diarrhea
- Abdominal pain and cramping
- Fever
- Bleeding—bright red blood in the toilet, dark blood in the stools, or occult blood (Chapter 34)
- Appetite: loss of
- Weight loss

IBD is often diagnosed before 30 years of age. Risk factors include a family history of IBD, cigarette smoking, some drugs, and a diet high in fat and refined foods.

Serious complications can result. They include bowel obstruction, ulcers in the GI tract (including the mouth and anus), colon cancer, osteoporosis, and liver disease. Treatment involves diet changes and drug therapy for inflammation, infection, diarrhea, pain, and nutrition. Surgery may be needed to remove damaged parts of the small intestine or colon. A colostomy or ileostomy (Chapter 26) may be necessary.

Gallstones

Bile is a liquid made in the liver. It is stored in the gallbladder until needed to digest fat. Gallstones form when the bile hardens into stone-like pieces (Fig. 46-4).

Bile is carried from the liver to the gallbladder through ducts (tubes). From the gallbladder, bile enters the small intestine through the common bile duct. Gallstones can lodge in any duct (Fig. 46-5). Bile flow is blocked. The gallbladder and ducts become inflamed. The liver and pancreas may be involved. Severe infections or damage can cause death.

Gallstones can be as small as a grain of sand or as big as a golf ball. A person may have 1 large stone or several that vary in size. Persons at risk include those who are:

- Women—especially women who:
  - Are pregnant
  - Use hormone replacement therapy
  - Take birth control pills
- Over age 40
- American Indians or Mexican Americans
- Over-weight or obese or have had rapid weight loss
- Diabetics

Signs and symptoms of a "gallbladder attack" or "gallstone attack" usually occur suddenly after eating. Signs and symptoms include nausea, vomiting, and pain in the abdomen, back, or right underarm. Surgical removal of the gallbladder is common.

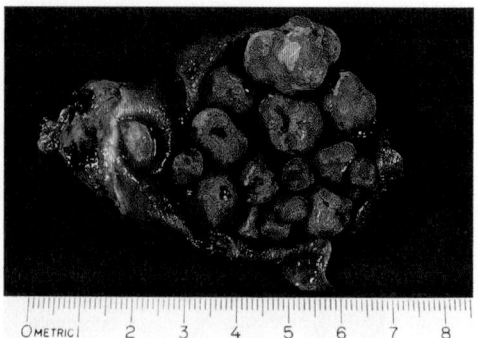

FIGURE 46-4 Inflamed gallbladder full of gallstones. (From Thompson JM, Wilson SF: *Health assessment for nursing practice,* St Louis, 1996, Mosby.)

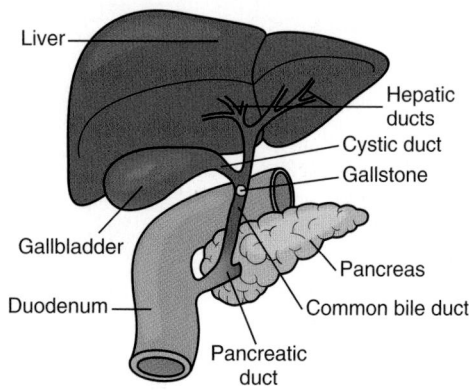

FIGURE 46-5 The gallbladder and ducts that carry bile from the liver, gallbladder, and pancreas to the small intestine. (Modified from National Institute of Diabetes and Digestive and Kidney Diseases, *Gallstones,* NIH Publication No. 13-2897, Bethesda, Md, updated November 27, 2013, National Institutes of Health.)

PROMOTING SAFETY AND COMFORT

Hepatitis

Safety

Hepatitis is contagious. Protect yourself and others. Practice hand-washing and follow Standard Precautions and the Bloodborne Pathogen Standard. Transmission-Based Precautions are ordered as necessary (Chapter 16). Assist the person with hygiene and hand-washing after BMs, before preparing or eating food, and as needed. Also, people should avoid sharing personal items with an infected person—toothbrush, razor, nail clippers, and so on.

Hepatitis

Hepatitis is inflammation (*itis*) and infection of the liver (*hepat*) caused by a virus. See Box 46-1 for signs and symptoms and persons at risk. Some people have no symptoms. There are 5 major types of hepatitis.

See *Promoting Safety and Comfort: Hepatitis.*

BOX 46-1	**Hepatitis**

Signs and Symptoms
- *Jaundice—yellowish color of the skin or whites of the eyes* (Fig. 46-6)
- Fatigue
- Pain: abdominal, joint
- Appetite: Loss of
- Nausea and vomiting
- Diarrhea
- Bowel movements (BMs): light, clay-colored
- Urine: dark
- Fever
- Headache
- Itching
- Weight loss
- Skin rash

Persons at Risk
Hepatitis A
- International travelers (especially to developing countries)
- People who live with or have sex with an infected person
- People living in areas where children are not routinely vaccinated against hepatitis A
- Day-care children and staff (during outbreaks)
- Men who have sex with men
- Users of illegal drugs

Hepatitis B
- People who live with or have sex with an infected person
- Men who have sex with men
- People who have multiple sex partners

Persons at Risk—cont'd
Hepatitis B—cont'd
- Injection drug users
- Immigrants and children of immigrants from areas with high rates of hepatitis B
- Infants born to infected mothers
- Hemodialysis patients (Chapter 47)
- People who received blood or blood products before 1987
- International travelers

Hepatitis C
- Injection drug users
- People who have sex with an infected person
- People who have multiple sex partners
- Health care workers
- Infants born to infected mothers
- People who received tattoos or piercings with non-sterile equipment
- Hemodialysis patients
- People who received blood or blood products before 1992
- People who received blood clotting factors made before 1987

Hepatitis D
- People who live with or have sex with an infected person
- People who received blood or blood products before 1987

Hepatitis E
- International travelers (especially to developing countries)
- People living in areas where hepatitis E outbreaks are common
- People who live with or have sex with an infected person

Modified from National Institute of Diabetes and Digestive and Kidney Diseases: Viral hepatitis: A through E and beyond, *NIH Publication No. 08-4762, Bethesda, Md, 2008, updated April 23, 2012, National Institutes of Health.*

Hepatitis A. This type is spread by food or water contaminated with feces from an infected person. Hepatitis A is spread through:
- Eating or drinking food or water contaminated with feces
- Eating or drinking from a contaminated vessel
- Eating raw shellfish from sewage-polluted water
- Having close contact or sex with an infected person

Treatment involves rest, a healthy diet, fluids, and no alcohol. The person should not prepare food for others. Recovery takes several weeks.

Persons with fecal incontinence, confusion, and dementia can cause contamination. Carefully look for contaminated items and areas.

Handle bedpans, toilets, diapers, and rectal thermometers carefully. The hepatitis A vaccine provides protection against the disease.

See *Focus on Children and Older Persons: Hepatitis A.*

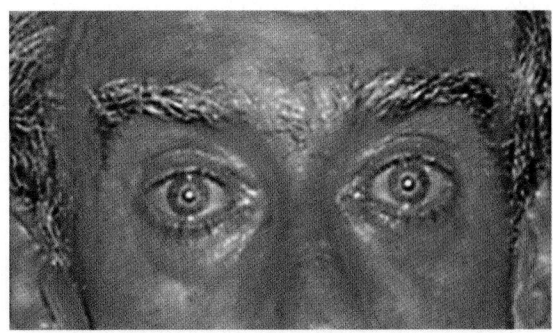

FIGURE 46-6 Jaundice. (From Butcher GP: *Gastroenterology: an illustrated colour text,* London, 2004, Churchill Livingstone.)

FOCUS ON CHILDREN AND OLDER PERSONS

Hepatitis A

Children
Pre-school and school-age children are at risk for hepatitis A. Children in day care also are at risk. Poor hygiene after BMs leads to contaminated eating and drinking vessels. Also, young children often put their hands in their mouths.

Hepatitis B. The hepatitis B virus (HBV) is the cause. It is spread through infected blood and body fluids (saliva, semen, vaginal secretions).
- By sharing blood-contaminated IV (intravenous) needles and syringes
- By accidental needle-sticks
- By sex without a condom, especially anal sex
- During childbirth from mother to baby

For the HBV vaccine, see Chapter 16. Drugs are ordered for chronic hepatitis B.

Hepatitis C. This type is spread by blood infected with the hepatitis C virus. A person may have no symptoms but can spread the disease. Serious liver disease and damage may appear years later. Hepatitis C is treated with drugs. The virus can be spread mainly through:
- Sharing blood-contaminated IV needles and syringes
- Contaminated tools used for tattoos or body piercings

Hepatitis D and Hepatitis E. Hepatitis D occurs only in people infected with hepatitis B. It is spread the same way as HBV.

Hepatitis E is spread through food or water contaminated by feces from an infected person. This disease is not common in the United States.

Cirrhosis

Cirrhosis is a liver condition caused by chronic liver damage (Fig. 46-7). *(Cirrho* means *yellow-orange. Osis* means *condition.)* Scar tissue blocks blood flow through the liver. Normal liver functions are affected.
- Fighting infection
- Processing, storing, and delivering nutrients to the body
- Cleaning the blood of toxins, fats, cholesterol, and drugs
- Making proteins for blood clotting
- Producing bile for fat digestion

Chronic alcohol abuse, chronic hepatitis B and C, and extra fat in the liver are common causes. Obesity is becoming a common cause. Signs and symptoms do not appear early in the disease. These may occur as the disease progresses.
- Weakness and fatigue
- Loss of appetite and weight loss
- Nausea
- *Ascites*—abdominal bloating from fluid buildup in the abdomen (Fig. 46-8)
- Edema (swelling) in the feet and legs
- Itching
- Spider-like blood vessels on the skin
- Jaundice

Cirrhosis has many serious complications. Infection, bruising, and bleeding occur. Blood vessels in the esophagus and stomach enlarge and burst. Gallstones may develop. Toxins build up in the brain, causing confusion, personality changes, and memory loss. Diabetes and liver cancer are risks.

Treatment is aimed at preventing scar tissue. Complications are treated. A low-sodium diet is needed for edema and ascites. Diuretic drugs (water pills) are ordered to remove fluid. Antibiotics are ordered for infection. The person must avoid alcohol and may need a liver transplant.

The measures listed in Box 46-2 may be part of the person's care plan.

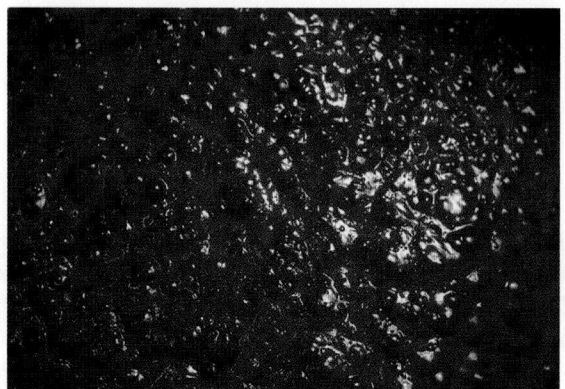

FIGURE 46-7 Liver damage from alcohol. (From Patton KT, Thibodeau GA: *The human body in health & disease,* ed 6, St Louis, 2014, Mosby.)

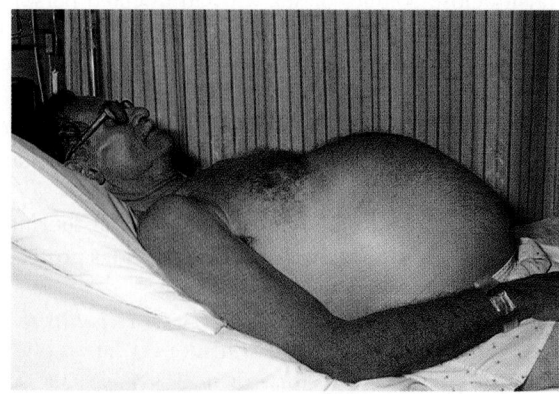

FIGURE 46-8 Fluid in the membrane lining the abdominal cavity *(ascites).* (From Swartz MH: *Textbook of physical diagnosis,* ed 5, Philadelphia, 2006, Saunders.)

BOX 46-2	Cirrhosis

General Care
- Follow the care plan to prevent complications from bedrest—pneumonia, blood clots, pressure ulcers.
- Provide good skin care.
  - Use warm water with baking soda for bathing. This decreases itching.
  - Apply lotion to the skin.
  - Discourage the scratching of itchy skin.
- Provide mouth care before meals and every 2 hours.
- Follow fluid restriction orders.
- Turn the person at least every 2 hours or as noted on the care plan.
- Promote comfort and the ability to breathe.
  - Semi-Fowler's or Fowler's position
  - Pillows under the arms for support
  - Coughing and deep-breathing exercises
- Assist with activities of daily living (ADL) as needed.

Measurements and Observations
- Observe vomitus, urine, and BMs for blood.
- Observe for signs of decreased mental function—confusion, memory loss, behavior changes, and so on.
- Measure vital signs every 2 to 4 hours.
- Measure intake and output (I&O).
- Measure weight daily.

Safety
- Use bed rails according to the care plan.
- Keep the call light and other needed items within reach.
- Complete a safety check before leaving the room. (See the inside of the front cover.)

ENDOCRINE DISORDERS

The endocrine system is made up of glands. The endocrine glands secrete hormones that affect other organs and glands. Diabetes, the most common endocrine disorder, involves the pancreas.

See *Body Structure and Function Review: The Endocrine System (Pancreas).*

Diabetes

In diabetes, the body cannot produce or use insulin properly. Without enough insulin, sugar builds up in the blood. Blood glucose (sugar) is high. Cells do not have enough sugar for energy and cannot function.

Types of Diabetes. A family history of the disease is a common risk factor for the 3 types of diabetes.
- *Type 1 diabetes.* Occurs most often in children and teenagers but can develop in adults. The pancreas produces little or no insulin. Onset is rapid.
- *Type 2 diabetes.* This type can occur at any age, even in children. Being over-weight and lack of exercise are risk factors. The pancreas secretes insulin. However, the body cannot use it well. Onset is slow. Infections are frequent. Wounds heal slowly. These ethnic groups are at risk.
  - American Indians
  - Blacks
  - Asian-Americans
  - Hispanics
- *Gestational diabetes.* Develops during pregnancy. (*Gestation* comes from *gestare.* It means *to bear.*) This type usually goes away after the baby is born. However, the mother is at risk for type 2 diabetes later in life.

BODY STRUCTURE AND FUNCTION REVIEW

The Endocrine System (Pancreas)

The *endocrine glands* (Fig. 46-9) secrete chemical substances called *hormones* into the bloodstream. Hormones regulate the activities of other organs and glands in the body.

The *pancreas* secretes *insulin.* Insulin regulates the amount of sugar in the blood available for use by the cells. Insulin is needed for sugar to enter the cells. With too little insulin, sugar cannot enter the cells. If sugar cannot enter the cells, excess amounts build up in the blood. This condition is called *diabetes.*

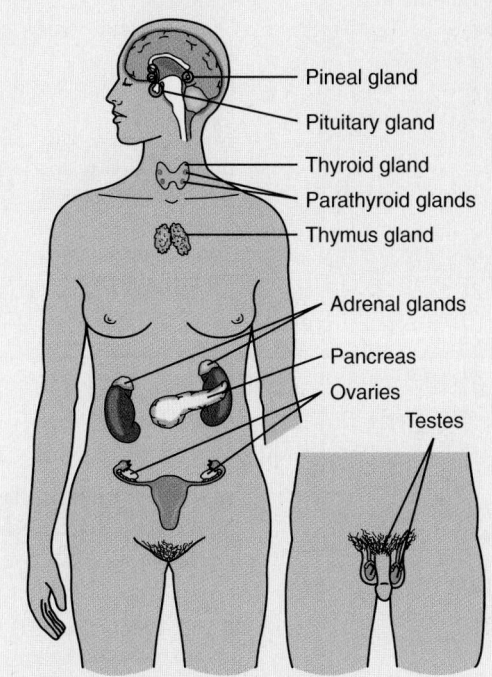

- Pineal gland
- Pituitary gland
- Thyroid gland
- Parathyroid glands
- Thymus gland
- Adrenal glands
- Pancreas
- Ovaries
- Testes

FIGURE 46-9 The endocrine system.

Signs and Symptoms. Signs and symptoms of diabetes are:

- Being very thirsty
- Frequent urination
- Feeling very hungry or tired
- Weight loss without trying
- Sores that heal slowly
- Dry, itchy skin
- Tingling or loss of feeling in the feet
- Blurred vision

Complications. Diabetes must be controlled to prevent complications. Diabetes can damage the heart, blood vessels, eyes, kidneys, and nerves. Heart and blood vessel damage can lead to stroke, heart attack, and slow healing. Foot and leg wounds and ulcers are very serious (Chapter 36). Infection and gangrene can occur. Sometimes amputation is necessary.

Treatment. Type 1 diabetes is treated with daily insulin therapy, healthy eating (Chapter 27), and exercise. Type 2 diabetes is treated with healthy eating, exercise, and weight loss if needed. The person with type 2 may take oral drugs or need insulin. Types 1 and 2 involve controlling blood pressure, cholesterol, and the risk factors for coronary artery disease.

Good foot care is needed. Corns, blisters, calluses, and other foot problems can lead to an infection and amputation. See Chapters 23 and 36.

The person's blood sugar level can fall too low or go too high. Blood glucose is monitored daily or 3 or 4 times a day for:

- *Hypoglycemia means low* (hypo) *sugar* (glyc) *in the blood* (emia).
- *Hyperglycemia means high* (hyper) *sugar* (glyc) *in the blood* (emia).

See Table 46-1 for the causes, signs, and symptoms of hypoglycemia and hyperglycemia. Both can lead to death if not corrected. Call for the nurse at once.

See *Focus on Children and Older Persons: Diabetes.*

TABLE 46-1	Hypoglycemia and Hyperglycemia		
Hypoglycemia (Low Blood Sugar)		**Hyperglycemia (High Blood Sugar)**	
Causes	Signs and Symptoms	Causes	Signs and Symptoms
Too much insulin or diabetic drugs	Fatigue; weakness	Not enough insulin or diabetic drugs	Weakness
Increased exercise	Dizziness; faintness	Too little exercise	Drowsiness
Omitting or missing a meal	Vision changes	Eating too much food	Vision: blurred
Delayed meal	Hunger	Emotional stress	Hunger; thirst
Eating too little food	Tingling around the mouth	Infection or sickness	Dry mouth (very)
Vomiting	Headache	Undiagnosed diabetes	Headache
Drinking alcohol	Skin: cold and clammy		Skin: dry
	Sweating		Face: flushed
	Respirations: rapid and shallow		Respirations: rapid, deep, and labored
	Pulse: rapid		Pulse: rapid, weak
	Blood pressure: low		Blood pressure: low
	Motions: clumsy and jerky		Breath odor: sweet
	Trembling; shakiness		Leg cramps
	Confusion		Urination: frequent
	Convulsions		Nausea; vomiting
	Unconsciousness		Convulsions
			Coma

FOCUS ON CHILDREN AND OLDER PERSONS

Diabetes

Children
Your assignment may include preparing meals for a child with diabetes. Follow the child's diet carefully. Also prepare snacks for the child to take to school. The snack is needed in case the child's blood sugar level drops.

FOCUS ON **PRIDE**

The Person, Family, and Yourself

Personal and Professional Responsibility

Understanding health problems allows you to safely assist with care. You may want to know more about a health problem. Or a person may have a disorder you did not learn about in your training. Ask the nurse to explain the problem and the care required. You can also look up the problem in a medical dictionary or on the Internet. Take pride in learning more.

Rights and Respect

For some health problems, family history is a risk factor. Others result from life-style choices. Poor diet, lack of exercise, drug abuse, unsafe sex, and alcohol abuse are examples. The cause must not affect how you treat the person. Always show dignity and respect.

Independence and Social Interaction

Many digestive and endocrine disorders require dietary changes. Dietary practices are cultural and personal. Adjusting to changes can be hard. The person may feel loss of control over an important part of his or her life-style. The person and family need education, support, and encouragement.

Delegation and Teamwork

The health team plans care to treat disorders and meet the person's needs. As needs change, the care plan changes. Good communication and teamwork are needed. Assist with the person's care as directed. Follow the person's care plan.

Ethics and Laws

Some problems need attention right away. Delays in care can cause harm. For example, a person who is vomiting uses the call light to signal for help. Minutes pass before anyone responds. The person aspirates. Vomitus obstructs the airway. The person dies.

The health team must promptly respond to needs. Otherwise negligence, neglect, and other legal problems can result (Chapter 5).

FOCUS ON **PRIDE**: *Application*

Choose a disorder in this chapter. What life-style changes are needed? Discuss the impact on the person and family. How does the health team help the person and family adjust?

REVIEW QUESTIONS

Circle the BEST answer.

1 A person has gastro-esophageal reflux disease. Which should you question?
   a Loose clothing
   b Supine position after meals
   c Small meals
   d No smoking or alcohol

2 A person with gastro-esophageal reflux disease has these food choices. Which is *best* for the person?
   a Baked chicken
   b Pasta with tomato sauce
   c Fried ravioli
   d Chicken wings with hot sauce

3 A person is vomiting. You should
   a Position the person supine
   b Leave to get the nurse
   c Do nothing
   d Turn the person's head to the side

4 Vomiting is dangerous because of
   a Aspiration
   b Diverticular disease
   c Ascites
   d Jaundice

5 Vomitus looks like coffee grounds. This signals
   a Gastro-esophageal reflux disease
   b Gallstones
   c Bleeding
   d A ruptured pouch

6 A person has diverticular disease. You will likely assist with
   a Giving antibiotics
   b Promoting normal bowel elimination
   c Dietary teaching and planning
   d Blood glucose monitoring

7 Gallbladder attacks usually occur
   a On awakening
   b During a fast
   c Suddenly after eating
   d When the person is lying down

8 Which is a sign of gallstones?
   a Extreme thirst
   b Abdominal pain
   c Black, tarry stools
   d Hoarseness and choking sensation

9 Hepatitis is inflammation of the
   a Liver
   b Gallbladder
   c Pancreas
   d Stomach

10 Which is spread by food or water contaminated with feces from an infected person?
   a Hepatitis A   c Hepatitis C
   b Hepatitis B   d Hepatitis D

11 Hepatitis requires
   a Sterile gloving
   b Double-bagging
   c Standard Precautions
   d Masks, gowns, and goggles

12 Which is a common cause of cirrhosis?
   a Diabetes
   b Alcohol abuse
   c Gallstones
   d GERD

13 A person has cirrhosis. Which should you question?
   a Measure I&O.
   b Weigh the person daily.
   c Use warm water with baking soda for bathing.
   d Encourage fluids.

Continued

REVIEW QUESTIONS—cont'd

14 A person has cirrhosis. You should observe stools and vomitus for blood.
    a   True
    b   False

15 Which is a sign of diabetes?
    a   Decreased urine output
    b   Weight gain
    c   Hunger
    d   Jaundice

16 A person with diabetes needs
    a   A sodium-controlled diet
    b   Fluid restriction
    c   Surgery
    d   Good foot care

17 A person with diabetes is vomiting after a meal. The person is at risk for
    a   Hypoglycemia
    b   Hyperglycemia
    c   Jaundice
    d   Bleeding

18 A person has diabetes. Blood glucose is monitored daily or
    a   2 or 3 times a day
    b   3 or 4 times a day
    c   4 or 5 times a day
    d   5 or 6 times a day

Answers to Chapter 46 questions are on p. 872.

FOCUS ON PRACTICE

Problem Solving

A resident with diabetes is confused, weak, and shaky. What do you do? What might these signs and symptoms indicate? How does understanding the person's health problems help you give better care?

Urinary and Reproductive Disorders

Urinary and reproductive disorders are common. Understanding the disorders gives meaning to the required care.

URINARY SYSTEM DISORDERS

Disorders can occur in urinary system structures—kidneys, ureters, bladder, and urethra. Men can develop prostate problems.

See *Body Structure and Function Review: The Urinary System*, p. 750.

BODY STRUCTURE AND FUNCTION REVIEW

The Urinary System

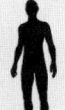

The urinary system (Fig. 47-1):
* Removes waste products from the blood.
* Maintains water balance.
* Maintains electrolyte balance. *Electrolytes* are substances that dissolve in water—sodium, potassium, and calcium. (See Chapter 10.)
* Maintains acid-base balance. (See Chapter 10.)

The *kidneys* are 2 bean-shaped organs in the upper abdomen. They lie against the back muscles on each side of the spine.

Each kidney has over a million tiny *nephrons*—the basic working unit of the kidney. Each nephron has a cluster of capillaries called a *glomerulus*. Blood passes through the glomeruli and is filtered by the capillaries. Most of the water and other needed substances are re-absorbed by the blood. The rest of the fluid and the waste products form *urine* in the tubule that drains into the *renal pelvis* in the kidney.

A *ureter* is attached to the renal pelvis of the kidney. The ureters carry urine from the kidneys to the *bladder*. Urine is stored in the bladder until there is a need to urinate. This usually occurs when there is about a half pint (250 mL) of urine in the bladder. Urine passes from the bladder through the *urethra*. The opening at the end of the urethra is called the *meatus*. Urine passes from the body through the meatus.

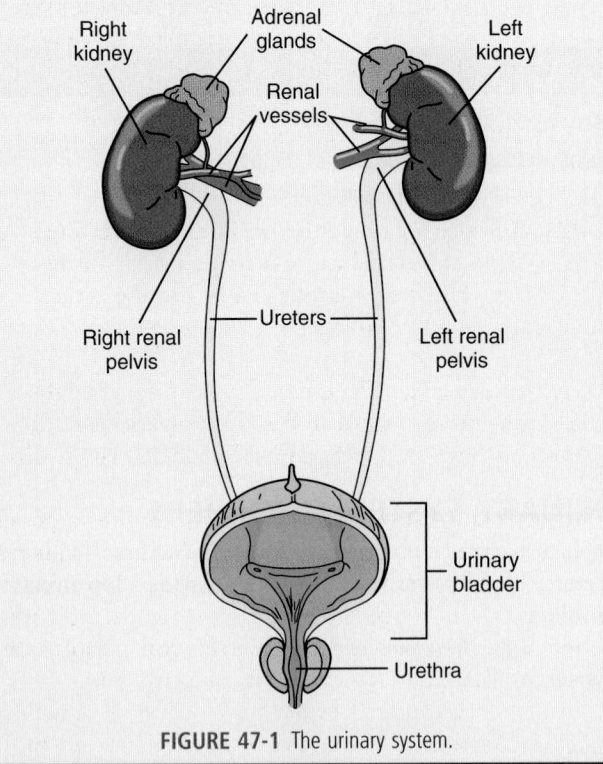

FIGURE 47-1 The urinary system.

Common Signs and Symptoms
* Urinary frequency
* *Oliguria—scant* (olig) *urine* (uria)
* Urgency
* *Dysuria—difficult or painful* (dys) *urination* (uria)
* Pain or burning on urination
* *Hematuria—blood* (hemat) *in the urine* (uria)
* *Pyuria—pus* (py) *in the urine* (uria)
* Cloudy urine
* Urine odor
* Pelvic pain—women
* Rectal pain—men

Cystitis—a bladder *(cyst)* infection *(itis)* caused by bacteria
* Additional symptoms
  * Pelvic pressure
  * Lower abdominal discomfort

Pyelonephritis—inflammation *(itis)* of the kidney *(nephr)* pelvis *(pyelo)*
* Additional symptoms
  * Back and side pain
  * High fever
  * Nausea and vomiting
  * Shaking and chills

Urinary Tract Infections

Urinary tract infections (UTIs) are common. Infection in 1 area can spread through the urinary tract. Microbes can enter the system through the urethra. Urological exams, intercourse, poor perineal hygiene, immobility, and poor fluid intake are common causes. Persons with urinary catheters are at high risk (Chapter 25). UTI is a common healthcare-associated infection (Chapter 16).

Women are at high risk. Microbes can easily enter the short female urethra. Prostate gland secretions help protect men from UTIs. However, an enlarged prostate increases the risk of UTI.

See Box 47-1 for the types of UTIs and their signs and symptoms. UTIs are treated with antibiotics. Fluids are encouraged—usually 2000 mL (milliliters) a day. Normal elimination is promoted. The person should urinate when the urge is felt. For prevention and treatment, proper perineal care and catheter care are needed.

Prostate Enlargement

The prostate is a walnut-shaped gland in men. It lies in front of the rectum and just below the bladder (Fig. 47-2, *A*). The prostate surrounds the urethra. The prostate grows larger (enlarges) as the man grows older (Fig. 47-2, *B*). This is called benign prostatic hyperplasia (BPH). *Benign* means *non-malignant. Hyper* means *excessive. Plasia* means *formation* or *development.* Benign prostatic hypertrophy is another name for enlarged prostate. (*Trophy* means *growth.*)

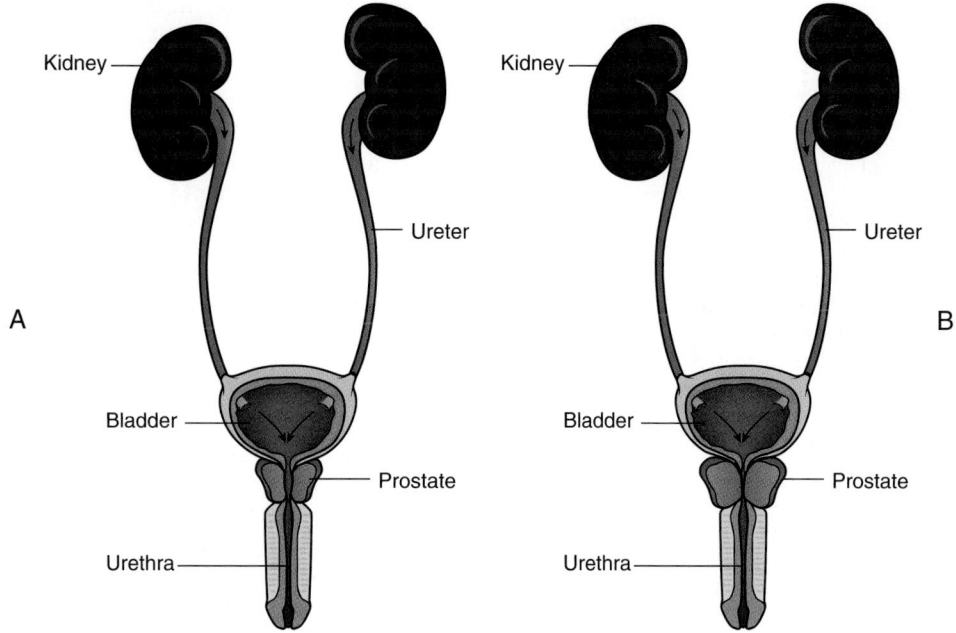

FIGURE 47-2 A, Normal prostate. **B,** Enlarged prostate. The prostate presses against the urethra. Urine flow is obstructed.

BPH is common in older men. The enlarged prostate presses against the urethra, obstructing urine flow. Bladder function is gradually lost. These problems are common.

- Trouble starting a urine stream
- A weak urine stream
- Frequent voidings of small amounts of urine
- Urgency and leaking or dribbling of urine
- Frequent voiding at night *(nocturia)*
- Urinary retention (The man cannot void. Urine remains in the bladder.)
- Urinary incontinence
- Pain during urination

For mild BPH, drugs can shrink the prostate or stop its growth. Some microwave and laser treatments destroy excess prostate tissue.

Transurethral resection of the prostate (TURP) is a common surgical procedure for severe BPH. Inserted through the penis, a lighted scope with a wire loop is used to cut tissue and seal blood vessels. The removed tissue is flushed out of the bladder. Flushing fluid enters the bladder through a catheter. Urine and the flushing fluid flow out of the bladder through the same catheter. Some bleeding and blood clots are normal. The person's care plan may include:

- No straining or sudden movements
- Drinking a least 8 cups of water daily
- No straining to have a bowel movement
- A balanced diet to prevent constipation
- No heavy lifting

Urinary Diversion

Cancer and bladder injuries are common reasons for surgical removal of the bladder. With the bladder removed, urine must still leave the body. A *urinary diversion is a surgically created pathway for urine to leave the body.*

Often an ostomy is involved. A *urostomy is a surgically created opening* (stomy) *that connects to the urinary tract* (uro). The 2 main types of urostomies are:

- *Ileal conduit.* A small section of the small intestine *(ileal)* is re-positioned to serve as a channel *(conduit)* for urine. The ureters are connected to the conduit and the conduit is connected to a stoma (Fig. 47-3, p. 752).
- *Cutaneous ureterostomy.* Ureters *(ureter)* are brought through the abdominal wall and a stoma *(ostomy)* is created on the skin *(cutaneous)*. This type may involve 1 or 2 stomas (Fig. 47-4, p. 752).

Urine drains constantly from the stoma into a pouch applied over the stoma (Fig. 47-5, p. 752). Empty pouches every 3 to 4 hours. Or empty them when becoming ⅓ (one-third) full. Pouches become heavy as they fill with urine. A heavy pouch can loosen the seal between the pouch and the skin. Urine can leak onto the skin.

Pouches are changed every 5 to 7 days. A pouch is replaced any time it leaks. Urine on the skin can cause irritation, breakdown, and infection.

Good skin care is needed. You must help prevent skin breakdown. Observe and report skin changes around the stoma. See "The Person With an Ostomy" in Chapter 26.

See *Promoting Safety and Comfort: Urinary Diversion*, p. 752.

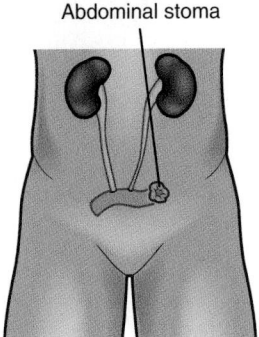

FIGURE 47-3 Ileal conduit. (Modified from Lewis SL and others: *Medical-surgical nursing: assessment and management of clinical problems*, ed 9, St Louis, 2014, Mosby.)

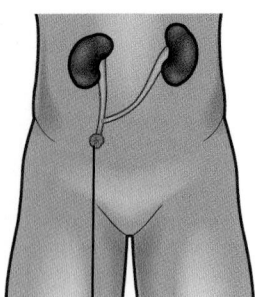

FIGURE 47-4 Cutaneous ureterostomy. The left ureter is connected to the right ureter. One stoma is needed. (Modified from Lewis SL and others: *Medical-surgical nursing: assessment and management of clinical problems*, ed 9, St Louis, 2014, Mosby.)

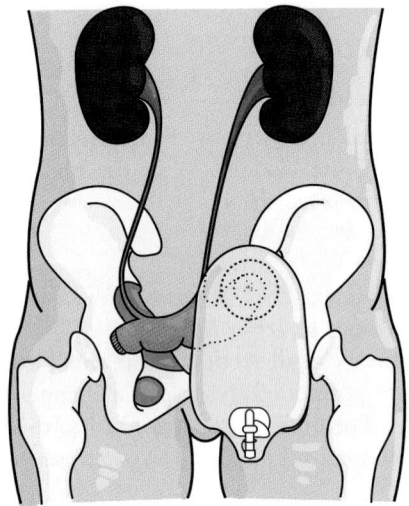

FIGURE 47-5 Urostomy pouch.

PROMOTING SAFETY AND COMFORT

Urinary Diversion

Safety

Urine may contain microbes and blood. And you have contact with mucous membranes. Follow Standard Precautions and the Bloodborne Pathogen Standard.

Comfort

The best time to change a pouch is after sleep and before eating or drinking. Urine flow is less when the person has not had anything to eat or drink for 2 to 3 hours.

The stoma does not have sensation. Touching the stoma does not cause pain or discomfort.

Kidney Stones

Kidney stones *(calculi)* are more common in men than in women. Stones vary in size from grains of sand to golf ball–sized (Fig. 47-6). Bedrest, immobility, and poor fluid intake are risk factors. Signs and symptoms include:

- Severe, cramping pain in the back and side just below the ribs (Fig. 47-7)
- Pain in the lower abdomen, thigh, and urethra
- Nausea and vomiting
- Fever and chills
- *Dysuria*—difficult or painful *(dys)* urination *(uria)*
- Urinary urgency
- Pain on urination
- *Hematuria*—blood *(hemat)* in the urine *(uria)*
- Cloudy urine
- Foul-smelling urine

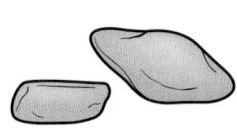

Smooth

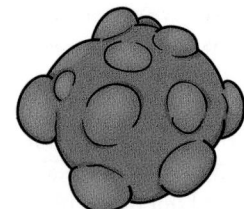

Golf ball–sized and brown

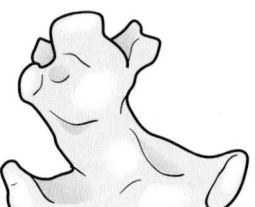

Staghorn

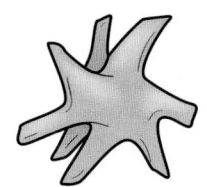

Jagged and yellow

FIGURE 47-6 Kidney stones.

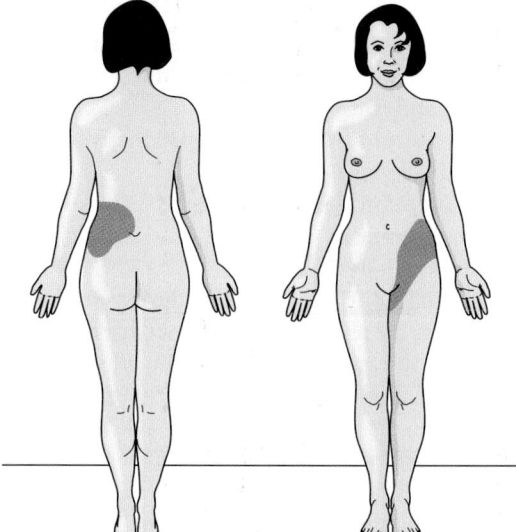

FIGURE 47-7 Shaded areas show where the pain from a left kidney stone is located.

Drugs are given for pain relief. The person needs to drink 2000 to 3000 mL a day. The fluids help flush stones out through the urine. All urine is strained (Chapter 34). Medical or surgical removal of the stone may be necessary. Diet changes may prevent stones.

Kidney Failure

In kidney failure (renal failure), the kidneys do not function or are severely impaired. Waste products are not removed from the blood. Fluid is retained. Heart failure and hypertension easily result. The person is very ill and can die.

Acute Kidney Failure. Acute kidney failure (acute kidney injury, acute renal failure) is sudden. Blood flow to the kidneys is severely decreased. Causes include severe injury or bleeding, heart attack, burns, infection, and severe allergic reactions.

At first, *oliguria* (scant amount of urine) occurs. Urine output is less than 400 mL in 24 hours. This phase lasts a few days to 2 weeks or longer. Then *diuresis* occurs—*the process* (esis) *of passing* (di) *urine* (ur). *Large amounts are produced—1000 to 3000 mL or more a day.* Kidney function improves and returns to normal during the recovery phase. This can take up to 1 year. Some persons develop chronic kidney failure.

Treatment involves drugs, restricted fluids, and diet therapy. The care plan may include the measures in Box 47-2. Urinary output is measured hourly. Report less than 30 mL per hour at once.

Chronic Kidney Disease. In chronic kidney disease (CKD; chronic kidney failure), kidney function is gradually lost. Nephrons are destroyed over many years. Hypertension and diabetes are common causes. Infections, urinary tract obstructions, and cancer are other causes.

CKD can affect every body system. Signs and symptoms are listed in Box 47-3.

Treatment includes fluid restriction, diet therapy, drugs, and dialysis. *Dialysis is the process of removing waste products from the blood.*

- *Hemodialysis* removes waste and fluid by filtering the blood (*hemo*) through an artificial kidney (Fig. 47-8, p. 754).
- *Peritoneal dialysis* uses the lining of the abdominal cavity (*peritoneal membrane*) to remove waste and fluid from the blood (Fig. 47-9, p. 754).

You will assist in the person's care. See Box 47-2.

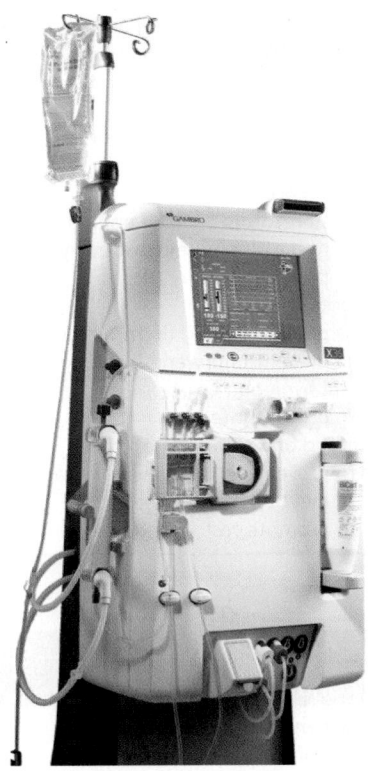

FIGURE 47-8 Dialysis machine. (Courtesy Baxter Healthcare Corp., Deerfield, Ill.)

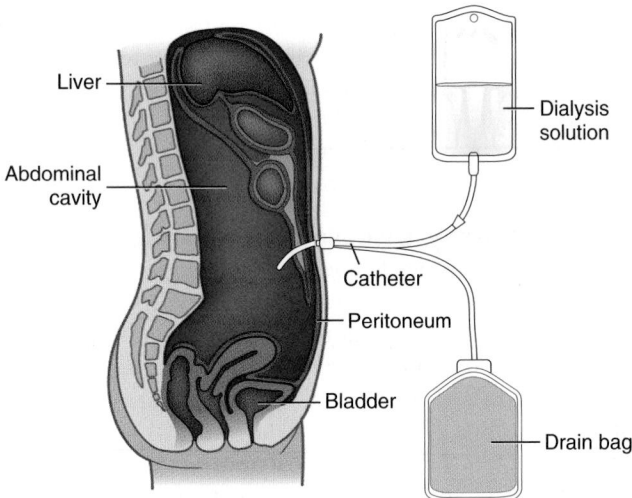

FIGURE 47-9 Peritoneal dialysis system. (Modified from Lewis SL and others: *Medical-surgical nursing: assessment and management of clinical problems*, ed 9, St Louis, 2014, Mosby.)

REPRODUCTIVE DISORDERS

Sexual activities involve the structures and functions of the reproductive system. The male reproductive system:

- Produces and transports sperm.
- Deposits sperm in the female reproductive tract.
- Secretes hormones.
  The female reproductive system:
- Produces eggs *(ova)*.
- Secretes hormones.
- Protects and nourishes the fetus during pregnancy.
  Aging affects the reproductive system (Chapters 12 and 51). Many injuries, diseases, and surgeries can affect reproductive structures and functions.

Sexually Transmitted Diseases

A sexually transmitted disease (STD) is spread by oral, vaginal, or anal sex (Table 47-1). Some people have no signs and symptoms or are not aware of an infection. Others know but do not seek treatment because of embarrassment.

STDs often occur in the genital and rectal areas. They also occur in the ears, mouth, nipples, throat, tongue, eyes, and nose. Condom use helps prevent the spread of STDs, especially the human immunodeficiency virus (HIV) and acquired immunodeficiency syndrome (AIDS). Some STDs are also spread through skin breaks, by contact with infected body fluids (blood, semen, saliva), or by contaminated blood or needles.

Standard Precautions and the Bloodborne Pathogen Standard are followed.

See *Focus on Children and Older Persons: Sexually Transmitted Diseases.*

FOCUS ON CHILDREN AND OLDER PERSONS

Sexually Transmitted Diseases

Older Persons

Many older people are sexually active. They get and can spread STDs in the same ways that younger persons do. However, many do not think they are at risk. Always practice Standard Precautions and follow the Bloodborne Pathogen Standard. Do not assume that older people are too old to have sex.

FIGURE 47-10 Herpes. **A,** Sores on the penis. **B,** Sores on the female perineum. (Courtesy United States Public Health Service, Washington, DC.)

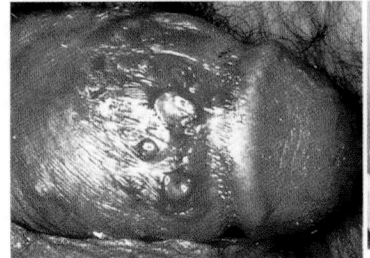
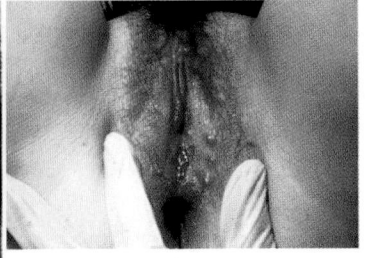

A
B

TABLE 47-1	**Sexually Transmitted Diseases**	
Disease	**Signs and Symptoms**	**Treatment**
Herpes	Painful, blister-like sores on or near the genitals, mouth, or anus (Fig. 47-10) Sores may have a watery discharge Pain, itching, burning, and tingling in the affected area Vaginal discharge Pain during urination or intercourse Fever Swollen glands	No known cure Anti-viral drugs
Genital warts	*Male*—Warts in or on the penis, anus, genitalia, mouth, or throat *Female*—Warts in or on the vagina, cervix, labia, anus, mouth, or throat	Application of an ointment that causes the warts to dry up and fall off Surgical removal may be necessary if the ointment is not effective
HIV/AIDS	See Chapter 43	See Chapter 43
Gonorrhea	Burning and pain on urination Urinary frequency and urgency Genital discharge (vagina, urethra, rectum)	Antibiotic drugs
Chlamydia	May not show symptoms Discharge from the penis or vagina Burning or pain on urination Testicular pain or swelling Vaginal bleeding Rectal inflammation and/or discharge Pain during intercourse Diarrhea Nausea Abdominal pain Fever	Antibiotic drugs
Pubic lice	Intense itching	Over-the-counter or prescription lice treatment Washing or dry-cleaning all exposed clothing, bedding, and towels
Trichomoniasis (occurs in women; men are carriers)	No symptoms in men Frothy, thick, foul-smelling, yellow vaginal discharge Genital itching and irritation Burning and pain on urination Genital swelling	Metronidazole
Syphilis	*Stage 1*—10 to 90 days after exposure • Painless sores (chancres)—penis, vagina, genitalia, lips, mouth, or anywhere on the body *Stage 2*—About 3 to 6 weeks after the sores • General fatigue, loss of appetite, nausea, fever, headache, rash, swollen glands, sore throat, bone and joint pain, hair loss, lesions on the lips and genitalia • Symptoms may come and go for many years *Stage 3*—3 to 15 years after infection • Central nervous system damage (including paralysis), heart damage, blindness, liver damage, mental health problems, death	Penicillin and other antibiotic drugs

FOCUS ON **PRIDE**

The Person, Family, and Yourself

Personal and Professional Responsibility

UTIs are a common healthcare-associated infection. Females are at high risk. Proper perineal care can prevent UTIs. Always clean the female perineum from front to back (top to bottom). Use a clean part of the washcloth for each stroke. Use more than 1 washcloth if needed.

You are responsible for providing care in a way that protects the person's health and safety. Take pride in performing safe and careful perineal care.

Rights and Respect

An STD can make the person feel embarrassed, ashamed, or guilty. Do not judge the person. Treat the person with dignity and respect.

Independence and Social Interaction

Persons with CKD cannot survive without dialysis. Hemodialysis is often done 3 times a week. Each session can take 4 hours or more. Peritoneal dialysis is often done in the home setting. Dialysis is done 4 to 6 times a day.

Dialysis takes a lot of time. Work, family time, and other activities are limited by the need for dialysis. These social changes affect quality of life. The person and family need support and encouragement.

Delegation and Teamwork

Kidney stone pain is severe. The pain can cause rude behavior. Once comfort needs are met, behavior returns to normal. The person is often sorry for being rude.

Promote comfort. Be patient, kind, and understanding. Treat the person well even if you are not treated well. Accept offered apologies. Tell the nurse if you need help dealing with the person's behavior.

Ethics and Laws

Urinary and reproductive disorders are personal. The person does not want information shared with others. Give information only to those directly involved in the person's care. Take pride in protecting the person's right to privacy and confidentiality.

FOCUS ON **PRIDE**: *Application*

Pain, coping with a disorder, and the stress of treatments affect behavior. What other factors affect the person? You cannot control the person's reactions. You can control yours. List helpful responses. What responses are not helpful?

REVIEW QUESTIONS

Circle the BEST answer.

1 A person has cystitis. This is a
   a Kidney infection
   b Kidney stone
   c Urinary diversion
   d Bladder infection

2 The person with cystitis needs to drink about
   a 500 mL daily
   b 1000 mL daily
   c 1500 mL daily
   d 2000 mL daily

3 BPH causes urinary problems because
   a The person has a weak urine stream
   b The person voids frequently at night
   c The enlarged prostate presses against the urethra
   d Voidings are in small amounts

4 Mr. Jones had a TURP. Which measure should you question?
   a No sudden movements
   b No oral fluids
   c No heavy lifting
   d No straining to have a bowel movement

5 A person with a urostomy
   a Has a new pathway for urine to exit the body
   b Needs dialysis
   c Had surgery for an enlarged prostate
   d Has pyuria

6 A person has kidney stones. You need to
   a Strain all urine
   b Empty the pouch
   c Collect a urine specimen
   d Change the urinary drainage bag

7 A person has kidney failure. Which is *true*?
   a Waste products are removed from the blood.
   b The body retains fluid.
   c Urinary diversion is needed.
   d Oliguria follows diuresis.

8 Chronic kidney disease care includes
   a A diet high in protein, potassium, and sodium
   b Encouraging fluids
   c Measuring weight daily
   d Straining the urine

9 Which statement about STDs is *true*?
   a Older persons do not get them.
   b They only affect the genital area.
   c Some persons have no signs or symptoms.
   d STDs cannot cause death.

10 STDs require
   a Masks and protective eyewear
   b Gowns
   c Double-bagging
   d Standard Precautions

Answers to Chapter 47 questions are on p. 872.

FOCUS ON PRACTICE

Problem Solving

Mrs. Fowler has a urinary catheter. Does this affect her UTI risk? Describe the care measures for perineal care and catheter care that help lower the risk of UTI.

Mental Health Disorders

- Define the key terms and key abbreviations in this chapter.
- Explain the difference between mental health and mental illness.
- List the causes of mental health disorders.
- Describe anxiety disorders and the defense mechanisms used to relieve anxiety.
- Explain schizophrenia.
- Describe bipolar disorder and depression.
- Describe personality disorders.
- Describe substance abuse and addiction.
- Describe suicide and the persons at risk.
- Describe the care required by persons with mental health disorders.
- Explain how to promote PRIDE in the person, the family, and yourself.

KEY TERMS

alcohol abuse When drinking leads to problems but the person is not dependent on alcohol

alcoholism Alcohol dependence that involves craving, loss of control, physical dependence, and tolerance

anxiety A vague, uneasy feeling in response to stress

compulsion Repeating an act over and over again (a ritual)

defense mechanism An unconscious reaction that blocks unpleasant or threatening feelings

delusion A false belief

delusion of grandeur An exaggerated belief about one's importance, wealth, power, or talents

delusion of persecution A false belief that one is being mistreated, abused, or harassed

drug abuse Using a drug for non-medical or non-therapy effects

drug addiction A strong urge or craving to use the substance and cannot stop using; tolerance develops

flashback Reliving a trauma in thoughts during the day and in nightmares during sleep

hallucination Seeing, hearing, smelling, or feeling things that are not real

mental Relating to the mind; something that exists in the mind or is done by the mind

mental health The person copes with and adjusts to everyday stresses in ways accepted by society

mental health disorder A disturbance in the ability to cope with or adjust to stress; behavior and function are impaired; mental illness, psychiatric disorder

mental illness See "mental health disorder"

obsession A recurrent, unwanted thought, idea, or image

panic An intense and sudden feeling of fear, anxiety, terror, or dread

personality The set of attitudes, values, behaviors, and traits of a person

phobia An intense fear

psychiatric disorder See "mental health disorder"

psychosis A state of severe mental impairment

stress The response or change in the body caused by any emotional, physical, social, or economic factor

stressor The event or factor that causes stress

suicide To kill oneself on purpose

suicide contagion Exposure to suicide or suicidal behaviors within one's family, one's peer group, or media reports of suicide

withdrawal syndrome The physical and mental response after stopping or severely reducing the use of a substance that was used regularly

KEY ABBREVIATIONS

AUD	Alcohol use disorder	**OCD**	Obsessive-compulsive disorder
BPD	Borderline personality disorder	**OTC**	Over-the-counter
CDC	Centers for Disease Control and Prevention	**PTSD**	Post-traumatic stress disorder
GAD	Generalized anxiety disorder		

The whole person has physical, social, psychological (mental), and spiritual parts. Each part affects the other.
- A physical problem can have social, mental, and spiritual effects.
- A mental health problem can have physical, social, and spiritual effects.
- A social problem can have physical, mental, and spiritual effects.

BASIC CONCEPTS

Mental relates to the mind. It is something that exists in the mind or is done by the mind. Therefore mental health involves the mind. Mental health and mental health disorders involve stress.
- *Stress—the response or change in the body caused by any emotional, physical, social, or economic factor.*
- *Mental health—the person copes with and adjusts to everyday stresses in ways accepted by society.*
- *Mental health disorder—a disturbance in the ability to cope with or adjust to stress. Behavior and function are impaired.* **Mental illness** and **psychiatric disorder** are other names.

Causes of mental health disorders include:
- Not being able to cope with or adjust to stress.
- Chemical imbalances.
- Genetics. Many mental health disorders tend to run in families. Generalized anxiety disorder, schizophrenia, bipolar disorder, and depression are examples.
- Physical, biological, or psychological factors.
- Drug or substance abuse.
- Social and cultural factors.
- Abuse.

Personality

Personality is the set of attitudes, values, behaviors, and traits of a person. Personality development starts at birth. Influencing factors include genes, culture, environment, parenting, and social experiences.

Maslow's theory of basic needs (Chapter 9) affects personality development. Physical needs are met before safety and security, love and belonging, self-esteem, and self-actualization needs. Children who grow up hungry, neglected, cold, or abused will not feel safe and secure. Higher-level needs cannot be met. Unmet needs at any age affect personality development.

Growth and development also affect personality development (Chapter 11). They occur in a sequence, order, and pattern. Certain tasks must be achieved at each stage. Each stage is the basis for the next stage.

ANXIETY DISORDERS

Anxiety is a vague, uneasy feeling in response to stress. The person senses danger or harm—real or imagined. The person acts to relieve the unpleasant feeling. Often anxiety occurs when needs are not met.

BOX 48-1	Anxiety—Signs and Symptoms

- Appetite: loss of
- Apprehension
- Attention span: poor
- Blood pressure: increased
- "Butterflies" in the stomach
- Diarrhea
- Directions: difficulty following
- "Lump" in the throat
- Mouth: dry
- Nausea
- Pulse: rapid
- Respirations: rapid
- Sleep: difficulty
- Speech: rapid, voice changes
- Sweating
- Tiredness
- Trembling
- Urinary frequency and urgency
- Weakness

Some anxiety is normal. Persons with mental health disorders have higher levels of anxiety. Signs and symptoms depend on the degree of anxiety (Box 48-1).

Anxiety level depends on the stressor. A *stressor is the event or factor that causes stress.* It can be physical, emotional, social, or economic. Past experiences and the number of stressors affect how a person reacts. A stressor may cause mild anxiety. Or it can cause higher anxiety at another time.

Coping and defense mechanisms may help relieve anxiety. Unhealthy coping includes over-eating, drinking, smoking, and fighting. Healthy coping includes discussing the problem, exercising, playing music, taking a hot bath, and wanting to be alone.

Defense mechanisms are unconscious reactions that block unpleasant or threatening feelings (Box 48-2). (*Unconscious reactions* are experiences and feelings that cannot be recalled.) Some use of defense mechanisms is normal. In mental health disorders, they are used poorly.

Anxiety disorders last at least 6 months. They often occur with other physical illnesses or mental health disorders. Depression, eating disorders, and substance abuse are examples. Persons 18 years of age and older are at risk. However, anxiety disorders can develop in childhood.

Generalized Anxiety Disorder

Some worry and anxiety are normal. However, the person with generalized anxiety disorder (GAD) has extreme worry for little or no reason. The person has extreme anxiety. He or she worries about health, money, or family problems. Getting through the day can be difficult. Worry can prevent the person from normal function.

BOX 48-2	Defense Mechanisms

Compensation. *Compensate* means *to make up for, replace, or substitute.* The person makes up for or substitutes a strength for a weakness.
  EXAMPLE: Not good in sports, a child develops another talent.

Conversion. *Convert* means *to change.* An emotion is shown as a physical symptom or changed into a physical symptom.
  EXAMPLE: Not wanting to read out loud in school, a child complains of a headache.

Denial. *Deny* means *refusing to accept or believe something that is true.* The person refuses to face or accept unpleasant or threatening things.
  EXAMPLE: After a heart attack, a person continues to smoke.

Displacement. *Displace* means *to move or take the place of.* An individual moves behaviors or emotions from 1 person, place, or thing to a safe person, place, or thing.
  EXAMPLE: Angry at your boss, you yell at a friend.

Identification. *Identify* means *to relate* or *recognize.* A person assumes the ideas, behaviors, and traits of another person.
  EXAMPLE: A neighbor is a high school cheerleader. A little girl practices cheerleading in her backyard.

Projection. *Project* means *to blame another.* An individual blames another person or object for unacceptable behaviors, emotions, ideas, or wishes.
  EXAMPLE: Sleeping too long, a worker blames the traffic when late for work.

Rationalization. *Rational* means *sensible, reasonable,* or *logical.* An acceptable reason or excuse is given for behaviors or actions. The real reason is not given.
  EXAMPLE: Often late for work, an employee does not get a raise. The employee thinks: "My boss doesn't like me."

Reaction formation. A person acts in a way opposite to what he or she truly feels.
  EXAMPLE: A worker does not like his boss. He buys the boss a gift.

Regression. *Regress* means *to move back* or *to retreat.* The person retreats or moves back to an earlier time or condition.
  EXAMPLE: A 3-year-old wants a baby bottle when a new baby comes into the family.

Repression. *Repress* means *to hold down* or *keep back.* The person keeps unpleasant or painful thoughts or experiences from the conscious mind. They cannot be recalled or remembered.
  EXAMPLE: A child was sexually abused. Now 33 years old, there is no memory of the event.

Panic Disorder

Panic is an intense and sudden feeling of fear, anxiety, terror, or dread. Onset is sudden with no obvious reason. The person cannot function. Signs and symptoms of anxiety are severe (see Box 48-1). The person may also have:
- Chest pain
- Shortness of breath
- Numbness and tingling in the hands
- Dizziness
- A smothering feeling
- Feeling of impending doom or loss of control

The person may feel that he or she is having a heart attack, losing his or her mind, or on the verge of death. Attacks can occur at any time, even during sleep.

Panic attacks can last for 10 minutes or longer. They can occur during sleep.

Many people avoid places where panic attacks occurred. For example, a person had a panic attack in a shopping mall. Malls are avoided.

Phobias

Phobia means an intense fear. The person has an intense fear of an object, situation, or activity that has little or no actual danger. Common phobias are fear of:
- Being in an open, crowded, or public place (*agoraphobia—agora* means *marketplace*)
- Being in pain or seeing others in pain (*algophobia—algo* means *pain*)
- Water (*aquaphobia—aqua* means *water*)
- Being in or trapped in an enclosed or narrow space (*claustrophobia—claustro* means *closing*)
- The slightest uncleanliness (*mysophobia—myso* means *anything that is disgusting*)
- Night or darkness (*nyctophobia—nycto* means *night* or *darkness*)
- Fire (*pyrophobia—pyro* means *fire*)
- Strangers (*xenophobia—xeno* means *strange*)

The person avoids what is feared. When faced with the fear, the person has high anxiety and cannot function.

Obsessive-Compulsive Disorder

The person with obsessive-compulsive disorder (OCD) has obsessions and compulsions. An *obsession is a recurrent, unwanted thought, idea, or image.* Some people are obsessed with microbes, dirt, violent thoughts, sexual acts, or things forbidden by religion. *Compulsion is repeating an act over and over again (a ritual).* The act may not make sense. Anxiety is great if the act is not done.

Common rituals are hand-washing, cleaning, counting things to a certain number, or touching things in a certain order. Such rituals can take over an hour every day. Hoarding is another OCD behavior. OCD behaviors are very distressing and affect daily life.

BOX 48-3	Post-Traumatic Stress Disorder—Signs and Symptoms

- Affection: problems with
- Aggressive and violent behaviors
- Anger: gets mad easily; outbursts
- Avoidance of situations that remind of the harmful event
- Closeness: problems with
- Difficulty around the anniversary of the harmful event
- Emotionally numb: especially to those with whom the person used to be close
- Flashbacks
- Guilt: intense
- Irritability
- Loss of interest in things he or she used to enjoy
- Physical symptoms:
  - Headache
  - Gastro-intestinal (GI) distress
  - Immune system problems
  - Dizziness
  - Chest pain
  - Discomfort in other body parts
- Sleeping: problems with
- Startles easily
- Trusting people: problems with

Post-Traumatic Stress Disorder

Post-traumatic stress disorder (PTSD) occurs after a terrifying event. There was physical harm or the threat of physical harm. PTSD can develop at any age. See Box 48-3 for signs and symptoms. PTSD can develop:

- After being harmed or after a loved one was harmed
- After seeing a harmful event happen to a loved one or stranger

PTSD can result from many traumatic events. They include:

- War, terrorist attack, bombing
- Abuse, mugging, rape, torture
- Kidnapping, being held captive
- Crashes—vehicle, train, plane
- Natural disasters—flood, tornado, hurricane, earthquake

Flashbacks are common. A *flashback is reliving the trauma in thoughts during the day and in nightmares during sleep.* Flashbacks may involve images, sounds, smells, or feelings. Everyday things can trigger them. A door slamming is an example. During a flashback, the person may believe that the trauma is happening all over again.

Signs and symptoms usually develop about 3 months after the event. Some people recover within 6 months. PTSD lasts longer in other people. The condition may become chronic.

SCHIZOPHRENIA

Schizophrenia means split (*schizo*) mind (*phrenia*). The person's thinking and emotions are not in balance. A severe, chronic, disabling brain disorder, schizophrenia involves:

- *Psychosis—a state of severe mental impairment.* The person does not view the real or unreal correctly.
- *Hallucinations—seeing, hearing, smelling, or feeling things that are not real.* A person may see animals, insects, or people that are not real. Hearing voices is the most common type of hallucination. "Voices" may comment on behavior or order the person to do things, warn of danger, or talk to other voices.
- *Delusions—false beliefs.* For example, the person believes that a radio station is airing the person's thoughts or that he or she is being harmed. The person may have:
  - *Delusions of grandeur—exaggerated beliefs about one's importance, wealth, power, or talents.* For example, a man believes he is Superman. Or a woman believes she is the Queen of England.
  - *Delusions of persecution—false beliefs that one is being mistreated, abused, or harassed.* For example, a person believes that someone is "out to get" him or her. Or a person thinks others are cheating, harassing, poisoning, spying on, or plotting against him or her.
- *Thought disorders.* The person has trouble organizing thoughts or connecting thoughts logically. Speech may be garbled and hard to understand. The person may suddenly stop speaking in the middle of a thought. Some persons make up words that have no meaning.
- *Movement disorders.* These include:
  - Agitated body movements
  - Repeating motions over and over
  - Sitting for hours without moving, speaking, or responding
- *Emotional and behavioral problems.* Normal functions are impaired or absent. The person may:
  - Lose motivation or interest in daily activities.
  - Be unable to plan or do activities.
  - Seem to lack emotions.
  - Neglect personal hygiene.
  - Withdraw socially.
- *Cognitive problems. Cognitive* relates to *understanding, remembering,* and *reasoning.* The person may have trouble paying attention or understanding or remembering information. Symptoms make it hard for the person to perform daily tasks.

The person with schizophrenia has severe mental impairment *(psychosis)*. Thinking and behavior are disturbed with false beliefs *(delusions)* and hallucinations. That is, the person sees, hears, smells, or feels things that are not real. The person has problems relating to others. The person may have difficulty organizing thoughts and may make up words. Responses are not appropriate. Communication is disturbed. The person may ramble or repeat what another says. Sometimes speech cannot be understood. The person may withdraw. That is, the person lacks interest in others and is not involved with people or society.

Some persons regress. To *regress* means *to retreat or move back to an earlier time or condition.* For example, a 5-year-old wets the bed when there is a new baby. This is normal. Healthy adults do not act like infants or children.

Symptoms usually begin between the ages of 16 and 30. The onset tends to be earlier in men than in women. In rare cases, it can appear in childhood. People with schizophrenia do not tend to be violent. However, if a person becomes violent, it is often directed at family members in the home setting. Some persons with schizophrenia attempt suicide (p. 765).

See *Focus on Communication: Schizophrenia.*

FOCUS ON COMMUNICATION

Schizophrenia

Delusions and hallucinations can frighten a person. Good communication is important.
- Speak slowly and calmly.
- Do not pretend you experience what the person does. Help the person focus on reality.
- Do not try to convince the person that the experience is not real. To the person, it is real.
  For example, a person hears voices. You can say: "I don't hear the voices but I believe you do. Try to listen to my voice and not the other voices."

BIPOLAR DISORDER

Bipolar means 2 *(bi)* poles or ends *(polar)*. The person with bipolar disorder has severe extremes in mood, energy, and function. There are emotional highs or "ups" *(mania)* and emotional lows or "downs" *(depression)*. Therefore the disorder is also called manic-depressive illness.

The disorder runs in families. It usually develops during the late teens or early adulthood. Life-long management is required. The person may have problems in school or keeping a job.

Signs and symptoms range from mild to severe (Box 48-4). Mood changes are called "episodes." Some people are suicidal.

DEPRESSION

Depression involves the body, mood, and thoughts (see Box 48-4). The person has prolonged sadness. With *major depression,* severe and prolonged feelings of sadness, loss, anger, or frustration interfere with daily life. Work, study, sleep, eating, and other activities are affected.

Some physical disorders can cause depression. Cancer and long-term pain are examples. Hormonal factors may cause depression. Thyroid problems, pregnancy, miscarriage, childbirth (post-partum depression), and menopause involve hormonal changes. A stressful event such as death of a partner, parent, or child may cause depression. So can divorce or job loss.

Depression in Older Persons

Depression is common in older persons. They have many losses—death of family and friends, loss of body functions, loss of independence. See Box 48-5, p. 762 for the signs and symptoms of depression in older persons.

Some medical conditions and drug side effects can cause symptoms of depression. Depression in older persons is often overlooked or a wrong diagnosis is made. Often the person is thought to have a cognitive disorder (Chapter 49). Therefore depression is often not treated.

BOX 48-4 Bipolar Disorder—Signs and Symptoms

Mania (Manic Episode)
- Increased energy, activity, and restlessness
- Excessively "high," overly happy, "up" mood
- Extreme irritability
- Feeling "jumpy" or "wired"
- Racing thoughts and rapid speech
- Jumping from 1 idea to another
- Easily distracted, problems concentrating
- Little sleep needed
- Unrealistic beliefs in one's abilities and powers
- Poor judgment
- Spending sprees
- A lasting period of behavior that is different from usual
- Increased sex drive
- Drug or alcohol abuse
- Aggressive behavior
- Denial that anything is wrong

Depression (Depressive Episode)
- Sadness; "down" mood
- Hopelessness
- Empty mood
- Worry and anxiety
- Guilt
- Loss of interest in sex or activities once enjoyed
- Feeling tired or "slowed down"
- Problems concentrating, remembering, or making decisions
- Restlessness or irritability
- Sleep problems
- Change in appetite: low or increased
- Chronic pain or other symptoms without a cause
- Thoughts of death or suicide
- Suicide attempts

BOX 48-5	Depression in Older Persons—Signs and Symptoms

- Fatigue
- Pleasure: inability to experience
- Feelings of uselessness, hopelessness, or helplessness
- Sexual interest: decreased
- Dependency: increased
- Anxiety
- Memory: slow, unreliable
- Paranoia
- Agitation
- Focus on the past
- Thoughts of death or suicide
- Activities of daily living: difficulty completing
- Sleep patterns: changes in
- Grooming: poor
- Withdrawal from people or interests
- Muscle aches, abdominal pain, and headaches
- Nausea and vomiting
- Dry mouth
- Loss of appetite
- Weight loss
- Alcohol or drugs: increased use of

PERSONALITY DISORDERS

Personality disorders involve rigid and maladaptive behaviors. To *adapt* means *to change* or *adjust. Mal* means *bad, wrong,* or *ill. Maladaptive* means *to change or adjust in the wrong way.* Because of their behavior, persons with personality disorders cannot function well in society.

Antisocial Personality Disorder

The person has a long-term pattern of thinking and behaviors that violates the rights of others. The person has no regard for the safety of others. Often angry, the person has no guilt. The person lies, charms, or cons others for personal gain or pleasure. Stealing, fighting, and drug abuse are common criminal acts.

Borderline Personality Disorder

Borderline personality disorder (BPD) involves unstable moods, behaviors, and relationships. The person has a long-term pattern of at least 5 of the following.
- Extreme reactions. These involve panic, depression, and rage.
- Intense and stormy relationships with loved ones, family, and friends. The person has extremes from love and closeness to dislike and anger.
- Unstable self-image. The person has sudden changes in feelings, opinions, values, and goals.
- Impulsive and dangerous behaviors. Spending sprees, unsafe sex, substance abuse, reckless driving, and binge eating are examples.
- Suicidal behaviors or threats of self-harm. Self-harm behaviors include cutting, burning, and hitting oneself; head banging; and hair pulling.
- Intense and changing moods.
- Feelings of emptiness or boredom.

- Intense anger or anger control problems.
- Paranoid thoughts or severe dissociative symptoms. *Paranoia* is a disorder *(para)* of the mind *(noia).* Paranoid thoughts include delusions and suspicions about a person or situation. *Dissociate* means *to disconnect* or *separate.* The person feels cut off from oneself, observes oneself from outside the body, or loses touch with reality.

SUBSTANCE ABUSE DISORDER

Substance abuse disorder is when a person needs alcohol or a drug (legal or illegal) to function normally. Substance abuse or addiction occurs when a person over-uses or depends on alcohol or drugs. Physical and mental health are affected. So is the welfare of others.

The substances involved affect the nervous system. Some depress the nervous system. Others stimulate it. All affect the mind and thinking.

Alcohol Use Disorder

Alcohol slows down brain activity. It affects alertness, judgment, coordination, and reaction time. Over time, heavy drinking damages the brain, central nervous system, liver, kidneys, heart, blood vessels, and stomach. It also can cause forgetfulness and confusion.

Alcohol use disorder (AUD) is when drinking causes serious problems yet the person continues to drink. The person needs more and more alcohol to feel drunk. Withdrawal symptoms may occur if the person stops drinking. AUD involves alcoholism and alcohol abuse.
- *Alcoholism* is alcohol dependence that involves:
  - *Craving*—a strong need or urge to drink.
  - *Loss of control*—cannot stop drinking once started.
  - *Physical dependence*—withdrawal symptoms (nausea, sweating, shakiness, anxiety) when drinking is stopped.
  - *Tolerance*—greater amounts of alcohol are needed to feel the same effect.
- *Alcohol abuse is when drinking leads to problems but the person is not dependent on alcohol.*

Alcoholism is a chronic disease. It lasts throughout life. Life-style and genetics are risk factors. Alcoholism can be treated but not cured. Alcohol recovery and support programs and drug therapy can help the person stop drinking. The person must avoid all alcohol to prevent a relapse.

Problems linked to alcoholism and alcohol abuse include:
- Not being able to meet work, school, home, family, or relationship responsibilities
- Motor vehicle crashes
- Drunk-driving arrests
- Drinking-related medical conditions

Occasional or regular drinking does not mean a drinking problem. However, even a few symptoms in Box 48-6 can signal alcohol use disorder.

See *Focus on Children and Older Persons: Alcohol Use Disorder.*

| BOX 48-6 | Alcohol Use Disorder—Signs and Symptoms |

- Drinking more or longer than intended to
- Wanting to or trying to cut down or stop drinking, but could not
- Spending time drinking or trying to get alcohol
- Spending time recovering from the effects of alcohol
- Craving alcohol or having a strong need or urge to drink
- Missing school or work because of drinking or being sick from drinking
- Continuing to drink even when it harms relationships with family and friends
- Avoiding activities once enjoyed
- Being involved in situations that increased the risk of harm—driving, swimming, using machines, unsafe sex, and so on
- Continuing to drink despite health problems caused by drinking—anxiety, depression, physical problems, memory problems (blackouts)
- Needing more and more alcohol to feel the effects or to get drunk
- Having withdrawal symptoms when the effects of alcohol wear off—trouble sleeping, shaking, irritability, anxiety, depression, restlessness, nausea, sweating

Modified from MedlinePlus, Alcohol use disorder, Bethesda, Md, updated September 9, 2015, U.S. Library of Medicine, National Institutes of Health and MedlinePlus, Alcoholism and Alcohol Abuse, Bethesda, Md, updated September 28, 2015, U.S. Library of Medicine, National Institutes of Health.

FOCUS ON CHILDREN AND OLDER PERSONS

Alcohol Use Disorder

Children

Alcohol is the most commonly abused substance among teenagers. According to a 2013 survey of high school students, the Centers for Disease Control and Prevention (CDC) reported that:
- Among high school students during the past 30 days:
  - 35% drank some alcohol.
  - 21% binge drank (4 or 5 or more drinks in about 2 hours).
  - 10% drove after drinking.
  - 22% rode with a driver who had been drinking.
  According to the CDC, under-age drinking is more likely to result in:
- School problems—absences, failing grades
- Social problems—fighting, not taking part in activities
- Legal problems—driving arrests, hurting someone while drunk
- Physical problems—hang-overs, illness
- Unwanted, unplanned, unprotected sexual activity
- Disrupted normal growth and sexual development
- Physical and sexual assault
- Risk for suicide and homicide
- Alcohol-related car crashes
- Alcohol-related injuries—burns, falls, drowning
- Memory problems
- Drug abuse
- Changes in brain development with life-long effects
- Death from alcohol poisoning

Older Persons

Even small amounts of alcohol can make older persons feel "high." Older persons are at risk for falls, vehicle crashes, and other injuries from drinking. They have:
- Slower reaction times
- Hearing and vision problems
- A lower tolerance for alcohol
  Mixing alcohol with some prescribed drugs can be harmful, even fatal. Alcohol also makes some health problems worse. High blood pressure is an example.

Drug Abuse and Addiction

Drugs affecting the nervous system affect normal brain function. While they create intense feelings of pleasure, they have long-term effects on the brain. Changes in the brain can turn drug abuse into addiction.

Drug abuse and addiction can involve illegal drugs or the mis-use of legal drugs—prescription drugs or over-the-counter (OTC) drugs. Legal drugs are approved for use in the United States. Illegal drugs are not approved for use. They are obtained through illegal means. Some people also obtain legal drugs through illegal means.

- *Drug abuse—using a drug for non-medical or non-therapy effects.*
- *Drug addiction—a strong urge or craving to use the substance and cannot stop using. Tolerance develops—*a higher dose is needed to get the same effect. A diagnosis is based on 2 or more of the following during a 12-month period. The person:
  - Takes the drug in larger amounts. Or it is taken longer than intended.
  - Tries to cut down or stop using the drug.
  - Spends much time using the drug or recovering from its effects. Or a great deal of time is spent getting the drug.
  - Has an intense urge for the drug. The person can think of nothing else.
  - Does not meet responsibilities or obligations.
  - Continues to use the drug despite knowing that health problems are caused by or made worse by using the drug.
  - Gave up or reduced social, job, or recreational events because of the drug.
  - Uses the drug in unsafe situations. Driving and using machines are examples.
  - Has tolerance to the drug.
    - The drug has less and less effect on the person.
    - More of the drug is needed to get high.
  - Has withdrawal symptoms (*withdraw* means *to stop, remove,* or *take away*).
    - *Withdrawal syndrome is the physical and mental response after stopping or severely reducing the use of a substance that was used regularly.* The body responds with anxiety, restlessness, insomnia, irritability, impaired attention, and physical illness.
  - The same (or similar) drug is taken to relieve or avoid withdrawal symptoms.

Drug abuse and addiction affect social and mental function. They are linked to crimes, violence, car crashes, and suicide. Family, work, school, legal, and financial issues can result. Physical effects can occur from 1 use, high doses, or prolonged use—HIV and AIDS, cardiovascular disease, stroke, sudden death, hepatitis, lung disease, cancer.

A drug treatment program combines various therapies and services to meet the person's needs. Drug abuse and addiction are chronic problems. Relapses can occur. A short-term, 1-time treatment is often not enough. Treatment is a long-term process.

See *Focus on Children and Older Persons: Drug Abuse and Addiction*.

EATING DISORDERS

An eating disorder involves extremes in eating patterns. The person has a severe disturbance in eating behavior. Eating disorders often develop during the teen years. However, they can develop during childhood, young adulthood, or later in life. The person may have other mental health disorders.

- *Anorexia nervosa. Anorexia* means no *(a)* appetite *(orexis). Nervosa* relates to *nerves* or *emotions*. The person has an intense fear of gaining weight. A fat body image is felt despite being quite thin (Fig. 48-1). The person eats in small amounts and only certain foods. Forced vomiting and intense exercise are common. So is enema and laxative use to rid the body of food. Laxatives are drugs that promote defecation. Diuretic abuse also may occur. These drugs cause the kidneys to produce large amounts of urine. Extra fluid in the body is lost. Weight loss results. Serious health problems can result. Death is a risk from cardiac arrest or suicide.
- *Bulimia nervosa.* Binge eating occurs. That is, the person eats large amounts of food. Then the body is purged (rid) of the food to prevent weight gain. Vomiting, laxatives, enemas, diuretics, fasting, and intense exercise are some methods used.
- *Binge eating disorder.* The person often eats large amounts of food. Eating is out of control. Binge eating is not followed by purging, fasting, or exercise. Often the person is over-weight or obese. High blood pressure, heart disease, diabetes, and joint pain can occur.

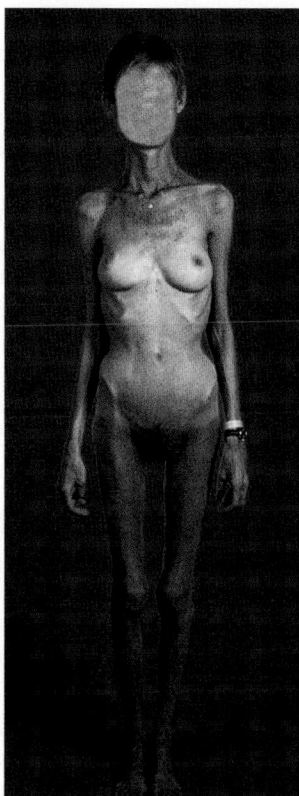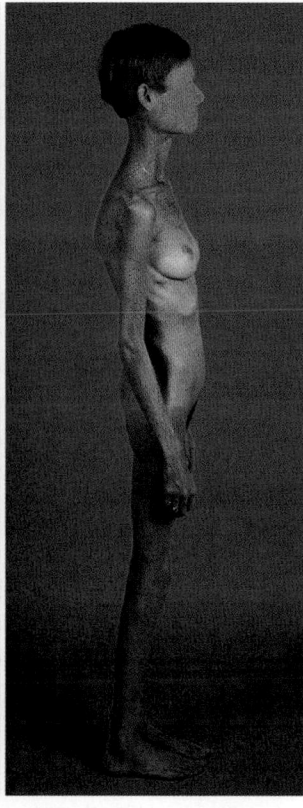

FIGURE 48-1 A person with anorexia nervosa. (Courtesy George D. Comerci, MD, Tucson. From Jarvis C: *Physical examination and health assessment,* ed 4, Philadelphia, 2004, Saunders.)

SUICIDE

Suicide means to kill oneself on purpose. According to a 2015 CDC report:

- Suicide is the 10th leading cause of death in the United States.
- There were more than 41,100 suicides in 2013.
- Women are more likely to have suicidal thoughts than men.
- More men than women die from suicide.
- Firearms are the most common method for men. For women, poison is the most common method.
- American Indians and Alaskan Natives have high rates of suicide.
- Suicide was the third leading cause of death among persons aged 10 to 14 and second among persons aged 15 to 34.

Risk factors are listed in Box 48-7. *If a person mentions or talks about suicide, take the person seriously. Call for the nurse at once. Do not leave the person alone.*

Agencies treating persons with mental health disorders must identify persons at risk for suicide. They must:

- Identify specific factors or features that increase or decrease the risk for suicide.
- Meet the person's immediate safety needs.
- Provide the most appropriate setting to treat the person.
- Provide crisis information to the person and family. A crisis "hotline" phone number is an example.

See *Focus on Communication: Suicide.*

See *Focus on Children and Older Persons: Suicide,* p. 766.

See *Focus on Long-Term Care and Home Care: Suicide,* p. 766.

BOX 48-7	**Suicide Risk Factors**

- Depression and other mental health disorders
- Substance abuse disorder
- Prior suicide attempt
- Family history of a mental health disorder or substance abuse
- Family history of suicide
- Family violence (including physical or sexual abuse)
- Firearms in the home
- Incarceration (prison or jail)
- Exposure to the suicidal behavior of others (family, friends, media figures)

Modified from National Institute of Mental Health: Suicide in America: frequently asked questions, NIH publication No. TR 14-6389, Bethesda, Md, National Institutes of Health.

FOCUS ON **COMMUNICATION**

Suicide

Some people talk about their thoughts of suicide. A person may say:

- "I just don't want to live anymore."
- "I wish I was dead."
- "I wish I had never been born."
- "Everyone would be better off without me."

Call for the nurse at once if a person talks about suicide.

A person may ask you not to tell anyone about the suicidal thoughts. Protecting personal information is important. But the person's safety is the priority. Never promise that you will not tell anyone. Report the statement to the nurse at once.

Suicide

Children

Suicide is a leading cause of death among children and young adults. Warning signs and risk factors include:

- Talking about wanting to die or killing oneself
- Focusing on death in conversations, writings, or drawings—feeling hopeless, having no reason to live, feeling trapped, being a burden to others
- Giving away personal items
- Withdrawing from family and friends
- Showing rage or having aggressive or hostile behaviors
- Running away from home
- Having access to guns
- Experiencing a romantic break-up
- Having a history of suicide in the family
- Having a history of hurting oneself, neglect, or abuse
- Being a victim of bullying or being bullied
- Being exposed to suicide among other people (see "Suicide Contagion")

Older Persons

According to the National Institute of Mental Health, older adults are at risk for suicide. Many older persons suffer from depression (p. 761). Depression often occurs with other serious illnesses. Heart disease, stroke, diabetes, cancer, and Parkinson's disease are examples. The person also may have social and financial problems.

Most older victims did not report depression to their doctors. Or depression was not diagnosed.

FOCUS ON **LONG-TERM CARE AND HOME CARE**

Suicide

Home Care

Access to firearms and other weapons is a risk factor for suicide. If a patient talks about suicide, find out if there are firearms or other weapons in the home. Find out what kind, how many, and where they are located. Tell the nurse at once. If the person is in danger, call 911.

Suicide Contagion

Suicide contagion is exposure to suicide or suicidal behaviors within one's family, one's peer group, or media reports of suicide. The exposure has led to suicides and suicidal behaviors in persons at risk. Adolescents and young adults are at risk for suicide contagion.

Following suicide exposure, those close to the victim need evaluation by a mental health professional. They include family, friends, peers, and co-workers. Persons at risk for suicide need mental health services.

CARE AND TREATMENT

Treatment of mental health disorders involves having the person explore thoughts and feelings. Psychotherapy and behavior, group, occupational, art, and family therapies are used. Often drugs are ordered.

The care plan reflects the needs of the total person. This includes physical, safety and security, and emotional needs.

Communication is important. Be alert to nonverbal communication. This includes the person's nonverbal communication and your own.

Persons with mental health disorders may respond to stress with anxiety, panic, or anger. Some become violent. You must protect yourself. Once you are safe, the health team can protect the person and others. To protect yourself:

- Call for help. Do not try to handle the situation on your own.
- Keep a safe distance between you and the person.
- Be aware of your setting. Do not let the person between you and the exit.

See *Focus on Communication: Care and Treatment.*

FOCUS ON **COMMUNICATION**

Care and Treatment

Nonverbal communication involves eye contact, tone of voice, facial expressions, body movements, and posture. Persons with depression often have little eye contact, poor posture, and speak softly. Some do not speak much at all. Facial expressions may not change. Some persons cry.

Persons with anxiety feel uneasy. They may be restless, unable to sit still, and talk fast. Eye contact may be prolonged and intense. Others have poor eye contact. The eyes may dart about. Be alert to nonverbal cues. Report what you observe.

Your nonverbal communication is also important. When interacting with persons with mental health disorders:

- Face the person.
- Maintain eye contact.
- Position yourself near the person but not too close. Do not invade the person's space.
- Crouch, sit, or stand at the person's level if safe to do so.
- Show interest and concern through your posture and facial expressions.
- Speak calmly.

FOCUS ON **PRIDE**

The Person, Family, and Yourself

P ersonal and Professional Responsibility

People do not choose to have physical or mental health problems. Just as a person does not choose to have diabetes, a person does not choose anxiety or depression. How you view the illness affects how you treat the person. Treat the person with kindness, respect, and compassion. Provide quality care.

R ights and Respect

Agencies have strict rules to protect the person's rights to privacy and confidentiality (Chapter 2). Do not talk about the person with your family or friends. This violates the person's rights. Never give information to someone not involved in the person's care. This includes the person's family. Direct questions to the nurse. Follow agency policies and procedures. Take pride in protecting the person's rights.

I ndependence and Social Interaction

Social support is important in the treatment of mental health disorders. Interacting with others is a healthy way to manage stress. Family and friends provide a sense of worth and belonging. The care plan includes how they are involved in the person's care.

Providing support for a person with a mental health disorder can be demanding. The family needs support. Many communities offer support groups. You can also offer encouragement. Tell the family that you value the support they give.

D elegation and Teamwork

Caring for persons with mental health disorders requires great teamwork. A person may become hostile or violent. Or the person may threaten or attempt suicide. The team must react quickly to protect the person and others. If someone calls for help, respond at once. Assist as the nurse directs. Take pride in working as a team to ensure safety.

E thics and Laws

Mental health disorders can affect the person's judgment. Unsafe actions can cause harm. The person must be protected. In this case, failure to protect the person resulted in patient harm and charges of negligence.

A patient sued a hospital after she set her bed and herself on fire. The patient was in the hospital for alcohol abuse and mental illness. She had a history of mental illness, suicide threats, and alcohol abuse.

While in the hospital:
- *Many packs of cigarettes were taken from her.*
- *Arm, leg, and waist restraints were applied when she became agitated. She was also given a sedative.*
- *After she calmed down, some restraints were removed at her request. They were removed from her right wrist, left ankle, and waist.*
- *She asked to go outside to smoke. A nurse left after asking her to wait a few minutes.*
- *While the nurse was out of the room, the patient set her bed on fire with a cigarette and lighter.*
- *The patient suffered severe burns to her left arm and chest. (The burns required skin grafting. Scars were left at the burn and skin graft sites.)*
- *The patient's lawsuit claimed negligence because:*
  - *The nurse left her.*
  - *Restraints were removed.*
  - *The cigarettes and lighter were not found.*

The jury found in favor of the patient. She was awarded $350,000 for past and future pain, suffering, and disfigurement.

(Wilson v Boscobel Area Health Care Center.)

FOCUS ON **PRIDE**: *Application*

Why are persons with mental health disorders at risk for violation of their rights? How must the health team protect the person's rights?

REVIEW QUESTIONS

Circle T if the statement is TRUE and F if it is FALSE.

1 T F Personality is how a person copes with stress.
2 T F Some anxiety is normal.
3 T F Anxiety is an intense and sudden feeling of fear or dread.
4 T F Panic occurs suddenly for no obvious reason.
5 T F Depression is common in older persons.
6 T F Sudden death can occur from 1 use of a substance.
7 T F The person with binge eating disorder is at risk for obesity.
8 T F A person is talking about suicide. You can leave the person alone to get the nurse.

Circle the BEST answer.

9 Stress is
  a A way to cope with or adjust to everyday living
  b A response or change in the body caused by some factor
  c A mental health disorder
  d An unwanted thought or idea

10 Defense mechanisms are used to
  a Blame others
  b Make excuses for behavior
  c Return to an earlier time
  d Block unpleasant feelings

11 These statements are about defense mechanisms. Which is *true?*
  a Using them signals a mental health disorder.
  b They relieve anxiety.
  c They prevent mental health disorders.
  d Persons with mental health disorders use them well.

12 A phobia is
  a The event that causes stress
  b A false belief
  c An intense fear of something
  d A feeling or emotion

13 A person cleans and cleans. This behavior is
  a A delusion
  b A hallucination
  c A compulsion
  d An obsession

Continued

REVIEW QUESTIONS—cont'd

14 A person has nightmares about a trauma. The person is having
  a Flashbacks
  b Phobias
  c Panic attacks
  d Anxiety

15 A woman believes she is married to a rock singer. This is called a
  a Fantasy
  b Delusion of grandeur
  c Delusion of persecution
  d Hallucination

16 A man believes someone is trying to kill him. This is called a
  a Fantasy
  b Delusion of grandeur
  c Delusion of persecution
  d Hallucination

17 Schizophrenia
  a Involves obsessions and compulsions
  b Can be cured with drugs and therapy
  c Usually begins in late adulthood
  d Is a disabling brain disorder

18 Bipolar disorder means that the person
  a Is very suspicious
  b Has anxiety
  c Is very unhappy and feels unwanted
  d Has severe extremes in mood

19 In bipolar disorder, an "emotional high" is called
  a Depression
  b A hallucination
  c Mania
  d An obsession

20 Which is a sign of depression in older persons?
  a Hallucinations
  b Withdrawal from people and interests
  c Increased energy and activity
  d Weight gain

21 In antisocial personality disorder, the person
  a Lacks regard for the rights and safety of others
  b Has a sad, anxious, or empty mood
  c Withdraws from people and interests
  d Is paranoid and avoids social situations

22 Substances involved in abuse and addiction affect the
  a Circulatory system
  b Respiratory system
  c Nervous system
  d Immune system

23 These statements are about alcoholism? Which is *true?*
  a The person has a strong craving for alcohol.
  b The disease can be cured.
  c After treatment, the person can have a social drink.
  d The person can control the amount and time spent drinking.

24 With drug addiction,
  a Physical and social function are not affected
  b The person cannot stop using the drug
  c Lower doses are needed for the effect
  d The person can stop taking the drug without treatment

25 A person has withdrawal syndrome. This means that
  a The person has a physical and mental response when the drug is not taken
  b The person needs higher doses of the drug
  c The effect is reduced with the same amount of drug
  d The person has a relapse after treatment

26 Binge eating followed by purging occurs in
  a Anorexia nervosa
  b Binge eating disorder
  c Bulimia nervosa
  d Borderline personality disorder

27 For men, the most common method of suicide involves
  a Suffocation
  b Poisoning
  c Alcoholism
  d Firearms

28 Suicide risk
  a Decreases with aging
  b Increases with mental health disorders
  c Decreases with suicide contagion
  d Is low for young adults

29 A person talks about suicide. What should you do?
  a Call for the nurse.
  b Identify factors that increase the risk of suicide.
  c Ask what method the person intends to use.
  d Restrain the person.

30 A person is becoming violent. You should
  a Ask the person to sit and talk
  b Use touch to comfort the person
  c Call for help
  d Let the person block the exit

Answers to Chapter 48 questions are on p. 872.

FOCUS ON PRACTICE

Problem Solving

Ms. Ellis is being treated for bipolar disorder. At 0300 she is pacing in her room. She appears restless. You ask if she needs anything. She begins to talk very fast about work that needs to be done at home. She says: "I don't need to be here. I'm leaving and you can't stop me!" What will you do? How will you protect yourself if she becomes violent?

Confusion and Dementia

OBJECTIVES

- Define the key terms and key abbreviations in this chapter.
- Describe confusion and its causes.
- List the measures that help confused persons.
- Explain the differences between delirium, depression, and dementia.
- Describe the signs, symptoms, and behaviors of Alzheimer's disease (AD).
- Explain the care required by persons with AD and other dementias.
- Describe the effects of AD on the family.
- Explain validation therapy.
- Explain how to promote PRIDE in the person, the family, and yourself.

KEY TERMS

cognitive function Involves memory, thinking, reasoning, ability to understand, judgment, and behavior
confusion A mental state of being disoriented to person, time, place, situation, or identity
delirium A state of sudden, severe confusion and rapid changes in brain function
delusion A false belief
dementia The loss of cognitive function that interferes with routine personal, social, and occupational activities

elopement When a person leaves the agency without staff knowledge
hallucination Seeing, hearing, smelling, or feeling something that is not real
paranoia A disorder *(para)* of the mind *(noia);* false beliefs (delusions) and suspicion about a person or situation
pseudodementia False *(pseudo)* dementia
sundowning Signs, symptoms, and behaviors of AD increase during hours of darkness

KEY ABBREVIATIONS

AD	Alzheimer's disease	**NIA**	National Institute on Aging
ADL	Activities of daily living		

Changes in the brain and nervous system occur with aging and certain diseases (Box 49-1, p. 770). Cognitive function may be affected. *(Cognitive* relates to *knowledge.)* Quality of life is affected. *Cognitive function involves memory, thinking, reasoning, ability to understand, judgment, and behavior.*

CONFUSION

Confusion is a mental state of being disoriented to person, time, place, situation, or identity. Disoriented means to be apart from (dis) *one's awareness* (oriented). Disease, brain injury, infections, hearing and vision loss, and drug side effects are some causes of confusion. Reduced blood flow to the brain with aging can cause personality and mental changes.

With confusion, memory and ability to make good judgments are lost. A person may not know people, the time, or the place. Daily activities may be affected. Behavior changes are common—anger, restlessness, depression, irritability.

Treatment is aimed at the cause. Confusion may be temporary or permanent. Some measures help improve function (Box 49-2, p. 770). You must meet the person's basic needs.

BOX 49-1   Nervous System Changes From Aging

- Nerve cells are lost.
- Nerve conduction slows.
- Reflexes, responses, and reaction times are slower.
- Vision, hearing, taste, smell, and touch decrease.
- Sensitivity to pain decreases.
- Blood flow to the brain is reduced.
- Sleep patterns change.
- Memory is shorter; forgetfulness occurs.
- Dizziness can occur.

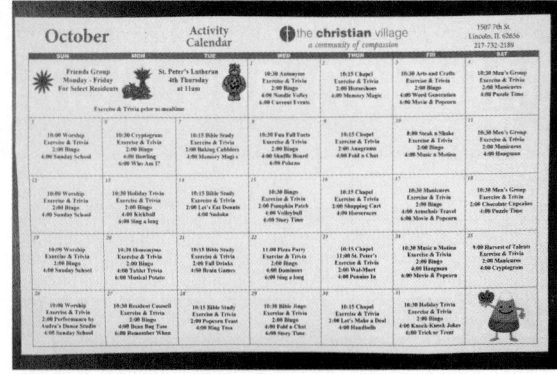

FIGURE 49-1 A large calendar can help persons who are confused.

BOX 49-2   Caring for Persons With Confusion

- Follow the care plan.
- Provide for safety.
- Face the person. Speak clearly.
- Call the person by name every time you have contact with him or her.
- State your name. Show your name tag.
- Give the date and time each morning. Repeat as needed during the day or evening.
- Explain what you are going to do and why.
- Give clear, simple directions and answers to questions.
- Break tasks into small steps when helping the person.
- Ask clear and simple questions. Allow time to respond.
- Keep calendars and clocks with large numbers in the person's room and in nursing areas (Fig. 49-1). Remind the person of holidays, birthdays, and other events.
- Have the person wear eyeglasses and hearing aids as needed.
- Use touch to communicate (Chapter 9).
- Place familiar objects and pictures within view.
- Provide newspapers, magazines, TV, and radio. Read to the person if appropriate.
- Discuss current events with the person.
- Maintain the day-night cycle.
  - Open window coverings during the day. Close them at night.
  - Use night-lights in rooms, bathrooms, hallways, and other areas at night.
  - Have the person wear regular clothes during the day—not sleepwear.
- Provide a calm, relaxed, and peaceful setting. Prevent loud noises, rushing, and crowded hallways and dining rooms.
- Be consistent. Follow the person's routine. Meals, bathing, exercise, TV, bedtime, and other activities have a schedule. This promotes a sense of order and what to expect.
- Do not re-arrange furniture or the person's belongings.
- Encourage the person to take part in self-care.

Delirium

Delirium is a state of sudden, severe confusion and rapid changes in brain function. Usually temporary and reversible, it occurs with physical or mental illness. Causes include acute or chronic illness, surgery, drug or alcohol abuse, drug side effects, and infections. Delirium often lasts for about 1 week. However, it may take several weeks for normal mental function to return.

Delirium signals physical illness. It is an emergency. The cause must be found and treated. See Box 49-3 for signs and symptoms.

BOX 49-3   Delirium—Signs and Symptoms

- Alertness: changes in (usually more alert in the morning and less alert a night)
- Sensation: changes in
- Awareness: changes in
- Movement: very active or slow moving
- Drowsiness
- Confusion about time or place
- Memory:
  - Decreased short-term memory and recall. Cannot remember events since the delirium began.
  - Cannot remember past events.
- Thinking and behavior are without purpose
- Problems concentrating
- Speech: does not make sense
- Incontinence
- Emotional changes:
  - Agitation
  - Anger
  - Depression
  - Euphoria
  - Irritability

Modified from MedlinePlus, Delirium, Bethesda, Md, February 10, 2014, U.S. National Library of Medicine, National Institutes of Health. Updated September 2015.

BOX 49-4	Causes of Dementia

Treatable Causes of Dementia
- Drug and alcohol abuse and drug side effects
- Thyroid problems and hypoglycemia
- Head injuries; bleeding in the brain
- Heart, lung, and blood vessel problems
- Hypoxia
- Infections
- Nutritional problems
- Poisoning
- Tumors

Causes of Permanent Dementia
- Alcohol-related dementia
- Alzheimer's disease
- AIDS-related dementia
- Brain tumors
- Huntington's disease—a genetic brain disorder
- Multi-infarct dementia (MID)—many *(multi)* strokes leave areas of damage *(infarct)*
- Multiple sclerosis
- Parkinson's disease
- Stroke
- Syphilis
- Traumatic brain injury

DEMENTIA

Dementia is the loss of cognitive function that interferes with routine personal, social, and occupational activities. (De means from. Mentia means mind.) Changes in personality, mood, behavior, and communication are common. Dementia is a group of symptoms, not a specific disease.

Dementia is caused by damage to brain cells. Causes are listed in Box 49-4. Some dementias can be reversed. When the cause is removed, so are the signs and symptoms. Permanent dementias result from changes in the brain. There is no cure. Function declines over time.

Dementia is not a normal part of aging. Most older people do not have dementia. Early warning signs include:
- Memory loss (losing things, forgetting names)
- Problems with common tasks (for example, dressing, cooking, driving)
- Problems with language and communication; forgetting simple words
- Getting lost in familiar places
- Misplacing things and putting things in odd places (for example, putting a watch in the oven)
- Personality, mood, and behavior changes
- Poor or decreased judgment (for example, going outdoors in the snow without shoes)

Pseudodementia means false (pseudo) *dementia.* The person has signs and symptoms of dementia. However, there are no changes in the brain. This can occur with delirium and depression. Both can be mistaken for dementia.

See *Focus on Children and Older Persons: Dementia.*

FOCUS ON CHILDREN AND OLDER PERSONS

Dementia

Older Persons

Depression is the most common mental health disorder in older persons. It is often overlooked or mistaken for dementia. Dementia, depression, aging, and some drug side effects have similar signs and symptoms. See Chapter 48 for signs and symptoms of depression in older persons.

Mild Cognitive Impairment

Mild cognitive impairment (MCI) causes slight changes in memory, language, thinking, and judgment. Changes are greater than those with normal aging. The person or others may notice problems. However, the problems do not interfere with daily life. The person is at risk for dementia.

ALZHEIMER'S DISEASE

Alzheimer's disease (AD) is the most common type of permanent dementia. Many brain cells are destroyed and die. Over time, the brain shrinks from nerve cell death and tissue loss (Fig. 49-2). Two abnormal structures are thought to cause damage.
- Plaques—protein pieces that build up in the spaces between nerve cells.
- Tangles—twisted protein fibers that build up inside cells.

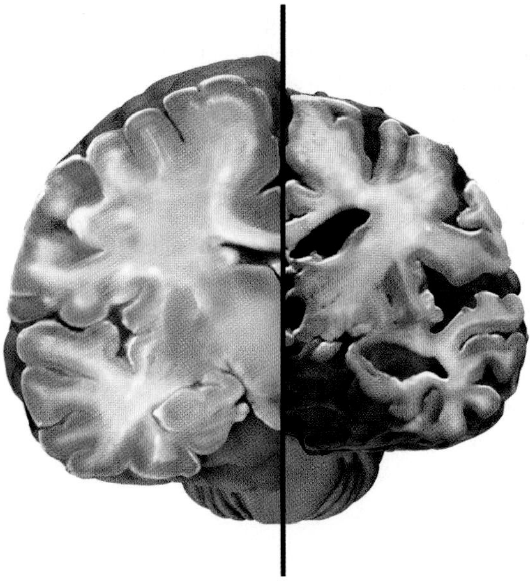

FIGURE 49-2 Nerve cell death and tissue loss shrink the brain in the person with AD. (From Alzheimer's Association, Brain Tour, 2011 www.alz.org/braintour/healthy_vs_alzheimers.asp.)

BOX 49-5	Signs of Alzheimer's Disease

Warning Signs
- Asks the same question over and over again.
- Repeats the same story—word for word, again and again.
- Forgets activities that were once done regularly and with ease—cooking, repairs, playing cards, and so on.
- Loses the ability to pay bills or balance a checkbook.
- Gets lost in familiar places.
- Misplaces household items.
- Neglects to bathe. Or wears the same clothes over and over again.
- Relies on someone else to make decisions or answer questions that he or she would have handled.

Other Signs
- Forgets recent events, conversations, and appointments.
- Forgets simple directions.
- Forgets names of family members and the names of everyday things (clock, TV, and so on).
- Forgets words, cannot find the right word, loses train of thought.
- Substitutes unusual words and names for what is forgotten.
- Speaks in a native language.
- Curses or swears.
- Forgets important dates and events.

Other Signs—cont'd
- Takes longer to do things.
- Misplaces things. Puts things in odd places.
- Has problems keeping track of bills and writing checks.
- Gives away large amounts of money.
- Does not recognize or understand numbers.
- Has problems following conversations.
- Has problems reading and writing.
- Has problems driving to familiar places.
- Forgets where he or she is.
- Forgets how he or she got to a certain place.
- Does not know how to get back home.
- Wanders from home.
- Cannot tell or understand time or dates.
- Cannot solve everyday problems (iron is left on, stove burners left on, food burning on the stove, and so on).
- Cannot perform everyday tasks (dressing, bathing, brushing teeth, and so on).
- Distrusts others.
- Is stubborn.
- Does not want to do things and withdraws socially.
- Is restless.
- Becomes suspicious and fearful.
- Sleeps more than usual.

Warning signs modified from Eric Pfeiffer, MD, The seven warning signs of Alzheimer's disease, University of South Florida Suncoast Alzheimer's and Gerontology Center. Reprinted with permission.

With aging, most people develop some plaques and tangles. In people with AD, plaque and tangle development is severe. Memory areas of the brain are often affected before other areas.

The onset of AD is gradual. Usually symptoms first appear after age 60. Persons with AD can live for 3 to 10 years or longer. More persons with AD are women because women live longer than men.

AD is not a normal part of aging. However, the greatest risk factor is increasing age. The risk increases after age 65. Nearly half the people aged 85 and older have AD. A family history of AD increases the risk of developing the disease.

Signs of AD

According to the Alzheimer's Association, the most common early symptom of AD is difficulty remembering newly learned information. *The classic sign is a gradual loss of short-term memory.* At first, the only symptom may be forgetfulness.

With AD there is a slow, steady decline in mental functions, including:
- Memory
- Thinking
- Reasoning
- Judgment
- Language
- Behavior
- Mood
- Personality

BOX 49-6	Alzheimer's Disease and Normal Aging

Signs of AD	Normal Age-Related Changes
• Poor judgment and decision making.	• Makes a bad decision once in a while.
• Cannot manage a budget.	• Misses a monthly payment.
• Loses track of the date or season.	• Forgets which day it is but remembers later.
• Problems having a conversation.	• Sometimes forgets which word to use.
• Misplaces things. Cannot retrace steps to find them.	• Loses things from time to time.

Modified from Alzheimer's Association, 10 early signs and symptoms of Alzheimer's, 2015.

The person has problems with work and everyday functions. Problems with family and social relationships occur.

Box 49-5 lists the warning and other signs of AD. See Box 49-6 for the differences between AD and normal age-related changes.

Stages of AD

Signs and symptoms become more severe as the disease progresses. The disease ends in death. AD is described in 3 stages (Box 49-7; Fig. 49-3).

BOX 49-7	Three Stages of Alzheimer's Disease

Mild AD
- Memory problems
- Getting lost
- Problems handling money and paying bills
- Repeating questions
- Taking longer to complete daily tasks
- Poor judgment
- Losing things or misplacing them in odd places
- Mood and personality changes

Moderate AD
- Increased memory loss and confusion
- Problems recognizing family and friends
- Cannot learn new things
- Problems with tasks having multiple steps—getting dressed is an example
- Problems coping with new situations
- Hallucinations, delusions, and paranoia (p. 775)
- Impulsive behavior

Severe AD
- Depends on others for care
- Cannot communicate
- Weight loss
- Seizures
- Skin infections
- Difficulty swallowing
- Groaning, moaning, or grunting
- Increased sleeping
- In bed most or all of the time
- Lack of bowel and bladder control

Modified from National Institute on Aging: About Alzheimer's disease: symptoms, National Institutes of Health.

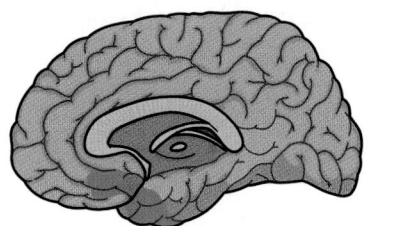

Very Early AD

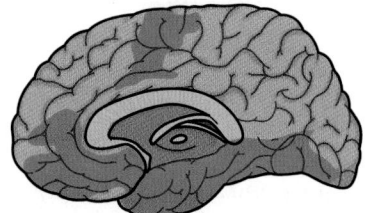

Mild to Moderate AD

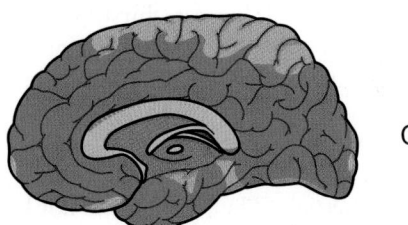

Severe AD

FIGURE 49-3 A, Very early AD. **B,** Mild to moderate AD. **C,** Severe AD. (NOTE: Blue shading shows the areas of the brain affected.) (Redrawn from Alzheimer's Disease Education & Referral Center: *Alzheimer's disease: Unraveling the mystery*, Bethesda, Md, September 2008, updated January 22, 2015, National Institutes of Health.)

Behaviors and Changes in Function

AD changes how a person behaves and acts. Besides the signs and symptoms in Boxes 49-5 and 49-7, these behaviors and changes are common.

- Wandering and getting lost
- Sundowning
- Hallucinations
- Delusions
- Paranoia
- Catastrophic reactions (p. 776)
- Agitation and aggression (p. 776)
- Communication changes (p. 776)
- Screaming (p. 777)
- Repetitive behaviors (p. 777)
- Rummaging and hiding things (p. 777)
- Changes in intimacy and sexuality (p. 777)

Besides changes in the brain, the following can affect the person's behavior.

- Health problems—illness, pain, infection, drugs, lack of sleep, constipation, hunger, thirst, poor vision or hearing, alcohol abuse, too much caffeine
- Emotions—sadness, fear, feeling overwhelmed, stress, anxiety
- Changes in routine
- Problems in the person's setting:
  - A strange setting. The person does not know the setting well.
  - Too much noise (TV, radio, music, people talking at once) can cause confusion and frustration.
  - Not understanding signs. The person may think that a WET FLOOR sign means to urinate on the floor.
  - Mirrors. The person may think that a mirror image is another person in the room.

See *Promoting Safety and Comfort: Behaviors and Changes in Function.*

PROMOTING SAFETY AND COMFORT
Behaviors and Changes in Function

Safety

Some behaviors are not caused by AD. They may be caused by illness, injury, or drugs. If the cause is not treated, it may threaten the person's life. Always report changes in behavior to the nurse.

Wandering and Getting Lost. Persons with AD are not oriented to person, time, and place. They may wander away and not find their way back. Wandering may be by foot, car, bike, or other means. They may be with you one moment and gone the next.

Judgment is poor. They cannot tell what is safe or dangerous. Life-threatening accidents are great risks. They can walk into traffic or into a nearby river, lake, ocean, or forest. If not properly dressed, heat or cold exposure is a risk.

Wandering may have no cause. Or the person may be looking for something or someone—the bathroom, the bedroom, a child, or a partner. Pain, drug side effects, stress, restlessness, too much stimulation, and anxiety are possible causes. A wandering pattern may be linked to a life-long routine—leaving work, getting children from school, and so on. Sometimes finding the cause prevents wandering.

See *Teamwork and Time Management: Wandering and Getting Lost.*

TEAMWORK AND TIME MANAGEMENT
Wandering and Getting Lost

Patients and residents may try to wander to another nursing unit or out of the agency. *Leaving the agency without staff knowledge is called elopement.* Serious injury and death have resulted from elopement. State and federal guidelines to prevent elopement are followed.

All staff must be alert to persons who wander. They are allowed to wander in safe areas (Fig. 49-4). Unsafe areas include kitchens, shower rooms, and utility rooms.

Tell your team members when you are caring for a person who wanders. You cannot be with the person all the time. The team can assist and monitor the person. Help your team members in the same way. If you see a person wandering into an unsafe area, gently guide the person to a safe place (Fig. 49-5). Report the problem to the nurse.

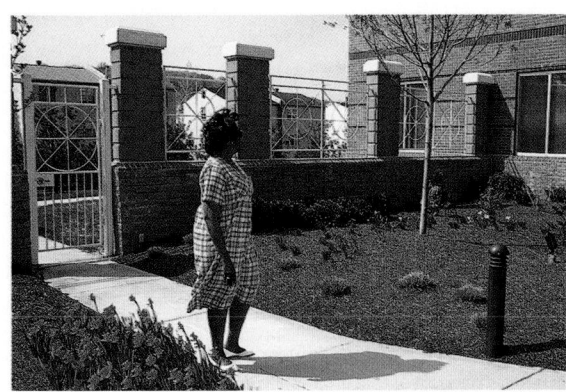

FIGURE 49-4 An enclosed garden allows persons with AD to wander in a safe setting.

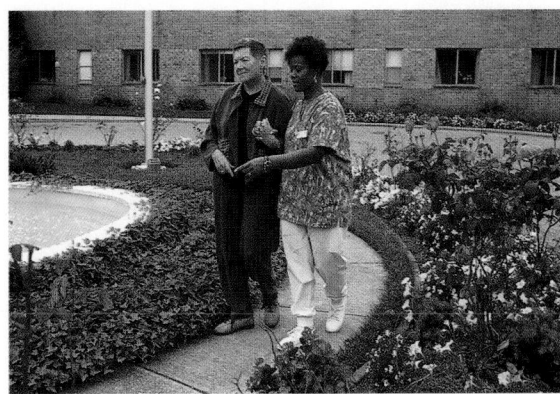

FIGURE 49-5 Guide the person who wanders to a safe area.

MedicAlert® + Alzheimer's Association Safe Return®. *MedicAlert® + Alzheimer's Association Safe Return®* is a 24-hour emergency service for persons who wander or have a medical emergency. The program is nationwide.

The purpose is to find and safely return persons who wander and become lost. A small fee is charged. A family member completes a form and provides a photo. These are entered into a national database. The person receives an ID (wallet card and bracelet or necklace).

When reported missing, the person's information is sent to the police. When the person is found, someone calls the toll-free number on the ID. *MedicAlert® + Alzheimer's Association Safe Return®* then calls the family member or caregiver. The person is returned home safely.

Sundowning. With *sundowning, signs, symptoms, and behaviors of AD increase during hours of darkness.* As daylight ends and darkness starts, confusion and restlessness increase. So do anxiety, agitation, and other symptoms. Behavior is worse after the sun goes down. It may continue throughout the night.

Sundowning may relate to being tired or hungry. Poor light and shadows may cause the person to see things that are not there. The person may be afraid of the dark.

Hallucinations and Delusions. A *hallucination is seeing, hearing, smelling, or feeling something that is not real.* Senses are dulled. Affected persons see animals, insects, or people that are not present. Some hear voices. They may feel bugs crawling or feel that they are being touched.

The problem may be caused by poor vision or hearing. The person needs to wear eyeglasses and hearing aids as prescribed. Other causes include infection, pain, and drugs.

Delusions are false beliefs. To the person, the beliefs are real. People with AD may think they are some other person. Some believe that they are in jail, are being killed, or are being attacked. A person may believe that the caregiver is someone else. Many other false beliefs can occur.

Paranoia. *Paranoia is a disorder* (para) *of the mind* (noia). *The person has false beliefs (delusions) and suspicion about a person or situation.* Paranoia is a type of delusion. The person believes that others are mean, lying, not fair, or "out to get" him or her. The person may be suspicious, fearful, or jealous.

Paranoia may worsen as memory loss gets worse. The National Institute on Aging (NIA) uses these examples.
* The person forgets where he or she put something. The person thinks someone is taking his or her things.
* The person forgets that you are a caregiver. The person thinks you are a stranger and does not trust you.
* The person forgets people whom he or she has met. The person believes that strangers are harmful.
* The person forgets directions that you give. The person thinks that you are trying to trick him or her.

The person may express loss through paranoia. Reasons for the loss do not make sense. Therefore the person blames or accuses others.

See *Promoting Safety and Comfort: Paranoia*, p. 776.

PROMOTING SAFETY AND COMFORT
Paranoia

Safety

The person's behaviors may not mean paranoia. Fears of harm, strangers, stealing, mistreatment, and so on may be real. Some people take advantage of vulnerable adults (Chapter 5). This includes sexual abuse and financial abuse.

The abuse may be by phone, mail, e-mail, or in person. The abuser may be a friend or family member. According to the NIA, financial abuse occurs when money or belongings are stolen. Financial abuse can include:

- Forging checks or cashing checks without permission
- Taking retirement and social security benefits
- Using the person's credit cards or bank accounts
- Changing names on wills, bank accounts, insurance policies, or titles to homes or cars
- "Scams" such as identity theft, phone prizes, and threats
- Borrowing money and not paying it back
- Giving away or selling the person's property without permission
- Forcing the person to sign over property

You must protect the person from harm, abuse, and mistreatment. Report the following at once.

- What the person is saying
- The person seems afraid or worried about money
- Some of the person's items are missing
- The person's behaviors
- Signs and symptoms of problems
- Visitors or family members acting strangely

Catastrophic Reactions. These are extreme responses to normal events or things. The person reacts as if there is a disaster or tragedy. The person may scream, cry, or be agitated or combative (ready to fight). These reactions are common from too many stimuli. Eating, music or TV playing, and being asked questions all at once can overwhelm the person.

Agitation and Aggression. When agitated, the person is restless or worried and cannot settle down. The person may pace, move about, or be unable to sleep. Agitation may lead to aggressive behaviors. The person may yell, scream, swear, hit, pinch, grab, or try to hurt someone. Common causes are:

- Pain or discomfort.
- Anxiety, depression, or stress.
- Drug interactions.
- Fatigue.
- Too many or too few stimuli.
- Hunger or thirst.
- Elimination needs, constipation, and incontinence.
- Feeling lost or abandoned.
- Care measures (bathing, dressing) that upset or frighten the person.
- Change in routine, caregiver, or setting.
- Caregivers. A caregiver may rush the person or be impatient. Or mixed verbal and nonverbal messages are sent. For example, a caregiver talks too fast or too loud. Always consider how your behaviors affect the person.

Communication Changes. Communication skills gradually decline. The person has trouble expressing thoughts and emotions. Communication changes include:

- Struggling to find the right word
- Forgetting what he or she wants to say
- Repeating familiar words
- Relying on gestures more than words
- Problems understanding the meaning of words
- Attention problems during conversations
- Losing one's train of thought when talking
- Problems blocking background noises—radio, TV, music, phones, and so on
- Frustration with problems communicating
- Being sensitive to touch, tone, and voice volume

In time, the person cannot understand others and communicate verbally.

See *Caring About Culture: Communication Changes.*
See *Focus on Communication: Communication Changes.*

CARING ABOUT CULTURE
Communication Changes

For some people, English is a second language. For example, the first language learned may be Spanish, Italian, French, Russian, Chinese, Japanese, and so on. With AD, the person may forget or no longer understand English. He or she may use and understand only the first language learned.

FOCUS ON COMMUNICATION
Communication Changes

To promote communication with the person with AD, see Box 49-8. Avoid:

- *Giving orders.* For example: "Sit down and eat." The statement is bossy. It does not show respect. Instead you can say: "Let me help you sit down."
- *Wanting the truth.* For example, do not say: "Don't you remember?" or "What day is it?" Instead you can say: "Today is Friday."
- *Correcting errors.* For example, do not say: "I just told you that it's time to get dressed. You already had breakfast." Instead you can say: "Let me help you get dressed."
- *Pointing out errors.* Instead of saying: "You missed a button," say: "Let's try it this way."
- *Giving many choices.* For example, "What would you like for dinner?" involves many choices. Instead, limit choices. You can say: "Do you want potatoes or rice?"
- *Asking open-ended questions.* For example, do not say: "How did you sleep last night?" Instead, ask "yes" or "no" questions. You can say: "Did you sleep okay last night?"

BOX 49-8	Communication—Persons With AD or Other Dementias

- Treat the person with dignity and respect.
- Approach the person in a calm, quiet manner.
- Approach the person from the front—not from the side or the back. This avoids startling the person.
- Make eye contact to get the person's attention. Then maintain eye contact.
- Have the person's attention before you start speaking.
- Identify yourself and other people by name.
- Call the person by name.
- Avoid pronouns (he, she, them, it, and so on). For example, instead of saying "She is here," say "Mary is here."
- Follow the rules of communication (Chapters 7 and 9).
- Practice measures to promote communication (Chapters 7 and 9).
- Control distractions and noise. TV, radio, and music are examples.
- Speak in a calm, gentle voice.
- Be aware of your body language. Smile and avoid frowning, grimacing, or other negative actions.
- Use gestures or cues. Point to objects.
- Comfort the person with touch. Hold the person's hand while you talk.
- Speak slowly. Use simple words and short sentences.
- Ask or say 1 thing at a time. Present 1 idea, statement, or question at a time.
- Give simple, step-by-step instructions.

- Provide explanations of all procedures and activities.
- Repeat instructions as needed. Give the person time to respond or react.
- Ask simple questions with simple answers. Do not ask complex questions.
- Do not "baby talk" or use a "baby voice."
- Let the person speak. Do not interrupt or rush the person.
- Give the person time to respond.
- Try other words if the person does not seem to understand.
- Provide the word the person is looking for if he or she is struggling to communicate a thought.
- Do not criticize, correct, interrupt, argue, or try to reason with the person.
- Give consistent responses.
- Practice the measures in Chapter 42.
  - To promote hearing
  - To communicate with speech-impaired persons
  - For blind and visually impaired persons
- Try these measures for the screaming person.
  - Provide a calm, quiet setting.
  - Play soft music.
  - Have the person wear hearing aids and eyeglasses.
  - Have a family member or favorite caregiver comfort and calm the person.
  - Use touch to calm the person.

Screaming. At first, persons with AD have a hard time finding the right words. As AD progresses, they speak in short sentences or in just words. Often speech is not understandable.

Screaming to communicate is common in persons who are very confused and have poor communication skills. They may scream a word or a name. Or they just make screaming sounds.

Possible causes include hearing and vision problems, pain or discomfort, fear, and fatigue. Too much or not enough stimulation is another cause. A person may react to a caregiver or family member by screaming. See Box 49-8.

Repetitive Behaviors. *Repetitive* means *to do over and over.* Persons with AD repeat the same motions, words, or questions over and over. For example, the person folds the same napkin over and over. Or the person says the same words or asks the same question over and over. Such behaviors do not harm the person. However, they can annoy caregivers and the family.

Rummaging and Hiding Things. To *rummage* means *to search for things by moving things around, turning things over, or looking through something such as a drawer or closet.* The behavior may not have meaning. Or the person may be looking for a certain item but cannot tell you what or why.

The person may hide things, throw things away, or lose things. Eyeglasses, hearing aids, and dentures must stay with the person. Always make sure these items are safe. Money, jewelry, and other important items usually are sent home with the family.

Changes in Intimacy and Sexuality. *Intimacy* is a special bond between people who love and respect each other. It includes the way people talk and act toward each other. *Sexuality* involves the way partners physically express their feelings for each other (Chapter 51). The person with AD may:

- Depend on and cling to his or her partner.
- Not remember life with his or her partner.
- Not remember feelings for his or her partner.
- Fall in love with another person.
- Have side effects from drugs that affect sexual interest.
- Have memory loss, brain changes, or depression that affects sexual interest.
- Have abnormal sexual behaviors.

Sexual behaviors are labeled abnormal because of how and when they occur. Sexual behaviors may involve the wrong person, the wrong place, and the wrong time. Also, persons with AD cannot control behavior.

Healthy persons do not undress or expose themselves in front of others. They do not masturbate or engage in sexual acts in public. They know their sexual partners. Persons with AD often mistake someone else for a sexual partner. The person kisses and hugs the other person.

Being overly *(hyper)* interested in sex is called *hypersexuality.* The person may try to seduce others. Or the person may masturbate often. These behaviors are symptoms of AD. They may not mean that the person wants to have sex. When a person masturbates in public, lead the person to his or her room. Provide for privacy and safety.

The nurse encourages the person's partner to show affection. Their normal practices are encouraged. Examples include hand holding, hugging, kissing, touching, and dancing.

Some behaviors are not sexual. Touching, scratching, and rubbing the genitals can signal infection, pain, or discomfort in the urinary or reproductive systems. Poor hygiene and incontinence are other causes. Good hygiene prevents itching. Clean the person quickly and thoroughly after elimination. Do not let the person stay wet or soiled. The nurse assesses the person for urinary or reproductive system problems.

CARE OF PERSONS WITH AD AND OTHER DEMENTIAS

The person may be cared for at home until symptoms become severe. Adult day care may help. Often assisted living or nursing center care is required. Other illnesses may require hospital care. You may care for persons with AD or other dementias in such settings. The person and family need your support and understanding.

People with AD do not choose to have the behaviors, signs, and symptoms of the disease. They cannot control what is happening to them. *The disease is responsible, not the person.*

Currently AD has no cure. Symptoms worsen over many years. Over time, the person depends on others for care. Safety, hygiene, food and fluids, elimination, and activity needs must be met. So must comfort and sleep needs. Good skin care and alignment prevent skin breakdown and contractures. The person's care plan will include many of the measures listed in Box 49-9.

BOX 49-9	Care of Persons With AD and Other Dementias

Environment
- Follow set routines.
- Avoid changing rooms or roommates.
- Place picture signs by room doors, bathrooms, dining rooms, and other areas (Fig. 49-6, p. 780).
- Keep personal items where the person can see and reach them.
- Stay within the person's sight to the extent possible.
- Place memory aids (large clocks and calendars) where the person can see them.
- Keep noise levels low.
- Play music and show movies from the person's past.
- Select tasks and activities that fit the person's abilities and interests.

Safety
- Reassure the person that you are there to help.
- Remove harmful, sharp, and breakable items from the area. This includes knives, scissors, glasses, dishes, razors, and tools.
- Provide plastic eating and drinking utensils. They help prevent breakage and cuts.
- Place safety plugs in electrical outlets. Or cover outlets with safety plates.
- Keep cords and electrical items out of reach.
- Remove electric appliances from the bathroom. Hair dryers, curling irons, make-up mirrors, and electric shavers are examples.
- Provide safe storage for:
  - Personal care items (shampoo, deodorant, lotion, and so on)
  - Household cleaners and drugs
  - Dangerous equipment and tools
  - Cigarettes, cigars, pipes, matches, and other smoking materials
  - Car keys
- Keep childproof caps on drug containers and household cleaners.
- Remove knobs from stoves or place safety covers on the knobs (Fig. 49-7, p. 780).

Safety—cont'd
- Remove dangerous appliances, power tools, and firearms and weapons from the home.
- Supervise the person who smokes.
- Practice safety measures to prevent:
  - Falls (Chapter 14)
  - Fires (Chapter 13)
  - Burns (Chapter 13)
  - Poisoning (Chapter 13)
- Lock doors to kitchens, utility rooms, and housekeeping closets. Keep them locked.

Wandering
- Follow agency policy for locking doors and windows. Locks are often at the top and bottom of doors (Fig. 49-8, p. 781). The person is not likely to look for a lock in such places.
- Keep door alarms and electronic doors turned on. Respond to alarms at once.
- Follow agency policy for fire exits. Everyone must be able to leave the building for a fire.
- Make sure the person wears an ID bracelet or *MedicAlert® + Alzheimer's Association Safe Return®* ID at all times.
- Know the times of day the person is more likely to wander.
- Follow the person's care plan for daily routines, activities, and exercise. Make sure food, fluid, and elimination needs are met.
- Involve the person in activities—folding napkins, dusting a table, sorting socks, rolling yarn, sweeping, sanding blocks of wood, or watering plants.
- Do not use restraints. Restraints require a doctor's order. They also tend to increase confusion and disorientation.
- Do not argue with the person who wants to leave. The person will not understand.
- Go with the person who insists on going outside. Make sure he or she is properly dressed. Guide the person inside after a few minutes.
- Let the person wander in enclosed areas. The agency may have enclosed areas for walking about. They provide a safe place for the person to wander.

BOX 49-9 Care of Persons With AD and Other Dementias—cont'd

Sundowning

- Complete treatments and activities early in the day.
- Encourage exercise and activity early in the day.
- Keep the person on a schedule. Waking up, meal times, and bedtime should involve a set routine.
- Avoid caffeine (coffee, tea, colas, chocolate), sweets, and alcohol late in the day. Provide a calm, quiet setting late in the day.
- Do not restrain the person.
- Meet nutrition and elimination needs. Unmet needs can increase restlessness.
- Use night-lights at night.
- Do not try to reason with the person. He or she will not understand.
- Do not ask the person to explain the problem. Communication changes impair understanding and speech.

Hallucinations and Delusions

- Have the person wear eyeglasses and hearing aids as needed.
- Do not argue with the person. He or she will not understand.
- Reassure the person. Say that you will provide protection from harm.
- Distract the person with some item or activity. Go to another room. Taking the person for a walk may be helpful.
- Turn off TV or movies when violent and disturbing programs are on. The person may believe the story is real.
- Comfort the person if he or she seems afraid. Use touch to calm and reassure the person (Fig. 49-9, p. 781).
- Eliminate noises that the person could misinterpret. TV, radio, music, furnaces, air conditioners, and other things could affect the person.
- Check lighting. Make sure there are no glares, shadows, or reflections.
- Cover or remove mirrors. The person could misinterpret his or her reflection.
- Make sure the person cannot reach anything that could be used to hurt the self or others.
- Report behavior changes. They may signal a physical illness.

Paranoia

- Do not react if the person blames you for something.
- Do not argue with the person.
- Let the person know that he or she is safe.
- Use touch or gently hug the person to show that you care.
- Search for missing things. This helps distract the person. Talk about what you found. For example, you find a photo. Talk about the photo.

Catastrophic Reactions

- Approach the person from the front. Do not startle the person from behind or the side.
- Be calm. Do not appear rushed. Allow the person time to calm down.
- Use touch appropriately. Know how the person responds to touch. Touch can comfort some people. Others do not like being touched.
- Explain in simple terms what you would like the person to do. For example: "It's time for bed. I'll help you into bed."
- Do not argue with the person.
- Follow the person's daily routine, including naps and bedtime.
- Distract the person with an activity.

Agitation and Aggression

- Look at how your behaviors affect the person.
- Provide a calm, quiet setting.
- Follow the person's care plan and a set routine for ADL (activities of daily living). Meet the person's basic needs.
- Observe for early signs of agitation and aggression. Try to remove the cause before the behaviors worsen.
- Do not ignore the problem. Try to find the cause.
- Allow personal choice. Let the person decide things to the extent possible.
- Try to distract the person. A snack, safe object, or an activity may help.
- Reassure the person.
  - Speak calmly.
  - Listen to concerns.
  - Try to show that you understand the person's anger or fears.
- Keep personal items within the person's sight. Photos and treasures are examples.
- Reduce glares, noise, and clutter.
- Limit the number of people in the room.
- Use gentle touch.
- Provide soothing music.
- Read to the person using a gentle voice.
- Provide quiet times.
- Limit the amount of caffeine (coffee, tea, colas, chocolate) and sweets that the person eats or drinks.
- See Chapter 9 for dealing with the angry person.
- See Chapter 13 for workplace violence.

Repetitive Behaviors

- Allow harmless acts. Holding a purse, folding napkins, and petting a stuffed animal are examples.
- Distract the person. Music, picture books, exercise, and movies may provide distraction.
- Take the person for a walk.
- Know when repetitive behaviors are likely to occur. For example, a person constantly calls for a nurse at bedtime.
- Use a calm voice and gentle touch.
- Do not argue with the person.
- Answer the person's question. You may have to answer the same question several times.
- Use memory aids according to the care plan. Clocks, calendars, and photos are examples.

Rummaging and Hiding Things

- Keep harmful items and products out of the person's sight and reach.
- Remove spoiled items from refrigerators and cabinets. The person may look for food and snacks. He or she may not know or be able to taste spoiled food.
- Guide the person away from other patient or resident rooms.
- Keep wastebaskets covered or out of sight. The person may rummage through a wastebasket or throw things away.
- Check wastebaskets before you empty them. Look for items thrown away or hidden. Do the same before discarding linens or returning food trays.
- Keep bathroom doors closed and toilet seats down. This helps prevent the person from flushing things down the toilet.
- Allow the person to rummage in a safe place. The agency may have a drawer, closet, bag, box, basket, or chest with safe items.

Continued

BOX 49-9   Care of Persons With AD and Other Dementias—cont'd

Sleep
- Develop a regular bedtime. Bedtime should be the same each evening.
- Provide a quiet, peaceful mood in the evening—dimmed lights, low noise level, and soft music.
- Follow bedtime rituals.
- Use night-lights so the person can see. Use them in rooms, hallways, bathrooms, and other areas. They help prevent accidents and disorientation.
- Limit caffeine during the day.
- Limit naps during the day.
- Follow the person's exercise plan. Play music to the exercise.
- Reduce noises.

Personal Hygiene and Grooming
- Provide good skin care. Keep the person's skin free of urine and feces.
- Promote personal hygiene.
  - Use the person's preferred bathing method (tub bath, shower).
  - Make sure the bathroom is warm and well-lit.
  - Do not force the person into a shower or tub. Do not argue with the person. People with AD are often afraid of bathing. Try bathing the person when he or she is calm.
  - Provide privacy and keep the person warm.
  - Check for a comfortable water temperature.
  - Place a towel over the person's shoulders or lap. The person feels less exposed.
  - Do not rush the person.
  - Tell the person what you will do step-by-step.
  - Allow the person to do as much as possible.
  - Give the person a washcloth to hold.
- Provide oral hygiene.
  - Allow the person to do as much as possible.
  - Explain what to do 1 step at a time. For example: "Pick up the toothpaste. Take off the cap. Squeeze the toothpaste on the toothbrush. Put the toothbrush in your mouth. Brush."

Personal Hygiene and Grooming—cont'd
- Assist with dressing and undressing.
  - Choose clothing that is comfortable and simple to put on. Front opening garments are easy to put on. Pullover tops are harder to put on. And the person may become frightened when his or her head is inside a garment.
  - Select clothing that closes with Velcro. Such items are easy to put on and take off. Buttons, zippers, snaps, and other closures can frustrate the person.
  - Offer simple clothing choices (Fig. 49-10). Let the person choose between 2 shirts or 2 blouses, 2 pants or 2 slacks, and so on.
  - Lay clothing out in the order it will be put on. Hand the person 1 item at a time. Tell or show the person what to do. Do not rush him or her.

Other Basic Needs
- Follow a daily routine. This helps the person know when certain things will happen.
- Meet food and fluid needs. Provide finger foods. Cut food and pour liquids as needed. Watch for signs of dysphagia. See Chapter 27.
- Promote urinary and bowel elimination and prevent incontinence.
- Provide incontinence care as needed.
- Promote exercise and activity during the day. This helps reduce wandering and sundowning behaviors. The person may also sleep better.
- Reduce intake of coffee, tea, and cola drinks. These contain caffeine. Caffeine is a stimulant. It can increase restlessness, confusion, and agitation.
- Provide a quiet, restful setting. Soft music is better than loud TV programs.
- Play music during care activities such as bathing and during meals.
- Have equipment ready for any procedure. This reduces the amount of time the person is involved in care measures.
- Observe for signs and symptoms of health problems (Chapter 8).
- Prevent infection.

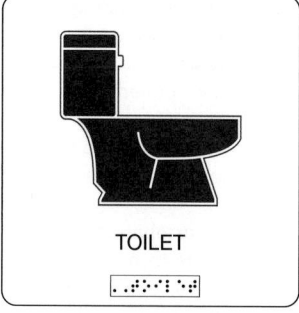

FIGURE 49-6 Signs give cues to persons with dementia.

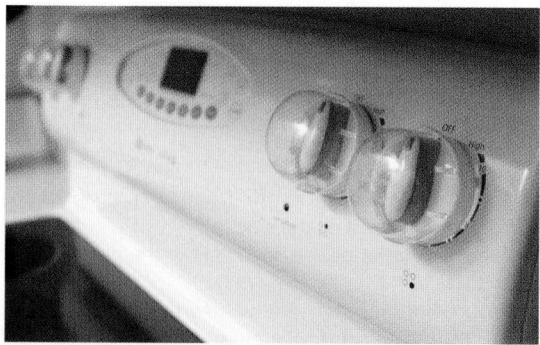

FIGURE 49-7 Safety covers are on stove knobs.

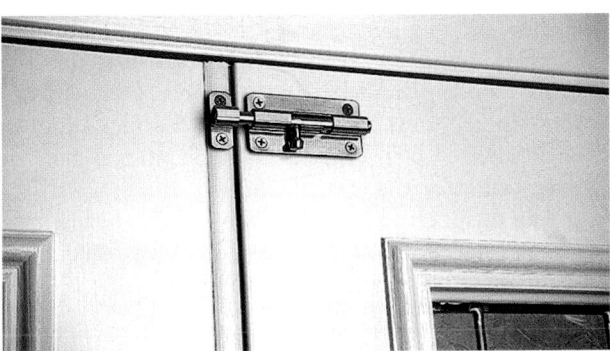

FIGURE 49-8 A slide lock is at the top of the door.

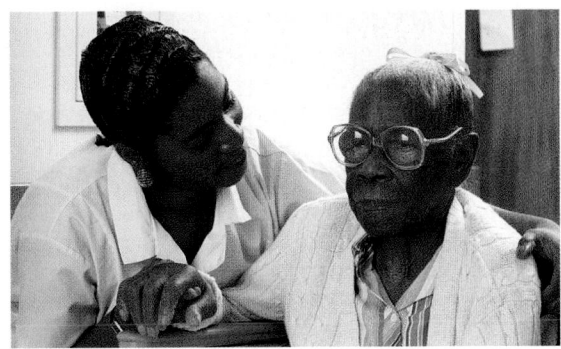

FIGURE 49-9 Use touch to calm the person.

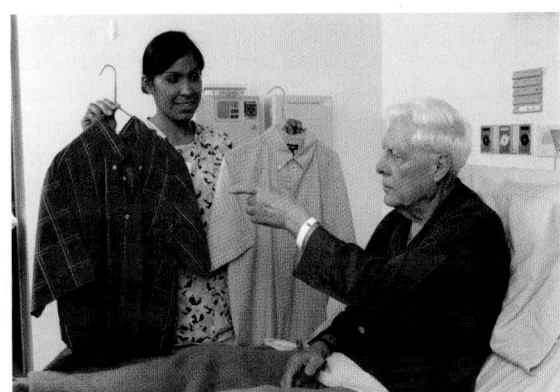

FIGURE 49-10 The person is offered simple clothing choices.

The person can have other health problems and injuries. However, the person may not be aware of pain, fever, constipation, incontinence, or other signs and symptoms. Carefully observe the person. Report any change in the person's usual behavior.

Infection is a risk. The person cannot fully tend to self-care. Infection can occur from poor hygiene. This includes poor skin care, oral hygiene, and perineal care after bowel and bladder elimination. Inactivity and immobility can cause pneumonia and pressure ulcers.

The person needs to feel useful, worthwhile, and active. This promotes self-esteem. Therapies and activities focus on the person's strengths and past successes. For example:

- A woman used to cook. She helps clean fruit.
- A man was a good dancer. Activities are planned so he can dance.
- A man likes to clean. He helps with dusting.

Supervised activities meet the person's needs and cognitive abilities. Activities are based on what the person enjoys and can do. Some people like crafts, exercise, gardening, and listening and moving to music. Others like sing-alongs, board games, and reminiscing. (*Reminiscence* or *to reminisce* is *to talk about or recall past events.*) Some like to string beads, fold towels, or roll dough.

You must treat these persons with dignity and respect. They have the same rights as everyone else. Speak in a calm voice. Always explain what you are going to do. Massage, soothing touch, music, and aromatherapy are comforting and relaxing. The person may need hospice care as death nears (Chapter 55).

See *Focus on Long-Term Care and Home Care: Care of Persons With AD and Other Dementias*, p. 782.

See *Teamwork and Time Management: Care of Persons With AD and Other Dementias*, p. 782.

See *Focus on Surveys: Care of Persons With AD and Other Dementias*, p. 782.

FOCUS ON LONG-TERM CARE AND HOME CARE

Care of Persons With AD and Other Dementias

Long-Term Care

Many nursing centers provide secure Alzheimer's environments (settings). This means that entrances and exits are locked. Residents cannot wander away. They have a safe setting to move about. Some persons have aggressive behaviors that disrupt or threaten others. They need a secured unit.

According to the *Omnibus Budget Reconciliation Act of 1987 (OBRA)*, secured units are physical restraints. The center must follow OBRA rules and use the least restrictive approach. A dementia diagnosis and a doctor's order are needed for placement on a secured unit. At least every 90 days, the health team reviews the person's need for a secured unit. The person's rights are always protected.

At some point, the secured unit is no longer needed for safe care. For example, a person's condition progresses to severe AD (see Box 49-7). The person cannot sit or walk. Wandering is not a concern. The person is transferred to another unit.

Licensing and accrediting agencies have standards of care for special care units. Staff must have special training in the care of persons with dementia. The unit must have programs that promote dignity, personal freedom, and safety.

TEAMWORK AND TIME MANAGEMENT

Care of Persons With AD and Other Dementias

The entire staff must protect the person from harm. Look for dangers in the person's room and in hallways, lounges, and dining and other areas. Remove the danger if you can and tell the nurse at once. If you cannot remove the danger, also tell the nurse at once.

FOCUS ON SURVEYS

Care of Persons With AD and Other Dementias

To ensure quality of life, surveyors will look at all aspects of dementia care. For example:
- Are bathing, dressing, and grooming needs met?
- Is independence promoted? For example, does the staff give cues so the person can dress himself or herself?
- Is the person reminded to use the toilet at regular times?
- Is the person in a calm, quiet setting for meals?
- Are enough fluids offered to prevent dehydration?
- Does the staff respond to the person in a dignified manner?
- Is a safe setting provided?
- Does the staff provide supervision for safe behaviors?

Federal laws require that nursing assistant education and training include dementia management and preventing abuse. Annual in-service training also is required. Surveyors will review employee records to make sure these requirements are met.

The Family

The person may live at home or with a partner, children, or other family members. Or someone stays with the person. Home health care may help for a while. Adult day care and assisted living are options (Chapters 1 and 53). Nursing center care is needed when:
- Family members cannot meet the person's needs.
- The person no longer knows the caregiver.
- Family members have health problems.
- Money problems occur.
- The person's behavior presents dangers to self and others.

Doctor's visits, drugs, home care, and assisted living are costly. So is nursing center care. The person's medical care can drain family finances.

Home care and nursing center care are stressful. The family has physical, emotional, social, and financial stresses. Adult children are in the *sandwich generation*. Their own children need attention while an ill parent needs care. Caring for 2 families is stressful. Often adult children have jobs too.

Caregivers can suffer from anger, anxiety, guilt, depression, and sleep problems. Some cannot concentrate or are irritable. Health problems can develop. They need to focus on their own health. They need a healthy diet, exercise, and plenty of rest. Asking family members and friends for help is important. However, asking for help is hard for some people.

Caregivers need much support and encouragement. The NIA suggests ways that family members can take care of themselves. See Box 49-10. AD support groups are sponsored by hospitals, nursing centers, and the Alzheimer's Association. The Alzheimer's Association has chapters across the country. Support groups offer encouragement and advice. Members share their feelings, anger, frustration, guilt, and other emotions. They also share coping and caregiving ideas.

The family often feels hopeless. No matter what is done, the person gets worse. Much time, money, energy, and emotion are needed to care for the person. Anger and resentment may result. Guilt feelings are common. The family knows that the person did not choose the disease and its signs, symptoms, and behaviors. Sometimes behaviors are embarrassing. The family may be upset and angry that the loved one cannot show love or affection.

The family is an important part of the health team. They help plan care when possible. The nurse and support group help the family learn how to provide a safe home setting and give needed care. They learn how to bathe, feed, dress, and give oral hygiene to the person.

In nursing centers, some family members take part in unit activities. For many persons, family members provide comfort. They also need support and understanding from the health team.

See Focus on Long-Term Care and Home Care: The Family.

BOX 49-10	Family Caregivers—Taking Care of Yourself

- Ask for help when you need it. Asking for something specific may be useful. For example:
  - "Can you make Mom's dinner Sunday night?"
  - "Can you stay with Dad from 2 to 4 Monday afternoon?"
  - "Can Mom stay at your house Saturday afternoon?"
- Join a support group.
- Take breaks every day.
- Spend time with friends.
- Maintain hobbies and interests.
- Eat healthy foods and exercise often.
- See a doctor regularly.
- Keep health, legal, and financial information current.
- Remember that these feelings are normal—being sad, lonely, frustrated, confused, angry. Say to yourself:
  - "I'm doing the best I can."
  - "What I'm doing would be hard for anyone."
  - "I'm not perfect and that's okay."
  - "I can't control some things."
  - "I need to do what works for right now."
  - "Even when I do everything I can, there will still be problem behaviors. They are caused by the illness, not what I do."
  - "I will enjoy the times when we can be together in peace."
  - "I will get counseling if caregiving becomes too much for me."

- Meet spiritual needs—attending religious services, believing that larger forces or a higher power is at work.
  - Understand that you may feel powerless and hopeless about what is happening.
  - Understand that you may feel a sense of loss and sadness.
  - Understand that you are caring for a person with AD. Was the choice made out of love, loyalty, duty, religious obligation, money concerns, fear, habit, or self-punishment?
  - Let yourself feel "uplifts." Examples include good feelings about the person, support from caring people, and time for your own interests.
  - Keep connected to something "higher than yourself." This may be believing good comes from every experience.

Modified from National Institute on Aging: Caring for a person with Alzheimer's disease, NIH Publication No. 15-6173, Bethesda, Md, March 2010, updated May 2015, National Institutes of Health.

FOCUS ON **LONG-TERM CARE AND HOME CARE**

The Family

Home Care

Home care is an option for many families. They may need help with meeting the person's needs—preparing meals, bathing, elimination, and so on. Someone needs to supervise the person while family members work, do errands, and have alone time. The amount and kind of care depend on the person's needs and the family's ability to provide care.

Validation Therapy

The person's care plan may include validation therapy. *Validation therapy* is a way to communicate with persons with dementia. *Validate* means *to show that a person's feelings and needs are fair and have meaning.* Behaviors signal the person's need to express feelings and needs—safety, security, comfort, love and belonging, feeling useful, and so on. Caregivers help the person express feelings and needs verbally or non-verbally. With validation, the person's reality (what the person thinks is real and true) is accepted. The person is treated with dignity and self-worth.

Validation therapy is based on these principles.

- All behavior has meaning.
- A person may have unresolved issues and emotions from the past.
- A person's mind may return to the past to resolve issues and emotions.
- Caregivers need to listen and provide empathy.
- Attempts are not made to correct thoughts or bring the person back to reality (reality orientation). For example:
  - Ms. Clark talks about waiting for the bus to go to work. The caregiver does not remind her that she no long works. Instead, the caregiver says: "Tell me about where you worked."
  - Mrs. Brown says that she is at the train station waiting to meet her husband. Killed in a war, her husband never returned home. The caregiver does not remind Mrs. Brown of what happened. Instead, the caregiver asks Mrs. Brown about her husband.
  - Mr. Garcia was 3 years old when his father died. He holds a ball constantly. He calls for his father and repeats "play ball, play ball." The caregiver does not remind Mr. Garcia that his father is not alive. Instead, the caregiver says: "Tell me about playing ball."

Validation therapy is useful for some persons. If used in your agency, you will be trained to use validation therapy correctly.

FOCUS ON PRIDE

The Person, Family, and Yourself

Personal and Professional Responsibility

Everyone has different talents, abilities, and interests. Persons with dementia are no different. They still have emotional and social needs. Understanding the person's past and his or her hobbies, talents, family, and work can help you give better care.

Learn about the person. Engage the person in activities that were enjoyed in the past. Treat each person as unique with his or her own history, interests, strengths, and needs.

Rights and Respect

The person has the right to privacy and confidentiality. Protect the person from exposure. Only those involved in the person's care are present for care and procedures. The person is allowed to visit in private. Do not share information about the person with others.

The person has the right to keep and use personal items. A pillow, blanket, afghan, or sweater may have meaning to the person. The person may not know why or even recognize the item. Still, it is important and provides comfort. Keep personal items safe. Protect the person's property from loss or damage.

Independence and Social Interaction

Persons with dementia have problems with ADL. Eating, bathing, dressing, and elimination are examples. Maintaining routines can help the person remain independent as long as possible. For example, Mrs. Lund uses the bathroom, washes hands, brushes teeth, puts on make-up, brushes hair, and dresses in the morning. She is more independent when ADL are done in this order. Changing the order causes confusion.

You may need to break down tasks into simple steps. Kindly tell the person each step. Repeat directions as needed. Allow extra time for each task. Resist the urge to take over. Let the person do what is safely possible.

Delegation and Teamwork

Persons with dementia may respond better to certain staff or caregivers. This can vary by day or time of day. Do not be offended if someone else provides care. The team works together to meet the person's needs.

Sometimes the person resists care from everyone. Encouraging the person to allow care is often useless. Use a calm and caring approach. Try giving care at a different time. Never use force.

Ethics and Laws

Persons with AD often have changes in mood, behavior, and personality. The person may become easily agitated or angry. The person cannot control words and actions. Some behaviors are hard to deal with. The following is a real example of a poor response to the person's behavior.

While a licensed nursing assistant (LNA) was feeding a resident with AD, the resident threw the tray on the floor. The LNA called the resident a degrading name and swore at her.

The Board of Nursing concluded that the LNA abused and improperly cared for the resident. The unprofessional conduct violated the Administrative Rules of the Board of Nursing because of:

- *Abusing or neglecting a patient*
- *Performing unsafe or unacceptable patient care*
- *Failing to conform to acceptable standards of practice*
- *Engaging in conduct likely to harm the public*
  The nursing assistant's license was reprimanded.
  (Author note: A reprimand means that the Board considered her conduct to be improper. However, the Board did not limit her right to work as an LNA.)
  (State of Vermont Board of Nursing, 2000.)

You must control your reactions to stress. Be professional. Tell the nurse if you feel frustrated, angry, or impatient. You may need an assignment change. Never take out your anger on the person. The person must be protected from physical and verbal abuse and mistreatment.

FOCUS ON PRIDE: Application

Dementia caregivers affect the person's quality of life. Describe care that values the person. What qualities must the caregiver have? How must the caregiver treat the person?

REVIEW QUESTIONS

Circle T if the statement is TRUE and F if it is FALSE.

1 T F   Cognitive function involves memory, thinking, reasoning, understanding, judgment, and behavior.

2 T F   The onset of delirium is gradual.

3 T F   Depression can cause cognitive changes.

4 T F   A person with AD is agitated and restless. A caregiver may have caused the behaviors.

5 T F   A person with AD keeps moving an empty cup back and forth across the table. You should take the cup away.

6 T F   A person with AD hides things. You should check wastebaskets before emptying them.

7 T F   The person with AD can control behavior.

8 T F   The person with AD can tell you about pain, constipation, and other discomforts.

9 T F   The person with AD is at risk for infection from poor hygiene after elimination.

10 T F   A set routine is important for the person with AD.

11 T F   You can use gestures or point to things to communicate with persons who have AD.

12 T F   Restraints help improve the behaviors of AD.

13 T F   Family members continue their hobbies and holiday events. They are abusing the person with AD.

REVIEW QUESTIONS—cont'd

Circle the BEST answer.

14 A person is confused after surgery. The confusion is likely to be
   a Permanent
   b Temporary
   c Caused by dementia
   d Caused by a brain injury

15 A person is confused. Which measure should you question?
   a Restrain in bed at night.
   b Give clear, simple directions.
   c Use touch to communicate.
   d Open drapes during the day.

16 A person has AD. Which is *true?*
   a AD is a normal part of aging.
   b Diet and drugs can cure the disease.
   c AD and delirium are the same.
   d AD ends in death.

17 A person is in the final stage of AD. The person is likely to
   a Wander and become lost
   b Follow simple commands
   c Need total assistance with ADL
   d Repeat questions over and over

18 Which is common in persons with AD?
   a Paralysis
   b Dyspnea
   c Headache
   d Sleep disturbances

19 A person has AD. To communicate, you should
   a Give orders
   b Limit the person's choices
   c Correct the person's mistakes
   d Ask open-ended questions

20 A person with AD is screaming. You know that this is
   a A way to communicate
   b An agitated reaction
   c Caused by a delusion
   d A repetitive behavior

21 Which statement about sundowning is *true?*
   a AD behaviors improve at night.
   b Encouraging activity late in the day can help.
   c Being tired or hungry can increase restlessness.
   d Dim lighting or darkness is calming.

22 A person has delusions. Which measure should you question?
   a Distract the person with an activity.
   b Tell the person you will provide protection.
   c Tell the person the beliefs are not real.
   d Use touch to calm the person.

23 Which can cause delusions in persons with AD?
   a Mirrors
   b Eyeglasses
   c Hearing aids
   d Night-lights

24 A person with AD keeps telling you that someone is stealing things. What should you do?
   a Nothing. The person suffers from paranoia.
   b Tell the nurse. Someone could be abusing the person.
   c Replace missing items.
   d Send other items home with the family.

25 A person with AD is at risk for elopement. Which measure should you question?
   a Make sure door alarms are turned on.
   b Make sure an ID bracelet is worn.
   c Assist with exercise as ordered.
   d Remind the person not to wander.

26 Which measure can help with rummaging?
   a Keep the person's room locked.
   b Provide safe places to rummage.
   c Ask the person to explain the behavior.
   d Hide items the person looks for.

27 Safety is important for persons with AD. Which measure is unsafe?
   a Safety plugs are placed in electrical outlets.
   b Cleaners and drugs are kept locked up.
   c The person keeps smoking materials.
   d Sharp and breakable objects are removed from the person's setting.

28 A person with AD is upset. Which is a correct response?
   a Try to reason with the person.
   b Ask what is bothering the person.
   c Ignore the problem.
   d Provide reassurance and try to find the cause.

29 You are caring for a person with AD. You should avoid
   a Trying to bring the person back to reality.
   b Offering support to the person's family.
   c Following a set routine.
   d Providing a quiet setting.

30 Validation therapy involves
   a Support groups and counseling for persons with severe AD
   b Drugs to treat AD
   c Helping the person with AD express needs and feelings
   d Orienting the person with AD to reality

Answers to Chapter 49 questions are on p. 872.

FOCUS ON **PRACTICE**

Problem Solving

Mr. Rosin has moderate AD. While preparing him for a bath, he becomes restless and upset. He repeats: "Go away" over and over. How will you respond? How might you meet his hygiene needs?

OBJECTIVES

- Define the key terms and key abbreviations in this chapter.
- Identify the areas of function limited by intellectual and developmental disabilities.
- Explain how intellectual and developmental disabilities affect the person and family across the life-span.
- Explain when intellectual and developmental disabilities occur and their causes.

- Identify the types of support and services available to persons with intellectual and developmental disabilities.
- Describe the intellectual and developmental disabilities presented in this chapter.
- Explain how to promote PRIDE in the person, the family, and yourself.

KEY TERMS

birth defect A problem that develops during pregnancy, often during the first 3 months; it may involve a body structure or function

developmental disabilities A group of conditions caused by physical, learning, language, or behavior impairments

disability Any lost, absent, or impaired physical or mental function

inherited That which is passed down from parents to children

intellectual disability Involves severe limits in intellectual function and adaptive behavior occurring before age 18

spastic Uncontrolled contractions of skeletal muscles

KEY ABBREVIATIONS

ADA	Americans With Disabilities Act of 1990	**IDD**	Intellectual and developmental disability
CP	Cerebral palsy	**IQ**	Intelligence quotient
DS	Down syndrome	**SB**	Spina bifida
Fragile X	Fragile X syndrome		

A *disability* is any lost, absent, or impaired physical or mental function. Intellectual and developmental disabilities (IDDs) affect physical, intellectual, and emotional development. An IDD can be a physical or mental impairment or both.

- *Developmental disabilities*—*a group of conditions caused by physical, learning, language, or behavior impairments.*
- *Intellectual disability*—*involves severe limits in intellectual function and adaptive behavior occurring before age 18.*

Occurring during the developmental period (Chapter 11), IDDs begin before, during, or after birth or during childhood. They may affect day-to-day function and usually last throughout life. IDDs can be mild to severe. Causes are listed in Box 50-1.

Some IDDs involve birth defects. A *birth defect is a problem that develops during pregnancy, often during the first 3 months. It may involve a body structure or function.* Spina bifida (p. 790) is an example of a structural defect. Down syndrome (p. 788) is a functional (developmental) defect. Birth defects may affect how a body looks, functions, or both.

| **BOX 50-1** | **Intellectual and Developmental Disabilities—Causes and Warning Signs** |

Causes
- Genetics
  - Abnormal genes may be inherited from 1 or both parents. *Inherited means to be passed down from parents to children.* See "Fragile X Syndrome," p. 789.
  - Problems when genes combine during fertilization. See "Down Syndrome," p. 788.
- The mother's health or behaviors during pregnancy:
  - Smoking.
  - Substance abuse or addiction (alcohol, drugs).
  - Infection with rubella (German measles).
  - Untreated or uncontrolled diabetes.
  - Contact with dangerous chemicals or toxins. Lead is an example.
  - Poor nutrition.
- Head injury during or after birth
- Lack of oxygen to the brain
- Problems at birth
  - Low birthweight
  - Premature birth
  - Multiple birth
  - Lack of oxygen to the brain
- Blood disease

Causes—cont'd
- Problems after birth
  - Infections—whooping cough, chicken pox, measles, Hib disease, meningitis, encephalitis
  - Head injuries
  - Near drowning
  - Poisoning—lead, alcohol, ammonia, bleaches, detergent, household products, gasoline, kerosene, lighter fluid, drugs, lye, paint thinners and removers, pesticides, turpentine, weed killers, mercury, and so on
  - Shaken baby syndrome
  - Poor nutrition
  - Dehydration
  - Reye's syndrome (a disease caused by drugs containing aspirin)
  - Poor health care

Warning Signs
- Delays in sitting up, crawling, or walking
- Delays in talking or having difficulty speaking
- Trouble remembering things
- Trouble understanding the rules of social behavior
- Trouble "seeing" or "understanding" the outcomes of actions
- Trouble solving problems

"Causes" modified from The Arc of the United States: Causes and prevention of intellectual disabilities, Silver Springs, Md, revised March 1, 2011. "Warning Signs" modified from National Institute of Child Health and Human Development: What are the signs of IDDs? Bethesda, Md, updated November 30, 2012.

Developmentally disabled children become adults. *Independence to the extent possible* is the goal for these persons. This includes having a job and living in the community. They need life-long help, support, and special services.

- Personal services:
  - Self-care
  - Assistive (adaptive) devices for eating, dressing, bathing, mobility, and other needs
  - Health care including drug therapy or surgery
  - Home and vehicle needs
  - Therapies: physical, occupational, speech and language, respiratory, recreation, and other
  - Hearing and vision aids
- Housing—family, independent living, group homes, or long-term care centers
- Finances and employment
- Education:
  - Understanding and expressing language
  - Job training
- Protection of their rights:
  - The *Americans With Disabilities Act of 1990 (ADA)*
  - The *Developmental Disabilities Assistance and Bill of Rights Act of 2000*

FOCUS ON LONG-TERM CARE AND HOME CARE

Intellectual and Developmental Disabilities

Long-Term Care
Changes from aging (Chapter 12) may occur earlier when IDDs are severe. Some adults with IDDs need nursing center care. They are further protected by the *Omnibus Budget Reconciliation Act of 1987 (OBRA)*. OBRA requires that centers provide age-appropriate activities. Staff must have special training to meet care needs.

Some severely disabled children live in centers for the developmentally disabled.

An IDD affects the family throughout life. The infant or child may become a teenager, young adult, middle-age adult, and older. Both the child and parents grow older. Often it is hard to provide care, handle, move, or financially support the disabled person. A parent may become ill, injured, or disabled or may die. Still the disabled person needs care.

See *Focus on Long-Term Care and Home Care: Intellectual and Developmental Disabilities.*

INTELLECTUAL DISABILITIES

Intellectual function relates to *learning, thinking, reasoning, and solving problems. Adapt* means *to change or adjust.* The person has low intellectual function. Adaptive behavior is impaired (Box 50-2). Adaptive behaviors are skills needed to function in everyday life—to live, work, and play.

The Arc of the United States is a national organization focusing on people with intellectual and related disabilities. The Arc describes an intellectual disability as:

- An IQ score between 70 and 75 or below. *(IQ means intelligence quotient.)* The person learns at a slower rate than normal. Learning ability is less than normal.
- A significant limit in at least 1 adaptive behavior.
- Onset before age 18.

Brain development is impaired. According to the Arc, alcohol is the leading preventable cause of intellectual disabilities. See Box 50-1 for other causes.

Intellectual disabilities can be mild to severe. Persons mildly affected are slow to learn in school. As adults, they can function in society with some support. For example, they need help finding a job. Support is not needed every day. Others need much support every day at home and at work. Still others need constant support in all areas.

See *Focus on Communication: Intellectual Disabilities.*

BOX 50-2	Adaptive Behaviors

- Communication
- Reading
- Writing
- Money concepts and managing money
- Social skills—interpersonal skills, responsibility, not being tricked by others, following rules, obeying laws
- Activities of daily living—eating, dressing, mobility, elimination, preparing meals, taking drugs, using the phone, using transportation, housekeeping, job skills, and maintaining a safe setting

---

FOCUS ON COMMUNICATION

Intellectual Disabilities

Mental retardation was a common term for intellectual disabilities. However, the term is offensive and out-dated. *Intellectual disabilities* is the preferred term.

In June 2003, the President's Committee on Mental Retardation was changed to the "President's Committee for People with Intellectual Disabilities." The name was changed to:

- Update and improve the image of people with intellectual disabilities.
- Help reduce discrimination against such persons.
- Reduce confusion between "mental illness" and "mental retardation."

Do not use "mental retardation" and "mentally retarded." Use "intellectual disabilities" and "intellectually disabled."

Sexuality

Persons with IDDs may have physical, emotional, and social needs and desires. Reproductive organs develop. Some have life partners. Others marry and have children. Some persons can control sexual urges. Others cannot. The type and site of sexual responses may be inappropriate.

The Arc's beliefs about sexuality include the right to:

- Develop friendships and emotional and sexual relationships. This involves the right to:
  - Love and be loved.
  - End a relationship if he or she chooses.
- Dignity and respect.
- Privacy and confidentiality.
- Freely choose associations.
- Sexual expression.
- Learn about sex, marriage and family, abstinence, safe sex, sexual orientation, sexual abuse, and emotional abuse.
- Be protected from sexual harassment and abuses—physical, sexual, emotional.
- Decide about having and raising children.
- Make birth control decisions.
- Have control over one's own body.
- Protection from sterilization because of the disability. *Sterilization* means to remove or block sex organs so the person cannot have children.

DOWN SYNDROME

Down syndrome (DS) is named for the doctor who identified the syndrome. DS is a genetic cause of mild to moderate intellectual disabilities. At fertilization, a male sex cell (sperm) unites with a female sex cell (ovum). Each cell has 23 chromosomes. The fertilized cell has 46 chromosomes. In DS, an extra chromosome is present. The fertilized cell has 47 chromosomes.

The DS child has certain features caused by the extra chromosome (Fig. 50-1).

- Small head, ears, and mouth
- Eyes that slant upward
- Flat face and wide, flat nose
- Short, wide neck
- Large tongue
- Short stature
- Short, wide hands with short fingers
- Poor muscle tone

Many children with DS have heart defects and thyroid gland problems. They tend to have hearing and vision problems and to be over-weight. They are at risk for ear and respiratory infections. Dementia may appear in adults with DS.

Persons with DS need the support and services listed on p. 787. Most learn self-care skills. They also need health and sex education. Weight gain and constipation are problems. They need a healthy diet and regular exercise.

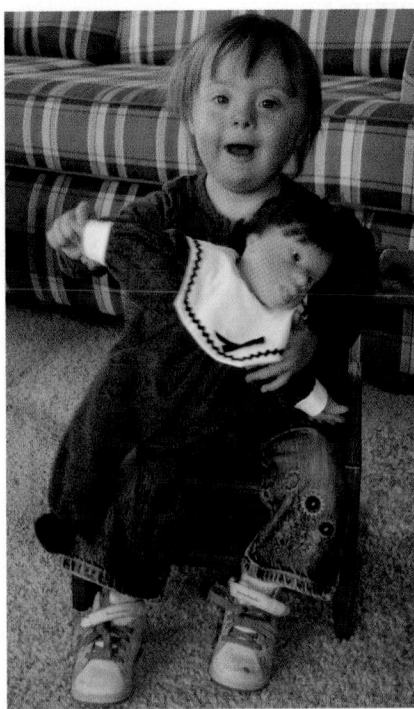

FIGURE 50-1 A child with Down syndrome. (From Hockenberry MJ, Wilson D: *Wong's nursing care of infants and children*, ed 10, St Louis, 2015, Mosby.)

FRAGILE X SYNDROME

Fragile X syndrome (Fragile X) is the most common form of inherited IDD. There is a change in the gene that makes a protein needed for brain development. The body makes little or none of the protein.

Girls have milder symptoms than boys. Fragile X has no cure. The following signs and symptoms are treated with educational, behavior, physical, and drug therapies.

- *Learning.* Learning disabilities range from mild to severe.
- *Physical.* The person may have a long or large face, ears, and jaws. Joints may be loose and flexible. This allows extending the elbow, thumb, and knee further than normal. Poor muscle tone, flat feet, and large body size are other signs.
- *Social and emotional.* Behavior problems are common.
  - Boys: attention problems, aggression
  - Girls: shyness
- *Speech and language.* Boys have more severe delays than girls.

AUTISM

Autism (*autos* means *self*) appears during the first 3 years. A brain disorder with no cure, autism affects social skills and communication. Signs of delayed development are seen at about 18 months of age (Box 50-3).

BOX 50-3   Signs of Autism

Communication
- Cannot start or maintain a social conversation.
- Uses gestures instead of words.
- Develops language slowly or not at all.
- Does not look at objects that others are looking at.
- Does not refer to self correctly. For example, may say "you want water" instead of "I want water."
- Does not point to objects.
- Repeats words or phrases. TV commercials are an example.

Social Interaction
- Does not make friends.
- Is withdrawn.
- May not respond to smiles or eye contact; may avoid eye contact.
- May treat others as objects.
- Prefers to spend time alone.
- Shows a lack of empathy.

Sensory
- Does not startle at loud noises.
- Has high or low senses of sight, hearing, touch, taste, or smell.
- May find normal noises painful. Holds the hand over the ears.
- May withdraw from physical contact that is over-stimulating or overwhelming.
- Rubs surfaces.
- Mouths or licks objects.
- Seems to have a high or low response to pain.

Play
- Does not imitate the actions of others.
- Prefers to play alone.
- Shows little pretend or imaginary play.

Behaviors
- Has intense tantrums.
- Gets stuck on 1 topic or task.
- Has a short attention span.
- Has narrow interests.
- Is over-active or passive.
- Shows aggression toward self or others.
- Shows a strong need for things to remain the same.
- Repeats body movements.

Modified from MedlinePlus: Autism spectrum disorder, Bethesda, Md, 2012, National Institutes of Health, updated May 14, 2014.

Autism is more common in boys than in girls. The cause is unknown. Genetics and environmental factors may be involved.

The disorder ranges from mild to severe. With therapy, the person can learn to change or control behaviors. The therapies include:

- Behavior modification
- Speech, language, and communication therapies
- Music therapy
- Auditory and sensory therapies
- Physical, occupational, and recreation therapies
- Drug therapy
- Diet therapy

Social and work skills are needed. As adults, some work and live independently. Others need family support and community services. Some live in group homes or residential facilities.

Other disorders are common with autism. They include Fragile X and seizures.

CEREBRAL PALSY

Cerebral palsy (CP) is a group of disorders involving paralysis *(palsy)* and injuries or abnormalities in the brain *(cerebral)*. Movement, learning, hearing, seeing, and thinking can be affected.

CP results from brain damage or poor brain development before, during, or within 2 years after birth. There is no cure. See Box 50-1 for causes.

There are different types of CP. Spastic CP is the most common type. **Spastic** *means uncontrolled contractions of skeletal muscles.* Muscles contract or shorten. They are stiff and cannot relax. One arm or leg, 1 side of the body, both legs, or both arms and legs may be involved. Posture, balance, and movement are affected. When arms are affected, there are problems with eating, writing, dressing, and other activities of daily living.

Other problems can occur with CP.

- Abnormal movements—twisting, jerking, writhing of the hands, feet, arms, or legs while awake. Such movements worsen during stress.
- Tremors.
- Unsteady gait.
- Loss of coordination.
- Floppy muscles and joints that move too much.
- Learning disabilities. However, some persons with CP are very smart.
- Speech, hearing, or vision problems.
- Seizures.
- Pain.
- Eating and swallowing problems.
- Vomiting or constipation.
- Drooling.
- Delayed growth.
- Breathing problems.
- Urinary incontinence.

Physical and intellectual disabilities range from mild to severe. Life-long help, support, and special services are needed (p. 787).

SPINA BIFIDA

Spina bifida (SB) is a defect of the spinal column. *(Spina* means *backbone. Bifid* means *split in 2 parts.)* The defect occurs during the first month of pregnancy. Hydrocephalus often occurs with SB.

Spinal column bones *(vertebrae)* protect the spinal cord. In SB, vertebrae and the membranes protecting the spinal cord do not form and close properly. This leaves a split in the vertebrae and the spinal cord unprotected. If the spinal cord is not protected, nerve damage occurs. Affected body parts do not function properly. Paralysis may occur. Bowel and bladder problems are common. Infection is a threat.

The lower back is a common site for SB. Types of SB include:

- *Spina bifida occulta. Occult* means *hidden.* Vertebrae are closed. A defect occurs in the vertebrae closure. In other words, the defect is hidden. The spinal cord and nerves are not damaged. The person has a dimple or tuft of hair on the back (Fig. 50-2). Often there are no symptoms. Foot weakness and bowel and bladder problems can occur.
- *Meningocele. Meningo* means *membrane. Cele* means *hernia or swelling.* Meninges are the connective tissue that cover and protect the brain and spinal cord. A sac of fluid without the spinal cord comes through an opening in the back (Fig. 50-3, *A* and Fig. 50-4). The sac does not contain nerve tissue. The spinal cord and nerves are usually normal with no damage. Surgery corrects the defect.
- *Myelomeningocele (or meningomyelocele). Myelo* means *spinal cord.* A sac of fluid containing nerves and part of the spinal cord comes through an opening in the back (see Fig. 50-3, *B*). Nerve damage occurs. Loss of function occurs below the level of damage. Leg paralysis and lack of sensation are common. So is the lack of bowel and bladder control. The defect is closed with surgery.

Children with SB are at high risk for bladder, bowel, and mobility problems. Skin breakdown, depression, and social and sexual issues are other risks. Some children have learning problems.

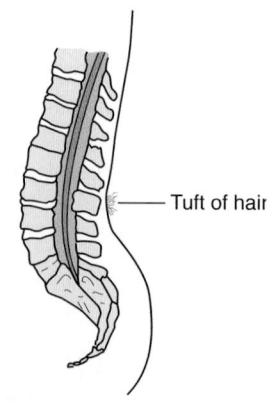

FIGURE 50-2 Spina bifida occulta.

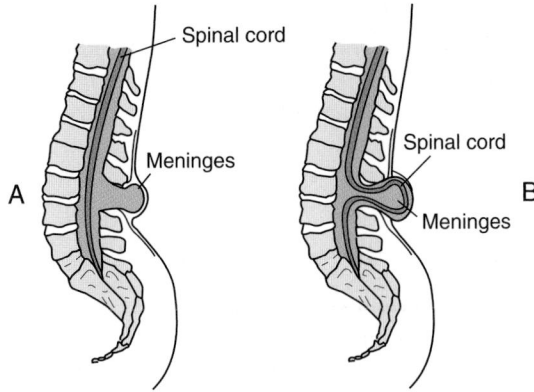

FIGURE 50-3 A, Meningocele. **B,** Meningomyelocele.

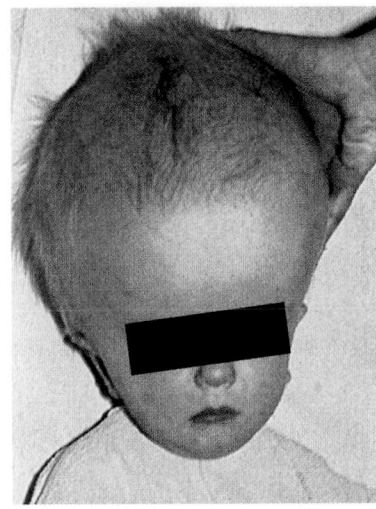

FIGURE 50-5 Hydrocephalus. (From Hart CA, Broadhead RL: *Color atlas of pediatric infectious diseases,* London, 1992, Mosby-Wolfe.)

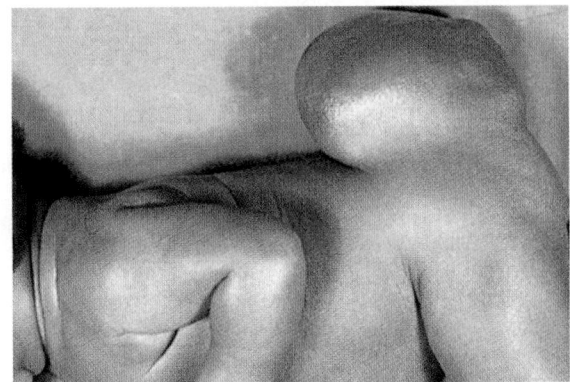

FIGURE 50-4 Meningocele. (From Vitelli BJ, Davis HW: *Atlas of pediatric physical diagnosis,* St Louis, 1987, Gower Medical Publishing.)

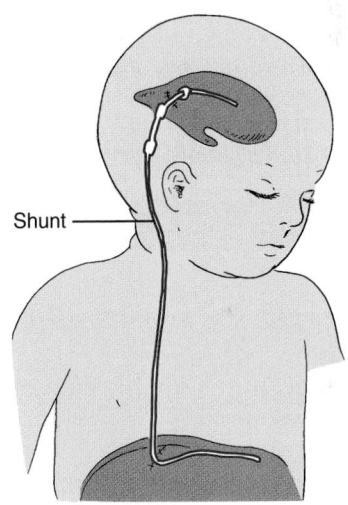

FIGURE 50-6 A shunt drains fluid from the brain. (Modified from Hockenberry MJ, Wilson D: *Wong's nursing care of infants and children,* ed 10, St Louis, 2015, Mosby.)

HYDROCEPHALUS

With hydrocephalus, cerebrospinal fluid collects in and around the brain. *(Hydro* means *water. Cephalo* means *head.)* The head enlarges (Fig. 50-5). Pressure inside the head increases. Intellectual disabilities and neurological damage occur without treatment. Vision problems, seizures, and learning disabilities can occur.

A shunt is placed in the brain. It allows cerebrospinal fluid to drain from the brain. The shunt is a long flexible tube. It goes from the brain into a body cavity to drain (Fig. 50-6). The shunt must remain open *(patent).* If blocked, the cerebrospinal fluid cannot drain from the brain.

Hydrocephalus can be present at birth. Genetic problems and problems with fetal development are causes. Hydrocephalus also can occur at any age after birth. Injury, stroke, infections, tumors, and bleeding in the brain are causes.

FOCUS ON PRIDE

The Person, Family, and Yourself

Personal and Professional Responsibility

Caring for persons with IDDs is a joy and a challenge. The person may struggle with speech, learning, mobility, or self-care. Care needs can be great. Even with these challenges, the person often has a positive outlook on life and brings joy to others.

Your attitude affects your life and work. A positive attitude brings joy, patience, and kindness. It builds teamwork and work ethics (Chapter 6). And it improves the person's quality of life.

Do not allow challenges to affect your attitude. Instead, let your attitude overcome the challenges. Take pride in your decision to have a positive attitude.

Rights and Respect

Persons with IDDs have the right to enjoy and maintain a good quality of life. Such a life involves friendships, health and safety, and the right to make choices and take risks. Your care affects the person's quality of life. Treat the person with dignity and respect. Allow personal choice. Always provide quality care.

Independence and Social Interaction

The Arc of the United States believes that children with IDDs should live in a family. They should learn and play with children without disabilities. As adults, they should control their lives as much as possible. They should speak, make choices, and act for themselves. They should live in a home, have friends, do meaningful work, and enjoy adult activities. Independence to the greatest extent possible is the goal.

Delegation and Teamwork

Some persons respond better to care from certain people. For example, Ms. Hawn has CP. You are patient and kind but she refuses to eat. Ms. Hawn's brother comes to visit. He is able to feed Ms. Hawn.

Do not be offended if the person responds to another person. It does not mean you have done something wrong. And it does not mean the person does not like you. The person may prefer another person at that time.

Do not let your pride get in the way of meeting the person's needs. Another caregiver may need to assist the person. Learn from the person. Ask for advice. He or she may take a different approach or know the person's preferences. Thank him or her for the help.

Ethics and Laws

Persons with IDDs must be protected from abuse, mistreatment, and neglect (Chapters 2 and 5). They may have limited ability to communicate. Or they may fear what will happen if they tell. Changes in mood or behavior, frequent injuries, poor hygiene, weight loss, and anxiety around the caregiver are signs of abuse. See Chapter 5 for others. Tell the nurse right away if you suspect abuse. Take pride in protecting the person's safety and well-being.

FOCUS ON PRIDE: Application

What factors affect quality of life? Are these the same for persons with IDDs? How do family members, caregivers, friends, and others affect the person's quality of life and self-worth?

REVIEW QUESTIONS

Circle the BEST answer.

1 All IDDs
a Are preventable
b Occur from trauma
c Are caused by birth defects
d Begin before, during, or after birth or in childhood

2 These statements are about IDDs. Which is *true?*
a Self-care, learning, and mobility are always affected.
b The disability is permanent.
c Physical and intellectual impairments are mild.
d The person cannot hold a job.

3 The person with an intellectual disability
a Has delayed development of sexual organs
b Does not have the skills to live, work, and play
c Learns at a slower rate than normal
d Needs care in a special setting

4 Intellectual disabilities
a Are always severe
b Begin before 18 years of age
c Are caused by an extra chromosome
d Affect the motor region of the brain

5 Down syndrome occurs
a At fertilization
b During the first month of pregnancy
c Any time before, during, or after birth
d From trauma

6 Down syndrome always involves some degree of
a Cerebral palsy
b Autism
c Impaired mobility
d Intellectual disability

7 Fragile X syndrome is
a The result of brain injury
b Caused by drug and alcohol use
c Inherited from parents
d Caused by an infection

8 Autism begins
a At fertilization
b During pregnancy
c At birth
d In early childhood

9 The person with autism has
a Impaired movement
b Paralysis and brain damage
c Social and communication problems
d Intellectual disabilities

10 Which statement about cerebral palsy is *true?*
a CP is caused by brain damage or abnormal brain development.
b Children with CP have distinct facial features.
c Drugs and therapies can cure CP.
d CP affects girls and boys differently.

11 The spastic type of cerebral palsy involves problems with
a Learning
b Drooling
c Posture, balance, and movement
d Weaving motions of the trunk, arms, and legs

12 Spina bifida involves
a Brain damage
b A defect in the spinal column
c Seizures
d Intellectual disabilities

13 Which is common in spina bifida?
a Bowel and bladder problems
b Short attention span
c Hearing and vision problems
d Seizures

14 Hydrocephalus often occurs with
a Down syndrome
b Cerebral palsy
c Spina bifida
d Autism

15 Hydrocephalus is treated with
a Braces and crutches
b A shunt
c Drugs
d Social services

Answers to Chapter 50 questions are on p. 872.

FOCUS ON **PRACTICE**

Problem Solving

Ms. Andrews has autism. She uses gestures and few words to communicate. Lately when helping her change clothing, she seems fearful and holds on to her clothing. Today she began crying. What will you do? Is this behavior expected? If not, what may be the cause?

OBJECTIVES

- Define the key terms and key abbreviations in this chapter.
- Describe sex, sexuality, and sexual relationships.
- Explain why sexuality is important throughout life.
- Explain how aging, injury, and illness can affect sexuality.
- Explain how the nursing team can promote sexuality.

- Explain why some persons become sexually aggressive.
- Describe how to deal with sexually aggressive persons.
- Explain how to promote PRIDE in the person, the family, and yourself.

KEY TERMS

bisexual A person who is attracted to both sexes

erectile dysfunction (ED) See "impotence"

gender identity A person's sense or feelings of being male, female, or transgender

heterosexual A person who is attracted to members of the other sex

homosexual A person who is attracted to members of the same sex

impotence The inability of the male to have an erection; erectile dysfunction

sex Physical activities involving the body and reproductive organs

sexual orientation The gender (male or female) to which a person is emotionally, romantically, and physically attracted

sexuality The physical, emotional, social, cultural, and spiritual factors that affect a person's feelings and attitudes about his or her sex

transgender Describes people who express their sexuality or gender in ways that do not fit with the sex (male, female) assigned at birth; see "transsexual" and "transvestite"

transsexual Refers to a person whose gender identity is different from the assigned sex at birth; persons who are undergoing hormone therapy or surgery for sexual re-assignment (female to male; male to female)

transvestite A person who dresses and behaves like the other sex for emotional and sexual relief

KEY ABBREVIATIONS

ED	Erectile dysfunction	**OBRA**	Omnibus Budget Reconciliation Act of 1987

Patients and residents are viewed as whole persons with basic needs. Their physical, emotional, social, and spiritual needs are considered. Sexuality involves the whole person. Illness, injury, and aging can affect sexuality.

See *Body Structure and Function Review: The Reproductive System.*

SEX AND SEXUALITY

Sex is the physical activities involving the body and reproductive organs. Sexuality is the physical, emotional, social, cultural, and spiritual factors that affect a person's feelings and attitudes about his or her sex. Sexuality involves the personality and the body—how a person behaves, thinks, dresses, and responds to others.

Sexuality development begins when a baby's sex (gender) is known. People choose names, colors, and toys based on gender. Blue is for boys. Pink is for girls. Dolls are for girls.

BODY STRUCTURE AND FUNCTION REVIEW
The Reproductive System

The Male Reproductive System
The male reproductive system is shown in Figure 51-1. The 2 *testes (testicles)* are the male sex glands. Male sex cells *(sperm)* are produced in the testes. So is *testosterone,* the male hormone. This hormone is needed for reproductive organ function and for the development of male secondary sex characteristics (Chapter 10).

The *prostate gland* lies just below the bladder. The *urethra* runs through the prostate gland. The urethra is contained within the penis.

The *penis* is outside of the body. The penis has *erectile* tissue. When a man is sexually excited, blood fills the erectile tissue. The penis enlarges and becomes hard and erect for sexual activity.

The Female Reproductive System
Figures 51-2 and 51-3 show the female reproductive system. The female sex glands are called *ovaries.* The 2 ovaries contain *ova* or eggs—the female sex cells. The ovaries secrete the female hormones *estrogen* and *progesterone.* These hormones are needed for reproductive system function and the development of female secondary sex characteristics (Chapter 10).

The uterus is a hollow, muscular organ. The uterus serves as a place for the *fetus* (unborn baby) to grow and receive nourishment. The cervix of the uterus projects into a muscular canal called the *vagina.* The vagina opens to the outside of the body. The vagina receives the penis during intercourse. It also is part of the birth canal. Glands in the vaginal wall keep it moistened with secretions.

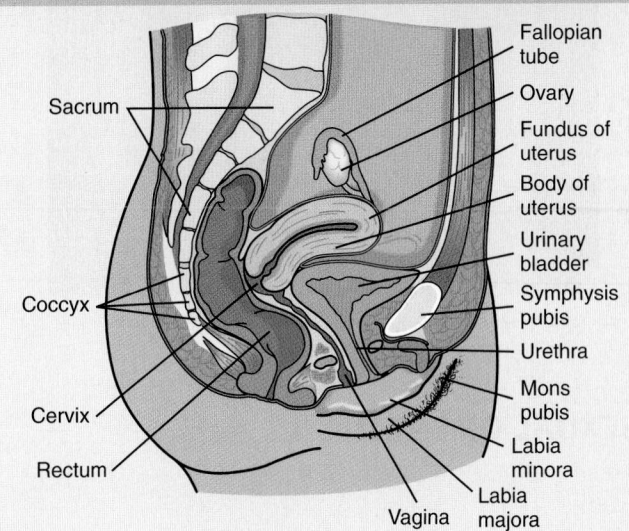

FIGURE 51-2 Female reproductive system.

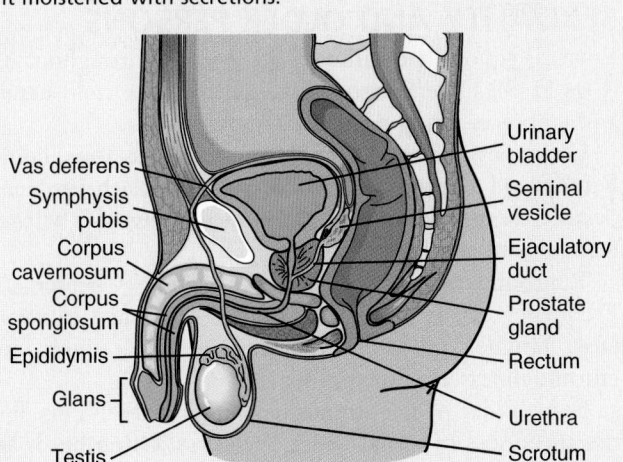

FIGURE 51-1 Male reproductive system.

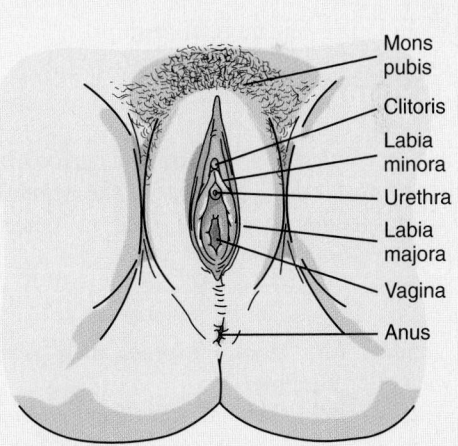

FIGURE 51-3 External female genitalia.

Trains are for boys. By the age of 2, children know their own sex. Three-year-olds know the sex of other children. They learn gender roles from adults (Fig. 51-4, p. 796). Children learn that boys and girls behave in certain ways.

As children grow older, interest increases about the body and how it works. Teens are more aware of sex and the body. Their bodies respond to stimulation. They engage in sexual behaviors. They kiss, embrace, pet, or have intercourse. Pregnancy and sexually transmitted diseases (Chapter 47) are great risks.

Sex has more meaning as young adults mature. Attitudes and feelings are important. Partners are selected. They decide about sex before marriage and birth control.

Sexuality is important throughout life. Attitudes and sex needs change with aging. They are affected by life events. These include divorce, death of a partner, injury, illness, and surgery.

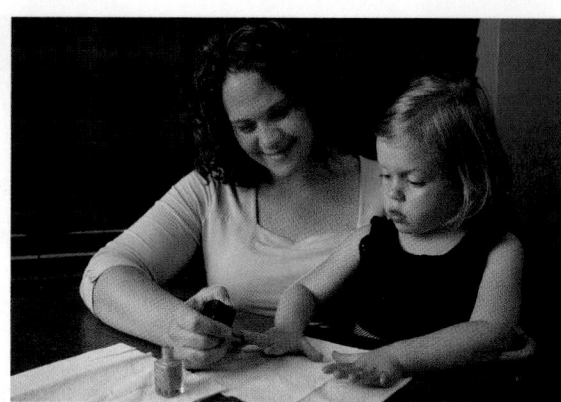

FIGURE 51-4 This little girl is learning female roles from her mother.

SEXUAL ORIENTATION

Sexual orientation refers to the gender (male or female) to which a person is emotionally, romantically, and physically attracted.

- *Heterosexual—a person who is attracted to members of the other sex.* Men are attracted to women. Women are attracted to men. Sexual behavior is male-female.
- *Homosexual—a person who is attracted to members of the same sex.* Men are attracted to men. Women are attracted to women. *Gay* refers to homosexuality. Homosexual men are called *gay men. Lesbian* refers to a female homosexual.
- *Bisexual—a person who is attracted to both sexes.* They have same-gender relationships (male-male or female-female) and male-female relationships.

Gender Identity

Gender identity refers to a person's sense or feelings of being male, female, or transgender. Sometimes a person's biological sex (male or female) does not fit with the person's gender identity. Transgender is a term used to describe such persons. *Transgender describes people who express their sexuality or gender in ways that do not fit with the sex (male, female) assigned at birth.*

Transgenders (or "trans") express their sexuality in various ways. For example:

- *Transsexual refers to a person whose gender identity is different from the assigned sex at birth.* A male believes he is a female in a man's body. A female believes she is a male in a woman's body. The term also describes *persons who are undergoing hormone therapy or surgery for sexual re-assignment (female to male; male to female).*
- *Transvestites are persons who dress and behave like the other sex for emotional and sexual relief.* They are commonly called cross-dressers.

INJURY, ILLNESS, AND SURGERY

Injury, illness, and surgery can affect sexual function. Sometimes the nervous, circulatory, and reproductive systems are involved. Sexual ability may change. Most chronic illnesses affect sexual function. Heart disease, stroke, diabetes, and chronic obstructive pulmonary disease are examples.

Reproductive system surgeries have physical and mental effects. Removal of the uterus, ovaries, or a breast affects women. Prostate or testes removal affects erections.

Impotence (erectile dysfunction; ED) is the inability of the male to have an erection. The many causes include diabetes, spinal cord injuries, prostate problems, alcoholism, cardiovascular disorders, drug abuse, and psychological factors. Some drugs for high blood pressure cause ED. So do other drugs. Some drugs treat ED.

Emotional changes are common. The person may feel unclean, unwhole, unattractive, or mutilated. The person may feel unfit for closeness and love. Therefore some problems are emotional. Time and understanding are helpful. So is a caring partner. Some persons need counseling.

Changes in sexual function greatly affect the person. Fear, anger, worry, and depression are seen in behavior and comments. The person's feelings are normal and expected. The care plan has measures to help the person deal with his or her feelings.

SEXUALITY AND OLDER PERSONS

Love, affection, and intimacy are needed throughout life (Fig. 51-5). Older persons love, fall in love, hold hands, and embrace. Many have intercourse.

Older persons have many losses. Children leave home. Family and friends die. People retire. Health problems occur. Strength decreases. Appearance changes. It helps to feel close to another person.

Reproductive organs change with aging (Chapter 12). Frequency of sex may decrease. Reasons relate to weakness, fatigue, and pain. Reduced mobility, aging, and chronic illness are other factors.

Some older people do not have intercourse. This does not mean loss of sexual needs or desires. Often needs are expressed in other ways. They hold hands, touch, caress, and embrace. These bring closeness and intimacy.

Sexual partners are lost through death, divorce, and relationship break-ups. Or a partner needs hospital or nursing center care. These situations occur in adults of all ages.

MEETING SEXUAL NEEDS

The nursing team promotes the meeting of sexual needs. The measures in Box 51-1 may be part of the person's care plan.

See *Focus on Long-Term Care and Home Care: Meeting Sexual Needs.*

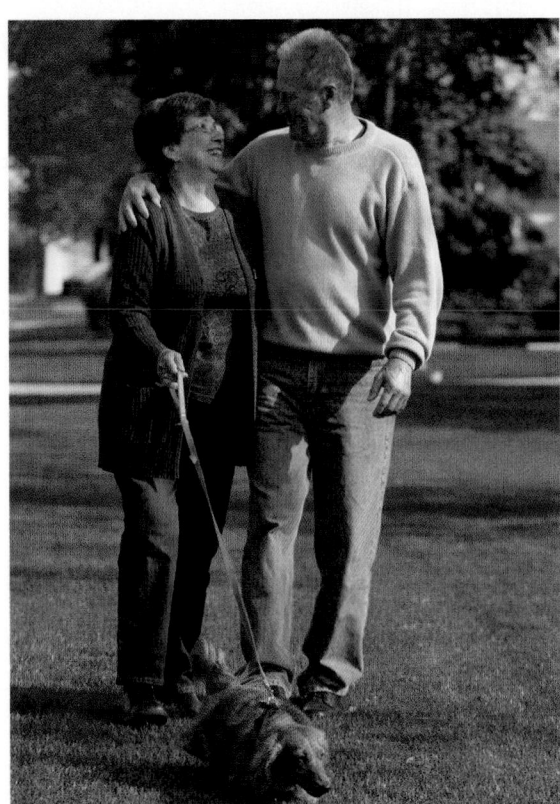

FIGURE 51-5 Love and affection are important to persons of all ages.

FOCUS ON LONG-TERM CARE AND HOME CARE

Meeting Sexual Needs

Long-Term Care
Married couples in nursing centers can share the same room. This is a requirement of the *Omnibus Budget Reconciliation Act of 1987 (OBRA)*. The couple has lived together a long time. Long-term care is no reason to keep them apart (Fig. 51-6). They can share the same bed if their conditions permit. A double, queen-sized, or king-sized bed is provided by the couple or the center.

Sometimes relationships develop between residents. They are allowed time together, not kept apart.

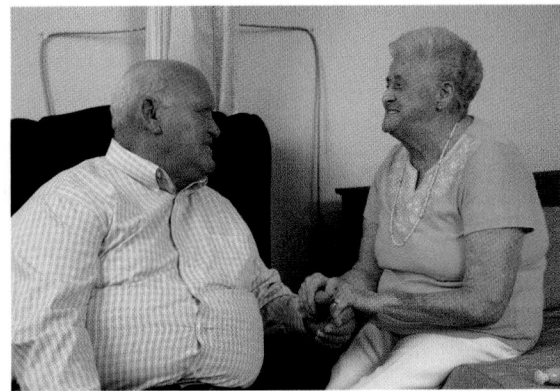

FIGURE 51-6 Relationships continue even when nursing center care is needed.

BOX 51-1	Promoting Sexuality

- Let the person practice grooming routines. Assist as needed. See Chapter 23.
- Let the person choose clothing. Patient gowns can embarrass the person. Street clothes are worn if the person's condition permits.
- Protect the right to privacy. Do not expose the person. Drape and screen the person.
- Treat the person with dignity and respect. The person may not share your sexual attitudes, values, or practices. The person may have a premarital or extramarital relationship. Do not judge or gossip about the person.
- Allow privacy. If the person has a private room, close the door for privacy. Some agencies have DO NOT DISTURB signs for doors. Let the person and partner know how much time they have alone. For example, remind them about meal times and care measures. Tell other staff that the person wants time alone.
- Knock before you enter any room. This simple courtesy shows respect for privacy.
- Consider the person's roommate. Privacy curtains do not block sound. Arrange for privacy when the roommate is out of the room. A roommate may offer to leave for a while. Or the nurse finds a private area.
- Allow privacy for masturbation. It is a normal form of sexual expression. Close the privacy curtain and the door. Knock before you enter the room. This saves you and the person embarrassment. Sometimes confused persons masturbate in public areas. Lead the person to a private area. Or distract him or her with an activity.

THE SEXUALLY AGGRESSIVE PERSON

Some persons want the health team to meet their sexual needs. They flirt or make sexual advances or comments. Some expose themselves, masturbate, or touch other staff. This can anger and embarrass the staff member. These reactions are normal. Often there are reasons for the person's behavior. Understanding this helps you deal with the matter.

Sexually aggressive behaviors have many causes. They include:
- Nervous system disorders
- Confusion, disorientation, and dementia
- Drug side effects
- Fever
- Poor vision

The person may confuse someone with his or her partner. Or the person cannot control the behavior. The healthy person controls sexual urges. Changes in the brain and mental function make control difficult. Sexual behavior in these cases is usually innocent.

Sometimes touch is used to gain attention. For example, Mr. Green cannot speak or move his right side. Your buttocks are near him. To get your attention, he touches your buttocks. His behavior is not sexual.

Some persons engage in masturbation. That is, they touch and fondle their own genitals for sexual pleasure. Sometimes masturbation is a sexually aggressive behavior. However, touching the genitals may signal a health problem. Urinary or reproductive system disorders can cause genital soreness and itching. So can poor hygiene and being wet or soiled from urine or feces.

Touch can have a sexual purpose. For example, a man wants to prove he is attractive and can perform sexually. You must be professional about the matter.

- Ask the person not to touch you. State the places where you were touched.
- Tell the person that you will not do what he or she wants.
- Tell the person what behaviors make you uncomfortable. Politely ask the person not to act that way.
- Allow privacy if the person is becoming aroused. Provide for safety. Complete a safety check of the room (see the inside of the front cover). Tell the person when you will return.
- Discuss the matter with the nurse. The nurse can help you understand the behavior.
- Follow the care plan. It has measures to deal with sexually aggressive behaviors. They are based on the cause of the behavior.

See *Focus on Communication: The Sexually Aggressive Person*.

FOCUS ON COMMUNICATION

The Sexually Aggressive Person

Confronting the sexually aggressive person is hard. This is true for young and older staff and for new and experienced staff. Ask yourself these questions.

- Does the person have a health problem that affects impulse control? If yes, the behavior may not have a sexual purpose.
- Is the person's behavior on purpose? Is the intent sexual? If yes, you must confront the behavior. Be direct and matter-of-fact. For example, you can say:
  - "You brushed your hand across my breast (or other body part) twice this morning. Please don't do that again."
  - "No, I cannot kiss you. It would be unprofessional."
  - "You exposed yourself to me again today. Please do not do that again."

The sexually aggressive person needs the nurse's attention. Report what happened and when. Also report what you said and did. The nurse must deal with the problem. If other staff report such behaviors, the nurse views the problem in a broader way.

Protecting the Person

The person must be protected from unwanted sexual comments and advances. This is sexual abuse (Chapter 5). Tell the nurse right away. No one is allowed to sexually abuse another person. This includes staff members, patients, residents, family members or other visitors, and volunteers.

SEXUALLY TRANSMITTED DISEASES

Some diseases are spread by sexual contact. They are discussed in Chapter 47.

FOCUS ON **PRIDE**

The Person, Family, and Yourself

Personal and Professional Responsibility
Touching a person's body without his or her consent is abuse and a crime (Chapter 5). You must take extra caution when care involves the genitals, buttocks, or breasts. Without consent, you may be accused of sexual abuse.

To obtain consent, explain what you will do before starting procedures and step-by-step. If the person asks you to stop, you must stop. Follow agency policies when caring for persons of the opposite sex. The nurse may need to ask the person's permission or delegate the task to staff of the same gender.

Obtaining consent and explaining procedures are professional responsibilities. The person has control over care, knows what to expect, and is more at ease. The person's rights are protected. And you protect yourself from being accused of sexual abuse.

Rights and Respect
Each member of the health team must maintain an appropriate relationship with the person. Professional sexual misconduct is a serious violation of the person's rights (Chapters 2 and 5). Report any suspected sexually inappropriate behavior. Take pride in protecting the person from mistreatment and abuse.

Independence and Social Interaction
Sexuality includes emotional, social, cultural, spiritual, and physical factors. To promote sexuality:

- Assist the person with hygiene and grooming before visitors arrive.
- Compliment the person's appearance. Comment on a woman's hair, clothing, jewelry, nails, and so on. Compliment men after shaving.
- Talk with the person about his or her family. Years of marriage and number of children are common topics. Respect privacy if the person does not want to talk.
- Use touch to show you care. A touch on the arm, shoulder, or upper back can communicate care without crossing boundaries (Chapter 5).

Delegation and Teamwork
The health team must try to determine the cause of sexually aggressive behaviors. If the cause can be fixed, the behavior may stop. When the cause cannot be fixed, the care plan includes measures to manage the behavior. A professional response is always needed.

Tell the nurse about sexually aggressive behaviors. The problem cannot be ignored. Rely on the nursing team for advice, guidance, and support.

FOCUS ON PRIDE—cont'd

The Person, Family, and Yourself

Ethics and Laws

All persons must be protected from sexual abuse. The following is a real case of a nursing assistant who violated the person's right to freedom from abuse and mistreatment.

A certified nursing assistant (CNA) had his certificate revoked by the Arizona State Board of Nursing. The Board found that he violated the state's Nurse Practice Act because of the following actions.

- He was convicted of "Driving Under the Influence" in 2002.
- He agreed to a $150 penalty on his CNA certificate for several incidents of resident abuse. He also admitted to removing an impaction from a female resident, which he knew was not within the scope of CNA duties.

- While employed at a nursing home in 2005:
  - A female resident reported that he was "rough with her and 'hurt her groin.'" The resident demanded a transfer to another facility.
  - An alert and oriented resident reported that the CNA "'raped' her by placing his hand inside her private parts." The resident also stated that she "could smell alcohol on his breath."
  - His employment was terminated for policy violation and "causing a resident undue stress and fear when he assisted her to expel an impaction."
- While employed in a group home in 2005, it was reported that he violated agency policy regarding alcohol use. (Arizona State Board of Nursing, 2006.)

No one is allowed to sexually abuse another person. Report concerns of abuse to the nurse.

FOCUS ON PRIDE: Application

Self-image affects sexuality. Identify ways you can promote the person's self-image.

REVIEW QUESTIONS

Circle the BEST answer.

1 Sex involves
   a The organs of reproduction
   b Attitudes and feelings
   c Cultural and spiritual factors
   d Masturbation

2 Sexuality is important to
   a Small children
   b Teenagers and young adults
   c Middle-age adults
   d Persons of all ages

3 Impotence is
   a A sexually aggressive behavior
   b A reaction to illness
   c Not being able to achieve an erection
   d No sexual activity

4 Reproductive organs change with aging.
   a True   b False

5 Mrs. Green lives in a nursing center. To promote her sexuality
   a Stay in the room while she talks to Mr. Green
   b Help her to dress in a patient gown
   c Help her style her hair
   d Convince her that shaving her legs is not needed

6 Two residents are holding hands. Nursing staff should keep them apart.
   a True   b False

7 Mr. and Mrs. Green want some time alone. Which measure would you question?
   a Close the room door.
   b Put a DO NOT DISTURB sign on the door.
   c Tell other staff that they want some time alone.
   d Close the privacy curtain so no one can hear them.

8 Mr. and Mrs. Green should each have a room. This is an OBRA requirement.
   a True   b False

9 A person is masturbating in the dining room. You should
   a Do nothing
   b Scold the person
   c Quietly take the person to his or her room
   d Restrain the person

10 A person touches you sexually and asks for a kiss. You should
   a Ignore the behavior
   b Do what the person asks
   c Tell your co-workers
   d Ask the person not to touch you

Answers to Chapter 51 questions are on p. 872.

FOCUS ON PRACTICE

Problem Solving

You are a student in the clinical setting. You need to practice the bathing skill. A nursing assistant and an older resident are preparing for a bath. You introduce yourself and ask if you can assist. The resident says: "Cindy always gives me my bath." The nursing assistant says: "You don't have any modesty left at your age. The student can give your bath today." The resident is quiet. What will you do?

OBJECTIVES

- Define the key terms and key abbreviations in this chapter.
- Describe how to meet the safety and security needs of infants and children.
- Identify the signs and symptoms of illness in infants.
- Explain how to help mothers with breast-feeding.
- Describe 3 forms of baby formulas.
- Explain how to bottle-feed babies.
- Explain how to burp a baby.
- Describe how to give cord care.

- Describe the purposes of circumcision, needed observations, and the required care.
- Explain how to bathe infants.
- Explain why infants are weighed.
- Describe the care needed by mothers after childbirth.
- Perform the procedures described in this chapter.
- Explain how to promote PRIDE in the person, the family, and yourself.

KEY TERMS

breast-feeding Feeding a baby milk from the mother's breasts; nursing
circumcision The surgical removal of foreskin from the penis
episiotomy Incision *(otomy)* into the perineum
lochia The vaginal discharge that occurs after childbirth
meconium A dark green to black, tarry bowel movement
nursing See "breast-feeding"

postpartum After *(post)* childbirth *(partum)*
prenatal care The health care a woman receives while pregnant
umbilical cord The structure that connects the mother and fetus (unborn baby); it carries blood, oxygen, and nutrients from the mother to the fetus

KEY ABBREVIATIONS

BM	Bowel movement		F	Fahrenheit
C	Centigrade		SIDS	Sudden infant death syndrome
C-section	Cesarean section		SUID	Sudden unexpected infant death

Mothers and newborns usually have short hospital stays. Some need home care after discharge. The mother or baby may need home care because of:
- Complications before or after childbirth
- Health problems
- Needing help with other young children
- A multiple birth (twins, triplets, and so on)
- Needing help with meals and housekeeping

Babies depend on others for basic needs—physical, safety and security, and love and belonging. A review of growth and development will help you care for babies (Chapter 11).

SAFETY AND SECURITY

Babies cannot protect themselves. They need to feel safe and secure. They feel secure when warm and when wrapped and held snugly. Babies cry to communicate. They cry when wet, hungry, hot or cold, tired, uncomfortable, or in pain. To promote safety and security, respond to their cries—feed them, change diapers as needed, comfort them, talk to them, and so on.

Follow the infant safety measures in Box 52-1. Follow the measures in Chapters 13 and 14 to protect children from burns, poisoning, choking and suffocation, and falls. Also see Appendix D, p. 877.

See *Focus on Long-Term Care and Home Care: Safety and Security*, p. 802.

BOX 52-1	Infant Safety

General Safety

- Keep the baby warm. Check windows for drafts. Close windows securely.
- Keep your fingernails short. Do not wear fake nails. Long nails can scratch the baby.
- Do not wear rings or bracelets. Jewelry can scratch the baby.
- Respond to the baby's crying. They communicate by crying. Responding to their cries helps them feel safe and secure.
- Keep 1 hand on a child lying in a crib or on a scale, bed, table, or other surface or furniture (Fig. 52-1).
- Keep pins and small objects out of the baby's reach.
- Do not shake powder directly over the baby. The powder can get into the baby's eyes and lungs. Shake some on your hand away from the baby.
- Do not tie a pacifier around the baby's neck.

Holding a Baby

- Use both hands to lift a newborn. Use 1 hand to support the head and upper back. Use your other hand to support the legs. Do not lift a newborn by the arms.
- Hold the baby securely. Use the cradle hold, football hold, or shoulder hold (Fig. 52-2).
- Support the baby's head and neck when lifting or holding the baby. Neck support is necessary for the first 3 months after birth.
- Handle the baby with gentle, smooth movements. Avoid sudden or jerking movements. Do not startle the baby.
- Hold and cuddle infants. It is comforting and helps them learn to feel love and security.

Crib and Furniture Safety

- Make sure the crib is within hearing distance of the caregivers.
- Do not put a pillow, quilts, bumper pads, or soft toys in the crib. They can cause suffocation.
- Place infants on a firm surface to sleep. Do not lay an infant on soft bedding products. This includes fluffy, plush products such as sheepskin, quilts, comforters, pillows, and toys. Soft products can cause suffocation.
- Report crib or furniture problems at once. Loose nuts, bolts, screws or bent, broken, or open mattress hooks are examples.
- See Appendix D, p. 877 for nursery equipment safety.

Sleep

- Remove bibs and necklaces before sleep.
- Lay babies on their backs for sleep. *Do not lay babies on their stomachs for sleep. This can interfere with chest expansion and breathing. The baby can suffocate.* Infants can lie on their sides and stomachs when awake and supervised.
- Make sure there is no soft bedding under the baby.
- Maintain a comfortable temperature. Babies must not get too hot during sleep. Avoid clothing that may cover the infant's head or cause over-heating.

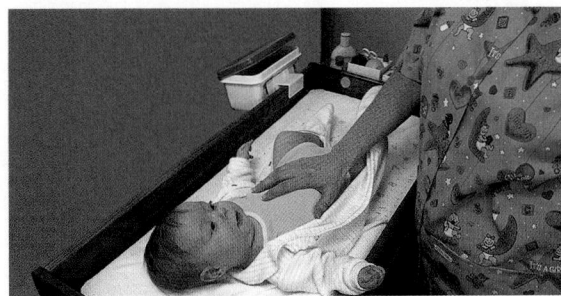

FIGURE 52-1 Keep 1 hand on a child lying on a raised surface.

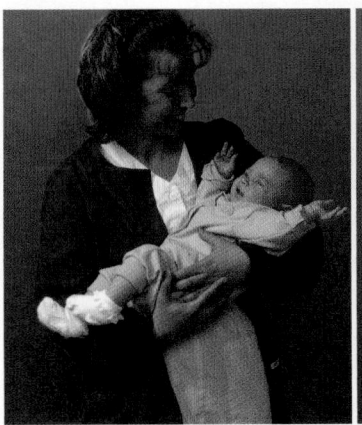 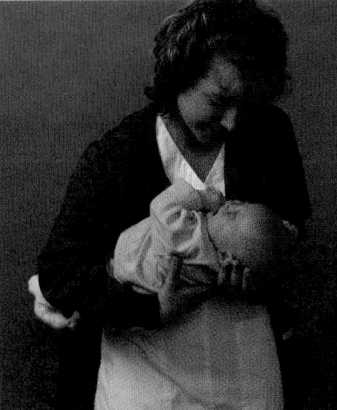 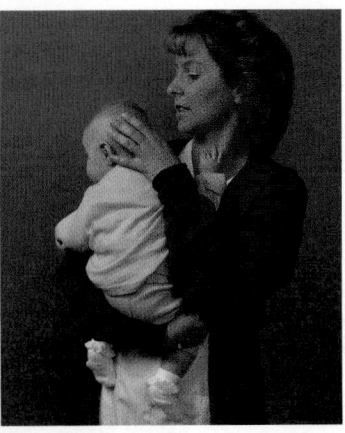

A   B   C

FIGURE 52-2 Holding a baby. A, The cradle hold. **B,** The football hold. **C,** The shoulder hold.

FOCUS ON LONG-TERM CARE AND HOME CARE

Safety and Security

Home Care

Injuries in the home are preventable. Safety measures can protect infants and children from harm.

- Supervise infants and children at all times.
- Use childproof locks or door knob covers leading to non-childproof areas (Fig. 52-3).
- Use safety gates at the top and bottom of stairs.
- Do not let children climb on furniture. Also prevent furniture from tipping.
- Remove or pad furniture with sharp or rough edges.
- Check that the crib meets federal safety standards.
- Store harmful items where children cannot reach them. Keep items in locked storage areas.
- Keep child-resistant caps on drugs and other harmful substances.
- Keep cords and strings out of reach and away from cribs and playpens.
- Use outlet safety covers or outlet plugs on electrical outlets (Chapter 13). A choking hazard, use outlet plugs with caution. The plug must not be easily removed by children.
- Keep the hot water heater temperature below 120°F (Fahrenheit) (48°C [centigrade]) to prevent burns.
- Supervise children in or near water. Prevent children from entering areas that contain water.
- Use federally approved car safety seats that fit the child's size and weight (Fig. 52-4). Follow the manufacturer's instructions for weight and height limits.
- Use car safety seats correctly. Seats are kept rear-facing as long as possible—usually until age 2 (Fig. 52-5).
- Check that the child's clothing is safe and fits well. Drawstrings, ribbons, and cords are hazards (Fig. 52-6). Loose clothing, long clothing, and items around the neck are dangerous.
- Check that all toys are age-appropriate and are not damaged.
- Keep small items away from children. Make sure the child cannot fit items in the mouth.
- Follow the safety measures in Appendix D (p. 877).

Nursery equipment must be safe and in good repair. Use the guidelines in Appendix D (p. 877) to check nursery equipment.

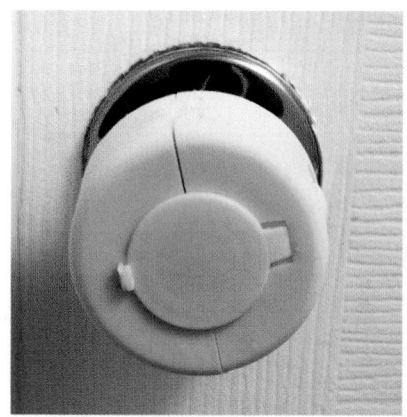

FIGURE 52-3 Door knob cover.

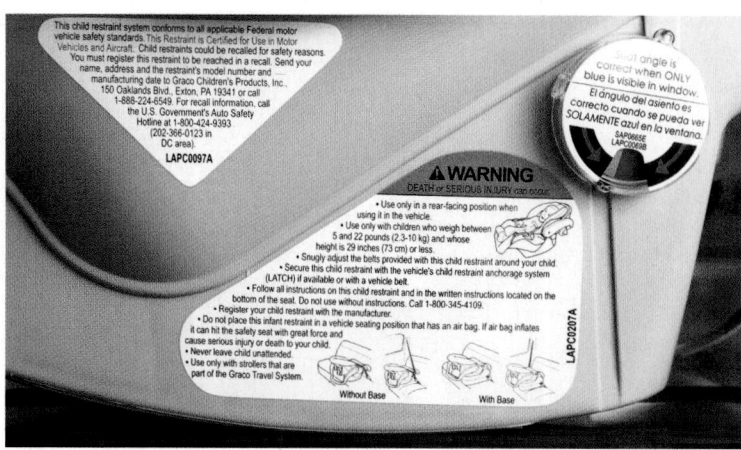

FIGURE 52-4 Federally approved car safety seats carry this label.

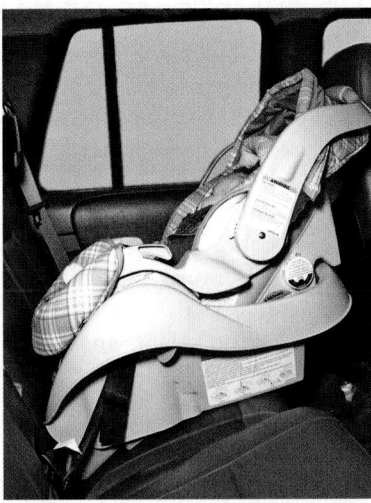

FIGURE 52-5 Car safety seat that is rear-facing.

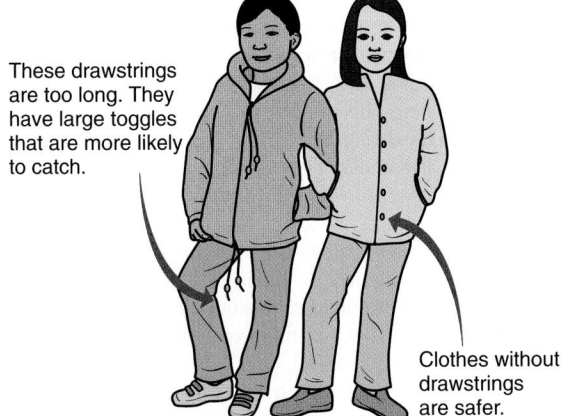

These drawstrings are too long. They have large toggles that are more likely to catch.

Clothes without drawstrings are safer.

Crib Safety

Cribs and crib linens present safety hazards. They can strangle and suffocate the baby. Mattresses, linens, and bumper pads pose many dangers.

- Bumper pads are not used.
- The mattress is covered with a crib sheet. The crib sheet fits snugly.
- Only fitted crib sheets that fit snugly are used. Sheets for larger beds are not used.
- Sheets are not used if they are frayed, worn, or have loose threads or stitching.
- Pillows, blankets, comforters, quilts, sheepskin, sleep positioners, and pillow-like stuffed toys and other soft products are not placed in the crib.
- Plastic trash bags, dry-cleaning bags, or plastic packaging materials are not used to protect the mattress. The plastic can cling to the baby's face, nose, and mouth. This prevents breathing and causes suffocation.

Report any hazard to the nurse.

See *Focus on Long-Term Care and Home Care: Crib Safety.*

FIGURE 52-6 Drawstrings, ribbons, and cords can get caught in many things and strangle the child.

FOCUS ON **LONG-TERM CARE AND HOME CARE**

Crib Safety

Home Care

The *Consumer Product Safety Improvement Act of 2008 (CPSIA)* created safety standards for new and used full-sized cribs effective June 28, 2011. The law applies to cribs in homes, childcare facilities, family childcare homes, and other businesses providing cribs. The law also applies to the re-sale of used and antique cribs at garage, yard, rummage, and similar sales; on-line auction sites; and donations to thrift stores. Because they are medical devices, the law does not apply to hospital cribs.

According to the American Academy of Pediatrics, new children's furniture should bear the Juvenile Products Manufacturers Association (JPMA) safety certification seal (Fig. 52-7, p. 804). This seal means that the product meets required safety testing standards.

The CPSIA full-sized crib standard:

- Bans the manufacture and sale of drop-side rail cribs. Drop-side cribs have been linked to infant suffocation and strangulation deaths.
- The mattress thickness must not be greater than 6 inches.

- The crib mattress must be firm. It must not sag from the infant's weight. A soft mattress can cover the baby's nose and mouth. This prevents breathing.
- The mattress must fit tight into the crib. There must be no gaps or space between the mattress and the crib. The baby can get trapped in such gaps or spaces between the mattress and the crib.
- Crib slats (bars) are no more than $2\frac{3}{8}$ inches apart—the width of a soda can. The baby's head can get caught between larger spaces, causing suffocation and death.
- The bottom of the 6-inch mattress is at least 26 inches lower than the top of the crib sides. This prevents the baby from falling out of the crib. The mattress is lowered to the lowest level when the baby starts to stand in the crib.
- The head-boards and foot-boards must not have cut-outs. The baby's head can get trapped in cut-outs.
- Corner posts (spindles) must be no higher than $\frac{1}{16}$ of an inch above the end-panels. This prevents the baby's clothing from getting caught on the corner posts.

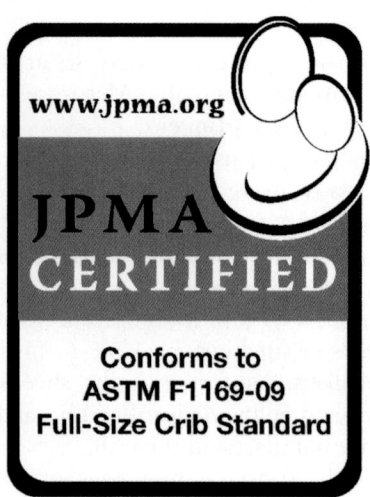

FIGURE 52-7 Juvenile Products Manufacturers Association safety certification seal. NOTE: ASTM stands for American Society for Testing and Materials. (From JPMA [Juvenile Products Manufacturers Association], Mt. Laurel, New Jersey.)

Sudden Unexpected Infant Death

Sudden unexpected infant death (SUID) is any sudden and unexpected death in an infant younger than 1 year old. The death may be explained or unexplained. The most common causes of SUID are:

* Sudden infant death syndrome (SIDS)—the sudden, unexplained death of an infant younger than 1 year old. SIDS is the leading cause of death in children between 1 month and 1 year of age. Most SIDS deaths occur between 1 and 4 months of age. It usually occurs during sleep.
* Accidental suffocation or strangulation in bed.
* Unknown causes.

Crib and sleep safety help prevent sudden infant death. See Box 52-1. *Lay babies on their backs for sleep.* These measures also reduce the risk.

* Place babies to sleep in the same room as the parents but not the same bed. Parents who share a bed with a baby can roll onto the child during sleep. Or the baby can suffocate in blankets or sheets.
* Breast-feed.
* Offer a pacifier for sleep. For breast-fed babies, wait until the baby feeds well before giving a pacifier.
* Keep babies away from smoke. This includes people who smoke and places where smoking occurs.
* Avoid home products such as wedges, positioning devices, special mattresses, and heart and lung monitors that claim to reduce SIDS risk.

Regular wellness visits are important for infant and child health. Vaccines may protect against sudden infant death.

The mother's health during pregnancy affects the baby's risk. Women should receive regular prenatal care. *Prenatal care is the health care a woman receives while pregnant.* Mothers must avoid smoking, alcohol, and illegal drug use during pregnancy.

SIGNS AND SYMPTOMS OF ILLNESS

Babies can become ill quickly. Signs and symptoms may be sudden. You must be very alert. Report any of the signs and symptoms in Box 52-2 at once. Be alert to any change in the baby's behavior—sleep pattern, cry, appetite, or activity.

Tell the nurse when a sign or symptom began. You may need to measure the baby's temperature, pulse, and respirations (Chapter 29). The nurse tells you what temperature site to use—tympanic, rectal, temporal artery, or axillary. Apical pulses are taken on infants and young children.

BOX 52-2	Illness in Babies—Signs and Symptoms

* The baby has *jaundice*—a yellowish color to the skin and whites of the eyes.
* The baby looks sick.
* The baby has redness or drainage around the cord stump (p. 813) or circumcision (p. 813).
* The baby has a fever (Chapter 29).
* The baby is limp and slow to respond.
* The baby is hard to wake up.
* The baby is less active than usual.
* The baby cries all the time or does not stop crying.
* The baby is flushed, pale, or perspiring.
* The baby has noisy, rapid, difficult, or slow respirations.
* The baby is coughing or sneezing.
* The baby has reddened or irritated eyes.
* The baby turns his or her head to 1 side or puts a hand to 1 ear (signs of an earache).
* The baby screams for a long time.
* The baby is feeding poorly or has skipped feedings.
* The baby has vomited most of the feeding or vomits between feedings.
* The baby has watery stools or hard, formed stools.
* Stools are light-colored, green, or foul-smelling.
* The baby has fewer wet diapers.
* The baby has a rash.

HELPING MOTHERS BREAST-FEED

Breast-feeding (nursing) is feeding a baby milk from the mother's breasts.

- The baby can feed at the mother's breast.
- The mother can pump milk from her breasts. The baby is fed breast-milk from a bottle.

Babies usually breast-feed every 2 to 3 hours during the first month (8 to 12 times a day). They are fed on demand. That is, they are fed when hungry, not on a schedule. Breast-milk is digested faster than formula. Therefore nursing is needed more often.

Babies nurse for a short time the first few days (5 to 10 minutes at each breast). Eventually nursing time takes 10 to 20 minutes at each breast. The rate varies for each baby.

A feeding ends when:
- The baby's sucking slows.
- The baby pulls off the breast.
- The baby is no longer interested in feeding.

Nurses help new mothers learn to breast-feed and about breast care. Tell the nurse if the mother or baby is having problems nursing.

Mothers may need help getting ready to nurse. They may need help with hand-washing and positioning. Provide for privacy and make sure the call light is within reach before leaving the room. Follow the care plan and the measures in Box 52-3.

See *Focus on Long-Term Care and Home Care: Helping Mothers Breast-Feed*, p. 806.

BOX 52-3	Assisting With Breast-Feeding

- Practice hand hygiene and Standard Precautions. Remember, the human immunodeficiency virus (HIV) can be transmitted through breast-milk (Chapter 43).
- Place milk, juice, or water near the mother. Most mothers become thirsty while breast-feeding.
- Help the mother wash her hands. She needs clean hands before handling her breasts.
- Help the mother to a comfortable position. The cradle position, side-lying position, and football hold are the basic positions for breast-feeding (Fig. 52-8, p. 806).
- Change the baby's diaper if necessary. Bring the baby to the mother.
- Make sure the mother holds the baby close to her breast.
- Have the mother use her nipple to stroke the baby's cheek or lower lip. This stimulates the *rooting reflex*. The baby turns his or her head toward the breast and starts to suck.
- Make sure the baby's nose is not blocked by the mother's breast. One nostril must be clear for breathing. If the nose seems blocked, have the mother do 1 of the following.
  - Re-position the baby. She can raise the baby's hips. Or she can move the baby's head back slightly.
  - Use her thumb to keep breast tissue away from the baby's nose with her thumb (Fig. 52-9, p. 806).
- Give her a baby blanket to cover the baby and her breast. This promotes privacy.
- Encourage nursing from both breasts at each feeding. If the last feeding ended at the right breast, the next feeding is started at the right breast. The mother can use a ribbon or diaper pin on her bra strap to remind her which breast to start with.

- Remind her how to remove the baby from the breast. To break the suction between the baby and the breast, she can insert a finger into a corner of the baby's mouth (Fig. 52-10, p. 806).
- Help the mother burp the baby (p. 809). The baby is burped after nursing at 1 breast. Then the baby is burped after nursing at the other breast.
- Remind the mother to air-dry her nipples after a feeding.
- Change the baby's diaper after the feeding.
- Lay the baby in the crib if he or she has fallen asleep. *Lay the baby on his or her back. Do not lay the baby on the stomach.*
- Help the mother prevent dry and cracked nipples. Follow the nurse's directions and the care plan.
  - Milk is left on the nipple after a feeding. The milk is allowed to air-dry.
  - The mother applies prescribed ointment or cream after each feeding if the nipples are cracked. If directed, remind her to wash her breasts with water before a feeding to remove the ointment or cream.
  - Soap is not used to clean the breasts and nipples.
  - Breasts and nipples are washed and dried gently.
- Help the mother straighten clothing after the feeding if necessary.
- Remind the mother to wash her breasts with a clean washcloth and warm water. Soap is not used. It can cause the nipples to dry and crack. Nipples are air-dried after washing to prevent cracking and soreness.
- Encourage the mother to wear a nursing bra day and night. The bra supports the breasts and promotes comfort.
- Encourage the mother to place nursing pads in the bra. The pads absorb leaking milk.

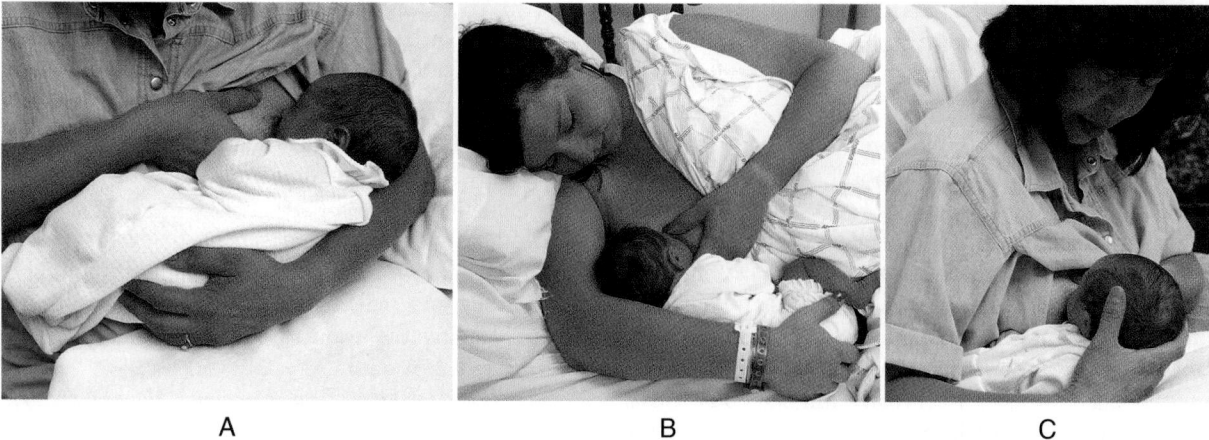

A   B   C

FIGURE 52-8 Basic breast-feeding positions. **A,** Cradle position. **B,** Side-lying position. **C,** Football hold. (From James SR and Ashwill JW: *Nursing Care of Children: Principles and Practice*, ed 3, St Louis, 2007, Saunders.)

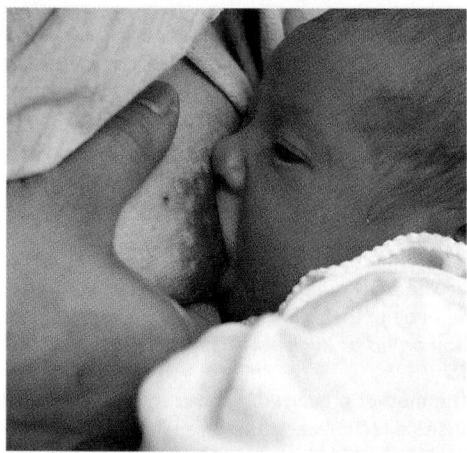

FIGURE 52-9 The mother supports her breast with 1 hand. The thumb is on top of the breast to keep breast tissue away from the baby's nose. (From James SR and Ashwill JW: *Nursing Care of Children: Principles and Practice*, ed 3, St Louis, 2007, Saunders.)

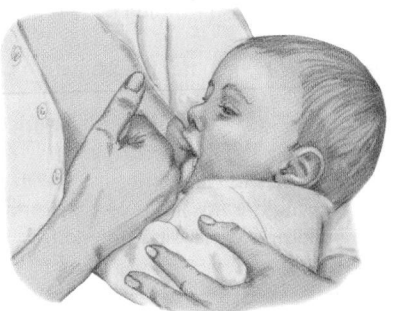

FIGURE 52-10 The mother inserts a finger into the corner of the baby's mouth to remove the baby from the breast. (From James SR, Ashwill JW, Droske SC: *Nursing Care of Children: Principles and Practice*, ed 2, Philadelphia, 2002, Saunders.)

FOCUS ON LONG-TERM CARE AND HOME CARE

Helping Mothers Breast-Feed

Home Care

When the mother is nursing, stay within hearing distance. She may need help.

The nursing mother needs good nutrition. When planning meals or grocery shopping, remember that:

- Calorie intake may increase. The nurse tells you what the mother's calorie intake needs to be.
- She should have 3 servings a day from the dairy group. The nurse tells you if more servings are needed.
- She needs foods high in calcium.
- She can eat the foods she likes. A certain food may cause the baby to be fussy or gassy or have cramping or diarrhea. She should avoid that food for a while. Onions, garlic, spices, cabbage, Brussels sprouts, asparagus, and beans are examples.
- Caffeine is used in moderation. Chocolate, coffee, tea, soda, and energy drinks contain caffeine. Caffeine can cause the baby to be fussy or gassy, become agitated, or have sleep problems.
- She should not drink alcohol.

BOTTLE-FEEDING BABIES

Babies who are not breast-fed use formula. The doctor prescribes the formula. It provides the nutrients the infant needs.

Formula comes in 3 forms.

- *Ready-to-feed.* Ready to use, it is poured from the can into a baby bottle (Fig. 52-11). The can may have more than 1 feeding. Refrigerate the can after opening it. Use the contents within 24 hours.
- *Powdered.* Container directions tell how much powder and water to use.
- *Liquid concentrate.* Container directions tell you how much liquid and water to use.

Bottles are prepared 1 at a time or in batches for the whole day. To prepare a bottle:

- Boil water as directed by the nurse.
- Follow the container directions carefully. Measure exact amounts.
- Pour the correct amount of water and formula into the bottle.
- Gently shake or swirl the bottle to mix.
- Place the bottle under cold water to cool the formula. Or place the bottle in cold or ice water. Keep the level of the cooling water below the bottle's lid to avoid contaminating the formula.
- Dry the outside of the bottle.
- Check the temperature by placing drops on the inside of your wrist. The formula should feel warm, not hot.
- Cap extra bottles (Fig. 52-12). Store them in the refrigerator. Use stored bottles within 24 hours.

Cleaning Baby Bottles

Protect the baby from infection. Baby bottles, caps, nipples, and other items must be as clean as possible. Disposable equipment is used in hospitals. Reusable equipment is common in homes. It is carefully washed in hot, soapy water or in a dishwasher. Complete rinsing is needed to remove all soap. Some bottles have plastic liners that are discarded after 1 use.

See *Focus on Long-Term Care and Home Care: Cleaning Baby Bottles.*

See *Promoting Safety and Comfort: Cleaning Baby Bottles.*

See procedure: *Cleaning Baby Bottles,* p. 808.

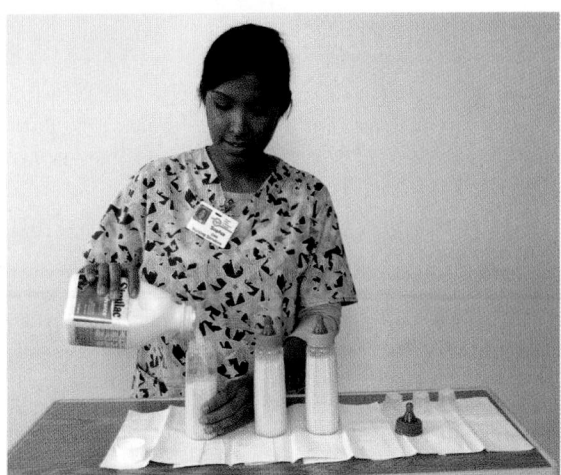

FIGURE 52-11 Ready-to-feed formula is poured from the container into the bottle.

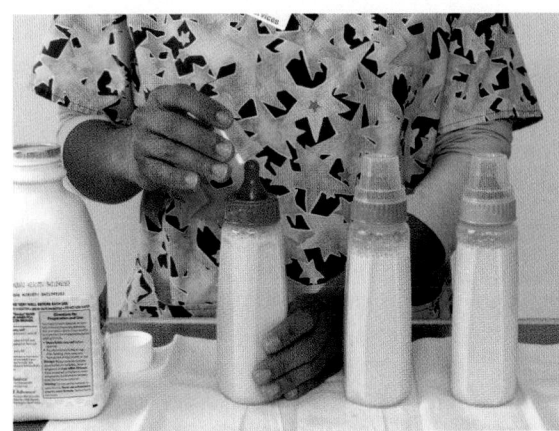

FIGURE 52-12 Bottles are capped for storage in the refrigerator.

FOCUS ON **LONG-TERM CARE AND HOME CARE**

Cleaning Baby Bottles

Home Care

Some homes have well water. The nurse may have you do 1 of the following.

- Place baby bottles, caps, and nipples in boiling water for 5 to 10 minutes.
- Use "terminal heating."
  - Fill the bottles with prepared formula.
  - Cap the bottles loosely.
  - Place the filled bottles in a pan of water. The water should reach half-way up the bottles.
  - Bring the water to a gentle boil for about 25 minutes.

PROMOTING SAFETY AND COMFORT

Cleaning Baby Bottles

Safety

Baby bottles, caps, nipples, and other items must be thoroughly rinsed to remove all soap. Otherwise, the baby takes in soap with the feeding. This can cause serious stomach and intestinal irritation.

Cleaning Baby Bottles

PRE-PROCEDURE

1 See *Promoting Safety and Comfort: Cleaning Baby Bottles*, p. 807.
2 Practice hand hygiene.
3 Collect the following.
- Bottles, nipples, and caps
- Funnel

- Can opener
- Bottle brush
- Dishwashing soap
- Other items used to prepare formula
- Towel

PROCEDURE

4 Wash the bottles, nipples, caps, funnel, and can opener in hot, soapy water. Wash other items used to prepare formula.
5 Clean inside baby bottles with the bottle brush (Fig. 52-13).
6 Squeeze hot, soapy water through the nipples (Fig. 52-14). This removes formula.

7 Rinse all items thoroughly in hot water. Squeeze hot water through the nipples to remove soap.
8 Lay a clean towel on the counter.
9 Stand bottles upside down to drain. Place nipples, caps, and other items on the towel. Let the items dry.

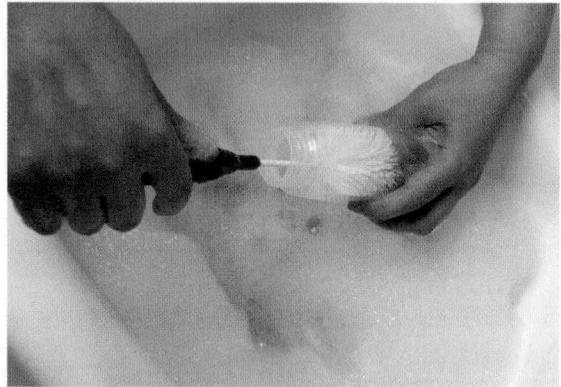

FIGURE 52-13 A bottle brush is used to clean inside a baby bottle.

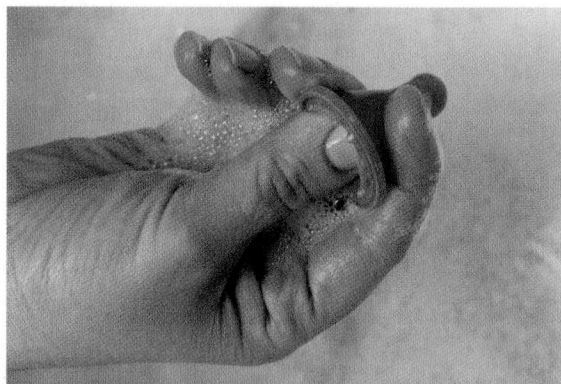

FIGURE 52-14 Water is squeezed through the nipple during washing and rinsing.

Feeding the Baby

Bottle-fed babies usually want to be fed every 2 to 4 hours. They are fed on demand. The amount of formula taken increases as they grow older. The nurse or the mother tells you how much formula a baby needs at each feeding. Babies usually take as much formula as they need. The baby stops sucking and turns away from the bottle when satisfied.

Most babies do not like cold formula out of the refrigerator. Warm a bottle before the feeding. Do 1 of the following.

- Warm it in a pan of water on the stove. Use low heat. Turn the bottle often.
- Hold the bottle under warm running tap water or in a container of warm water. Turn the bottle to warm the formula evenly.

The formula should feel warm. To test the temperature, sprinkle a few drops on the inside of your wrist (Fig. 52-15). Allow formula to cool if it is hot. The guidelines in Box 52-4 will help you bottle-feed babies.

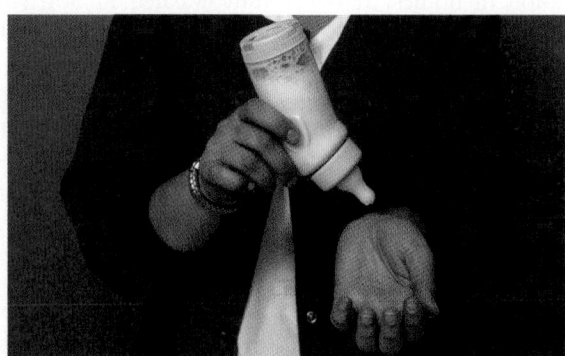

FIGURE 52-15 Formula should feel warm on the inside of your wrist.

Solid foods are given at 4 to 6 months. Usually baby rice cereal is the first solid food given. The cereal is mixed with breast-milk or formula to a thin consistency. Other solid foods are added as the baby grows. The nurse tells you what foods the baby can have.

See *Promoting Safety and Comfort: Feeding the Baby*.

BOX 52-4	Bottle-Feeding Babies

- Warm a refrigerated bottle. The formula should feel warm to the inside of your wrist.
- Assume a comfortable position for the feeding.
- Hold the baby close to you. Relax and snuggle the baby.
- Stroke the baby's cheek or lip with the nipple. The baby's head will turn to the nipple.
- Tilt the bottle so that the neck of the bottle and the nipple are always full (Fig. 52-16). Otherwise some air is in the neck or nipple. The baby sucks air into the stomach, causing cramping and discomfort.
- Do not prop the bottle and lay the baby down for the feeding (Fig. 52-17).
- Burp the newborn after every $\frac{1}{2}$ to 1 ounce of formula. Older babies are burped less often—after every 2 to 3 ounces. Also burp the baby at the end of the feeding.
- Do not leave the baby alone with a bottle.
- Do not force the baby to finish the bottle.
- Discard remaining formula. Do not save or reheat it for another feeding.
- Wash the bottle, cap, and nipple after the feeding (see procedure: *Cleaning Baby Bottles*).

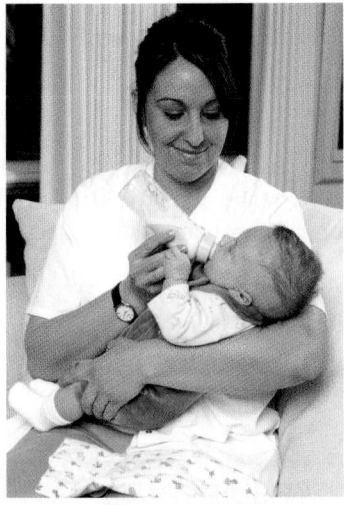

FIGURE 52-16 The bottle is tilted so that formula fills the bottle neck and nipple.

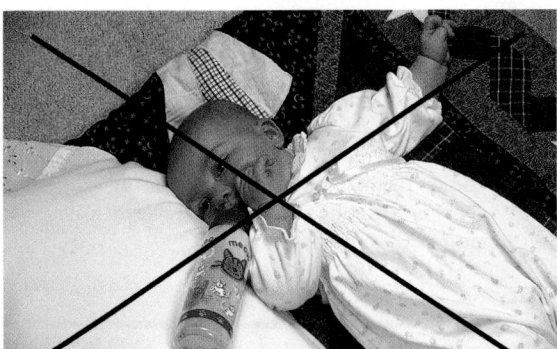

FIGURE 52-17 Do NOT prop the bottle to feed the baby.

PROMOTING SAFETY AND COMFORT
Feeding the Baby

Safety
Do not set the bottle out to warm at room temperature. This takes too long and allows the growth of microbes. Do not heat formula in microwave ovens. The formula can heat unevenly and burn the baby's mouth.

BURPING THE BABY

Babies take in air during feedings. Air in the stomach and intestines causes cramping and discomfort. This can lead to vomiting. Burping helps to get rid of the air. Most babies burp mid-way and after a feeding.

Burping a baby also is called *bubbling*. You pat or rub the baby's back with circular motions. Do this for 2 or 3 minutes. Figure 52-18, p. 810, shows how to position the baby for burping.

- *Over the shoulder.* First place a clean diaper or towel over your shoulder. This protects your clothing if the baby "spits up." Then hold the infant over your shoulder.
- *On your lap.* Support the baby in a sitting position on your lap. Hold the towel or diaper in front of the baby. *Remember to support the infant's head and neck for the first 3 months after birth.*
- *On the baby's stomach.* First place a clean diaper or towel on your lap where the baby's head will be. Position the baby on your lap with his or her stomach down.

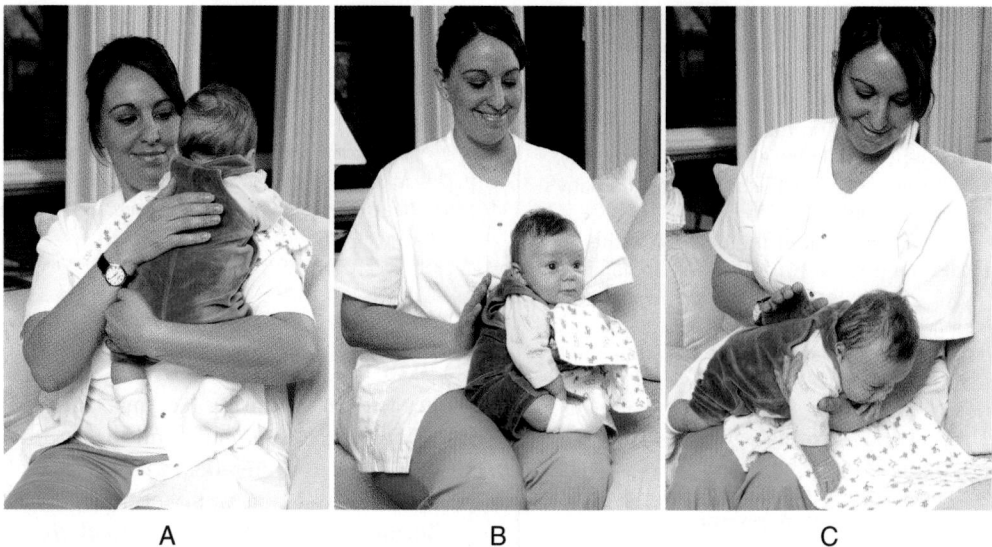

FIGURE 52-18 Burping a baby. **A,** The baby is held over the shoulder. **B,** The baby is supported in the sitting position. **C,** The baby is laid on the stomach.

DIAPERING

In the first 1 or 2 days after birth, newborns have meconium stools. *Meconium is a dark green to black, tarry bowel movement.* By day 3 or 4, stools are greenish brown to yellowish brown in color and less sticky. By day 4 or 5:

- *Breast-fed babies*—have yellow and seedy-looking stools. They are soft or runny. Breast-fed babies usually have a bowel movement (BM) with every feeding.
- *Bottle-fed babies*—have yellow to brown stools. Bottle-fed babies have fewer stools than breast-fed babies and their stools are firmer. They may have 1 or 2 stools a day.

Over time, an elimination pattern develops. Some babies have 1, 2, or 3 stools a day. Stools are usually soft and unformed. Hard, formed stools signal constipation. Watery stools mean diarrhea. Diarrhea is very serious in infants. Their fluid balance is upset quickly (Chapter 27). Tell the nurse at once if you suspect constipation or diarrhea.

Babies wet at least 6 to 8 times a day. Diapers are changed when wet or when stools are present.

Cloth diapers are re-used. With Velcro fasteners, no diaper pins are needed. The danger of sticking the baby or yourself with a diaper pin is avoided. To care for cloth diapers:

- Rinse a soiled cloth diaper. Rinse feces into the toilet.
- Store soiled diapers in a diaper pail.
- Wash them daily or every 2 days.
- Do not wash them with other laundry items.
- Wash them in hot water. Use a baby laundry detergent.
- Put them through the wash cycle a second time without detergent. This helps remove all soap.
- Hang them outside to dry if possible for a fresh, clean smell. Otherwise, dry them in the dryer.

Disposable diapers are secured with Velcro or tape strips. Fold soiled diapers so the soiled area is on the inside. Then discard the diaper in the trash container. Do not flush it down the toilet. Using disposable diapers costs more than using cloth ones.

Changing diapers often helps prevent diaper rash. Moisture, stools, and urine irritate the baby's skin. When changing diapers, make sure the baby is clean and dry before applying a clean diaper. If a diaper rash develops, tell the nurse at once.

See *Delegation Guidelines: Diapering a Baby.*
See *Promoting Safety and Comfort: Diapering a Baby.*
See procedure: *Diapering a Baby.*

DELEGATION GUIDELINES

Diapering a Baby

Before changing a baby's diaper, you need this information from the nurse and the care plan.

- The size and type of diaper to use (cloth or disposable)
- If you need to give cord care (p. 813) or circumcision care (p. 813)
- What lotion or cream to use
- What observations to report and record:
  - Color and amount of urine—small, medium, large
  - Color, amount, consistency, and odor of stools
  - Condition of the baby's skin and genital area
  - Redness or irritation of the skin or genital area
  - Blood or discharge on the diaper
- When to report observations
- What concerns about the baby to report at once

PROMOTING SAFETY AND COMFORT

Diapering a Baby

Safety

Disposable diapers present safety hazards to babies. Babies can choke on tab papers that cover the tape strips. Keep the tab papers away from the baby. Discard them as soon as possible.

Older babies can tear and pull disposable diapers apart. They can choke or suffocate on the plastic if they put the plastic in their noses or mouths. Observe babies closely. Change any torn or damaged diaper at once.

Keep the baby safe during diapering. The baby may squirm, wiggle, or kick and cry. To prevent falls:

- Gather all needed supplies before you begin.
- Place the baby on a firm surface. If the baby is on a table, make sure it is sturdy.
- Always keep 1 hand on a baby who is on a table or other raised surface.
- Never look away from the baby.
  Diaper pins for cloth diapers must point away from the abdomen. If a pin opens toward the abdomen, it can pierce the skin and damage organs.

Diapering a Baby

QUALITY OF LIFE

- Knock before entering the baby's room.
- Address the baby and parents by name.
- Introduce yourself by name and title.

- Explain the procedure to the parents before starting and during the procedure.
- Protect the baby's rights during the procedure.
- Handle the baby gently during the procedure.

PRE-PROCEDURE

1 Follow *Delegation Guidelines: Diapering a Baby*. See *Promoting Safety and Comfort: Diapering a Baby*.
2 Practice hand hygiene.
3 Collect the following.
   - Gloves
   - Clean diaper
   - Waterproof changing pad
   - Washcloth
   - Disposable wipes or cotton balls
   - Basin of warm water
   - Baby soap
   - Baby lotion or cream

PROCEDURE

4 Put on the gloves.
5 Place the changing pad under the baby.
6 Unfasten the dirty diaper. Place diaper pins out of the baby's reach.
7 Wipe the genital area with the front of the diaper (Fig. 52-19, *A*, p. 812). Wipe from the front to the back (top to bottom).
8 Note the color and amount of urine and feces. Fold the diaper so urine and feces are inside. Set the diaper aside.
9 Clean the genital area from front to back (top to bottom). Use a wet washcloth, disposable wipes, or cotton balls (Fig. 52-19, *B*, p. 812). Wash with mild soap and water for a large amount of feces or if the baby has a rash. Rinse thoroughly and pat the area dry.
10 Clean the circumcision (p. 813). Give cord care (p. 813).
11 Apply cream or lotion to the genital area and buttocks. Do not use too much. Caking can occur.
12 Raise the baby's legs. Slide a clean diaper under the buttocks.

13 Fold a cloth diaper as follows.
   a *For a boy:* the extra thickness is in the front (Fig. 52-20, *A*, p. 812).
   b *For a girl:* the extra thickness is at the back (Fig. 52-20, *B*, p. 812).
   c Bring the diaper between the baby's legs.
14 Make sure the diaper is snug around the hips and abdomen.
   a It is loose near the penis if the circumcision has not healed.
   b It is below the umbilicus if the cord stump has not healed.
15 Secure the diaper in place. Use the tape strips or Velcro on disposable diapers (Fig. 52-21, *A*, p. 812). Make sure the tabs stick in place. Use baby pins or Velcro for cloth diapers. Pins point away from the abdomen (Fig. 52-21, *B*, p. 812). Keep the tab papers away from the baby.
16 Apply a diaper cover or plastic pants if cloth diapers are worn.
17 Put the baby in the crib, infant seat, or other safe place.

POST-PROCEDURE

18 Rinse feces from the cloth diaper into the toilet and flush.
19 Store used cloth diapers in a covered pail. Put a disposable diaper and paper tabs in the trash.
20 Remove and discard the gloves. Practice hand hygiene.
21 Put on clean gloves.

22 Clean, rinse, dry, and return other items to their proper place.
23 Remove and discard the gloves. Practice hand hygiene.
24 Report and record your observations.

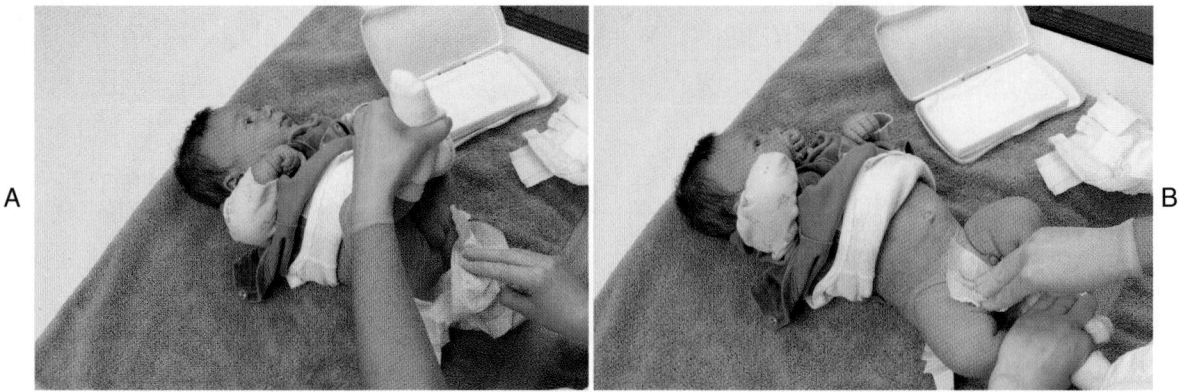

FIGURE 52-19 A, The front of the diaper is used to wipe the genital area from front (top) to back (bottom). **B,** A disposable wipe is used to clean the genital area from front (top) to back (bottom).

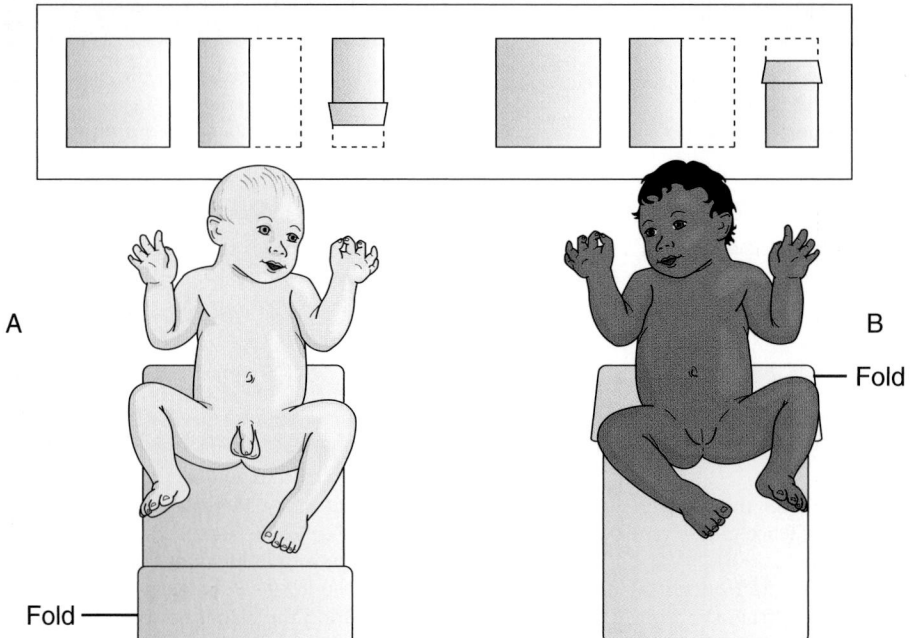

FIGURE 52-20 A, A cloth diaper is folded in front for boys. **B,** The diaper has a fold in the back for girls.

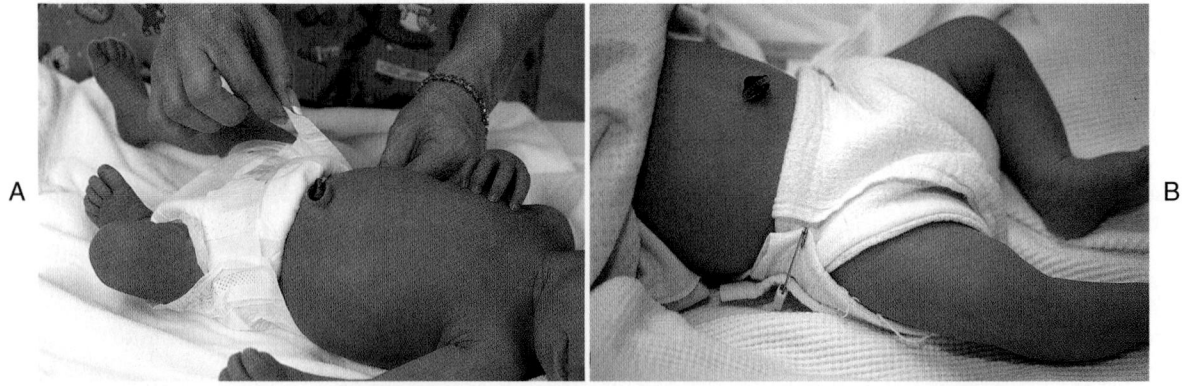

FIGURE 52-21 Securing a diaper. A, A disposable diaper is secured in place with tape strips. **B,** Diaper pins secure a cloth diaper. Pins point away from the abdomen. NOTE: The diapers in A and B are below the cord.

UMBILICAL CORD CARE

The *umbilical cord connects the mother and fetus (unborn baby). It carries blood, oxygen, and nutrients from the mother to the fetus* (Fig. 52-22). The cord is not needed after birth. Shortly after delivery, the doctor clamps and cuts the cord. A cord stump is left on the baby (see Fig. 52-21). The stump dries up and falls off usually within 2 weeks after birth. Slight bleeding can occur when the cord comes off.

The cord provides a place for microbes to grow. Keep the cord clean and dry. Cord care is done at each diaper change. Cord care is continued for 1 or 2 days after the cord comes off. It involves the following.

- Do not get the stump wet.
- Keep the diaper below the cord as in Figure 52-21. This prevents the diaper from irritating the stump. It also keeps the cord from becoming wet from urine.
- Give sponge baths until the cord falls off. Then the baby can have a tub bath.
- Do not pull the cord off—even if it looks ready to fall off.
- Report the following.
  - Swelling, redness, odor, or drainage from the stump
  - Bleeding from the cord or navel area
  - Fever
  - Crying when the cord or skin near the cord is touched.

See *Promoting Safety and Comfort: Umbilical Cord Care.*

PROMOTING SAFETY AND COMFORT
Umbilical Cord Care

Safety

For cord care, a common practice involved wiping the base of the stump with alcohol at every diaper change. The alcohol promoted drying. It is now thought that the stump heals faster if left to air-dry. When giving cord care, follow the nurse's directions. The nurse may have you wash the stump with water if it is dirty or sticky. If so, dry it thoroughly after washing.

CIRCUMCISION CARE

Boys are born with foreskin on the penis. *The surgical removal of foreskin from the penis is called a* **circumcision** (Chapter 22). The procedure is optional. The parents decide whether or not to circumcise.

Circumcision is thought to:
- Allow for easier hygiene.
- Prevent urinary tract infections in infants.
- Lower the risk of cancer of the penis.
- Prevent problems with foreskin retraction. Some foreskin is too tight to be pulled back (retracted) over the penis.
- Decrease the risk of sexually transmitted diseases.

The procedure is usually done within 1 to 10 days after birth. Circumcision is a religious ceremony in the Jewish faith.

The tip of the penis will look red, swollen, and sore. However, the entire penis should not be swollen. And the circumcision should not interfere with voiding. Carefully observe for signs of bleeding and infection. There should be no odor, drainage, or fever. A slight yellowish discharge or crust at the tip of the penis is normal. It does not signal infection. Report any concerns at once. The area should heal in 7 to 10 days.

Circumcision care involves the following.
- Clean the penis at each diaper change. This is very important after a BM.
- Use mild soap and water, plain water, or commercial wipes as the nurse directs.
- Apply a petrolatum gauze dressing or petrolatum jelly to the penis as the nurse directs. This protects the penis from urine and feces. It also prevents the penis from sticking to the diaper. Use a cotton swab to apply the petrolatum jelly (Fig. 52-23, p. 814).
- Apply the diaper loosely. This prevents the diaper from irritating the penis.

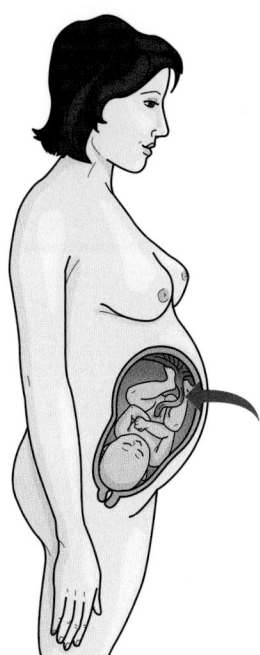

FIGURE 52-22 The umbilical cord connects the mother and fetus.

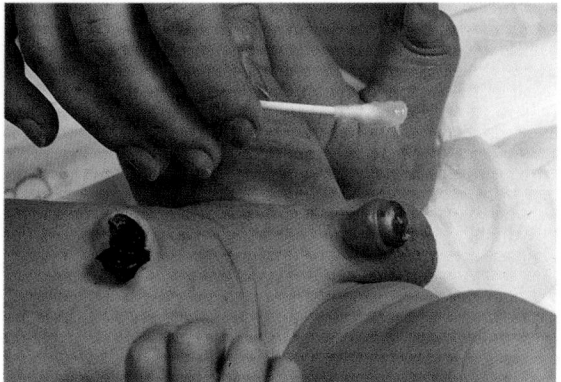

FIGURE 52-23 Petrolatum jelly is applied to the circumcised penis.

FOCUS ON LONG-TERM CARE AND HOME CARE

Bathing an Infant

Home Care

Families have routines. Some babies are bathed in the morning. The baby is more alert and ready to interact at this time. Others bathe in the evening. Evening baths:

- Comfort and relax the baby. This helps some babies sleep longer at night.
- Allow a parent who works during the day to be involved in the bath.

Sometimes fathers bathe babies so mothers can rest or tend to other children. Follow the family's routine when working in the home.

▣ BATHING AN INFANT

Infants do not need a bath every day. Bathing too often can cause dry skin. Bathing 3 times a week is common. Areas with creases need special attention—under the arms, behind the ears, around the neck, and the genital area. Also wash and dry well between the fingers and toes.

Baths comfort and relax babies. They provide a wonderful time to hold, touch, and talk to babies. Stimulation is important for development. Being touched and held helps babies learn safety, security, and love and belonging.

Planning for the bath is important. You cannot leave the baby alone if you forget something. Gather needed equipment, supplies, and the baby's clothes before you start the bath. Everything you need must be within your reach.

There are 2 bath procedures for babies. Sponge baths are given until the cord stump falls off and the umbilicus and circumcision heal. *The cord must not get wet.* The tub bath is given after the cord site and circumcision heal (Fig. 52-24).

See *Focus on Long-Term Care and Home Care: Bathing an Infant.*

See *Delegation Guidelines: Bathing an Infant.*

See *Promoting Safety and Comfort: Bathing an Infant.*

See procedure: *Giving a Baby a Sponge Bath.*

See procedure: *Giving a Baby a Tub Bath*, p. 817.

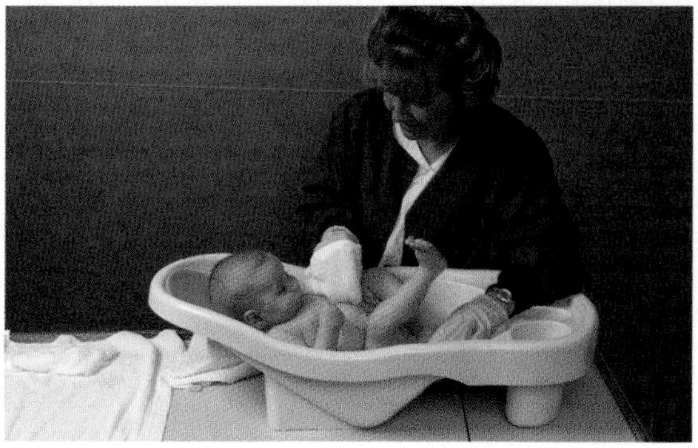

DELEGATION GUIDELINES

Bathing an Infant

Before bathing an infant, you need this information from the nurse and the care plan.

- How often to bathe the baby.
- What type of bath to give—sponge bath or tub bath.
- What water temperature to use—usually 100°F to 105°F (37.7°C to 40.5°C).
- When to bathe the infant.
- If you should use baby soap or plain water. Usually soap is not used unless the baby is dirty or smells.
- If you should apply lotion after the bath.
- What observations to report and record:
  - Bruising
  - Rashes
  - Skin irritation
  - Redness
  - Swelling
  - Open skin areas
  - See "Umbilical Cord Care," p. 813
  - See "Circumcision Care," p. 813
- When to report observations.
- What concerns about the baby to report at once.

FIGURE 52-24 The baby is given a tub bath in a baby bathtub.

PROMOTING SAFETY AND COMFORT

Bathing an Infant

Safety

To protect an infant during a bath, follow these safety measures.

- Turn up the thermostat and close windows and doors about 20 minutes before the bath. Room temperature should be 75°F to 80°F for the bath. The room may be too warm for you. Remove a sweater or lab coat or roll up your sleeves before starting the bath.
- Measure bath water temperature with a bath thermometer. The nurse tells you what temperature to use (usually 100°F to 105°F [37.7°C to 40.5°C]). Or test water temperature with the inside of your wrist (Fig. 52-25). The water should feel warm and comfortable. Babies have delicate skin and are easily burned.
- Never leave the baby alone on a table or in the bathtub.
- Always keep 1 hand on the baby if you must look away for a moment.
- Hold the baby securely during the bath. Babies are slippery when they are wet. A wet, squirming baby is hard to hold.
- Keep the baby's face out of the water.

Comfort

Keep the baby warm and comfortable during the bath. For a sponge bath, cover the table or other bathing surface with a towel. You can also wrap the baby in a towel and expose only the body parts being washed. For a tub bath, pour warm water over the baby's body during the bath.

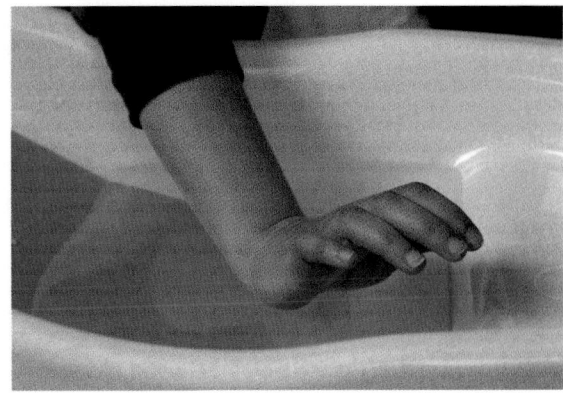

FIGURE 52-25 The inside of the wrist is used to test bath water temperature.

Giving a Baby a Sponge Bath

QUALITY OF LIFE

- Knock before entering the baby's room.
- Address the baby and parents by name.
- Introduce yourself by name and title.

- Explain the procedure to the parents before starting and during the procedure.
- Protect the baby's rights during the procedure.
- Handle the baby gently during the procedure.

PRE-PROCEDURE

1 Follow *Delegation Guidelines: Bathing an Infant.* See *Promoting Safety and Comfort: Bathing an Infant.*
2 Practice hand hygiene.
3 Place the following items in your work area.
  - Baby bathtub
  - Bath thermometer
  - Bath towel
  - 2 hand towels
  - Receiving blanket
  - Washcloth
  - Clean diaper

  - Clean clothing for the baby
  - Cotton balls
  - Baby soap (if needed)
  - Baby shampoo
  - Baby lotion
  - Gloves
4 Identify the baby. Check the ID bracelet against the assignment sheet. Use 2 identifiers (Chapter 13). Follow agency policy.
5 Provide for privacy.

PROCEDURE

6 Fill the baby bathtub with 2 to 3 inches of warm water. Water temperature should be 100°F to 105°F (37.7°C to 40.5°C). Measure water temperature with the bath thermometer or use the inside of your wrist. The water should feel warm and comfortable.
7 Put on gloves.
8 Undress the baby. Leave the diaper on.

9 Wash the baby's eye lids (Fig. 52-26, p. 816).
  a Dip a cotton ball into the water.
  b Squeeze out excess water.
  c Wash 1 eye lid from the inner part to the outer part.
  d Repeat this step for the other eye with a new cotton ball.

Continued

Giving a Baby a Sponge Bath—cont'd

PROCEDURE—cont'd

10 Moisten the washcloth and make a mitt (Chapter 22). Clean the outside of the ear and then behind the ear. Repeat this step for the other ear. Be gentle.

11 Rinse and squeeze out the washcloth. Make a mitt with the washcloth.

12 Wash the baby's face (Fig. 52-27). Clean inside the nostrils with the washcloth. *Do not use cotton swabs to clean inside the nose.* Pat the face dry.

13 Pick up the baby. Hold the baby over the baby bathtub using the football hold. Support the baby's head and neck with your wrist and hand.

14 Wash the baby's head (Fig. 52-28).

  a Squeeze a small amount of water from the washcloth onto the baby's head. Or bring water to the baby's head using a cupped hand.

  b Apply a small amount of baby shampoo to the head.

  c Wash the head with circular motions.

  d Rinse the head by squeezing water from a washcloth over the baby's head. Or bring water to the baby's head using a cupped hand. Rinse thoroughly. Do not get soap in the baby's eyes.

  e Use a small hand towel to dry the head.

15 Lay the baby on the table.

16 Remove the diaper.

17 Wash the front of the body with a washcloth or your hands. Do not get the cord wet. Also wash the arms, hands, fingers, legs, feet, and toes. Wash the genital area and all creases and folds. Rinse thoroughly. Pat dry.

18 Give cord care. Clean the circumcision.

19 Turn the baby to the prone position. Wash the back and buttocks. Use a washcloth or your hands. Rinse thoroughly. Pat dry.

20 Apply baby lotion as directed by the nurse.

21 Remove and discard the gloves. Practice hand hygiene.

22 Put a clean diaper and clean clothes on the baby.

23 Wrap the baby in the receiving blanket. Put the baby in the crib or other safe area.

POST-PROCEDURE

24 Practice hand hygiene. Put on gloves.

25 Clean, rinse, dry, and return equipment and supplies to the proper place. Do this step when the baby is settled.

26 Remove and discard the gloves. Practice hand hygiene.

27 Complete a safety check of the room. (See the inside of the front cover.)

28 Report and record your observations.

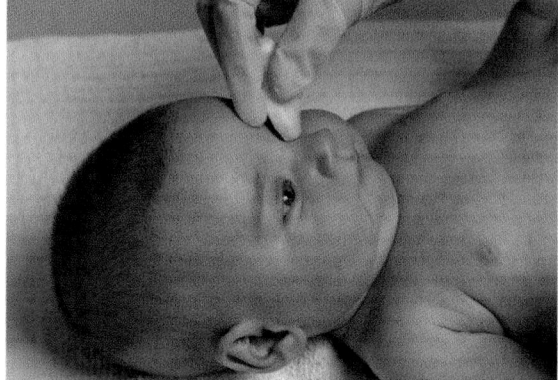

FIGURE 52-26 Wash the baby's eyes with cotton balls. The eye lids are cleaned from the inner to the outer part.

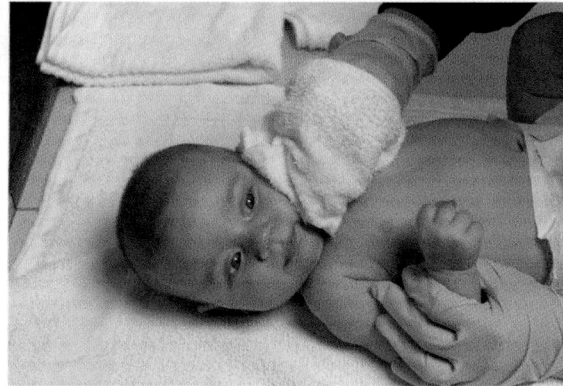

FIGURE 52-27 The baby's face is washed with a mitted washcloth.

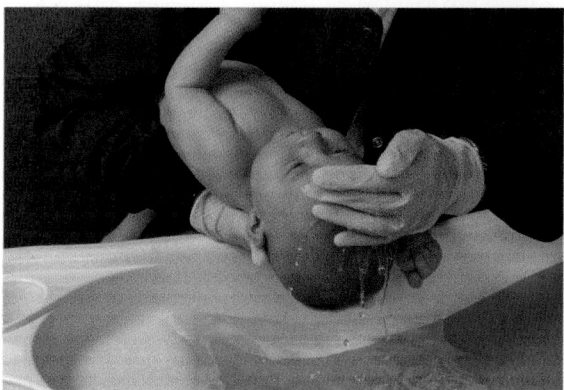

FIGURE 52-28 The baby's head is washed over the bath basin.

Giving a Baby a Tub Bath

QUALITY OF LIFE

- Knock before entering the baby's room.
- Address the baby and parents by name.
- Introduce yourself by name and title.

- Explain the procedure to the parents before beginning and during the procedure.
- Protect the baby's rights during the procedure.
- Handle the baby gently during the procedure.

PROCEDURE

1 Follow steps 1 through 16 in procedure: *Giving a Baby a Sponge Bath* (p. 815).
2 Hold the baby as in Figure 52-29.
  a Place 1 hand under the baby's shoulders. Your thumb should be over the baby's shoulder. Your fingers should be under the arm.
  b Support the buttocks with your other hand. Slide your hand under the thighs. Hold the far thigh with your other hand.
3 Lower the baby into the water feet first.
4 Wash the front of the baby's body. Also wash the arms, hands, fingers, legs, feet, and toes. Wash the genital area and all creases and folds.

5 Reverse your hold. Use your other hand to hold the baby. Keep the baby's face out of the water.
6 Wash the baby's back and buttocks. Rinse thoroughly.
7 Reverse your hold again. Hold the baby with your other hand.
8 Lift the baby out of the water and onto a towel.
9 Wrap the baby in the towel. Also cover the baby's head.
10 Pat the baby dry. Dry all creases and folds.
11 Follow steps 20 through 28 in procedure: *Giving a Baby a Sponge Bath*.

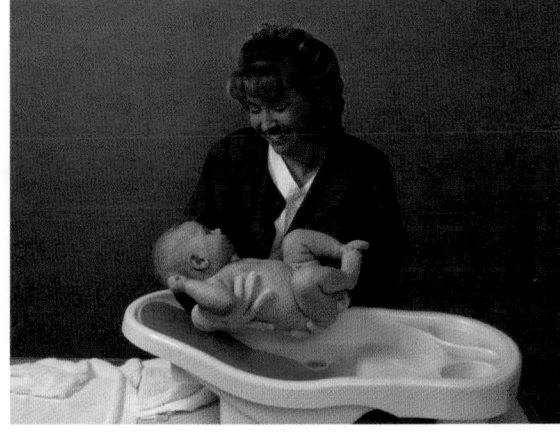

FIGURE 52-29 The baby is held for lowering into the baby bathtub.

NAIL CARE

The baby's fingernails and toenails are kept short. Otherwise, the baby can scratch himself or herself and others. Nails are best cut after a bath or when the baby is sleeping. The sleeping baby is quiet and will not squirm or fuss. Use infant nail clippers and a soft emery board.

- Hold the finger or toe with 1 hand.
- Press the skin under the nail. This moves the skin out of the way to avoid pinching or cutting the skin.
- Trim the nails with an infant nail clipper.
  - *Fingernails:* clip following the natural shape of the nail.
  - *Toenails:* clip straight across as for an adult (Chapter 23).
- Smooth rough or sharp edges with a soft emery board.

WEIGHING INFANTS

The infant's birth weight is a baseline for measuring growth. The nurse uses weight measurements in the assessment step of the nursing process. They also are used to measure the amount of breast-milk taken in during breast-feeding. The baby is weighed before and after breast-feeding. The difference in the weights is the amount of milk taken in during breast-feeding. It tells the nurse if the baby is getting enough milk.

See *Focus on Math: Weighing Infants.*
See *Delegation Guidelines: Weighing Infants,* p. 818.
See *Promoting Safety and Comfort: Weighing Infants,* p. 818.
See procedure: *Weighing an Infant,* p. 818.

FOCUS ON **MATH**

Weighing Infants

For a "before" and "after" feeding weight, subtract the infant's "before" weight from the "after" weight.
  The nurse uses the weight difference to calculate the amount of breast-milk taken in.
  For example, a baby's "before" feeding weight is 2720 grams. (A gram is a measurement of weight.) After feeding, the baby weighs 2750 grams. You report a weight change of 30 grams.

2750 grams (after feeding) – 2720 grams (before feeding)
= 30 grams (weight change)

DELEGATION GUIDELINES

Weighing Infants

Before weighing an infant, you need this information from the nurse and the care plan.
- When to weigh the baby.
- If the baby is breast-fed or bottle-fed. Breast-fed babies wear the same diaper for "before" and "after" feeding weight measurements. The clothes and blanket are removed.
- When to report the weight measurement.
- What concerns about the baby to report at once.

PROMOTING SAFETY AND COMFORT

Weighing Infants

Safety
You must meet the baby's safety needs. Protect the baby from chills. Keep the room warm and free of drafts. Also protect the baby from falling. Always keep a hand over the baby when measuring weight. Remember to keep 1 hand on the baby if you need to look away.

Weighing an Infant

QUALITY OF LIFE

- Knock before entering the baby's room.
- Address the baby and parents by name.
- Introduce yourself by name and title.
- Explain the procedure to the parents before beginning and during the procedure.
- Protect the baby's rights during the procedure.
- Handle the baby gently during the procedure.

PRE-PROCEDURE

1 Follow *Delegation Guidelines: Weighing Infants*. See *Promoting Safety and Comfort: Weighing Infants*.
2 Practice hand hygiene.
3 Collect the following.
   - Baby scale (Fig. 52-30)
   - Paper for the scale
   - Items for diaper changing (see procedure: *Diapering a Baby*, p. 811)
   - Gloves
4 Identify the baby. Check the ID bracelet against the assignment sheet. Use 2 identifiers (Chapter 13). Follow agency policy.

PROCEDURE

5 Place the paper on the scale. Adjust the scale to zero (0).
6 Put on the gloves.
7 Undress the baby and remove the diaper. Clean the genital area.
8 Remove and discard the gloves and practice hand hygiene. Put on clean gloves.
9 Lay the baby on the scale. Keep 1 hand over the baby to prevent falling.
10 Read the digital display or move the weights until the scale is balanced (Chapter 32).
11 Note the measurement.
12 Take the baby off of the scale.
13 Diaper and dress the baby. Lay the baby in the crib.
14 Discard the paper and soiled diaper.
15 Disinfect the scale following agency policy.
16 Remove and discard the gloves. Practice hand hygiene.

POST-PROCEDURE

17 Return the scale to its proper place.
18 Practice hand hygiene.
19 Report and record your observations.

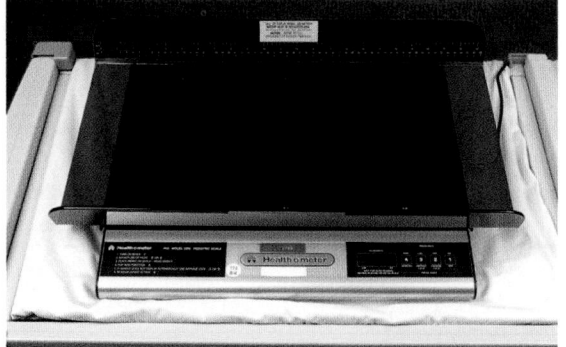

FIGURE 52-30 Digital infant scale.

CARE OF THE MOTHER

Postpartum means after (post) *childbirth* (partum). The postpartum period starts with birth of the baby. It ends 6 weeks later. The mother's body returns to its normal state during this time. The mother adjusts physically and emotionally to childbirth.

The uterus returns almost to its pre-pregnant size. This is called *involution of the uterus.* If the mother does not breast-feed, she can expect a menstrual period within 4 to 6 weeks. Breast-feeding is not an effective method of birth control. Without birth control measures, the mother can get pregnant again.

After childbirth, a vaginal discharge called **lochia** *occurs.* (*Lochia* comes from the Greek word *lochos.* It means *child-birth.*) Lochia consists of blood and other matter left in the uterus from childbirth. The lochia changes color and decreases in amount during the postpartum period.

* *Lochia rubra*—is dark or bright red (*rubra*) discharge. Mainly blood, it is seen during the first 3 to 4 days.
* *Lochia serosa*—is pinkish-brown (*serosa*) drainage. It lasts until about 10 days after birth.
* *Lochia alba*—is whitish (*alba*) drainage. It continues for 10 to 14 days or more after birth.

Lochia increases with breast-feeding and activity. When she stands after lying or sitting, the mother may feel a gush of lochia. She wears a sanitary napkin to absorb the lochia. Normally lochia smells like menstrual flow. Foul-smelling lochia signals infection.

Good perineal care is important. Sanitary pads are changed often. When wiping after elimination, the mother wipes from front (top) to back (bottom). Sanitary napkins are applied and removed from front to back (top to bottom). Good hand-washing is essential after perineal care, changing sanitary napkins, and elimination. Standard Precautions and the Bloodborne Pathogen Standard are followed.

Some mothers have episiotomies. An *episiotomy is an incision* (otomy) *into the perineum.* (*Episeion* means *pubic region.*) The doctor performs this procedure during child-birth. It increases the size of the vaginal opening for the baby. The incision is sutured after delivery. The doctor may order sitz baths for comfort and hygiene (Chapter 38). Like other incisions, complications can develop. These include infection and wound separation (*dehiscence*). Tell the nurse at once if the mother complains of pain, discomfort, or a discharge.

Some mothers deliver by *cesarean section (C-section).* The baby is delivered through an incision made into the abdominal wall. The doctor performs a C-section when:

* The baby must be delivered to save the baby's or mother's life.
* The baby is too large to pass through the birth canal or is in an abnormal position.
* The mother has a vaginal infection that could be transmitted to the baby.
* A normal vaginal delivery will be difficult for the baby or mother.

The C-section incision needs to heal. See Chapter 36 for wound healing and wound care.

The mother has emotional reactions after childbirth. Hormone changes, life-style changes, and lack of sleep can cause mood swings. So can frequent visits and phone calls from family and friends. Some interfere or offer advice and opinions about parenting. The mother can help herself by resting when the baby sleeps. She needs time for herself and her partner. She may feel better after a shower, hair care, and getting dressed.

Complications can occur during pregnancy, labor, and delivery. They also can occur in the postpartum period. Report any sign or symptom listed in Box 52-5 at once.

BOX 52-5	**Postpartum Complications—Signs and Symptoms**

* Temperature of 100.4°F or greater
* Pain: abdominal or perineal
* Discharge:
  * Foul smelling from the vagina
  * From an episiotomy
  * From a C-section incision
* Bleeding from an episiotomy or C-section incision
* Redness, swelling: episiotomy or C-section incision
* Saturating a sanitary napkin within 1 hour of application
* Lochia:
  * Red lochia after lochia has changed color to pinkish-brown or white
  * Lochia with large clots
* Urination: burning
* Leg pain, tenderness, or swelling
* Sadness or feelings of depression
* Breast pain, tenderness, or swelling

FOCUS ON **PRIDE**

The Person, Family, and Yourself

P ersonal and Professional Responsibility

Newborns do not spend every moment in the mother's room. A newborn may go to the nursery while the mother rests or when a test or procedure is needed. A circumcision is an example.

Identification of the newborn is important. You must return the baby to the correct parent. You must not rely on the parent to identify the baby. Safe identification of the baby is a professional responsibility. Follow agency policy to identify the mother and newborn.

R ights and Respect

A parent's preferences for newborn care may differ from yours. For example, a mother wants to bottle-feed. You believe babies should be breast-fed. Your opinion must not affect the care you give. Respect parent preferences.

I ndependence and Social Interaction

Parents must learn to care for their baby. The nurse teaches parents about newborn care. They watch the nurse. Then they try it on their own. Parents gain confidence by performing care independently.

Parents who rely on the staff may not know how to provide care at home. Avoid doing everything for the parents. Tell the nurse if the parents rely on the staff too much.

D elegation and Teamwork

Alarm systems are used to protect the security of newborns. The baby wears an electronic security bracelet. An alarm sounds when the baby is carried toward an exit. Alarms and exits are checked at once. All staff members respond. If a baby is missing, security sends out a message to the entire agency. Procedures are followed to find the baby. The entire agency works as a team to protect the newborn.

E thics and Laws

Having a baby is usually a happy time. However, this is not always the case. The health team must monitor closely for signs of mistreatment. A parent may not be interested in the baby. Or the parent may be unwilling to learn how to care for the baby. The baby must be protected from abuse and neglect. Tell the nurse about any concerns at once.

FOCUS ON **PRIDE**: *Application*

New parents have to adjust to many new things. Explain the health team's role in helping parents adjust. How can you provide support and encouragement?

REVIEW QUESTIONS

Circle T if the statement is TRUE and F if it is FALSE.

1 **T   F**   A baby's crib should be within hearing distance of caregivers.

2 **T   F**   A baby needs a pillow for sleep.

3 **T   F**   A baby is placed on his or her back for sleep.

4 **T   F**   A yellowish crust at the tip of a circumcised penis is a sign of infection.

5 **T   F**   A baby's diapers are changed whenever they are wet.

6 **T   F**   A baby's cord and circumcision have not healed. The baby should have a sponge bath.

7 **T   F**   Cotton swabs are used to clean a baby's ears.

8 **T   F**   A breast-fed baby needs a "before" and "after" feeding weight. The baby is weighed with the diaper on.

Circle the BEST answer.

9 A baby's head and neck are supported for the first
   a 7 to 10 days
   b Month
   c 3 months
   d 6 months

10 Which is unsafe when holding a newborn?
   a Holding the infant securely
   b Cuddling the infant
   c Using 2 hands
   d Lifting the infant by the arms

11 You see the following in an infant's home. Which is unsafe?
   a Electrical outlets have safety covers.
   b A cord hangs near the crib.
   c Drugs have child-resistant caps.
   d Cleaning supplies are in locked cabinets.

12 Which is safe?
   a A crib without bumper pads
   b A crib with a loose crib sheet
   c A crib with a soft blanket and stuffed toys
   d A crib with a drop-side rail

13 You observe the following. Which is normal?
   a The baby looks flushed and is perspiring.
   b The baby has watery stools.
   c The baby's eyes are red and irritated.
   d The baby spits up a small amount when burped.

14 A breast-feeding mother should
   a Nurse the infant every 4 to 6 hours
   b Avoid wearing a bra
   c Clean her breasts with soap and water
   d Stimulate the rooting reflex

15 A breast-fed baby is burped
   a Every 5 minutes
   b After nursing from a breast
   c After 1 ounce of breast milk
   d After half the formula is taken

REVIEW QUESTIONS—cont'd

16 You are shopping for baby formula. Which should you buy?
   a The one that is on sale
   b The ready-to-feed type
   c The one ordered by the doctor
   d The powdered form

17 When warming a baby bottle
   a Warm the bottle in the microwave
   b Leave the formula out to warm at room temperature
   c Check that the formula is warm on the inside of your wrist
   d Boil the formula in a pan for 5 minutes

18 When bottle-feeding a baby
   a Tilt the bottle so the formula fills the neck of the bottle and the nipple
   b Save remaining formula for the next feeding
   c Burp the baby every 5 minutes
   d Leave the baby alone with the bottle

19 A newborn's cord has not yet healed. The diaper should be
   a Loose over the cord
   b Snug over the cord
   c Below the cord
   d Disposable

20 A circumcision is cleaned
   a Once a day
   b When the baby has a BM
   c 3 times a day
   d At every diaper change

21 Bath water for a newborn should be
   a 85°F to 90°F
   b 90°F to 95°F
   c 95°F to 100°F
   d 100°F to 105°F

22 Which should you use to wash a baby's nose?
   a A mitted washcloth
   b Alcohol wipes
   c A cotton swab
   d Cotton balls

23 A mother has a red vaginal discharge the first few days after childbirth. This
   a Is a menstrual period
   b Signals a postpartum complication
   c Is lochia rubra
   d Is from her episiotomy

24 A cesarean delivery involves
   a A vaginal incision
   b A perineal incision
   c An abdominal incision
   d A normal delivery through the birth canal

Answers to Chapter 52 questions are on p. 872.

FOCUS ON PRACTICE

Problem Solving

Mrs. Crawford had a vaginal delivery yesterday. She just finished breast-feeding and stands to the lay the baby down. You enter the room to measure her vital signs. As she stands, she says: "I just felt a gush of blood. Is that normal?" How will you respond? What will you do? Describe normal and abnormal vaginal discharge after birth.

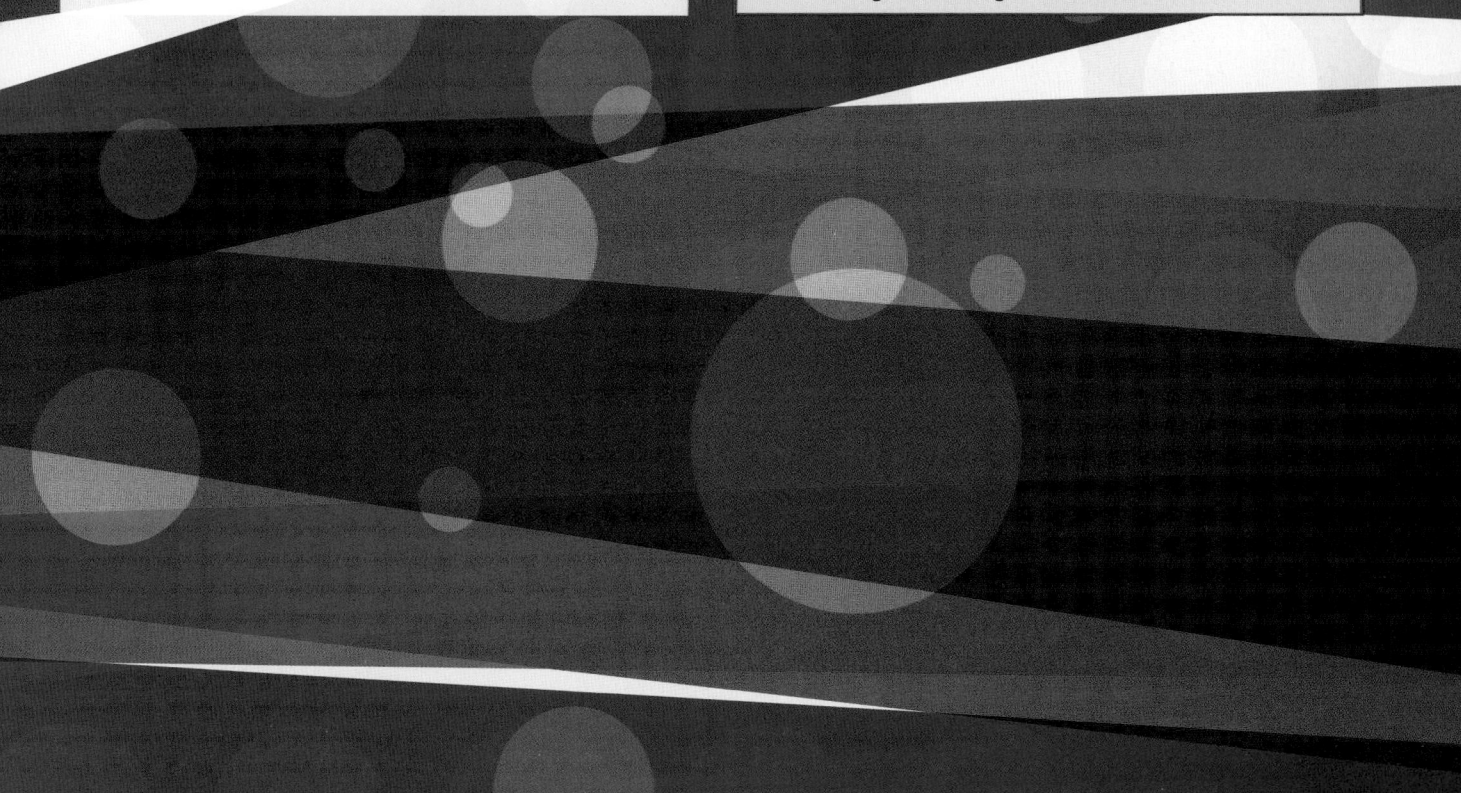

OBJECTIVES

- Define the key terms and key abbreviations in this chapter.
- Describe the purpose of assisted living.
- Describe assisted living residents and their rights.
- Identify the types of assisted living residences and the living areas offered.
- Describe requirements and features of assisted living units.
- Describe the requirements for assisted living staff.
- Describe the usual needs and abilities of assisted living residents.

- Describe an assisted living service plan.
- Explain how to safely assist with meals, housekeeping, and laundry.
- Explain how to assist with drugs.
- Identify the reasons for transferring, discharging, or evicting a person.
- Explain how to promote PRIDE in the person, the family, and yourself.

KEY TERMS

assisted living A housing option for older persons who need help with activities of daily living but do not need constant care
medication reminder Reminding the person to take drugs, observing them being taken as prescribed, and recording that they were taken

service plan A written plan listing the services needed, how much help is needed, and who provides services

KEY ABBREVIATIONS

ADL Activities of daily living

ALR Assisted living residence

Many older people cannot or do not want to live alone. Some need help with self-care or taking drugs. Some have physical or cognitive problems and disabilities. *Assisted living is a housing option for older persons who need help with activities of daily living (ADL) but do not need constant care.*

Assisted living residences (ALRs) offer quality of life with independence, companionship, and social involvement. A home-like setting is provided.

ALRs may be part of a retirement community, nursing center, senior citizen housing, or a stand-alone facility. Licensing requirements and residents' rights vary from state to state.

See *Promoting Safety and Comfort: Assisted Living.*

PROMOTING SAFETY AND COMFORT

Assisted Living

Safety

Residents have the same diseases and illnesses as persons at home, in hospitals, and in nursing centers. Infections are risks. This includes sexually transmitted and other communicable diseases. Follow Standard Precautions and the Bloodborne Pathogen Standard when in contact with blood, body fluids, secretions, and excretions, or when contact with potentially contaminated items and surfaces is likely.

ASSISTED LIVING RESIDENTS

Assisted living residents do not have complex medical problems and do not need 24-hour nursing care. However, they usually need some help with 1 or more ADL.

- Personal care—bathing, dressing, grooming, elimination
- Meals—cooking, eating
- Taking drugs
- Housekeeping
- Personal safety
- Transportation

Mobility is often a requirement. The person walks or uses a wheelchair or motor scooter. The person is able to leave the building in an emergency. Stable health also is required. Only limited health care or treatment is needed.

Resident Rights

ALR residents have rights and liberties as United States citizens. They also gain special rights under state laws and rules (Box 53-1) for ALRs. Such rights are similar to those in Chapter 2. If unable to exercise his or her rights, family members, legal representatives, or ombudsmen act on the person's behalf.

ALR SERVICES AND LIVING AREAS

Assisted living residences usually offer:

- 3 meals a day
- Help with ADL—bathing, dressing, grooming, toileting, eating, walking
- Housekeeping, laundry, and maintenance
- A 24-hour communications system for an emergency or to call for help
- 24-hour security and supervision
- Transportation
- Social, educational, recreational, and spiritual services
- Help with shopping, banking, and money management
- Some health services
- Exercise and wellness programs
- Medication (drug) management or help taking drugs
- Supervision for persons with Alzheimer's disease (AD), dementia, or other disabilities

Living areas vary. A small apartment has a bedroom, bathroom, living area, kitchen, and laundry areas (Figs. 53-1 and 53-2). Some people just want a bedroom and bathroom. Box 53-2, p. 824 lists the requirements and features of assisted living units.

See *Focus on Long-Term Care and Home Care: ALR Services and Living Areas*, p. 824.

BOX 53-1	Assisted Living Resident Rights

A resident has the right to:

- Not be discriminated against based on race, national origin, religion, gender, sexual orientation, age, disability, marital status, or diagnosis.
- Receive ALR services that support and respect the person's individuality, choices, strengths, and abilities.
- Receive privacy in:
  - Personal care
  - Correspondence, communication, and visits
  - Financial and personal matters
- Maintain, use, and display personal items. Such items must not pose a safety hazard.
- Take part in or refuse to take part in activities—social, recreational, rehabilitative, religious, political, community.
- Review his or her medical record.
- Take part in developing a service plan. The resident may have his or her family or representative involved.
- Have help from others (family, representative) in understanding, protecting, or exercising resident rights.

Modified from Resident Rights, Arizona Administrative Code (R9-10-810).

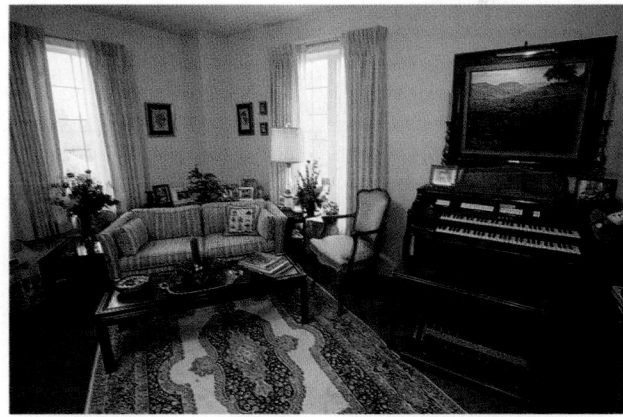

FIGURE 53-1 A living area in an assisted living apartment.

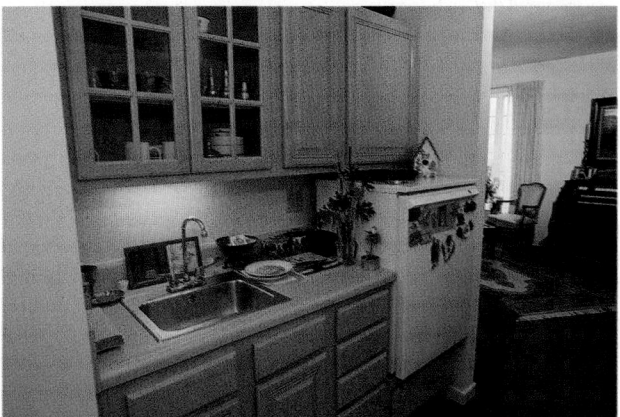

FIGURE 53-2 A kitchen in an assisted living apartment.

BOX 53-2	Assisted Living Units

Required Features

- A door that locks; the person keeps a key
- A telephone jack
- A 24-hour emergency communication system in the person's room
- A window or door that provides natural light
- Wheelchair access
- Lighted common areas
- A window or door that allows safe exit in an emergency
- A mailbox for each person
- A bathroom that provides privacy
  - A sink in the bathroom or in the next room
  - A bathtub or shower that has a shower curtain and non-slip surfaces
  - Ventilation or a window that opens
  - Grab bars for the toilet and bathtub or shower
  - Other assistive devices needed for safety and identified in the service plan
- Smoke alarms and a fire sprinkler system
- A bed (frame and mattress) that is clean and in good repair
- General and task lighting
- An easy chair
- A table and chair for meals
- Adjustable window covers that provide privacy
- A dresser or storage space for clothing and personal items
- Appliances for food—sink, stove, refrigerator with freezer, and storage for food and cooking items

Environment Requirements

- The ALR is clean, safe, orderly, odor-free, and in good repair.
- The ALR is free of insects and rodents.
- Garbage is stored in covered containers lined with plastic bags. Bags are removed at least once a week.
- Hot water temperatures are no higher than 120°F (Fahrenheit).
- The hot and cold water supply meets hygiene needs.
- Bathrooms have toilet paper, soap, and cloth towels, paper towels, or a hand dryer.
- Clean linens are handled, transported, and stored to prevent contamination.
- Soiled linen and clothing are stored in closed containers away from food, kitchen, and dining areas.
- Oxygen containers are stored according to the manufacturer's instructions.
- Cleaning solutions, insecticides, and other hazardous substances are stored in their original containers. They are in locked cabinets in rooms separate from food, dining areas, and drugs.
- Pets and animals are controlled to protect residents and maintain sanitation.
- Employees have access to a first aid kit.

FOCUS ON LONG-TERM CARE AND HOME CARE

ALR Services and Living Areas

Home Care

Unlike assisted living residents, home care patients may still need medical care. They may need help with:

- Prescribed exercises
- Changing wound dressings
- Taking drugs, fluids, or feedings intravenously
- Measuring vital signs
- Managing urinary catheters or ostomies
- Taking drugs correctly
- Personal care, dressing, and grooming
- Getting in and out of bed, showers or bathtubs, and cars

The home care patient may need help with meals, food safety, housekeeping, and laundry. The measures described in this chapter apply to the home setting. So do the measures for medication assistance if that role is allowed by your state and agency.

STAFF REQUIREMENTS

Staff requirements vary among states. Some require a nursing assistant training and competency evaluation program (NATCEP). Besides a NATCEP, staff may need additional training in these areas.

- The needs and goals of ALR residents
- Using service plans
- Menu planning and food preparation, service, and storage
- Housekeeping and sanitation
- Assisting with drugs

Criminal background and fingerprint checks are common requirements. The ALR cannot employ a person with a criminal record.

SERVICE PLANS

Similar to a care plan, a *service plan is a written plan listing:*

- *The services needed*
- *How much help is needed*
- *Who provides the services*

The plan relates to ADL, activities and social services, dietary needs, taking drugs, and special needs.

For example, the service plan states that you will help the person get dressed. For physical therapy after a hip fracture, a physical therapist will visit. And a family member will assist with the person's drugs.

The plan is reviewed when the person's condition, wants, or service needs change. Services are added or reduced as needed.

Meals

Three meals a day and snacks are provided. Special dietary needs are met. Menus are posted for residents to see.

Dining options range from cafeteria style to fine dining. Residents eat in the dining room with others. Or they can eat in their rooms if they wish.

Food Safety

Certain measures are needed to handle, prepare, and store food. They protect against infection. See Chapter 27. Also practice these safety measures.

- Follow the safe handling instructions on food labels (Fig. 53-3).
- Use liquid detergent and hot water to wash eating and cooking items. Wash glasses and cups first. Follow with silverware, bowls, and then pots and pans. Rinse well with hot water.
- Place washed items in a drainer to dry. Air-drying is more aseptic than towel drying.
- Rinse dishes before loading them into a dishwasher. Use dishwasher soap.
- Do not wash pots and pans and cast iron, wood, and some plastic items in a dishwasher.
- Clean appliances, counters, tables, and other surfaces after each meal. Use hot, soapy water and paper towels or clean cloths.
- Remove grease spills and splashes. Use a liquid surface cleaner.
- Clean sinks with a sink cleaner.
- Save or discard left-overs.
- Dispose of garbage and other soiled supplies after each meal. Use a garbage disposal for food and liquid garbage but not bones.
- Recycle paper, boxes, cans, and plastic containers according to ALR policy.
- Empty garbage at least once a day.

Housekeeping

Housekeeping measures help prevent infection. And they keep living units neat and clean.

- Wipe up spills right away.
- Use a dust mop or broom to sweep. Use a dustpan to collect dust and crumbs.
- Sweep daily or more often as needed.
- Make sure toilets flush after each use.
- Rinse the sink after washing, shaving, or oral hygiene.
- Clean the tub or shower after each use.
- Remove and dispose of hair from the sink, tub, or shower.
- Hang towels to dry. Or place them in a hamper.

Safe Handling Instructions

This product was prepared from inspected and passed meat and/or poultry. Some food products may contain bacteria that could cause illness if the product is mishandled or cooked improperly. For your protection, follow these safe handling instructions.

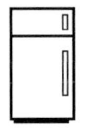 Keep refrigerated or frozen. Thaw in refrigerator or microwave.

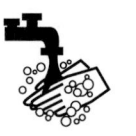 Keep raw meat and poultry separate from other foods. Wash working surfaces (including cutting boards), utensils, and hands after touching raw meat or poultry.

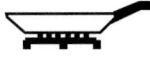 Cook thoroughly.

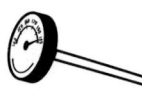 Keep hot foods hot. Refrigerate leftovers immediately or discard.

FIGURE 53-3 Safe handling instructions for meat and poultry. They are required by the U.S. Department of Agriculture. (Redrawn from [USDA] United States Department of Agriculture, Food Safety and Inspection Service.)

- Clean bathroom surfaces every day. Use a disinfectant or water and detergent to clean all surfaces.
  - The toilet bowl, seat, and outside areas of the toilet
  - The floor
  - The sides, walls, and curtain or door of the tub or shower
  - Towel racks and toilet tissue, toothbrush, and soap holders
  - The sink and mirror
  - Window sills
- Mop or vacuum the bathroom floor every day.
- Empty bathroom wastebaskets every day.
- Put out clean towels and washcloths every day.
- Wash bath mats, the wastebasket, and laundry hamper every week.
- Replace toilet and facial tissues as needed.
- Open bathroom windows for a short time. Also use air fresheners.
- Dust furniture at least weekly.
- Vacuum floors at least weekly and as needed.

Laundry

Clean linens may be provided. For personal laundry, residents can use a washer, dryer, iron, and ironing board. When assisting with laundry:

- Wear gloves to handle soiled laundry (see *Promoting Safety and Comfort: Assisted Living*, p. 822).
- Separate white, colored, and dark items. Separate sturdy and delicate fabrics.
- Empty pockets.
- Fasten buttons, zippers, snaps, hooks, and other closures.
- Wash heavily soiled items separately.
- Follow detergent directions.
- Follow care label directions and the person's preferences for the correct:
  - Wash cycle and water temperature
  - Drying temperature and cycle
- Fold, hang, or iron clothes as the person prefers.

See *Teamwork and Time Management: Laundry.*

TEAMWORK AND TIME MANAGEMENT

Laundry

Residents may share washers and dryers. If assisting with laundry, remove clothes from washers and dryers promptly. Others may want to use the machines.

Sometimes laundry is left in a washer or dryer. First, try to find the person who left the laundry. Politely tell the person that the machine is done and that you have laundry to do. Offer to remove the laundry if the other person is busy. If you cannot find that person, do the following.

- If left in a washer—place wet items on a clean surface, not in the dryer. Some items may need to dry flat, hang to dry, or need certain dryer settings. Or the resident may have drying preferences.
- If left in a dryer—fold and place items on a clean surface.

While laundry is in the washer or dryer, tend to other tasks. Assist with ADL, do housekeeping, prepare meals, and so on.

Nursing Services

Some ALRs provide limited nursing services. The nurse assesses each person and monitors health. The nurse supervises tasks delegated to you. If a person cannot manage his or her own drugs, the nurse gives them.

Medication Assistance

Drugs must be taken as prescribed. The 6 rights of drug administration are:

- The right drug
- The right dose (amount)
- The right route (by mouth, injection, applied to the skin, inhalation, vaginally, or rectally)
- The right time
- The right person
- The right documentation (recording)

Your role depends on your state's laws, ALR policy, and your training and education. *Remember, you do not give drugs (Chapter 3). Also remember that the person has the right to refuse to take prescribed drugs.* Your role may involve:

- Reminding the person to take a drug
- Reading the drug label to the person
- Opening containers if the person cannot do so
- Checking the dosage against the drug label
- Providing water, juice, milk, crackers, applesauce, or other food and fluids
- Making sure the person takes the right drug, the right amount, at the right time, and in the right way (route)
- Recording that the person took or refused to take the drug (right documentation)
- Storing drugs

Self-directed medication management is when residents manage and take their own drugs. The person knows drugs by name, color, or shape. The person knows what drugs to take, the correct doses, and when and how to take them. The person questions changes in the usual drug routine. For example, a pill is not broken in half. Or a pill looks different. Report comments or questions to the nurse.

Pill organizers (Fig. 53-4) have sections for days and times. They are for a week or month. The person, a family member or representative, or a nurse prepares the pill organizer. Drugs are taken on the right day and at the right time.

You may need to remind some people. A *medication reminder means reminding the person to take drugs, observing them being taken as prescribed, and recording that they were taken.* Setting clock or wireless phone alarms for when to take drugs is useful for some people.

See *Focus on Communication: Medication Assistance.*

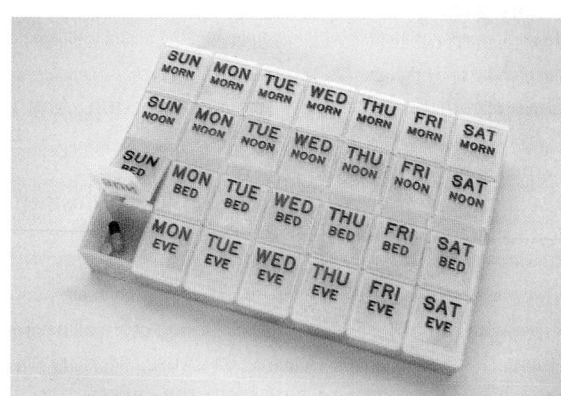

FIGURE 53-4 Pill organizer.

Medication Record. A medication record is kept. The record includes:
- The person's name
- Drug name, dose, directions, and route of administration
- Date and time to take the drug
- Date and time help was given
- Signature or initials of the person assisting

Drug Errors. Report any drug error to the nurse. Also complete an incident report. An error means 1 or more of the following.
- Taking another person's drugs
- Taking the wrong drug
- Taking the wrong dose
- Taking an extra dose
- Missing or skipping a dose
- Taking a drug at the wrong time
- Taking a drug by the wrong route
- Not taking a drug when ordered
- Not recording that a drug was taken

Storing Drugs. Drugs are kept in a secure place. This prevents others from taking them. The ALR may keep drugs in a locked place. Some persons store their own drugs. If sharing a room, each person's ability to safely have drugs is assessed. Drugs are in a locked container if safety is a factor.

Drugs must have the original pharmacy label. They are stored as directed on the label. For example, some drugs are refrigerated. Others are kept away from light. The label also has an expiration date. The ALR has procedures for disposing of expired or discontinued drugs.

Activities and Recreation

Residents are urged to take part in activity and recreational programs. Social, physical, and community activities promote well-being and independence. An activities director plans, organizes, and conducts the ALR's activity program. ALR and community events and activities are noted on a calendar.

Special Services and Safety Needs

Sometimes emergencies occur. Some people need help getting out of bed or transferring to a wheelchair. Then they can leave the building with little or no help.

Other people cannot walk or use a wheelchair. They need attendants 24 hours a day. The ALR and the person agree on how and who will meet the person's needs.

TRANSFER, DISCHARGE, AND EVICTION

Residents can be transferred, discharged, or evicted. The ALR must tell the person about the action. Reasons are:
- The ALR can no longer meet the person's needs. The person is a threat to the health and safety of self or others. Or the ALR cannot provide needed care.
- The person fails to pay for services.
- The person fails to comply with ALR policies or rules.
- The person wants to transfer.
- The ALR closes.

Continued

FOCUS ON P R I D E—cont'd

The Person, Family, and Yourself

D elegation and Teamwork

Residents are allowed to have personal belongings. This helps the apartment or room feel home-like. Good teamwork is needed when new residents arrive. The person and family should see that the staff is helpful and works together to meet the person's needs.

E thics and Laws

How you assist with drugs depends on your state's laws, ALR policy, and your training. There are legal limits to your role. If you act beyond those limits, you could be practicing nursing without a license. You can lose your job and your ability to work as a nursing assistant. Follow the limits for your state and agency.

FOCUS ON **PRIDE**: *Application*

Identify the changes a new ALR resident faces. How might the person respond? Describe positive and negative feelings. How do the following affect the transition?
* The person's attitude
* The family's involvement and support level
* The ALR's appearance
* The ALR staff's conduct

REVIEW QUESTIONS

Circle T *if the statement is TRUE and* F *if it is FALSE.*

1 T F   ALRs provide 24-hour nursing care.

2 T F   Some ALR residents have Alzheimer's disease.

3 T F   ALR residents must have stable health.

4 T F   ALR residents must speak English.

5 T F   ALRs provide 24-hour security.

6 T F   ALR residents can refuse care.

7 T F   ALR residents must organize their own activities.

8 T F   Resident apartment doors must remain unlocked.

9 T F   ALRs provide an emergency communication system.

10 T F   Food safety involves following safe handling instructions on food labels.

Circle the BEST answer.

11 Which violates an ALR resident's rights?
   a Covering the person during personal care
   b Giving the person opened mail
   c Keeping information confidential
   d Not allowing the use of harmful personal items

12 A person wants to attend a concert. Which is *true?*
   a The ALR must approve the concert.
   b The person must return by 10 PM.
   c An attendant must go with the person.
   d The ALR must respect the person's choice.

13 Assisted living staff must
   a Complete a nursing assistant training and evaluation program
   b Meet state requirements
   c Assist with drugs
   d Provide transportation for residents

14 A service plan
   a Describes nursing care needs
   b Lists the drugs the person needs to take
   c Describes needed services and who provides them
   d Lists service fees and charges

15 Which statement about ALR dining is *true?*
   a Residents are allowed to eat in their rooms.
   b Residents must cook their own meals.
   c The family provides meals if a special diet is needed.
   d Eating in the dining room is discouraged.

16 When assisting with housekeeping
   a Dust and vacuum daily
   b Wipe up spills right away
   c Clean the bathroom only as needed
   d Put out clean washcloths and towels weekly

17 You assist with laundry. Which is *true?*
   a Care label directions are followed.
   b Clothes are washed in hot water.
   c Clothes are ironed.
   d Gloves are not needed for soiled laundry.

18 Usually ALR nursing assistants are allowed to
   a Give drugs
   b Give medication reminders
   c Refill drugs
   d Prepare pill organizers

19 Drugs are kept
   a In the person's closet
   b In the person's drawer
   c In a secure place
   d With the family

20 The ALR cannot provide a person with all needed services. Which is *true?*
   a The ALR must hire more staff.
   b The family must provide the needed care.
   c The ALR can ask the person to transfer.
   d The person's service plan needs to change.

Answers to Chapter 53 questions are on p. 872.

FOCUS ON PRACTICE

Problem Solving

Your state and ALR allow you to assist with drugs. The roles on p. 826 are allowed. Mr. Boyd asks you to help put in his eye drops and apply a "patch for his heart." What do you do? Explain what you can and cannot do.

Basic Emergency Care

OBJECTIVES

- Define the key terms and key abbreviations in this chapter.
- Describe the rules of emergency care.
- Identify the signs of cardiac arrest and the emergency care required.
- Describe emergency care for poisoning.
- Describe emergency care for hemorrhage, fainting, and shock.
- Describe emergency care for stroke.
- Explain how to care for a person during a seizure.
- Describe emergency care for concussions.
- Describe emergency care for burns.
- Perform the procedures described in this chapter.
- Explain how to promote PRIDE in the person, the family, and yourself.

KEY TERMS

anaphylaxis A life-threatening sensitivity to an antigen

cardiac arrest See "sudden cardiac arrest"

convulsion See "seizure"

fainting The sudden loss of consciousness from an inadequate blood supply to the brain

first aid Emergency care given to an ill or injured person before medical help arrives

hemorrhage The excessive loss of blood in a short time

respiratory arrest Breathing stops but heart action continues for several minutes

seizure Violent and sudden contractions or tremors of muscle groups caused by abnormal electrical activity in the brain; convulsion

shock Results when tissues and organs do not get enough blood

sudden cardiac arrest (SCA) The heart stops suddenly and without warning; cardiac arrest

KEY ABBREVIATIONS

AED	Automated external defibrillator		**EMS**	Emergency Medical Services
AHA	American Heart Association		**MET**	Medical Emergency Team
BLS	Basic Life Support		**RRT**	Rapid Response Team
CPR	Cardiopulmonary resuscitation		**SCA**	Sudden cardiac arrest
ECC	Emergency Cardiovascular Care		**VF; V-fib**	Ventricular fibrillation

Emergencies can occur anywhere. Sometimes you can save a life if you know what to do. First aid and Basic Life Support (BLS) courses prepare you to give emergency care.

The BLS procedures in this chapter are given as basic information. They do not replace certification training. You need a BLS course for health care providers.

BLS guidelines are updated as new information becomes available. You are responsible for following current guidelines. Emergency Cardiovascular Care (ECC) updates can be found on-line at ECCguidelines.heart.org.

EMERGENCY CARE

First aid is the emergency care given to an ill or injured person before medical help arrives. The goals of first aid are to:

- Prevent death.
- Prevent injuries from becoming worse.

In an emergency, the Emergency Medical Services (EMS) system is activated. Emergency personnel (paramedics, emergency medical technicians) rush to the scene. They treat, stabilize, and transport persons with life-threatening problems. They have guidelines for care and communicate with doctors in hospital emergency rooms. The doctors can direct their care. Their ambulances have emergency drugs, equipment, and supplies. To activate the EMS system, do 1 of the following.

- Dial 911.
- Call the local fire or police department.
- Call the phone operator.

Each emergency is different. The rules in Box 54-1 apply to any emergency. Hospitals and other agencies have procedures for emergencies. Rapid Response Teams (RRTs) or Medical Emergency Teams (METs) are called when a person shows warning signs of a life-threatening condition. An RRT (MET) may include a doctor, a nurse, and a respiratory therapist. The RRT's (MET's) goal is to prevent death.

See *Focus on Communication: Emergency Care.*

See *Focus on Long-Term Care and Home Care: Emergency Care.*

See *Promoting Safety and Comfort: Emergency Care.*

BOX 54-1   Emergency Care Rules

- Wait for help to arrive if the scene is not safe enough for you to approach.
- Know your limits. Do not do more than you are able. Do not perform an unfamiliar procedure. Do what you can under the circumstances.
- Stay calm. This helps the person feel more secure.
- Know where to find emergency supplies.
- Follow Standard Precautions and the Bloodborne Pathogen Standard to the extent possible.
- Check for life-threatening problems. Check for breathing, a pulse, and bleeding.
- Keep the person lying down or as you found him or her. Moving the person could make an injury worse.
- Move the person only if the setting is unsafe. Examples include:
  - A burning car or building
  - A building that might collapse
  - Stormy conditions with lightning
  - In water
  - Near electrical wires
- Perform necessary emergency measures.
- Call for help. Or have someone activate the EMS system. *Do not hang up until the operator has hung up.* Give the following information.
  - Your location—street address and city, cross streets or roads, and landmarks
  - Phone number you are calling from
  - What seems to have happened (for example: heart attack, crash, fire)—police, fire equipment, and ambulances may be needed
  - How many people need help
  - Conditions of victims, obvious injuries, and life-threatening situations
  - What aid is being given
- Do not remove clothes unless you have to. If you must remove clothing, tear or cut garments along the seams. (For CPR, remove clothing or move it out of the way. See p. 832.)
- Keep the person warm. Cover the person with a blanket, coats, or sweaters.
- Reassure the person. Explain what is happening and that help was called.
- Do not give the person fluids.
- Keep on-lookers away. They invade privacy and tend to stare, give advice, and comment about the person's condition. The person may think the situation is worse than it is.

FOCUS ON COMMUNICATION

Emergency Care

Some illnesses and injuries are life-threatening. To find out what happened and the person's condition, you can say:
- "Are you okay?"
- "Tell me what's wrong."
- "Where does it hurt?"
- "If you can, please point to where it hurts."
- "Can you move your arms and legs?"

FOCUS ON LONG-TERM CARE AND HOME CARE

Emergency Care

Long-Term Care

In nursing centers, a nurse decides when to activate the EMS system. The nurse tells you how to help. If a person has stopped breathing or is in sudden cardiac arrest, the nurse may start cardiopulmonary resuscitation (CPR). Some centers allow nursing assistants to start CPR. Others do not. Know your center's policy about CPR.

Death is expected in persons with terminal illnesses. Usually these persons are not resuscitated (Chapter 55). This information is in the care plan.

PROMOTING SAFETY AND COMFORT

Emergency Care

Safety

During emergencies, contact with blood, body fluids, secretions, and excretions is likely. Follow Standard Precautions and the Bloodborne Pathogen Standard to the extent possible.

When an emergency occurs in an agency, call for the nurse at once. You may need to activate the EMS system or the RRT (MET). Or you take the person's vital signs (Chapter 29). Assist as instructed by the nurse.

Comfort

Mental comfort is important during emergencies. Help the person feel safe and secure. Give reassurance. Explain the care you provide. Use a calm approach.

BLS FOR ADULTS

When the heart and breathing stop, the person is clinically dead. Blood is not circulated through the body. Heart, brain, and other organ damage occurs within minutes. The American Heart Association's (AHA's) BLS procedures support circulation and breathing.

Sudden Cardiac Arrest

Sudden cardiac arrest (SCA) or *cardiac arrest is when the heart stops suddenly and without warning.* Within moments, breathing stops as well. Permanent brain and other organ damage occurs unless circulation and breathing are restored.

There are 3 major signs of SCA.
* No response.
* No breathing or no normal breathing. The person may have *agonal gasps* or *agonal respirations* early during SCA. (*Agonal* means *to struggle*. Agonal is used in relation to death and dying.) Agonal gasps do not bring enough oxygen into the lungs. Agonal gasps are not normal breathing.
* No pulse.

The person's skin is cool, pale, and gray. The person is not coughing or moving.

SCA is a sudden, unexpected, and dramatic event. It can occur anywhere and at any time—while driving, shoveling snow, playing golf or tennis, watching TV, eating, or sleeping. Common causes include heart disease, heart attack, enlarged heart, heart valve problems, dysrhythmias (arrhythmias), and congenital heart defects (Chapter 45). Electrical shock, chest trauma, and illegal drug use are other causes. These causes lead to an abnormal heart rhythm called ventricular fibrillation (p. 835). The heart cannot pump blood. A normal rhythm must be restored. Otherwise the person will die.

Chains of Survival. The AHA's BLS courses teach *Chains of Survival*. The Chains of Survival identify the different pathways of care for in-hospital and out-of-hospital cardiac arrests (Box 54-2). Care is provided as soon as possible. Any delay reduces the person's chance of surviving.

See *Focus on Communication: Chains of Survival.*

Respiratory Arrest

Respiratory arrest is when breathing stops but heart action continues for several minutes. If breathing is not restored, cardiac arrest occurs. Respiratory arrest can occur from:
* Problems affecting nerves, muscles, or areas of the brain that control breathing—amyotrophic lateral sclerosis (ALS), spinal cord injuries, stroke (Chapter 44); drug or alcohol over-dose; drug side-effects
* Damage to the lungs—injury to the chest
* Lung disorders and problems—pneumonia, chronic obstructive pulmonary disease (Chapter 45), pulmonary embolism (Chapter 35)
* Blocked airflow—choking (Chapter 13 and p. 844), drowning, suffocation
* Inhaling harmful substances—smoke, chemicals, fumes

Rescue Breathing. Rescue breaths are given when there is a pulse but no breathing or only agonal gasping. To give rescue breaths:
* Open the airway (p. 833).
* Give 1 breath every 5 to 6 seconds for adults.
* Give 1 breath every 3 to 5 seconds for infants and children.
* Give each breath over 1 second. The chest should rise when breaths are given.
* Check the pulse every 2 minutes. If there is no pulse, begin CPR. If the pulse is 60 or less in an infant or child, begin CPR (p. 839).

BOX 54-2   Chains of Survival

In-Hospital Chain of Survival
1. Surveillance and prevention.
2. Recognizing cardiac arrest and activating the EMS system.
3. Immediate high-quality CPR.
4. Rapid defibrillation. See p. 835.
5. Advanced life support and post-arrest care. This is care given to improve survival following cardiac arrest.

Out-of-Hospital Chain of Survival
1. Recognizing cardiac arrest and activating the EMS system.
2. Immediate high-quality CPR.
3. Rapid defibrillation.
4. Basic and advanced EMS. Care is given by EMS staff, doctors, nurses, and respiratory therapists. They give drugs and perform life-saving measures.
5. Advanced life support and post-arrest care.

FOCUS ON COMMUNICATION

Chains of Survival

Getting help is a critical step. If alone, activate the EMS system using your wireless phone while continuing to give care. If alone with no wireless phone, leave the adult to activate the EMS system and get an AED yourself before giving care. (AED stands for automated external defibrillator. See p. 835.) Guidelines for children and infants differ from adult guidelines. See p. 839.

If others are around, tell a certain person to activate the EMS system. You may not know the person's name. Point to the person. Make eye contact. You can say: "Call 911 and get an AED." Begin care. Follow up soon. Make sure the person was able to call for help.

Adult CPR

When the heart and breathing stop, blood and oxygen are not supplied to the body. Brain and other organ damage occurs within minutes.

CPR must be started at once when a person has SCA. CPR supports circulation and breathing. It provides blood and oxygen to the heart, brain, and other organs until advanced emergency care is given. CPR involves:
* Chest compressions
* Airway
* Breathing
* Defibrillation

CPR procedures require speed, skill, and efficiency. See *Promoting Safety and Comfort: Adult CPR*, p. 832.

Chest Compressions. The heart, brain, and other organs must receive blood. Otherwise, permanent damage results. In cardiac arrest, the heart has stopped beating. Blood must be pumped through the body another way. Chest compressions force blood through the circulatory system.

Before starting chest compressions, check for a pulse. Use the carotid artery on the side near you. To find the carotid pulse, place 2 or 3 fingertips on the trachea (windpipe). Then slide your fingers down off the trachea to the groove of the neck (Fig. 54-1). Check for a pulse for no more than 10 seconds. While checking for a pulse, look for signs of circulation. See if the person has started breathing or is coughing or moving.

The heart lies between the sternum (breastbone) and the spinal column. When pressure is applied to the sternum, the sternum is depressed (moved down). This compresses the heart between the sternum and spinal column (Fig. 54-2). For effective chest compressions, the person must be supine on a hard, flat surface—floor or back-board. You are positioned at the person's side.

Hand position is important for effective chest compressions (Fig. 54-3). You use the heels of your hands—1 on top of the other—for chest compressions. For proper placement:

- Expose the person's chest. Remove clothing or move it out of the way. You need to see the person's bare skin for proper hand position.
- Place the heel of 1 hand (usually your dominant hand) in the center of the bare chest. The heel of this hand is placed between the nipples on the lower half of the sternum.
- Place the heel of your other hand on top of the heel of the first hand.

To give chest compressions, your arms are straight. Your shoulders are directly over your hands. And your fingers are interlocked (Fig. 54-4). Exert firm downward pressure to depress the average adult sternum at least 2 inches. According to AHA guidelines, avoid pressing down more than 2.4 inches. Then release pressure without removing your hands from the chest. Avoid leaning on the chest between compressions. Releasing pressure allows the chest to recoil—to return to its normal position. Recoil lets the heart fill with blood.

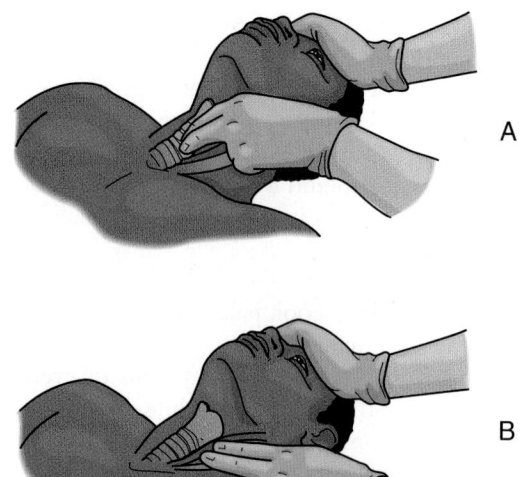
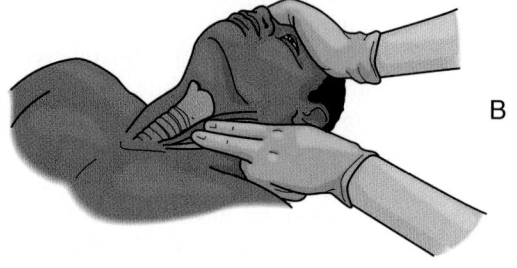

FIGURE 54-1 Locating the carotid pulse. **A,** Two fingers are placed on the trachea. **B,** The fingertips are moved down into the groove of the neck to the carotid artery.

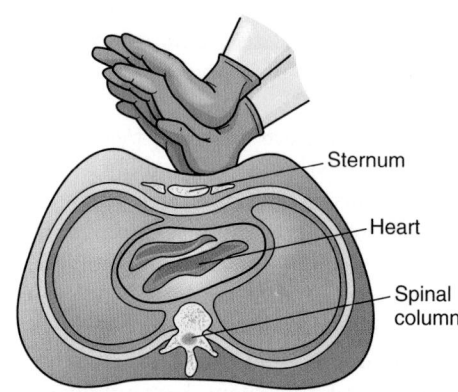

FIGURE 54-2 The heart lies between the sternum and the spinal column. The heart is compressed when pressure is applied to the sternum.

The AHA recommends that you:
- Give compressions at a rate of 100 to 120 per minute.
- Interrupt chest compressions only when necessary. Interruptions should be less than 10 seconds. When there are no chest compressions, blood does not flow to the heart, brain, and other organs.

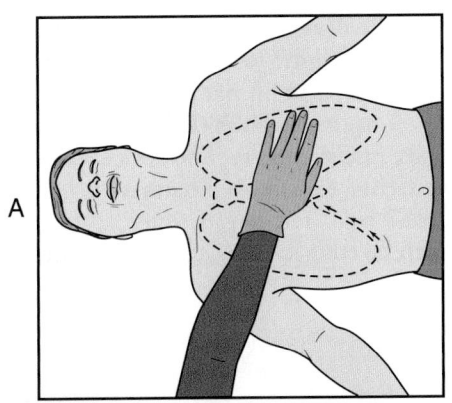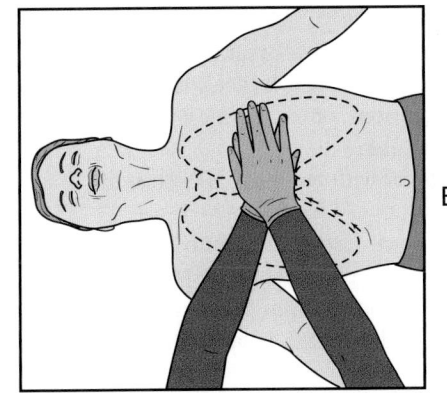

FIGURE 54-3 Proper hand position for CPR. **A,** The heel of the dominant hand is placed in the center of the chest. It is between the nipples and on the lower half of the sternum. **B,** The heel of the non-dominant hand is placed on top of the dominant hand.

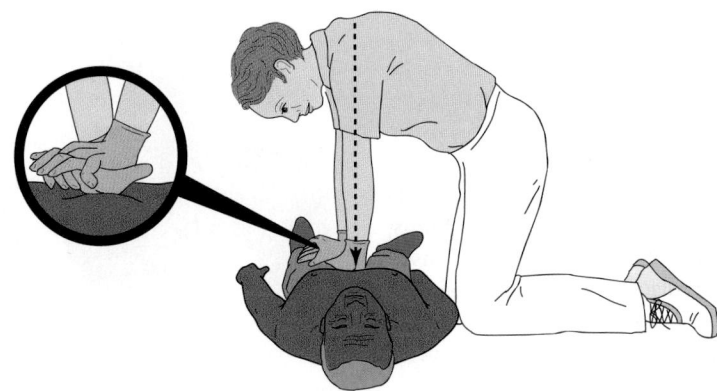

FIGURE 54-4 Giving chest compressions. The arms are straight. The shoulders are over the hands. The fingers are interlocked.

Airway. The respiratory passages (airway) must be open to restore breathing. The airway is often obstructed (blocked) during SCA. The person's tongue falls toward the back of the throat and blocks the airway. The head tilt–chin lift method opens the airway (Fig. 54-5).

- Place the palm of 1 hand on the forehead.
- Tilt the head back by pushing down on the forehead with your palm.
- Place the fingers of your other hand under the lower jaw. Use your index and middle fingers. Do not use your thumb.
- Lift the jaw. This brings the chin forward.
- Do not close the person's mouth. The mouth should be slightly open.

Breathing. Air is not inhaled when breathing stops. The person must get oxygen. If not, permanent heart, brain, and other organ damage occurs. The person is given *breaths*. That is, a rescuer inflates the person's lungs.

Each breath should take 1 second. *You should see the chest rise with each breath.* Two breaths are given after every 30 chest compressions.

See *Focus on Children and Older Persons: Breathing.*

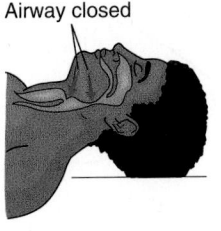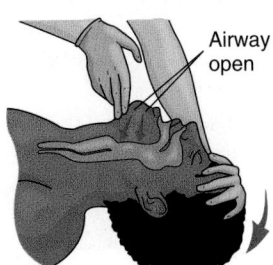

Airway closed

Airway open

FIGURE 54-5 The head tilt–chin lift method opens the airway. One hand is on the person's forehead. Pressure is applied to tilt the head back. The chin is lifted with the fingers of the other hand.

FOCUS ON CHILDREN AND OLDER PERSONS

Breathing

Children
When 2 rescuers perform CPR on an infant or child, 2 breaths are given after every 15 compressions (p. 839).

Mouth-to-Mouth Breathing. Mouth-to-mouth breathing (Fig. 54-6) is one way to give breaths. You place your mouth over the person's mouth. Contact with the person's blood, body fluids, secretions, or excretions is likely. To give mouth-to-mouth breathing:

1. Keep the airway open with the head tilt–chin lift method.
2. Pinch the nostrils shut. Use your thumb and index finger. Use the hand on the forehead. Shutting the nostrils prevents air from escaping through the nose.
3. Take a breath. A regular breath is needed, not a deep breath.
4. Place your mouth tightly over the person's mouth. Seal the mouth with your lips.
5. Blow air into the person's mouth. You should see the chest rise as the lungs fill with air.
6. Repeat the head tilt–chin lift method if the chest did not rise.
7. Remove your mouth from the person's mouth. Then take in a quick breath.
8. Give another breath. You should see the chest rise.

Barrier Device Breathing. A barrier device is used for giving breaths whenever possible. The device prevents contact with the person's mouth and blood, body fluids, secretions, or excretions. A face shield may be used (Fig. 54-7). A face shield is replaced with a face mask as soon as possible (Fig. 54-8, *A*). The mask is placed over the person's mouth and nose (Fig. 54-8, *B*). When using a barrier device, seal the device against the person's face. The seal must be tight. Then open the airway with the head tilt–chin lift method.

A bag valve mask (Fig. 54-9) is another device used to give rescue breaths. The device consists of a hand-held bag attached to a mask. The mask is held securely to the person's face. The bag is squeezed to give breaths. The bag can be connected to an oxygen source.

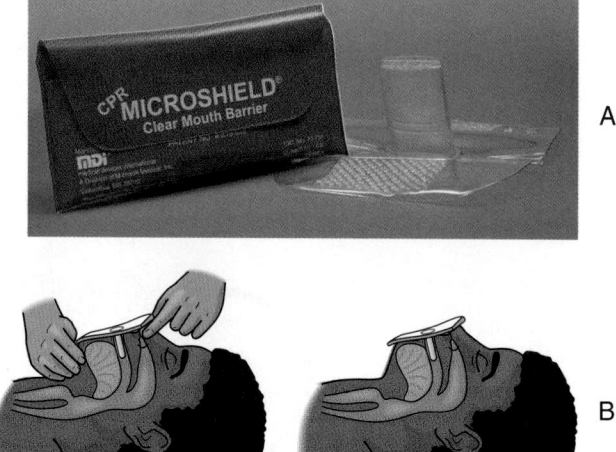

FIGURE 54-7 A, Face shield. **B,** The face shield is in place.

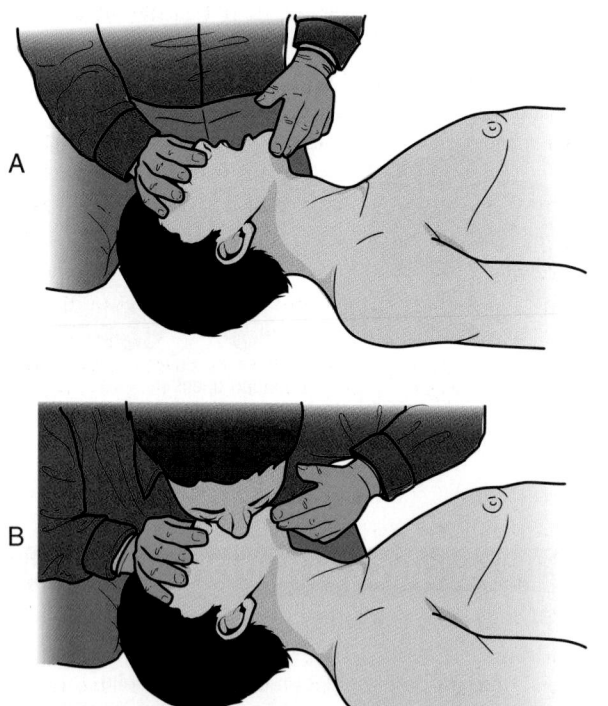

FIGURE 54-6 Mouth-to-mouth breathing. **A,** The person's airway is opened. The nostrils are pinched shut. **B,** The person's mouth is sealed by the rescuer's mouth.

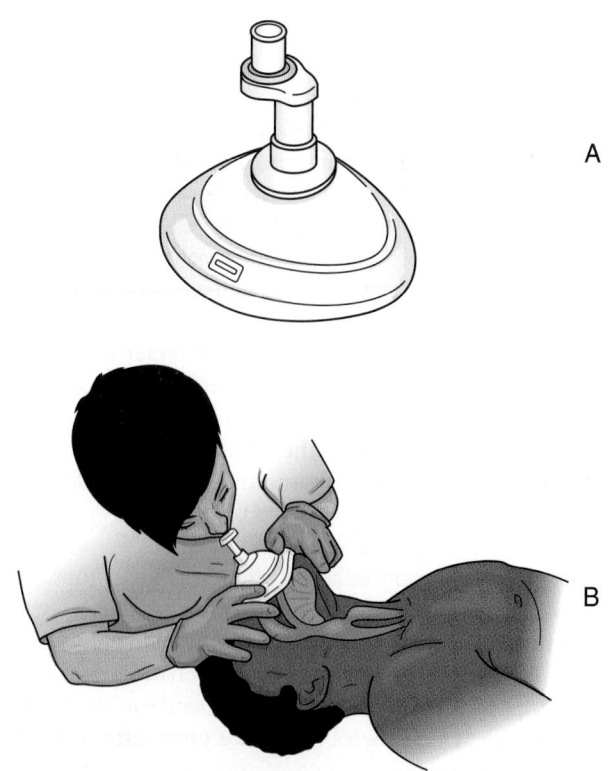

FIGURE 54-8 A, Mask for giving breaths. **B,** The mask is in place.

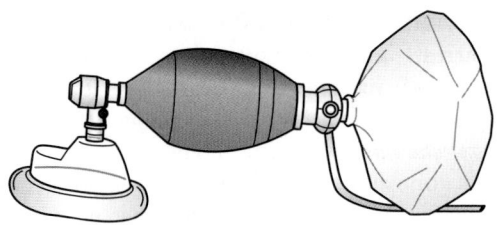

FIGURE 54-9 A bag valve mask.

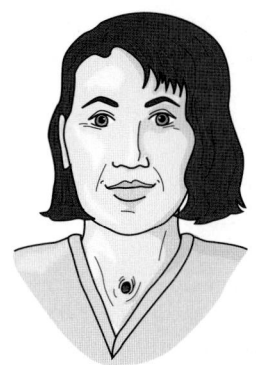

FIGURE 54-11 A stoma in the neck. The person breathes in and out of the stoma.

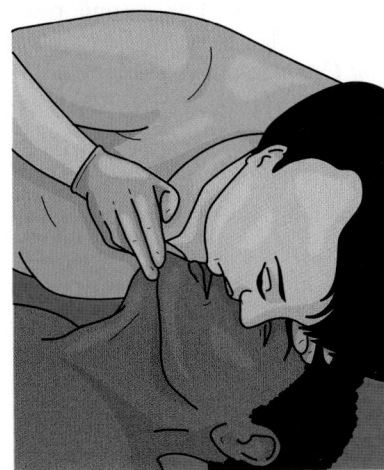

FIGURE 54-10 Mouth-to-nose breathing.

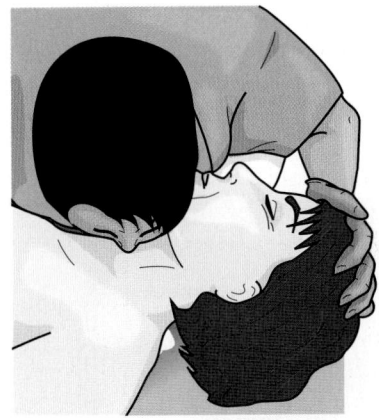

FIGURE 54-12 Mouth-to-stoma breathing.

Mouth-to-Nose Breathing. Mouth-to-nose breathing is used when:
- You cannot breathe through the person's mouth.
- You cannot open the mouth.
- Your mouth is too small to make a tight seal for mouth-to-mouth breathing.
- The mouth or jaw is severely injured.
- The person is bleeding from the mouth.

The mouth is closed for mouth-to-nose breathing. The head tilt–chin lift method opens the airway. Pressure is placed on the chin to close the mouth. To give a breath, place your mouth over the person's nose and blow air into the nose (Fig. 54-10). After giving a breath, remove your mouth from the person's nose.

Mouth-to-Stoma Breathing. Some people breathe through stomas (openings) in their necks (Fig. 54-11). To give mouth-to-stoma breathing:
1. Keep the person's mouth closed.
2. Do not tilt the person's head back.
3. Seal your mouth around the stoma.
4. Blow air into the stoma (Fig. 54-12).

If the person's chest does not rise, you may need to pinch the nostrils shut.

Before giving mouth-to-mouth or mouth-to-nose breathing, always check to see if the person has a stoma. Other rescue breathing methods are not effective if the person has a stoma.

Defibrillation. *Ventricular fibrillation (VF, V-fib)* is an abnormal heart rhythm (Fig. 54-13, p. 836). It causes sudden cardiac arrest. Rather than beating in a regular rhythm, the heart shakes and quivers like a bowl of Jell-O. The heart does not pump blood. The heart, brain, and other organs do not receive blood and oxygen.

A *defibrillator* is used to deliver a shock to the heart. The shock stops the VF (V-fib). This allows the return of a regular heart rhythm. Defibrillation as soon as possible after the onset of VF (V-fib) increases the person's chance of survival.

For adults, the AHA recommends that rescuers:
- Use an AED as soon as possible.
- Minimize interruptions in chest compressions before and after a shock is given. CPR is given while the AED pads are applied and until the AED is ready to check the rhythm.
- Give 1 shock. Then resume CPR at once. Begin with chest compressions.
- Check for a heart rhythm again after about 2 minutes of CPR (when prompted by the AED).

AEDs are found in health care agencies (Fig. 54-14, p. 836). They are on airplanes and in airports, health clubs, malls, and other public places. Some people have them in their homes.

You will learn more about using an AED in the AHA's *BLS for Healthcare Providers* course.

See *Focus on Children and Older Persons: Defibrillation,* p. 836.

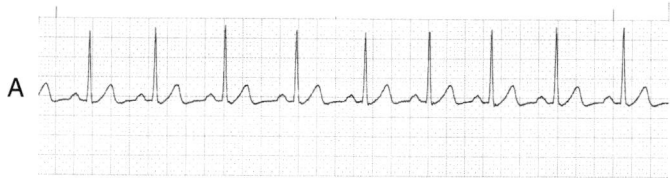

A

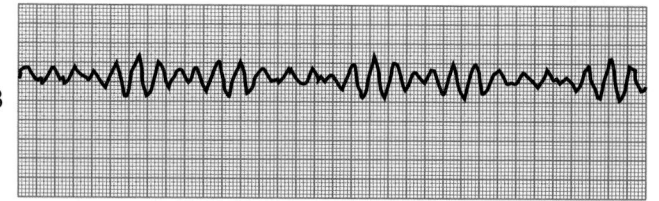

B

FIGURE 54-13 A, Normal rhythm. **B,** Ventricular fibrillation. (From Ignatavicius DD, Workman ML: *Medical-surgical nursing: patient-centered collaborative care,* ed 7, St Louis, 2013, Saunders.)

Performing Adult CPR. CPR is done only for cardiac arrest. You must determine if cardiac arrest or fainting (p. 845) has occurred. *CPR is done if the person does not respond, is not breathing or only gasping (has no normal breathing), and has no pulse.*

CPR is done alone or with another person. When done alone, chest compressions and breaths are given by 1 rescuer. With 2 rescuers, 1 person gives chest compressions and the other gives breaths (Fig. 54-15). Rescuers switch tasks about every 2 minutes to avoid fatigue and inadequate compressions. The second rescuer uses the AED if one is available.

See *Focus on Communication: Performing Adult CPR.*
See *Promoting Safety and Comfort: Performing Adult CPR.*
See procedure: *Adult CPR—1 Rescuer.*
See procedure: *Adult CPR With AED—2 Rescuers.*

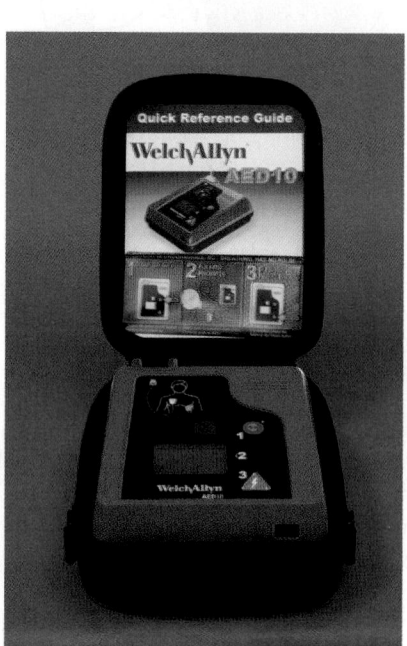

FIGURE 54-14 An automated external defibrillator (AED).

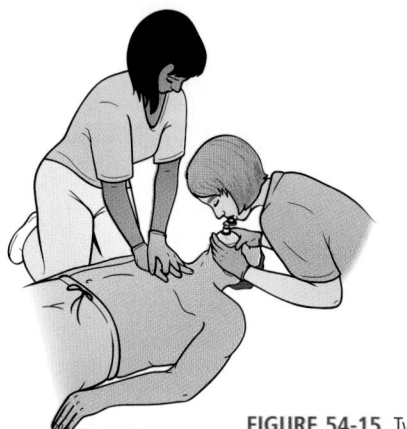

FIGURE 54-15 Two people perform CPR.

FOCUS ON COMMUNICATION

Performing Adult CPR

Good communication is needed when 2 rescuers perform CPR. The rescuer giving compressions must count out loud so the other rescuer is ready to give breaths. Clear communication prevents delays and minimizes interruptions in chest compressions.

FOCUS ON CHILDREN AND OLDER PERSONS

Defibrillation

Children

Some AEDs are designed for adults and children. A key or switch is used to change the dosage. Or child pads are used. Always follow the manufacturer's instructions.

The shock dosage for children 8 years and older is the same as the adult dosage. Lower shock dosages are used for children younger than 8 years. For infants, a manual defibrillator is best. Trained staff and EMS use the defibrillator. If one is not available, an AED with child dosages may be used. If neither is available, adult dosages may be used. If adult pads are used, the pads must not touch or over-lap.

PROMOTING SAFETY AND COMFORT

Performing Adult CPR

Safety

Never practice CPR on another person. Serious damage can be done. Mannequins are used to learn and practice CPR.

Make sure you have a safe setting for CPR. Move the person only if the setting is unsafe (see Box 54-1). Do not approach the person if the scene is unsafe for you.

The person must be on a hard, flat surface for CPR. Logroll the person so there is no twisting of the spine. Place the arms alongside the body. If the person is in bed, you may need to place a board under the person. Or move the person to the floor.

Basic Life Support guidelines are updated as new information becomes available. You are responsible for following current guidelines. Updates can be found on-line at ECCguidelines.heart.org.

Adult CPR—1 Rescuer

PROCEDURE

1 Make sure the scene is safe.
2 Check for a response. Tap or gently shake the person. Call the person by name, if known. Shout: "Are you okay?"
3 Shout for help if the person does not respond.
4 Activate the EMS system or the agency's RRT (MET).
   a *If alone with a wireless phone,* use it while continuing to give care.
   b *If alone without a wireless phone,* leave the person to activate the EMS system before starting CPR.
   c *If help arrives,* send him or her to activate the EMS system.
5 Get an AED.
   a *If alone,* get the AED before starting CPR.
   b *If help arrives,* ask him or her to get the AED.
6 Check for breathing and a carotid pulse at the same time. Look for no breathing or only gasping. Start CPR for no breathing (or only gasping) and no definite pulse within 10 seconds.
7 Position the person for CPR if not already done. The person is supine on a hard, flat surface.
8 Expose the person's chest.
9 Give CPR.
   a Place 2 hands on the lower half of the sternum. Give 30 chest compressions at a rate of 100 to 120 per minute. Establish a regular rhythm. Count out loud. Allow the chest to recoil between compressions.
   b Open the airway. Use the head tilt–chin lift method.
   c Give 2 breaths. Each breath should take only 1 second. The chest should rise. If the first breath does not make the chest rise:
      1) Open the airway. Use the head tilt–chin lift method.
      2) Give another breath.
10 Continue CPR with 30 chest compressions followed by 2 breaths. Limit compression interruptions to less than 10 seconds. Use the AED when available. See procedure: *Adult CPR With AED—2 Rescuers.*
11 Continue CPR until help takes over or the person begins to move. If movement occurs, place the person in the recovery position (p. 838).

Adult CPR With AED—2 Rescuers

PROCEDURE

1 Make sure the scene is safe.
2 *Rescuer 1:*
   a Check for a response. Tap or gently shake the person. Call the person by name, if known. Shout: "Are you okay?"
   b Shout for help if the person does not respond.
3 *Rescuer 2:*
   a Activate the EMS system or the agency's RRT (MET) using a wireless phone (if available) or leave to do so.
   b Get an AED.
4 *Rescuer 1:*
   a Check for breathing and a carotid pulse at the same time. Look for no breathing or only gasping. Start CPR for no breathing (or only gasping) and no definite pulse within 10 seconds.
   b Position the person for CPR if not already done. The person is supine on a hard, flat surface.
   c Expose the person's chest.
   d Place 2 hands on the lower half of the sternum. Give 30 chest compressions at a rate of 100 to 120 per minute. Establish a regular rhythm. Count out loud. Allow the chest to recoil between compressions.
   e Open the airway. Use the head tilt–chin lift method.
   f Give 2 breaths. Each breath should take only 1 second. The chest should rise. If the first breath does not make the chest rise:
      1) Open the airway. Use the head tilt–chin lift method.
      2) Give another breath.
   g Continue CPR with 30 chest compressions followed by 2 breaths. Limit compression interruptions to less than 10 seconds.
5 *Rescuer 2:*
   a Open the AED case.
   b Turn on the AED (Fig. 54-16, *A*, p. 838).
   c Apply adult electrode pads to the chest (Fig. 54-16, *B*, p. 838). Follow the AED's instructions and diagram.
   d Attach the connecting cables to the AED (Fig. 54-16, *C*, p. 838).
   e Clear away from the person. Make sure no one is touching the person (Fig. 54-16, *D*, p. 838).
   f Let the AED check the heart rhythm.
   g Make sure everyone is clear of the person if the AED advises a "shock" (see Fig. 54-16, *D*, p. 838). Loudly tell others not to touch the person. Say: "I am clear, you are clear, everyone is clear!" Look to make sure no one is touching the person.
   h Press the SHOCK button if the AED advises a "shock" (Fig. 54-16, *E*, p. 838).
6 *Rescuers 1 and 2—perform 2-rescuer CPR.*
   a Begin with compressions. One rescuer gives 30 chest compressions. The rescuer pauses for the other rescuer to give 2 breaths.
   b The other rescuer gives 2 breaths after every 30 chest compressions.
7 Pause for a rhythm check when prompted by the AED (after about 2 minutes of CPR). Repeat step 5 e-h. Change positions and continue CPR. Begin with compressions.
8 Continue CPR and use of the AED until help takes over or the person begins to move. If movement occurs, place the person in the recovery position (p. 838).

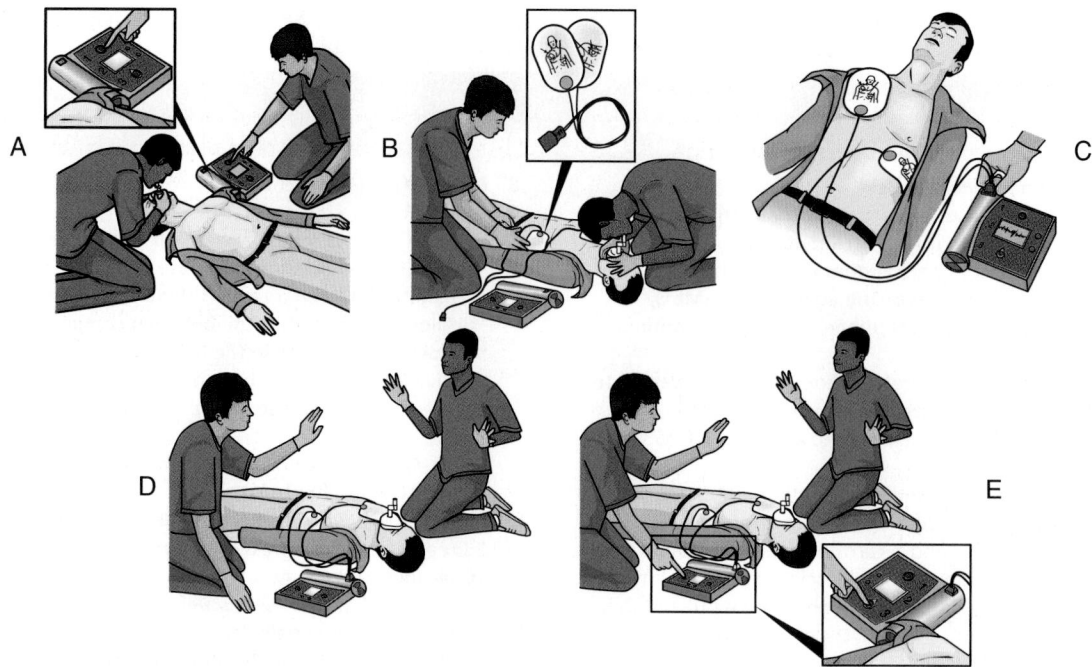

FIGURE 54-16 **A,** The rescuer turns on the AED. **B,** Electrode pads are placed on the person's chest. **C,** The cables are connected to the AED. **D,** The rescuer "clears" the person. The rescuer makes sure no one is touching the person. **E,** The SHOCK button is pressed to deliver a shock.

Hands-Only CPR. With cardiac arrest, the person's survival depends on others nearby. Outside of the health care setting, persons trained in BLS are often not available. Bystanders may worry that they will not do CPR correctly or that they may injure the person.

The AHA developed "Hands-Only CPR" (compression-only CPR) to improve the response of bystanders who witness an adult or adolescent collapse suddenly in the out-of-hospital setting. In "Hands-Only CPR," CPR involves 2 steps.
1. Call 911.
2. Push hard and fast in the center of the chest.

"Hands-Only CPR" is used to educate persons *not* trained in BLS. As a health care provider, use the CPR method presented in this chapter and in a BLS course.

See *Focus on Children and Older Persons: Hands-Only CPR.*

FOCUS ON CHILDREN AND OLDER PERSONS

Hands-Only CPR

Children
CPR with compressions and breaths should be done for infants and children. However, if the rescuer is unable or unwilling to deliver breaths, "Hands-Only CPR" may be done.

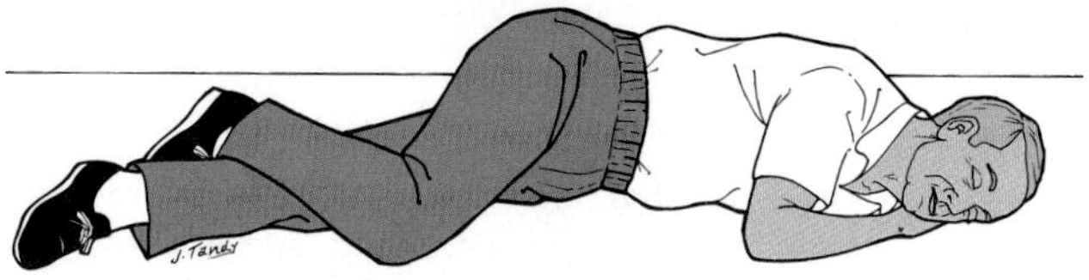

FIGURE 54-17 Recovery position.

Recovery Position

The recovery position is used when the person is breathing and has a pulse but is not responding (Fig. 54-17). The position helps keep the airway open and prevents aspiration.

Logroll the person into the recovery position. Keep the head, neck, and spine straight. A hand supports the head. *Do not use this position if the person might have neck injuries or other trauma.*

BLS FOR CHILDREN AND INFANTS

The AHA defines a child and an infant as follows.
- *Child*—from 1 year of age to puberty. Puberty is marked by secondary sex characteristics in males and females (Chapter 11).
- *Infant*—from birth (outside of the delivery room) until 1 year (12 months) of age.

Cardiac Arrest in Children and Infants

Cardiac arrest caused by heart disease is rare in children. More common causes involve respiratory diseases or injuries that lead to respiratory arrest or circulatory failure. Motor vehicle crashes, drowning, suffocation, burns, smoke inhalation, falls, and poisoning are major death-producing injuries. Sudden infant death syndrome (SIDS) is the leading cause of death in children between 1 month and 1 year of age (Chapter 52).

CPR for Children and Infants

The AHA's CPR guidelines for children and infants differ from adult guidelines (Box 54-3). The procedures also differ.

If you are alone, the timing of activating the EMS system or the agency's RRT (MET) and getting an AED differs for children and infants.

Compressions are given if the pulse is 60 beats per minute or less and the child or infant has signs of poor circulation—pale, mottled (blotchy), or bluish skin.

See *Focus on Math: CPR for Children and Infants.*

FOCUS ON MATH

CPR for Children and Infants

You count the pulse for no more than 10 seconds. To calculate the number of beats per minute:

- Multiply the number counted by 12 when you count for 5 seconds.
- Multiply the number counted by 6 when you count for 10 seconds.

For example, when checking for a child's pulse you count 4 beats in 5 seconds. Multiply 4 beats (the number of beats in 5 seconds) by 12 to calculate the number of beats per minute.

4 (number of beats in 5 seconds) × 12 = 48 beats per minute

You calculate 48 beats per minute. This is less than 60 beats per minute. You give compressions.

As a quick guide, give compressions if the number of beats counted is less than or equal to the number of seconds counted. For example:

- Give compressions if you count 10 beats or less in 10 seconds.
- Give compressions if you count 9 beats or less in 9 seconds, and so on.

BOX 54-3 CPR—Children and Infants

Children and Infants

- If you are alone:
  - *If the arrest was sudden and witnessed*—follow the steps for adults for activating the EMS system or the agency's RRT (MET) and getting an AED. See steps 4 and 5 in the procedure: *Adult CPR—1 Rescuer,* p. 837.
  - *If the arrest was not witnessed*—give about 2 minutes of CPR. Then activate the EMS system or the agency's RRT (MET) and get an AED.
- Check breathing and pulse at the same time. This should take less than 10 seconds.
- Start CPR if the child's heart rate is 60 beats per minute or less with signs of poor circulation. See *Focus on Math: CPR for Children and Infants.*
- Give compressions at a rate of 100 to 120 per minute.
- Release pressure and allow the chest to recoil after each compression. Do not lean on the chest after each compression.
- Change chest compressions and breathing when 2 rescuers are present.
  - 1 rescuer—30 compressions followed by 2 breaths
  - 2 rescuers—15 compressions followed by 2 breaths
- Give only enough air to make the chest rise. If the child or infant is very small, use less air than for larger children and adults.

Children and Infants—cont'd

- Give 2 breaths that make the chest rise. If a breath does not make the chest rise:
  - Try again to open the airway.
  - Give a breath. The breath should make the chest rise.
- Use an AED as soon as possible. Use child pads and a child system for children younger than 8 years if possible.

Children

- Use the carotid artery to check for a pulse. See p. 832 and Figure 54-1. Or use the femoral artery (Chapter 29). If a pulse is not definitely felt within 10 seconds, begin CPR.
- Use the same hand position for chest compressions as for adults (p. 833).
- Use 1 or 2 hands for chest compressions if the child is very small (Fig. 54-18, p. 840).
- Give chest compressions with enough pressure to press down at least ⅓ (one-third) the depth of the chest (about 2 inches).

Infants

- Use the brachial artery to check for a pulse (Fig. 54-19, p. 840).
  - Place the index and middle fingers on the inside of the infant's upper arm. Finger placement is between the elbow and shoulder.
  - Press gently for no more than 10 seconds.

Continued

BOX 54-3   CPR—Children and Infants—cont'd

Infants—cont'd

- Locate hand position for chest compressions. Imagine a line between the nipples. Find the sternum (breastbone) in the center of the chest.
  - *For 1-rescuer CPR*—place 2 fingers on the sternum just below the imaginary line (Fig. 54-20).
  - *For 2-rescuer CPR*—use the 2 thumb-encircling hands method (Fig. 54-21).
    - Place both thumbs just below the imaginary line. The thumbs are side by side in the center of the chest. (Thumbs may overlap. The infant may be small. Or you may have large hands.)
    - Encircle the infant's chest with your hands.
    - Support the infant's back with your fingers. Use both hands.
    - Press down on the sternum with your thumbs. Squeeze the chest with your fingers.
- Give chest compressions as follows.
  - Press on the lower half of the sternum. Do not press on the bottom of the sternum.
  - Use enough pressure to press down at least $\frac{1}{3}$ (one-third) the depth of the chest (about $1\frac{1}{2}$ inches).

Infants—cont'd

- Use the head tilt–chin lift method to open the airway. Often the tongue obstructs the airway when it falls into the throat (Fig. 54-22).
  - Place 1 hand on the infant's forehead.
  - Use your palm to push the head back.
  - Place the fingers of your other hand under the bony part of the lower jaw. This is near the chin. Do not press in deep.
  - Use your fingers (not your thumb) to lift the jaw to bring the chin forward. The head should be in a neutral ("sniffing") position.
  - Do not close the infant's mouth completely.
- Use the mouth-to-mouth-and-nose method to give breaths (Fig. 54-23). This is the preferred method. Use the mouth-to-mouth method if you cannot cover the infant's nose and mouth with your mouth. To give mouth-to-mouth-and-nose breaths:
  - Keep the airway open with the head tilt–chin lift method.
  - Cover the infant's nose and mouth with your mouth. Make sure you have a tight seal.
  - Blow air into the infant's nose and mouth.

Adapted from American Heart Association: Highlights of the 2015 American Heart Association guidelines update for CPR and ECC, copyright 2015.

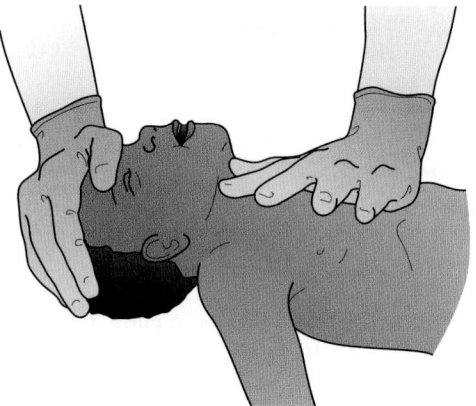

FIGURE 54-18 The heel of 1 hand can be used for CPR if the child is very small. The fingers are off the chest.

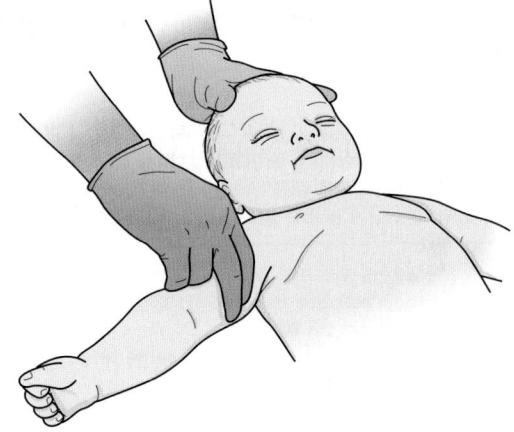

FIGURE 54-19 Locating the infant's brachial pulse.

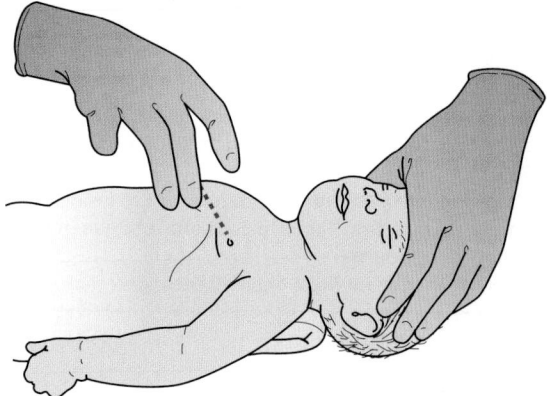

FIGURE 54-20 Locating hand position for infant chest compressions. Imagine a line between the nipples. Find the sternum (breastbone). For 1-rescuer CPR, place 2 fingers on the sternum just below the imaginary line.

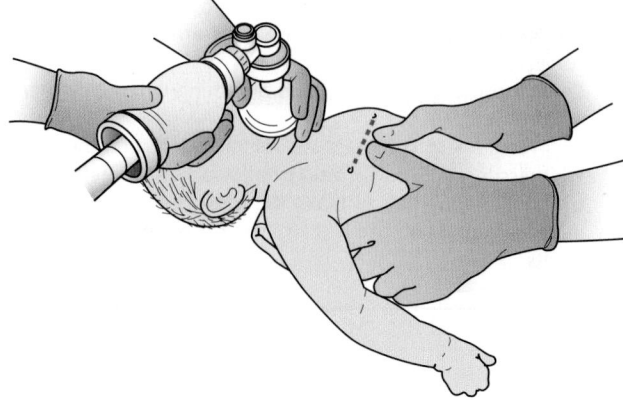

FIGURE 54-21 The 2-thumb-encircling hands method for chest compressions. This method is used when 2 rescuers perform CPR on an infant.

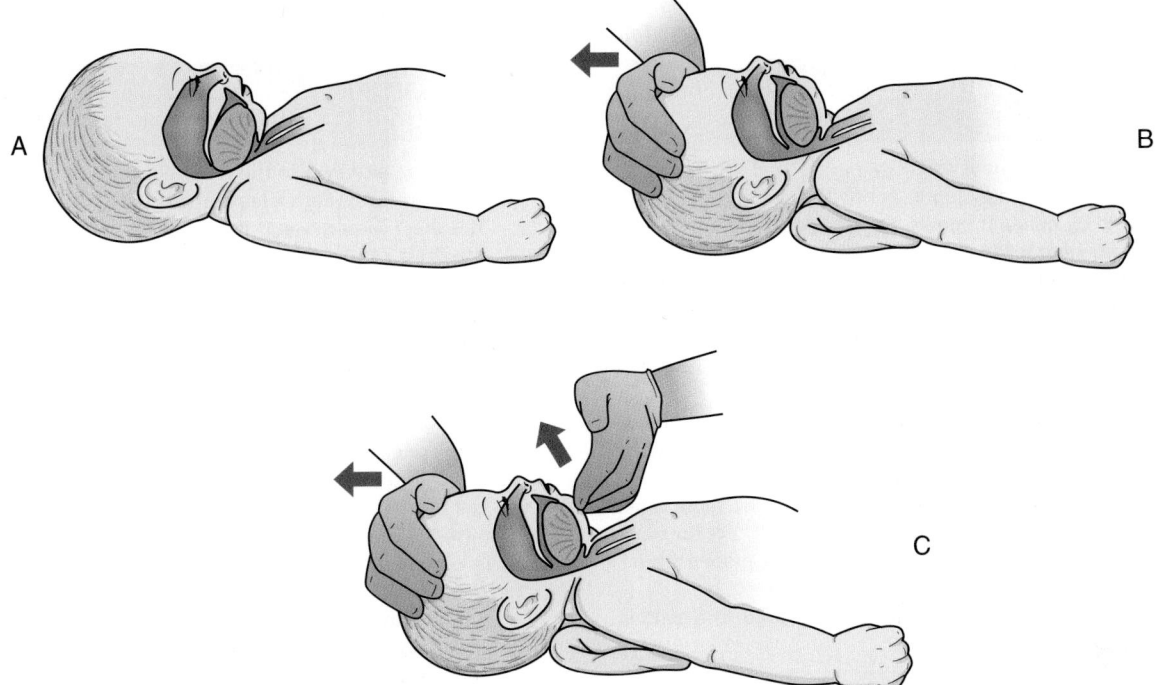

FIGURE 54-22 The head tilt–chin lift method for infants. A, The tongue is at the back of the throat, obstructing the airway. **B,** One hand is on the infant's forehead. The palm is used to push the head back. **C,** The fingers of the other hand are under the bony part of the lower jaw. This is near the chin. The fingers are used to lift the jaw to bring the chin forward. The head is in a neutral ("sniffing") position.

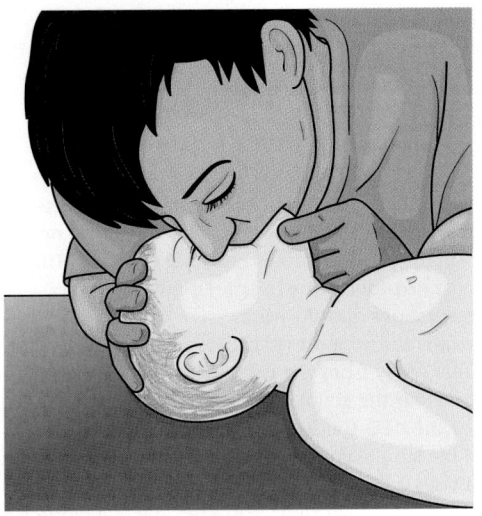

FIGURE 54-23 Mouth-to-mouth-and-nose breathing. The infant's nose and mouth are covered to give breaths.

Child CPR. When 1 rescuer gives child CPR, 30 compressions are given followed by 2 breaths. When 2 rescuers are present, 15 compressions are given followed by 2 breaths. An AED is used as soon as 1 is available.

See procedure: *Child CPR—1 Rescuer*, p. 842.

See procedure: *Child CPR With AED—2 Rescuers*, p. 842.

Infant CPR. The guidelines and procedures for infant CPR differ from adult and child CPR. See Box 54-3.

See procedure: *Infant CPR—1 Rescuer*, p. 843.

See procedure: *Infant CPR With AED—2 Rescuers*, p. 843.

Basic Life Support guidelines are updated as new information becomes available. You are responsible for following current guidelines. Updates can be found on-line at ECCguidelines.heart.org.

Child CPR—1 Rescuer

PROCEDURE

1 Make sure the scene is safe.
2 Check for a response. Tap or gently shake the child. Call the child by name, if known. Shout, "Are you okay?"
3 Shout for help if the child does not respond.
4 Activate the EMS system or the agency's RRT (MET). Get an AED.
    a *If the collapse is sudden and witnessed*—follow steps 4 and 5 in the procedure: *Adult CPR—1 Rescuer*, p. 837.
    b *If the collapse is unwitnessed*—give about 2 minutes of CPR before leaving the child to activate the EMS system or RRT (MET) and get the AED.
5 Check for breathing and a carotid pulse at the same time. Look for no breathing or only gasping. Start CPR for no breathing (or only gasping) and no definite pulse within 10 seconds.
6 Position the child for CPR if not already done. The child is supine on a hard, flat surface.
7 Expose the child's chest.
8 Give CPR.
    a Place 2 hands on the lower half of the sternum. (Use 1 or 2 hands for a very small child.) Give 30 chest compressions at a rate of 100 to 120 per minute. Establish a regular rhythm. Count out loud. Allow the chest to recoil between compressions.
    b Open the airway. Use the head tilt–chin lift method.
    c Give 2 breaths. Each breath should take only 1 second. The chest should rise. If the first breath does not make the chest rise:
       1) Open the airway. Use the head tilt–chin lift method.
       2) Give another breath.
9 Continue CPR with 30 chest compressions followed by 2 breaths. Limit compression interruptions to less than 10 seconds.
10 Do the following after about 2 minutes of CPR if not already done.
    a Activate the EMS system or the agency's RRT (MET).
    b Get an AED.
11 Use the AED. See step 5 in the procedure: *Child CPR With AED—2 Rescuers.*
    a *If a shock is advised*—give 1 shock. Then start CPR. Begin with compressions.
    b *If the rhythm is not shockable*—start CPR. Begin with compressions.
12 Pause for a rhythm check when prompted by the AED (after about 2 minutes of CPR).
13 Continue CPR and use of the AED until help takes over or the child begins to move.

Child CPR With AED—2 Rescuers

PROCEDURE

1 Make sure the scene is safe.
2 Rescuer 1:
    a Check for a response. Tap or gently shake the child. Call the child by name if known. Shout, "Are you okay?"
    b Shout for help if the child does not respond.
3 Rescuer 2:
    a Activate the EMS system or the agency's RRT (MET) using a wireless phone (if available) or leave to do so.
    b Get an AED.
4 Rescuer 1:
    a Check for breathing and a carotid pulse at the same time. Look for no breathing or only gasping. Start CPR for no breathing (or only gasping) and no definite pulse within 10 seconds.
    b Position the child for CPR if not already done. The child is supine on a hard, flat surface.
    c Expose the child's chest.
    d Begin 1-rescuer CPR until the AED is ready. (See procedure: *Child CPR—1 Rescuer*, steps 8 and 9.)
5 Rescuer 2:
    a Open the AED case.
    b Turn on the AED.
    c Apply child electrode pads if available. Or use the key or switch to change to the child setting. If neither is available, use the adult pads and settings. The pads must not touch or overlap. Follow the AED's instructions and diagram.
    d Attach the connecting cables to the AED.
    e Clear away from the child. Make sure no one is touching the child.
    f Let the AED check the heart rhythm.
    g Make sure everyone is clear of the child if the AED advises a "shock." Loudly tell others not to touch the child. Say: "I am clear, you are clear, everyone is clear!" Look to make sure no one is touching the child.
    h Press the "SHOCK" button if the AED advises a "shock."
6 Rescuers 1 and 2—perform 2-rescuer CPR.
    a Begin with chest compressions. One rescuer gives 15 chest compressions. The rescuer pauses for the other rescuer to give 2 breaths.
    b The other rescuer gives 2 breaths after every 15 chest compressions.
7 Allow a rhythm check when prompted by the AED (after about 2 minutes of CPR). Repeat step 5 e-h. Change positions and continue CPR. Begin with compressions.
8 Continue CPR and use of the AED until help takes over or the child begins to move.

Basic Life Support guidelines are updated as new information becomes available. You are responsible for following current guidelines. Updates can be found on-line at ECCguidelines.heart.org.

Infant CPR—1 Rescuer

PROCEDURE

1 Make sure the scene is safe.
2 Check for a response. Tap the infant's foot. Shout, "Are you okay?" (Note: Infants cannot answer you. However, shouting should startle the responsive infant.)
3 Shout for help if the infant does not respond.
4 Activate the EMS system or the agency's RRT (MET). Get an AED.
   a *If the collapse is sudden and witnessed*—follow steps 4 and 5 in the procedure: *Adult CPR—1 Rescuer,* p. 837.
   b *If the collapse is unwitnessed*—give about 2 minutes of CPR before leaving the infant to activate the EMS system or RRT (MET) and get the AED.
5 Check for breathing and a brachial pulse at the same time. Look for no breathing or only gasping. See Box 54-3 and Figure 54-19. Start CPR for no breathing (or only gasping) and no definite pulse within 10 seconds.
6 Position the infant supine on a hard, flat surface if not already done.
7 Expose the infant's chest.

8 Give CPR.
   a Place 2 fingers on the sternum just below the nipple line. See Box 54-3 and Figure 54-20. Give 30 chest compressions at a rate of 100 to 120 per minute. Establish a regular rhythm. Count out loud. Allow the chest to recoil between compressions.
   b Open the airway. Use the head tilt–chin lift method. The head should be in a neutral ("sniffing") position. See Box 54-3 and Figure 54-22.
   c Give 2 breaths. Each breath should take only 1 second. The chest should rise. If the first breath does not make the chest rise:
      1) Open the airway. Use the head tilt–chin lift method.
      2) Give another breath.
9 Continue CPR with 30 chest compressions followed by 2 breaths. Limit compression interruptions to less than 10 seconds.
10 Do the following after about 2 minutes of CPR if not already done.
   a Activate the EMS system or the agency's RRT (MET).
   b Get an AED.
11 Use the AED. See step 5 in the procedure: *Infant CPR With AED—2 Rescuers.*
   a *If a shock is advised*—give 1 shock. Then start CPR beginning with compressions.
   b *If the rhythm is not shockable*—start CPR beginning with compressions.
12 Allow a rhythm check when prompted by the AED (after about 2 minutes of CPR).
13 Continue CPR and use of the AED until help takes over or the infant begins to move.

Infant CPR With AED—2 Rescuers

PROCEDURE

1 Make sure the scene is safe.
2 Rescuer 1:
   a Check for a response. Tap the infant's foot. Shout, "Are you okay?" (Note: Infants cannot answer you. However, shouting should startle the responsive infant.)
   b Shout for help if the infant does not respond.
3 Rescuer 2:
   a Activate the EMS system or the agency's RRT (MET) using a wireless phone (if available) or leave to do so.
   b Get an AED.
4 Rescuer 1:
   a Check for breathing and a brachial pulse at the same time. Look for no breathing or only gasping. Start CPR for no breathing (or only gasping) and no definite pulse within 10 seconds.
   b Position the infant supine on a hard, flat surface if not already done.
   c Expose the infant's chest.
   d Begin 1-rescuer CPR until the AED is ready. (See procedure: *Infant CPR—1 Rescuer,* steps 8 and 9.)

5 Rescuer 2—use the AED. Follow step 5 in the procedure: *Child CPR With AED—2 Rescuers.*
6 Rescuers 1 and 2—perform 2-rescuer CPR.
   a Begin with compressions. One rescuer uses the 2 thumb-encircling hands method to give 15 compressions at a rate of 100 to 120 per minute in a regular rhythm and counting out loud. See Box 54-3 and Figure 54-21. The rescuer pauses for the other rescuer to give 2 breaths.
   b The other rescuer gives 2 breaths after every 15 chest compressions.
7 Allow a rhythm check when prompted by the AED (after about 2 minutes of CPR). Follow step 5 e-h in the procedure: *Child CPR With AED—2 Rescuers.* Change positions and continue CPR. Begin with compressions.
8 Continue CPR and use of the AED until help takes over or the infant begins to move.

CHOKING

Foreign bodies can obstruct the airway. This is called *choking* or *foreign-body airway obstruction (FBAO)*. Air cannot pass through the airways into the lungs. The body does not get enough oxygen. It can lead to cardiac arrest.

Airway obstruction can be mild or severe. With severe airway obstruction, air does not move in and out of the lungs. If the obstruction is not removed, the person will die. Abdominal thrusts are used to relieve severe airway obstruction. See Chapter 13 for emergency care of the choking person.

POISONING

A poison is any substance harmful to the body when ingested, inhaled, injected, or absorbed through the skin. See Chapter 13 for measures to prevent poisoning.

Some common signs and symptoms of poisoning are:
- Burns or redness around the mouth and lips
- A chemical odor to the breath
- Burns, stains, or odors on the person, on clothing, or around the person
- Empty drug bottles or spilled drugs
- Vomiting
- Dyspnea
- Drowsiness
- Confusion

If you think a person has had contact with a poison, call the Poison Control Center. The number is 1-800-222-1222. Also follow these emergency measures.
- *Poison in the eyes*—rinse the eyes with running water.
- *Poison on the skin*—remove any clothing in contact with the poison. Rinse the skin with running water.
- *Inhaled poison*—leave the area. Get the person to fresh air at once.
- *Swallowed poison*—do not have the person try to vomit or give the person anything to cause vomiting. Do not give the person anything to eat or drink unless told to do so by the Poison Control Center.
- Activate the EMS system if the person stops breathing, collapses, or has a seizure (p. 829). Provide BLS if the person is not responding or breathing. See p. 846 for emergency care for seizures.
- Follow the rules in Box 54-1. Also follow the directions given by the Poison Control Center.

HEMORRHAGE

Life and body functions require an adequate blood supply. If a blood vessel is cut or torn, bleeding occurs. The larger the blood vessel, the greater the bleeding and blood loss. *Hemorrhage is the excessive loss of blood in a short time.* If bleeding is not stopped, the person will die.

Hemorrhage is internal or external. You cannot see internal hemorrhage. The bleeding is inside body tissues and body cavities. Pain, shock, vomiting blood, coughing up blood, cold and moist skin, and loss of consciousness signal internal hemorrhage. There is little you can do for internal bleeding.
- Follow the rules in Box 54-1. This includes activating the EMS system.
- Keep the person warm, flat, and quiet until help arrives.
- Do not give fluids.

If not hidden by clothing, external bleeding is usually seen. Bleeding from an artery occurs in spurts. There is a steady flow of blood from a vein. To control bleeding:
- Follow the rules in Box 54-1. This includes activating the EMS system.
- Do not remove any objects that have pierced or stabbed the person.
- Place a sterile dressing directly over the wound. Or use any clean material (handkerchief, towel, cloth, or sanitary napkin).
- Apply firm pressure directly over the bleeding site (Fig. 54-24). Do not release pressure until the bleeding stops. If needed, wrap an elastic bandage firmly over the dressing or material.
- Do not remove the dressing or material. If bleeding continues, apply more on top and apply more pressure.
- Bind the wound when bleeding stops. Tape or tie the dressing in place. You can tie the dressing with such things as clothing, a scarf, or a necktie.

See *Promoting Safety and Comfort: Hemorrhage.*

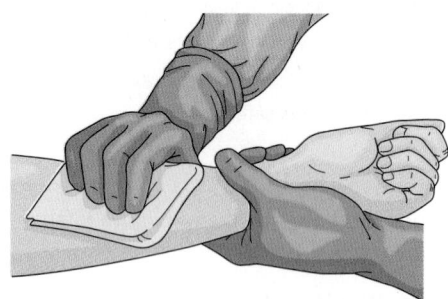

FIGURE 54-24 Direct pressure is applied to the wound to stop bleeding.

PROMOTING SAFETY AND COMFORT
Hemorrhage

Safety

Contact with blood is likely with hemorrhage. Follow Standard Precautions and the Bloodborne Pathogen Standard to the extent possible. Wear gloves if possible. Practice hand hygiene as soon as you can.

FAINTING

Fainting is the sudden loss of consciousness from an inadequate blood supply to the brain. Hunger, fatigue, fear, and pain are common causes. Some people faint at the sight of blood or injury. Standing in 1 position too long and being in a warm, crowded room are other causes. Hemorrhage and other serious problems can cause fainting.

Dizziness, perspiration (sweating), and blackness before the eyes are warning signals. The person looks pale. The pulse is weak. Respirations are shallow if consciousness is lost.

Emergency care includes the following.

- Have the person sit or lie down before fainting occurs.
- If sitting, the person bends forward and places the head between the knees (Fig. 54-25).
- If the person is lying down, raise the legs.
- Loosen tight clothing (belts, ties, scarves, collars, and so on).
- Keep the person lying down if fainting has occurred. Raise the legs about 12 inches.
- Do not let the person get up quickly.
- Help the person to a sitting position after recovery from fainting. Observe for fainting.
- Provide BLS if there is no response or breathing.

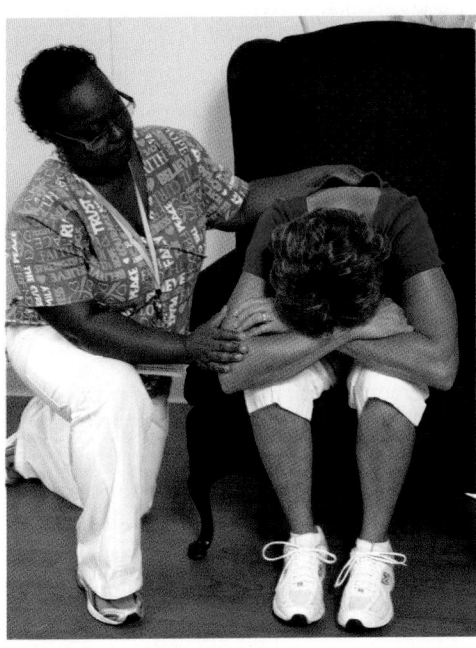

FIGURE 54-25 The person bends forward and lowers her head to prevent fainting.

SHOCK

Shock results when tissues and organs do not get enough blood. Blood loss, allergic reaction, poisoning, heart attack (myocardial infarction), burns, and severe infection are causes. Signs and symptoms include:

- Low or falling blood pressure
- Rapid and weak pulse
- Rapid respirations
- Cold, moist, and pale skin
- Thirst
- Nausea and vomiting
- Restlessness
- Confusion and loss of consciousness as shock worsens

Shock is possible in any person who is acutely ill or severely injured. Follow the rules in Box 54-1. Keep the person lying down. If the person does not have injuries from trauma, raise the legs about 12 inches. Lower the feet if the position causes pain. Maintain an open airway and control bleeding. Begin CPR if cardiac arrest occurs.

Anaphylactic Shock

Some people are allergic or sensitive to foods, insects, chemicals, and drugs. For example, many people are allergic to the drug *penicillin*. An *antigen* is a substance that the body reacts to. The body releases chemicals to fight or attack the antigen. The person may react with an area of redness, swelling, or itching. Or the reaction may involve the entire body.

Anaphylaxis is a life-threatening sensitivity to an antigen. (*Ana* means *without*. *Phylaxis* means *protection*.) The reaction can occur within seconds. Signs and symptoms include:

- An itchy rash
- Flushed or pale skin
- Feeling warm
- Dyspnea or wheezing from airway narrowing or a swollen tongue or throat
- Feeling that there is a "lump" in the throat
- A fast and weak pulse
- Nausea, vomiting, or diarrhea
- A feeling of dread or doom
- Dizziness or fainting
- Signs and symptoms of shock

Anaphylactic shock is an emergency. The EMS system must be activated. The person needs special drugs to reverse the allergic reaction. Keep the person lying down and the airway open. Start CPR if cardiac arrest occurs.

Some persons carry *epinephrine*. Epinephrine is a drug used to treat life-threatening allergic reactions. The person injects the drug into the outer thigh. One dose is given for anaphylaxis. The person may give himself or herself a second dose if:

- There is no response to the first dose.
- EMS arrival will take longer than 5 to 10 minutes.

STROKE

Stroke (cerebrovascular accident) occurs when the brain is suddenly deprived of its blood supply (Chapter 44). Usually only part of the brain is affected. A stroke may be caused by a thrombus, an embolus, or hemorrhage if a blood vessel in the brain ruptures.

Signs of stroke vary (Chapter 44). They depend on the size and location of brain injury. The National Institute of Neurological Disorders and Stroke lists these major signs.

* Sudden numbness or weakness of the face, arm, or leg, especially on 1 side of the body
* Sudden confusion or trouble speaking or understanding speech
* Sudden trouble seeing in 1 or both eyes
* Sudden trouble walking, dizziness, or loss of balance or coordination
* Sudden, severe headache with no known cause

If you suspect a stroke, activate the EMS system at once. The most effective stroke treatments must be given within 3 hours of the onset of symptoms. Find out when the person's symptoms began. Tell the EMS staff the time. Follow the rules in Box 54-1. Keep the person comfortable, warm, and quiet. Provide BLS and emergency care for seizures if necessary.

SEIZURES

Seizures (convulsions) are violent and sudden contractions or tremors of muscle groups caused by abnormal electrical activity in the brain. Movements are uncontrolled. The person may lose consciousness. Causes include head injury during birth or from trauma, high fever, brain tumors, poisoning, and nervous system disorders or infections. Lack of blood flow to the brain can also cause seizures.

Epilepsy

Epilepsy is a brain disorder in which clusters of nerve cells sometimes signal abnormally. There are brief changes in the brain's electrical function. The person can have strange sensations, emotions, and behavior. Sometimes there are seizures, muscle spasms, and loss of consciousness.

A single seizure does not mean epilepsy. In epilepsy, seizures recur from a permanent brain injury or defect.

Epilepsy develops more often in children and older adults. However, epilepsy can begin at any age. It can occur with any problem affecting the brain. Such causes include:

* Brain injury during or after birth (Chapter 50)
* Problems with brain development before birth
* The mother having an injury or infection during pregnancy
* Traumatic brain injury (accidents, gunshot wounds, sports injuries, falls, blows to the head)
* Brain tumor
* Poison—such as lead and alcohol
* Infection—such as meningitis and encephalitis
* Stroke
* Dementia

There is no cure at this time. Drugs control seizures in many people. For others, drug therapy does not work.

When controlled, epilepsy usually does not affect learning and activities of daily living. Activity and job limits occur in severe cases. For example, a person has seizures at any time. The person may not be allowed to drive. This may limit job choices. Also, the person is at risk for accidents and injuries. Safety measures are needed. They are needed for the home, workplace, transportation, and recreation.

Types of Seizures

The major types of seizures are:

* *Partial seizure.* Only 1 part of the brain is involved. A body part may jerk. Or the person has a hearing or vision problem or stomach discomfort. The person does not lose consciousness.
* *Generalized tonic-clonic (grand mal) seizure.* This type has 2 phases. In the *tonic* phase, the person loses consciousness. If standing or sitting, the person falls to the floor. The body is rigid because all muscles contract at once. The *clonic* phase follows. Muscle groups contract and relax. This causes jerking and twitching movements. Urinary and fecal incontinence may occur. A deep sleep is common after the seizure. Confusion and headache may occur on awakening.
* *Generalized absence (petit mal) seizure.* This type usually lasts a few seconds. There is loss of consciousness, twitching of the eyelids, and staring. No first aid is necessary. However, you should guide the person away from dangers—stairs, streets, a hot stove, fireplaces, and so on.

Emergency Care for Seizures

You cannot stop a seizure. However, you can protect the person from injury.

* Follow the rules in Box 54-1. This includes activating the EMS system.
* Do not leave the person alone.
* Lower the person to the floor. This protects the person from falling.
* Note the time the seizure started.
* Place something soft under the person's head (Fig. 54-26). It prevents the person's head from striking the floor. You can use a pillow, a cushion, or a folded blanket, towel, or jacket. Or cradle the person's head in your lap.
* Remove eyeglasses and loosen tight jewelry and clothing around the person's neck. Ties, scarves, collars, and necklaces are examples.
* Turn the person onto his or her side. Make sure the head is turned to the side. See Fig. 54-26.
* Do not put any object or your fingers between the person's teeth. The person can bite down on your fingers or injure his or her teeth or jaw.
* Do not try to stop the seizure or control the person's movements.

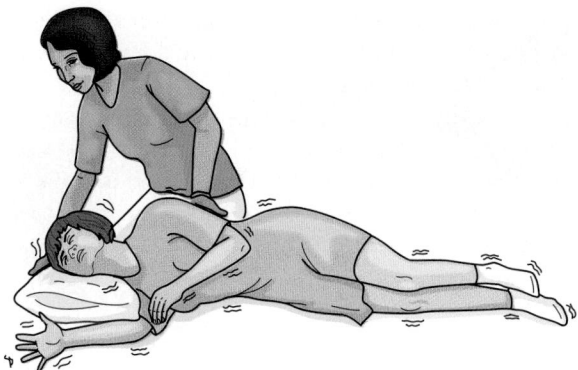

FIGURE 54-26 A pillow protects the person's head during a seizure.

- Move furniture, equipment, and sharp objects away from the person. He or she may strike these objects during the seizure.
- Note the time when the seizure ends.
- Make sure the mouth is clear of food, fluids, and saliva after the seizure.
- Provide BLS if the person is not breathing after the seizure.

CONCUSSIONS

Head injuries can be minor or serious and life-threatening. Concussion is the most common brain injury. Concussion comes from the Latin word *concutere* that means *to shake violently*. A concussion results from a bump or blow to the head or jolt to the head or body. The head and brain move quickly back and forth.

Symptoms can last for days, weeks, or longer. Symptoms affect:

- Thinking—difficulty thinking clearly, concentrating, remembering new information
- Physical function—headache, fuzzy or blurred vision, nausea and vomiting, dizziness, sensitivity to noise or light, balance problems, tired feeling, no energy
- Mood—irritability, sadness, nervousness, anxiety
- Sleep—more or less sleep than usual, trouble falling asleep

Some people have repeated concussions. Football players are examples. Long-term effects from repeated concussions include chronic problems with concentration, memory, headaches, and balance.

Emergency Care for Concussions

The following danger signs in adults signal the need for emergency care.

- Headache—gets worse or does not go away
- Stiff neck
- Weakness, numbness, or decreased coordination
- Nausea or vomiting more than once
- Slurred speech
- Very sleepy; drowsy; cannot be awakened
- One eye pupil is larger than the other
- Convulsions or seizures
- Cannot recognize people, places, or things
- Increased confusion, restlessness, or agitation
- Unusual behavior
- Loss of consciousness

Emergency care for a concussion includes the following.

- Follow the rules in Box 54-1. This includes activating the EMS system.
- Provide BLS if the person is not responding or breathing.
- Place your hands on both sides of the head to keep the head aligned with the spine. Prevent movement.
- Apply firm pressure with a clean cloth to a bleeding area. See "Hemorrhage" on p. 844. Be careful not to move the person's head.
- Do not apply direct pressure to the skull if the skull may be fractured. Cover the wound with sterile gauze dressing.
- Do not remove any object from a wound.
- Logroll the person as a unit onto the side if vomiting occurs.
- Apply ice packs to swollen areas.

See *Focus on Children and Older Persons: Emergency Care for Concussions.*

FOCUS ON **CHILDREN AND OLDER PERSONS**

Emergency Care for Concussions

Children

Children can receive a bump, blow, or jolt to the head or body. Emergency care is needed if the child:

- Has the danger signs listed for adults.
- Will not stop crying.
- Cannot be consoled (comforted).
- Will not nurse or eat.

BURNS

Burns can severely disable a person. They can also cause death. Most burns occur in the home. Infants, children, and older persons are at risk. Common causes of burns and fires are:

- Scalds from hot liquids
- Playing with matches and lighters
- Electrical injuries
- Cooking accidents (barbecues, microwave ovens, stoves, ovens)
- Falling asleep while smoking
- Fireplaces
- Space heaters
- No smoke alarms or non-functioning smoke alarms
- Sunburn
- Chemicals

The skin has 2 layers: the epidermis and dermis. Burns are described as:

- *Superficial (first degree) burns*—involve the epidermis only. They are painful, but the burn is not severe.
- *Partial thickness (second degree) burns*—involve the epidermis and part of the dermis. They are very painful. Nerve endings are exposed.
- *Full thickness (third degree) burns*—involve the entire epidermis and dermis. Fat, muscle, and bone may be injured or destroyed. These burns are not painful. Nerve endings are destroyed.

Some burns are minor; others are severe (Fig. 54-27). Severity depends on burn size and depth, the body part involved, and age. Burns to the face, hands, feet, groin, buttocks, or over a joint are more serious than burns to an arm or leg. Infants, young children, and older persons are at high risk for death.

Emergency care for severe burns includes the following.

- Follow the rules in Box 54-1. This includes activating the EMS system.
- Do not touch the person if he or she is in contact with an electrical source. Have the power source turned off. Do not approach the person or try to remove the electrical source with any object until the power source is turned off.

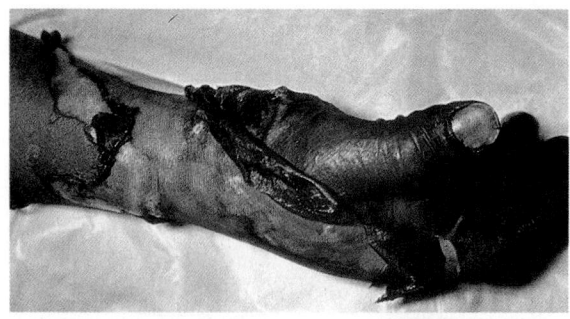

FIGURE 54-27 Full thickness burn. (From Ignatavicius DD, Workman ML: *Medical-surgical nursing: patient-centered collaborative care,* ed 7, St Louis, 2013, Saunders.)

- Remove the person from the fire or burn source.
- Stop the burning process. Put out flames with water or roll the person in a blanket. Or smother flames with a coat, sheet, or towel.
- Apply cold or cool water (59°F to 77°F [15°C to 25°C]) for 10 to 15 minutes. Do not apply ice directly to the burn.
- Remove hot clothing that is not sticking to the skin. If you cannot remove hot clothing, cool the clothing with water.
- Remove jewelry and any tight clothing that is not sticking to the skin.
- Provide rescue breathing and CPR as needed.
- Cover burns with sterile, dry dressings. Or use a sheet or any other clean cloth.
- Do not put oil, butter, salve, or ointments on the burns.
- Keep blisters intact. Do not break blisters.
- Elevate the burned area above heart level if possible.
- Cover the person with a blanket or coat to prevent heat loss.

FOCUS ON PRIDE

The Person, Family, and Yourself

Personal and Professional Responsibility

Understanding emergency care allows you to safely assist during an emergency. This chapter includes basic information. BLS courses for health care providers offer further training. The courses allow you to practice emergency procedures. CPR and the use of an AED are examples.

Most agencies require nursing assistants to be certified in BLS. Certification courses often involve a written and skills test. During the skills test, you show you can provide BLS. Take the course seriously. And take pride in this training. What you learn can save a life.

Rights and Respect

Protect the right to privacy. Do not expose the person unnecessarily. You may be in a place where you cannot close doors or window coverings. The person may be in a lounge, dining area, or public place. Do what you can to provide privacy. As always, treat the person with dignity and respect.

Independence and Social Interaction

Promoting quality of life and independence is important. Choices may be few. However, they are given when possible. Hospital care may be required. The person has the right to choose a hospital.

Some persons refuse care. The EMS staff has guidelines for refusing care. For example, the person must be competent and able to legally make medical decisions. The person must also be informed of the risks, benefits, and alternatives to the care recommended.

Delegation and Teamwork

In public areas, on-lookers can threaten privacy and confidentiality. Your main concern is the person's illness or injuries. You cannot give care and manage on-lookers at the same time. Ask someone else to deal with on-lookers. If someone else is giving care, keep on-lookers away from the person. Work together to protect the person's privacy.

Ethics and Laws

People are curious. They want to know what happened, the extent of injuries or illness, and if the person will be okay. Do not discuss the situation. Do not offer ideas of what is wrong with the person. Information about the person's care, treatment, and condition is confidential. Keep the person's information private. It is the right thing to do.

FOCUS ON PRIDE: Application

Emergencies are stressful. A calm, professional approach helps the person and family feel more secure. Describe professional conduct during an emergency. Explain how you will prepare yourself to respond in an emergency.

REVIEW QUESTIONS

Circle the BEST answer.

1 The goals of first aid are to
   a Call for help and keep the person warm
   b Prevent death and prevent injuries from becoming worse
   c Stay calm and give emergency care
   d Calm the person and keep bystanders away

2 When giving first aid, you should
   a Know your own limits
   b Move the person
   c Give the person fluids
   d Keep the person cool

3 Sudden cardiac arrest is
   a The same as stroke
   b The sudden stopping of heart action
   c The sudden loss of consciousness
   d When organs and tissues do not get enough blood

4 The signs of sudden cardiac arrest are
   a Restlessness, rapid breathing, and a weak pulse
   b Confusion, hemiplegia, and slurred speech
   c No response, no normal breathing, and no pulse
   d Dizziness, pale skin, and slow breathing

5 Rescue breathing for an adult involves
   a Giving each breath over 2 seconds
   b Watching the abdomen rise with each breath
   c Giving a breath every 3 to 5 seconds
   d Giving a breath every 5 to 6 seconds

6 Which hand placement is correct for adult chest compressions?
   a 1 hand in the center of the chest
   b 2 hands below the sternum
   c 2 hands on the lower half of the sternum
   d 2 fingers on the lower half of the sternum

7 When checking for breathing
   a Use the head tilt–chin lift method to open the airway
   b Look for no breathing or agonal gasping
   c Look, listen, and feel for air moving in and out of the lungs
   d Take 10 to 15 seconds to listen for breathing

8 Which pulse is used during adult CPR?
   a The carotid pulse
   b The apical pulse
   c The brachial pulse
   d The femoral pulse

9 Which compression rate is used for adult, child, and infant CPR?
   a 30 compressions per minute
   b 100 to 120 compressions per minute
   c 15 compressions per minute
   d 60 to 100 compressions per minute

10 When doing adult CPR
   a Give 2 breaths after every 15 compressions
   b Give 2 breaths after every 30 compressions
   c Give 1 breath after every 5 compressions
   d Give 2 breaths when you are tired from giving compressions

Continued

REVIEW QUESTIONS—cont'd

11 Two rescuers are giving adult CPR. When should the AED be used?
a After 5 cycles of CPR
b After 2 minutes of CPR
c As soon as the AED arrives
d When EMS staff arrives

12 Two rescuers are giving child CPR. Breaths are given
a After every compression
b After every 5 compressions
c After every 15 compressions
d After every 30 compressions

13 When performing 2-rescuer CPR on an infant
a Use the 2-thumb-encircling hands method for compressions
b Give 30 compressions followed by 2 breaths
c Check for a carotid pulse
d Give CPR if the heart rate is less than 100 beats per minute

14 A person swallowed a chemical. You should
a Have the person drink a glass of water
b Have the person try to vomit
c Call the Poison Control Center
d Contact the chemical's manufacturer

15 Arterial bleeding
a Cannot be seen
b Oozes from the wound
c Is dark red
d Occurs in spurts

16 A person is hemorrhaging from the left forearm. Your *first* action is to
a Lower the arm
b Apply pressure to the brachial artery
c Tape a dressing in place
d Apply direct pressure to the wound

17 A person is about to faint. What should you do?
a Have the person sit or lie down.
b Take the person outside for fresh air.
c Have the person stand very still.
d Raise the head if the person is lying down.

18 Which is a sign of shock?
a High blood pressure
b Slow pulse
c Slow and deep respirations
d Cold, moist, and pale skin

19 A person in shock needs
a Rescue breathing
b Clothes removed
c To be kept lying down
d The recovery position

20 A person is having a stroke. Emergency care involves
a Asking when the person's symptoms began
b Giving the person sips of water
c Controlling bleeding
d Positioning the person bent forward with the head lowered

21 A person is having a tonic-clonic (grand mal) seizure. You should
a Place an object between the person's teeth
b Loosen tight jewelry and clothing around the neck
c Try to stop the person's movements
d Place the person's head on a firm surface

22 After falling down stairs, a person is confused and has a headache. You should
a Place the person in the recovery position
b Give the person a pain-relief drug
c Prevent movement of the head and neck
d Help the person to bed to lie down

23 A person was burned. There are no complaints of pain. You know that
a The burn is minor
b The burn is partial thickness
c The burn is full thickness
d Nerve endings are exposed

24 While waiting for help to arrive, cover a severe burn with
a A sterile, dry dressing or clean cloth
b Butter or oil
c Salve or an ointment
d Nothing

Answers to Chapter 54 questions are on p. 872.

FOCUS ON PRACTICE

Problem Solving

A resident has a seizure during an activity. What emergency care will you provide? After the seizure, the person is only gasping. Explain what you would do step-by-step. How will you and the nursing team provide for the person's privacy?

End-of-Life Care

OBJECTIVES

- Define the key terms and key abbreviations in this chapter.
- Describe terminal illness.
- Describe palliative care and hospice care.
- Describe the factors affecting attitudes about death.
- Describe how different age-groups view death.
- Describe the 5 stages of dying.
- Explain how to meet the needs of the dying person and family.

- Explain the purposes of the Patient Self-Determination Act.
- Explain what is meant by a "Do Not Resuscitate" order.
- Identify the signs of approaching death and the signs of death.
- Explain how to assist with post-mortem care.
- Perform the procedure in this chapter.
- Explain how to promote PRIDE in the person, the family, and yourself.

KEY TERMS

advance directive A document stating a person's wishes about health care when that person cannot make his or her own decisions
autopsy The examination of the body after death
end-of-life care The support and care given during the time surrounding death
palliative care Care that involves relieving or reducing the intensity of uncomfortable symptoms without producing a cure
post-mortem care Care of the body after (post) death (mortem)

reincarnation The belief that the spirit or soul is reborn in another human body or in another form of life
rigor mortis The stiffness or rigidity (rigor) of skeletal muscles that occurs after death (mortis)
terminal illness An illness or injury from which the person will not likely recover

KEY ABBREVIATIONS

DNR	Do Not Resuscitate	**OBRA**	Omnibus Budget Reconciliation Act of 1987
ID	Identification		

End-of-life care describes the support and care given during the time surrounding death. Sometimes death is sudden. Often it is expected. Some people gradually fail. End-of-life care may involve days, weeks, or months.

Most people die in hospitals or nursing centers. Hospice care is a common option. You may see death and dying often. Death and dying cause staff discomfort because they mean helplessness and failure to cure. They also remind us that our loved ones and we will die.

Your feelings about death affect the care you give. You will help meet the dying person's physical, psychological, social, and spiritual needs. Therefore you must understand the dying process. Then you can approach the dying person with caring, kindness, and respect.

See *Teamwork and Time Management: End-of-Life Care.*

TEAMWORK AND TIME MANAGEMENT
End-of-Life Care

Dying persons need a lot of time from nurses. Often it is a busy time before and after someone dies. Offer to take equipment and supplies to and from the room. Also help with other patients or residents.

TERMINAL ILLNESS

Many illnesses and diseases have no cure. The body cannot function after some injuries. Recovery is not expected. The disease or injury ends in death. *An illness or injury from which the person will not likely recover is a* **terminal illness**.

Doctors cannot predict the time of death. A person may have days, months, weeks, or years to live. People expected to live for a short time have lived for years. Others have died before expected to do so.

Modern medicine has found cures or has prolonged life in many cases. Research will bring new cures. However, hope and the will to live strongly influence living and dying. Many people have died for no apparent reason after losing hope or the will to live.

Types of Care

Terminally ill persons can choose palliative care or hospice care. The person may opt for palliative care and then change to hospice care.

- *Palliative care. Palliate* means *to soothe or relieve.* ***Palliative care*** *involves relieving or reducing the intensity of uncomfortable symptoms without producing a cure.* The focus is on relieving symptoms and treating the illness. The intent is to improve quality of life and provide family support. This care is for anyone with a long-term illness that will cause death. Settings include hospitals, nursing centers, and home settings.
- *Hospice care.* The focus is on the physical, emotional, social, and spiritual needs of dying persons and their families (Chapter 1). Often the person has less than 6 months to live. Cure or life-saving measures are not concerns. Pain relief and comfort are stressed. The goal is to improve quality of life. Hospital, nursing centers, and home care agencies offer hospice care. A hospice may be a separate agency. Follow-up care and support groups for survivors are hospice services. Hospice also provides support for the health team to help deal with a person's death.

ATTITUDES ABOUT DEATH

Experiences, culture, religion, and age influence attitudes about death. Many people fear death. Others do not believe they will die. Some look forward to and accept death. Attitudes about death often change as a person grows older and with changing needs.

The family is often involved in the person's care. They usually gather at the bedside to comfort the person and each other. When death occurs, the funeral director is called. The body is taken to the funeral home to prepare for funeral practices.

Many adults and children have had no contact with a dying person. Nor have they been present at the time of death. Some have not attended a visitation (wake) or funeral. They have not seen the process of dying and death. Therefore it is frightening, morbid, and a mystery.

Cultural and Spiritual Needs

Practices and attitudes about death differ among cultures. See *Caring About Culture: Death Rites.* In some cultures, dying people are cared for at home by the family. Some families prepare the body for burial.

Spiritual needs relate to the human spirit and to religion and religious beliefs. They involve finding meaning in one's life. Some people need to resolve issues with family and friends. Many people strengthen their religious beliefs when dying. Religion provides comfort for the dying person and the family.

Attitudes about death are closely related to religion. Some believe that life after death is free of suffering and hardship. They also believe in reunion with loved ones. Many believe sins and misdeeds are punished in the after-life. Others do not believe in the afterlife. To them, death is the end of life.

There are also religious beliefs about the body's form after death. Some believe the body keeps its physical form. Others believe that only the spirit or soul is present in the afterlife. ***Reincarnation*** *is the belief that the spirit or soul is reborn in another human body or in another form of life.*

✿ CARING ABOUT CULTURE

Death Rites

In *Vietnam,* dying persons are helped to recall past good deeds and to achieve a fitting mental state. Death at home is preferred. In some areas, a coin or jewels (a wealthy family) or rice (a poor family) is put in the dead person's mouth. The belief is that they will help the soul go through encounters with gods and devils and the soul will be born rich in the next life.

The *Chinese* have an aversion to death and anything concerning death. Autopsy and disposal of the body are not prescribed by religion. Donating body parts is encouraged. The eldest son makes all arrangements. The body is buried in a coffin. After 7 years, the body is exhumed and cremated. The urn, with the ashes, is buried in the family tomb. White, yellow, or black clothing is worn for mourning.

In *India,* Hindu persons are often accepting of God's will. The person's desire to be clear-headed as death nears must be assessed in planning treatment. A time and place for prayer are essential for the family and the person. Prayer helps them deal with anxiety and conflict. The Hindu priest reads from Holy Sanskrit books. Some priests tie strings (meaning a blessing) around the neck or waist. After death, the son pours water into the mouth of the deceased. Blood transfusions, organ transplants, and autopsies are allowed. Cremation is preferred.

From D'Avanzo CE: Pocket guide to cultural health assessment, ed 4, St Louis, 2008, Mosby.

Many religions practice rites and rituals during the dying process and at the time of death. Prayers, blessings, scripture readings, and religious music are common sources of comfort. So are visits from a cleric.

See *Focus on Communication: Cultural and Spiritual Needs.*

Age

Adults fear pain and suffering, dying alone, and the invasion of privacy. They also fear loneliness and separation from loved ones. They worry about the care and support of those left behind. Adults often resent death because it affects plans, hopes, dreams, and ambitions.

See *Focus on Children and Older Persons: Age.*

FOCUS ON **COMMUNICATION**

Cultural and Spiritual Needs

Your cultural or religious practices and beliefs about death may differ from those of patients and residents. Do not judge the person by your standards. Do not make negative comments or insult the person's beliefs. Respect the person as a whole. This includes his or her beliefs and customs.

FOCUS ON **CHILDREN AND OLDER PERSONS**

Age

Children

Infants and toddlers do not understand the nature or meaning of death. They know or sense that something is different. They sense a caregiver's absence or a different caregiver. They also sense changes in when and how their needs are met. They may feel a sense of loss.

Between 2 and 6 years old, children think death is temporary. It can be reversed. The dead person continues to live and function in some ways and can come back to life. These ideas come from fairy tales, cartoons, movies, video games, and TV. Children this age often blame themselves when someone or something dies. To them, death is punishment for being bad. They know when family members or pets die. They notice dead birds or bugs. Answers to questions about death often cause fear and confusion. Children who are told "He is sleeping" may be afraid to go to sleep.

Between 6 and 11 years, children learn that death is final. They do not think they will die. Death happens to others, especially adults. It can be avoided. Children relate death to punishment and body mutilation. It also involves witches, ghosts, goblins, and monsters. Understanding increases as children grow older and have more experiences with death.

By age 11, death is more fully understood. Death is still viewed as something that happens to other people. One's own death is an event in the distant future. Without correct information, they may have some wrong ideas.

Older Persons

Older persons know death will occur. They have more experiences with dying and death. Many have lost family and friends. Some welcome death as freedom from pain, suffering, and disability. Death also means reunion with those who have died. Like younger adults, many fear dying alone.

THE STAGES OF DYING

Dr. Elisabeth Kübler-Ross described 5 stages of dying. They also are called the "stages of grief." *Grief* is the person's response to loss.

- *Stage 1: Denial.* The person refuses to believe that he or she is dying. "No, not me" is a common response. The person believes a mistake was made. Information about the illness or injury is not heard. The person cannot deal with any problem or decision about the matter. This stage can last for a few hours, days, or much longer. Some people are still in denial when they die.
- *Stage 2: Anger.* The person thinks "Why me?" There is anger and rage. Dying persons envy and resent those with life and health. Family, friends, and the health team are often targets of anger. The person blames others and finds fault with those who are loved and needed the most. It can be hard to deal with the person during this stage. Anger is normal and healthy. Do not take the person's anger personally. Control any urge to attack back or avoid the person.
- *Stage 3: Bargaining.* Anger has passed. The person now says: "Yes, me but..." The person may bargain with God or a higher power for more time. Promises are made in exchange for more time. The person may want to see a child marry, see a grandchild, have another Christmas, or live for a special event. Usually more promises are made as the person makes "just one more" request. Bargaining is usually private and spiritual.
- *Stage 4: Depression.* The person thinks "Yes, me" and is very sad. The person mourns lost things and the future loss of life. The person may cry or say little. Sometimes the person talks about people and things that will be left behind.
- *Stage 5: Acceptance.* The person is calm, at peace, and accepts death. The person has said what needs to be said. Unfinished business is complete. This stage may last for many months or years. Reaching the acceptance stage does not mean death is near.

Dying persons do not always pass through each stage. A person may never get beyond a certain stage. Some move back and forth between stages. For example, Mr. Jones moves from acceptance back to bargaining. Then he moves forward to acceptance. Some people stay in 1 stage.

COMFORT NEEDS

Comfort is part of end-of-life care. It involves physical, mental and emotional, and spiritual needs. For spiritual needs, see "Cultural and Spiritual Needs" on p. 852. Comfort goals are to:

- Prevent or relieve suffering to the extent possible.
- Respect and follow end-of-life wishes.

Dying persons may want family and friends present. They may want to talk about their fears, worries, and anxieties. Some want to be alone. Often they need to talk during the night. Things are quiet, distractions are few, and there is more time to think. You need to listen and use touch.

- *Listening.* The person needs to talk and share worries and concerns. Let the person express feelings and emotions in his or her own way. Do not worry about saying the wrong thing or finding comforting words. You do not need to say anything. Being there for the person is what counts.
- *Touch.* Touch shows care and concern when words cannot. Sometimes the person does not want to talk but needs you nearby. Do not feel that you need to talk. Silence, along with touch, is a powerful and meaningful way to communicate.

Some people may want to see a spiritual leader. Or they want to take part in religious practices. Provide privacy during prayer and spiritual times. Be courteous to the spiritual leader. The person has the right to have religious objects nearby—medals, pictures, statues, writings, and so on. Handle them with care and respect.

See *Focus on Communication: Comfort Needs.*

See *Focus on Children and Older Persons: Comfort Needs.*

FOCUS ON COMMUNICATION

Comfort Needs

You may not know what to say to the dying person. That is hard for many health team members. Unless you have been near death yourself, do not say: "I understand what you are going through." The statement is a communication barrier. Instead you can say:

- "Would you like to talk? I have time to listen."
- "You seem sad. How can I help?"
- "Is it okay if I quietly sit with you for a while?"

FOCUS ON CHILDREN AND OLDER PERSONS

Comfort Needs

Older Persons

Persons with Alzheimer's disease (AD) become more and more disabled. Those with advanced AD cannot share their concerns, discomforts, or problems. And it is hard to provide emotional and spiritual comfort.

Focus on the person's senses—hearing, touch, sight—to promote comfort. Comforting touch or massage can be soothing. So can soft music or sounds from nature—birds chirping, gentle breezes, ocean waves, and so on.

Physical Needs

Dying may take a few minutes, hours, days, or weeks. Body processes slow. The person is weak. Changes occur in levels of consciousness. The person remains independent to the extent possible. As the person weakens, basic needs are met by others. Every effort is made to promote physical and psychological comfort. The person is allowed to die in peace and with dignity.

Pain. Pain can range from none to severe. Report signs and symptoms of pain at once (Chapter 31). Pain management is important. The nurse can give pain-relief drugs to prevent or control pain. Preventing and controlling pain are easier than relieving pain.

Skin care, personal and oral hygiene, back massages, and good alignment promote comfort. So do frequent position changes and supportive devices. Turn the person slowly and gently. Follow the care plan to prevent and control pain.

Breathing Problems. Shortness of breath and difficulty breathing *(dyspnea)* are common end-of-life problems. Semi-Fowler's position and oxygen (Chapter 39) are helpful. An open window for fresh air may be helpful. So might a fan circulating air.

Noisy breathing—called the *death rattle*—is common as death nears. This is caused by mucus collecting in the airway. These measures may help.

- The side-lying position
- Suctioning by the nurse
- Drugs to reduce the amount of mucus

Vision, Hearing, and Speech. Vision blurs and gradually fails. The person turns toward light. A darkened room may frighten the person. The eyes may be half-open. Secretions may collect in the eye corners.

Because of failing vision, explain who you are and what you are doing to the person or in the room. The room should be well lit. Avoid bright lights and glares.

Good eye care is needed (Chapter 22). If the eyes stay open, a nurse may apply a protective ointment. Then the eyes are covered with moist pads to prevent injury.

Hearing is one of the last functions lost. Many people hear until the moment of death. Even unconscious persons may hear. Always assume that the person can hear. Speak in a normal voice. Provide reassurance and explanations about care. Offer words of comfort. Avoid upsetting topics. Do not talk about the person.

Speech becomes harder. It may be hard to understand the person. Sometimes the person cannot speak. Anticipate the person's needs. Do not ask questions with long answers. Ask a few "yes" or "no" questions. Despite speech problems, you must talk to the person.

Mouth, Nose, and Skin. Oral hygiene promotes comfort. Give routine mouth care if the person can eat and drink. Give frequent oral hygiene as death nears and when taking oral fluids is difficult. Oral hygiene is needed if mucus collects in the mouth and the person cannot swallow. A lip balm may help dry lips.

Crusting and irritation of the mouth can occur. Nasal secretions, an oxygen cannula, and a naso-gastric tube are common causes. Carefully clean the nose. Apply lubricant as directed by the nurse and the care plan.

Circulation fails. Body temperature rises as death nears although the skin is cool, pale, and mottled (blotchy). Sweating increases. Skin care, bathing, and preventing pressure ulcers are necessary. Linens and gowns are changed as needed. Although the skin feels cool, only light bed coverings are needed. Blankets may cause warmth and restlessness. However, observe for signs of cold—shivering, hunching shoulders, and pulling covers. Prevent drafts and provide more blankets.

Nutrition. Nausea, vomiting, and loss of appetite are common at the end of life. The doctor can order drugs for nausea and vomiting.

Some persons are too tired or weak to eat. You may need to feed them. Favorite foods may help loss of appetite. So may small, frequent meals.

As death nears, loss of appetite is common. The person may choose not to eat or drink. Do not force the person to eat or drink. Tell the nurse.

Elimination. Urinary and fecal incontinence may occur. Use incontinence products or waterproof bed protectors as directed. Give perineal care as needed. Constipation and urinary retention are common. Enemas and catheters may be needed. Follow the care plan for catheter care.

The Person's Room. Provide a comfortable and pleasant room. It should be well lit and well ventilated. Remove unnecessary equipment. Some equipment is upsetting to look at (suction machines, drainage containers). If possible, keep these items out of the person's sight.

Mementos, pictures, cards, flowers, and religious items provide comfort. The person and family arrange the room as they wish. This helps meet love, belonging, and esteem needs. The room should reflect the person's choices.

Mental and Emotional Needs

Mental and emotional needs are very personal. Some persons are calm and at peace. Others are anxious or depressed or have specific fears and concerns. Examples include:

- Severe pain
- When and how death will occur
- What will happen to loved ones
- Dying alone

The doctor may order drugs for anxiety or depression. Simple measures may be soothing—touch, holding hands, back massage, soft lighting, music at a low volume.

THE FAMILY

This is a hard time for the family. It may be hard to find comforting words. To show you care, use touch and be available, courteous, and considerate.

Family members usually can stay as long as they wish. Sometimes the family keeps a vigil. That is, someone is always with the person even at night. They watch over or pray for the person. Help make the family as comfortable as possible.

Respect the right to privacy. The person and family need time together. However, do not neglect care because the family is present. Most agencies let family members help give care. Or you can suggest that they take a beverage or meal break.

The family may be very tired, sad, and tearful. Watching a loved one die is very painful. So is dealing with the eventual loss of that person. The family goes through stages like the dying person. They need support, understanding, courtesy, and respect. A spiritual leader may provide comfort. Communicate this request to the nurse at once.

LEGAL ISSUES

Much attention is given to the right to die. Many people do not want machines or other measures keeping them alive. Consent is needed for any treatment. When able, the person makes care decisions. Some people make end-of-life wishes known.

Advance Directives

The *Patient Self-Determination Act* and the *Omnibus Budget Reconciliation Act of 1987 (OBRA)* give persons the right to accept or refuse treatment. They also give the right to make advance directives. An ***advance directive*** *is a document stating a person's wishes about health care when that person cannot make his or her own decisions.* It identifies the care wanted if seriously ill or dying. Advance directives usually forbid certain care if there is no hope of recovery. Quality of care cannot be less because of the person's advance directives.

Agencies must inform all persons of the right to advance directives on admission. This information is in writing. The medical record documents whether or not the person has made them.

Living wills and durable power of attorney for health care are common advance directives.

See *Focus on Surveys: Advance Directives*, p. 856.

Living Wills. A living will is about measures that support or maintain life when death is likely. Tube feedings, ventilators, and resuscitation are examples. A living will may instruct doctors:

- Not to start measures that prolong dying
- To remove measures that prolong dying

Durable Power of Attorney for Health Care. This advance directive gives the power to make health care decisions to another person. That person is often called a *health care proxy*. Usually this is a family member, friend, or lawyer. When a person cannot make health care decisions, the health care proxy can do so. This advance directive does not cover property or financial matters.

"Do Not Resuscitate" Orders

When death is sudden and unexpected, efforts are made to save the person's life. See Chapter 54.

For terminally ill persons, doctors often write "Do Not Resuscitate" (DNR) or "No Code" orders. The person will not be resuscitated. The person is allowed to die with peace and dignity. The orders are written after consulting with the person and family. The family and doctor make the decision if the person is not mentally able to do so. Some advance directives address resuscitation.

You may not agree with care and resuscitation decisions. However, you must follow the person's or family's wishes and the doctor's orders. These may be against your personal, religious, and cultural values. If so, talk to the nurse. You may need an assignment change.

SIGNS OF DEATH

In the weeks before death, the dying process may involve:
- Restlessness and agitation
- Shortness of breath; pauses in breathing
- Depression
- Anxiety
- Drowsiness
- Confusion
- Constipation or incontinence
- Nausea and loss of appetite
- Healing problems
- Swelling in the hands, feet, or other body areas

As death nears, these signs may occur fast or slowly.
- Movement, muscle tone, and sensation are lost. This usually starts in the feet and legs. Mouth muscles relax, the jaw drops. The mouth may stay open. The facial expression is often peaceful.
- Peristalsis and other gastro-intestinal functions slow down. Abdominal distention, fecal incontinence, nausea, and vomiting are common.
- Body temperature rises. The person feels cool or cold, looks pale, and perspires heavily.
- Circulation fails. The pulse is fast or slow, weak, and irregular. Blood pressure starts to fall.
- The respiratory system fails. Slow or rapid and shallow respirations are observed. Mucus collects in the airway. Breathing sounds are noisy and gurgling—commonly called the *death rattle*.
- Pain decreases as the person loses consciousness. However, some people are conscious until the moment of death.

The signs of death include *no pulse, no respirations*, and *no blood pressure*. The pupils are fixed and dilated. A doctor determines that death has occurred. He or she pronounces the person dead. In nursing centers, a nurse calls the doctor to report the signs of death. The time and place are noted for the death certificate.

CARE OF THE BODY AFTER DEATH

Care of the body after (post) *death* (mortem) *is called* **post-mortem care.** You may be asked to assist the nurse. Post-mortem care begins when the person is pronounced dead.

Post-mortem care is done to maintain a good appearance of the body. Discoloration and skin damage are prevented. Valuables and personal items are gathered for the family.

Within 2 to 4 hours after death, rigor mortis develops. **Rigor mortis** *is the stiffness or rigidity* (rigor) *of skeletal muscles that occurs after death* (mortis). The body is positioned in normal alignment before rigor mortis sets in. The family may want to see the body. The body should appear in a comfortable and natural position.

In some agencies, the body is prepared only for viewing by the family. The funeral director completes post-mortem care.

Sometimes an autopsy is done. An **autopsy** *is the examination of the body after death.* (*Autos* means *self. Opsis* means *view.*) It is done to determine the cause of death. Post-mortem care is not done. Doing so could remove or destroy evidence.

Post-mortem care involves moving the body. For example, soiled areas are bathed and the body is placed in good alignment. Moving the body can cause air in the lungs, stomach, and intestines to be expelled. When air is expelled, sounds are produced. Do not let those sounds alarm or frighten you. They are normal and expected.

See *Delegation Guidelines: Care of the Body After Death.*

See *Promoting Safety and Comfort: Care of the Body After Death.*

See procedure: *Assisting With Post-Mortem Care.*

DELEGATION GUIDELINES
Care of the Body After Death

To assist with post-mortem care, you need this information from the nurse.

- If dentures are inserted or placed in a denture cup
- If tubes and dressings are removed or left in place
- If rings are removed or left in place
- If the family wants to view the body
- Special agency policies and procedures

PROMOTING SAFETY AND COMFORT
Care of the Body After Death

Safety
Standard Precautions and the Bloodborne Pathogen Standard are followed. You may have contact with blood, body fluids, secretions, and excretions.

Assisting With Post-Mortem Care

PRE-PROCEDURE

1 Follow *Delegation Guidelines: Care of the Body After Death*. See *Promoting Safety and Comfort: Care of the Body After Death*.
2 Practice hand hygiene.
3 Collect the following.
   - Post-mortem kit (shroud or body bag, gown, ID [identification] tags, gauze squares, safety pins)
   - Waterproof bed protectors
   - Wash basin
   - Bath towel and washcloths
   - Denture cup
   - Items for shaving facial hair (Chapter 23)
   - Tape
   - Dressings
   - Gloves
   - Cotton balls
   - Valuables envelope
4 Provide for privacy.
5 Raise the bed for body mechanics.
6 Make sure the bed is flat.

PROCEDURE

7 Put on the gloves.
8 Position the body supine. Arms and legs are straight. A pillow is under the head and shoulders. Or raise the head of the bed 15 to 20 degrees if this is agency policy.
9 Close the eyes. Gently pull the eyelids over the eyes. Apply moist cotton balls gently over the eyelids if the eyes will not stay closed.
10 Insert dentures if it is agency policy to do so. If not, put them in a labeled denture cup.
11 Close the mouth. If necessary, place a rolled towel under the chin to keep the mouth closed.
12 Follow agency policy for jewelry. Remove all jewelry, except for wedding rings if this is agency policy. List the jewelry that you removed. Place the jewelry and the list in a valuables envelope.
13 Place a cotton ball over the rings. Tape them in place.
14 Remove drainage containers.
15 Remove tubes and catheters. Use the gauze squares as needed.
16 Shave facial hair if this is agency policy or desired by the family.
17 Bathe soiled areas with plain water. Dry thoroughly.
18 Place a waterproof bed protector under the buttocks.
19 Remove soiled dressings. Replace them with clean ones.
20 Put a clean gown on the body. Position the body as in step 8.
21 Brush and comb the hair if necessary.
22 Cover the body to the shoulders with a sheet if the family will view the body.
23 Gather the person's belongings. Put them in a bag labeled with the person's name. Make sure you include eyeglasses, hearing aids, and other valuables.
24 Remove supplies, equipment, and linens. Straighten the room. Provide soft lighting.
25 Remove and discard the gloves. Practice hand hygiene.
26 Let the family view the body. Provide for privacy. Return to the room after they leave.
27 Practice hand hygiene. Put on gloves.
28 Fill out the ID tags. Tie 1 to the ankle or to the right big toe.
29 Place the body in the body bag or cover it with a sheet. Or apply a shroud (Fig. 55-1, p. 858).
   a Position the shroud under the body.
   b Bring the top down over the head.
   c Fold the bottom up over the feet.
   d Fold the sides over the body.
   e Pin or tape the shroud in place.
30 Attach the second ID tag to the shroud, sheet, or body bag.
31 Leave the denture cup with the body.
32 Pull the privacy curtain around the bed. Or close the door.

POST-PROCEDURE

33 Remove and discard the gloves. Practice hand hygiene.
34 Strip the unit after the body has been removed. Wear gloves for this step.
35 Remove and discard the gloves. Practice hand hygiene.
36 Report the following.
   - The time the body was taken by the funeral director
   - What was done with jewelry, other valuables, and personal items
   - What was done with dentures

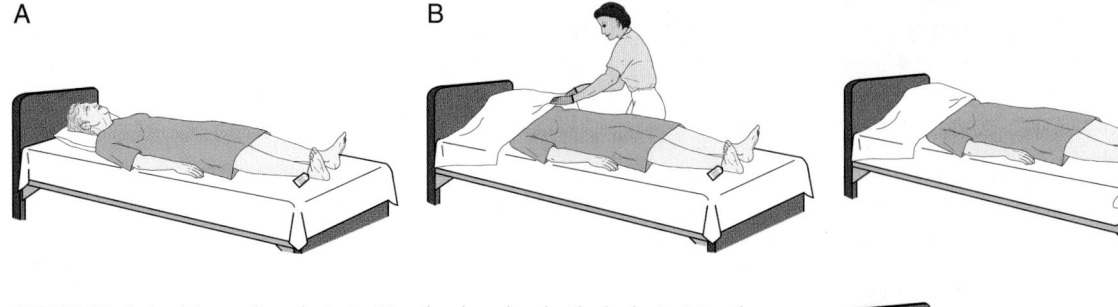

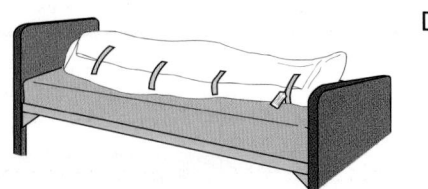

FIGURE 55-1 Applying a shroud. **A,** Position the shroud under the body. **B,** Bring the top of the shroud down over the head. **C,** Fold the bottom up over the feet. **D,** Fold the sides over the body. Tape or pin the sides together. Attach the ID tag.

FOCUS ON **PRIDE**

The Person, Family, and Yourself

Personal and Professional Responsibility

You may assist with the dying person's care. To give quality care:

- Promote comfort. Report the person's complaints or signs of pain at once. Follow the comfort measures in the care plan.
- Protect the person's privacy.
- Provide support to the person and family. Be kind. Show compassion and respect.
- Offer the family time alone with the person.

Take pride in supporting the person and family during a difficult time.

Rights and Respect

Understanding the person's needs and desires allows you to give better care. Box 55-1 contains the dying person's bill of rights. Respect these rights. Respect the person's right to die in peace and with dignity. The right to privacy and the right to be treated with dignity and respect apply after death.

Independence and Social Interaction

The person is encouraged to take part in his or her care to the extent possible. Some days the person can do more than other days. Follow the nurse's directions and the care plan. Do not force the person to do more than he or she can physically or mentally do.

Delegation and Teamwork

Over time, the health team often bonds with the person. This is common in hospice and long-term care. The person's death is difficult for the staff. Sadness and grief may occur.

Tell the nurse if you have trouble coping with a person's death. Support others who need help. A kind word, a hug, or taking time to listen show concern. Take pride in being a part of a caring and supportive team.

Ethics and Laws

The dying person has rights under OBRA.

- *The right to privacy before and after death.* The person has the right not to have his or her body seen by others. Proper draping and screening are important.
- *The right to visit others in private.* If the person is too weak to leave the room, the roommate may have to do so. The nurse and social worker develop a plan that satisfies everyone. Moving the dying person to a private room provides privacy. The family can also stay as long as they like.
- *The right to confidentiality before and after death.* The final moments and cause of death are kept confidential. So are statements, conversations, and family reactions.
- *The right to be free from abuse, mistreatment, and neglect.* The person has the right to receive kind and respectful care before and after death. Report signs of abuse, mistreatment, or neglect to the nurse at once.
- *Freedom from restraint.* Restraints are used only if ordered by the doctor. Dying persons are often too weak to be dangerous to themselves or others.
- *The right to have personal possessions.* The person may want photos and religious items nearby. Protect the person's property from loss or damage before and after death. They may be family treasures or mementos.
- *The right to a safe and home-like setting.* Dying persons depend on others for safety. Everyone must keep the setting safe and home-like. Try to keep equipment and supplies out of view. The room also should be free from unpleasant odors and noises. Do your best to keep the room neat and clean.
- *The right to personal choice.* The person has the right to be involved in treatment and care. The dying person may refuse treatment. Advance directives are common. The health team must respect choices to refuse treatment or not prolong life.

FOCUS ON **PRIDE**: *Application*

Genuine concern for the dying person is reflected in the care you give. Identify ways you can show respect at the end of life and with post-mortem care. How can you show care and concern for the grieving family?

BOX 55-1 A Dying Patient's Bill of Last Rights

- *The Right to BE IN CONTROL.* Grant me the right to make as many decisions as possible regarding my care. Please do not take choices from me. Let me make my own decisions.
- *The Right to HAVE A SENSE OF PURPOSE.* I have lost my job. I can no longer fulfill my role in my family. Please help me find some sense of purpose in my last days.
- *The Right to REMINISCE.* There has been pleasure in my life, moments of pride, moments of love. Please give some time to recollect those moments. And please listen to my recollections.
- *The Right to TOUCH AND BE TOUCHED.* Sometimes I need distance. Yet sometimes I have a strong need to be close. When I want to reach out, please come to me and hold me as I hold you.
- *The Right to LAUGH.* People often—far too often—come to me wearing masks of seriousness. Although I am dying, I still need to laugh. Please laugh with me and help others to laugh as well.

- *The Right to BE ANGRY AND SAD.* It is difficult to leave behind all my attachments and all that I love. Please allow me the opportunity to be angry and sad.
- *The Right to HAVE A RESPECTED SPIRITUALITY.* Whether I am questioning or affirming, doubting or praising, I sometimes need your ear, a non-judging ear. Please let my spirit travel its own journey, without judging its direction.
- *The Right to HEAR THE TRUTH.* If you withhold the truth from me, you will treat me as if I am no longer living. I am still living, and I need to know the truth about my life. Please help me find that truth.
- *The Right to BE IN DENIAL.* If I hear the truth and choose not to accept it, that is my right.
  Honor these Rights. One day you too will want the same Rights.

Modified from The Hospice RN: Patient's bill of rights: a dying patient's bill of last rights.

REVIEW QUESTIONS

Circle the BEST answer.

1 Which is *true?*
   a Death from terminal illness is sudden.
   b Doctors know when death will occur.
   c An illness is terminal when recovery is not likely.
   d All severe injuries end in death.

2 Which statement is *true?*
   a Attitudes about death change as a person ages.
   b Culture does not influence attitudes about death.
   c Young children understand death well.
   d A family member's death does not affect a toddler.

3 Reincarnation is the belief that
   a There is no afterlife
   b The spirit or soul is reborn into another human body or form of life
   c The body keeps its physical form in the afterlife
   d Only the spirit or soul is present in the afterlife

4 A 5-year-old views death as
   a Temporary   c Adults do
   b Final   d Going to sleep

5 Adults and older persons usually fear
   a Reincarnation   c Advance directives
   b The 5 stages of dying d Dying alone

6 Persons in the stage of denial
   a Are angry
   b Are calm and at peace
   c Refuse to believe they are dying
   d Are sad and quiet

7 A person tries to gain more time during the stage of
   a Anger   c Depression
   b Bargaining   d Acceptance

8 When caring for the dying person, you should
   a Use touch and listen
   b Do most of the talking
   c Ask questions with long answers
   d Speak in a loud voice

9 As death nears, the last sense lost is
   a Sight   c Smell
   b Taste   d Hearing

10 The dying person's care includes the following. Which should you question?
   a Eye care
   b Mouth care
   c Active range-of-motion exercises
   d Position changes

11 The dying person is positioned in
   a The supine position
   b The Fowler's position
   c Good body alignment
   d The dorsal recumbent position

12 A "DNR" order means that
   a CPR will not be done
   b The person has a living will
   c Life-prolonging measures will be carried out
   d The person is kept alive as long as possible

13 Which signals approaching death?
   a Increased pain
   b Slow and shallow respirations
   c Increased blood pressure
   d Warm and dry skin

14 The signs of death are
   a Convulsions and incontinence
   b No pulse, respirations, or blood pressure
   c Loss of consciousness and convulsions
   d The eyes stay open, no muscle movements, and the body is rigid

15 Post-mortem care is done
   a After rigor mortis sets in
   b When the funeral director arrives for the body
   c After the family has viewed the body
   d After the doctor pronounces the person dead

Answers to Chapter 55 questions are on p. 872.

FOCUS ON PRACTICE

Problem Solving

Mr. Perez is near the end of his life. You want to provide mouth care. His family enters his room. Is this a good time to give care? What will you say to his family?

OBJECTIVES

- Define the key terms and key abbreviations in this chapter.
- Identify the sources for jobs and places to work.
- Describe what employers look for when hiring staff.
- Describe the qualities and traits needed to work in home care settings.
- Describe how you can prove completion of a nursing assistant training and competency evaluation program (NATCEP).
- Explain how to complete a job application.
- Identify the documents to keep in an education and work history file.

- Describe in-person, phone, and video interviews.
- Explain how to prepare and dress for an interview.
- Identify common interview questions.
- Explain how to conduct yourself during an interview.
- Describe the questions you cannot be asked during an interview or on a job application.
- Explain what to do after an interview.
- Explain how to accept or decline a job offer.
- Explain how to promote PRIDE in the person, the family, and yourself.

KEY TERMS

job application An agency's official form listing questions that require factual answers

job interview When an employer asks a job applicant questions about his or her education and career

KEY ABBREVIATIONS

EEOC Equal Employment Opportunity Commission
NATCEP Nursing assistant training and competency evaluation program

OBRA Omnibus Budget Reconciliation Act of 1987

Successfully completing a nursing assistant training and competency evaluation program (NATCEP) gives you a valuable credential for employment. And it may be a step toward becoming a registered nurse (RN) or licensed practical nurse/licensed vocational nurse (LPN/LVN).

During your NATCEP or after, you will likely focus on getting a job. This chapter will help you do so in a professional and efficient manner.

SOURCES OF JOBS

There are easy ways to find out about jobs and places to work.

- Newspaper ads
- Local and state employment services
- Agencies you would like to work at
- Phone book yellow pages
- People you know—instructor, family, and friends
- The Internet
- Your school's or college's job placement counselors
- Your clinical experience site
- Job fairs

Your clinical experience site is an important source. The staff observe students as future employees. They look for good work ethics. They watch how students treat patients, residents, and co-workers. They look for the qualities and traits described in Chapter 6—being caring, dependable, considerate, cheerful, trustworthy, respectful courteous, conscientious, honest, cooperative, enthusiastic, self-aware, and patient and having empathy. If your clinical agency is not hiring, the staff may suggest other places to apply.

WHAT EMPLOYERS LOOK FOR

If you owned a business, who would you hire? Your answer helps you better understand the employer's point of view. Employers want staff who:

- Are dependable
- Are well-groomed
- Have needed job skills and training
- Have values and attitudes that fit with the agency

To function well, you need good work ethics. Review Chapter 6 and the "Ethics and Laws" sections in the *Focus on PRIDE* boxes at the end of each chapter to help you develop positive attitudes and work practices.

Being dependable is important. You must be at work on time and when scheduled. Undependable people cause everyone problems. Other staff have extra work. Fewer staff give care. Quality of care suffers. Supervisors spend time trying to find out if the person is coming to work. They also have to find someone to cover for the absent employee. You want co-workers to work when scheduled. Otherwise, you have extra work. You have less time to spend with patients and residents. Likewise, co-workers expect you to work when scheduled.

Applicants who look good communicate many things to the employer. You have 1 chance to make a good first impression. A well-groomed person will likely get the job. A sloppy person with wrinkled or dirty clothes may not get the job. Nor will someone with body or breath odors. See p. 865 for how to dress for an interview.

See *Focus on Long-Term Care and Home Care: What Employers Look For.*

FOCUS ON LONG-TERM CARE AND HOME CARE

What Employers Look For

Home Care
Besides the qualities and traits already described and those in Chapter 6, home care requires:
- *The ability to work alone.* Usually a nurse is not with you in the home. If problems occur, you can reach the nurse by phone. You must provide skillful and safe care.
- *Self-discipline.* You must arrive at homes on time. Plan activities so personal care needs and housekeeping tasks get done. Avoid temptations. This includes watching TV, talking on the phone, visiting, and stopping for a cup of coffee.
- *Honesty.* You might need to shop for the person. Be honest and thrifty with the person's money. Accurately report what you bought, the cost with receipts, amount spent, and amount of money returned.
- *Respect for the person's property.* You will handle valuables and personal property in health care settings. Access to the person's property is greater in the home. You use furnishings, appliances, linens, and household items to give care and for housekeeping. Treat personal and family property with respect. Prevent damage. Read the manufacturer's instructions before using any appliance. Clean the appliance after use.

Job Skills and Training

Employers need to know that you have the required job skills. The employer checks the nursing assistant registry and requests proof of successful NATCEP completion. To prove NATCEP completion, an employer will accept 1 or more of the following.
- A certificate of course completion
- A high school, college, or technical school transcript
- An official grade report (report card)

Give the employer a *copy* of your certificate, transcript, or grade report. Never give the original to anyone. Keep originals in a safe place for future use. Some employers want a transcript sent directly from the school or college.

See *Focus on Long-Term Care and Home Care: Job Skills and Training.*

FOCUS ON LONG-TERM CARE AND HOME CARE

Job Skills and Training

Long-Term Care
To work in long-term care, you must complete a state-approved NATCEP. This is a requirement of the *Omnibus Budget Reconciliation Act of 1987 (OBRA)*. The employer requests proof of training. The nursing assistant registry is checked. Nursing centers cannot hire persons convicted of abuse, neglect, or mistreatment. This also is an OBRA requirement.

Home Care
Home care agencies that receive Medicare funds must meet OBRA requirements. You must complete a NATCEP outlined by OBRA. Some states have additional training requirements for working in home care.

JOB APPLICATIONS

A *job application* is an agency's official form listing questions that require factual answers (Fig. 56-1, pp. 862-863). Personal information (legal name, address, phone number), employment history, education, qualifications, and references are examples.

You get a job application from the *personnel office (human resources office)* or on-line. If the application is on paper, you use a pen to complete the form. You can complete the application at the agency. Or you can take it home for return by mail or in person. You must be well-groomed and behave pleasantly when seeking or returning a job application. It may be your first chance to make a good impression.

On-line job applications require a computer. Follow the agency's instructions for completing an on-line application.

Text continued on p. 864.

EMPLOYMENT APPLICATION

APPLICANT INSTRUCTIONS

If you need help filling out this application form or for any phase of the employment process, please notify the person that gave you this form and every effort will be made to accommodate your needs in a reasonable amount of time.

1. Please read "APPLICANT NOTE" below.
2. Complete both sides of this page.
3. If more space is needed to complete any question, use comments section at the bottom of this page.
4. Print clearly: incomplete or illegible applications will not be processed. PLEASE NOTE "NOT APPLICABLE" IF NOT ANSWERING A QUESTION.
5. Provide only requested information. Failure to do so may result in disqualification of your application.
6. Some packets may include an AFFIRMATIVE ACTION QUESTIONNAIRE. This information is being gathered for affirmative action under Section 503 of the Rehabilitation Act of 1973. The information requested is voluntary and will be kept confidential. An applicant will not be subject to any adverse treatment for refusing to complete the questionnaire.
7. DO NOT FILL OUT ANY OTHER ATTACHED FORMS OR PAGES UNTIL INSTRUCTED.

TODAY'S DATE: _____

NAME: _____
LAST   FIRST   MI

SOCIAL SECURITY NUMBER: _____

HOME PHONE: _____ WORK PHONE: _____

CURRENT ADDRESS: _____
STREET

_____
CITY   STATE   ZIP

PRIOR ADDRESS: _____
STREET

_____
CITY   STATE   ZIP

APPLICANT NOTE

This application form is intended for use in evaluating your qualifications for employment. This is not an employment contract. Please answer all appropriate questions completely and accurately. False or misleading statements during the interview and on this form are grounds for terminating the application process or, if discovered after employment, terminating employment. All qualified applicants will receive consideration without discrimination based on sex, marital status, race, color, age, creed, national origin, sexual orientation, military reserve membership, ancestry, religion, height, weight, use of a guide or support animal because of blindness, deafness or physical handicap, or the presence of disabilities. A conviction will not necessarily bar an applicant from employment. Additional testing of job-related skills and for the presence of drugs in your body may be required prior to employment. After an offer of employment, and prior to reporting to work, you may be required to submit to a medical review. Depending on company policy and the needs of the job, you will be required to complete a medical history form and may be required to be examined by a medical professional designated by the company.

AVAILABILITY

For which position are you applying? _____

What date can you start? _____ What category would you prefer? ❑ Full time ❑ Part time ❑ Temporary ❑ Labor pool

For which schedules are you available?* ❑ Weekdays ❑ Weekends ❑ Evenings ❑ Nights ❑ Overtime ❑ Shift ❑ Other_____

*reasonable efforts will be made to accommodate sincerely held moral and ethical beliefs, (WI) religious beliefs and practices (All other States)

JOB-RELATED SKILLS

NOTE: Do not fill out any part of this section you believe to be non-job related.

❑ Yes ❑ No If the job requires, do you have the appropriate valid drivers license?
Name on license _____ DL# _____ Type _____ State of Issue_____

❑ Yes ❑ No Have you had any moving violations within the last seven years? Please describe._____
Please list any other skills, licenses or certificates that may be job-related or that you feel would be of value to this job or company. _____

❑ Yes ❑ No Have you been given a job description or had the essential functions of the job explained to you?

❑ Yes ❑ No Do you understand these essential functions?

❑ Yes ❑ No Can you perform the essential functions of this job with or without reasonable accommodation?

SECURITY

List states and counties of residence for the past seven years: _____

❑ Yes ❑ No Have you used any names or Social Security Numbers other than given above? If so, please list in comments, below.

❑ Yes ❑ No Have you been convicted of a crime in the past seven years? If so, please describe in the boxes below. (Conviction will not necessarily be a bar to employment. In accordance with company policy and applicable state and federal laws, factors such as age at time of the offense, remoteness of the offense, time since last conviction, nature of the job sought and rehabilitation effort will be reviewed.)

INCIDENT	CITY/STATE	CHARGE
1.		
2.		

COMMENTS (ASK FOR AN ADDITIONAL PAGE IF NECESSARY)

_____
_____
_____
_____

FIGURE 56-1 A sample job application. (Courtesy ADP Screening and Selection Services, Ft. Collins, Colo.)

PREVIOUS EMPLOYERS

PLEASE NOTE: Your application will not be considered unless every question in this section is answered. Since we will make every effort to contact previous employers, the **correct telephone numbers of past employers are critical.** Ask for a phone book or call information if necessary. FOR EMPLOYERS OUTSIDE THE U.S., A CURRENT FAX NUMBER IS MANDATORY.

MOST RECENT EMPLOYER

☐ Yes   ☐ No   Are you currently working for this employer?
☐ Yes   ☐ No   If yes, may we contact?

PHONE ( )
FAX ( )

COMPANY NAME _____ CITY _____ STATE _____

FROM _____ TO _____
DATES EMPLOYED   JOB TITLE _____ SUPERVISOR NAME _____

DUTIES _____

PER
SALARY _____ (HOUR, WEEK, MONTH)   REASON FOR LEAVING _____

SECOND MOST RECENT EMPLOYER

PHONE ( )
FAX ( )

COMPANY NAME _____ CITY _____ STATE _____

FROM _____ TO _____
DATES EMPLOYED   JOB TITLE _____ SUPERVISOR NAME _____

DUTIES _____

PER
SALARY _____ (HOUR, WEEK, MONTH)   REASON FOR LEAVING _____

THIRD MOST RECENT EMPLOYER

PHONE ( )
FAX ( )

COMPANY NAME _____ CITY _____ STATE _____

FROM _____ TO _____
DATES EMPLOYED   JOB TITLE _____ SUPERVISOR NAME _____

DUTIES _____

PER
SALARY _____ (HOUR, WEEK, MONTH)   REASON FOR LEAVING _____

REFERENCES

Include only individuals familiar with your work ability. Do not include relatives.

NAME	ADDRESS/PHONE	YEARS KNOWN/RELATIONSHIP
1.		
2.		

EDUCATION

NOTE: Do not fill out any part of this section you believe to be non-job related.
Please circle highest grade completed.   7   8   9   10   11   12   13   14   15   16   16+

If your school records are under a different name than listed on page 1, please enter that name_____

NAME	CITY/STATE	GRADUATED	DEGREE?
HIGH SCHOOL			
COLLEGE			
OTHER			

CERTIFICATION AND RELEASE

I certify that I have read and understand the applicant note on page one of this form and that the answers given by me to the foregoing questions and the statements made by me are complete and true to the best of my knowledge and belief. I understand that any false information, omissions or misrepresentations of facts called for in this application, whether on this document or not, may result in rejection of my application or discharge at any time during my employment. I authorize the company and/or its agents, including consumer reporting bureaus, to verify any of this information. I authorize all former employers, persons, schools, companies and law enforcement authorities from any liability for any damage whatsoever for issuing this information. I also understand that the use of illegal drugs is prohibited during employment. If company policy requires, I am willing to submit to drug testing to detect the use of illegal drugs prior to and during employment.

SIGNATURE _____   DATE _____

FIGURE 56-1, cont'd

BOX 56-1	Guidelines for Completing a Job Application

- Read and follow the directions. They may ask you to print using black ink. Employers look at job applications to see if you can follow directions. Following directions on the job application gives the employer insight about your ability to follow directions on the job.
- Write neatly. Writing must be readable. A messy application gives a bad image. Readable writing gives the correct information. The agency cannot contact you if unable to read your phone number. You may miss getting the job.
- Complete the entire form. Something may not apply to you. If so, write "N/A" for non-applicable. Or draw a line through the space. This shows that you read the section. It also shows that you did not skip the item on purpose.
- Report any felony convictions as directed. Write "no" or "none" as appropriate. Criminal background and fingerprint checks are common requirements.
- Give information about employment gaps. If you did not work for a time, the employer wonders why. Providing this information shows you are honest. Some reasons are an illness, going to school, raising your children, or caring for an ill or older family member.

- Tell why you left a job, if asked. Be brief but honest. People leave jobs for one that pays better. Some leave for career advancement. Others leave for reasons given for employment gaps. If you were fired from a job, give an honest but positive answer. Do not talk badly about a former employer.
- Provide references. Be prepared to give names, titles, addresses, and phone numbers of at least 4 non-family references. Have this information written down before completing an application. (Always ask references if an employer can contact them.) You may get the job faster if the employer can check references quickly. If they are missing or not complete, the employer waits for all the information. This wastes your time and the employer's time. Also, the employer wonders if you are hiding something with incomplete reference information.
- Be prepared to provide the following.
  - Social Security number
  - Proof of the legal right to work in the United States
  - Proof of successful NATCEP completion
  - Identification—driver's license or government-issued ID card
- Give honest answers. Lying on an application is fraud. It is grounds for being fired.

Completing a Job Application

To complete a job application, follow the guidelines in Box 56-1. How you fill out the application may mean getting or not getting the job. Often the application is your first chance to impress the employer. A neat, readable, and complete application gives a good image. A sloppy or incomplete one does not. A job application is easier to complete if you have a file of your education and work history. The file should contain:

- A copy of your high school diploma or general equivalency diploma (GED).
- A copy of any grade reports, degrees, certificates, or military training.
- A copy of your NATCEP certificate of completion.
- Nursing assistant registry information for each state in which you are registered or licensed.
- Copies of communications with your state's nursing assistant registry agency.
- Copies of court records for criminal convictions.
- A copy of your Social Security card.
- Names, addresses, and phone numbers of references.
- Names, addresses, and phone numbers of current and past employers. Include:
  - Your job title
  - Dates employment started and ended
  - Your supervisor's name
  - Hourly salary
- Proof of in-services attended and continuing education units (CEUs).

When requesting a job application, also ask for the agency's nursing assistant job description (Chapter 3).

THE JOB INTERVIEW

A *job interview is when an employer asks a job applicant questions about his or her education and career.* The employer gets to know and evaluate you. You learn about the agency.

The interview may be at the time when you complete the job application. Some agencies schedule interviews after reviewing applications. An interview may be conducted by 1 person or 2 or more people.

When an interview is scheduled, write down the interviewer's name and the interview date and time. If you need directions to the agency, ask for them when the interview is scheduled.

When expecting a call from the agency, answer your phone. Do not let your phone go to an answering machine or voice mail. If circumstances are such that the caller has to leave a message, make sure your greeting is appropriate and professional.

Types of Interviews

Interviews may be in-person, by phone, or by video. You need good communication skills. (See Chapters 7 and 9.)

- *In-person interview.* You and the interviewer meet in the same room face-to-face. Appropriate dress and body language are needed.
- *Phone interview.* A phone interview may be your only interview or it may be used to decide if an in-person interview will follow. If distance is a factor, a phone interview may be efficient for the agency and you.
- *Video interview.* You use a computer at home or other site. Appropriate dress and body language are needed.

BOX 56-2 **Common Interview Questions**

What the Interviewer May Ask You
- Tell me about yourself.
- Tell me about your career goals.
- What are you doing to reach these goals?
- Describe what *professional* behavior means to you.
- Tell me about your last job. Why did you leave?
- What did you like the most about your last job? What did you like the least?
- What would your supervisor and co-workers tell me about you? Your dependability? Your skills? Your flexibility?
- Which functions are the hardest for you? How do you handle this difficulty?
- How do you set your priorities?
- How have your experiences prepared you for this job?
- What would you like to change about your last job?
- How do you handle problems with patients, residents, families, and co-workers?
- Why do you want to work here?
- Why should this agency hire you?

Questions You May Ask the Interviewer
- Which job functions do you think are the most important?
- What employee qualities and traits are the most important to you?
- What nursing care pattern is used here (Chapter 1)?
- Who will I work with?
- When are performance evaluations done? Who does them? How are they done?

Questions You May Ask the Interviewer—cont'd
- What performance factors are evaluated?
- How does the supervisor handle problems?
- What are the most common reasons that nursing assistants lose their jobs here?
- What are the most common reasons that nursing assistants resign from their jobs here?
- How do you see this job in the next year? In the next 5 years?
- What is the greatest reward from this job?
- What is the greatest challenge from this job?
- What do you like the most about nursing assistants who work here? What do you like the least?
- Why should I work here rather than in another agency?
- How much will I make an hour?
- What hours will I work?
- What uniforms are required?
- What benefits do you offer?
  - Health and dental insurance?
  - Continuing education?
  - Vacation time?
- Does the agency have a new employee orientation program? How long is it?
- May I have a tour of the agency and the unit I will work on? Will you introduce me to the nurse manager and unit staff?
- Can I have a few minutes to talk to the nurse manager?

For phone and video interviews:
- Use a quiet room. Turn off phones, music, TV, and other electronic devices. Do not use a room where phones will ring, people are talking, or where there are pets.
- Be ready to answer the phone or turn on the computer at the scheduled time.
- Make sure your wireless phone or computer is charged. Consider plugging into a power source to prevent dropped calls or your computer turning off.
- Speak clearly and slowly. Do not shout.
- Listen carefully. Let the interviewer finish a question before you answer.
- Smile. Smile even for a phone interview. Attitude and facial expression affect your voice tone.

Preparing for the Interview

Box 56-2 lists common interview questions. Prepare your answers ahead of time. Also prepare a list of your skills. Give the list to the interviewer.

You must present a good image. You need to be neat, clean, and well-groomed. How you dress is important. Follow the guidelines in Box 56-3.

BOX 56-3 **Grooming and Dressing for an Interview**

- Bathe and brush your teeth. Wash your hair. Men should shave facial hair or groom beards and mustaches.
- Use deodorant or antiperspirant.
- Make sure your hands and fingernails are clean.
- Apply make-up in a simple, attractive manner.
- Style your hair in a neat and attractive way. Wear it as you would for work.
- Do not wear jeans, shorts, tank tops, halter tops, or other casual clothing.
- Iron clothing. Sew on loose buttons and mend garments as needed.
- Wear clothing that covers tattoos (body art).
- Wear a simple dress, skirt or slacks and blouse, or suit (women). Wear a suit or slacks and a shirt (men). A jacket or tie is optional. A long-sleeved white or light blue shirt is best. See Figure 56-2, p. 866.
- Wear socks (men and women) or hose (women). Hose should be free of runs and snags.
- Make sure shoes are clean and in good repair.
- Avoid heavy perfumes, colognes, and after-shave lotions. A light fragrance is okay.
- Wear only simple jewelry that complements your clothes. Avoid adornments in body piercings. If you have multiple ear piercings, wear only 1 set of earrings.
- Stop in the restroom when you arrive for the interview. Check your hair, make-up, and clothes.

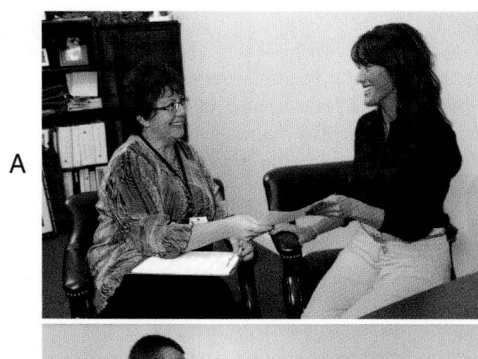

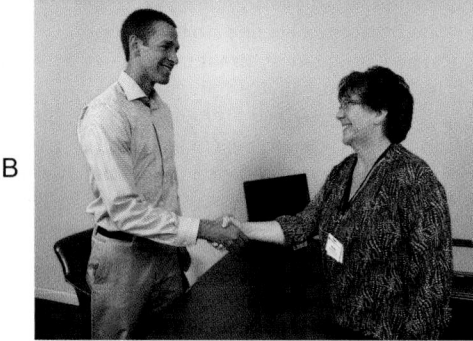

FIGURE 56-2 A, This woman wears a simple blouse and slacks for a job interview. **B,** This young man wears a simple shirt and slacks for a job interview.

Be on time for in-person, phone, or video interviews. It shows you are dependable. For an in-person interview, go to the agency some day before your interview. Note how long it takes to get there and where to park. Also find the personnel office. A dry run (practice run) gives an idea of the time needed to get from your home to the personnel office.

When you arrive for an interview, turn off your phone and other electronic devices. Tell the receptionist your name and why you are there. Also give the interviewer's name. Then sit quietly in the waiting area. Do not smoke, chew gum, or use your phone for calls, e-mails, text messages, or other reasons. While you wait, review your answers to the common interview questions. Waiting may be part of the interview. The interviewer may ask the receptionist about how you acted while waiting. Smile and be polite and friendly.

During the Interview

Politely greet the interviewer. Address the interviewer as Miss, Mrs., Ms., Mr., or Doctor. For an in-person interview, a firm hand-shake is correct for men and women. Stand until asked to sit. Sit with good posture and in a professional way. If offered a beverage, you may accept. Be sure to thank the person.

Good eye contact is needed for in-person and video interviews. Look directly at the interviewer when you answer or ask questions. Poor eye contact sends negative information—being shy, insecure, dishonest, or lacking interest.

Also watch your body language (Chapter 9). Body language involves facial expressions, gestures, posture, and body movements. What you say is important. However, how you use and move your body also tells a great deal. Avoid distracting habits—biting nails; playing with jewelry, clothing, or your hair; crossing your arms; and crossing and swinging legs back and forth. Focus on the interview. Do not touch or read things on the person's desk.

The interview lasts 15 to 20 minutes. Give complete and honest answers. Speak clearly and with confidence. Avoid short and long answers. "Yes" and "no" answers give little information. Briefly explain "yes" and "no" responses (Chapter 9).

The interviewer will ask about your skills. Share your skills list. You may be asked about a skill not on your list. Explain that you are willing to learn if your state allows nursing assistants to perform the skill.

Find the right job for you. An employer wants to hire someone who will be happy in the job and the agency. Box 56-2 lists some questions for you to ask at the end of the interview. The person's answers will help you decide if the job is right for you.

Review the job description with the interviewer. Ask any questions at this time. Advise the interviewer of functions you cannot perform because of training, legal, ethical, or religious reasons. Honesty now prevents problems later.

The interviewer signals the end of the interview. You may be offered a job at this time. Or you are told when to expect a call or letter. Follow-up is acceptable. Ask when you can check on your application. Always thank the interviewer. Say that you look forward to hearing from him or her. Shake the person's hand before leaving an in-person interview.

See *Focus on Long-Term Care and Home Care: During the Interview.*

Questions You Cannot Be Asked. The U.S. Equal Employment Opportunity Commission (EEOC) is an agency of the United States government. To guard against discrimination in hiring, the EEOC has guidelines for questions that cannot be asked of a job applicant during an interview or on a job application. See Box 56-4.

See *Focus on Communication: Questions You Cannot Be Asked.*

FOCUS ON LONG-TERM CARE AND HOME CARE

During the Interview

Home Care
You need to ask more questions when interviewing with a home care agency.

- What part of the community does the agency serve?
- What neighborhoods will you go to?
- How far will you have to travel between homes?
- Do you use your own car or an agency car?
- If you use your own car, how are you paid for mileage and tolls?
- Will you use public transportation? If yes, who pays for bus or train fares? If the agency pays, are you given fare money beforehand or repaid later?

BOX 56-4	Interview Questions Not Allowed by the EEOC

- *Age.* Generally, you cannot be asked your age, your birth date, or any question that refers to your age. However, OBRA requires that you be at least 16 years of age. Some states have limits on the tasks allowed for persons under 18 years of age.
- *Color, race, gender, or national origin.* This includes questions related to your place of birth or that of your parents; language spoken; or how you learned to read, write, or speak a language.
- *Religion or spiritual beliefs.* You cannot be asked about your religion, religious practices, church, priest or pastor, or religious holidays observed.
- *Sex.* You cannot be asked any question about sex or your sexuality.
- *Disabilities.* You cannot be asked if you have disabilities or what they are. This includes treatment for alcoholism. However, you can be asked if you can perform the job with reasonable accommodation.
- *Pregnancy or plans for pregnancy.* You cannot be asked if you are pregnant, planning to get pregnant, or about your pregnancy history or number of children.

- *Marital status.* You cannot be asked if you are married, single, divorced, separated, engaged, or widowed.
- *Children.* You cannot be asked if you have children, how many children or their ages, or who will care for children while you are at work.
- *Arrest record.* You cannot be asked about arrests. However, you can be asked about criminal convictions.
- *Finances.* You cannot be asked about credit cards or bank accounts or if you own your home or car.
- *Number of sick days used in the last year.* You cannot be asked about your medical history. However, you may have to take a medical exam or have some tests done after a job offer is made.
- *Citizenship.* You cannot be asked if you are a United States citizen. You cannot be asked to provide proof of citizenship. However, if hired, you can be asked to provide proof of the legal right to work in the United States.

FOCUS ON COMMUNICATION

Questions You Cannot Be Asked

If asked a question listed in Box 56-4, you have the right to decline to answer. Decline politely. You can say: "I'm sorry, but the EEOC does not allow you to ask that question. What else can I answer for you?"

After the Interview

A thank-you letter or note is advised (Fig. 56-3). Write this within 24 hours after the interview. Write neatly and clearly. Use a computer or typewriter if your writing is hard to read. The thank-you note should include:

- The date
- The interviewer's formal name using Miss, Ms., Mrs., Mr., or Dr.
- A statement thanking the person for the interview
- Comments about the interview, the agency, and your eagerness to hear about the job
- Your signature, using your first and last names

ACCEPTING OR DECLINING A JOB OFFER

You can apply to many places and have many interviews. Think about all offers before accepting one. You might have more questions about an agency. Ask them before accepting a job. To help you decide, discuss the offer with a family member, friend, co-worker, or your instructor.

When you accept a job, agree on a starting date, pay rate, and work hours. Ask where to report on your first day. Ask for such information in writing. That way you and the agency have the same understanding of the job offer. Use the written offer later if questions arise. Also ask for the employee handbook and other agency information. Read everything before you start working.

December 12

Dear Ms. O'Neal,

Thank you for the interview yesterday. I enjoyed meeting you and learning more about the nursing center. I was impressed by the friendliness of the staff and would enjoy working in that environment.

Again, thank you. I look forward to hearing from you soon.

Sincerely,
Alison M. Teal

FIGURE 56-3 Sample thank-you note written after a job interview.

Accept a job that is best for you. You may want to decline a job offer. If so, thank the person for offering you a job. If asked why you are refusing, give a positive response. For example: "Thank you for offering me a job. I've decided to accept a job that is closer to my home."

Sometimes a job is not offered. You may not hear back from the agency. Or the agency calls, writes, or e-mails telling you that you will not be offered the job. If this happens, thank the person for letting you know. Ask that the agency keep you in mind for the future. For example: "Thank you for letting me know. I'm disappointed but please keep me in mind for other openings."

DRUG TESTING

State laws vary about drug testing. Drug testing may be part of the application process. If so, review the job application before signing it. The application usually states 1 of the following.

- Drug testing is part of the application screening process for new staff.
- A job offer depends on passing a drug test.

FOCUS ON PRIDE

The Person, Family, and Yourself

P ersonal and Professional Responsibility

Employers invest much time and money in new staff. Changing jobs often can reflect poorly on you. Before an interview, find out about the agency. Plan questions to ask the interviewer. See Box 56-2. This helps you decide if the agency is a good fit for you. Also, your interest in the agency can make a good impression during an interview.

R ights and Respect

You have the right to protection from discrimination. *Discrimination* involves unjust treatment based on age, race, sex, and other personal qualities. Employers must limit questions to those that relate to your ability to do the job. See Box 56-4 for questions that are not allowed.

Job-related questions are allowed if asked to all applicants, regardless of age or gender. The following questions are appropriate.

- What languages do you read, write, and speak fluently?
- Can you perform the duties of this job? Do you need any special accommodations to perform the job?
- Have you ever been convicted of a crime?

Know your rights. Plan how to respond if you suspect a question violates your rights.

I ndependence and Social Interaction

Some employers perform social media backgrounds checks. State laws vary about what information can be accessed—public or private. Age, sex, disability, color, race, gender, national origin, or religion must not be considered in hiring decisions. Employers must focus only on information related to the job.

Show good judgment when using social media (Chapter 5). Facebook, Twitter, Instagram, and LinkedIn are examples. Be professional. Employers may view these during the hiring process.

D elegation and Teamwork

This may be your first job in health care. Other work experiences, education, and training are important. They give employers information about your dependability, teamwork, and the quality of your work. Draw from your experiences. Be prepared with examples of how you showed positive work ethics.

E thics and Laws

Patient and resident safety is of great importance. Employers watch for safe and ethical conduct. They must act when conduct is unsafe or unethical. Background checks, drug testing, and interview questions help employers decide if a job applicant will meet safety and ethical standards. This is a real example of a nursing assistant who did not meet standards for safe and ethical behavior.

A certified nursing assistant (CNA) began working at an Arizona hospital. While employed, she received Employee Corrective Action reports for:

- *Poor communication with co-workers*
- *Arguing with an RN who gave her instructions*
- *Not being able to work in a team environment*
- *Excess time off the nursing unit for breaks*
- *Not taking the initiative in answering call lights, collecting equipment, or transferring patients' belongings*
- *Excess socializing with staff in other departments*
- *Not meeting standards relating to customer service relations*

She was terminated from the hospital in January 2000.

Four years later she applied for a job at another Arizona hospital. A pre-employment urine drug screen was positive for benzodiazepine. The CNA reported the drug test to the Arizona State Board of Nursing. The CNA reported that she had a headache the night before her interview at the hospital. She admitted taking Valium (benzodiazepine) that was prescribed for her mother. The CNA explained that "she knew this was wrong, that this was a one-time occurrence and that it would not happen again."

The Board requested that the CNA submit to a urine drug screen. It was positive for benzodiazepine. The CNA did not have a prescription for that drug.

The Board revoked the CNA's certificate for unprofessional conduct. The Arizona State Board of Nursing found that the CNA's actions violated these aspects of the state's Nurse Practice Act.

- *Conduct or a practice that is or might be harmful or dangerous to the health of a patient or the public*
- *Committing an act that deceives, defrauds, or harms the public*
- *Obtaining, possessing, using, or selling any narcotic, controlled substance, or illegal drug in violation of any federal or state criminal law, or in violation of the policy of any employer*
- *Using violent or abusive behavior in any work setting*
- *Failing to cooperate with the Board during an investigation*
- *Practicing in any other manner that gives the Board reasonable cause to believe that the health of a patient or the public may be harmed*

(Arizona State Board of Nursing, 2005.)

Poor conduct outside of work can affect your job. Take pride in making good choices inside and outside the workplace.

FOCUS ON PRIDE: *Application*

Job interviews can be stressful. You may be nervous about what questions will be asked, how you will answer, and if you will make a good impression. Being prepared helps. Describe how you will prepare yourself for a job interview. How will you respond to a question not allowed by the EEOC?

REVIEW QUESTIONS

Circle the BEST answer.

1 When should you ask questions about your job description?
a After completing the job application
b Before completing the job application
c When your interview is scheduled
d During the interview

2 Lying on a job application is
a Negligence
b Fraud
c Libel
d Defamation

3 When completing a job application
a Use pencil
b Leave spaces blank that do not apply to you
c Give information about employment gaps
d List family members as references

4 Which of the following do employers look for the *most?*
a Cooperation
b Courtesy
c Empathy
d Dependability

5 What should you wear to a job interview?
a A uniform
b Party clothes
c Slacks and a shirt or blouse
d What is most comfortable

6 For a phone interview you should
a Shout answers so they are heard
b Take another call during the interview
c Have the interviewer leave a message
d Use a quiet room

7 Which is poor behavior during a job interview?
a Crossing your arms and legs
b Good eye contact with the interviewer
c Shaking hands with the interviewer
d Asking the interviewer questions

8 Which is the *best* response to an interview question?
a Brief explanations
b "Yes" or "no"
c Long answers
d A written response

9 An interviewer asks the following. Which should you decline to answer?
a Tell me about yourself.
b Are you married?
c Have you ever been convicted of a crime?
d What are your career goals?

10 After an interview
a Ask if the employer plans to hire you
b Ask to be paid for your time at the interview
c Write a thank-you note
d Do not apply to any other agencies

11 When accepting a job offer, avoid discussing
a Starting date
b Personal finances
c Pay rate
d Work hours

12 A long-term care employer can legally
a Require a drug test before hiring employees
b Ask job applicants for a record of past arrests
c Hire a person convicted of abuse
d Hire a 14-year-old as a nursing assistant

Answers to Chapter 56 questions are on p. 872.

FOCUS ON PRACTICE

Problem Solving

You are asked the following questions at a job interview. How will you respond to each?
• Why did you decide to become a nursing assistant?
• What are your strengths and weaknesses?
• Describe a problem you faced in your clinical training. How did you resolve it?
• Describe a situation where you had to prioritize. How did you decide what to do first, second, and so on?

Review Question Answers

CHAPTER 1:
INTRODUCTION
TO HEALTH CARE
AGENCIES
1. d
2. b
3. a
4. c
5. b
6. b
7. a
8. d
9. a
10. b
11. a
12. a
13. c
14. c
15. b
16. d

CHAPTER 2: THE
PERSON'S RIGHTS
1. F
2. T
3. T
4. F
5. T
6. F
7. T
8. F
9. T
10. F
11. F
12. a
13. d
14. b
15. c
16. d
17. b
18. a
19. a
20. d
21. b
22. c
23. d
24. a
25. b
26. d
27. c
28. b

CHAPTER 3:
THE NURSING
ASSISTANT
1. T
2. F
3. T
4. F
5. F
6. F
7. b
8. d
9. c
10. c
11. b
12. a
13. c
14. b
15. d

CHAPTER 4:
DELEGATION
1. F
2. F
3. T
4. T
5. T
6. F
7. T
8. c
9. a
10. d
11. b
12. d
13. c
14. d
15. a

CHAPTER 5:
ETHICS AND
LAWS
1. b
2. c
3. d
4. a
5. b
6. a
7. c
8. a
9. d
10. c
11. c
12. b
13. a
14. d
15. b
16. d
17. a
18. a
19. c
20. b
21. a
22. c
23. b
24. c
25. a

CHAPTER 6:
STUDENT AND
WORK ETHICS
1. T
2. T
3. F
4. T
5. T
6. T
7. F
8. F
9. T
10. F
11. d
12. c
13. a
14. b
15. b
16. a
17. d
18. a
19. c
20. a

21. b
22. a
23. d
24. a
25. c
26. d

CHAPTER 7:
COMMUNICATING
WITH THE HEALTH
TEAM
1. T
2. T
3. F
4. T
5. F
6. T
7. F
8. F
9. d
10. c
11. a
12. c
13. b
14. b
15. d
16. a
17. b
18. c
19. d
20. a
21. b
22. b
23. a
24. c

CHAPTER 8:
ASSISTING WITH THE
NURSING PROCESS
1. c
2. d
3. b
4. c
5. d
6. b
7. a
8. c
9. c
10. d
11. b
12. c
13. d
14. a

CHAPTER 9:
UNDERSTANDING
THE PERSON
1. c
2. d
3. b
4. a
5. c
6. c
7. d
8. c
9. d
10. d
11. b
12. a

13. b
14. a
15. d
16. c
17. d
18. b
19. a
20. b
21. c
22. a

CHAPTER 10:
BODY
STRUCTURE
AND FUNCTION
1. a
2. b
3. a
4. c
5. c
6. a
7. b
8. c
9. d
10. d
11. c
12. b
13. a
14. b
15. b
16. b
17. c
18. d
19. a
20. d
21. a
22. b

CHAPTER 11:
GROWTH AND
DEVELOPMENT
1. b
2. d
3. b
4. a
5. b
6. c
7. b
8. a
9. c
10. c
11. c
12. b
13. d
14. d
15. a
16. c
17. b
18. d
19. c
20. a

CHAPTER 12: CARE
OF THE OLDER
PERSON
1. b
2. c
3. a
4. b
5. c

6. d
7. c
8. a
9. c
10. a
11. d
12. b
13. c
14. c
15. b
16. a
17. d
18. b
19. a
20. b
21. a
22. c
23. a

CHAPTER 13:
SAFETY
1. a
2. d
3. c
4. a
5. b
6. c
7. d
8. b
9. a
10. c
11. c
12. d
13. b
14. a
15. c
16. b
17. c
18. b
19. a
20. d
21. d
22. b
23. c
24. c
25. c
26. d
27. b
28. d

CHAPTER 14:
FALL PREVENTION
1. a
2. c
3. c
4. a
5. b
6. c
7. d
8. b
9. c
10. b
11. a
12. c
13. c
14. b
15. d

CHAPTER 15:
RESTRAINT
ALTERNATIVES
AND SAFE
RESTRAINT USE
1. F
2. T
3. T
4. F
5. F
6. T
7. T
8. T
9. F
10. F
11. T
12. F
13. F
14. T
15. F
16. d
17. c
18. b
19. c
20. a
21. b
22. a
23. c
24. d

CHAPTER 16:
PREVENTING
INFECTION
1. F
2. T
3. T
4. F
5. F
6. T
7. F
8. F
9. T
10. T
11. F
12. F
13. b
14. b
15. a
16. c
17. a
18. b
19. d
20. c
21. c
22. a
23. d
24. c
25. d
26. c
27. b
28. a
29. a
30. c
31. d
32. b

CHAPTER 17: BODY
MECHANICS
1. a
2. b

3. c
4. a
5. a
6. c
7. b
8. a
9. d
10. c
11. b
12. b
13. c
14. a

CHAPTER 18: SAFELY MOVING THE PERSON
1. b
2. a
3. c
4. a
5. b
6. c
7. d
8. b
9. a
10. d
11. d
12. c

CHAPTER 19: SAFELY TRANSFERRING THE PERSON
1. b
2. d
3. c
4. a
5. b
6. c
7. a
8. b
9. d
10. b
11. c
12. b
13. c
14. a

CHAPTER 20: THE PERSON'S UNIT
1. T
2. T
3. F
4. T
5. F
6. T
7. T
8. T
9. F
10. T
11. d
12. c
13. b
14. d
15. c
16. a
17. b
18. a
19. b
20. c
21. b
22. c

CHAPTER 21: BEDMAKING
1. F
2. F
3. T

4. F
5. T
6. T
7. F
8. T
9. d
10. b
11. a
12. b
13. a
14. c

CHAPTER 22: PERSONAL HYGIENE
1. T
2. T
3. F
4. T
5. F
6. F
7. F
8. F
9. T
10. F
11. T
12. F
13. T
14. F
15. F
16. T
17. T
18. T
19. a
20. c
21. d
22. c
23. b
24. a
25. d
26. c
27. a
28. d
29. b
30. b

CHAPTER 23: GROOMING
1. T
2. F
3. F
4. T
5. T
6. F
7. T
8. F
9. F
10. d
11. b
12. c
13. a
14. d
15. c
16. b
17. d
18. b
19. a
20. c

CHAPTER 24: URINARY ELIMINATION
1. c
2. d
3. a
4. a

5. b
6. b
7. a
8. d
9. c
10. c
11. d
12. a

CHAPTER 25: URINARY CATHETERS
1. c
2. d
3. a
4. a
5. c
6. b
7. d
8. c
9. a
10. b
11. a
12. d

CHAPTER 26: BOWEL ELIMINATION
1. b
2. a
3. b
4. c
5. c
6. a
7. c
8. d
9. b
10. d
11. a
12. d
13. c
14. d

CHAPTER 27: NUTRITION AND FLUIDS
1. T
2. F
3. T
4. F
5. F
6. F
7. F
8. T
9. T
10. b
11. b
12. d
13. c
14. d
15. a
16. a
17. c
18. a
19. d
20. b
21. c
22. b
23. c
24. a
25. d
26. b
27. c
28. d
29. c
30. a

31. b
32. d

CHAPTER 28: NUTRITIONAL SUPPORT AND IV THERAPY
1. c
2. a
3. a
4. b
5. d
6. a
7. a
8. c
9. c
10. d
11. b
12. b
13. a
14. d
15. b
16. c
17. b
18. a

CHAPTER 29: MEASURING VITAL SIGNS
1. b
2. a
3. b
4. c
5. a
6. d
7. c
8. b
9. d
10. c
11. c
12. a
13. c
14. d
15. b

CHAPTER 30: EXERCISE AND ACTIVITY
1. T
2. F
3. T
4. F
5. F
6. T
7. T
8. T
9. b
10. b
11. c
12. d
13. c
14. a
15. c
16. a
17. d
18. a
19. b
20. a

CHAPTER 31: COMFORT, REST, AND SLEEP
1. T
2. T
3. F
4. T

5. T
6. T
7. T
8. F
9. F
10. T
11. F
12. T
13. F
14. T
15. T
16. c
17. d
18. c
19. d
20. a
21. b
22. d
23. c
24. b
25. a

CHAPTER 32: ADMISSIONS, TRANSFERS, AND DISCHARGES
1. T
2. F
3. T
4. F
5. F
6. T
7. T
8. T
9. F
10. T
11. F
12. T
13. b
14. a
15. c
16. c
17. a
18. d

CHAPTER 33: ASSISTING WITH THE PHYSICAL EXAMINATION
1. b
2. c
3. c
4. d
5. a

CHAPTER 34: COLLECTING AND TESTING SPECIMENS
1. d
2. b
3. a
4. a
5. c
6. b
7. a
8. d
9. a
10. b
11. c
12. a
13. d
14. b

CHAPTER 35: THE PERSON HAVING SURGERY
1. F
2. T
3. F
4. F
5. F
6. T
7. T
8. F
9. T
10. T
11. c
12. b
13. b
14. a
15. d
16. c
17. c
18. a
19. b
20. c
21. a
22. a
23. d
24. b
25. d
26. a

CHAPTER 36: WOUND CARE
1. a
2. c
3. a
4. c
5. b
6. d
7. b
8. c
9. c
10. b
11. a
12. c
13. b
14. d
15. a
16. c

CHAPTER 37: PRESSURE ULCERS
1. F
2. T
3. T
4. T
5. T
6. T
7. F
8. T
9. F
10. T
11. F
12. F
13. T
14. b
15. d
16. a
17. a
18. c
19. c
20. b
21. b
22. d
23. a
24. b
25. a

26. d
27. c
28. c
29. d
30. b

CHAPTER 38:
HEAT AND COLD
APPLICATIONS
1. d
2. b
3. b
4. a
5. c
6. a
7. b
8. c
9. a
10. b
11. d
12. c
13. a
14. b

CHAPTER 39:
OXYGEN NEEDS
1. a
2. c
3. c
4. b
5. b
6. d
7. c
8. d
9. a
10. b
11. a
12. b
13. d
14. c
15. d
16. b
17. a
18. c

CHAPTER 40:
RESPIRATORY
SUPPORT AND
THERAPIES
1. c
2. d
3. d
4. b
5. b
6. a
7. d
8. c
9. a
10. b
11. c
12. b

CHAPTER 41:
REHABILITATION
AND RESTORATIVE
NURSING CARE
1. T
2. T
3. T
4. F
5. F
6. T
7. F
8. T

9. T
10. c
11. b
12. a
13. d
14. c
15. c

CHAPTER 42:
HEARING, SPEECH,
AND VISION
PROBLEMS
1. b
2. c
3. d
4. b
5. a
6. c
7. c
8. d
9. a
10. b
11. a
12. c
13. a
14. b
15. c
16. a
17. d
18. d
19. c
20. b

CHAPTER 43:
CANCER, IMMUNE
SYSTEM, AND
SKIN DISORDERS
1. F
2. T
3. T
4. T
5. T
6. F
7. T
8. T
9. T
10. F
11. b
12. a
13. b
14. a
15. c
16. d
17. a
18. c
19. d
20. b

CHAPTER 44:
NERVOUS SYSTEM
AND MUSCULO-
SKELETAL
DISORDERS
1. a
2. b
3. d
4. c
5. d
6. b
7. a
8. a
9. c
10. b
11. a
12. c

13. a
14. d
15. b
16. a
17. b
18. d
19. d
20. a
21. c

CHAPTER 45:
CARDIOVASCULAR,
RESPIRATORY, AND
LYMPHATIC
DISORDERS
1. d
2. a
3. b
4. b
5. c
6. b
7. a
8. c
9. a
10. a
11. b
12. d
13. a
14. c
15. d
16. a
17. a
18. c
19. c
20. a
21. a
22. d

CHAPTER 46:
DIGESTIVE AND
ENDOCRINE
DISORDERS
1. b
2. a
3. d
4. a
5. c
6. b
7. c
8. b
9. a
10. a
11. c
12. b
13. d
14. a
15. c
16. d
17. a
18. b

CHAPTER 47:
URINARY AND
REPRODUCTIVE
DISORDERS
1. d
2. d
3. c
4. b
5. a
6. a
7. b
8. c
9. c
10. d

CHAPTER 48:
MENTAL HEALTH
DISORDERS
1. F
2. T
3. F
4. T
5. T
6. T
7. T
8. F
9. b
10. d
11. b
12. c
13. c
14. a
15. b
16. c
17. d
18. d
19. c
20. b
21. a
22. c
23. a
24. b
25. a
26. c
27. d
28. b
29. a
30. c

CHAPTER 49:
CONFUSION AND
DEMENTIA
1. T
2. F
3. T
4. T
5. F
6. T
7. F
8. F
9. T
10. T
11. T
12. F
13. F
14. b
15. a
16. d
17. c
18. d
19. b
20. a
21. c
22. c
23. a
24. b
25. d
26. b
27. c
28. d
29. a
30. c

CHAPTER 50:
INTELLECTUAL AND
DEVELOPMENTAL
DISABILITIES
1. d
2. b
3. c
4. b

5. a
6. d
7. c
8. d
9. c
10. a
11. c
12. b
13. a
14. c
15. b

CHAPTER 51:
SEXUALITY
1. a
2. d
3. c
4. a
5. c
6. b
7. d
8. b
9. c
10. d

CHAPTER 52: CARING
FOR MOTHERS AND
BABIES
1. T
2. F
3. T
4. F
5. T
6. T
7. F
8. T
9. c
10. d
11. b
12. a
13. d
14. d
15. b
16. c
17. c
18. a
19. c
20. d
21. d
22. a
23. c
24. c

CHAPTER 53: ASSISTED
LIVING
1. F
2. T
3. T
4. F
5. T
6. T
7. F
8. F
9. T
10. T
11. b
12. d
13. b
14. c
15. a
16. b
17. a
18. b
19. c
20. c

CHAPTER 54: BASIC
EMERGENCY CARE
1. b
2. a
3. b
4. c
5. d
6. c
7. b
8. a
9. b
10. b
11. c
12. c
13. a
14. c
15. d
16. d
17. a
18. c
19. c
20. a
21. b
22. c
23. c
24. a

CHAPTER 55:
END-OF-LIFE CARE
1. c
2. a
3. b
4. a
5. d
6. c
7. b
8. a
9. d
10. c
11. c
12. a
13. b
14. b
15. d

CHAPTER 56: GETTING
A JOB
1. d
2. b
3. c
4. d
5. c
6. d
7. a
8. a
9. b
10. c
11. b
12. a

National Nurse Aide Assessment Program (NNAAP®)
Written Examination Content Outline

The NNAAP® Written Examination is comprised of seventy (70) multiple choice questions. Ten (10) of these questions are pre-test (non-scored) questions on which statistical information will be collected.

I. Physical Care Skills
   A. Activities of Daily Living   14% of exam
     1. Hygiene
     2. Dressing and Grooming
     3. Nutrition and Hydration
     4. Elimination
     5. Rest/Sleep/Comfort
   B. Basic Nursing Skills   39% of exam
     1. Infection Control
     2. Safety/Emergency
     3. Therapeutic/Technical Procedures
     4. Data Collection and Reporting
   C. Restorative Skills   7% of exam
     1. Prevention
     2. Self Care/Independence

II. Psychosocial Care Skills
   A. Emotional and Mental Health Needs   11% of exam
   B. Spiritual and Cultural Needs   2% of exam

III. Role of the Nurse Aide
   A. Communication   8% of exam
   B. Client Rights   7% of exam
   C. Legal and Ethical Behavior   3% of exam
   D. Member of the Health Care Team   9% of exam

National Nurse Aide Assessment Program (NNAAP®)
Skills Evaluation

List of Skills

1. Hand hygiene (hand washing)
2. Applies one knee-high elastic stocking
3. Assists to ambulate using transfer belt
4. Assists with use of bedpan
5. Cleans upper or lower denture
6. Counts and records radial pulse
7. Counts and records respirations
8. Donning and removing PPE (gown and gloves)
9. Dresses client with affected (weak) right arm
10. Feeds client who cannot feed self
11. Gives modified bed bath (face and one arm, hand and underarm)
12. Measures and records blood pressure
13. Measures and records urinary output
14. Measures and records weight of ambulatory client
15. Performs modified passive range of motion (PROM) for one knee and one ankle
16. Performs modified passive range of motion (PROM) for one shoulder
17. Positions on side
18. Provides catheter care for female
19. Provides foot care on one foot
20. Provides mouth care
21. Provides perineal care (peri-care) for female
22. Transfers from bed to wheelchair using transfer belt

Appendix B

MINIMUM DATA SET—SELECTED PAGES

Resident _____ Identifier _____ Date _____

Section G	Functional Status

G0110. Activities of Daily Living (ADL) Assistance
Refer to the ADL flow chart in the RAI manual to facilitate accurate coding

Instructions for Rule of 3

- When an activity occurs three times at any one given level, code that level.
- When an activity occurs three times at multiple levels, code the most dependent, exceptions are total dependence (4), activity must require full assist every time, and activity did not occur (8), activity must not have occurred at all. Example, three times extensive assistance (3) and three times limited assistance (2), code extensive assistance (3).
- When an activity occurs at various levels, but not three times at any given level, apply the following:
  - When there is a combination of full staff performance, and extensive assistance, code extensive assistance.
  - When there is a combination of full staff performance, weight bearing assistance and/or non-weight bearing assistance code limited assistance (2).

If none of the above are met, code supervision.

1. ADL Self-Performance

Code for **resident's performance** over all shifts - not including setup. If the ADL activity occurred 3 or more times at various levels of assistance, code the most dependent - except for total dependence, which requires full staff performance every time

Coding:

Activity Occurred 3 or More Times

0. **Independent** - no help or staff oversight at any time
1. **Supervision** - oversight, encouragement or cueing
2. **Limited assistance** - resident highly involved in activity; staff provide guided maneuvering of limbs or other non-weight-bearing assistance
3. **Extensive assistance** - resident involved in activity, staff provide weight-bearing support
4. **Total dependence** - full staff performance every time during entire 7-day period

Activity Occurred 2 or Fewer Times

7. **Activity occurred only once or twice** - activity did occur but only once or twice
8. **Activity did not occur** - activity did not occur or family and/or non-facility staff provided care 100% of the time for that activity over the entire 7-day period

2. ADL Support Provided

Code for **most support provided** over all shifts; code regardless of resident's self-performance classification

Coding:

0. **No** setup or physical help from staff
1. **Setup** help only
2. **One** person physical assist
3. **Two+** persons physical assist
8. ADL activity itself **did not occur** or family and/or non-facility staff provided care 100% of the time for that activity over the entire 7-day period

	1. Self-Performance	2. Support
	↓ Enter Codes in Boxes ↓	
A. Bed mobility - how resident moves to and from lying position, turns side to side, and positions body while in bed or alternate sleep furniture	☐	☐
B. Transfer - how resident moves between surfaces including to or from: bed, chair, wheelchair, standing position (**excludes** to/from bath/toilet)	☐	☐
C. Walk in room - how resident walks between locations in his/her room	☐	☐
D. Walk in corridor - how resident walks in corridor on unit	☐	☐
E. Locomotion on unit - how resident moves between locations in his/her room and adjacent corridor on same floor. If in wheelchair, self-sufficiency once in chair	☐	☐
F. Locomotion off unit - how resident moves to and returns from off-unit locations (e.g., areas set aside for dining, activities or treatments). **If facility has only one floor,** how resident moves to and from distant areas on the floor. If in wheelchair, self-sufficiency once in chair	☐	☐
G. Dressing - how resident puts on, fastens and takes off all items of clothing, including donning/removing a prosthesis or TED hose. Dressing includes putting on and changing pajamas and housedresses	☐	☐
H. Eating - how resident eats and drinks, regardless of skill. Do not include eating/drinking during medication pass. Includes intake of nourishment by other means (e.g., tube feeding, total parenteral nutrition, IV fluids administered for nutrition or hydration)	☐	☐
I. Toilet use - how resident uses the toilet room, commode, bedpan, or urinal; transfers on/off toilet; cleanses self after elimination; changes pad; manages ostomy or catheter; and adjusts clothes. Do not include emptying of bedpan, urinal, bedside commode, catheter bag or ostomy bag	☐	☐
J. Personal hygiene - how resident maintains personal hygiene, including combing hair, brushing teeth, shaving, applying makeup, washing/drying face and hands (**excludes** baths and showers)	☐	☐

Resident _____   Identifier _____   Date _____

Section G	Functional Status

G0120. Bathing

How resident takes full-body bath/shower, sponge bath, and transfers in/out of tub/shower (**excludes** washing of back and hair). Code for **most dependent** in self-performance and support

Enter Code [ ]
A. Self-performance
0. **Independent** - no help provided
1. **Supervision** - oversight help only
2. **Physical help limited to transfer only**
3. **Physical help in part of bathing activity**
4. **Total dependence**
8. **Activity itself did not occur** or family and/or non-facility staff provided care 100% of the time for that activity over the entire 7-day period

Enter Code [ ]
B. Support provided
(Bathing support codes are as defined in item **G0110 column 2, ADL Support Provided**, above)

G0300. Balance During Transitions and Walking

After observing the resident, **code the following walking and transition items for most dependent**

Coding:
0. **Steady at all times**
1. **Not steady, but able to stabilize without staff assistance**
2. **Not steady, only able to stabilize with staff assistance**
8. **Activity did not occur**

↓ Enter Codes in Boxes

[ ] **A. Moving from seated to standing position**

[ ] **B. Walking** (with assistive device if used)

[ ] **C. Turning around** and facing the opposite direction while walking

[ ] **D. Moving on and off toilet**

[ ] **E. Surface-to-surface transfer** (transfer between bed and chair or wheelchair)

G0400. Functional Limitation in Range of Motion

Code for limitation that interfered with daily functions or placed resident at risk of injury

Coding:
0. **No impairment**
1. **Impairment on one side**
2. **Impairment on both sides**

↓ Enter Codes in Boxes

[ ] **A. Upper extremity** (shoulder, elbow, wrist, hand)

[ ] **B. Lower extremity** (hip, knee, ankle, foot)

G0600. Mobility Devices

↓ Check all that were normally used

[ ] **A. Cane/crutch**

[ ] **B. Walker**

[ ] **C. Wheelchair** (manual or electric)

[ ] **D. Limb prosthesis**

[ ] **Z. None of the above were used**

G0900. Functional Rehabilitation Potential
Complete only if A0310A = 01

Enter Code [ ]
A. Resident believes he or she is capable of increased independence in at least some ADLs
0. **No**
1. **Yes**
9. **Unable to determine**

Enter Code [ ]
B. Direct care staff believe resident is capable of increased independence in at least some ADLs
0. **No**
1. **Yes**

From Centers for Medicare & Medicaid Services: MDS 3.0, http://www.cms.gov/Medicare/Quality-Initiatives
-Patient-Assessment-Instruments/NursingHomeQualityInits/MDS30RAIManual.html.

Appendix C

CARE AREA ASSESSMENT (CAA)—SAMPLE PAGE

Resident _____ Identifier _____ Date _____

Section V	Care Area Assessment (CAA) Summary

V0200. CAAs and Care Planning

1. Check column A if Care Area is triggered.
2. For each triggered Care Area, indicate whether a new care plan, care plan revision, or continuation of current care plan is necessary to address the problem(s) identified in your assessment of the care area. The Care Planning Decision column must be completed within 7 days of completing the RAI (MDS and CAA(s)). Check column B if the triggered care area is addressed in the care plan.
3. Indicate in the Location and Date of CAA Documentation column where information related to the CAA can be found. CAA documentation should include information on the complicating factors, risks, and any referrals for this resident for this care area.

A. CAA Results

Care Area	A. Care Area Triggered	B. Care Planning Decision	Location and Date of CAA documentation
	↓ Check all that apply ↓		
01. Delirium	☐	☐	
02. Cognitive Loss/Dementia	☐	☐	
03. Visual Function	☐	☐	
04. Communication	☐	☐	
05. ADL Functional/Rehabilitation Potential	☐	☐	
06. Urinary Incontinence and Indwelling Catheter	☐	☐	
07. Psychosocial Well-Being	☐	☐	
08. Mood State	☐	☐	
09. Behavioral Symptoms	☐	☐	
10. Activities	☐	☐	
11. Falls	☐	☐	
12. Nutritional Status	☐	☐	
13. Feeding Tube	☐	☐	
14. Dehydration/Fluid Maintenance	☐	☐	
15. Dental Care	☐	☐	
16. Pressure Ulcer	☐	☐	
17. Psychotropic Drug Use	☐	☐	
18. Physical Restraints	☐	☐	
19. Pain	☐	☐	
20. Return to Community Referral	☐	☐	

B. Signature of RN Coordinator for CAA Process and Date Signed

1. Signature

2. Date ☐☐ – ☐☐ – ☐☐☐☐
Month   Day   Year

C. Signature of Person Completing Care Plan Decision and Date Signed

1. Signature

2. Date ☐☐ – ☐☐ – ☐☐☐☐
Month   Day   Year

From Centers for Medicare & Medicaid Services: MDS 3.0, http://www.cms.gov/Medicare/Quality-Initiatives
-Patient-Assessment-Instruments/NursingHomeQualityInits/MDS30RAIManual.html.

INFANT AND CHILD SAFETY
Home Safety*
The following home safety measures can protect infants and children from harm.

Kitchen
- Knives, forks, scissors, and other sharp tools are kept in a drawer with a childproof latch.
- The stove has a lock and knob protectors.
- A dishwasher lock is installed.
- Childproof latches are installed on all cabinet doors.
- Chairs and step stools are away from the stove.
- When cooking, pot handles on the stove are turned inward or placed on back burners where children cannot reach them.
- Tablecloths and placemats are not used. Infants and children can pull things off the table and onto themselves.
- Glass objects and appliances with sharp blades are stored out of reach.
- The garbage can is behind a cabinet door with a childproof latch.
- Appliances are unplugged when not in use, with cords out of reach.
- Matches and lighters are stored in a locked cabinet.
- Hazardous chemicals such as cleaning supplies, bug sprays, dishwasher detergent, and dishwashing liquids are out of children's reach.
- Bottles containing alcohol are stored out of reach.
- Plastic garbage bags and sandwich bags are out of reach.
- Cords or wires from wall telephones or cable TV are out of reach.
- Refrigerator magnets and other small objects are out of reach.
- There is a working fire extinguisher. Family members know how to use it.

Bathroom
- The thermostat on the hot water heater is set below 120°F (49°C).
- Razors, nail clippers, and other sharp items are stored in a locked cabinet.
- Drug bottles are closed tightly with child-resistant caps and stored out of children's reach.
- Childproof latches are installed on all drawers and cabinets.

Bathroom—cont'd
- Toilets are closed and have toilet-lid locks.
- Sinks, tubs, and basins are empty when not in use.
- Outlets have ground fault circuit interrupters. These protect against electrical injuries if an electrical appliance gets wet.
- Hair dryers, curling irons, and electric razors are unplugged when not in use.
- There are non-skid strips on the bottoms of bathtubs.
- There are non-slip pads under rugs to hold them securely to the floor.
- Cosmetics and cleaners are stored in a locked cabinet.
- Bottles of mouthwash, perfumes, hair dyes, hair sprays, nail polishes, and nail polish removers are stored in a locked cabinet.

Doors, Windows, Walls, and Floors
- Doors have finger-pinch guards.
- Rubber tips are removed from door stops or 1-piece door stops are installed.
- Doorknob covers or childproof locks are used on doors leading outside and to non-childproof areas.
- Glass doors have decorative markers so they are not mistaken for open doors.
- Sliding doors have childproof locks.
- Safety bars or window guards are installed on upper-story windows.
- Window stops are present to keep windows from closing all the way.
- Window blind and curtain cords are kept out of reach.
- Cribs, playpens, beds, or other furniture are not placed near a window.
- Window guards are placed on windows that are not emergency exits.
- Windows are opened from the top down.
- Walls are in good condition with no peeling or cracking paint.
- Mirrors and frames are hung securely.
- Rugs are secured to floors, fitted with anti-slip pads underneath, or removed.

Furniture
- Bookshelves and other furniture are secured with wall brackets to prevent tipping.
- Children are not allowed to climb on furniture. This includes using shelves as steps.
- Toys or things that attract children are not placed on the top of furniture.

---

*Home Safety modified and adapted from kidshealth.org: *Household safety checklists.*

Furniture—cont'd

- Protective padding is placed on corners of coffee tables, furniture, and countertops with sharp edges.
- Baby equipment has not been recalled.
- Flatscreen TVs are mounted securely on the wall. Older, heavy TVs are on low, stable furniture.
- Stops are on all removable drawers to prevent them from falling out.

Stairways

- Hardware-mounted safety gates are at the top and bottom of every stairway.
- Stairways are clear of tripping hazards such as loose carpeting or toys.
- Banisters and railings have guards if a child can fit through the rails.
- The railings and banisters are secure.
- The door to the basement steps is kept locked.
- There is enough light in the stairway.
- Children are supervised around stairs.

Child's Bedroom and Clothing

- The changing table has a safety belt.
- Painted cribs, bassinets, and high chairs made before 1978 are not used. (Paint was lead based before 1978.)
- The crib meets federal safety standards. See "Cribs," p. 882 and Chapter 52.
- There are no soft pillows, large stuffed animals, bumper pads, and soft bedding in the crib.
- Infants are not put to sleep on an adult or child's bed, water bed, couch, pillow, or other soft surface. Death from entrapment and suffocation are risks.
- Strings or ribbons have been removed from hanging mobiles and crib toys.
- The top bunk of a bunk bed has guard-rails. Children younger than 6 years are not allowed on the top bunk.
- Dressers are secured to walls with drawers closed.
- Night-lights do not touch any fabric such as bedspreads or curtains.
- Sleepwear is flame-retardant.
- Drawstrings are removed from clothing.
- Children are not allowed to wear necklaces, strings, cords, ribbons, or other such items around the neck.
- Bibs are removed before naptime and bedtime.
- Clothing fits well. Clothing is not loose and does not touch or drag the floor.

Garage and Laundry Area

- Gardening, automotive, and lawn care tools and supplies are stored safely away from children.
- Hazardous automotive, pool, and gardening products are in a locked area.
- Recycling containers storing glass and metal are out of reach.
- Garbage cans are securely covered.
- Cleaning products are out of reach.
- Laundry chutes are locked with childproof locks. Laundry room doors are kept closed.

Outdoors, Backyard, and Pool

- Walkways and outdoor stairways are well lit. They are clear of toys, objects, or things blocking a clear path.
- Sidewalks and outdoor stairways are without cracks and missing pieces.
- Playground equipment is safe with no loose parts, splinters, sharp edges, or rust.
- The surface beneath playground equipment is cushioned with material such as sand, mulch, wood chips, or approved rubber surfacing mats to absorb the shock of a fall.
- Outdoor toys are in a secure, dry place when not used.
- Toys are kept away from pools, spas, hot tubs, or whirlpools. Children playing with such toys could fall into the water.
- Toys are removed from pools after swimming.
- Climb-proof fencing is at least 4 feet high on all sides of the pool. The fence has a self-closing gate with a childproof lock.
- The ladder is removed from an above-ground pool when not in use.
- Door, window, and pool alarms are on. They alert you if a child wanders into an unsafe area.
- Inflatable flotation devices are not relied on to keep a child afloat. Children near water must be constantly supervised.
- Buckets, pails, containers, and wading pools are empty and upside down when not in use.

Vehicle Safety

- Children are not left alone in any vehicle even if the windows are down. They can develop heat-related illness, suffocate, and die from high temperatures within minutes.
- Seat-belt laws are followed.
- Children do not ride as passengers on tractors, mowers, mini-bikes, or all-terrain vehicles.
- Vehicle doors and the trunk are locked. Keys are kept out of children's sight and reach.
- Trunk access is kept closed.
- Children are not allowed to play in vehicles.

Electrical

- Un-used outlets are covered.
- Electrical items are unplugged when not in use.
- Major electrical appliances are grounded.
- Cord holders keep cords fastened against walls.
- There are no potential electrical fire hazards such as over-loaded electrical sockets and electrical wires running under carpets.
- Equipment with old or frayed cords and damaged extension cords are removed.
- Computers, TVs, and stereo equipment are against walls. This prevents children from touching cords.
- Electronic toys are checked for signs of danger. Toys that spark, feel hot, or smell unusual are repaired or discarded.

Heating and Cooling Elements

- Radiators and baseboard heaters are covered with childproof screens.
- Gas fireplaces are secured with a valve cover or key.
- Working fireplaces have a screen and other barriers in place when in use.
- Chimneys have been cleaned recently.
- Electric space heaters are at least 3 feet from beds, curtains, or anything flammable.

Emergency Equipment and Numbers

- A list of emergency phone numbers is near each phone in the home.
- Fire extinguishers are on every floor and in the kitchen.
- Upper floors of the home have an emergency ladder.
- Smoke alarms are on each floor of the home and in hallways between all bedrooms.
- Smoke alarms are tested monthly and batteries changed every 6 months.
- The home has a carbon monoxide alarms. (See Chapter 13.)

Firearm Safety

- Guns are stored in a securely locked case out of children's reach. All firearms are stored unloaded and in the un-cocked position.
- Ammunition is stored in a separate place and in a securely locked container out of reach.
- Keys for gun storage, ammunition, and gun-cleaning supplies are kept where children cannot find them.
- Trigger locks or other childproof devices are used.
- Gun safety is practiced. Adults have taken a firearm safety course to use the firearm safely and correctly.
- Children are taught that guns are not toys, they are not to touch or play with guns, and they should tell an adult if they find one.
- Gun-cleaning supplies are locked up. Cleaning supplies are often poisonous.

General Safety

- Infants and children are supervised at all times.
- Medication bottles, loose pills, coins, scissors, and any other small or sharp objects are out of reach.
- Smoking is not allowed in the home.
- Testing has been done for lead, radon, asbestos, mercury, mold, and carbon monoxide when such substances may be present.
- There are no potentially poisonous houseplants.
- Children are supervised around dogs and other pets.

Nursery Equipment Safety*

Nursery equipment must be safe, in good repair, and used properly. Use the following guidelines to check nursery equipment in an agency or home setting.

Carriers

- The carrier has:
  - Straps that prevent the baby from falling or crawling out
  - A firm, padded head support
  - Durable fabric with strong stitching or large, heavy fasteners to prevent slipping
- There is enough depth to support the baby's back.
- Leg openings are small enough to prevent the baby from slipping out but large enough to prevent chafing.
- A framed carrier has a kickstand that locks in the open position. The folding mechanism is free of pinch points that could pinch the baby's fingers. There is padding on the metal frame around the baby's face.
- Follow these safety measures when using carriers.
  - Never use a framed carrier before an infant is 4 to 5 months old. Do not use it as an infant seat. It can tip over without warning.
  - Use restraining straps at all times if the carrier has them.
  - If you need to lean over, bend from the knees rather than the waist to prevent the baby from falling out of the carrier.
  - Check the carrier often for loose fasteners or ripped seams.

Infant Seats

- The seat has a wide, sturdy base for stability.
- The item has non-skid feet to prevent slipping.
- Locking mechanisms are secure. Push down on the unit to make sure it is sturdy.
- Supporting devices lock securely.
- The seat has a crotch and waist strap. The buckle or strap is easy to use.
- The seat belt is secure and the fabric is washable.
- Follow these safety measures when using infant seats.
  - Never place the baby in an infant seat on a table or other raised surface.
  - Use the safety belt every time you place the baby in the seat.
  - Do not place the seat on soft surfaces such as beds or sofas. The seat may tip over and the baby can suffocate.
  - The seat is never used to transport a baby in a vehicle.

---

*Nursery Equipment Safety modified and adapted from U.S. Consumer Product Safety Commission: *The safe nursery,* CPSC 202, Washington, DC, and kidshealth.org.

Baby Bathtubs

- The bathtub has slip-resistant backing to keep it from moving.
- There are no rough edges that can scratch the baby.
- The tub stays firm in the center when filled with water.
- Bath rings, baby flotation devices, and bath seats are avoided. The baby can drown if the device tips.
- Foam cushions are avoided. Pieces can be torn off and swallowed.
- Follow these bathing safety measures.
  - Always check the water temperature before putting the baby in the bathtub. Water that is too hot can burn babies.
  - Only adults should give babies baths. Baths can be dangerous. Babies can drown in less than 1 inch of water.
  - Always keep 1 hand on the baby while he or she is in water.
  - Always take the baby with you if you step away from the bathtub.
  - Gather bathing supplies ahead of time, including shampoo, soap, washcloth, towel, clean clothes, a clean diaper, and wipes.
  - Always empty the bathtub and turn it upside down when it is not being used. A plug at the bottom of the tub makes draining easier.

Changing Tables

- The table is sturdy. The base is wide enough to prevent tipping.
- The table has safety straps to prevent falls.
- The table has drawers or shelves that are easy to reach without leaving the baby unattended. Supplies are within your reach but out of the baby's reach.
- A flat changing surface is surrounded on all 4 sides by a guard-rail that is at least 2 inches high. The surface is lower in the middle than on the sides to keep the baby from rolling.
- Follow these safety measures.
  - Use the safety belt when you change the baby.
  - Never leave the infant unattended, even if you think he or she is secure.
  - Stop using the changing table when the baby reaches the manufacturer's age or weight limit. Age 2 or 30 pounds is common.

Gates

- The gate has a pressure bar or other fastener that will resist forces exerted by a child.
- A hardware-mounted gate is used at the top of stairs. Pressure-mounted or free-standing gates can fall if the child pushes hard enough.
- The gate has a straight top edge with rigid bars or a tight mesh screen.
- There is less than 2 inches between the floor and the gate bottom to prevent a child from going underneath.

Gates—cont'd

- Rigid vertical slats or rods are no more than $2\frac{3}{8}$ inches apart to prevent head entrapment between the slats.
- There are no sharp edges or pieces that could cut a child's hand. Wooden gates are smooth to prevent splinters.
- There are no openings to use for climbing.
- The gate should be at least three quarters ($\frac{3}{4}$) of the child's height.
- Accordion-style gates are not used. They can trap a child's head.
- Follow these safety measures when using gates.
  - Keep large toys away from the gate. A child can use the toy to climb over.
  - Pressure-mounted gates may be used for doors between rooms unless there are stairs between the rooms. Place the pressure bar away from the child.
  - Gates that swing out are never to be used at the top of stairways.
  - Stop using the gate when the child is about 2 years old.

Hook-on Chairs

- The chair has a restraining strap.
- The chair has a clamp that locks onto the table for added security.
- Caps or plugs on tubing are firmly attached and cannot be pulled off and choke a child.
- The hook-on chair has a warning never to place the chair where the child can push off with the feet.

High Chairs

- The high chair has a "crotch" strap that must be used when restraining a child in a high chair.
- The high chair has restraining straps that are independent of the tray.
- The tray locks securely.
- Buckles on straps are easy to fasten and unfasten.
- The high chair has a wide, stable base.
- Caps or plugs on tubing are firmly attached and cannot be pulled off and choke a child.
- A folding high chair has an effective locking device that keeps the chair from collapsing.

Playpens

- Playpens or travel cribs have top rails that automatically lock when lifted into the normal-use position.
- The playpen does not have a rotating hinge in the center of the top rails.
- The locks for lowering a side are out of the baby's reach.
- The sides are at least 20 inches high, measured from the floor of the playpen.

Playpens—cont'd

- Playpen mesh has small weave (less than $\frac{1}{4}$-inch openings).
- The mesh has no tears, holes, or loose threads.
- The mesh is securely attached and checked regularly for breaks and tears.
- A wooden playpen has slats spaced no more than $2\frac{3}{8}$ inches apart.
- The playpen has well-protected hinges and supports.
- There is padding on the tops of the rails.
- The bottom of the playpen has a 1-inch firm mattress or pad.
- Follow these safety measures when using playpens.
  - Never leave a baby in a mesh playpen with the side lowered. Entrapment between the mesh side and floor board is a risk.
  - Never use soft bedding or pillows.
  - Do not replace the mattress or pad. The new mattress may not fit the playpen well.
  - Check all padded parts regularly for tears. Cover or repair tears.
  - Do not place the playpen near windows. Cords on window coverings can strangle the baby.
  - Do not use a playpen with large diamond-shaped openings. Entrapment is a risk.
  - Never tie or string toys from the sides of the playpen.
  - Stop using the playpen when the child can easily climb out—when the child is 34 inches tall or weighs 30 pounds.

Strollers and Carriages

- There is a wide base to prevent tipping.
- The seat belt and crotch strap securely attach to the frame. A 5-point harness is safest.
- The seat-belt buckle is easy to use.
- Brakes securely lock the wheels.
- The shopping basket is low on the back. It is located directly over or in front of the rear wheels.
- When used in the carriage position, the leg openings can be closed.
- No stroller parts can pinch a child's fingers or are a choking hazard.
- The leg openings are small enough to prevent an infant from slipping through.
- Follow these safety measures.
  - Never leave a child unattended.
  - Avoid using a pillow or blanket as a mattress.
  - Always apply the brakes when not moving.
  - Never hang purses or diaper bags on the handles.
  - Fold and unfold the stroller or carriage away from children to avoid pinching fingers.

Walkers

- Walkers are not used. Walkers are a leading cause of injury in babies. Injury risks include:
  - Falling over objects or down stairs
  - Rolling into dangerous objects or areas—hot stoves, heaters, and pools are examples
  - Reaching higher than normal and touching dangerous items—stovetops, kitchen knives, and hot coffee cups are examples

Toys and Toy Chests

- Small toys are kept away from children. Make sure toys are too large to fit into the child's mouth. Objects should have a diameter of $1\frac{3}{4}$ inches or more. This includes marbles, balls, and games with balls.
- Battery cases on battery-operated toys are secured with screws.
- Toys are strong and durable. They do not have:
  - Sharp ends, small parts, and small ends that can extend into the back of a baby's mouth
  - Strings longer than 7 inches
  - Parts that can pinch fingers
- Toys with loud, sharp, or shrill noises are avoided.
- Squeeze toys do not contain a squeaker that could detach and choke a baby.
- Rattles do not have ball-shaped ends.
- Riding toys are stable and secure to prevent tipping.
- Safety gear is worn for bicycles, skateboards, scooters, in-line skates, and other devices with wheels. A helmet and hand, wrist, and shin guards are examples.
- Follow these safety measures for toys.
  - Follow manufacturers' age recommendations.
  - Read all warning labels.
  - Make sure used toys have not been recalled for safety reasons.
  - Never give balloons or latex gloves to children younger than 8 years.
  - Never give a baby vending machine toys. They often contain small parts.
  - Keep older children's toys away from infants and younger children.
  - Check toys and play equipment for cracks, chips, breaks, sharp edges, loose parts, and other damage.
  - Have children put away their toys.
- The toy chest has no latch to entrap the child within the chest.
- The toy chest has a spring-loaded lid support that will not require frequent adjustment. It supports the lid in any position to prevent lid slam.
- The chest has ventilation holes or spaces in case the child gets caught inside.

Pacifiers

- The item has no ribbons, strings, cords, or yarn attached.
- The shield is large and firm enough so it cannot fit into the child's mouth.
- The guard or shield has ventilation holes to allow the baby to breathe if the shield does get into the mouth.
- The pacifier nipple has no holes or tears that might cause it to break off in the baby's mouth.

Crib Toys

- Strings or cords do not dangle into the crib.
- A crib gym or mobile has a label warning to remove the device from the crib when 1 of the following occur.
  - The child can push on the hands and knees.
  - The child reaches 5 months of age.
- Toy parts are too large to be a choking hazard.

Cribs

- Side rails are fixed and not adjustable. The U.S. Consumer Product Safety Commission (CPSC) banned the sale of drop-side cribs.
- Slats are spaced no more than $2\frac{3}{8}$ inches apart.
- No slats are missing, loose, or cracked.
- The mattress fits snugly—less than a 2-finger width between the edge of the mattress and crib side.
- The mattress support is securely attached to the head and foot-boards.
- The mattress pad fits tightly and the plastic mattress packaging is removed.
- There are no cut-outs in the head-board or foot-board. Cut-outs allow head entrapment.
- Crib corner posts are either flush with the top of the head-board and foot-board or are over 16 inches.
- The crib meets federal safety standards for strength, durability, and testing.
- Follow these safety measures when using cribs.
  - Always place a baby on his or her back to sleep.
  - Remove a baby's bib when in the crib.
  - Check that all screws and hardware are present and tight.
  - Never place soft bedding or soft toys in the crib.
  - Bumper pads are not used.
  - Never place a crib near a window or drapes. A baby can become entangled in window covering cords.

Bassinets and Cradles

- The item has a sturdy bottom and a wide base for stability.
- The item has smooth surfaces. There are no protruding staples or other hardware that can injure the baby.
- Legs have strong, effective locks to prevent folding while in use.
- The mattress is firm and fits snugly.
- Wood or metal cradles have slats spaced no more than $2\frac{3}{8}$ inches apart.

Child Safety Seats (Car Seats)

- The car seat is federally approved and fits the child's size and weight.
- Parts and manufacturer labels, including the manufacturer's name, model number, and date made, are intact.
- The seat has not been in a motor vehicle accident.
- The seat is less than 6 years old. Check the manufacturer's recommended expiration date.
- Follow these safety measures for using car seats.
  - Do not use a car seat that does not have the manufacturer's instructions.
  - Infants and toddlers ride rear-facing until 2 years of age or until they have reached the weight and height limits recommended by the manufacturer.
  - Children in forward-facing seats are harnessed in until they reach the weight or height for that seat.
  - A booster seat is used for children who have outgrown the forward-facing harness seat. Booster seats are for children between the ages of 4 and 8 years (about 40 and 80 pounds). The child is secured with the lap-and-shoulder belts according to the manufacturer's instructions.
  - Children use a booster seat until the vehicle's lap-and-shoulder belt fits properly. This usually occurs when the child has reached 4 feet, 9 inches in height—between 8 and 12 years of age.
  - Children less than 12 years ride in the back seat.
  - Do not use a rear-facing car seat or convertible seat in the front seat of a vehicle with an air bag.
  - Do not use a car safety seat that has cracks, missing parts, or torn or loose harnesses and buckles.

Glossary

A

abbreviation A shortened form of a word or phrase

abduction Moving a body part away from the mid-line of the body

abrasion A partial-thickness wound caused by the scraping away or rubbing of the skin

abuse The willful infliction of injury, unreasonable confinement, intimidation, or punishment that results in physical harm, pain, or mental anguish; depriving the person (or the person's caregiver) of the goods or services needed to attain or maintain well-being

accountable Being responsible for one's actions and the actions of others who performed the delegated tasks; answering questions about and explaining one's actions and the actions of others

acetone See "ketone"

activities of daily living (ADL) The activities usually done during a normal day in a person's life

acute illness A sudden illness from which a person is expected to recover

acute pain Pain that is felt suddenly from injury, disease, trauma, or surgery

adduction Moving a body part toward the mid-line of the body

admission Official entry of a person into a health care setting

adolescence The time between puberty and adulthood; a time of rapid growth and physical, sexual, emotional, and social changes

advance directive A document stating a person's wishes about health care when that person cannot make his or her own decisions

afebrile Without (*a*) a fever (*febrile*)

alcohol abuse When drinking leads to problems but the person is not dependent on alcohol

alcoholism Alcohol dependence that involves craving, loss of control, physical dependence, and tolerance

allergy A sensitivity to a substance that causes the body to react with signs and symptoms

alopecia Hair loss

AM care See "early morning care"

ambulation The act of walking

amputation The removal of all or part of an extremity

anaphylaxis A life-threatening sensitivity to an antigen

anesthesia The loss of all sensation, especially pain, produced by a drug

anorexia The loss of appetite

anterior At or toward the front of the body or body part; ventral

antibiotic A drug that kills certain microbes that cause infection

anticoagulant A drug that prevents or slows down (*anti*) blood clotting (*coagulate*)

antisepsis The processes, procedures, and chemical treatments that kill microbes or prevent them from causing an infection; *anti* means *against* and *sepsis* means *infection*

anxiety A vague, uneasy feeling in response to stress

aphasia The total or partial loss (*a*) of the ability to use or understand language (*phasia*); parts of the brain responsible for language are damaged

apical-radial pulse Taking the apical and radial pulses at the same time

apnea The lack or absence (*a*) of breathing (*pnea*)

arrhythmia See "dysrhythmia"

arterial ulcer An open wound on the lower legs or feet caused by poor arterial blood flow

artery A blood vessel that carries blood away from the heart

arthritis Joint (*arthr*) inflammation (*itis*)

arthroplasty The surgical replacement (*plasty*) of a joint (*arthro*)

asepsis The absence (*a*) of disease-producing microbes (*sepsis* means *infection*)

aspiration Breathing fluid, food, vomitus, or an object into the lungs

assault Intentionally attempting or threatening to touch a person's body without the person's consent

assessment Collecting information about the person; a step in the nursing process

assisted living A housing option for older persons who need help with activities of daily living but do not need constant care

assisted living residence (ALR) Provides housing, personal care, support services, health care, and social activities in a home-like setting to persons needing help with daily activities

atelectasis The collapse of a portion of a lung

atrophy Shrink; the decrease in size or wasting away of tissue

autopsy The examination of the body after death

avoidable pressure ulcer A pressure ulcer that develops from the improper use of the nursing process

B

bariatrics The field of medicine focused on the treatment and control of obesity

base of support The area on which an object rests

battery Touching a person's body without his or her consent

bedfast Confined to bed

bed mobility How a person moves to and from a lying position, turns from side to side, and re-positions in a bed or other furniture

bed rail A device that serves as a guard or barrier along the side of the bed; side rail

benign tumor A tumor that does not spread to other body parts

biohazardous waste Items contaminated with blood, body fluids, secretions, or excretions; *bio* means *life* and *hazardous* means *dangerous* or *harmful*

Biot's respirations Rapid and deep respirations followed by 10 to 30 seconds of apnea

birth defect A problem that develops during pregnancy, often during the first 3 months; it may involve a body structure or function

bisexual A person who is attracted to both sexes

blindness The absence of sight

blood pressure (BP) The amount of force exerted against the walls of an artery by the blood

body alignment The way the head, trunk, arms, and legs are aligned with one another; posture

body language Messages sent through facial expressions, gestures, posture, hand and body movements, gait, eye contact, and appearance

body mechanics Using the body in an efficient and careful way

body temperature The amount of heat in the body that is a balance between the amount of heat produced and the amount lost by the body

bony prominence An area where the bone sticks out or projects from the flat surface of the body; pressure point

boundary crossing A brief act or behavior of being over-involved with the person; the intent of the act or behavior is to meet the person's needs

boundary sign Acts, behaviors, or thoughts that warn of a boundary crossing or violation

boundary violation An act or behavior that meets your needs, not the person's

bradycardia A slow (*brady*) heart rate (*cardia*); less than 60 beats per minute

bradypnea Slow (*brady*) breathing (*pnea*); respirations are fewer than 12 per minute

braille A touch reading and writing system that uses raised dots for each letter of the alphabet; the first 10 letters also represent the numbers 0 through 9

breast-feeding Feeding a baby milk from the mother's breasts; nursing

Broca's aphasia See "expressive aphasia"

bullying Repeated attacks or threats of fear, distress, or harm by a bully toward a victim

burnout A job stress resulting in being physically or mentally exhausted, having doubts about your abilities, and having doubts about the value of your work

C

calorie The fuel or energy value of food

cancer See "malignant tumor"

capillary A tiny blood vessel; food, oxygen, and other substances pass from the capillaries into the cells

cardiac arrest See "sudden cardiac arrest (SCA)"

carrier A human or animal that is a reservoir for microbes but does not develop the infection

case management A nursing case manager coordinates the care of specific groups of patients from admission through discharge and into the home or long-term care setting

catheter A tube used to drain or inject fluid through a body opening

catheterization The process of inserting a catheter

cell The basic unit of body structure

certification Official recognition by a state that standards or requirements have been met

cerumen Earwax

chairfast Confined to a chair

chart See "medical record"

chemical restraint Any drug that is used for discipline or convenience and not required to treat medical symptoms

Cheyne-Stokes respirations Respirations gradually increase in rate and depth and then become shallow and slow; breathing may stop (*apnea*) for 10 to 20 seconds

child abuse and neglect The intentional harm or mistreatment of a child under 18 years old; it involves any recent act or failure to act on the part of a parent or caregiver; it results in death, serious physical or emotional harm, sexual abuse, or exploitation; and it presents a likely or immediate risk for harm

cholesterol A soft, waxy substance found in the bloodstream and all body cells

chronic illness An ongoing illness, slow or gradual in onset; it has no known cure; it can be controlled and complications prevented with proper treatment

chronic pain Pain that continues for a long time (months or years) or occurs off and on; persistent pain

chronic wound A wound that does not heal easily

circadian rhythm Daily rhythm based on a 24-hour cycle; the day-night cycle or body rhythm

circulatory ulcer An open sore on the lower legs or feet caused by decreased blood flow through the arteries or veins; vascular ulcer

circumcised The fold of skin (foreskin) covering the glans of the penis was surgically removed

circumcision The surgical removal of foreskin from the penis

civil law Laws concerned with relationships between people

clean-contaminated wound Occurs from the surgical entry of the reproductive, urinary, respiratory, or gastro-intestinal system

clean technique See "medical asepsis"

clean wound A wound that is not infected

clinical record See "medical record"

closed fracture The bone is broken but the skin is intact

closed wound Tissues are injured but the skin is not broken

code of ethics Rules, or standards of conduct, for group members to follow

cognitive function Involves memory, thinking, reasoning, ability to understand, judgment, and behavior

colonized The presence of bacteria on the wound surface or in wound tissue; the person does not have signs and symptoms of an infection

colostomy A surgically created opening (*stomy*) between the colon (*colo*) and the body's surface

coma A state of being unaware of one's setting and being unable to react or respond to people, places, or things

comatose Being unable to respond to stimuli

comfort A state of well-being; the person has no physical or emotional pain and is calm and at peace

communicable disease A disease caused by pathogens that spread easily; contagious disease

communication The exchange of information—a message sent is received and correctly interpreted by the intended person

competent Having the necessary ability, knowledge, or skill to perform a task safely and successfully

compound fracture See "open fracture"

compress A soft pad applied over a body area

compulsion Repeating an act over and over again (a ritual)

condom catheter A soft sheath that slides over the penis and is used to drain urine

confidentiality Trusting others with personal and private information

conflict A clash between opposing interests or ideas

confusion A mental state of being disoriented to person, time, place, situation, or identity

congenital To be born with

constipation The passage of a hard, dry stool

constrict To narrow

contagious disease See "communicable disease"

contaminated wound A wound with a high risk of infection

contamination The process of becoming unclean

contracture The lack of joint mobility caused by abnormal shortening of a muscle

contusion A closed wound caused by a blow to the body; a bruise

convenience Any action taken to control or manage a person's behavior that requires less effort by the staff; the action is not in the person's best interest

convulsion See "seizure"

cotton drawsheet A drawsheet made of cotton; it helps keep the mattress and bottom linens clean

courtesy A polite, considerate, or helpful comment or act

crime An act that violates a criminal law

criminal law Laws concerned with offenses against the public and society in general

cross-contamination Passing microbes from 1 person to another by contaminated hands, equipment, or supplies

culture The characteristics of a group of people—language, values, beliefs, habits, likes, dislikes, customs—passed from 1 generation to the next

cyanosis Bluish (*cyano*) color; bluish color (*cyano*) to the skin, lips, mucous membranes, and nail beds

D

dandruff Excessive amounts of dry, white flakes from the scalp

deafness Hearing loss in which it is impossible for the person to understand speech through hearing alone

deconditioning The loss of muscle strength from inactivity

defamation Injuring a person's name and reputation by making false statements to a third person

defecation The process of excreting feces from the rectum through the anus; a bowel movement

defense mechanism An unconscious reaction that blocks unpleasant or threatening feelings

dehiscence The separation of wound layers

dehydration The excessive loss of water from tissues; a decrease in the amount of water in body tissues

delegate To authorize another person to perform a nursing task in a certain situation

delirium A state of sudden, severe confusion and rapid changes in brain function

delusion A false belief

delusion of grandeur An exaggerated belief about one's importance, wealth, power, or talents

delusion of persecution A false belief that one is being mistreated, abused, or harassed

dementia The loss of cognitive and social function caused by changes in the brain; the loss of cognitive function that interferes with routine personal, social, and occupational activities

denture An artificial tooth or a set of artificial teeth

development Changes in mental, emotional, and social function

developmental disabilities A group of conditions caused by physical, learning, language, or behavior impairments

developmental task A skill that must be completed during a stage of development

diabetic foot ulcer An open wound on the foot caused by complications from diabetes

dialysis The process of removing waste products from the blood

diaphoresis Profuse (excessive) sweating

diarrhea The frequent passage of liquid stools

diastole The period of heart muscle relaxation; the heart is at rest

diastolic pressure The pressure in the arteries when the heart is at rest

digestion The process that breaks down food physically and chemically so it can be absorbed for use by the cells

dilate To expand or open wider

dirty wound See "infected wound"

disability Any lost, absent, or impaired physical or mental function

disaster A sudden, catastrophic event in which people are injured and killed and property is destroyed

discharge Official departure of a person from a health care setting

discipline Any action taken by the agency to punish or penalize a patient or resident

discomfort See "pain"

disinfectant A liquid chemical that can kill many or all pathogens except spores.

disinfection The process of killing pathogens

distal The part farthest from the center or from the point of attachment

distraction To change the person's center of attention

diuresis The process (*esis*) of passing (*di*) urine (*ur*); large amounts of urine are produced—1000 to 3000 mL (milliliters) or more a day

dorsal See "posterior"

dorsal recumbent position The back-lying or supine position; the supine position with the legs together (*dorsal* means *the back of something; recumbent* means *to lie down*); horizontal recumbent position

dorsiflexion Bending the toes and foot up at the ankle

drawsheet A small sheet placed over the middle of the bottom sheet

drug abuse Using a drug for non-medical or non-therapy effects

drug addiction A strong urge or craving to use the substance and cannot stop using; tolerance develops

dysphagia Difficulty (*dys*) swallowing (*phagia*)

dyspnea Difficult, labored, or painful (*dys*) breathing (*pnea*)

dysrhythmia An abnormal (*dys*) heart rhythm (*rhythmia*); arrhythmia

dysuria Painful or difficult (*dys*) urination (*uria*); burning on urination

E

early morning care Routine care given before breakfast; AM care

edema The swelling of body tissues with water; swelling caused by fluid collecting in tissues

ejaculation The release of semen

elder abuse Any knowing, intentional, or negligent act by a caregiver or any other person to an older adult; the act causes harm or serious risk of harm

elective surgery Surgery done by choice to improve life or well-being

electrical shock When electrical current passes through the body

electronic health record (EHR) An electronic version of a person's medical record; electronic medical record

electronic medical record (EMR) See "electronic health record (EHR)"

elopement When a patient or resident leaves the agency without staff knowledge

embolus A blood clot that travels through the vascular system until it lodges in a blood vessel

emergency surgery Surgery done at once to save life or function

emesis See "vomitus"

enabler A device that limits freedom of movement but is used to promote independence, comfort, or safety

end-of-life care The support and care given during the time surrounding death

end-of-shift report A report that the nurse gives at the end of the shift to the on-coming shift; change-of-shift report

endorsement A state recognizes the certificate, license, or registration issued by another state; reciprocity or equivalency

enema The introduction of fluid into the rectum and lower colon

enteral nutrition Giving nutrients into the gastro-intestinal (GI) tract (*enteral*) through a feeding tube

entrapment Getting caught, trapped, or entangled in spaces created by the bed rails, the mattress, the bed frame, the head-board, or the foot-board

enuresis Urinary incontinence in bed at night

epidermal stripping Removing the epidermis (outer skin layer) as tape is removed from the skin

episiotomy Incision (*otomy*) into the perineum

equivalency See "endorsement"

erectile dysfunction (ED) See "impotence"

ergonomics The science of designing the job to fit the worker; *ergo* means *work*, *nomos* means *law*

eschar Thick, leathery dead tissue that may be loose or adhered to the skin; it is often black or brown

esteem The worth, value, or opinion one has of a person

ethics Knowledge of what is right conduct and wrong conduct

evaluation To measure if goals in the planning step were met; a step in the nursing process

evening care Care given in the evening at bedtime; PM care

evisceration The separation of the wound along with the protrusion of abdominal organs

excoriation Loss of the epidermis (top skin layer) caused by scratching or when skin rubs against skin, clothing, or other material

expressive aphasia Difficulty expressing or sending out thoughts through speech or writing; motor aphasia, Broca's aphasia

extension Straightening a body part

external rotation Turning the joint outward

F

fainting The sudden loss of consciousness from an inadequate blood supply to the brain

false imprisonment Unlawful restraint or restriction of a person's freedom of movement

febrile With a fever

fecal impaction The prolonged retention and buildup of feces in the rectum

fecal incontinence The inability to control the passage of feces and gas through the anus

feces The semi-solid mass of waste products in the colon that is expelled through the anus; also called a *stool* or *stools*

fever Elevated body temperature

first aid Emergency care given to an ill or injured person before medical help arrives

flashback Reliving a trauma in thoughts during the day and in nightmares during sleep

flatulence The excessive formation of gas or air in the stomach and intestines

flatus Gas or air passed through the anus

flexion Bending a body part

flow rate The number of drops per minute (*gtt/min*) or milliliters per hour (*mL/hr*)

Foley catheter See "indwelling catheter"

footdrop The foot falls down at the ankle; permanent plantar flexion

Fowler's position A semi-sitting position; the head of the bed is raised between 45 and 60 degrees

fracture A broken bone

fraud Saying or doing something to trick, fool, or deceive a person

freedom of movement Any change in place or position of the body or any part of the body that the person is able to control

friction The rubbing of 1 surface against another

full-thickness wound The dermis, epidermis, and subcutaneous tissue are penetrated; muscle and bone may be involved

full visual privacy Having the means to be completely free from public view while in bed

functional incontinence The person has bladder control but cannot use the toilet in time

functional nursing A nursing care pattern focusing on tasks and jobs; each nursing team member has certain tasks and jobs to do

functional status The person's ability to perform the activities of daily living (ADL) required to meet basic needs and required for health and well-being

G

gait belt See "transfer belt"

gangrene A condition in which there is death of tissue

gastrostomy tube A feeding tube inserted through a surgically created opening (*stomy*) in the stomach (*gastro*); stomach tube

gavage The process of giving a tube feeding

gender identity A person's sense or feelings of being male, female, or transgender

general anesthesia A treatment with certain drugs that produces a deep sleep and the absence of all sensation, especially pain

genupectoral position See "knee-chest position" (*genu* means *knee*; *pectoral* refers to the *chest*)

geriatrics The field of medicine concerned with the problems and diseases of old age and older persons; the care of aging people

gerontology The study of the aging process

global aphasia Difficulty expressing or sending out thoughts and difficulty understanding language; mixed aphasia

glucometer A device for measuring (*meter*) blood glucose (*gluco*); glucose meter

glucosuria Sugar (*glucose*) in the urine (*uria*); glycosuria

glycosuria Sugar (*glycos*) in the urine (*uria*); glucosuria

goal That which is desired for or by a person as a result of nursing care

gossip To spread rumors or talk about the private matters of others

graduate A measuring container for fluid

ground That which carries leaking electricity to the earth and away from an electrical item

growth The physical changes that are measured and that occur in a steady, orderly manner

guided imagery Creating and focusing on an image

H

hallucination Seeing, hearing, smelling, or feeling things that are not real

harassment To trouble, torment, offend, or worry a person by one's behavior or comments

hazard Any thing in the person's setting that may cause injury or illness

hazardous chemical Any chemical that is a health hazard or a physical hazard

healthcare-associated infection (HAI) An infection that develops in a person cared for in any setting where health care is given; the infection is related to receiving health care

health team The many health care workers whose skills and knowledge focus on the person's total care; interdisciplinary health care team

hearing loss Not being able to hear the normal range of sounds associated with normal hearing

heartburn A burning sensation in the chest or throat

hematoma A swelling (*oma*) that contains blood (*hemat*)

hematuria Blood (*hemat*) in the urine (*uria*)

hemiplegia Paralysis (*plegia*) on 1 side (*hemi*) of the body

hemoglobin The substance in red blood cells that carries oxygen and gives blood its red color

hemoptysis Bloody (*hemo*) sputum (*ptysis* means *to spit*)

hemorrhage The excessive loss (*rrhage*) of blood (*hemo*) in a short time

hemothorax Blood (*hemo*) in the pleural space (*thorax*)

heterosexual A person who is attracted to members of the other sex

high blood pressure See "hypertension"

high-Fowler's position A semi-sitting position; the head of the bed is raised 60 to 90 degrees

hirsutism Excessive body hair

holism A concept that considers the whole person; the whole person has physical, social, psychological, and spiritual parts that are woven together and cannot be separated

homosexual A person who is attracted to members of the same sex

horizontal recumbent position See "dorsal recumbent position"

hormone A chemical substance secreted by the endocrine glands into the bloodstream

hospice A health care agency or program for persons who are dying

hospital bed system The bed frame and its parts; the parts include the mattress, bed rails, head- and foot-boards, and bed attachments

hydration Having an adequate amount of water in body tissues

hyperextension Excessive straightening of a body part

hyperglycemia High (*hyper*) sugar (*glyc*) in the blood (*emia*)

hypertension When the systolic pressure is 140 mm Hg or higher (*hyper*) or the diastolic pressure is 90 mm Hg or higher; high blood pressure

hyperthermia A body temperature (*thermia*) that is much higher (*hyper*) than the person's normal range

hyperventilation Breathing (*ventilation*) is rapid (*hyper*) and deeper than normal

hypoglycemia Low (*hypo*) sugar (*glyc*) in the blood (*emia*)

hypotension When the systolic pressure is below (*hypo*) 90 mm Hg or the diastolic pressure is below 60 mm Hg

hypothermia A very low (*hypo*) body temperature (*thermia*)

hypoventilation Breathing (*ventilation*) is slow (*hypo*), shallow, and sometimes irregular

hypoxemia A reduced amount (*hypo*) of oxygen (*ox*) in the blood (*emia*)

hypoxia Cells do not have enough (*hypo*) oxygen (*oxia*)

I

ileostomy A surgically created opening (*stomy*) between the ileum (small intestine [*ileo*]) and the body's surface

immunity Protection against a disease or condition; the person will not get or be affected by the disease

implementation To perform or carry out nursing interventions (nursing measures or nursing actions) in the care plan; a step in the nursing process

impotence The inability of the male to have an erection; erectile dysfunction

incident An event that has harmed or could harm a patient, resident, visitor, or staff member

incision A cut produced surgically by a sharp instrument; it creates an opening into an organ or body space

indwelling catheter A catheter left in the bladder so urine drains constantly into a drainage bag; retention or Foley catheter

infancy The first year of life

infected wound A wound containing large amounts of microbes that shows signs of infection; a dirty wound

infection A disease state resulting from the invasion and growth of microbes in the body

infection control Practices and procedures that prevent the spread of infection

infestation Being in or on a host

inherited That which is passed down from parents to children

insomnia A chronic condition in which the person cannot sleep or stay asleep all night

intact skin Normal skin and skin layers without damage or breaks

intake The amount of fluid taken in; input

intellectual disability Involves severe limits in intellectual function and adaptive behavior occurring before age 18

intentional wound A wound created for therapy

internal rotation Turning the joint inward

intimate partner violence (IPV) Physical, sexual, or psychological harm by a current or former partner or spouse

intravenous (IV) therapy Giving fluids through a needle or catheter inserted into a vein; IV and IV infusion

intubation Inserting an artificial airway

invasion of privacy Violating a person's right not to have his or her name, photo, or private affairs exposed or made public without giving consent

involuntary seclusion Separating a person from others against his or her will, keeping the person to a certain area, or keeping the person away from his or her room without consent

J

jaundice Yellowish color of the skin or whites of the eyes

jejunostomy tube A feeding tube inserted into a surgically created opening (*stomy*) in the *jejunum* of the small intestine

job application An agency's official form listing questions that require factual answers

job description A document that describes what the agency expects you to do

job interview When an employer asks a job applicant questions about his or her education and career

joint The point at which 2 or more bones meet to allow movement

K

Kardex A type of card file that summarizes information found in the medical record—drugs, treatments, diagnoses, routine care measures, equipment, and special needs

ketone A substance appearing in urine from the rapid breakdown of fat for energy; acetone, ketone body

ketone body See "ketone"

knee-chest position The person kneels and rests the body on the knees and chest; the head is turned to 1 side, the arms are above the head or flexed at the elbows, the back is straight, and the body is flexed about 90 degrees at the hips; genupectoral position

Kussmaul respirations Very deep and rapid respirations

L

laceration An open wound with torn tissues and jagged edges

laryngeal mirror An instrument used to examine the mouth, teeth, and throat

lateral Away from the mid-line; at the side of the body or body part

lateral position The person lies on 1 side or the other; side-lying position

lateral transfer When a person moves between 2 horizontal surfaces

law A rule of conduct made by a government body

libel Making false statements in print, in writing (including e-mail and text messages), through pictures or drawings, through broadcast (radio, TV, or video), posted on-line on websites, or through video sites and social media sites

lice See "pediculosis"

licensed practical nurse (LPN) A nurse who has completed a practical nursing program and has passed a licensing test; called *licensed vocational nurse (LVN)* in California and Texas

licensed vocational nurse (LVN) See "licensed practical nurse (LPN)"

lithotomy position The woman lies on her back with the hips at the edge of the exam table, her knees are flexed, her hips are externally rotated, and her feet are in stirrups

local anesthesia The loss of sensation, produced by a drug, in a small area

lochia The vaginal discharge that occurs after childbirth

logrolling Turning the person as a unit, in alignment, with 1 motion

low vision Vision loss that cannot be corrected with eyeglasses, contact lenses, drugs, or surgery; vision loss interferes with every-day activities

lymphedema A buildup of lymph in the tissues causing edema (swelling)

M

malignant tumor A tumor that invades and destroys nearby tissues and can spread to other body parts; cancer

malpractice Negligence by a professional person

mechanical ventilation Using a machine to move air into and out of the lungs

meconium A dark green to black, tarry bowel movement

medial At or near the middle or mid-line of the body or body part

medical asepsis Practices used to reduce the number of microbes and prevent their spread from 1 person or place to another person or place; clean technique

medical diagnosis The identification of a disease or condition by a doctor

medical record The legal account of a person's condition and response to treatment and care; chart or clinical record

medical symptom An indication or characteristic of a physical or psychological condition

medication reminder Reminding the person to take drugs, observing them being taken as prescribed, and recording that they were taken

melena A black, tarry stool

menarche The first menstruation and the start of menstrual cycles

menopause The time when menstruation stops and menstrual cycles end

menstruation The process in which the lining of the uterus (*endometrium*) breaks up and is discharged from the body through the vagina

mental Relating to the mind; something that exists in the mind or is done by the mind

mental health The person copes with and adjusts to everyday stresses in ways accepted by society

mental health disorder A disturbance in the ability to cope with or adjust to stress; behavior and function are impaired; mental illness, psychiatric disorder

mental illness See "mental health disorder"

metabolism The burning of food for heat and energy by the cells

metastasis The spread of cancer to other body parts

microbe See "microorganism"

microorganism A small (*micro*) living thing (*organism*) seen only with a microscope; microbe

micturition See "urination"

mite A very small spider-like organism

mixed aphasia See "global aphasia"

mixed incontinence The combination of stress incontinence and urge incontinence

mole A brown, tan, or black spot on the skin that is flat or raised and round or oval

morbid obesity The person weighs 100 pounds or more over his or her normal weight

morning care Care given after breakfast; hygiene measures are more thorough at this time

motor aphasia See "expressive aphasia"

N

nasal speculum An instrument (*speculum* means *mirror*) used to examine the inside of the nose (*nasal*)

naso-enteral tube A feeding tube inserted through the nose (*naso*) into the small bowel (*enteral*)

naso-gastric (NG) tube A feeding tube inserted through the nose (*naso*) into the stomach (*gastro*)

need Something necessary or desired for maintaining life and mental well-being

neglect The failure of responsible persons to provide food, shelter, health care, or protection for a vulnerable elder

negligence An unintentional wrong in which a person did not act in a reasonable and careful manner and a person or the person's property was harmed

nocturia Frequent urination (*uria*) at night (*noc*)

non-pathogen A microbe that does not usually cause an infection

nonverbal communication Communication that does not use words

normal flora Microbes that live and grow in a certain area

NREM sleep The phase of sleep with *no rapid eye movement*; non-REM sleep

nursing See "breast-feeding"

nursing assistant A person who has passed a nursing assistant training and competency evaluation program; performs delegated nursing tasks under the supervision of a licensed nurse

nursing care plan A written guide about the person's nursing care; care plan

nursing diagnosis Describes a health problem that can be treated by nursing measures; a step in the nursing process

nursing intervention An action or measure taken by the nursing team to help the person reach a goal; nursing action, nursing measure

nursing process The method nurses use to plan and deliver nursing care; its 5 steps are assessment, nursing diagnosis, planning, implementation, and evaluation

nursing task Nursing care or a nursing function, procedure, activity, or work that can be delegated to nursing assistants when it does not require a nurse's professional knowledge or judgment

nursing team Those who provide nursing care—RNs, LPNs/LVNs, and nursing assistants

nutrient A substance that is ingested, digested, absorbed, and used by the body

nutrition The processes involved in the ingestion, digestion, absorption, and use of foods and fluids by the body

O

obesity Having an excess amount of total body fat; body weight is 20% or more above what is normal for the person's height and age

objective data Information that is seen, heard, felt, or smelled by an observer; signs

observation Using the sense of sight, hearing, touch, and smell to collect information

obsession A recurrent, unwanted thought, idea, or image

obstetrics The field of medicine concerned with the care of women during pregnancy, labor, and childbirth and for 6 to 8 weeks after birth

oliguria Scant amount (*olig*) of urine (*uria*); less than 500 mL in 24 hours

ombudsman Someone who supports or promotes the needs and interests of another person

open fracture The broken bone has come through the skin; compound fracture

open wound The skin or mucous membrane is broken

ophthalmoscope A lighted instrument (*scope*) used to examine the internal eye (*ophthalmo*) structures

opposition Touching an opposite finger with the thumb

optimal level of function A person's highest potential for mental and physical performance

oral hygiene Mouth care

organ Groups of tissue with the same function

orthopnea Breathing (*pnea*) deeply and comfortably only when sitting (*ortho*)

orthopneic position Sitting up (*ortho*) and leaning over a table to breathe (*pneic*)

orthostatic hypotension Abnormally low (*hypo*) blood pressure when the person suddenly stands up (*ortho* and *static*); postural hypotension

orthotic device A device used to support a muscle, promote a certain motion, or correct a deformity; *ortho* means *to straighten*

ostomy A surgically created opening that connects an internal organ to the body's surface; see "colostomy" and "ileostomy"

otoscope A lighted instrument (*scope*) used to examine the external ear (*oto*) and the eardrum (tympanic membrane)

output The amount of fluid lost

over-active bladder See "urge incontinence"

over-flow incontinence Small amounts of urine leak from a full bladder

oxygen concentration The amount (percent) of hemoglobin containing oxygen

P

pack Wrapping a body part with a wet or dry application

padded waterproof drawsheet A drawsheet made of an absorbent top and waterproof bottom used to protect the mattress and bottom linens from dampness and soiling

pain To ache, hurt, or be sore; discomfort

palliative care Care that involves relieving or reducing the intensity of uncomfortable symptoms without producing a cure

panic An intense and sudden feeling of fear, anxiety, terror, or dread

paralysis Loss of muscle function, sensation, or both

paranoia A disorder (*para*) of the mind (*noia*); false beliefs (delusions) and suspicion about a person or situation

paraphrasing Re-stating the person's message in your own words

paraplegia Paralysis in the legs, lower trunk, and pelvic organs (*para* means *beyond*; *plegia* means *paralysis*)

parenteral nutrition Giving nutrients through a catheter inserted into a vein; *para* means *beyond*; *enteral* relates to the bowel

partial-thickness wound The dermis and epidermis of the skin are broken

patent Open and unblocked

pathogen A microbe that is harmful and can cause an infection

patient-focused care A nursing care pattern; services are moved from departments to the bedside

pediatrics The field of medicine concerned with the growth, development, and care of children—newborns to teenagers

pediculosis Infestation with wingless insects; lice

pediculosis capitis Infestation of the scalp (*capitis*) with lice

pediculosis corporis Infestation of the body (*corporis*) with lice

pediculosis pubis Infestation of the pubic (*pubis*) hair with lice

peer A person of the same age-group and background

penetrating wound An open wound that breaks the skin and enters a body area, organ, or cavity

percussion hammer An instrument used to tap body parts to test reflexes (*percussion* means *to strike hard*); reflex hammer

percutaneous endoscopic gastrostomy (PEG) tube A feeding tube inserted into the stomach (*gastro*) through a small incision (*stomy*) made through (*per*) the skin (*cutaneous*); a lighted instrument (*scope*) is used to see inside a body cavity or organ (*endo*)

pericare See "perineal care"

perineal care Cleaning the genital and anal areas; pericare

peristalsis Involuntary muscle contractions in the digestive system that move food down the esophagus through the alimentary canal; the alternating contraction and relaxation of intestinal muscles

persistent pain See "chronic pain"

personality The set of attitudes, values, behaviors, and traits of a person

person's unit The personal space, furniture, and equipment provided for the person by the agency

phantom pain Pain felt in a body part that is no longer there

phlebitis Inflammation (*itis*) of a vein (*phleb*)

phobia An intense fear

physical restraint Any manual method or physical or mechanical device, material, or equipment attached to or near the person's body that he or she cannot remove easily and that restricts freedom of movement or normal access to one's body

pivot To turn one's body from a set standing position

planning Setting priorities and goals; a step in the nursing process

plantar flexion The foot (*plantar*) is bent (*flexion*); bending the foot down at the ankle

plaque A thin film that sticks to the teeth; it contains saliva, microbes, and other substances

pleural effusion The escape and collection of fluid (*effusion*) in the pleural space

PM care See "evening care"

pneumonia Inflammation and infection of lung tissue

pneumothorax Air (*pneumo*) in the pleural space (*thorax*)

poison Any substance harmful to the body when ingested, inhaled, injected, or absorbed through the skin

pollutant A harmful chemical or substance in the air or water

polyuria Abnormally large amounts (*poly*) of urine (*uria*)

posterior At or toward the back of the body or body part; dorsal

post-mortem care Care of the body after (*post*) death (*mortem*)

post-operative After surgery

postpartum After (*post*) childbirth (*partum*)

postural hypotension See "orthostatic hypotension"

posture See "body alignment"

prefix A word element placed before a root; it changes the meaning of the word

pre-hypertension When the systolic pressure is between 120 and 139 mm Hg or the diastolic pressure is between 80 and 89 mm Hg

prenatal care The health care a woman receives while pregnant

pre-operative Before surgery

pressure point See "bony prominence"

pressure ulcer A localized injury to the skin and/or underlying tissue, usually over a bony prominence, resulting from pressure or pressure in combination with shear; any lesion caused by unrelieved pressure that results in damage to underlying tissues

primary caregiver The person mainly responsible for providing or assisting with the child's basic needs

primary nursing A nursing care pattern; a registered nurse (RN) is responsible for the person's total care

priority The most important thing at the time

professional boundary That which separates helpful behaviors from behaviors that are not helpful

professionalism Following laws, being ethical, having good work ethics, and having the skills to do your work

professional sexual misconduct An act, behavior, or comment that is sexual in nature

progress note Describes the care given and the person's response and progress

pronation Turning the joint downward

prone position Lying on the abdomen with the head turned to 1 side

prosthesis An artificial replacement for a missing body part

protected health information Identifying information and information about the person's health care that is maintained or sent in any form (paper, electronic, oral)

proximal The part nearest to the center or to the point of attachment

pseudodementia False (pseudo) dementia

psychiatric disorder See "mental health disorder"

psychiatry The field of medicine concerned with mental health disorders

psychosis A state of severe mental impairment

puberty The period when reproductive organs begin to function and secondary sex characteristics appear

pulse The beat of the heart felt at an artery as a wave of blood passes through the artery

pulse deficit The difference between the apical and radial pulse rates

pulse oximetry Measures (metry) the oxygen (oxi) concentration in arterial blood

pulse rate The number of heartbeats or pulses in 1 minute

puncture wound An open wound made by a sharp object

purulent drainage Thick green, yellow, or brown drainage

pyuria Pus (py) in the urine (uria)

Q

quadriplegia Paralysis in the arms, legs, trunk, and pelvic organs (quad means 4; plegia means paralysis); tetraplegia

R

radiating pain Pain felt at the site of tissue damage and in nearby areas

range of motion (ROM) The movement of a joint to the extent possible without causing pain

receptive aphasia Difficulty understanding language; Wernicke's aphasia

reciprocity See "endorsement"

recording The written account of care and observations; charting, documentation

reflex An involuntary movement

reflex incontinence Urine is lost at predictable intervals when the bladder is full

regional anesthesia The loss of sensation, produced by a drug, in a large area

registered nurse (RN) A nurse who has completed a 2-, 3-, or 4-year nursing program and has passed a licensing test

regurgitation The backward flow of stomach contents into the mouth

rehabilitation The process of restoring the person to his or her highest possible level of physical, psychological, social, and economic function

reincarnation The belief that the spirit or soul is reborn in another human body or in another form of life

relaxation To be free from mental and physical stress

religion Spiritual beliefs, needs, and practices

REM sleep The phase of sleep with rapid eye movement

remove easily The manual method, device, material, or equipment used to restrain the person that can be removed intentionally by the person in the same manner it was applied by the staff

reporting The oral account of care and observations

representative A person with the legal right to act on the patient's or resident's behalf when he or she cannot do so for himself or herself

reservoir The environment in which a microbe lives and grows; host

respiration The process of supplying the cells with oxygen and removing carbon dioxide from them; breathing air into (inhalation) and out of (exhalation) the lungs

respiratory arrest When breathing stops; breathing stops but heart action continues for several minutes

respiratory depression Slow, weak respirations at a rate of fewer than 12 per minute

responsibility The duty or obligation to perform some act or function

rest To be calm, at ease, and relaxed with no anxiety or stress

restorative aide A nursing assistant with special training in restorative nursing and rehabilitation skills

restorative nursing care Care that helps persons regain health, strength, and independence

retention catheter See "indwelling catheter"

reverse Trendelenburg's position The head of the bed is raised and the foot of the bed is lowered

rigor mortis The stiffness or rigidity (rigor) of skeletal muscles that occurs after death (mortis)

root A word element containing the basic meaning of the word

rotation Turning the joint

S

sanguineous drainage Bloody (sanguis) drainage

scabies A skin disorder caused by the female mite—a very small spider-like organism

sedation A state of quiet, calmness, or sleep produced by a drug

seizure Violent and sudden contractions or tremors of muscle groups caused by abnormal electrical activity in the brain; convulsion

self-actualization Experiencing one's potential

self-esteem Thinking well of oneself and seeing oneself as useful and having value

self-neglect A person's behaviors and way of living that threaten his or her health, safety, and well-being

semi-Fowler's position The head of the bed is raised 30 degrees; or the head of the bed is raised 30 degrees and the knee portion is raised 15 degrees

semi-prone side position See "Sims' position"

serosanguineous drainage Thin, watery drainage (sero) that is blood-tinged (sanguineous)

serous drainage Clear, watery fluid (serum)

service plan A written plan listing the services needed, how much help is needed, and who provides services

sex Physical activities involving the body and reproductive organs

sexual orientation Sexual arousal or romantic attraction to persons of the other gender (heterosexual), the same gender (homosexual), or both genders (bisexual); the gender (male or female) to which a person is emotionally, romantically, and physically attracted

sexuality The physical, emotional, social, cultural, and spiritual factors that affect a person's feelings and attitudes about his or her sex

shear When layers of the skin rub against each other; when the skin remains in place and underlying tissues move and stretch, tearing underlying capillaries and blood vessels and causing tissue damage

shearing When skin sticks to a surface while muscles slide in the direction the body is moving

shock Results when tissues and organs do not get enough blood

side-lying position See "lateral position"

signs See "objective data"

simple fracture The bone is broken in 1 place

Sims' position A left side-lying position in which the upper leg (right leg) is sharply flexed so it is not on the lower leg (left leg) and the lower arm (left arm) is behind the person; semi-prone side position

skin breakdown Changes or damage to intact skin—normal skin and skin layers

skin tear A break or rip in the outer layers of the skin; the epidermis (top skin layer) separates from the underlying tissues

slander Making false statements through the spoken word, sounds, sign language, or gestures

sleep A state of unconsciousness, reduced voluntary muscle activity, and lowered metabolism

sleep apnea Pauses (*a*) in breathing (*pnea*) that occur during sleep

sleep deprivation The amount and quality of sleep are reduced

sleepwalking When the person leaves the bed and walks about

slough Dead tissue that is shed from the skin; it is usually light colored, soft, and moist; may be stringy at times

spastic Uncontrolled contractions of skeletal muscles

sphygmomanometer A cuff and measuring device used to measure blood pressure (*sphygmo* means *pulse*; *manometer* is *a device for measuring pressure*)

spore A bacterium protected by a hard shell

sputum Mucus from the respiratory system that is expectorated (expelled) through the mouth

standard of care The skills, care, and judgments required by a health team member under similar conditions

stasis ulcer See "venous ulcer"

sterile The absence of *all* microbes

sterile field A work area free of *all* pathogens and non-pathogens (including spores)

sterile technique See "surgical asepsis"

sterilization The process of destroying *all* microbes

stethoscope An instrument used to listen to the sounds produced by the heart, lungs, and other body organs

stoma A surgically created opening seen on the body's surface; see "colostomy" and "ileostomy"

stomatitis Inflammation (*itis*) of the mouth (*stomat*)

stool Excreted feces

straight catheter A catheter that drains the bladder and then is removed

stress The response or change in the body caused by any emotional, physical, social, or economic factor

stress incontinence When urine leaks during exercise and certain movements that cause pressure on the bladder

stressor The event or factor that causes stress

subjective data Things a person tells you about that you cannot observe through your senses; symptoms

suction The process of withdrawing or sucking up fluid (secretions)

sudden cardiac arrest (SCA) The heart stops suddenly and without warning; cardiac arrest

suffix A word element placed after a root; it changes the meaning of the word

suffocation When breathing stops from the lack of oxygen

suicide To kill oneself on purpose

suicide contagion Exposure to suicide or suicidal behaviors within one's family, one's peer group, or media reports of suicide

sundowning Signs, symptoms, and behaviors of Alzheimer's disease increase during hours of darkness

supination Turning the joint upward

supine position The back-lying or dorsal recumbent position

suppository A cone-shaped, solid drug that is inserted into a body opening; it melts at body temperature

surgical asepsis The practices used to remove *all* microbes; sterile technique

surveyor a person who collects information by observing and asking questions

symptoms See "subjective data"

syncope A brief loss of consciousness; fainting

system Organs that work together to perform special functions

systole The period of heart muscle contraction; the heart is pumping blood

systolic pressure The pressure in the arteries when the heart contracts

T

tachycardia A rapid (*tachy*) heart rate (*cardia*); more than 100 beats per minute

tachypnea Rapid (*tachy*) breathing (*pnea*); respirations are more than 20 per minute

tartar Hardened plaque

team nursing A nursing care pattern; a team of nursing staff is led by a registered nurse (RN) who decides the amount and kind of care each person needs

teamwork Staff members work together as a group; each person does his or her part to give safe and effective care

teen dating violence The physical, sexual, psychological, or emotional violence within a dating relationship as well as stalking

terminal illness An illness or injury from which the person will not likely recover

tetraplegia See "quadriplegia" (*tetra* means *4*; *plegia* means *paralysis*)

thermometer A device used to measure (*meter*) temperature (*thermo*)

thrombus A blood clot

tinnitus A ringing, roaring, hissing, or buzzing sound in the ears or head

tissue A group of cells with similar functions

tort A wrong committed against a person or the person's property

tracheostomy A surgically created opening (*stomy*) into the trachea (*tracheo*)

transfer How a person moves to and from surfaces—bed, chair, wheelchair, toilet, or standing position: moving the person to another health care setting; moving the person to a new room

transfer belt A device applied around the waist used to support a person who is unsteady or disabled; gait belt

transgender Describes people who express their sexuality or gender in ways that do not fit with the sex (male, female) assigned at birth; see "transsexual" and "transvestite"

transient incontinence Temporary or occasional incontinence that is reversed when the cause is treated

transsexual Refers to a person whose gender identity is different from the assigned sex at birth; persons who are undergoing hormone therapy or surgery for sexual re-assignment (female to male; male to female)

transvestite A person who dresses and behaves like the other sex for emotional and sexual relief

trauma An accident or violent act that injures the skin, mucous membranes, bones, and organs

treatment The care provided to maintain or restore health, improve function, or relieve symptoms

Trendelenburg's position The head of the bed is lowered and the foot of the bed is raised

tumor A new growth of abnormal cells that is benign or malignant

tuning fork An instrument vibrated to test hearing

U

ulcer A shallow or deep crater-like sore of the skin or mucous membrane

umbilical cord The structure that connects the mother and fetus (unborn baby); it carries blood, oxygen, and nutrients from the mother to the fetus

unavoidable pressure ulcer A pressure ulcer that occurs despite efforts to prevent one through proper use of the nursing process

uncircumcised The male has foreskin covering the head of the penis

unintentional wound A wound resulting from trauma

urge incontinence The loss of urine in response to a sudden, urgent need to void; the person cannot get to a toilet in time; over-active bladder

urgent surgery Surgery needed for the person's health; it can be delayed for a few days

urinary diversion A surgically created pathway for urine to leave the body

urinary frequency Voiding at frequent intervals

urinary incontinence The involuntary loss or leakage of urine

urinary retention The inability to void

urinary urgency The need to void at once

urination The process of emptying urine from the bladder; micturition or voiding

urostomy A surgically created opening (*stomy*) that connects to the urinary tract (*uro*)

V

vaccination Giving a vaccine to produce immunity against an infectious disease

vaccine A preparation containing dead or weakened microbes

vaginal speculum An instrument (*speculum*) used to open the vagina (*vaginal*) to examine it and the cervix

vascular ulcer See "circulatory ulcer"

vector A carrier (animal, insect) that transmits disease

vehicle Any substance that transmits microbes

vein A blood vessel that returns blood to the heart

venous ulcer An open sore on the lower legs or feet caused by poor venous blood flow; stasis ulcer

ventral See "anterior"

verbal communication Communication that uses written or spoken words

vertigo Dizziness

vital signs Temperature, pulse, respirations, and blood pressure; and pain in some agencies

voiding See "urination"

vomitus Food and fluids expelled from the stomach through the mouth; emesis

vulnerable adult A person 18 years old or older who has a disability or condition that makes him or her at risk to be wounded, attacked, or damaged

W

weight-bearing To put weight on one's legs

Wernicke's aphasia See "receptive aphasia"

will A legal document of how a person wants property distributed after death

withdrawal syndrome The physical and mental response after stopping or severely reducing the use of a substance that was used regularly

word element A part of a word

work ethics Behavior in the workplace

workplace violence Violent acts (including assault and threat of assault) directed toward persons at work or while on duty

work-related musculo-skeletal disorder Injuries and disorders of the muscles, tendons, ligaments, joints, and cartilage; they are caused or made worse by the work setting

wound A break in the skin or mucous membrane

Key Abbreviations

AD Alzheimer's disease
ADA American Dental Association
ADA Americans With Disabilities Act of 1990
ADL Activities of daily living
ADU Accessory dwelling unit
AE Anti-embolism; anti-embolic
AED Automated external defibrillator
AHA American Heart Association
AIDS Acquired immunodeficiency syndrome
ALR Assisted living residence
ALS Amyotrophic lateral sclerosis
AMD Age-related macular degeneration
ASL American Sign Language
AUD Alcohol use disorder

BLS Basic Life Support
BM Bowel movement
BP Blood pressure
BPD Borderline personality disorder
BPH Benign prostatic hyperplasia

C Centigrade
CAA Care Area Assessment
CAD Coronary artery disease
CBC Complete blood count
CCRC Continuing care retirement community
CDC Centers for Disease Control and Prevention
CHF Congestive heart failure
CKD Chronic kidney disease
cm Centimeter
CMS Centers for Medicare & Medicaid Services
CNA Certified nursing assistant; certified nurse aide
CNS Central nervous system
CO Carbon monoxide
CO$_2$ Carbon dioxide
COPD Chronic obstructive pulmonary disease
CP Cerebral palsy
CPR Cardiopulmonary resuscitation
C-section Cesarean section
CVA Cerebrovascular accident

DNR Do Not Resuscitate
DON Director of nursing
DS Down syndrome
DUS Doppler ultrasound stethoscope

ECC Emergency Cardiovascular Care
ECG Electrocardiogram
ECHO Elder Cottage Housing Opportunity

ED Erectile dysfunction
EEOC Equal Employment Opportunity Commission
EHR Electronic health record
EKG Electrocardiogram
EMR Electronic medical record
EMS Emergency Medical Services
EPA Environmental Protection Agency
EPHI; ePHI Electronic protected health information
ET Endotracheal
EV-D68 Enterovirus D68

F Fahrenheit
FBAO Foreign-body airway obstruction
FDA Food and Drug Administration
Fragile X Fragile X syndrome
ft Feet

GAD Generalized anxiety disorder
GERD Gastro-esophageal reflux disease
GI Gastro-intestinal
gtt Drops
gtt/min Drops per minute

HAI Healthcare-associated infection
HBV Hepatitis B virus
HCS Hazard Communication Standard
Hg Mercury
HIPAA Health Insurance Portability and Accountability Act of 1996
HIV Human immunodeficiency virus

IBD Inflammatory bowel disease
ID Identification
IDCP Interdisciplinary care planning
IDD Intellectual and developmental disability
in Inch; inches
I&O Intake and output
IPV Intimate partner violence
IQ Intelligence quotient
IV Intravenous

JRA Juvenile rheumatoid arthritis

lb Pound
L/min Liters per minute
LNA Licensed nursing assistant
LPN Licensed practical nurse
LVN Licensed vocational nurse

MDRO Multidrug-resistant organism
MDS Minimum Data Set
MET Medical Emergency Team
mg Milligram
MI Myocardial infarction
mL Milliliter
mL/hr Milliliters per hour
mm Millimeter
mm Hg Millimeters of mercury
MRSA Methicillin-resistant *Staphylococcus aureus*
MS Multiple sclerosis
MSD Musculo-skeletal disorder

NATCEP Nursing assistant training and competency evaluation program
NCSBN National Council of State Boards of Nursing
NG Naso-gastric
NIA National Institute on Aging
NPO *Non per os;* nothing by mouth
NPUAP National Pressure Ulcer Advisory Panel
NREM No rapid eye movement

O$_2$ Oxygen
OASIS Outcome and Assessment Information Set
OBRA Omnibus Budget Reconciliation Act of 1987
OCD Obsessive-compulsive disorder
OPIM Other potentially infectious materials
OR Operating room
OSHA Occupational Safety and Health Administration
OTC Over-the-counter
oz Ounce

PACU Post-anesthesia care unit
PASS *Pull* the safety pin, *aim* low, *squeeze* the lever, *sweep* back and forth
PEG Percutaneous endoscopic gastrostomy
PHI Protected health information
post-op Post-operative
PPE Personal protective equipment
pre-op Pre-operative
PTSD Post-traumatic stress disorder

RA Rheumatoid arthritis
RACE Rescue, alarm, confine, extinguish

RBC Red blood cell
REM Rapid eye movement
RN Registered nurse
RNA Registered nurse aide
ROM Range-of-motion
RRT Rapid Response Team
RT Respiratory therapist

SB Spina bifida
SCA Sudden cardiac arrest
SCD Sequential compression device
SDS Safety data sheet
SIDS Sudden infant death syndrome
SNF Skilled nursing facility
SpO$_2$ Saturation of peripheral oxygen (oxygen concentration)
SRNA State registered nurse aide
SSE Soapsuds enema
STD Sexually transmitted disease
STNA State tested nurse aide
SUID Sudden unexpected infant death

TB Tuberculosis
TBI Traumatic brain injury
TED Thrombo-embolic disease
TIA Transient ischemic attack
TJC The Joint Commission
TPN Total parenteral nutrition
TPR Temperature, pulse, and respirations
TRS Telecommunications Relay Service
TURP Transurethral resection of the prostate

U/A Urinalysis
USDA United States Department of Agriculture
UTI Urinary tract infection

VF; V-fib Ventricular fibrillation
VHF Viral hemorrhagic fever
VRE Vancomycin-resistant *Enterococci*

WBC White blood cell

A

Abandonment
    child, 49
    elder, 46
Abbreviations, 67, 77-80
Abdominal binders, 618, 618*f*
Abdominal regions, 79, 80*f*
Abdominal thrusts, 165, 166*b*, 167*f*
    hand positioning for, 166*b*, 167*f*
    self-administered, 165*b*
Abduction, 513
Ablation, 730
Abrasions, 604, 605*b*, 606*f*
Absence: reporting, 59*b*
Abuse, 44
    alcohol abuse, 757, 762
    child abuse and neglect, 38, 48-49
    definition of, 16, 38, 44
    drug abuse, 757, 763-764
    elder abuse, 38, 46-47, 47*b*-48*b*, 47*f*, 146*b*
    emotional or mental, 46
    financial, 776*b*
    freedom from, 16
    physical, 46, 46*b*
    preventing, 45*b*
    reporting, 44-52, 45*b*, 52*b*-53*b*
    right to freedom from, 16, 673*b*-674*b*
    sexual, 46, 776*b*, 798, 798*b*-799*b*
    substance abuse disorder, 762-764
    verbal, 46
Acceptance (stage of dying), 853
Accessory dwelling units (ADUs), 148
Accidents
    equipment accidents, 169-171
    risk factors for, 156, 156*b*
Accountability, 31, 81*b*
Accreditation standards, 9
Acetone. *See* Ketone
Acoustic nerve, 115, 676*b*
Acquired immunodeficiency syndrome (AIDS),
    700-702, 701*b*. *See also* Human
    immunodeficiency virus (HIV) infection
ACTH. *See* Adrenocorticotropic hormone
Activities directors, 5*t*-6*t*
Activities of daily living (ADLs), 666-667
    basic observations, 85*b*
    Minimum Data Set form, 874*f*
Activity(ies), 17, 513-530
    in assisted living, 827
    and BMs, 425
    communication that promotes, 17*b*
    helping residents with, 18*b*, 18*f*
    meaningful, 17
    at nursing centers, 151*b*
    in older persons, 514*b*
    right to activities that enhance well-being, 17
    in surveys, 18*b*
    teamwork that promotes, 18*b*
    time management for, 18*b*
    ways to promote, 529*b*
Acute illness, 1-2
Acute kidney failure, 753
Acute pain, 531, 533
Acute problems, 666
AD. *See* Alzheimer's disease
Adaptive behaviors, 788*b*
Adaptive devices
    for eating, 449, 450*f*
    grooming aids, 366, 367*f*
    for hygiene, 337*b*, 337*f*
Addiction, 757, 763-764
Addressing the person, 93

Adduction, 513
ADEAR. *See* Alzheimer's Disease Education and
    Referral Center
Adenoids, 118, 735*b*
ADH. *See* Antidiuretic hormone
Admission forms, 307*f*
Admission records, 69
Admissions, 545-546, 546*b*
    admitting the person, 306, 306*b*
    comfort measures, 546*b*
    definition of, 545
    guidelines for, 547*b*
    in long-term care, 546*b*, 547
    procedure for, 306-316
    safety measures, 546*b*
Adolescence, 126, 128*b*, 135-136, 135*f*
Adrenal cortex, 123
Adrenal glands, 123
Adrenal medulla, 123
Adrenocorticotropic hormone (ACTH), 122
Adult care facilities, 149
Adult day care, 146*b*, 148, 148*f*
Adult foster care, 149
Adulthood
    late, 128*b*, 137
    middle, 128*b*, 137, 137*f*-138*f*
    young, 128*b*, 136-137, 137*f*
ADUs. *See* Accessory dwelling units
Advance directives, 69, 851, 855-856, 856*b*
AE (anti-embolism or anti-embolic) stockings, 598
AEDs. *See* Automated external defibrillators
Affection, 796, 797*f*
African-Americans, 100*b*
Afternoon care, 338*b*
Age
    accident risk factors, 156, 156*b*
    and attitudes about death, 853
    and blood pressure, 506*b*
    and food practices, 449
    and hip fractures, 719
    and sleep, 540
Age spots, 144
Age-related macular degeneration, 684
Aggression, 104, 776, 778*b*-780*b*
    accident risk factors, 156
    safety measures for, 179*b*
    sexual, 797-798, 798*b*
Aging, 141*b*
    and arthritis, 713
    and BMs, 425
    coping with, 140
    myths about, 141*b*
    nervous system changes of, 770*b*
    normal changes of, 772*b*
    and oxygen needs, 643
    physical changes of, 142-147, 143*b*, 450*b*
Agitation, 776, 778*b*-780*b*
    accident risk factors, 156
    safety measures for, 179*b*
Agoraphobia, 759
AIDS. *See* Acquired immunodeficiency syndrome
AIIRs. *See* Airborne infection isolation rooms
Air flotation beds, 628, 629*f*
Airborne infection isolation rooms (AIIRs), 230*b*
Airborne precautions, 230*b*
Airway obstruction
    foreign-body (FBAO), 163
    head tilt–chin lift method to open, 833, 833*f*
    mild, 163
    severe, 163
Airways
    artificial, 658-660, 659*b*, 659*f*
    suctioning, 660-661, 661*f*
Alarms and call lights, 188*b*-189*b*
    bed and chair alarms, 190, 190*f*
    call lights, 313, 313*f*-314*f*

Alarms and call lights *(Continued)*
    call systems, 313-315, 314*b*, 314*f*
    in home care, 314*b*, 314*f*
    IV pump alarms, 484*b*
    safety measures for, 315
    smoke alarms, 158*b*
Alcohol, 57
    and blood pressure, 506*b*
    and cancer, 697
    liver damage from, 744*f*
    and oxygen needs, 643
Alcohol abuse, 757, 762
    in children, 763*b*
    and hip fractures, 719
    in older persons, 763*b*
    problems linked to, 762
    signs and symptoms of, 763*b*
    under-age drinking, 763*b*
Alcohol treatment, 671
Alcohol use disorder, 762
Alcohol-based hand rub, 225*b*, 226*f*
Alcoholism, 757, 762
    in children, 763*b*
    in older persons, 763*b*
    problems linked to, 762
Alert, oriented persons, 97*b*
Algophobia, 759
Alimentary canal (GI tract), 119, 443*b*, 740*b*
Allergies, 642-643
Alopecia, 366, 368
ALRs. *See* Assisted living residences
ALS. *See* Amyotrophic lateral sclerosis
Alternative medicine, 698
Alveoli, 118, 504*b*, 643*b*, 731*b*
Alzheimer's Association, 773, 775, 778*b*-780*b*, 782
Alzheimer's disease, 771-778, 771*f*
    behaviors and changes in function in, 774-778,
        774*b*
    care of persons with, 778-783, 778*b*-780*b*, 782*b*
    communication changes in, 776-777
    communication with persons with, 776*b*-777*b*
    family of persons with, 782
    long-term care for persons with, 782*b*
    safety measures for persons with, 774*b*
    signs of, 772, 772*b*
    stages of, 773, 773*b*, 773*f*
    warning signs, 772*b*
Alzheimer's Disease Education and Referral Center
    (ADEAR), 97*b*, 464*b*
AM care. *See* Early morning care
Ambu bags, 661, 661*f*
Ambulation, 513, 522-528
    assisting with, 524*b*-525*b*, 525*f*
    early after surgery, 590, 601
Ambulatory (out-patient) care, 2
American Dental Association (ADA), 339, 339*b*
American Heart Association (AHA), 830, 832, 835,
    838
American Hospital Association (AHA), 13*b*
American Indians, 101*b*
American Nurses Association (ANA), 39
American Sign Language (ASL), 678, 679*f*
Americans with Disabilities Act of 1990, 680, 691*b*
Amputation, 705, 721, 722*f*
Amputee rehabilitation, 671
Amputee slings, 296
Amyotrophic lateral sclerosis, 709
Anal sphincter, 112
Anaphylactic shock, 845
Anaphylaxis, 829, 845
Anatomy, 108
Anesthesia, 588, 595
    general, 588, 595
    local, 588, 595
    regional, 588, 595
Anesthesiologists, 595

Page numbers followed by *b*, *t*, and *f* indicate boxes,
tables, and figures, respectively.

895

Anesthetists, 595
Anger, 104, 105b
  A Dying Patient's Bill of Last Rights, 859b
  stage of dying, 853
Angina, 728, 728f
Ankle exercises, 519b-520b, 522f
Ankle restraints, 205b-206b
Ankle-foot orthoses, 528, 528f
Anorexia, 442, 449
Anorexia nervosa, 764, 765f
Answering phones, 77b
Antibiotics, 217-218
Antibodies, 123, 699b
Anticoagulants, 366, 374
Antidiuretic hormone (ADH), 123
Anti-embolism or anti-embolic (AE) stockings, 598
Antigens, 123, 699b
Antisepsis, 217
Antisocial personality disorder, 762
Anus, 119, 443b, 740b
Anxiety, 757-758, 766b
  and pain, 533
  signs and symptoms of, 758b
Anxiety disorders, 758-760
Aorta, 116, 497b
Aphasia, 670, 675, 682
  expressive, 675, 682
  global, 675, 682
  receptive, 675, 682
Apical pulse
  location of, 501, 501f
  taking, 501, 502b
Apical-radial pulse, 486, 501, 502b-503b, 502f
Apnea, 642, 644, 724, 732-733
Appearance, 56-57, 57b, 58f
Appetite, 85b, 449
Apraxia, 681
Aquaphobia, 759
Aquathermia pads, 636, 636f, 638b
Aqueous chamber, 115, 682b
Aqueous humor, 115, 682b
Arabic culture, 102b
Arachnoid, 114
Arachnoid space, 114
Arc of the United States, the, 788, 792b
Armrests, elevated, 259, 259f
Arrhythmias. See Dysrhythmias
Arterial system, 497f, 726f
Arterial ulcers, 604, 609, 609f
Arteries, 108, 116, 117f, 497b, 725b-726b
Arterioles, 116, 725b-726b
Arthritis, 705, 712-713, 714b
Arthroplasty, 705, 713
Artificial airways, 658-660, 659b, 659f
Ascites, 744, 744f
Ascorbic acid (vitamin C), 447t
Asepsis, 217, 221, 226, 227b-228b, 228f
  common practices, 222, 222b
  home care practices, 222b
  medical, 217, 221-226
  surgical, 217, 221, 244
Ashtray safety, 174b
Asians, 101b-102b
ASL. See American Sign Language
Aspiration, 335, 342, 442, 473-474
  prevention of, 342, 454b, 477, 477b
Assault(s), 38, 43, 49, 178
Assessment, 83-84
  for delegation, 33
  in home care, 86b
  in long-term care, 86b
Assignment sheets, 89, 89b, 89f
Assisted living, 822-828
  home care, 824b
  living areas, 823, 823f, 824b
  resident rights, 823, 823b
  safety measures, 822b, 827
  services, 823, 824b, 827
Assisted living residences (ALRs), 1, 3, 149, 822,
    823f, 824b
Assisted living units, 824b
Assisted-living residents, 823, 823b
Assistive devices
  for arthritis, 713
  for eating, 449, 450f, 667, 668f

Assistive devices (Continued)
  hearing aids, 678-680, 680f
  hearing devices, 680
  moving the person up in bed with, 269
  self-help devices, 668f
Asthma, 732
Asthma attacks, 732
Atelectasis, 642, 648
Atherosclerosis, 727, 727f
Athlete's foot, 609b-610b, 610f
Atria, 116, 725b-726b
Atrophy, 140, 144, 513-514
Attendance, 58, 59b
Attention, 533
Attitude, 59, 852-853
AUD. See Alcohol use disorder
Audiologists, 5t-6t
Auditory canal, 115
Auricle, 115
Austria, 443b
Autism, 789-790, 789b
Autoclaves, 226, 227f
Autoimmune disorders, 699-700, 700f
Automated external defibrillators (AEDs), 835, 836f
  adult CPR, 837b, 838f
  child CPR, 836b, 842b
  infant CPR, 843b
Autonomic hyperreflexia, 712, 712b
Autonomic nervous system, 114, 706b
Autopsy, 851, 856
Axillary temperature, 488b, 488t, 492b, 493f

B
B cells (B lymphocytes), 123, 699b
Baby bathtubs, 880
Baby bottle tooth decay, 338f, 339b
Baby bottles
  cleaning, 807, 807b-808b, 808f
  preparing, 807, 807f
  warming, 808
Baby gates, 880
Back injuries, 254, 254b
Back massages, 537, 537b-538b, 538f
Backrests, 303, 309f
Backyard safety measures, 878
Bacteria, 218
Bag baths, 353
Bag valve masks, 834, 835f
Bagging items, 238, 239b, 239f
Balance scales, 307b, 308f, 309, 316
Ball-and-socket joints, 111, 111f, 251b, 251f, 713b,
    713f
Balloon safety, 164b
Bandages, elastic, 600
Barber shops, 367b
Bargaining, 853
Bariatric bedpans, 391, 391f
Bariatric beds, 310, 311b, 311f
Bariatric care, 96
  bathing, 349b
  falling persons, 196b
  moving the person up in bed with an assist device,
    269b
  personal hygiene, 349
Bariatric ceiling lifts, 295, 295f
Bariatric slings, 296
Bariatric stretchers, 293
Bariatrics, 92, 96
Bariatric-safe equipment, 169
Barrel chest, 732, 732f
Barrier device breathing, 834, 834f
Barriers, 188b-189b, 189f
Base of support, 250
Basic Life Support (BLS), 829-841
Basic needs, 239-240, 240b, 619
Bassinets, 882
Bat gio ("catch wind"), 94b
Bathing, 346-355, 363b-364b
  bag baths, 353
  comfort measures, 349b
  complete bed baths, 350, 350b-351b, 352f
  delegation guidelines for, 348b
  Minimum Data Set, 875f
  observations to report and record, 363b
  partial baths, 353, 353b-354b

Bathing (Continued)
  pre-operative, 591
  rules for, 347b
  safety measures, 349b, 354b
  shower safety, 354b
  showers, 354-355
  Sitz baths, 635
  towel baths, 353, 353b
  tub baths and showers, 354-355, 354b, 355f,
    356b-357b
Bathing bariatric persons, 349b
Bathing children, 348b
Bathing infants, 814
  guidelines for, 814b
  home care, 814b
  safety and comfort measures, 815b, 815f
  sponge baths, 814, 815b-816b, 816f
  tub baths, 814, 814f, 817b, 817f
Bathing older persons, 348b, 353b
Bathing slings, 296
Bathrooms
  home safety measures, 877
  options for older persons, 147b
  in person's room, 315, 315f
  safety measures to prevent falls, 188b-189b
Bathtubs for babies, 880
Battery, 38, 43
Beard care, 376
Beauty shops, 367b, 367f
Bed(s), 306-310, 307f
  bariatric, 310
  closed, 319, 320f, 324, 324b-325b, 325f-326f
  comfort measures, 307b, 324b
  electric, 306, 307f
  home care, 307b
  hospital bed systems, 303, 309
  making, 322-331, 323b-324b
  manually operated, 306, 307f
  occupied, 319, 320f, 324b, 328, 328b-330b, 331f
  open, 319, 320f, 328, 328b
  post-operative, 331
  recovery, 331
  safety measures, 188b-189b, 307b
  special beds, 628, 629f
  surgical, 319, 320f, 331, 331b-332b, 332f
  transferring persons from bed to chair or
    wheelchair, 287, 287b-288b, 289f
  types of, 319
Bed and chair alarms, 190, 190f
Bed angles, 257b, 257f
Bed baths, complete, 350, 350b-351b, 352f
Bed cradles, 515, 516f, 628
Bed linens, 320-322, 320f
Bed mobility, 262, 263b
Bed positions, 308, 309b
Bed protectors, 322f
Bed rail covers, 205b-206b, 208f
Bed rails, 186, 190-191, 191f
  for children, 191b
  in home care, 192b
  in long-term care, 192b
  safety and comfort measures, 192b
Bed safety, 309, 309b
Bed wheel locks, 192, 193f
Bed-boards, 515, 515f
Bedfast persons, 621, 624
Bedpans, 391
  bariatric, 391, 391f
  fracture, 391, 391f
  guidelines for, 391b
  procedure for giving, 392b, 393f
  recommended practices, 405b
  safety measures for, 391b
  standard, 391, 391f
Bedrest, 514-517, 515b
Bedrooms, 147b, 878
Bedside stands, 312, 312f
Behavioral health treatment, 671
Behavioral problems, 104, 105b-106b, 760, 789
Beliefs, health care, 94b
Belonging, 94, 539
Belt restraints, 205b-206b, 206f, 211, 211f, 212b-214b
Belted under-garments, 399, 399f
Belts. See Transfer belts
Benign prostatic hyperplasia, 750-751

Benign tumors, 693, 694f
Bicuspid valve (mitral valve), 116
Bile, 119, 443b, 740b
Bilevel positive airway pressure (BiPAP), 733
Binders and compression garments, 618, 618b
Binge eating disorder, 764
BIOHAZARD symbol, 238, 238f
Biohazardous waste, 217, 238
Biological therapy, 698
Biot's respirations, 642, 644
BiPAP. *See* Bilevel positive airway pressure
Bipolar disorder, 761, 761b
Birth defects, 786
Bisexual, 794, 796
Bladder, 85b, 120, 389b, 750b
    over-active. *See* Urge incontinence
Bladder cancer, 695b-696b
Bladder re-training, 404
Bladder training, 404
Bleeding
    basic observations, 85b
    external, 844
    internal, 844
    ways to control, 844, 844f
Blindness, 675, 682, 685-688, 686b-687b, 687f
Blisters, 609b-610b, 610f
Blood, 115-116, 241b, 725b-726b
    occult, 577, 578b-579b, 579f
    testing for, 574
Blood clots, 597, 597f
Blood flow, 117
Blood glucose testing, 582, 582b, 582f
    guidelines for, 582b
    procedure, 584b-585b, 585f-586f
    rules for, 583b
    safety and comfort measures, 583b
    sites for skin punctures, 582, 582f-583f, 583b
Blood pressure (BP), 486, 506-508, 506b
    in children, 507b
    communication about, 507b
    high. *See* Hypertension
    measuring, 508, 508b-510b, 510f-511f
    normal ranges, 506, 511b
    in older persons, 507b
Blood pressure equipment, 507, 507f, 508b
Blood vessels, 115-117, 497b, 725b-726b
Blood volume, 506b
Bloodborne Pathogen Standard, 240-243, 241b
Bloodborne pathogens, 241b
BLS. *See* Basic Life Support
Board and care homes (group homes), 149
Body alignment, 250, 252f
Body language, 92, 100
Body mechanics, 56, 250, 252f-253f, 253, 253b
Body structure and function, 108-125
    caring for yourself, 124b
    circulatory system, 115-117, 725b-726b
    digestive system, 443b, 740b, 740f
    ear, 676b, 676f
    endocrine system, 122-123, 745b, 745f
    eye, 682b, 682f
    female reproductive system, 795f
    gastro-intestinal tract, 423b
    heart and blood vessels, 497b
    immune system, 699b
    integumentary system, 702b, 702f
    lymphatic system, 735b, 735f
    male reproductive system, 795b, 795f
    musculo-skeletal system, 713b
    nervous system, 706b
    organization of the body, 108-109, 109f
    reproductive system, 795b
    respiratory system, 504b, 643b, 643f, 731b
    teeth, gums, and skin, 336b, 336f
    urinary system, 389b, 750b, 750f
Body temperature, 486, 488-494, 488b, 488t,
        491b-492b, 493f-494f, 494b-496b, 511b
Bomb threats, 173
Bones, 110-111, 111f, 251b, 713b
    flat, 110, 251b, 713b
    irregular, 110, 251b, 713b
    long, 110, 251b, 713b
    short, 110, 251b, 713b
Bony political regulations, 621
Bony prominences, 621, 622f

Borderline personality disorder, 762
Bottle-fed babies, 810
Bottle-feeding babies, 807-808, 808f-809f, 809b
Bottles, baby
    cleaning, 807, 807b-808b, 808f
    preparing, 807, 807f
    warming, 808
Boundaries, 38-40, 40b-41b, 40f, 52b-53b
Boundary crossings, 38, 40
Boundary signs, 38, 40, 41b
Boundary violations, 38, 40
Bowel elimination, 422-441, 426b
    in children, 424b
    comfort and privacy measures, 440b
    communication during, 426b
    factors affecting BMs, 425-426, 425b
    guidelines for, 423b
    normal, 423-424, 424b
    observations of, 85b, 424, 424b
    pre-operative, 590
    safety and comfort measures, 423b, 426, 426b
Bowel elimination records, 424b, 425f
Bowel training, 430
Bowman's capsule, 120
BPH. *See* Benign prostatic hyperplasia
Braces, 528, 528f
Braden Scale for Predicting Pressure Sore Risk, 630f,
        631
Bradycardia, 486, 498
Bradypnea, 642, 644
Braille, 675, 688, 688f
Brain, 114, 114f, 706b, 706f
Brain attack. *See* Stroke
Brain death, 710, 710f
Brain injury rehabilitation, 671
Brain tumors, 695b-696b
Brainstem, 114, 706b
Brazil: meal time practices, 443b
Breaks, 61
Breast binders, 618, 618f
Breast cancer, 695b-696b
Breast-fed babies, 810
Breast-feeding, 800, 805, 805b-806b, 806f
Breasts (mammary glands), 122, 122f
Breathing. *See also* Respiration(s)
    adult CPR, 833-835
    barrier device, 834, 834f
    deep, 648
    at end of life, 854
    infant or child CPR, 833b
    mouth-to-mouth, 834, 834f
    mouth-to-mouth-and-nose, 839b-840b, 841f
    mouth-to-nose, 835, 835f
    mouth-to-stoma, 835, 835f
    rescue breathing, 831
British Sign Language, 678
Broca's aphasia. *See* Expressive aphasia
Bronchioles, 118, 504b, 643b, 731b
Bronchitis, chronic, 732
Brujos (brujas), 94b
Brushing and combing hair, 369
    for children, 369b
    guidelines for, 369b
    procedure for, 370b, 370f
    safety and comfort measures, 369b
Brushing and flossing teeth, 340, 340b, 342f
Bubbling, 809
Building safety and security, 179b
Bulimia nervosa, 764
Bullying, 55, 64
Bunions, 609b-610b, 610f
Burnout, 55, 63, 63b
Burns, 848
    causes of, 848
    emergency care for, 848
    full-thickness (third degree), 159, 159t, 848,
        848f
    infection in, 220
    in older persons, 159b
    partial-thickness (second degree), 159, 848
    preventing, 158b-159b, 159
    severity of, 159
    superficial (first degree), 159, 848
Burping babies, 809, 810f
Butterfly rash, 700f

C
CAAs. *See* Care Area Assessments
Calcium, 448t
Calculi, renal, 752
Calendars, 770b, 770f
Call systems, 313-315, 314b
    call lights, 313, 313f-314f
    call lights and alarms, 188b-189b
    in home care, 314b, 314f
    safety measures for, 315
Calluses, 609b-610b
Calorie counts, 454
Calorie-controlled diet, 451t-452t
Calories, 442, 444
    calorie-controlled diet, 451t-452t
    high-calorie diet, 451t-452t
Cancer, 693-699, 695b-696b, 699b. *See also* Malignant
        tumors
Candles, 174b
Canes, 522-523, 522f-523f, 688
Cao gio ("rub wind"), 94b
Capillaries, 108, 116, 725b-726b
Car safety, 180b-181b
Car safety seats (car seats), 802b, 802f-803f, 879, 882
Carbohydrates, 447
Carbon monoxide poisoning, 161, 163b
Cardiac arrest
    in children and infants, 839
    sudden cardiac arrest (SCA), 829-831
Cardiac muscle, 112, 251b
Cardiac rehabilitation, 671, 728
Cardiopulmonary resuscitation (CPR), 166b
    adult, 831-838, 832b, 836f, 837b, 838f
    child CPR, 833b, 838b-840b, 839, 840f, 842b
    communication in, 836b
    hand position for, 832, 833f
    hands-only, 838, 838b
    infant CPR, 833b, 839-841, 839b-840b, 840f, 843b
Cardiovascular disorders, 725-731, 726b-727b
Cardiovascular system, 115
Cardioversion, 730
Care Area Assessments (CAAs), 88b, 876f
Care conferences, 88, 88b
Care equipment. *See* Equipment
Care summaries, 72f
Caregivers
    children as, 142
    family, 783b
    for older persons, 146b
    primary, 126, 138b
Caring for the person, 92-93
Carotid pulse, 832, 832f
Carriers, 217, 219, 879
Carrying persons, 177f-178f
Cartilage, 111
Case management, 1, 8, 146b
Cast care, 718b, 718f
Casts, 717, 717f
Cataracts, 683, 683f
Catastrophic reactions, 776, 778b-780b
Catering, 24-hour, 470b
Catheter care, 408, 409b-411b, 409f, 420b
Catheterization, 407
Catheters
    clamping, 404, 405f
    cleaning, 411b, 412f
    condom, 407, 418, 418b-419b, 418f, 420f
    definition of, 407
    indwelling, 407-408, 408f, 416-418, 416b-418b,
        416f-417f
    purposes of, 408
    securing, 409b, 410f
    straight, 407-408
    types of, 408
    urinary, 407-421
CCRCs. *See* Continuing care retirement communities
Celiac disease, 699
Cell membrane, 108
Cells, 108-109, 109f
Centers for Disease Control and Prevention (CDC)
    definition of intimate partner violence (IPV), 51
    recommendations for flu vaccine, 733
    recommendations for HIV testing, 702b
    recommendations to prevent lead poisoning,
        161b

Centers for Medicare and Medicaid Services (CMS), 12
  definition of bed mobility, 262
  definition of fall, 186*b*
  definition of pressure ulcer, 622
  environment requirements, 150, 150*b*
  requirements for assessment of nutritional status, 443*b*
  requirements for comprehensive care plans, 88*b*
  requirements for disaster plans, 176
  requirements for preventing abuse, 45*b*
  requirements for reporting deaths, 203
  requirements for resident care conferences, 88*b*
  requirements for resident rooms, 304*b*
  requirements for staff training in emergency procedures, 173*b*
  rules for using restraints, 200
Central lines, 480
Central nervous system (CNS), 113-114, 113*f*, 706*b*, 706*f*
Central venous catheter, 480
Central venous sites, 480
Cerebellum, 114, 706*b*
Cerebral cortex, 114
Cerebral palsy, 790
Cerebrospinal fluid, 114, 706*b*
Cerebrovascular accident (CVA). *See* Stroke
Cerebrum, 114, 706*b*
Certification, 9, 21, 23, 24*b*
Cerumen, 115, 675, 676*b*
Cervical cancer, 695*b*-696*b*
Cervical injuries, 711
Cervical traction, 719, 719*f*
Cesarean section (C-section), 819
Chains of Survival, 831, 831*b*
Chair alarms, 190, 190*f*
Chair position, 259
Chairfast persons, 621, 624
Chairs
  high, 880
  hook-on, 880
  in person's unit, 303*f*, 312
  re-positioning the person in, 279
  transfer to bed from, 290, 290*b*, 291*f*
Changing tables, 880
Charting, 191. *See also* Medical records; Recording
  rules for, 75*b*
  samples, 75*f*-76*f*, 191*f*, 209*f*, 277*f*, 511*f*, 526*f*, 631*f*, 650*f*
Check times, 316*b*-317*b*
Chemical restraints, 200, 203
Chemicals, hazardous, 154, 171-172
Chemotherapy
  for cancer, 697-698
  infection in patients on, 220
  safety measures for, 698*b*
Chest compressions, 832, 832*f*-833*f*
  2-thumb-encircling hands method, 839*b*-840*b*, 840*f*
  for children and infants, 839*b*-840*b*, 840*f*
  hand position, 832, 833*f*, 839*b*-840*b*, 840*f*
  recommendations for, 832
Chest pain, 644*b*
Chest thrusts, 165, 165*b*, 165*f*, 168*b*, 168*f*
Chest tubes, 663, 663*f*-664*f*, 664*b*
Chewing problems, 449
Cheyne-Stokes respirations, 642, 644
Child abuse and neglect, 38, 48-49, 50*b*
Child car seats, 882
Child pornography, 49
Child prostitution, 49
Child safety seats, 882
Childcare, 58
Childhelp National Child Abuse Hotline, 52*b*-53*b*
Children, 96, 96*f*, 138*b*, 838
  3-year-old, 132, 132*f*-133*f*
  4-year-old, 132-133, 133*f*
  5-year-old, 133, 133*f*
  9 or 10 to 12 years, 134-135, 134*f*
  accident risk factors, 156*b*
  alcoholism and alcohol abuse in, 763*b*
  applying dressings to, 616*b*
  applying restraints to, 212*b*
  arthritis in, 714*b*
  attitudes about death, 853*b*
  Basic Life Support (BLS) for, 838-841

Children *(Continued)*
  bathing, 348*b*
  bed rails for, 191*b*
  bed safety for, 309*b*
  blankets for, 640*b*
  blood pressure, 507*b*
  blood pressure equipment for, 508*b*
  bowel elimination, 424*b*
  bowel movements (BMs), 425*b*
  brushing and combing hair for, 369*b*
  cancer in, 696*b*
  cardiac arrest in, 839
  cardiovascular disorders in, 726*b*
  as caregivers, 142
  caring for mothers and babies, 800
  cleansing enemas for, 432*b*
  clothing for, 802*b*, 803*f*
  collecting sputum specimens from, 580*b*
  collecting stool specimens from, 577*b*
  collecting urine specimens from, 573, 573*b*-574*b*
  comfort measures for, 536*b*
  concussions in, 847*b*
  counting respirations in, 505*b*
  CPR for, 833*b*, 838*b*-840*b*, 839-841, 840*f*, 842*b*
  death of, 142
  deep-breathing exercises for, 648*b*, 648*f*
  defibrillation in, 836*b*
  developmental tasks, 128*b*
  diabetes in, 746*b*
  diarrhea in, 429*b*
  drug abuse and addiction in, 764*b*
  enema solutions for, 432*b*
  fecal incontinence in, 430*b*
  flossing in, 339*b*
  fluid requirements, 456*b*
  fractures in, 717*b*
  hearing checklist for, 678*b*-679*b*
  hearing loss in, 678*b*
  heat and cold applications for, 634*b*
  helping children eat vegetables and fruits, 445*b*
  hepatitis A in, 743*b*
  home safety measures, 802*b*, 877-879
  infection control with, 240*b*
  IV sites, 480*b*, 480*f*
  lead poisoning in, 162*b*
  oral hygiene for, 339*b*
  ostomy pouches for, 438*b*
  otitis media in, 676*b*
  oxygen therapy for, 654*b*
  pain in, 534*b*
  physical examination of, 565*b*
  physical examination preparation, 562*b*
  pneumonia in, 734*b*
  pre-operative care for, 590*b*
  preschool, 128*b*, 132-133, 132*f*
  pressure ulcers in, 624*b*
  preventing burns with, 158*b*
  preventing poisoning with, 160*b*
  preventing suffocating with, 164*b*
  pulse oximetry for, 645*b*
  pulse sites in, 498*b*
  range-of-motion exercises for, 518*b*
  recommendations for physical activity, 445*b*
  rehabilitation for, 667*b*
  relieving choking in, 166*b*
  safety measures for, 802*b*, 802*f*, 879
  school-age, 128*b*, 133-134, 134*f*
  shampooing, 371*b*
  suctioning for, 662*b*
  suicide in, 766*b*
  temperature sites, 488*b*
  touch with, 100*b*
  tracheostomy care for, 660*b*, 660*f*
  transport to the operating room, 595*b*
  traumatic brain injury in, 711*b*
  urinary incontinence in, 398*b*
  urination in, 390*b*
  vital signs in, 487*b*
China
  death rites, 852*b*
  family roles in sick care, 104*b*
  food practices, 448*b*
  pain reactions, 534*b*
  touch practices, 100*b*
Chlamydia, 755*t*

Choice, right to, 15
Choking, 163-165, 165*b*-166*b*, 165*f*, 168*b*, 844
Cholesterol, 442, 446
Choroid, 114, 682*b*
Chromosomes, 109
Chronic bronchitis, 732
Chronic illness, 1-2
Chronic kidney disease, 753, 753*b*, 756*b*
Chronic obstructive pulmonary disease, 732
Chronic pain, 531, 533
Chronic problems, 666
Chronic wounds, 604, 605*b*
Church of Jesus Christ of Latter-Day Saints (Mormons), 450*b*
Chyme, 119, 423*b*, 443*b*, 740*b*
Cigarette smoking, 56, 174*b*
  and blood pressure, 506*b*
  and cancer, 697
  and hip fractures, 719
  and oxygen needs, 643
  preventing burns, 158*b*
Ciliary muscle, 114, 682*b*
Circadian rhythms, 531, 539
Circulatory system, 115-117
  changes in aging, 143*b*, 145
  functions of, 115
  oxygen needs, 643
  preventing post-operative complications, 597-601, 597*f*
  structure and function of, 725*b*-726*b*
Circulatory ulcers, 604, 608-609, 608*b*
Circumcision, 335, 358, 358*f*, 800, 813
Circumcision care, 813, 814*f*
Cirrhosis, 744, 744*f*, 745*b*
Civil laws, 38, 41
Clarifying, 101
Claustrophobia, 759
Clean technique. *See* Medical asepsis
Clean wounds, 604, 605*b*
Clean-contaminated wounds, 604, 605*b*
Cleaning, 226, 468, 469*b*
Cleaning baby bottles, 807, 807*b*-808*b*, 808*f*
Cleaning dentures, 345*b*-346*b*
Cleanliness, 13*b*
Cleansing enemas, 431*b*-434*b*, 432, 433*f*
Clerics, 5*t*-6*t*
Clinical laboratory technicians, 5*t*-6*t*
Clinical nurse specialists, 5*t*-6*t*, 7
Clinical records. *See* Medical records
Clitoris, 121
Closed beds, 319, 320*f*, 324, 324*b*-325*b*
Closed fractures, 705, 716, 716*f*
Closed head injuries, 709
Closed wounds, 604
Closets, 315, 315*b*, 315*f*, 672*b*-673*b*
Clostridium difficile (*C. difficile*) infection, 429*b*
Cloth diapers, 810
Clothes dryers, 174*b*
Clothing
  changing a person's garments, 379-384
  children's, 802*b*, 803*f*, 878
  dressing and undressing, 379
  for job interviews, 865*b*, 866*f*
  personal choice in, 15, 15*f*
  safety measures for, 188*b*-189*b*, 878
  simple choices for, 778*b*-780*b*, 781*f*
CMS. *See* Centers for Medicare and Medicaid Services
Cochlea, 115, 676*b*
Code of conduct, 39*b*
Codes of ethics, 38-39
Cognitive function, 769
Cognitive impairment, 760
  and food practices, 449
  mild, 771
  after TBI, 710
Cold applications, 619, 634, 636-637, 640*b*
  applying, 637, 637*b*-639*b*
  for arthritis, 713
  comfort measures, 640*b*
  complications of, 636
  guidelines for, 638*b*
  in home care, 637*b*
  moist and dry, 637
  safety measures, 638*b*, 640*b*

Cold packs, 638b
Cold versus flu, 733t
Colitis, ulcerative, 742
Collecting random urine specimens, 569b, 569f
Collecting specimens, 239, 567-587, 567b-568b
Collecting tubules, 120
Colon. See Large intestine
Colonization, 621, 631
Color charts
    for stool, 424f
    for urine, 390, 390f
Color-coded wristbands, 182, 182f
Colorectal cancer, 695b-696b
Colostomy, 422, 436-437
Colostomy sites, 436-437, 437f
Coma, 154, 156, 710
Comatose persons, 103
Combat injuries, 710
Combing hair, 369, 369b-370b, 370f
Comfort, 531-532
Comfort measures, 536b, 543b
    for admissions, transfers, and discharges, 546b
    attitude, 386b
    back massages, 537b
    for bathing, 349b
    for bathing infants, 815b
    in bed, 307b
    with bed rails, 192b
    for bed-to-chair or wheelchair transfers, 287b
    with bedpans, 391b
    for blood glucose testing, 583b
    for blood pressure equipment, 508b
    for bowel elimination, 426, 426b
    for brushing and combing hair, 369b
    for catheter care, 410b
    for changing patient gowns, 384b
    for children, 536b
    for collecting sputum specimens, 580b
    for collecting urine specimens, 568b
    with commodes, 395b
    communication, 304b, 532b, 854b
    with condom catheters, 418b
    for dangling, 277b
    for denture care, 344b
    for dressings, 616b
    with elastic bandages, 600b
    with elastic stockings, 598b
    in emergency care, 830b
    in end-of-life care, 854-855, 854b
    for enteral nutrition, 477
    for feeding the person, 464b
    for giving enemas, 432b
    with gloves, 233b
    with hand hygiene, 223b
    for heat and cold applications, 638b
    for helping the person walk, 524b
    with ID bracelets, 157b
    with incontinence products, 400b
    for logrolling, 275b
    in long-term care, 532b
    for lymphedema, 736b
    for making occupied beds, 324b
    for measuring intake and output, 459b
    for measuring weight, 309b
    for mechanical lifts, 297b
    in mouth care for unconscious persons, 343b
    for moving the person, 263b
    for moving the person to the side of the bed, 271b
    for nail and foot care, 377b
    nursing measures, 536
    for occupied beds, 328b
    for older persons, 854b
    oral hygiene measures, 339b
    with ostomy pouches, 438b
    in perineal care, 359b
    in person's unit, 304-306
    for persons with AD and other dementias, 778b-780b, 781f
    for persons with feeding tubes, 477, 477f
    positioning the person, 256b
    in post-operative care, 602
    in preparing for meals, 460b
    in preparing the person for physical examination, 563b

Comfort measures (Continued)
    in preventing respiratory and circulatory complications, 597b
    for pulse oximetry, 646b
    for radiation therapy, 697b
    for range-of-motion exercises, 518b
    with restraints, 212b
    for serving meals, 462b
    for shampooing, 372b
    for shaving, 375b
    for stand and pivot transfers, 286b
    for sterile gloving, 245b
    for stethoscopes, 500b, 500f
    with stool specimens, 577b
    for taking temperatures, 491b
    with transfer belts, 194b
    for transferring persons, 282b
    for tub baths and showers, 356b
    for turning persons, 273b
    with urinals, 394b
    with urinary diversions, 752b
    with urine drainage systems, 413b
    wound care, 619b
Commercial hot and cold packs, 638b
Commodes, 395, 395b-396b, 395f
Communicable disease, 217, 228
Communication(s), 5b, 67-68, 100-101, 670b
    for activities, 17b
    addressing the person, 93
    in adult CPR, 836b
    aids for, 98, 98f-99f
    answering phones, 77b
    before applying tape, 615b
    with artificial airways, 659b
    asking for help, 783b
    assignment sheets for, 89b
    for assisting with the exam, 565b
    about bariatric beds, 311b
    barriers to, 102, 102b
    behavior issues, 105b
    with binders and compression garments, 618b
    with blind and visually impaired persons, 686b-687b
    about blood pressure, 507b
    body language, 100
    during bowel elimination, 426b
    call system, 314b
    in cases of harassment, 63b
    Chains of Survival, 831b
    changes in Alzheimer's disease, 776-777, 776b
    while checking rectal temperature, 488b
    for collecting midstream specimens, 570b
    for comfort, 304b, 532b, 600b
    for comfort in end-of-life care, 854b
    and confidentiality, 60b
    for cough etiquette, 648
    about culture and religion, 95b
    for delegation, 33-34, 34b, 34f
    for dressing and undressing, 379b
    effective, 97, 97b
    with elastic bandages, 600b
    electronic communications, 43, 43b-44b
    in emergency care, 830b
    facial expressions, 100b
    fall prevention programs, 189b
    for fire safety, 175b
    about food and fluids, 460b
    with foreign-speaking persons, 102b
    giving directions, 301b
    hazard statements, 171
    with health team, 67-82
    for heat and cold applications, 637b
    for helping the person walk, 524b
    identifying the person, 157b
    informed consent, 44b
    introducing yourself, 305, 307f
    job descriptions, 29b
    for making occupied beds, 328b
    for measuring vital signs, 487b
    for measuring weight and height, 309
    for medication assistance, 827b
    for meeting oxygen needs, 647b
    for moving the person, 262b
    for moving persons in bed, 265b
    for moving persons to a new room, 318

Communication(s) (Continued)
    nonverbal, 92, 99-100, 766b, 781f
    with older persons, 142b
    about pain, 532b, 535b
    paraphrasing, 92
    patient information, 589, 589b
    for perineal care, 358b
    with the person, 97-102
    during personal hygiene procedures, 336b
    with persons at risk for suicide, 765b
    with persons from other cultures, 102b
    with persons who have disabilities, 103
    with persons with Alzheimer's disease, 776b-777b
    with persons with cancer, 699b
    with persons with dementia, 777b
    with persons with hearing loss, 678
    with persons with mental health disorders, 766b
    with persons with schizophrenia, 761b
    pictograms, 171
    for positioning the person, 256b
    precautionary statements, 171
    while preparing the person for physical examination, 562b
    about pressure ulcers, 625b
    professional boundaries, 41b
    professional speech, 60
    to provide a sense of identity, worth, and belonging, 106b
    while providing drinking water, 466b
    for quality of life, 17b
    for range-of-motion exercises, 517b
    recording, 75b
    for refusing tasks, 36b
    rehabilitation, 670, 670b-671b
    when removing indwelling catheters, 416b
    reporting abuse, 45b
    reporting and recording time, 73b
    reporting your absence, 59b
    resigning from a job, 64
    with restraints, 208b, 211b
    rights to information, 14b
    role limits, 26b
    rules of, 97
    with sexually aggressive persons, 798b
    signal words, 171
    about skin and scalp conditions, 368b
    with speech-impaired persons, 681b
    statements that signal bad attitude, 59
    for stool specimens, 577b
    surgery consent, 594
    telephone, 77
    terms for incontinence products, 400b
    terms for intellectual disabilities, 788b
    terms for persons with hearing loss, 677b
    in training programs, 23b
    with transfer/gait belts, 193b
    for transferring the person, 281b
    for transmission-based precautions, 231b
    after traumatic brain injury, 710
    with unconscious persons, 343b
    with urinals, 394b
    about urination, 390b
    verbal, 92, 98
    ways to decrease noise, 306b
    ways to improve, 106b
    in workplace, 65b
Community-based services, 146b
Companionship services, 146b
Compensation, 759b
Competence, 24, 24b, 31
Competency evaluation, 23
Complementary and alternative medicine (CAM), 698
Complementary medicine, 698
Complete bed baths, 350, 350b-351b, 352f
Complete care, 97b
Compound fractures. See Open fractures
Comprehensive care plans, 88b
Compresses, 634-635
Compression garments, 618, 618f
Compressions. See Chest compressions
Compulsions, 757, 759
Computers, 75-77, 76b
Concussions, 847, 847b
Condom catheters, 407, 418, 418b-419b, 418f, 420f
Confidentiality, 15, 55, 59-60, 60b, 858b

Conflict, 55, 62
Conflict resolution, 62, 63b, 65b
Confused and disoriented persons, 97b
Confusion, 769-770, 770b
Congenital heart defects, 726b
Congestive heart failure, 729
Congregate housing, 149
Connective tissue, 109
Consciousness, altered, 710, 710f
Constipation, 422, 426
Constriction, 110, 112, 634-635, 635f
Consumer Product Safety Improvement Act of 2008
   (CPSIA), 803b
Contact lenses, 690
Contagious disease. *See* Communicable disease
Contaminated laundry, 242
Contaminated wounds, 604, 605b
Contamination, 217, 221
   bagging items, 238
   Bloodborne Pathogen Standard terms, 241b
   cross-contamination, 217, 221, 221f
Continuing care retirement communities (CCRCs),
   149
Continuous feedings, 476
Continuous positive airway pressure (CPAP), 733
Contraction, muscular, 112
Contractures, 513-514, 514f
Controlled substances, 49
Contusion, 604, 605b, 606f
Convenience, 200
Conversion, 759b
Converting inches into feet and inches, 307b
Converting measures, 456b
Convoluted tubules, 120
Convulsions. *See* Seizures
Cooking, 158b, 468, 469b
Cooling and warming blankets, 640b
Cooling elements, 879
Cooperation, 56b
COPD. *See* Chronic obstructive pulmonary disease
Coping, 140
Cord and ribbon safety, 164b
Cornea, 114, 682b
Cornrows (small braids), 369b
Corns, 609b-610b, 610f
Coronary arteries, 727
Coronary artery bypass surgery, 727, 728f
Coronary artery disease, 727-728
Corrective lenses, 688-690, 688b
Costs: reducing, 22
Cotton drawsheets, 319, 322, 322f
Cough, 644b, 732
Cough etiquette, 229b, 648, 648b
Coughing, 648
Coughing exercises, 597b, 648b-649b, 650f
Counseling
   cardiac rehabilitation, 728
   financial, 146b
Counting respirations, 504-505, 505b-506b
Courtesy, 17b, 55, 56b, 60
Cowper's glands, 121
CPAP. *See* Continuous positive airway pressure
CPR. *See* Cardiopulmonary resuscitation
Crabs, 368
Cradles, 882
Cramping, 432b
Cranial nerves, 114, 706b
Crib rails, 191b
Crib safety, 801b, 803-804, 803b
Crib toys, 882
Cribs, 882
Crime, 38
Criminal laws, 38, 41
Crohn's disease, 742
Cross-contamination, 217, 221, 221f
Cross-dressers, 796
Crutch gait, 526, 527f-528f
Crutches, 526, 526f-527f
Culture(s), 92, 94-95
   communication about, 95b
   communication with persons from other cultures,
      102b
   death rites, 852b
   dietary practices, 442
   end-of-life needs, 852-853, 853b

Culture(s) *(Continued)*
   eye contact practices, 101b
   facial expressions, 100b
   food practices, 448b, 449
   foreign-born persons, 141b
   hair care practices, 369b
   health care beliefs, 94b
   home care practices, 95b
   meal time practices, 443b
   and pain, 534
   pain reactions, 534b
   personal hygiene practices, 336b
   sick care practices, 94b
   touch practices, 100b
Curanderos (curanderas), 94b
Curtains, privacy, 312, 312b
Cushions, 628, 629f
Cutaneous ureterostomy, 751, 752f
Cuticles: pushing back, 378b, 379f
CVA (cerebrovascular accident). *See* Stroke
Cyanosis, 634, 638b, 642, 644b
Cystitis, 750b
Cytoplasm, 108

D

Daily care, 337, 338b
Daily Value (DV), 448
Dairy food group, 446, 453b
Dance (step) reflex, 128, 129f
Dandruff, 366, 368
Danger zone, 468, 468f
Dangling (sitting on the side of the bed), 276,
   276b-278b, 277f
Data, 83-84
Dating, teen, 136, 136b
Dating violence, 52b, 126, 136b
Deafness, 675, 677
Death, 142
   attitudes about, 852-853, 853b
   brain death, 710, 710f
   care of the body after, 856, 857b
   of children, 142
   reporting deaths, 203
   signs of, 856
   stages of dying, 853
Death rattle, 856
Death rites, 852b
Deconditioning, 513, 514b
Decontamination, 241b, 242
Deep-breathing exercises, 648, 648b-649b, 648f-649f
Defamation, 38, 42
Defecation, 422, 423b
Defense mechanisms, 757-758, 759b
Defibrillation, 730, 835, 836b
Defibrillators, 730, 835
Dehiscence, 604, 612, 612f, 819
Dehydration, 422, 429, 442, 456, 456b
Delegation, 29b, 31-37
   accepting tasks, 35
   communication for, 34, 34b, 34f
   definition of, 31
   example tasks that can and cannot be delegated to
      you, 32b
   Five Rights of Delegation (NCSBN), 35, 35b
   guidelines for, 34b
   guidelines for admissions, transfers, and discharges,
      547b
   guidelines for applying dressings, 616b
   guidelines for applying incontinence products, 400b
   guidelines for applying restraints, 212b
   guidelines for assisting with IV therapy, 483b
   guidelines for assisting with sterile procedures, 244b
   guidelines for assisting with tube feedings, 478b
   guidelines for back massage, 537b
   guidelines for bathing, 348b
   guidelines for bathing infants, 814b
   guidelines for bedpans, 391b
   guidelines for blood glucose testing, 582b
   guidelines for bowel elimination, 423b
   guidelines for brushing and combing hair, 369b
   guidelines for care of the body after death, 857b
   guidelines for catheter care, 410b
   guidelines for changing patient gowns, 384b
   guidelines for collecting sputum specimens, 580b
   guidelines for collecting stool specimens, 577b

Delegation *(Continued)*
   guidelines for commodes, 395b
   guidelines for condom catheters, 418b
   guidelines for counting respirations, 505b
   guidelines for dangling, 276b
   guidelines for deep-breathing and coughing
      exercises, 648b
   guidelines for diapering babies, 810b
   guidelines for dressing and undressing, 380b
   guidelines for elastic bandages, 600b
   guidelines for elastic stockings, 598b
   guidelines for enemas, 432b
   guidelines for eyeglasses, 688b
   guidelines for fecal impaction, 427b
   guidelines for feeding the person, 464b
   guidelines for heat and cold applications, 638b
   guidelines for helping the person walk, 524b
   guidelines for incentive spirometry, 651b
   guidelines for making beds, 323b
   guidelines for measuring blood pressure, 509b
   guidelines for measuring intake and output, 459b
   guidelines for measuring weight and height, 309b
   guidelines for moving persons in bed, 266b
   guidelines for nail and foot care, 377b
   guidelines for nutritional support and IV therapy,
      474b
   guidelines for oral hygiene, 339b
   guidelines for ostomy pouches, 438b
   guidelines for oxygen set-up, 655b
   guidelines for perineal care, 358b
   guidelines for positioning the person, 256b
   guidelines for preparing for meals, 460b
   guidelines for preparing the person for physical
      examination, 563b
   guidelines for preventing work-related injuries,
      264b
   guidelines for providing drinking water, 466b
   guidelines for pulse oximetry, 646b
   guidelines for range-of-motion exercises, 518b
   guidelines for removing indwelling catheters, 416b
   guidelines for serving meals, 462b
   guidelines for shampooing, 372b
   guidelines for shaving, 374b
   guidelines for stand and pivot transfers, 286b
   guidelines for suctioning, 662b
   guidelines for suppositories, 431b
   guidelines for taking pulses, 499b
   guidelines for taking temperatures, 491b
   guidelines for testing urine, 575b
   guidelines for transferring persons, 282b
   guidelines for transferring persons to stretchers,
      293b
   guidelines for transmission-based precautions, 231b
   guidelines for tub baths and showers, 356b
   guidelines for turning persons, 273b
   guidelines for urinals, 394b
   guidelines for urine drainage systems, 412b
   guidelines for urine specimens, 568b
   guidelines for using mechanical lifts, 296b
   guidelines for weighing infants, 818b
   in health care agencies, 10b
   in home care, 34b
   and preventing infection, 247b
   process of, 32-35, 33f
   protecting person's rights in, 19b
   refusing tasks, 35-36
   roles in, 35-36
   safe, 32, 32b, 32f
   teamwork in, 36b
   for wound care, 619b
Delirium, 769-770, 770b
Delusions, 757, 760-761, 761b, 769, 775, 778b-780b
   of grandeur, 757, 760
   of persecution, 757, 760
Dementia, 154, 156b, 769, 771, 771b
   pseudodementia, 769, 771
   risk factors for accidents, 156b
Dementia care, 778-783, 778b-780b, 782b
   infection control, 240b
   in long-term care, 782b
   recommendations for communication, 97b, 777b
Denial
   as defense mechanism, 759b
   A Dying Patient's Bill of Last Rights, 859b
   stage of dying, 853

Dental floss, 339
Dental hygienists, 5t-6t
Dentists, 5t-6t
Denture care, 344, 344b-346b, 346f
Dentures, 335, 344, 344f
    full, 344
    partial, 344
    pre-operative, 591
Dependability, 56b, 57-58
Dependence, total, 263b, 283b
Depression, 761
    in bipolar disorder, 761
    major, 761
    in older persons, 761, 762b
    signs and symptoms of, 761b-762b
    stage of dying, 853
Depressive episode, 761b
Dermis, 110, 336b, 702b
Detection of disease, 2
Development, 126
Developmental disabilities, 786, 792b
    causes of, 787b
    intellectual and developmental disabilities, 786-793
    long-term care for persons with, 787b
    safety measures for persons with, 183b
    warning signs, 787b
Developmental monitoring, 138b
Developmental tasks, 126-127, 128b
Diabetes, 123, 745-746, 746b
Diabetes meal plan, 451t-452t, 453
Diabetic foot care, 609b-610b, 610f
Diabetic foot ulcers, 604, 609
Diabetic retinopathy, 683f, 684
Diagnosis
    medical, 83, 86
    nursing, 83, 86, 86b
Dialysis, 749, 753, 756b
    hemodialysis, 753, 754f
    peritoneal, 753, 754f
Dialysis machines, 754f
Diapering babies, 810, 810b-811b, 812f
Diaphoresis, 335
Diaphragm, 118, 504b, 731b
Diarrhea, 422, 429, 429b
Diastole, 116, 486, 497b, 506, 725b-726b
Diastolic pressure, 486, 506
Diet, 56, 451
    and blood pressure, 506b
    and BMs, 425
    calorie-controlled, 451t-452t
    and cancer, 697
    cultural practices, 442
    meal time practices, 443b
    religious practices, 450b
    sodium-controlled, 452
    special diets, 451-454, 451t-452t
    tips to help children eat vegetables and fruits, 445b
Dietary guidelines, 444
Dietary Guidelines for Americans, 2015, 444
Dietitians, 5t-6t
Digestion, 108, 119
Digestive disorders, 739-744
Digestive system, 119f, 423f, 443b, 443f, 740f
    changes in aging, 143b, 145-146
    structure and function of, 740b
Digital infant scale, 818b, 818f
Digital thermometers, 489, 489f
Dignity, 17b
Dilation, 110, 634-635, 635f
Dining programs, 462b
Directional terms, 79, 80f
Directions: giving, 301b
Director of nursing (DON), 6-7
Dirty wounds. See Infected wounds
Disability, 92, 95, 103, 666, 786
    and BMs, 425
    communication barriers, 102
    effects of, 95-96, 95b
    and food practices, 449
    intellectual and developmental disabilities, 786-793
    safety measures for persons with, 183b
    after TBI, 710
Disability etiquette, 103b
Disaster drills, 173b
Disaster plans, 173, 176

Disasters, 154, 173-176, 173b
Discharges, 545, 546b-547b, 558, 558b, 559f
    from assisted living, 827
    in long-term care, 546b
Discipline, 200
Discomfort, 85b. See also Pain
Disease
    communicable, 217, 228
    detection and treatment of, 2
    prevention of, 2
Disinfectants, 217, 226
Disinfection, 217, 226, 227b
Displacement, 759b
Disposable diapers, 810
Disposable incontinence products, 399f
Disposable oral thermometers, 490, 490f
Disposable sharps containers, 243b, 243f
Dissociative symptoms, 762
Distraction, 531, 536, 536f
Diuresis, 749, 753
Diverticular disease, 741
Diverticulitis, 741
Diverticulosis, 741, 741f
Diverticulum, 741
DNR ("Do Not Resuscitate") orders, 856
Documentation. See also Charting; Recording;
        Reporting
    assignment sheets, 89, 89b, 89f
    flow sheets, 71, 71b, 71f
    graphic sheets, 69, 70f
    health history (nursing history), 69
    intake and output (I&O) records, 456-457
    Kardex or care summaries, 72f
    personal hygiene, 363, 363b
    pressure ulcers, 631, 631f
    progress notes, 67, 69, 69b, 71f
    reporting and recording time, 73, 73b
    restraint use, 210
Domestic abuse. See Intimate partner violence (IPV)
Domestic violence. See Intimate partner violence
        (IPV)
DON. See Director of nursing
Door knob covers, 802b, 802f
Doors and windows, 672b-673b, 877
Doppler ultrasound stethoscope (DUS), 503, 504f
Dorsal recumbent position, 250, 259, 561, 564, 564f
Dorsiflexion, 513
Double-bagging, 238, 239b, 239f
Down syndrome, 786, 788, 789f
Drainage
    measurement of, 613
    purulent, 613, 614f
    sanguineous, 604, 613, 614f
    serosanguineous, 604, 613, 614f
    serous, 604, 613, 614f
    wound, 613, 614f
Draping, 564, 564b, 564f
Drawer space, 315
Drawers, 315b
Drawsheets, 270f, 319, 322, 322f, 323b
Dreams, wet (nocturnal emissions), 135
Dressing and undressing, 379, 778b-780b, 781f
    communication for, 379b
    guidelines for, 380b
    in home care, 379b
    in long-term care, 379b
    for older persons, 379b
    procedure for dressing the person, 382b-383b,
        383f-384f
    procedure for undressing the person, 380b-381b,
        381f-382f
    rules for, 379b
    safety measures, 380b
Dressings, 614-616
    applying, 616, 616b
    dry, 615
    dry, non-sterile, 617b, 617f
    for pressure ulcers, 631
    securing, 615, 615f
    types of, 614-615, 615f
    wet, 615
Drinking, 158b
Drinking alcohol. See Alcohol abuse
Drinking water: providing, 466, 466b-467b, 467f
Droplet precautions, 230b

Drug abuse, 757, 763-764, 764b
Drug addiction, 757, 763-764, 764b
Drug administration, 826
Drug and alcohol treatment, 671
Drug errors, 827
Drug testing, 65, 867
Drugs, 57
    accident risk factors, 156
    and blood pressure, 506b
    and BMs, 425
    and food practices, 449
    and hip fractures, 719
    immuno-suppressive, 697
    and oxygen needs, 643
    pre-operative, 595
    preventing poisoning with prescription drugs, 160b
    role limits, 26b
    and sleep, 540
    storing, 827
Dry and cracked skin, 609b-610b, 610f
Dry cold applications, 637
Dry dressings, 615
Dry heat applications, 636
Duodenum, 119, 443b
Dura mater, 114
Durable power of attorney for health care, 856
Dying: stages of, 853
A Dying Patient's Bill of Last Rights, 859b
Dying persons: rights of, 858b-859b
Dysarthria, 681
Dysphagia, 145, 442, 454, 454b, 670
Dysphagia diet, 454, 454b
Dyspnea, 145, 642, 644
Dysrhythmias, 724, 730, 730b
Dysuria, 388, 390t, 749, 750b

E
Ear(s), 115, 115f
    basic observations, 85b
    changes in aging, 145
    structure and function of, 676b, 676f
Ear disorders, 675-680
Eardrum, 115, 676b
Early morning care, 335, 337, 338b
Earwax, 677
East Indian Hindus, 336b
Eating
    devices for, 449, 450f, 667, 668f
    factors affecting, 449
    older persons, 450b
    preventing burns, 158b
Eating disorders, 764
Eating habits, 442, 443b
Eavesdropping, 60
Ebola (Ebolavirus), 731
ECHO homes. See Elder Cottage Housing
        Opportunity
ED (erectile dysfunction). See Impotence
Edema, 442, 456, 604, 608
    lymphedema, 724, 736, 736b, 736f
Education. See also Training
    cardiac rehabilitation, 728
Educational neglect, 49
EHRs. See Electronic health records (EHRs)
Ejaculation, 126, 135
Ejaculatory duct, 120
Elastic bandages, 600, 600b-601b, 601f
Elastic stockings, 598, 598b-599b, 599f
Elbow: range-of-motion exercises for, 519b-520b,
        521f
Elbow protectors, 628, 629f
Elbow splints, 212b-214b, 212f
Elder(s), 46
Elder abuse, 38, 46-47
    examples of, 47, 48b
    in home care, 48b
    in long-term care, 48b
    prosecuted cases, 48b
    reporting, 47, 48b
    required actions when abuse is suspected, 48b
    signs of, 46, 47b, 47f
Elder abuse prevention programs, 146b
Elder Cottage Housing Opportunity (ECHO), 148
Elective surgery, 588-589
Electric beds, 306, 307f

Electric shavers, 374, 374f
Electrical appliances, 672b-673b
Electrical equipment, 169, 169f
Electrical safety, 878
    home assessment checklist, 672b-673b
    outlet safety, 170b, 170f
    preventing accidents, 170b, 170f
    preventing burns, 158b
    preventing suffocating, 164b
    three-pronged plugs, 169, 169f
    warning signs, 169
Electrical shock, 154, 169
Electrocardiography, 590, 590f
Electrolytes, 119
Electronic communications, 43, 43b-44b, 76f
Electronic devices, 75-77, 76b
Electronic health records (EHRs), 67-68, 68f, 75
Electronic IV pumps, 481, 481f
Electronic medical records (EMRs). See Electronic
        health records (EHRs)
Electronic recordings, 75
Electronic thermometers, 489, 489b, 489f, 491, 492b,
        493f
Elevated armrests, 259, 259f
Elimination
    at end of life, 855
    post-operative, 602
    rehabilitation for, 667
Elopement, 154, 176, 769, 774b
Emancipated minors, 138b
Embolus, 588, 597
Emergency care, 829-830, 830b
    in long-term care, 146b
    for older persons, 146b
    requirements for staff training, 173b
    rules for, 830b
Emergency equipment, 879
Emergency Medical Services (EMS) system, 829
Emergency surgery, 588-589
Emesis. See Vomitus
Emotional abuse
    child abuse, 49, 50b
    elder abuse, 46
    intimate partner violence (IPV), 51
Emotional neglect, 49
Emotional problems, 760
    at end of life, 855
    in fragile X syndrome, 789
    and sleep, 540
    after TBI, 710
Empathy, 56b
Emphysema, 732, 732f
Employment
    accepting or declining job offers, 867
    getting a job, 860-869
    in home care, 861b
    job skills and training, 861, 861b
    in long-term care, 861b
    sources of jobs, 860
    what employers look for, 860-861, 861b
EMS system. See Emergency Medical Services
        system
Enablers, 200, 203
Endocardium, 116
Endocrine disorders, 745-746
Endocrine glands, 122, 745b
Endocrine system, 122-123, 122f, 745b, 745f
End-of-life care, 851-859, 851b, 853b-854b, 858b
End-of-shift reports, 67, 74, 74b
Endometrium, 121
Endorsement, 21, 24
Endotracheal (ET) tubes, 658, 659f, 664b-665b
Enemas, 422, 431-436
    for children, 432b
    cleansing, 431b-434b, 432, 433f
    comfort measures, 432b
    guidelines for, 432b
    observations to report and record, 432b
    oil-retention, 431, 436, 436b
    procedure for giving, 431b, 433f
    safety measures, 432b, 436b
    small-volume, 431, 434, 434f, 435b
    solutions for, 431, 432b
Engineering controls, 241b
English, 100b, 102b

Enteral nutrition, 473-477
    observations to report, 476
Enterococci, vancomycin-resistant (VRE), 218
Enterovirus D68 (EV-D68), 733
Entrapment, 303
Entrapment zones, 309, 310f
Enuresis, 531, 540b
Environment, 18
    and cancer, 697
    and care of persons with AD and other dementias,
        778b-780b
    resident rights to safe, clean comfortable, and
        home-like setting, 18
    and sleep, 540
Environmental care, 229b
Epidermal stripping, 621, 624b
Epidermis, 110, 336b, 702b
Epididymis, 120
Epiglottis, 118
Epilepsy, 846
Epinephrine, 123, 845
Episiotomy, 800, 819
Epithelial tissue, 109
Equal Employment Opportunity Commission
        (EEOC), 867b
Equipment. See also Adaptive devices; Assistive
        devices
    bariatric-safe, 169
    blood pressure, 507, 508b
    cleaning, 226
    contact precautions, 230b
    decontamination of, 242
    infection control, 226
    for IV therapy, 479f
    nursery equipment safety, 879-882
    for oral hygiene, 340
    personal protective equipment (PPE), 229b-230b,
        232-239, 232b, 241b, 242
    in person's unit, 306-316, 316f
    for physical examinations, 561, 562f
    pre-operative teaching about, 590
    preventing accidents with, 169-171, 170b
    preventing injuries with, 255b
    preventive measures for infection control, 242
    protective devices, 628
    safety measures to prevent falls, 188b-189b
    standard precautions, 229b
    transporting, 255b
Equivalency. See Endorsement
Erectile dysfunction (ED). See Impotence
Erectile tissue, 121
Ergonomics, 250, 254
Erythrocytes, 116, 725b-726b
Eschar, 621, 625b
Esophagus, 119, 443b, 740b
Esteem, 92, 94
Estrogen, 121, 123, 795b
Ethical aspects, 39-40
Ethics, 29b, 38-54, 106b
    codes of ethics, 38-39
    in delegating tasks, 36b
    in health care agencies, 10b
    in protecting person's rights, 19b
    student ethics, 55-66
    unethical student behavior, 65
    work ethics, 55-66
Etiquette
    cough, 229b
    disability, 103b
Eustachian tube, 115, 676b
Evacuation, 176
Evaluation, 35, 83, 90
    competency, 23
    of delegated tasks, 35
    drug testing, 65
Evening care, 335, 337, 338b
Eviction from assisted living, 827
Evisceration, 604, 612, 612f
Excoriation, 604, 605b, 606f
Exercise(s), 56, 517
    for arthritis, 713
    and blood pressure, 506b
    cardiac rehabilitation, 728
    coughing exercises, 649b, 650f
    deep-breathing exercises, 648, 649b, 649f

Exercise(s) (Continued)
    leg exercises, 598, 598f
    for older persons, 145, 145f, 514b
    and oxygen needs, 643
    range-of-motion exercises, 517, 517b-520b, 519f,
        521f-522f
    and sleep, 540
    ways to promote, 529b
Exhalation, 118, 504b, 731b
Expiration (breathing out), 118, 731b
Exploitation or misappropriation, financial, 46, 776b
Explosive blasts, 710
Exposure control plans, 240
Exposure incidents, 241b, 243
Expressive aphasia, 675, 682
Extended length slings, 296
Extension, 513
Extensive assistance (functional status), 263b, 283b
External ear, 115
External female genitalia, 121, 121f, 795f
External fixation, 716, 716f
External rotation, 513
Eye(s), 56, 114-115, 115f
    basic observations, 85b
    changes in aging, 145
    layers of, 114
    structure and function of, 682b, 682f
Eye contact practices, 101b
Eye disorders, 682-690, 683f
Eye protection, 229b
Eyeglasses, 688, 688b-689b, 689f

F
Face masks
    giving breaths with, 834, 834f
    oxygen masks, 653, 653f
    partial-rebreather masks, 653, 653f
Face shields, 232, 232b
    donning and removing, 234f-236f, 237b
    giving breaths with, 834, 834f
Facial expressions, 100b
Fainting, 829, 845, 845f
Fall(s), 186b, 710
    causes of, 187, 187b
    risk factors for, 187, 187b
Fall prevention, 186-199, 188b-189b, 192b
    with babies, 811b
Fall prevention programs, 188-192, 189b
Falling persons, 196-197, 196b-197b, 196f-197f
Fallopian tubes, 121
False imprisonment, 38, 42, 204
False teeth, 344
Family, 103-104, 138b, 148
    in end-of-life care, 855
    in home care, 104b, 783b
    of older persons, 104b
    of person with Alzheimer's disease, 782
    safety measures for, 179b
    in sick care, 104b
    ways to provide support, 664b-665b
    ways to show care and concern, 559
Family caregivers, 783b
Family dining, 462b
Family duties, 533
Family history, 713
Fat-controlled diet, 451t-452t
Fats, 447
Faxes, 76b
FBAO. See Foreign-body airway obstruction
FDA. See Food and Drug Administration
Fears about surgery, 589b
Fecal impaction, 422, 427, 427f
    checking for and removing, 428b
    guidelines for, 427b
    in long-term care, 427b
    safety measures, 427b
Fecal incontinence, 422, 429-430, 430b
Feces, 422, 423b, 740b
Federal laws, 22-25
Feedback, 35, 36b
Feeding
    of babies, 808, 809b
    bottle-feeding babies, 807-808, 808f-809f, 809b
    continuous, 476
    of older persons, 464b

Feeding (Continued)
    of the person, 463-464, 463f, 464b-465b, 465f
    safety and comfort measures, 464b
    scheduled, 476
    supplemental feedings, 466
    tube feedings, 476-477, 476f, 478b
    of visually impaired persons, 463, 463f
Feeding pumps, 476, 476f
Feeding times, 476
Feeding tubes, 474, 477, 477f, 484b
Female breast, 122, 122f
Female perineal care, 359b-360b, 361f
Female reproductive system, 121-122, 121f, 795f
    changes in aging, 143b, 147
    structure and function of, 795b
Fertilization, 122
Fetus, 121
Fever, 486, 488
    and oxygen needs, 643
    terms to describe persons with, 488
    viral hemorrhagic fevers, 731
Fiber, 425, 451t-452t
Financial counseling, 146b
Financial exploitation or misappropriation, 46, 776b
Financial issues
    and food practices, 449
    helping patients with bills and insurance claims, 13b
    paying for health care, 8-9
    reducing costs, 22
Finger cushions, 515, 516f
Fingernail clipping, 377b, 377f, 817
Fingers: range-of-motion exercises for, 519b-520b, 521f
Finland, 443b
Fire extinguishers, 174b, 176, 176b, 177f
Fire prevention, 175
Fire safety, 174-176, 174b
    communication for, 175b
    for home care, 174b
    RACE mnemonic for, 175, 175f
    what to do during fires, 175-176, 176b
Firearm safety, 879
First aid, 829-830
Five Rights of Delegation (NCSBN), 35, 35b
Fixation, 716
    external, 716, 716f
    internal, 716, 717f
Flank area, 409b, 410f
Flashbacks, 757, 760
Flat bones, 110, 251b, 713b
Flatulence, 422, 430
Flatus, 422, 430
Flexion, 513
Floor cushions, 188b-189b, 190f
Floors, 188b-189b, 877
Flora, normal, 217-218, 233
Flossing, 339-340, 339b-340b, 342f
Flow rate, IV, 473, 481, 481f-482f, 482b
Flow sheets, 71, 71b, 71f
Flu. See Influenza
Fluid balance, 456-457
Fluid orders, 456
Fluid restriction, 456
Fluid-filled pads and cushions, 628
Fluids, 442-472, 444b
    and BMs, 425
    communication with the person about, 460b
    meeting the person's needs, 460-466
    normal requirements for, 456, 456b
    at nursing centers, 151b
    post-operative, 602
    pre-operative, 590
    pre-operative teaching about, 590
Foam cushions, 628, 629f
Focusing, 101
Folate (folic acid), 447t
Folding linens, 329b-330b, 330f
Foley catheters. See Indwelling catheters
Folic acid (folate), 447t
Folk healers, 94b
Folk medicine, 94b
Food(s). See also Meals
    and BMs, 425
    communication with the person about, 460b

Food(s) (Continued)
    cultural practices, 448b
    dairy group, 446
    fruit group, 446
    grains group, 446
    high-fiber, 425
    high-sodium, 453b
    meeting the person's needs, 460-466
    mobile food carts, 470b
    at nursing centers, 151b
    pre-operative teaching about, 590
    protein foods group, 446
    serving sizes, 445t
    vegetable group, 446
Food and Drug Administration (FDA), 201
Food intake, 454, 455b, 455f
Food labels, 448, 448f
Food practices, 448b
Food safety, 825
    for preventing suffocating, 164b
    safe handling instructions, 825, 825f
    tips to keep food safe, 468, 469b
Food servings, 448
Food temperature, 468, 468f
Foodborne illness, 468, 468b
Foot care, 376, 376b, 378b, 379f
    guidelines for, 377b
    in home care, 377
    for persons with diabetes, 609b-610b
    range-of-motion exercises, 519b-520b, 522f
    safety and comfort measures, 377b
Foot elevators, 628
Foot ulcers, diabetic, 604, 609, 610b
Foot-boards, 515, 515f
Footdrop, 513, 515
Forearm: range-of-motion exercises for, 519b-520b, 521f
Forearm crutches, 526, 526f
Foreign-body airway obstruction (FBAO), 164
Foreign-born persons, 141b
Foreign-speaking persons, 102b
Foreskin, 121
Formula
    for bottle-feeding babies, 807, 807f
    for enteral nutrition, 475, 475b
Foster care, adult, 149
Fowler's position, 250, 256, 257b, 257f, 303, 308, 308f
Fracture pans, 391, 391f
Fractures, 705, 716-720, 716f, 717f
Fragile X syndrome, 789
Fraud, 43
Freedom
    from abuse, mistreatment, and neglect, 16, 673b-674b, 858b
    of movement, 200
    from restraints, 16
French culture, 102b
Friction, 262, 264, 621
Friends, 103-104, 104b
Fruits, 445b, 446, 453b
Full visual privacy, 303, 312b
Full-sling mechanical lifts, 299b, 300f
Full-slings, 296, 296f
Functional incontinence, 388, 397
Functional nursing, 1, 8
Functional rehabilitation, 875f
Functional status, 262-263, 263b, 283b
Fundus, 121
Fungal infections, 218, 609b-610b
Furniture
    changing tables, 880
    cribs, 882
    high chairs, 880
    home assessment checklist, 672b-673b
    home safety measures, 877-878
    hook-on chairs, 880
    infant safety measures, 801b
    room furniture, 306-316
    safety measures to prevent falls, 188b-189b

G
GAD. See Generalized anxiety disorder
Gait, crutch, 526, 527f-528f
Gait belts. See Transfer belts
Gallbladder, 119, 443b, 740b, 742f

Gallbladder attacks, 742
Gallbladder pain, 533f
Gallstone attacks, 742
Gallstones, 742, 742f
Gangrene, 604, 608, 705, 721, 721f
Gap protectors, 205b-206b
Garages, 878
Garments. See Clothing
Gastric juices, 119, 443b, 740b
Gastro-esophageal reflux disease, 740
Gastro-intestinal (GI) system, 443b, 450b, 740b
Gastro-intestinal tract, 423b, 443b
Gastrostomy tubes, 473-474, 475f
    percutaneous endoscopic gastrostomy (PEG) tubes, 473-474, 475f
Gates, 880
Gauze, 614
Gavage, 473
Gay men, 796
Gehrig, Lou, 709
Gel- or fluid-filled pads and cushions, 628, 629f
Gender identity, 794, 796
Gender roles, 794-795, 796f
General anesthesia, 588, 595
General diet, 451
Generalized anxiety disorder, 758
Genes, 109
Genital warts, 755t
Genupectoral position. See Knee-chest position
GERD. See Gastro-esophageal reflux disease
Geriatrics, 92, 96, 140
Germany, 443b
Gerontology, 140
Gestational diabetes, 745
GH. See Growth hormone
GI tract (alimentary canal), 119
Glans, 121
Glass thermometers, 490, 490f, 491b, 494b-496b, 494f
Glaucoma, 684-685, 684f
Global aphasia, 675, 682
Glomerulus, 120, 750b
Gloves, 233, 233b, 233f
    contact precautions, 230b
    donning and removing, 234f-236f, 238f
    standard precautions, 229b
    sterile gloving, 244, 245b-246b, 246f
Glucocorticoids, 123
Glucometer, 567
Glucose, 583f
    blood testing, 582, 582b-585b, 582f
    urine testing, 574
Glucosuria, 567, 574
Gluten-free diet, 451t-452t
Glycosuria, 567
Goals, 83, 86
Goggles, 232, 232b, 234f-236f, 237b
Gonads, 120, 123
Gonorrhea, 755t
Gossip, 55, 59
Gowns, 232
    changing patient gowns, 384, 385b, 385f
    contact precautions, 230b
    donning and removing, 234f-236f, 237b
    standard precautions, 229b
Grab bars, 192, 193f
Graduate (container), 442, 457, 458f
Grains, 446, 453b
Grand mal seizures, 846
Grandeur: delusions of, 757, 760
Graphic sheets, 69, 70f
Grasp reflex, palmar, 128, 129f
Graves' disease, 699, 700f
Greece, 443b
Greek Orthodox church, 450b
Grief, 853
Grievances, 16
Grieving, 142
Grooming, 366-387, 366b
    for job interviews, 865b, 866f
    personal, 58f
    for persons with AD and other dementias, 778b-780b
Grooming aids, 366, 367f
Ground (electrical), 154, 169
Group homes (board and care homes), 149

Group insurance, 8
Group settings for older persons, 149
Growth and development, 126-139, 127*f*
Growth hormone (GH), 122
Guide dogs, 688
Guided imagery, 531, 536
Guidelines for Isolation Precautions: Preventing Transmission of Infectious Agents in Healthcare Settings 2007, 228
Gums, 336*b*

H

Habit training/scheduled voiding, 404
HAI. *See* Healthcare-associated infection
Hair, 110
Hair care, 367-371
  brushing and combing hair, 369, 369*b*-370*b*, 370*f*
  cultural practices, 369*b*
  in long-term care, 367*b*
  pre-operative, 591
  shampooing, 371, 371*b*-373*b*, 371*f*
  shaving, 374-376, 374*b*-376*b*, 376*f*
Hallucinations, 757, 760, 761*b*, 769, 775
  in Alzheimer's disease, 775
  care of persons with, 778*b*-780*b*
Hammer toes, 609*b*-610*b*, 610*f*
Hand grips, 515, 516*f*
Hand hygiene, 223*b*
  alcohol-based hand rub, 225*b*, 226*f*
  rules of, 223*b*
  standard precautions, 229*b*
Hand position
  for CPR, 832, 833*f*
  for infant chest compressions, 839*b*-840*b*, 840*f*
Hand rails, 192, 192*f*
Hand rolls, 515
Handling
  safe handling instructions for meat and poultry, 825, 825*f*
  safe handling programs, 279*b*-280*b*
  of used linens, 333*b*
Hands-only CPR, 838, 838*b*
Hand-washing, 222*b*, 224*f*-225*f*, 225*b*
Hand-washing facilities, 241*b*
Harassment, 55, 63-64, 63*b*
Hashimoto's disease, 699
Hazard Communication Standard (HCS), 171, 172*f*
Hazard statements, 171
Hazardous chemicals, 154, 171-172
  labeling for containers, 171
  safety measures, 173*b*
Hazardous waste, household, 243*b*
Hazards, 154, 155*b*
HCS. *See Hazard Communication Standard*
Head: raising the person's head and shoulders, 266, 266*b*, 267*f*
Head injuries, 709-710
Head tilt–chin lift method, 166*b*, 167*f*, 833, 833*f*, 839*b*-840*b*, 841*f*
Health, 56-57
Health care, 2, 13*b*
  paying for, 8-9, 9*b*
  standards of care, 38, 41
Health care agencies, 1-11, 2*b*, 4*f*
Health care beliefs, 94*b*
Health care proxy, 856
Health care systems, 3, 3*f*, 4*b*, 22
Health history (nursing history), 69
Health information, protected, 38, 42
Health information technicians, 5*t*-6*t*
Health insurance, 8, 13*b*
Health insurance exchanges, 9
Health Insurance Portability and Accountability Act of 1996 (HIPAA), 42-43, 90*b*, 102*b*
Health promotion, 2
Health teams, 1, 5
  communication with, 5*b*, 67-82
  members of, 5*t*-6*t*, 7*f*
Healthcare-associated infection (HAI), 217, 220, 220*b*-221*b*, 223
Healthy life-style
  for arthritis, 713
  for GERDM, 740
  in retirement, 141
  and sleep, 540

Hearing, 114
  ear function, 676*b*, 676*f*
  measures to promote, 680*b*
Hearing, speech, and vision rehabilitation, 671
Hearing aids, 678-680, 680*f*
Hearing assistance dogs, 678
Hearing checklists, 678*b*-679*b*
Hearing devices, 680
Hearing disorders, 675
Hearing loss, 675, 677-680
  accident risk factors, 156
  in children, 678*b*
  effects of, 677-678, 678*b*
  at end of life, 854
  risk factors for, 677
  safety measures, 677*b*
  signs and symptoms of, 677*b*
  terms for persons with, 677*b*
Heart, 115-116, 497*b*, 725*b*-726*b*
  chambers of, 116
  layers of, 116
  location of, 116, 116*f*, 497*b*, 497*f*
  structures of, 116*f*, 725*b*-726*b*, 725*f*
Heart defects, congenital, 726*b*
Heart failure, 729-730, 730*b*
Heartburn, 739-740
Heat applications, 619, 634-637, 637*b*-640*b*
  for arthritis, 713
  for children, 634*b*
  complications of, 635
  dry, 636
  guidelines for, 638*b*
  in home care, 636*b*
  moist, 635-636, 635*f*
  for older persons, 634*b*
  safety and comfort measures, 638*b*, 640*b*
Heat stroke, 640
Heating elements, 879
Heating pads, 636*b*
Heavy lifting, 253
Heberden nodes, 713*f*
Heel elevators, 628, 629*f*
Heel protectors, 628, 629*f*
Height, 306*b*-307*b*, 308
Height measurement, 307*b*, 309, 309*b*, 309*f*-310*f*, 311*b*
Height rods, 307*b*, 308*f*-309*f*
Heimlich maneuver, 165
Hematoma, 567, 582*b*, 604
Hematuria, 388, 390*t*, 567, 574, 749, 750*b*
Hemiplegia, 154, 156, 705, 707
Hemodialysis, 753, 754*f*
Hemoglobin, 108, 116, 725*b*-726*b*
Hemoptysis, 567, 580*b*, 642, 644*b*
Hemorrhage, 604, 612, 724, 731, 829, 844
  external, 612
  internal, 612
  safety measures, 844*b*
Hemorrhagic fever, viral, 731
Hemothorax, 658, 663
Hemovac, 613, 614*f*
Hepatitis, 742-743, 742*b*-743*b*
Hepatitis A, 743, 743*b*
Hepatitis B, 743*b*, 744
Hepatitis B vaccination, 241
Hepatitis C, 743*b*, 744
Hepatitis D, 743*b*, 744
Hepatitis E, 743*b*, 744
Hernias, hiatal, 740, 741*f*
Herpes, 754*f*, 755*t*
Heterosexual, 794, 796
Hiatal hernia, 740, 741*f*
Hiding things, 777, 778*b*-780*b*
High blood pressure. *See* Hypertension
High chairs, 880
High-Fowler's position, 256, 303, 308, 308*f*
Hinduism, 450*b*, 852*b*
Hinge joints, 111, 111*f*, 251*b*, 251*f*, 713*b*, 713*f*
Hip abduction wedge, 515, 516*f*
Hip exercises, 519*b*-520*b*, 521*f*
Hip fractures, 719-720, 720*b*, 720*f*
Hip protectors, 201*b*, 202*f*
Hip replacement care, 714*b*, 715*f*
HIPAA. *See Health Insurance Portability and Accountability Act of 1996*

Hirsutism, 366, 368
Hispanic Americans, 100*b*
History, 21-22, 201
HIV. *See* Human immunodeficiency virus
Hoarding, 759
Hodgkin lymphoma, 736
Holding babies, 801*b*, 801*f*
Holism, 92
Holistic care, 93
Home assessment checklist, 672*b*-673*b*
Home care
  ALR services, 824*b*
  aseptic practices for, 222*b*
  assessment, 86*b*
  attendance for, 59*b*
  bathing infants, 814*b*
  bed making, 323*b*
  bed positions for, 309*b*
  bed rails in, 192*b*
  beds in, 307*b*
  call systems in, 314*b*, 314*f*
  cleaning baby bottles, 807*b*
  cold applications, 637*b*
  crib safety, 803*b*
  cultural practices, 95*b*
  delegation in, 34*b*
  for diabetic foot ulcers, 610*b*
  disasters in, 173*b*
  disinfection in, 227*b*
  drawsheets, 323*b*
  dressing and undressing, 379*b*
  for dysrhythmias, 730*b*
  elder abuse in, 48*b*
  employment in, 861*b*
  for families, 783*b*
  family and friends in, 104*b*
  fire safety, 174*b*, 189*b*
  flow sheets in, 71*b*
  food safety, 469*b*
  glass thermometers, 491*b*
  hazards in, 187*b*
  healthcare-associated infection (HAI) in, 221*b*
  heat applications for, 636*b*
  helping mothers breast-feed, 806*b*
  for hip fractures, 720*b*
  for impaired vision and blindness, 686*b*
  IV therapy, 481*b*
  job interviews for, 866*b*
  job skills and training for work in, 861*b*
  lead poisoning in, 161*b*
  linen changes, 321*b*
  mechanical ventilation in, 663*b*
  meeting nutritional needs, 449*b*
  for multiple sclerosis, 709*b*
  after myocardial infarction, 729*b*
  nail and foot care, 377
  for older persons, 146*b*-147*b*
  oxygen therapy, 652*b*
  personal safety measures for, 180*b*-181*b*
  for pressure ulcers, 626*b*
  preventing falls, 189*b*
  preventing poisoning, 159*b*
  privacy curtains in, 312*b*
  rehabilitation programs and services, 672*b*
  religious practices, 95*b*
  risk factors for falls, 187*b*
  risk factors for suicide, 766*b*
  roles and responsibilities in, 25*b*
  safety measures for, 181*b*, 189*b*, 802*b*, 802*f*
  shampooing, 372*b*
  sterilization, 227*b*
  stroke care, 708*b*
  telephone communications in, 77*b*
  tub baths and showers, 356*b*
  for tuberculosis, 734*b*
  for urinary incontinence, 399*b*
  for vulnerable adults, 45*b*
  waste disposal, 243*b*
  wound assessment, 613*b*
Home care agencies, 3
Home health aides, 5*t*-6*t*
Home needle destruction devices, 243*b*
Home repair and modification, 146*b*
Home safety, 181*b*, 189*b*, 802*b*, 802*f*, 877-879
Homemaker services, 146*b*

Homeostasis, 108
Home-sharing, 149
Homosexual, 794, 796
Honesty, 56b
Hook-on chairs, 880
Horizontal recumbent position, 561
Hormone therapy, 698
Hormones, 108, 122, 745b
Hospice, 1, 3, 146b, 852
Hospital bed systems, 303, 309, 310f
Hospital care
    Chains of Survival actions, 831b
    in-patient care, 2
    out-patient (ambulatory) care, 2
Hospital rooms, 2f
Hospitals, 2, 22
Hosts, susceptible, 219-220
Hot compresses, 635
Hot packs, 635-636, 638b
Hot soaks, 635
Hot-cold balance, 94b
House diet, 451
Household disposable sharps containers, 243b, 243f
Household hazardous waste, 243b
Housekeeping, 242, 825
Housing
    congregate, 149
    group settings, 149
    for older persons, 147-150, 147b
    rental options, 148-149
    senior citizen, 148
    shared, 149
Human immunodeficiency virus (HIV), 700-702
Human immunodeficiency virus (HIV) infection,
        700-702, 701b
    measures to prevent, 702
    testing for, 702b
Human resources, 861
Humidifiers, 654, 654f
Hydration, 442, 456, 470b
Hydrocephalus, 791, 791f
Hygiene, 56-57
    adaptive devices for, 337b, 337f
    hand hygiene, 222, 223b, 225b, 226f, 229b
    hand-washing procedure for, 224f-225f, 225b
    oral, 335, 338-344, 591
    personal, 146b, 335-365, 337b, 602, 778b-780b
    respiratory, 229b
Hymen, 121
Hyperalimentation, 478
Hyperextension, 513
Hyperglycemia, 739, 746, 746t
Hypertension, 486, 506, 724, 727
    pre-hypertension, 724, 727
Hyperthermia, 634, 640
Hyperthermia blankets, 640
Hyperventilation, 642, 644, 661
Hypoglycemia, 739, 746, 746t
Hypotension, 486, 506
    orthostatic, 513-514, 515b
Hypothermia, 634, 640
Hypothermia blankets, 640
Hypoventilation, 642, 644
Hypoxemia, 642, 644
Hypoxia, 642, 644, 644b

I
IBD. See Inflammatory bowel disease
ICDs. See Implantable cardiac defibrillators
Ice bags, 636, 636f
Ice packs, 637b
IDDs. See Intellectual and developmental disabilities
Identification, 759b
Identification (ID) bracelets, 156, 156f-157f, 157b
Identification of the person, 156-157, 157b, 157f
Identity, gender, 794, 796
Ileal conduits, 751, 752f
Ileostomy, 422, 437, 438f
Ileum, 119, 443b, 740b
Illness
    acute, 1-2
    in babies, 804, 804b
    chronic, 1-2
    communication barriers, 102
    effects of, 95-96, 95b

Illness (Continued)
    foodborne, 449, 468, 468b-469b
    in long-term care, 95b
    and pain, 534
    and sexual function, 796
    and sleep, 540
    terminal, 1-2, 851-852
Immune system, 123, 699b
Immune system disorders, 699-702
Immunity, 108, 123, 217, 241, 699b
Immuno-suppressive drugs, 697
Implantable cardiac defibrillators (ICDs), 730
Implementation, 83, 88-89
Impotence, 794, 796
Imprisonment, false, 38, 42, 204
Incentive spirometry, 590, 650-651, 651b
Incest, 49
Incidents, 154, 182, 183b
Incision, 604, 605b, 606f
Income, reduced, 141
Incontinence
    fecal, 422, 429-430, 430b
    urinary, 390t, 396-399
Incontinence products, 399, 399f, 400b-402b,
        402f-404f
Incus, 115, 676b
Independence, 2, 29b
    in delegated tasks, 36b
    functional status, 263b, 283b
    in health care agencies, 10b
    promoting, 17b, 19b, 215b, 279b-280b, 316b-317b,
        673b-674b, 722b
India, 100b, 448b, 852b
Indwelling catheter care, 409b, 409f
Indwelling catheters, 407-408, 408f
    parts of, 408f
    removing, 416-418, 416b-418b, 416f-417f
Infant carriers, 879
Infant seats, 879
Infant strollers and carriages, 881
Infants, 127-131, 130f-131f
    Basic Life Support (BLS) for, 838-841
    bathing, 814, 814b-817b, 814f-817f
    bottle-fed, 810
    bottle-feeding babies, 807-808, 808f-809f, 809b
    breast-fed, 810
    burping babies, 809, 810f
    cardiac arrest in, 839
    caring for mothers and babies, 800
    chest thrusts in, 168b, 168f
    collecting urine specimens from, 573, 573b-574b, 573f
    CPR for, 833b, 839-841, 839b-840b, 840f, 843b
    definition of, 126-127, 838
    developmental tasks, 128b
    diapering, 810, 811b, 812f
    feeding babies, 808, 809b
    holding babies, 801b, 801f
    home safety measures to protect, 802b, 877-879
    illness in, 804, 804b
    language development, 131, 131b
    nail care for, 817
    relieving choking in, 168b, 168f
    safety measures for, 131b, 800-804, 801b-802b,
        801f-802f, 879
    traumatic brain injury in, 711b
    weighing, 817, 817b-818b
Infected wounds, 604, 605b
Infection(s), 217-220, 612
    and cancer, 697
    chain of, 219-220, 219f
    fungal, 609b-610b
    healthcare-associated (HAI), 217, 220, 220b-221b
    local, 219
    methods of transmission of, 219, 220f
    nosocomial, 220
    in older persons, 219b
    preventing, 217-249, 409b, 733
    signs and symptoms of, 219b
    susceptible hosts, 219-220
    systemic, 219
    urinary tract, 750, 750b
Infection control, 217-218
    aseptic measures for, 226, 227b-228b, 228f
    aseptic practices for, 222, 222b
    for children, 240b

Infection control (Continued)
    isolation precautions, 228-240, 231b
    and meeting basic needs, 239-240, 240b
    for older persons, 240b
    preventive measures, 241-242
    standard precautions, 228, 229b
    transmission-based precautions, 230b-231b, 231
Inferior vena cava, 117, 725b-726b
Infestations, 366, 368
Inflammation, 611
Inflammatory bowel disease, 742
Influenza, 733, 733b, 733t
Information
    protected health information, 38, 42
    right to, 14, 14b
Informed consent, 44, 44b, 204
    surgery consent, 594
Ingrown toenails, 609b-610b, 610f
Inhalation, 118, 504b, 643b, 731b
    lead poisoning by, 161
Injury
    back injuries, 254
    combat injuries, 710
    head injuries, 709-710
    and sexual function, 796
    spinal cord injury, 711-712
    traumatic brain injury, 710
    work-related, 253-254, 255b
In-law apartments, 148
Inner ear, 115
In-patient care, 2, 588
In-service programs, 24b
In-service training, 24b
Insomnia, 531, 541
Inspiration (breathing in), 118, 504b, 643b, 731b
Insulin, 123, 745b
Intake, 442, 456
    measurement of, 456-457, 456b, 458b-459b, 458f
Intake and output (I&O) records, 456-457, 457f
Integumentary system, 110, 143b, 144, 702b
Intellectual and developmental disabilities, 786-793,
        787b
Intellectual disabilities, 786, 787b-788b, 788, 792b
Intensive care units, 96f
Intentional wounds, 604
Internal fixation, 716, 717f
Internal rotation, 513
International time, 73, 73f
Interventions, nursing, 83, 87
Interviews
    in-person, 864
    job interviews, 860, 864-867, 865b, 866f-867f, 867b
    phone, 864-865
    video, 864-865
Intimacy, 777-778
Intimate partner violence (IPV), 38, 51-52, 51b-52b
Intimidation, 44
Intravenous (IV) therapy, 473, 479-482
    assisting with, 482, 482b-484b, 482f-483f
    changing patient gowns on persons with IVs, 385b
    checking flow rate, 481, 481f-482f
    for children, 480b, 480f
    equipment for, 479f, 481, 481f
    flow rate, 473, 481
    guidelines for, 474b
    home care, 481b
    pump alarms, 484b
    safety measures, 482b
    signs and symptoms of complications, 482b
    sites, 479-480, 479f-480f, 480b
Introductions, 305, 306b, 307f
Intubation, 658
Invasion of privacy, 38, 42-43
Involuntary muscles, 112, 251b
Involuntary seclusion, 12, 16, 46
Iodine, 448t
IPV. See Intimate partner violence
Iran, 443b
Iraq, 101b
Ireland, 100b
Iris, 114
Irish, 100b
Iron, 448t, 451t-452t
Irregular bones, 110, 251b, 713b
Islam, 450b

Isolation precautions, 228-240, 231*b*
Italian Americans, 100*b*
IVs. *See* Intravenous (IV) therapy

J

Jacket restraints, 211, 211*f*, 212*b*-214*b*
Jackson-Pratt drainage system, 613, 614*f*
Jaundice, 739, 743*b*, 743*f*
Jejunostomy tubes, 473-474, 475*f*
Jejunum, 119, 443*b*, 740*b*
Jewelry, 591
Jewish Americans, 100*b*
Job applications, 860-864, 862*f*-863*f*, 864*b*
Job descriptions, 21, 26-29, 27*f*-28*f*, 29*b*
Job interviews, 860, 864-867, 866*b*
    common questions, 865*b*
    grooming and dressing for, 865*b*, 866*f*
    questions not allowed by EEOC, 867*b*
    questions you cannot be asked, 866, 867*b*
    thank-you letters or notes for, 867, 867*f*
Job offers, 867
Job safety, 61
Job skills and training, 861, 861*b*
Job titles, 29, 29*b*
Job-related questions, 868*b*
Jobs, 860
Joint care, 713
Joint Commission, The (TJC), 201
Joint injuries, 713
Joint replacement surgery, 713
    hip replacement care, 714*b*, 715*f*
    knee replacement care, 714*b*
Joints, 108, 111, 251*b*, 713*b*
    ball-and-socket, 111, 111*f*, 713*b*, 713*f*
    hinge, 111, 111*f*, 713*b*, 713*f*
    pivot, 111, 111*f*, 713*b*, 713*f*
    types of, 111, 111*f*, 251*b*, 251*f*, 713*f*
JPMA. *See* Juvenile Products Manufacturers
    Association
Judaism (Jewish faith), 450*b*, 813
Juvenile Products Manufacturers Association (JPMA)
    safety certification seal, 803*b*, 804*f*
Juvenile rheumatoid arthritis, 714*b*

K

Kardex or care summaries, 67, 72*f*
Kennedy terminal ulcers, 626, 626*f*
Ketone bodies. *See* Ketones
Ketones, 567, 574
Kidney cancer, 695*b*-696*b*
Kidney failure, 753, 753*b*
    acute, 753
    chronic kidney disease, 753
Kidney stones, 752-753, 752*f*-753*f*, 756*b*
Kidneys, 119, 389*b*, 389*f*, 750*b*
Kitchens, 147*b*, 158*b*, 877
Kneading, 537*b*-538*b*, 538*f*
Knee exercises, 519*b*-520*b*, 521*f*
Knee replacement care, 714*b*
Knee replacement prosthesis, 713, 714*f*
Knee-chest position, 561, 564, 564*f*
Kübler-Ross, Elisabeth: stages of dying, 853
Kussmaul respirations, 642, 644

L

Labeling
    on bariatric equipment, 169
    food labels, 448, 448*f*
    on hazardous chemical containers, 171
    warning labels, 171, 171*f*
Labia majora, 121
Labia minora, 121
Laboratory technicians, 5*t*-6*t*
Laceration, 604, 605*b*, 606*f*
Language
    abbreviations, 77-80
    body language, 92, 100
    common terms and phrases, 80, 80*b*
    communication barriers, 102
    directional terms, 79, 80*f*
    medical terminology, 77-80, 78*b*-79*b*
    professional, 60
    terms for incontinence products, 400*b*
    terms for intellectual disabilities, 788*b*
    words to describe pain, 535*b*

Language delays, 789
Language development, 131, 131*b*
Large intestine (large bowel or colon), 119, 423*b*,
    443*b*, 740*b*
Laryngeal cancer, 695*b*-696*b*
Laryngeal mirror, 561
Larynx (voice box), 118, 504*b*, 643*b*, 731*b*
Late adulthood, 128*b*, 137
Late childhood, 128*b*
Lateral position, 250, 258*f*, 259
Lateral transfer device with slide board, 292, 293*f*
Lateral transfers, 255*b*, 281, 292-293
Laughter, 859*b*
Laundry, 244*b*
    in assisted living, 826, 826*b*
    contaminated, 241*b*, 242
    standard precautions for, 229*b*
Laundry areas, 878
Law(s), 38-54
    criminal, 38, 41
    and delegation of tasks, 36*b*
    federal, 22-25
    for health care agencies, 10*b*
    nurse practice acts, 22
    for nursing assistants, 29*b*
    for protecting person's rights, 19*b*
    state, 22-25
Laxatives, 426
Lead poisoning, 161, 161*b*-162*b*
Learning disabilities, 789
Least restrictive methods, 204
Left atrium, 116, 497*b*, 725*b*-726*b*
Left bronchus, 118, 504*b*, 643*b*, 731*b*
Left lymphatic duct (thoracic duct), 118
Left ventricle, 497*b*, 725*b*-726*b*
Leg bags, 412, 413*b*-414*b*, 414*f*
Leg exercises, post-operative, 598, 598*f*
Leg prostheses, 722*f*
Legal aspects, 40-44
Legal assistance, 146*b*
Legal issues, 855-856
Legs: shaving, 376
Lens, 114, 682*b*
Lesbian, 796
Leukemia, 695*b*-696*b*
Leukocytes, 116, 725*b*-726*b*
Liability, 41
Libel, 38, 42
Lice. *See* Pediculosis
Licensed practical nurses (LPNs), 1, 5*t*-6*t*, 7
Licensed vocational nurses (LVNs), 1, 5*t*-6*t*, 7
Licensure, 9, 24*b*
Life-style changes
    for arthritis, 713
    for GERDM, 740
    in retirement, 141
    and sleep, 540
Lift teams, 282*b*
Lifting, 253, 255*b*
Lifts, mechanical, 295-296, 295*f*, 296*b*-299*b*, 298*f*,
    300*f*
Ligaments, 111
Lighting, 306, 306*b*
    call lights, 188*b*-189*b*, 313, 313*f*-314*f*
    home assessment checklist, 672*b*-673*b*
    safety measures to prevent falls, 188*b*-189*b*
Limbs: loss of, 721
Limited assistance (functional status), 283*b*
Linens, 320-322, 320*f*-321*f*, 321*b*, 329*b*-330*b*, 330*f*,
    333*b*
Lip cancer, 695*b*-696*b*
Liquid oxygen systems, 651, 652*f*
Listening, 100, 101*f*, 102, 854
Lithotomy position, 561, 564, 564*f*
Liver, 119, 443*b*, 740*b*
Liver damage, 744*f*
Liver spots, 144
Living wills, 855
Local anesthesia, 588, 595
Local infection, 219
Lochia, 800, 819
Lochia alba, 819
Lochia rubra, 819
Lochia serosa, 819
Locks, 778*b*-780*b*, 781*f*

Logrolling, 262, 275, 275*b*, 276*f*
Long bones, 110, 251*b*, 713*b*
Long-term care
    admissions, transfers, and discharges in, 546*b*, 547*b*
    assessment in, 86*b*
    bed rails in, 192*b*
    care conferences for, 88*b*
    comfort measures, 532*b*
    dressing and undressing in, 379*b*
    elder abuse in, 48*b*
    emergency care, 830*b*
    fecal impaction in, 427*b*
    flow sheets in, 71*b*
    hair care, 367*b*
    identifying the person in, 157*b*
    illness and disability in, 95*b*
    job skills and training for work in, 861*b*
    linens and linen changes, 321*b*
    mechanical ventilation in, 663*b*
    nutritional assessment in, 443*b*
    nutritional needs in, 449*b*
    personal belongings in, 182*b*
    person's unit in, 304*b*
    for persons with AD and other dementias, 782*b*
    for persons with intellectual and developmental
        disabilities, 787*b*
    persons you will care for in, 97*b*
    pressure ulcers in, 623*b*
    privacy curtains in, 312*b*
    progress notes in, 69*b*
    promoting sleep in, 542*b*
    range-of-motion exercises in, 518*b*
    rehabilitation in, 667*b*, 672*b*
    restorative care, 667*b*
    risk factors for falls in, 187*b*
    safety and security needs in, 94*b*
    serving meals, 462*b*, 462*f*
    sexual needs in, 797*b*, 797*f*
    shampooing, 372*b*
    stroke care, 708*b*
    for tuberculosis, 734*b*
    for victims of intimate partner violence, 52*b*
Long-term care centers, 3, 4*b*
Loss of limb, 721
Lost, getting, 774-775, 774*b*
Lotion, 537
Lou Gehrig's disease, 709
Love and affection, 796, 797*f*
Love and belonging, 94, 539
Low vision, 675, 685
LPNs. *See* Licensed practical nurses
Lumbar injuries, 711
Lung cancer, 695*b*-696*b*
Lungs, 731*b*
Lupus, 699, 700*f*
LVNs. *See* Licensed vocational nurses
Lymph, 117, 735*b*
Lymph nodes, 118, 735*b*
Lymphatic disorders, 735-736
Lymphatic system, 117-118, 117*f*, 735*b*, 735*f*
Lymphatic vessels, 118, 735*b*
Lymphedema, 724, 736, 736*b*, 736*f*
Lymphocytes, 117, 123, 699*b*, 735*b*
Lymphoma, 695*b*-696*b*, 736

M

MA-C. *See* Medication assistant-certified
Macula, 682*b*
Macular degeneration, 683*f*, 684
Mail-back programs, 243*b*
Major depression, 761
Male perineal care, 362*b*, 362*f*
Male reproductive system, 120-121, 121*f*, 754, 795*f*
    changes in aging, 143*b*, 146
    structure and function of, 795*b*, 795*f*
Malignant tumors, 693, 694*f*
Malleus, 115, 676*b*
Malpractice, 38, 41
Mammary glands (breasts), 122, 122*f*
Managed care, 22
Mandatory reporters, 52*b*-53*b*
Mania (manic episode), 761, 761*b*
Manometers, 509*b*-510*b*, 511*f*
Manual alphabet, 678, 679*f*
Manual beds, 306, 307*f*

Manual lifting, 255b
Masks, 232, 234f-236f, 237b, 238f
Massage, 537, 537b
Master gland, 122
Masturbation, 798
Material safety data sheets (MSDS), 172
Mathematics
    for counting respirations, 505b
    CPR for children and infants, 839b
    for giving enemas, 431b
    for measuring blood pressure, 509b
    for measuring food intake, 455b
    for measuring intake and output, 458b
    for measuring weight and height, 307b
    for removing indwelling catheters, 416b
    for taking apical and apical-radial pulses, 502b
    for taking radial pulses, 500b
    for taking temperatures with glass thermometers, 495b
    for weighing infants, 817b
MCI. See Mild cognitive impairment
MDROs. See Multidrug-resistant organisms
Meal programs, 146b
Meal time practices, 443b
Meal trays, 463b
Meals, 61
    in assisted living, 825
    preparing the person for, 460, 460b-461b
    serving, 462, 462b-463b, 462f, 470b
Measurement(s)
    converting measures, 307b, 456b
    post-operative, 596
Meatus, 120, 389b, 750b
Mechanical lifts, 295-296, 295f, 296b-299b, 298f, 300f
Mechanical ventilation, 658, 662, 662f, 663b, 670
Meconium, 800, 810
Medicaid, 8
Medical asepsis, 217, 221-226
Medical devices, 627b-628b
Medical diagnosis, 83, 86
Medical Emergency Teams (METs), 830
Medical laboratory technician, 5t-6t
Medical neglect, 49
Medical records, 67-71, 68f
Medical records technicians, 5t-6t
Medical symptoms, 200, 202
Medical terminology, 77-80, 78b-80b
MedicAlert®, 775, 778b-780b
Medicare, 8, 9b
Medication assistance, 826-827, 827b
Medication assistant-certified (MA-C), 5t-6t
Medication management, self-directed, 827
Medication records, 827
Medication reminders, 822, 826
Medications. See Drugs
Medulla, 114, 706b
Melanoma, 695b-696b
Melena, 567, 577
Menarche, 126, 135
Meniere's disease, 677
Meninges, 114
Meningocele, 790, 791f
Meningomyelocele, 790, 791f
Menopause, 126, 137
Menstrual cycle, 122
Menstruation, 108, 122
Mental abuse, 46
Mental health, 757-758
Mental health centers, 3
Mental health disorders, 96, 97b, 757-768, 766b, 855
Mental illness. See Mental health disorders
Mental retardation (term), 788b
Metabolism, 108, 123
Metastasis, 693, 694f
Methicillin-resistant Staphylococcus aureus (MRSA), 218
METs. See Medical Emergency Teams
Mexican Americans, 94b
Mexico, 100b-101b, 448b, 534b
Microbes, 218-219, 220f
Microorganisms, 217-218
Micturition. See Urination
Midbrain, 114, 706b
Middle adulthood, 128b, 137, 137f-138f
Middle ear, 115
Midstream urine specimens, 570, 570b-571b, 570f

Mild cognitive impairment, 771
Military time, 73, 73f
Mineralocorticoids, 123
Minerals, 447, 448t
Minimum Data Set, 874
Minors, 138b
Misappropriation, financial, 46, 776b
Misconduct, professional, 38, 40
Mistreatment. See also Abuse
    right to freedom from, 16, 673b-674b
Mitered corners, 324b-325b, 326f
Mites, 366, 368
Mitosis, 109
Mitral valve (bicuspid valve), 116, 725b-726b
Mitt restraints, 205b-206b, 210, 210f, 212b-214b
Mitted washcloths, 350b-351b, 351f
Mixed aphasia. See Global aphasia
Mixed incontinence, 388, 397
Mobile food carts, 470b
Mobility
    accident risk factors, 156
    bed mobility, 262, 263b
    with impaired vision and blindness, 688
    Minimum Data Set form, 875f
    rehabilitation for, 668, 669f-670f
Moist cold applications, 637
Moist heat applications, 635-636, 635f
Moles, 693, 695b-696b
Molestation, 49
Monitoring, 179b, 179f
Mons pubis, 121
Montgomery ties, 615, 615f
Morbid obesity, 92, 96
Morning care, 335, 337, 338b
Moro reflex, 128, 129f
Motor aphasia. See Expressive aphasia
Mothers, 96, 800, 805, 806b, 818-819, 820b
Mouth (oral cavity), 85b, 119, 423b, 443b, 740b
Mouth, nose, and eye protection, 229b
Mouth cancer, 695b-696b
Mouth care. See Oral hygiene
Mouth problems, 855
Mouth-to-mouth breathing, 834, 834f
Mouth-to-mouth-and-nose breathing, 839b-840b, 841f
Mouth-to-nose breathing, 835, 835f
Mouth-to-stoma breathing, 835, 835f
Movement, 85b
    freedom of, 200
Movement disorders, 760
Moving the person, 262-280, 262b-263b
    with assist devices, 269, 270b, 270f
    in bed, 255b, 265-271, 265b-266b
    communication for, 262b, 265b
    measures to prevent injuries, 255b, 263b-264b
    measures to promote comfort, 263b
    raising the person's head and shoulders, 266, 266b, 267f
    to the side of the bed, 271, 271f, 272b
    to a stretcher, 293b
    up in bed, 267, 267f, 268b, 269, 269f-270f, 270b
MRSA. See Methicillin-resistant Staphylococcus aureus
MSDs. See Musculo-skeletal disorders
MSDS. See Material safety data sheets
Multidrug-resistant organisms, 218
Multiple sclerosis, 709, 709b
Muscle atrophy, 514, 514f
Muscle tissue, 109
Muscles, 112, 112f, 251b, 252f
Musculo-skeletal disorders, 712-721
    preventing, 254
    risk factors for, 253-254
    work-related, 250, 253
Musculo-skeletal system, 110-112, 251b
    changes in aging, 143b, 144
    structure and function of, 713b
Mustaches, 376
Myelin sheath, 113, 706b
Myelomeningocele, 790, 791f
Myocardial infarction, 729, 729b, 729f
Myocardium, 116
MyPlate, 444-447, 444f, 445b, 445t
Mysophobia, 759
Myths, 140, 141b

N
Nail and foot care, 376-377, 376b-378b, 379f, 817
Nails, 110
Narcotics, 643
Nasal cannula, 653, 653f
Nasal speculum, 561
Naso-enteral tubes, 473-474, 475f
Naso-gastric (NG) tubes, 473-474, 474f
National Council of State Boards of Nursing (NCSBN), 23
    delegation process, 33, 33f
    Five Rights of Delegation, 35, 35b
    reasons for losing certification, a license, or registration, 24b
National Domestic Violence Hotline, 52b-53b
National Federation of Licensed Practical Nurses, 39
National Institute on Aging (NIA), 773b, 775
National Nurse Aide Assessment Program (NNAAP®), 873
National Pressure Ulcer Advisory Panel (NPUAP), 622
NCSBN. See National Council of State Boards of Nursing
Neck exercises, 519b-520b, 519f
Need(s), 92-93
    basic, 93-94, 93f, 239-240, 240b, 619
    at end of life, 852-855, 853b
    for love and belonging, 94
    for oxygen, 642-657
    physical, 93, 539, 854-855
    for safety and security, 93, 94b, 539
    for self-actualization, 94
    for self-esteem, 94
    special: persons with, 103
    spiritual, 783b, 852-853, 853b
Needle disposal, 243b
Neglect, 38
    child, 38, 48-49, 50b
    educational, 49
    elder, 46
    emotional, 49
    medical, 49
    physical, 49
    reporting, 52b-53b
    right to freedom from, 16
    self-neglect, 38
    after stroke, 707
Negligence, 38, 41, 405b
Neonates, 127. See also Newborns
Nephrons, 120, 120f, 750b
Nerve tissue, 109
Nervous system, 113-115
    changes in aging, 143b, 144-145, 770b
    disorders of, 705-712
    oxygen needs, 643
    structure and function, 706b
Newborns, 96, 127-129, 128f
    caring for mothers and babies, 800, 820b
NG tubes. See Naso-gastric tubes
Niacin (vitamin B3), 447t
Nipple, 122
NNAAP. See National Nurse Aide Assessment Program
"No Code" orders, 856
Nocturia, 388, 390t
Nocturnal emissions (wet dreams), 135
Noise, 305, 306b
Non-Hodgkin lymphoma, 736
Non-pathogens, 217-218
Non-rebreather masks, 653, 653f
Non-specific immunity, 123
Nonverbal communication, 92, 99-100, 766b
Norepinephrine, 123
Normal flora, 217-218, 233
North American Nursing Diagnosis Association International (NANDA-I), 86b
Northern Europeans, 100b
Nose, 85b, 118
Nose and eye protection, 229b
Nose problems, 855
Nosocomial infections, 220
Nothing by mouth (NPO) order, 456
NREM sleep, 531, 539, 540b
Nucleus of cell, 108
Nurse practice acts, 22
Nurse practitioners, 5t-6t, 7

Nurse supervisors or managers, 6
Nursery equipment safety, 879-882
Nursing: assisting with, 83-91
Nursing assistant registries, 23
Nursing assistants, 5t-6t, 8, 21-30
    certification for, 23
    code of conduct for, 39b
    competency evaluation for, 23
    current trends, 21-22
    definition of, 1
    history of, 21-22
    job descriptions, 26-29, 27f-28f, 29b
    job titles, 29, 29b
    laws for, 22
    maintaining competence, 24, 24b
    roles and responsibilities of, 25-29, 25b-26b, 35-36,
        90
    rules for, 25b
    standards for, 26, 26b
    training programs for, 22, 23f
    working in another state, 24-25
Nursing care. See also specific types of nursing
    assisting with, 83-91
    functional, 1, 8
    patterns of care, 8, 8f
    primary, 1, 8
    restorative, 666-674
    team, 1, 8
Nursing care plans, 83, 87, 87f
Nursing centers, 149-150, 149f, 152b
    barber shops in, 367b
    beauty shops in, 367b, 367f
    when care is needed, 782
    dining programs in, 462b
    environment requirements for, 150, 150b
    features of, 151b
    organization of, 4b
Nursing diagnoses, 83, 86, 86b
Nursing education staff, 7
Nursing history (health history), 69
Nursing interventions, 83, 87
Nursing mothers. See Breast-feeding
Nursing process, 83, 84f, 90b
    roles in, 90
    steps, 83
Nursing services, 6-7
    in assisted living, 826
Nursing tasks, 21, 31
    accepting, 35
    example tasks that can and cannot be delegated to
        you, 32b
    refusing, 35-36, 36b
Nursing team, 1, 7-8
Nursing team members, 306b, 307f
Nutrients, 442, 444, 447
Nutrition, 442-472, 444b
    basic, 444-448
    factors affecting, 449
    and hip fractures, 719
    meeting nutritional needs, 448-449
    and oxygen needs, 643
    rehabilitation for, 670
    and sleep, 540
Nutritional assessment, 443b
Nutritional support, 473-485
    end-of-life care, 855
    enteral nutrition, 473-477
    guidelines for, 474b
    in home care, 449b
    in long-term care, 449b
    for older persons, 450b
    parenteral nutrition, 473, 478-479, 478f
    post-operative care, 602
    pre-operative care, 590
    total parenteral nutrition (TPN), 478-479
Nutritionists, 5t-6t
Nyctophobia, 759

O

Obamacare (Patient Protection and Affordable Care
    Act), 9
Obesity, 92, 96
    and cancer, 697
    chest thrusts for obese persons, 165b
    morbid, 92, 96

Objective data, 83-84
OBRA. See Omnibus Budget Reconciliation Act of 1987
Observation(s), 83-84
    basic, 85b
    bowel elimination, 424b
    cast care, 718b
    with chest tubes, 664b
    of cirrhosis, 745b
    with dressings, 616b
    enteral nutrition, 476
    while giving enemas, 432b
    indwelling catheter care, 409b
    while inserting suppositories, 431b
    parenteral nutrition, 479
    personal hygiene, 363, 363b
    post-operative, 596, 596b
    to report at once, 712
    reporting, 84, 84b, 84f
    in umbilical cord care, 813
    urination, 390
    vital signs, 487
    wound, 613b
Obsessions, 757, 759
Obsessive-compulsive disorder, 759
Obstetrics, 92, 96
Occult blood, 577, 578b-579b, 579f
Occupational exposure, 241b
Occupational Safety and Health Administration
    (OSHA)
    Bloodborne Pathogen Standard, 240-243
    guidelines for preventing workplace violence, 178
    Hazard Communication Standard (HCS), 171
    recommendations for moving the person from the
        floor, 197, 197f
    recommendations for preventing work-related
        injuries, 263
    requirements for contaminated laundry, 242
    requirements for PPE, 242
    requirements for work practice controls, 242
    risk factors for MSDs, 253-254
Occupational therapist registration (OTR), 5t-6t
Occupational therapy assistant, 5t-6t
Occupied beds, 319, 320f, 328, 328b
    making, 329b-330b, 330f-331f
    safety and comfort measures for, 324b, 328b
Ocular prostheses, 690, 690f, 691b
Odors, 305
Oil glands, 110, 702b
Oil-retention enemas, 431, 436, 436b
Oils, 447
The Older American Act, 18
Older persons, 96, 104b, 137, 142f
    accident risk factors, 156b
    activity in, 514b
    alcoholism and alcohol abuse in, 763b
    applying dressings to, 616b
    applying restraints to, 212b
    aseptic practices with, 222b
    attitudes about death, 853b
    bathing, 348b, 353b
    bedroom options for, 147b
    blood pressure in, 507b
    body temperature, 488b
    care for, 140-153
    collecting sputum specimens from, 580b
    comfort measures for, 854b
    communication(s) with, 142b
    community-based services for, 146b
    dangling, 276b
    dementia in, 771b
    depression in, 761, 762b
    diarrhea in, 429b
    draping, 564b
    dressing and undressing, 379b
    drug abuse and addiction in, 764b
    eating, 450b
    exercise for, 514b
    factors affecting BMs, 425b
    falling, 196b
    family and friends of, 104b
    fecal incontinence in, 430b
    feeding, 464b
    flossing in, 339b
    fluid requirements, 456b
    heat and cold applications for, 634b

Older persons (Continued)
    HIV/AIDS in, 701b
    infection control with, 240b
    infection in, 219b
    influenza in, 733b
    in-home services for, 146b
    lighting needs, 306b
    living with family, 148
    nutrition for, 450b
    otitis media in, 676b
    pain in, 534b
    personal hygiene for, 337b
    physical examinations of, 562b, 565b
    pneumonia in, 734b
    positioning, 564b, 597b
    preparing for physical examination, 562b
    pressure ulcers in, 624b
    preventing aspiration in, 477b
    preventing burns with, 159b
    preventing respiratory and circulatory
        complications in, 597b
    preventing work-related injuries with, 263b
    promoting sleep in, 542b
    psychological changes in, 140-142
    rehabilitation for, 667b
    relieving choking in, 166b
    risk of skin tears in, 607b
    safe care measures for, 263b
    sensitivity to temperature and ventilation, 305b
    sexuality and, 796
    sexually transmitted diseases in, 754b
    shampooing, 371b
    shaving, 374b
    skin protection for, 265b
    social changes for, 140-142
    social relationships of, 141-142, 142b
    suicide in, 766b
    taking temperatures in, 491b
    tolerance for noise levels, 306b
    towel baths for, 353b
    transferring, 282b
    tuberculosis in, 734b
    urinary incontinence in, 398b
    vital signs in, 487b
Oliguria, 388, 390t, 749, 750b
Ombudsman, 12, 18
Ombudsman programs, 18
Ombudsman services, 18
Omnibus Budget Reconciliation Act of 1987 (OBRA), 12,
    22-24, 44, 150, 797b, 855
    required actions to promote dignity and privacy,
        17b
    required actions when abuse is suspected, 48b
    requirements for resident rooms, 304b
    requirements for summaries of care, 69b
One-rescuer carry, 178f
Open beds, 328, 328b
Open dining, 462b
Open fractures, 705, 716, 716f
Open head injuries, 709
Open wounds, 604
Operating rooms: transport to, 595
Ophthalmoscopes, 561
OPIM. See Other potentially infectious material
Opposition, 513
Optic nerve, 682b
Optimal level of function, 92, 96
    steps to help maintain, 124b
Oral cavity (mouth), 119, 443b
Oral hygiene, 335, 338-344, 339b, 363b
    pre-operative, 591
    for unconscious persons, 342, 342f, 343b-344b
Oral temperature, 488b, 488t, 511b
Oral thermometers, disposable, 490, 490f
Organs, 108-109, 114-115
Oro-pharyngeal airways, 658, 659f
Orthopedic rehabilitation, 671
Orthopnea, 642, 644
Orthopneic position, 642, 647, 647f
Orthostatic hypotension, 513-514, 515b
Orthotic devices, 513, 528
OSHA. See Occupational Safety and Health
    Administration
Ossicles, 115
Osteoarthritis, 712, 713f

Osteomyelitis, 631
Osteoporosis, 721
Ostomy, 422, 436-438
Ostomy pouches, 438, 438b-439b, 438f
Other potentially infectious material (OPIM), 241b
Otitis media, 676, 676b
Otoscopes, 561
Outdoor home safety measures, 878
Out-patient (ambulatory) care, 2
Output, 442, 456
    intake and output (I&O) records, 456-457, 457f
    measurement of, 456-457, 456b, 458-459b, 458f
Ova, 121
Ovaries, 121, 795b
Over-active bladder. See Urge incontinence
Over-bed tables, 312
Over-flow incontinence, 388, 397
Over-weight, 713
Ovulation, 121
Oxygen, 642
Oxygen concentrations, 642
Oxygen concentrators, 651, 652f
Oxygen flow rate, 654, 654f
Oxygen hoods, 654b, 654f
Oxygen masks
    non-rebreather masks, 653, 653f
    partial-rebreather masks, 653, 653f
    simple face masks, 653, 653f
    Venturi masks, 653, 653f
Oxygen needs, 642-657, 647b
Oxygen tanks, 651, 651f-652f
Oxygen therapy, 651-655, 652b, 656b
    for children, 654b
    fire safety with, 174b, 175
    home care, 652b
    oxygen devices, 653
    oxygen set-ups, 654, 654f, 655b
    oxygen sources, 651
    safety measures for, 175, 652b, 655, 656b
    setting up, 655b
Oxytocin, 123

P
PA. See Physician's assistant
Pacemakers, 730, 730f
Pacifier thermometers, 489, 489f
Pacifiers, 882
Packing, 634
    cold packs, 638b
    hot packs, 635-636, 638b
    ice packs, 637b
PACU. See Post-anesthesia care unit
Padded tongue blades, 342, 343f
Padded waterproof drawsheets, 319, 322, 322f
Pads and cushions, gel- or fluid-filled, 628
Pads and under-garments, 399, 399f, 401b-402b, 403f
Pain, 511, 531-537, 532b
    acute, 531, 533
    and blood pressure, 506b
    chronic, 531, 533
    communication about, 532b, 535b
    at end of life, 854
    factors affecting, 533-534, 534b
    gallbladder, 533f
    from kidney stones, 752, 753f, 756b
    nursing measures for, 536, 536b, 536f
    observations of, 85b
    and oxygen needs, 643
    phantom, 531, 533, 721
    pre-operative teaching about, 590
    radiating, 531, 533, 533f
    signs and symptoms of, 534, 535b
    after surgery, 602
    types of, 533
    value or meaning of, 533
    words to describe, 535b
Pain control, 713
Pain rating scales, 534, 534f
Pain reactions, 534b
Pakistan, 104b
Palliative care, 851-852
Palmar grasp reflex, 128, 129f
Pancreas, 119, 123, 443b, 740b, 745b
Pancreatic cancer, 695b-696b
Panic, 757, 759

Panic attacks, 759
Panic disorder, 759
Paper charting, 75b, 75f. See also Recording
Paralysis, 154, 156, 705, 711, 712b
Paranoia, 762, 769, 775, 776b, 778b-780b
Paraphrasing, 92, 101
Paraplegia, 154, 156, 705, 711, 711f
Parasympathetic nervous system, 114, 706b
Parathormone, 123
Parathyroid glands, 123
Parenteral nutrition, 473, 478-479, 478f
Parents, 126
Parking your car, 180b-181b
Parkinson's disease, 708, 708f
Partial baths, 353, 353b-354b
Partial-rebreather masks, 653, 653f
Partner abuse. See Intimate partner violence (IPV)
Past experience, 533
Pathogens, 217-218, 240-243, 241b
Patience, 56b
Patient care partnership, 13b
The Patient Care Partnership: Understanding
    Expectations, Rights, and Responsibilities, 12
Patient gowns: changing, 384, 384b-385b, 385f
Patient Protection and Affordable Care Act
    (Obamacare), 9
Patient rights, 12
Patient Self-Determination Act, 855
Patient-focused care, 1, 8, 22
Paying for health care, 8-9
Pedal pulses, 503, 503f-504f
Pediatrics, 92, 96
Pediculosis (lice), 366, 368
Pediculosis capitis (head lice), 366, 368, 368f
Pediculosis corporis (body lice), 366, 368
Pediculosis pubis (pubic lice), 366, 368, 755t
Peers, 126
PEG tubes. See Percutaneous endoscopic gastrostomy
    tubes
Penetrating wounds, 604, 605b, 606f
Penis, 120, 795b
    circumcised, 335, 358, 358f
    uncircumcised, 335, 358, 358f
Penrose drains, 613, 614f
Percussion hammers, 561
Percutaneous endoscopic gastrostomy (PEG) tubes,
    473-474, 475f
Pericardium, 116
Pericare. See Perineal care
Perineal care, 335, 358, 358b
    communication for, 358b
    female, 359b-360b, 361f
    male, 362b, 362f
    nursing measures for, 398b
    observations to report and record, 363b
    safety and comfort measures, 359b
Peripheral nervous system, 113-114, 113f, 706b
Peripherally inserted central catheters (PICCs), 480
Peristalsis, 108, 119, 422, 423b, 740b
Peritoneal dialysis, 753, 754f
Persecution: delusions of, 757, 760
Persistent pain. See Chronic pain
Person(s), 92-107, 93f
    with disabilities, 103
    persons you will care for, 96, 97b
Personal belongings, 182, 182b
Personal care, 591b. See also Personal hygiene
    pre-operative, 591
Personal care items, 313, 313f
Personal choice, 15
    in clothing, 15, 15f
    and food practices, 449
    OBRA-required actions to promote, 17b
    in person's unit, 316b-317b
    right to, 858b
Personal duties, 533
Personal grooming, 58f
Personal hygiene, 335-365
    adaptive devices for, 337b, 337f
    afternoon care, 338b
    communication during procedures, 336b
    cultural differences in, 336b
    daily care, 337, 338b
    early morning care, 337, 338b
    evening care, 335, 337, 338b

Personal hygiene (Continued)
    morning care, 335, 337, 338b
    observations to report and record, 363b
    for older persons, 146b, 337b
    oral hygiene, 335, 338-344
    perineal care, 335
    for persons with AD and other dementias,
        778b-780b
    for persons with bariatric needs, 349
    reporting and recording, 363
    right to refuse, 363b-364b
    safety measures, 337b
    after surgery, 602
    ways to promote, 778b-780b
Personal items, 16
Personal matters, 60-61
Personal possessions, 858b
Personal privacy, 15
Personal protective equipment (PPE), 232-239, 241b,
    242
    airborne precautions, 230b
    donning and removing, 233, 234b, 234f-236f, 237b
    droplet precautions, 230b
    requirements for, 242
    standard precautions, 229b
    time management with, 232b
Personal responsibility, 29b
    for delegation, 36b
    in health care agency work, 10b
    for protecting person's rights, 19b
    for reporting abuse and neglect, 52b-53b
    in workplace, 65b
Personal safety measures, 180b-181b, 181f
Personality, 757-758
Personality disorders, 762
Personnel offices, 861
Person's rights, 12-20
Person's unit, 303-318, 303f, 304b, 316b-317b
    in end-of-life care, 855
    preparing the person's room, 303f, 305, 306b, 589
Petit mal seizures, 846
pH, 119, 574
Phagocytes, 123, 123f, 699b
Phantom pain, 531, 533, 721
Pharmacists, 5t-6t
Pharynx (throat), 118-119, 443b, 504b, 643b, 731b,
    740b
Philippines, 100b, 448b, 534b
Phlebitis, 604, 608
Phobias, 757, 759
Phone communications, 77, 77b
    answering phones, 77b
    reassurance for older persons, 146b
Phone interviews, 864-865
Phosphorus, 448t
Physical abuse
    child abuse, 48, 50b
    elder abuse, 46
    examples, 46b
Physical activity, 444, 445b
    and cancer, 697
    recommendations for, 444, 445b
Physical disabilities, 789
Physical examinations, 561-566, 562b, 565b
    equipment for, 561, 562f
    positioning and draping for, 564, 564f
    preparing the person for, 562, 562b-563b
Physical needs, 93, 539, 854-855
Physical neglect, 49
Physical restraints, 200, 203
Physical therapists (PTs), 5t-6t
Physical violence
    intimate partner violence (IPV), 51
    threats of, 51
Physicians (doctors), 5t-6t
    orders from, 26b
Physician's assistant (PA), 5t-6t
Physiology, 108
Pia mater, 114
Pictograms, 171, 172f
Picture boards, 98, 99f
Picture signs, 778b-780b, 780f
Pigment, 702b
Pill organizers, 826, 826f
Pillowcases, 324b-325b, 327f

Pinna, 115
Pituitary gland, 122
Pivot, 281, 286
Pivot joints, 111, 111f, 251b, 251f, 713b, 713f
Planning, 83, 86-88, 87b
  for delegating work, 33
  your work, 61, 61b
Plantar flexion, 513, 515
Plantar warts, 609b-610b, 610f
Plaque, 335, 338
Plasma, 116, 725b-726b
Plastics safety, 164b
Platelets, 116, 725b-726b
Playpens, 880-881
Pleural effusion, 658, 663
PM care. See Evening care
Pneumonia, 643, 724, 733-734, 734b
Pneumothorax, 658, 663
Podiatrists, 5t-6t
Poison(s), 154, 159
Poison Control Center, 160b
Poisoning, 844
  carbon monoxide, 161, 163b
  emergency measures for, 844
  intentional, 159
  lead, 161, 161b-162b
  preventing, 159-161, 159b-160b, 161f
  signs and symptoms of, 844
  unintentional, 159
Poland, 448b
Policy books, 41, 42f
Pollutants, 642-643
Polyuria, 388, 390t
Pons, 114, 706b
Pornography, child, 49
Portable screens, 312, 312f
Portable tubs (shower trolleys), 355
Posey quick-release tie, 205b-206b, 207f
Positioning the person, 256-259
  in bed, 515
  and blood pressure, 506b
  for burping babies, 809
  cast care, 718b
  chair position, 259
  comfort measures, 256b
  communication for, 256b
  delegation guidelines for, 256b
  dorsal recumbent position, 250, 259, 561, 564, 564f
  droplet precautions, 230b
  exam positions, 564
  Fowler's position, 250, 256, 257b, 257f
  horizontal recumbent position, 561
  knee-chest position, 561, 564, 564f
  lateral position, 258f, 259
  lithotomy position, 561, 564, 564f
  for meeting oxygen needs, 647
  moving the person to the side of the bed, 271, 271f, 272f
  moving the person up in bed, 267, 267f, 268b
  for older persons, 564b, 597b
  orthopneic, 642, 647, 647f
  for physical examination, 564, 564f
  post-operative, 597
  for postural drainage, 580b, 580f
  pre-operative teaching about restrictions, 590
  pre-operative teaching about turning persons, 590
  for preventing pressure ulcers, 627b-628b
  prone position, 258f, 259
  raising the person's head and shoulders, 266, 266b, 267f
  recovery position, 838, 838f
  re-positioning, 273b-274b, 279, 279f, 590
  restrictions, 590
  safety measures, 256b
  Sims' position, 250, 258f, 259, 564, 564f
  standard precautions, 229b
  supine position, 258f, 259
  supportive devices for, 515
  30-degree lateral position, 627b-628b, 628f
  turn clock for, 628f
  turning persons, 273-275, 273b-274b, 274f, 590
Post-anesthesia care unit (PACU), 590, 590f
Posterior pituitary lobe, 122
Post-mortem care, 851, 856, 857b
Post-operative (post-op) beds, 331

Post-operative (post-op) care, 595-602
  comfort and rest, 602
  early ambulation, 601
  leg exercises, 598, 598f
  measurements and observations, 596, 596b
  nutrition and fluids, 602
  personal hygiene, 602
  preventing respiratory and circulatory complications, 597-601, 597b
Postpartum care, 800, 818
Postpartum complications, 819b
Post-traumatic stress disorder, 760, 760b
Postural drainage: positions for, 580b, 580f
Postural hypotension. See Orthostatic hypotension
Postural supports, 259, 260f
Posture, 250, 253. See also Body alignment
  body language, 92, 100
Potassium, 448t
PPE. See Personal protective equipment
PPSs. See Prospective payment systems
Pre-adolescence, 126
Precautionary statements, 171
Prefixes, 67, 77-79, 78b-79b
Pregnancy: chest thrusts for pregnant persons, 165b
Pre-hypertension, 724, 727
Prenatal care, 800, 804
Pre-operative (pre-op) care, 589-595, 589b
  checklist for, 594, 594f
  for children, 590b
  drugs, 595
  personal care, 591
  skin preparation, 591, 592f
  special tests, 590
  teaching, 590
Prepuce, 121
Preschoolers, 128b, 132-133, 132f
Prescription drugs. See Drugs
Pressure points. See Bony prominences
Pressure ulcers, 623f, 624b-625b, 627b
  avoidable, 621, 623, 623b
  Braden Scale for Predicting Pressure Sore Risk, 630f, 631
  preventing, 624b, 627-631, 627b-628b
  reporting and recording, 631, 631f
  risk factors for, 623, 624b, 624f
  stages of, 625-626, 625b-626b, 625f
  unavoidable, 621, 623, 623b
Primary caregivers, 126, 138b
Primary nursing, 1, 8
Priorities, 55, 61, 89b
Privacy, 15, 15f
  during bowel elimination, 425, 440b
  full visual privacy, 303, 312b
  invasion of, 38, 42-43
  OBRA-required actions to promote, 17b
  personal, 15
  protection of, 13b, 15
  right to, 673b-674b, 858b
  and sexuality, 797b
  ways to respect, 15, 42b, 586b, 640b, 673b-674b
Privacy curtains, 42b, 42f, 312, 312b
Private insurance, 8
Probiotics, 741
Problem solving, 62
Procedure manuals, 41, 42f
Professional appearance, 57f
Professional boundaries, 38-40, 40b-41b, 40f, 52b-53b
Professional responsibility, 29b, 90b
  for communicating with the health team, 81b
  for delegation, 36b
  in health care agency work, 10b
  for protecting person's rights, 19b
  for reporting abuse and neglect, 52b-53b
  in workplace, 65b
Professional sexual misconduct, 38, 40
Professionalism, 55
Progesterone, 121, 123, 795b
Progress notes, 67, 69, 69b, 71f
Projection, 759b
Prompted voiding, 404
Pronation, 513
Prone position, 250, 258f, 259
Property, personal, 16
Prospective payment systems (PPSs), 9
Prostate cancer, 695b-696b

Prostate enlargement, 750-751, 751f
Prostate gland, 120, 795b
Prostheses, 666, 668, 721
  knee, 713, 714f
  leg, 722f
  ocular, 690, 690f, 691b
  pre-operative, 591
Prostitution, child, 49
Protected health information, 38, 42
Protective devices, 628
Protein, 447
Protein foods, 446, 451t-452t, 453b
Protoplasm, 108
Protozoa, 218
Pseudodementia, 769, 771
Psychiatric disorders. See Mental health disorders
Psychiatry, 96
Psychological care, 589
Psychological violence, 51
Psychosis, 757, 760-761
PTSD. See Post-traumatic stress disorder
Puberty, 126-127
Public transportation, 180b-181b
Pull-on underwear, 399, 399f, 401b-402b, 404f
Pulse, 486, 497-503
  apical, 501, 502b
  apical-radial, 486, 501, 502b-503b, 502f
  normal ranges, 511b
  pedal, 503
  radial, 500b-501b, 500f
  taking pulses, 498-503, 499b
Pulse deficit, 486
Pulse force, 498
Pulse oximetry, 642, 645, 645b-646b, 645f
Pulse rate, 486, 498, 498f, 498t
Pulse rhythm, 498, 498f
Pulse sites, 497, 498, 498f
Puncture wounds, 604, 605b, 606f
Pupil, 114, 682b
Purulent drainage, 613, 614f
Pyelonephritis, 750b
Pyloric sphincter, 112, 113f
Pyrophobia, 759
Pyuria, 749, 750b

Q
Quadriplegia, 154, 156, 705, 711, 711f
Quality assurance, 13b
Quality of life, 16-18, 673
  ways to promote, 17b, 673
Questions
  direct, 101
  in job interviews, 865b, 866, 867b-868b
  open-ended, 101
Quick-release ties, 205b-206b, 207f

R
RA. See Rheumatoid arthritis
RACE mnemonic for fire safety, 175, 175f
Radial pulses, 500b-501b, 500f
Radiating pain, 531, 533, 533f
Radiation, 697
Radiation therapy, 697, 697b
Radio listening systems, 680
Radiographers, 5t-6t
Radiologic technologists, 5t-6t
Range of motion (ROM), 513, 517, 875f
Range-of-motion exercises, 517, 519b-520b, 519f, 521f-522f
  for children, 518b
  communication for, 517b
  guidelines for, 518b
  joint movements, 517b
  in long-term care, 518b
  safety and comfort measures for, 517b-518b
Rape or sexual assault, 49
Rapid Response Teams (RRTs), 830
Rationalization, 759b
RBCs. See Red blood cells
Reaction formation, 759b
Reagent strips
  testing blood glucose with, 583b-585b, 583f, 585f
  testing urine with, 574, 574f, 575b
Receptive aphasia, 675, 682
Reciprocity. See Endorsement

Recording, 67, 72-75, 75*b*, 81*b*. *See also*
    Documentation
    admission records, 69
    bowel elimination records, 424*b*, 425*f*
    electronic health records (EHRs), 67-68, 68*f*
    electronic recordings, 75
    intake and output (I&O) records, 456-457
    medical records, 67-71, 68*f*
    rules for, 75*b*
Recovery beds, 331
Recovery position, 838, 838*f*
Recreation, 827
Recreational therapists, 5*t*-6*t*
Rectal suppositories, 430, 430*f*
Rectal temperature, 488*b*-489*b*, 488*t*, 492*b*, 493*f*
Rectal thermometers, 490, 490*f*
Rectum, 119, 740*b*
Red blood cells (RBCs), 116, 643, 725*b*-726*b*
Reduction, 716
Reflex incontinence, 388, 397
Reflexes, 113, 126, 128, 706*b*
Reflux, gastro-esophageal, 740
Refusing care, 14-15
    personal hygiene, 363*b*-364*b*
    right to refuse treatment, 14-15
Refusing tasks, 35-36, 36*b*
Regional anesthesia, 588, 595
Registered nurses (RNs), 1, 5*t*-6*t*, 7
Registration, 24*b*
Regression, 759*b*, 761
Regular diet, 451
Regulated waste, 241*b*, 242
Regurgitation, 473, 477
Rehabilitation, 2-3, 666-674, 671*b*
    amputee, 671
    bladder, 404
    brain injury, 671
    cardiac, 671, 728
    for children, 667*b*, 671*b*
    communication during, 670*b*
    for complex medical and surgical conditions,
        671
    economic aspects, 670
    goals of, 666
    hearing, speech, and vision, 671
    home care programs and services, 672*b*
    in long-term care, 667*b*, 672*b*
    for older persons, 146*b*, 667*b*
    orthopedic, 671
    persons needing, 96
    problems requiring, 666*b*
    psychological aspects, 670, 670*b*
    respiratory, 671
    social aspects, 670, 670*b*
    spinal cord, 671
    stroke, 671
    for whole person, 667-670
Rehabilitation teams, 670-671
Reincarnation, 851-852
Relationships, 797*b*, 797*f*
Relaxation, 531, 536
Religion, 92, 94-95
    communication about, 95*b*
    dietary practices, 450*b*
    food practices, 449
    home care practices, 95*b*
Religious services, 94-95, 95*f*
REM sleep, 531, 539
Reminiscence, 781, 859*b*
Renal cell carcinoma, 695*b*-696*b*
Renal pelvis, 120, 750*b*
Renal tubules, 120
Renting, 148
Repetitive behaviors, 777, 778*b*-780*b*
Reporting, 67, 72-75, 73*b*, 74*f*. *See also*
    Documentation
    abuse and neglect, 44-52, 45*b*, 48*b*, 52*b*-53*b*
    end-of-shift reports, 67, 74, 74*b*
    incidents, 182, 183*b*
    observations, 84, 84*b*, 84*f*
    personal hygiene, 363, 363*b*
    pressure ulcers, 631, 631*f*
    restraint use, 210
    rules for, 74*b*
    safety issues, 155*b*

Re-positioning the person, 273*b*-274*b*. *See also*
    Positioning the person
    in a chair or wheelchair, 279, 279*f*
    pre-operative teaching about, 590
Representative, 12
Repression, 759*b*
Reprimands, 81*b*
Reproductive disorders, 754, 756*b*
Reproductive system, 120-122
    changes in aging, 143*b*, 146-147
    female, 121-122, 121*f*, 143*b*, 147, 795*b*, 795*f*
    male, 120-121, 121*f*, 143*b*, 146, 754, 795*b*, 795*f*
    structure and function of, 795*b*
Rescue breathing, 831
Reservoirs, 217-218, 227*b*-228*b*
Resident care conferences, 88*b*
Resident groups, 16
Resident rooms, 304*b*
Residential hotels, 149
Residential special waste pick-up services, 243*b*
Residents, 3
    assisted-living residents, 823
    life-long, 97*b*
    with mental health disorders, 97*b*
    short-term, 97*b*
    terminally ill, 97*b*
Residents' rights, 12-18, 13*b*-14*b*, 823, 823*b*
Resigning from a job, 64
Respect, 56*b*
    for co-workers, 65*b*
    in delegation, 36*b*
    A Dying Patient's Bill of Last Rights, 859*b*
    for fellow students, 65*b*
    in health care agencies, 10*b*
    for nursing assistants, 29*b*
    for persons, 106*b*, 183*b*
    for person's rights, 19*b*
Respectful treatment, 52*b*-53*b*
Respiration(s), 108, 118, 486, 504-505, 504*b*, 731*b*
    abnormal breathing problems, 644, 645*f*
    altered respiratory function, 644, 644*b*
    basic observations of, 85*b*
    Biot's respirations, 642, 644
    Cheyne-Stokes respirations, 642, 644
    counting respirations, 504-505, 505*b*-506*b*
    Kussmaul respirations, 642, 644
    normal ranges, 511*b*
    preventing complications in older persons, 597*b*
    preventing post-operative complications, 597-601
Respirators
    donning and removing, 234*f*-236*f*, 237*b*
    tuberculosis respirators, 232, 232*f*
Respiratory arrest, 642-643, 829, 831
Respiratory depression, 642-643
Respiratory disorders, 731-734
Respiratory hygiene, 229*b*
Respiratory protection, 232
Respiratory rehabilitation, 671
Respiratory support, 658-665, 658*b*
Respiratory system, 118, 118*f*, 504*b*, 504*f*, 643*b*, 643*f*,
    731*f*
    changes in aging, 143*b*, 145
    structure and function of, 731*b*
Respiratory tests, 645-647
Respiratory therapist (RT), 5*t*-6*t*
Respiratory therapy, 658-665
Respite care, 97*b*, 146*b*, 148
Responsibility, 25-29, 25*b*, 31. *See also* Personal
    responsibility; Professional responsibility
Rest, 56, 531-532, 539
    for arthritis, 713
    bedrest, 514-517, 515*b*
    and pain, 533
    post-operative, 602
    ways to promote, 539, 539*f*
Restorative aides, 666-667
Restorative care, 2, 666-667, 667*b*
Restraints, 210-211, 211*b*-215*b*
    alternatives to, 201, 201*b*, 203*f*
    chemical, 200, 203
    communication with, 208*b*, 211*b*
    history of use of, 201
    laws, rules, and guidelines for use of, 204
    physical, 200, 203
    reporting and recording, 210

Restraints *(Continued)*
    right to freedom from, 16, 858*b*
    risk from use of, 203, 203*b*
    safe use of, 200, 202-211, 202*b*, 205*b*-206*b*,
        206*f*-208*f*, 208*b*-209*b*, 212*b*
Retention catheters. *See* Indwelling catheters
Retina, 114, 682*b*
Retirement, 141, 141*f*
Retirement communities, 149
Reverse Trendelenburg's position, 303, 308, 308*f*
Rheumatoid arthritis, 712, 714*b*
Ribbon safety, 164*b*
Riboflavin (vitamin B2), 447*t*
Rickettsiae, 218
Right atrium, 116, 497*b*, 725*b*-726*b*
Right bronchus, 118, 504*b*, 643*b*, 731*b*
Right lymphatic duct, 118
Right ventricle, 116, 497*b*, 725*b*-726*b*
Rights
    to activities that enhance well-being, 17
    of assisted living residents, 823, 823*b*
    when communicating with the health team, 81*b*
    in delegation, 36*b*
    of drug administration, 826
    A Dying Patient's Bill of Last Rights, 859*b*
    of dying persons, 858*b*
    Five Rights of Delegation (NCSBN), 35, 35*b*
    to form and take part in resident groups, 16
    to freedom from abuse and mistreatment,
        673*b*-674*b*
    to grievances, 16
    in health care agency work, 10*b*
    to information, 14
    to keep and use personal items, 16
    to make choices, 15
    for nursing assistants, 29*b*
    patient rights, 12
    to personal privacy, 15
    person's rights, 12-20, 19*b*
    to privacy, 42*b*, 673*b*-674*b*
    to quality of life, 16
    to refuse treatment, 14-15
    resident rights, 12-18, 13*b*-14*b*
    to safe, clean comfortable, and home-like setting,
        18
    to safe settings, 673*b*-674*b*
    about sexuality, 788
    to work, 16
Rigor mortis, 851, 856
Risk management, 181-182
Rituals, 759*b*, 852*b*
RNs. *See* Registered nurses
Roll guards, 201*b*, 202*f*
Roman Catholic church, 450*b*
Room dividers, 312
Room furniture, 306-316
Rooting reflex, 128, 129*f*
Roots, 77-79
Rotation, 513
Rots, 78*b*-79*b*
RRTs. *See* Rapid Response Teams
RT. *See* Respiratory therapist
Rummaging, 777, 778*b*-780*b*
Russians, 94*b*, 102*b*

S
Sadness, 859*b*
Safe handling, 279*b*-280*b*
    of meat and poultry, 825, 825*f*
    of used linens, 333*b*
Safe Medical Devices Act, 203
Safe Return®, 775, 778*b*-780*b*
Safe settings, 155, 155*b*, 673*b*-674*b*, 858*b*
Safety, 154-185, 155*b*
    in admissions, transfers, and discharges, 546*b*
    adult CPR, 832*b*, 836*b*
    in arthritis, 713
    in assisted living, 822*b*, 827
    in back massages, 537*b*
    in bathing, 349*b*
    in bathing infants, 815*b*, 815*f*
    bed safety, 307*b*, 309, 309*b*
    in bedmaking, 324*b*
    with bedpans, 391*b*
    in blood glucose testing, 583*b*

Safety (Continued)
  with blood pressure equipment, 508b
  in bowel elimination, 423b, 426, 426b
  in brushing and combing hair, 369b
  building safety and security, 179b
  call system, 315
  in care of the body after death, 857b
  cast care, 718b
  in changing patient gowns, 384b
  in chemotherapy, 698b
  for children, 309b, 800-804, 879
  in cirrhosis, 745b
  in cleaning baby bottles, 807b
  closet and drawer space, 315b
  in collecting and testing specimens, 568b
  with commodes, 395b
  with condom catheters, 418b
  with corrective lenses, 688b
  cough etiquette, 648b
  crib safety, 801b, 803-804, 803b
  in dangling, 277b
  delegation for, 32, 32b, 32f
  denture care, 344b
  in diapering babies, 811b
  in diarrhea, 429b
  disinfection, 227b
  donning and removing PPE, 234b
  in dressing and undressing, 380b
  with dressings, 616b
  with drugs, 160b
  with elastic bandages, 600b
  with elastic stockings, 598b
  emergency care, 830b
  end-of-shift reports for, 74b
  with enemas, 432b
  face shields, 232b
  in fecal impaction, 427b
  in feeding, 464b
  in feeding babies, 809b
  fire safety, 174b, 176b
  flow rate, 482b
  food safety, 468, 469b, 825
  with glass thermometers, 491b
  gloves, 233b
  goggles, 232b
  hand hygiene, 223b
  with hazardous chemicals, 173b
  with heat and cold applications, 638b
  in helping the person walk, 524b
  in hemorrhage, 844b
  in hepatitis, 742b
  home care, 181b
  home safety measures to protect infants and
      children, 802b, 802f, 877-879
  identifying the person, 157b
  with incontinence products, 400b
  infant safety measures, 131b, 800-804, 801b, 801f,
      879
  job, 61
  logrolling, 275b
  in long-term care, 94b
  in lymphedema, 736b
  in measuring intake and output, 459b
  in measuring weight and height, 309b
  with mechanical lifts, 297b
  with midstream specimens, 570b
  for mothers and children, 800-804
  mouth care for unconscious persons, 343b
  in moving and transferring the person, 262-302,
      262b-263b, 282b
  in moving the person from bed to chair or
      wheelchair, 287b
  in moving the person to a stretcher, 293b
  in moving the person to the side of the bed, 271b
  in moving the person up in bed, 268b
  in moving the person up in bed with an assist
      device, 269b
  in moving the person to and from the toilet, 291b
  nail and foot care, 377b
  nursery equipment, 879-882
  in nursing centers, 151b
  with occupied beds, 328b
  with ocular prostheses, 691b
  with oil-retention enemas, 436b
  oral hygiene measures, 339b

Safety (Continued)
  with ostomy pouches, 438b
  oxygen, 652b, 655, 655b-656b
  patient care partnership for, 13b
  perineal care, 359b
  personal, 180b-181b, 181f
  personal care, 591b
  personal hygiene measures, 337b
  for persons with AD and other dementias, 774b,
      778b-780b, 780f
  for persons with developmental disabilities, 183b
  for persons with hearing loss, 677b
  for persons with paranoia, 776b
  in positioning the person, 256b
  in preparing for meals, 460b
  in preparing for physical examination, 563b
  to prevent carbon monoxide poisoning, 163b
  to prevent equipment accidents, 170b
  to prevent falls, 188b-189b, 192b
  to prevent lead poisoning, 162b
  to prevent poisonings, 160b
  to prevent suffocating, 164b
  to prevent workplace violence, 179b
  promotion of, 9b, 183b
  in providing drinking water, 466b
  in pulse oximetry, 646b
  in radiation therapy, 697b
  in range-of-motion exercises, 517b-518b
  in removing indwelling catheters, 417b
  in removing PPE, 234f-236f
  reporting issues, 155b
  in respiratory support, 658b
  with restraints, 202-211, 202b, 205b-206b,
      206f-208f, 208b-209b, 212b
  rules for electronic communications, 43b
  in serving meals, 462b
  in shampooing, 372b
  in shaving, 375b
  in skin preparation, 593b
  with sputum specimens, 580b
  staff measures, 179b
  in stand and pivot transfers, 286b
  standard precautions, 229b
  sterile gloving, 245b
  sterile procedures, 244b
  with stethoscopes, 500b
  with stool specimens, 577b
  with stretchers, 171, 283, 284b, 286f
  stroke care, 708b
  in suctioning, 662b
  surgical beds, 331b
  surveys of, 155b
  in taking pulses, 499b
  in taking temperatures, 489b, 491b
  teen dating, 136b
  in testing urine, 575b
  with tracheostomies, 660
  with transfer belts, 194b
  transmission-based precautions, 231b
  tub bath and shower safety, 354b, 356b
  in tube feedings, 478b
  in turning persons, 273b
  umbilical cord care, 813b
  with urinals, 394b
  with urinary catheters, 407b
  with urinary diversions, 752b
  with urinary elimination, 389b
  with urine drainage systems, 413b
  with urine specimens, 571b
  in vertigo, 677
  for victims of intimate partner violence, 52b
  with walkers, 523b
  for wanderers, 774b, 775f
  in weighing infants, 818b
  wheelchair, 171, 283
  with wheelchairs, 284b, 285f
  worker, 229b
  in wound care, 605b
Safety and security needs, 93, 539
Safety certification seals (JPMA), 803b, 804f
Safety covers, 778b-780b, 780f
Safety data sheets, 172
Safety devices, 179b, 179f, 672b-673b
Safety razors, 374, 374f, 375b-376b, 376f
Safety seats, 802b, 802f-803f

Saline enemas, 431-432, 433b-434b
Saliva, 119
Salivary glands, 119, 443b, 740b
Sandwich generation, 782
Sanguineous drainage, 604, 613, 614f
Scabies, 366, 368, 368f
Scales
  digital infant scale, 818b, 818f
  teamwork for using, 309b
  types of, 308f, 309
Scalp conditions, 368, 368b
SCDs. See Sequential compression devices
Scheduled feedings, 476
Scheduled voiding, 404
Schizophrenia, 760-761, 761b
School: preparing for, 57-58
School-age children, 128b, 133-134, 134f
Sclera, 114, 682b
Screaming, 777
Screens, portable, 312, 312f
Scrotum, 120
SDS. See Safety data sheets
Sebaceous glands, 110
Seclusion, involuntary, 12, 16, 46
Secondary sex characteristics, 135
Security, 93
  building safety and security, 179b
  for mothers and children, 800-804
Sedation, 588, 595
Seizures, 829, 846-847, 847f
Self-actualization, 92, 94
Self-administered abdominal thrusts, 165b
Self-awareness, 56b
Self-care, 667, 668b
Self-centered behavior, 104
Self-determination, 17b
Self-directed medication management, 827
Self-esteem, 92, 94, 386b, 539
  ways to promote, 781
Self-harm behaviors, 762
Self-help devices, 668f
Self-image, unstable, 762
Self-neglect, 38
Semen, 120
Semicircular canals, 115, 676b
Semi-Fowler's position, 256, 303, 308, 308f
Seminal vesicle, 120
Semi-prone side position. See Sims' position
Senior centers, 146b
Senior citizen housing, 148
Sense organs, 114-115
  changes in aging, 144-145
  problems after TBI, 710
Sequential compression devices (SCDs), 601, 601f
Serosanguineous drainage, 604, 613, 614f
Serous drainage, 604, 613, 614f
Service plans, 822, 824-827
Serving meal trays, 463b
Serving meals, 462, 462b, 462f, 470b
Seventh-Day Adventist church, 450b
Sex, 794-795
Sex hormones, 123
Sexting, 64
Sexual abuse, 776b, 798, 798b-799b
  child abuse, 49, 50b
  elder abuse, 46
Sexual assaults, 49
Sexual behavior, 104, 777
Sexual harassment, 64
Sexual misconduct, professional, 38, 40
Sexual orientation, 126, 135, 794, 796
Sexual violence, 51
Sexuality, 777, 794-795
  changes in Alzheimer's disease, 777-778
  injury, illness, and surgery and, 796
  in long-term care, 797b, 797f
  meeting sexual needs, 796, 797b, 797f
  for older persons, 796
  for persons with intellectual disabilities, 788
  rights about, 788
  ways to promote, 797b-799b
Sexually aggressive persons, 797-798, 798b-799b
Sexually transmitted diseases, 754, 754b, 755t, 756b,
    798
Shampoo caps, 371

Shampoo trays, 371, 371*f*
Shampooing, 371, 371*b*-373*b*, 371*f*, 591
Shared housing, 149
Sharps, 241*b*, 243*b*
Sharps containers, 243*b*, 243*f*
Shaving, 374-376, 374*b*-375*b*
  with safety razors, 375*b*-376*b*, 376*f*
  skin prep, 591, 591*b*, 593*f*
Shear, 621
Shearing, 262, 264, 264*f*
Shingles, 703, 703*f*
Shock, 604, 612, 829, 845
  anaphylactic, 845
  electrical, 154
  signs and symptoms of, 612, 845
Shoes, 188*b*-189*b*
Short bones, 110, 251*b*, 713*b*
Short-term residents, 97*b*
Shoulder exercises, 519*b*-520*b*, 519*f*
Shoulders: raising the person's head and shoulders,
  266, 266*b*, 267*f*
Shower benches, 354, 354*f*
Shower cabinets, 355, 355*f*
Shower chairs, 355, 355*f*
Shower stalls, 355
Shower trolleys (portable tubs), 355, 356*f*
Showers, 354-355, 354*b*, 356*b*-357*b*, 591
Shower/tub rooms, 188*b*-189*b*
Shrouds, 857*b*, 858*f*
Shunts, 791, 791*f*
Sick care, 94*b*, 104*b*
Side-lying position. *See* Lateral position
SIDS. *See* Sudden infant death syndrome
Sight, 114
Signs, 778*b*-780*b*, 780*f*. *See also* Objective data
Silence, 101, 102*b*
Simple fractures, 705
Sims' position, 250, 258*f*, 259, 564, 564*f*
Sinoatrial (SA) node, 725*b*-726*b*
Sitting on the side of the bed (dangling), 276,
  277*f*-278*f*, 278*b*
Sitz baths, 635, 638*b*
Skeletal muscles, 251*b*
Skeletal traction, 719, 719*f*
Skilled nursing facilities, 3
Skin, 110, 336*b*, 702*b*
  basic observations of, 85*b*
  dry and cracked, 609*b*-610*b*, 610*f*
  intact, 621, 623, 624*f*
  layers of, 110, 110*f*, 337*f*
  structures of, 702*b*, 702*f*
Skin breakdown, 621, 623, 623*b*
Skin cancer, 695*b*-696*b*
Skin care, 627*b*-628*b*
Skin care products, 347*t*
Skin conditions, 368, 368*b*, 702-703, 855
Skin failure, 626
Skin prep kits, 591, 593*f*
Skin preparation (skin prep), 591, 591*b*, 592*f*, 593*b*
Skin protection, 265*b*
  for lateral transfers, 292
  while moving persons, 264
Skin tears, 604, 607, 607*b*, 607*f*
Skin traction, 719
Slander, 38, 42
Sleep, 56, 531-532, 539-541
  factors affecting, 540
  guidelines for, 541*t*
  infant safety measures, 801*b*
  measures to prevent suffocating, 164*b*
  NREM sleep, 531, 539, 540*b*
  and pain, 533
  for persons with AD and other dementias,
    778*b*-780*b*
  REM sleep, 531, 539
  ways to promote, 541, 542*b*
Sleep apnea, 724, 732-733
Sleep cycles, 539, 540*b*, 540*f*
Sleep deprivation, 531, 541
Sleep disorders, 541, 541*b*
Sleepwalking, 531, 541, 541*b*
Slide locks, 778*b*-780*b*, 781*f*
Slide sheets, 269, 269*f*, 292, 293*f*
Sliding boards, 283*f*, 291-292, 293*f*
Slings, 296, 296*f*

Slough, 621, 625*b*
Small braids (cornrows), 369*b*
Small intestine (small bowel), 119, 423*b*, 443*b*
Small objects and toy safety, 164*b*
Small-volume enemas, 431, 434, 434*f*, 435*b*
Smell, 114, 145, 156
Smoke alarms, 158*b*
Smoke odors, 305
Smoker's cough, 732
Smoking safety, 174*b*. *See also* Cigarette smoking
Snacks, between-meal, 466
SNFs. *See* Skilled nursing facilities
Soaks, hot, 635
Soapsuds enemas (SSEs), 431-432, 433*b*-434*b*
Social considerations, 29*b*, 52*b*-53*b*
  in delegation, 36*b*
  in health care agencies, 10*b*
  for older persons, 141-142, 142*b*
  and protecting person's rights, 19*b*
  ways to promote relationships, 152*b*, 619*b*
  in workplace, 65*b*
Social dining, 462*b*, 462*f*
Social problems, 789
Social workers, 5*t*-6*t*
Sodium, 448*t*, 453*b*
Sodium-controlled diet, 451*t*-452*t*, 452
Solid fats, 447
Source individuals, 241*b*
Space heaters, 174*b*
Spanish culture, 102*b*
Special care units, 96
Special diets, 451-454, 451*t*-452*t*
Special fluid orders, 456
Special needs: persons with, 103
Special services, 827
Specific immunity, 123
Specimen collecting and testing, 239, 567-587
  blood glucose testing, 582, 582*b*, 582*f*
  sputum specimens, 647
  stool specimens, 577, 577*b*
  urine specimens, 568-576
Speculum
  nasal, 561
  vaginal, 561
Speech, professional, 60
Speech and vision rehabilitation, 671
Speech delays, 789
Speech disorders, 675, 681-682
  communicating with speech-impaired persons, 681*b*
  at end of life, 854
Speech therapists, 5*t*-6*t*
Speech-language pathologists, 5*t*-6*t*, 681
Sperm, 120, 795*b*
Sphincters, 112
Sphygmomanometers, 486, 507, 507*f*-508*f*
Spina bifida, 786, 790
Spina bifida occulta, 790, 790*f*
Spinal cord, 114, 706*b*
Spinal cord injury, 711-712
Spinal cord rehabilitation, 671
Spinal nerves, 114, 706*b*
Spirituality, 783*b*, 852-853, 853*b*, 859*b*
Spirometers, 650, 650*f*
Spirometry. *See* Incentive spirometry
Spleen, 118, 735*b*
Splints, 515, 516*f*
Sponge baths, 814, 815*b*-816*b*, 816*f*
Spores, 217, 226
Sports injuries, 710
Spousal abuse. *See* Intimate partner violence (IPV)
Sputum, 567, 580, 642, 644*b*, 647
Sputum specimens, 580, 580*b*-581*b*, 581*f*, 647
SSEs. *See* Soapsuds enemas
Staff
  assisted living requirements, 824
  cost reductions, 22
  at nursing centers, 151*b*
  safety measures for, 179*b*
  training in emergency procedures for, 173*b*
Stairways, 878
Stand and pivot transfers, 255*b*, 286-291, 286*b*
Standard precautions, 228, 229*b*
Standards
  for accreditation, 9
  for certification, 9

Standards (*Continued*)
  for health care agencies, 9
  for licensure, 9
  for nursing assistants, 26, 26*b*
Standards of care, 38, 41
Stand-assist bed attachments, 283*f*
Stand-assist mechanical lifts, 297*b*-298*b*, 298*f*
Standing scales, 307*b*, 308*f*, 309
Stapes, 115, 676*b*
Staphylococcus aureus ("staph"), 218
Startle reflex (Moro reflex), 128, 129*f*
Stasis ulcers. *See* Venous ulcers
State laws, 22-25
STDs. *See* Sexually transmitted diseases
Stem cell transplants, 698
Step (dance) reflex, 128, 129*f*
Sterile fields, 217, 244, 245*b*, 245*f*
Sterile gloving, 244, 245*b*-246*b*, 246*f*
Sterile procedures, 244, 244*b*
Sterile technique, 26*b*. *See also* Surgical asepsis
Sterilization, 217, 221, 226, 227*b*, 241*b*, 788
Stethoscopes, 486, 499, 499*b*-500*b*, 499*f*
  Doppler ultrasound (DUS), 503, 504*f*
  safety and comfort measures with, 500*b*, 500*f*
Stoma, 422, 436, 437*f*, 835, 835*f*
  mouth-to-stoma breathing, 835, 835*f*
Stomach, 443*b*, 740*b*
Stomatitis, 693, 698
Stones
  gallstones, 742, 742*f*
  kidney stones, 752-753, 752*f*, 756*b*
Stool softeners, 426
Stool specimens, 577, 577*b*-579*b*, 579*f*
Stools, 422, 423*b*, 424*f*
  after birth, 810
Storage areas, 315, 672*b*-673*b*. *See also* Closets
Storing drugs, 827
Straight catheters, 407
Straining urine, 576, 576*b*, 577*f*
Stress, 55, 62, 506*b*, 757-758
  post-traumatic stress disorder, 760
Stress incontinence, 388, 397
Stress management, 62-63
Stressors, 55, 62, 757-758
Stretchers, 283
  bariatric, 293
  moving the person to, 293, 293*b*-294*b*, 294*f*
  safety measures, 171, 283, 284*b*, 286*f*
Striated muscles, 251*b*
Stripping, epidermal, 621
Stroke, 707, 846
  effects of, 707, 707*f*, 708*b*
  safety precautions for, 708*b*
  warning signs of, 707, 707*b*
Stroke care, 708*b*
  emergency care, 846
  home care, 708*b*
  long-term care, 708*b*
Stroke rehabilitation, 671
Strollers and carriages, 881
Student ethics, 55-66
Student learning, 2
Sub-acute care, 96
Sub-acute care agencies, 3
Subcutaneous tissue, 110
Subjective data, 83-84
Substance abuse, 49
Substance abuse disorder, 762-764
Sucking reflex, 128
Suction, 658, 660
Suctioning the airway, 660-661, 661*b*-662*b*, 661*f*
Sudden cardiac arrest (SCA), 829-831
Sudden infant death syndrome (SIDS), 804, 839
Sudden unexpected infant death (SUID), 804
Sudoriferous glands, 110, 336*b*
Suffixes, 67, 77-79, 78*b*-79*b*
Suffocation, 154, 163
  preventing, 163-165, 164*b*
Suicide, 757, 765-766, 766*b*
  communication with persons at risk for, 765*b*
  risk factors for, 765*b*-766*b*
Suicide contagion, 757, 766
SUID. *See* Sudden unexpected infant death
Summaries of care, 69*b*, 72*f*
Sundowning, 769, 775, 778*b*-780*b*

Superior vena cava, 117, 725b-726b
Supervision, 34
Supination, 513
Supine position, 258f, 259
Supplemental feedings, 466
Supplies, 226
Support from others, 533
Suppositories, 422, 430, 430f, 431b
Surgery, 96, 588-603
    for cancer, 697
    complications of, 596b
    coronary artery bypass, 727, 728f
    elective, 588-589
    emergency, 588-589
    fears and concerns about, 589b
    joint replacement, 713
    patient information, 589, 589b
    post-operative (post-op) care, 595-602
    pre-operative (pre-op) care, 589-595, 589b
    psychological care for the person having, 589
    and sexual function, 796
    urgent, 588-589
Surgery consent, 594
Surgical asepsis, 217, 221, 244, 245b, 245f
Surgical beds, 319, 320f, 331, 331b-332b, 332f
Surgical sites: marking, 594
Surgical skin prep, 591b
Surgi-centers (surgery centers), 588
Surveillance, 34
Survey teams, 10b
Surveyors, 1, 10b
Surveys, 9, 10b, 81b, 152b
    of activities, 18b
    of advance directives, 856b
    of bed-to-chair or wheelchair transfers, 287b
    of dementia care, 782b
    disaster drills, 173b
    of fall prevention, 186b
    of feeding, 464b
    of hand hygiene, 223b
    of infection prevention, 219b
    of laundry, 244b
    of linen use, 321b
    of maintaining competence, 24b
    of management of incontinence, 399b
    of noise levels, 306b
    of nutrition and fluids, 444b
    of pain, 532b
    of planning, 87b
    of pressure ulcers, 627b
    of resident rights protection, 13b
    of safety, 155b
    of self-care, 668b
    of skin protection, 265b
    of transmission-based precautions, 231b
    of urinary catheters, 407b
Susceptible hosts, 219-220
Swallowing problems, 449, 454
Sweat glands, 110, 336b, 702b
Swimming pools, 878
Swing-carry technique, 177f
Swing-to gait, 526
Sympathetic nervous system, 114, 706b
Symphysis pubis, 121
Symptoms. See also Subjective data
    medical, 200, 202
Syncope, 513-514
Synovial fluid, 111
Synovial membrane, 111
Syphilis, 755t
Syringe-exchange programs, 243b
Syringes: disposal of, 243b
Systemic infection, 219
Systems, organ, 108-109
Systole, 116, 486, 497b, 506, 725b-726b
Systolic pressure, 486, 506

T
T cells (T lymphocytes), 123, 699b
Tables, over-bed, 312
Tachycardia, 486, 498
Tachypnea, 642, 644
Tap water enemas, 431-432, 433b-434b
Tape, 615, 615b, 615f
Tartar, 335, 338

Taste, 114, 145
Taste buds, 119, 443b
TB. See Tuberculosis
TBI. See Traumatic brain injury
Teaching, pre-operative, 590
Team nursing, 1, 8
Teamwork, 29b, 58-61
    for activities, 18b
    for AD and other dementias, 782b
    for admissions, transfers, and discharges, 546b
    for blood glucose testing, 582b
    in body, 124b
    call systems, 314b
    check times, 316b-317b
    communicating with the health team, 67-82
    for competence, 24b
    definition of, 55, 58
    delegating work, 36b
    for electronic thermometers, 489b
    for end-of-life care, 851b
    end-of-shift reports, 74b
    for formulas, 475b
    for grooming, 366b
    for handling used linens, 333b
    in health care agencies, 10b
    for IV therapy, 483b
    for laundry, 826b
    for making beds, 324b
    for measuring weight, 307b
    for moving the person up in bed, 268b, 269, 269f
    for oxygen set-ups, 655b
    for personal hygiene, 349b, 363b-364b
    personal safety measures for, 183b
    for physical examinations, 565b
    for pre-operative (pre-op) care, 589b
    for preventing falls, 187b, 198b
    for preventing pressure ulcers, 624b
    for preventing work-related injuries, 264b
    promoting, 59b
    for protecting person's rights, 19b
    for raising the person's head and shoulders, 266b, 267f
    for rehabilitation, 671b
    reporting, 73b
    with restraints, 209b
    for transferring persons, 282b
    for tub baths and showers, 356b
    for urination, 390b
    work ethics, 65b
TED (thrombo-embolic disease) hose, 598
Teen dating, 136, 136b
Teen dating violence, 52b, 126, 136b
Teen drug use, 764b
Teeth, 119, 336b, 336f
    brushing and flossing, 340, 340b, 342f
    false, 344
Telecommunications Relay Service (TRS), 680, 681f
Telephone amplifying devices, 680
Telephone calls, 15, 15f, 77
    answering phones, 77b
    in home care, 77b
    reassurance for older persons, 146b
Telephone interviews, 864-865
Television (TV) listening systems, 680
Temperature
    body. See Body temperature
    food danger zone, 468, 468f
    food temperature guide, 468f
    heat and cold ranges, 637t
    room, 305, 305b
Temperature-sensitive tape, 490, 490f
Temporal artery temperature, 488b, 488t
Temporal artery thermometers, 489, 489f
Tendons, 112
Terminal illness, 1-2, 97b, 851-852
Terminology
    Bloodborne Pathogen Standard terms, 241b
    common terms and phrases, 80, 80b
    to describe pain, 535b
    to describe persons with fever, 488
    directional, 79, 80f
    for incontinence products, 400b
    for intellectual disabilities, 788b
    medical, 77-80, 78b-79b
Testes (testicles), 120, 795b

Testing
    blood glucose testing, 582, 582b, 582f
    collecting and testing specimens, 239, 567-587
    drug testing, 65, 867
    urine testing, 574, 575b
Testosterone, 120, 123
Tetraplegia. See Quadriplegia
Textiles, 229b
TH. See Thyroid hormone (thyroxine)
Thank-you letters or notes, 867, 867f
The Arc of the United States, 788, 792b
Thermometers, 486, 489-490
    disposable oral thermometers, 490, 490f
    electronic, 489, 489f, 491, 492b, 493f
    glass, 490, 490f, 491b, 494b-496b, 494f
Thiamin (vitamin B1), 447t
30-degree lateral position, 627b-628b, 628f
Thoracic duct (left lymphatic duct), 118
Thoracic injuries, 711
Thought disorders, 760
Throat (pharynx), 118-119, 443b, 504b, 643b, 731b, 740b
Thrombocytes, 116, 725b-726b
Thrombo-embolic disease (TED) hose, 598
Thrombus, 588, 597
Thumb exercises, 519b-520b, 521f
Thymosin, 123
Thymus (thymus gland), 118, 123, 735b
Thyroid cancer, 695b-696b
Thyroid gland, 123
Thyroid hormone (TH) (thyroxine), 123
Thyroid-stimulating hormone (TSH), 122
Thyroxine, 123
TIA. See Transient ischemic attack
Time management, 59b
    for activities, 18b
    for applying dressings, 616b
    assignment sheets for, 89b
    and behavior issues, 105b
    for blood glucose testing, 582b
    for bowel elimination, 426b
    calendars, 770b, 770f
    call systems, 314b
    for collecting and testing specimens, 568b
    for competence, 24b
    with electronic thermometers, 489b
    for end-of-life care, 851b
    for fall prevention, 187b
    for formulas, 475b
    for grooming, 366b
    for heat and cold applications, 637b
    for laundry, 826b
    for making beds, 324b
    with mechanical lifts, 296b
    for nail and foot care, 376b
    for oxygen therapy, 652b
    for personal hygiene, 349b, 363b-364b
    with personal protective equipment (PPE), 232b
    for physical examinations, 565b
    for pre-operative (pre-op) care, 589b
    reporting and recording time, 73, 73b, 73f
    for serving meals, 462b
    for testing urine, 575b
    for transferring persons, 282b
    for tub baths and showers, 356b
    for urination, 390b
Tinnitus, 675-676
Tissue(s), 108-109
    connective, 109
    epithelial, 109
    erectile, 109
    muscle, 109
    nerve, 109
    subcutaneous, 110
TJC. See Joint Commission, The
Tobacco, 697. See also Cigarette smoking
Toddlerhood, 128b, 131-132, 132f
Toe exercises, 519b-520b, 522f
Toenails, 377b
    fungal infection of, 609b-610b
    ingrown, 609b-610b, 610f
    trimming infant nails, 817
Toes, hammer, 609b-610b, 610f
Toilet: transferring the person to and from, 291, 291b, 292f

Toileting slings, 296
Tongue, 119, 443b, 740b
Tongue blades, padded, 342, 343f
Tonsils, 118, 735b
Torts, 39, 41-43, 52b-53b
Total dependence (functional status), 263b, 283b
Total joint replacement care, 714b, 715f
Total parenteral nutrition (TPN), 478-479
Touch, 114, 778b-780b, 781f
    changes in aging, 144
    with children, 100b
    communication by, 99
    cultural practices, 100b
    A Dying Patient's Bill of Last Rights, 859b
    end-of-life care, 854
    impaired, 156
    masturbation, 798
    sexual, 798, 798b-799b
Towel baths, 353, 353b
Toy chests, 881
Toy safety, 164b
Toys and toy chests, 881-882
TPN. See Total parenteral nutrition
Trachea (windpipe), 118, 504b, 643b, 731b
Tracheostomies, 658-660
Tracheostomy care, 660, 660b, 660f
Tracheostomy tubes, 658-659, 659f
Traction, 719, 719b
    cervical, 719, 719f
    skeletal, 719, 719f
    skin, 719
Traction set-ups, 719, 719f
Traffic accidents, 710
Training
    cardiac rehabilitation, 728
    exposure control plan, 240
    for hazardous chemicals, 172
    in-service, 24b
    job skills and training, 861, 861b
    staff, 172, 173b, 824
Training programs, 22, 23b-24b, 23f
Transfer belts, 186, 193, 193b-195b, 193f-195f, 198b, 255b, 286
Transferring the person, 281-302, 545, 546b, 558
    from assisted living, 827
    from bed to chair or wheelchair, 287, 287b-288b, 289f
    from chair or wheelchair to bed, 290, 290b, 291f
    communication for, 281b
    definition of, 281, 545
    delegation guidelines for, 282b
    with full-sling mechanical lifts, 300f
    guidelines for, 547b
    lateral transfers, 255b, 292-293
    lifting or moving the person in bed, 255b
    in long-term care, 546b
    to a new room, 314b, 315, 557, 557b
    to the operating room, 595, 595b
    preparation for, 301b
    procedure for, 558b
    safety and comfort measures, 301b, 546b
    stand and pivot transfers, 255b, 286-291, 286b
    with stand-assist mechanical lifts, 297b-298b, 298f
    to a stretcher, 293, 293b-294b, 294f
    to and from the toilet, 291, 291b, 292f
    wheelchair safety, 284b
Transgender, 794, 796
Transient incontinence, 388
Transient ischemic attack (TIA), 707
Transmission-based precautions, 230b-231b, 231
Transparent adhesive film, 614
Transplant patients, 220
Transportation, 58, 180b-181b
Transporting equipment, 255b
Transporting persons, 239
    guidelines for infection control, 239
    guidelines for preventing injuries, 255b
    older persons, 146b
    to operating rooms, 595
    precautions, 230b
    wheelchair safety, 284b, 285f
Transsexual, 794, 796
Transurethral resection of the prostate (TURP), 751
Transvestite, 794, 796
Trapeze, 517, 517f

Trauma, 604-605
Traumatic brain injury, 710, 710b-711b
Treatment, 12, 14-15
    of disease, 2
    pre-operative teaching about, 590
    refusal of, 14-15
    respectful, 52b-53b
Tremors, 708
Trendelenburg's position, 269b, 303, 308, 308f
Trends, current, 21-22
Trichomoniasis, 755t
Tricuspid valve, 116, 725b-726b
Trochanter rolls, 515, 516f
Trustworthiness, 56b
Truth, 859b
TSH. See Thyroid-stimulating hormone
Tub baths, 354-355, 355f, 356b-357b
    for babies, 814, 814f, 817b, 817f
    pre-operative, 591
    safety and comfort measures, 354b, 356b
Tube feedings, 476-477, 476f, 478b
Tuberculosis (TB), 734, 734b
Tuberculosis respirators, 232, 232f
Tubes, 26b. See also specific types
Tumors, 693, 694f
    benign, 693, 694f
    malignant, 693, 694f
Tuning forks, 561
Turn clock, 628f
Turning pads, 265f
Turning persons, 273-275, 273b-274b, 274f
    guidelines for, 273b
    pre-operative teaching about, 590
TURP. See Transurethral resection of the prostate
TV listening systems, 680
24-hour clock (military time or international time), 73, 73b, 73f
Tympanic membrane, 115, 676b
Tympanic membrane temperature, 488b, 488t
Tympanic membrane thermometers, 489, 489f, 492b, 493f

U
Ulcerative colitis, 742
Ulcers, 604, 605b
    arterial, 604, 609, 609f
    circulatory, 604, 608-609
    diabetic foot ulcers, 604, 609, 610b
    pressure, 621-633, 623f
    venous, 604, 608
Ultrasound, Doppler, 503, 504f
Umbilical cord, 800, 813, 813f
Umbilical cord care, 812f, 813, 813b
Unconscious persons
    communication with, 343b
    mouth care for, 342, 342f, 343b-344b
    safety and comfort measures for, 343b
Underarm crutches, 526, 527f
Underarms: shaving, 376
Under-garments, 399, 399f, 401b-402b, 403f
Under-pads, 269b, 322f
Understanding the person, 92-107
Underwear, pull-on, 399, 399f, 401b-402b, 404f
United Kingdom, 100b-101b
United States, 100b, 448b
Ureterostomy, cutaneous, 751, 752f
Ureters, 120, 389b, 750b
Urethra, 120, 389b, 750b, 795b
Urethral sphincters, 112
Urge incontinence, 388, 397
Urgent surgery, 588-589
Urinals, 393, 394b-395b, 394f
Urinary catheters, 407-421, 407b
Urinary diversions, 749, 751, 752f
Urinary elimination, 388-406, 389b, 390t
    pre-operative, 591
Urinary frequency, 388, 390t
Urinary incontinence, 388, 390t, 396-399
    causes of, 397b
    functional, 388, 397
    management of, 397, 398b-399b
    mixed, 388, 397
    nursing measures for, 398b
    over-flow, 388, 397
    persistent, 397b

Urinary incontinence (Continued)
    reflex, 388, 397
    risk factors for, 397b
    stress, 388, 397
    temporary, 397b
    transient, 388, 397
    types of, 397
    urge, 388, 397
Urinary retention, 388, 390t
Urinary system, 119-120, 120f, 389b, 389f, 750f
    changes in aging, 143b, 146
    disorders of, 749-753, 756b
    structure and function of, 750b
Urinary tract infections, 750, 750b, 756b
    prevention of, 398b
Urinary urgency, 388, 390t
Urination, 388-395, 389b-390b
Urine, 120
    color chart for, 390, 390f
    measurement of, 409b
    normal, 390
    straining, 576, 576b, 577f
    testing, 574, 575b
Urine drainage systems, 408f, 412
    changing leg bags to standard drainage bags, 413b-414b, 414f
    emptying urine drainage bags, 415b, 415f
    guidelines for, 412b
    indwelling catheter care, 409b, 409f
    leg bags, 412
    re-connecting catheters and drainage tubes, 412b
    safety and comfort measures, 413b
    standard drainage bags, 412
    types of bags, 412
Urine specimens, 568-576
    24-hour, 571, 571b-572b
    clean-catch, 570
    clean-voided, 570
    comfort measures for, 568b
    guidelines for, 568b
    from infants or children, 573, 573b-574b, 573f
    midstream, 570, 570b-571b, 570f
    random, 568, 569b, 569f
Urostomy, 749, 751
Urostomy pouches, 751, 752f
U.S. Department of Agriculture (USDA)
    MyPlate, 444-447, 444f, 445b, 445t
    recommendations for physical activity, 444
    recommendations for sodium intake, 452
    safety tips to keep food safe, 468
    tips to help children eat vegetables and fruits, 445b
Uterine cancer, 695b-696b
Uterus, 121, 795b
    involution of, 818

V
Vaccines and vaccinations, 217, 241
    hepatitis B, 241
    recommendations for flu vaccine, 733
Vagina, 121, 795b
Vaginal speculum, 561
Validation therapy, 783
Valuables, 182
Valves, cardiac, 116, 725b-726b
Vancomycin-resistant enterococci (VRE), 218
Varicose veins, 608, 608f
Vas deferens, 120
Vascular ulcers. See Circulatory ulcers
Vectors, 217, 219
Vegetables, 445b, 446, 453b
Vegetative state, 710, 710f
Vehicle safety, 878
Vehicles, 217, 219
Veins, 108, 117, 117f, 497b, 725b-726b, 726f
Venous ulcers, 604, 608, 608f
Ventilation
    hyperventilation, 642, 644, 661
    hypoventilation, 642, 644
    mechanical, 658, 662, 662f, 663b, 670
    for older persons, 305b
    in person's unit, 305
    protecting persons from drafts, 305
Ventricles, 116, 497b, 725b-726b

Ventricular fibrillation (VF, V-fib), 835, 836f
Venturi masks, 653, 654f
Venules, 117, 725b-726b
Verbal abuse, 46
Verbal communication, 92, 98
Vertigo, 677
Vest restraints, 205b-206b, 206f, 211, 212b-214b
VHFs. See Viral hemorrhagic fevers
Video interviews, 864-865
Vietnam, 100b-101b, 104b, 534b, 852b
Vietnamese Americans, 94b
Villi, 119, 443b
Violence
    intimate partner violence (IPV), 38, 51-52
    TBIs due to, 710
    teen dating violence, 52b, 126, 136b
    workplace, 154, 178-179, 179b
Viral hemorrhagic fevers, 731
Viruses, 218
Vision disorders, 675
Vision loss, 683f, 685-688, 686b-687b, 687f
    accident risk factors, 156
    central vision, 684
    at end of life, 854
    feeding persons with, 463, 463f
    home care for, 686b
    signs and symptoms of, 685b
Vision rehabilitation, 671
Visitors, 179b
Visual privacy, full, 303, 312b
Vital signs, 486-512, 487b
    measuring and reporting, 487, 487b-488b
    normal ranges, 511b
    observations to report at once, 487
    and pain, 534
    pre-operative teaching about, 590
Vitamin A, 447t
Vitamin B1 (thiamin), 447t
Vitamin B2 (riboflavin), 447t
Vitamin B3 (niacin), 447t
Vitamin B12, 447t
Vitamin C (ascorbic acid), 447t
Vitamin D, 447t
Vitamin E, 447t
Vitamin K, 447t
Vitamins, 447, 447t
Vitreous humor, 115, 682b
Voice box (larynx), 118, 504b, 643b, 731b
Voiding. See Urination
Voluntary muscles, 112, 251b
Vomiting, 698b, 741
Vomitus (emesis), 739, 741
VRE. See Vancomycin-resistant enterococci
Vulnerable adults, 39, 45, 45b
Vulva, 121

W
Walkers, 522-523, 523b, 523f
    injury risks, 881
Walking
    with a cane, 523, 523f
    helping the person walk, 524, 524b-525b, 525f-526f
    personal safety measures, 180b-181b
Walking aids, 526-528
Wall oxygen outlets, 644, 651f
Wandering, 774-775, 774b, 775f, 778b-780b
Warming baby bottles, 808
Warming blankets, 640b
Warning labels, 171, 171f
Warts
    genital, 755t
    plantar, 609b-610b, 610f
Waste
    biohazardous, 217
    in home care, 243b
    preventive measures for infection control, 242
    regulated, 241b, 242
Waste disposal
    drop-off collection sites, 243b
    in home care, 243b
    needle disposal, 243b
    options for, 243b
    residential special waste pick-up services, 243b
Water, 447
    drinking water, 466, 466b-467b, 467f
    preventing burns, 158b
Water mugs, 466, 466f
Waterproof drawsheets, padded, 319, 322, 322f
WBCs. See White blood cells
Weapon safety, 179b, 879
Weighing infants, 817, 817b-818b
    guidelines for, 818b
    safety measures, 818b
Weight, 306b-307b, 308-309, 308f, 309b, 311b, 506b
Weight control, 713
Weight-bearing, 262, 263b
Wellness programs, 146b
Wernicke's aphasia. See Receptive aphasia
Wet dreams (nocturnal emissions), 135
Wet dressings, 615
Wheel locks, 192, 193f
Wheelchairs, 283, 283f
    positions for transfers to the toilet, 291b, 292f
    re-positioning the person in, 279, 279f
    safety measures, 171, 205b-206b, 207f, 283, 284b, 285f
Whirlpool tubs, 354
White blood cells (WBCs), 116, 725b-726b
Wills, 39, 52
Window safety, 672b-673b, 877

With special needs, 103
Withdrawal, 104
Withdrawal syndrome, 757, 763
Wong-Baker FACES Pain Rating Scale, 534, 535f
Work, 16
    accepting or declining job offers, 867
    getting a job, 860-869
    losing a job, 64, 64b
    preparing for, 57-58
    resigning from a job, 64
    right to, 16
    sources of jobs, 860
Work ethics, 55-66, 56b, 56f
Work practice controls, 241b, 242
Workplace violence, 154, 178-179, 179b
Work-related injuries, 253-254
    musculo-skeletal disorders, 250, 253
    preventing, 229b, 255b, 263, 263b-264b
Wound(s), 604-605
    appearance of, 612, 613b
    causes of, 605, 605b
    chronic, 604, 605b
    clean, 604, 605b
    clean-contaminated, 604, 605b
    closed, 604, 605b
    contaminated, 604, 605b
    full-thickness, 604, 605b
    infected, 604, 605b
    intentional, 604, 605b
    open, 604, 605b
    partial-thickness, 604, 605b
    penetrating, 604, 605b, 606f
    puncture, 604, 605b, 606f
    types of, 605b
    unintentional, 604, 605b
Wound care, 604-620, 619b
    cleaning wounds, 617b, 617f
    dressings, 614-616
    post-operative healing, 602
    safety and comfort measures, 619b
Wound drainage, 613, 614f
Wound healing, 611-613, 611f
Wound observations, 613b, 613f
Wrist exercises, 519b-520b, 521f
Wrist restraints, 205b-206b, 210, 210f, 213b-214b
Wristbands, color-coded, 182, 182f
Writing messages, 98

X
Xenophobia, 759

Y
Yankauer suction catheters, 661f
Yerberos, 94b
Young adulthood, 128b, 136-137, 137f